Fifth Edition

NURSING

A Human Needs Approach

D0142590

Janice R. Ellis
Elizabeth A. Nowlis

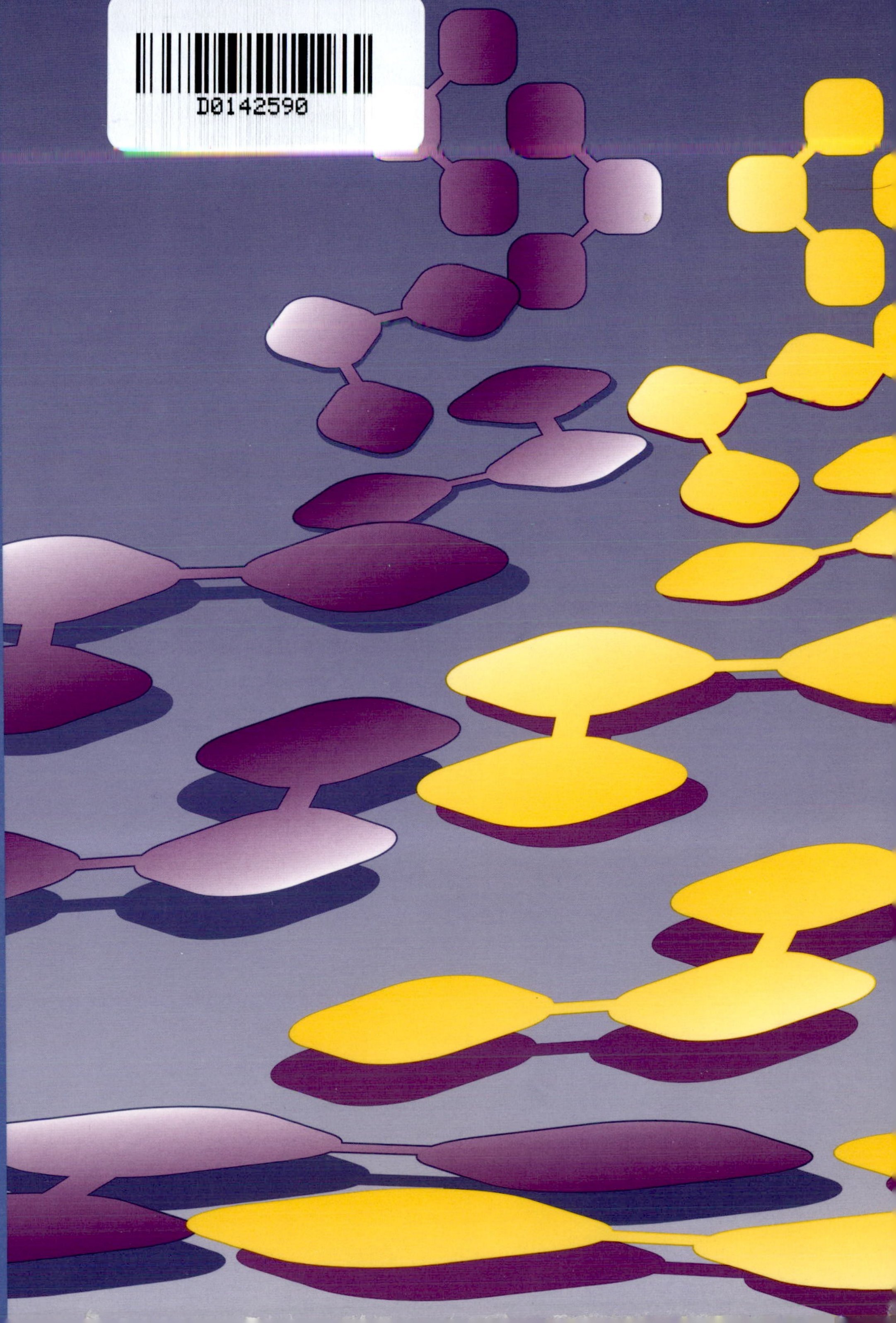

J. B. Lippincott Company

Contents

WITHDRAWN

Nursing

A
Human Needs
Approach

HobK
990
White

Nursing:

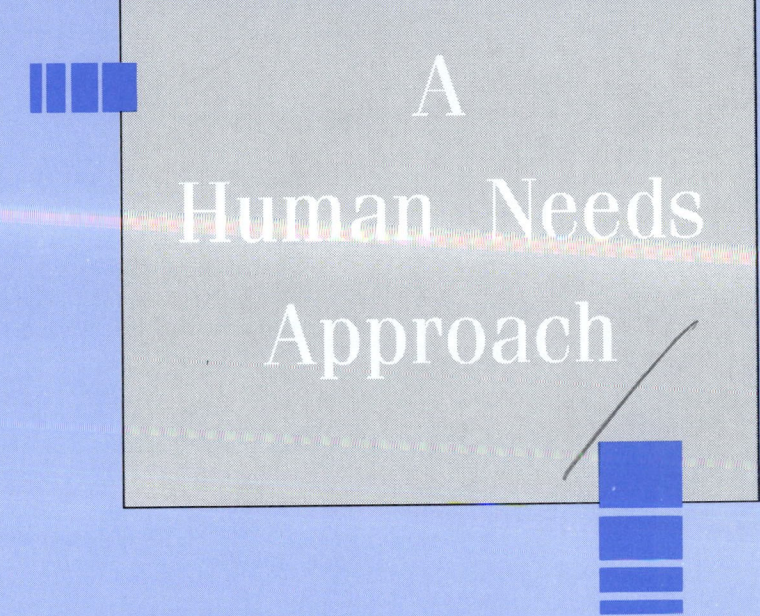

A Human Needs Approach

Janice Rider Ellis, RN, PhD

Elizabeth Ann Nowlis, RN, EdD

Fifth Edition

1792

J. B. Lippincott Company
Philadelphia

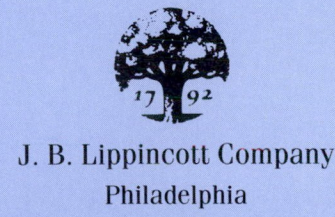

Sponsoring Editor: Donna L. Hilton, RN, BSN
Coordinating Editorial Assistant: Susan M. Keneally
Developmental Editor: Marian A. Bellus
Project Editor: Amy P. Jirsa
Indexer: Ellen Murray
Art Director: Susan Hermansen
Interior Design: Anne O'Donnell
Production Manager: Helen Ewan
Production Coordinator: Maura C. Murphy
Compositor: Pinetree Composition Inc.
Printer/Binder: Courier Book Company/Westford
Cover Printer: Lehigh Press

5th Edition

Copyright © 1994, by J. B. Lippincott Company.
Copyright © 1989, 1985, 1981, 1977 by Houghton Mifflin Company. All rights reserved. No part of this book may be used or reproduced in any manner whatsoever without written permission except for brief quotations embodied in critical articles and reviews. Printed in the United States of America. For information write J. B. Lippincott Company, 227 East Washington Square, Philadelphia, Pennsylvania 19106.

6 5 4 3 2 1

Library of Congress Cataloging in Publications Data

Ellis, Janice Rider.
Nursing, a human needs approach / Janice Rider Ellis, Elizabeth Ann Nowlis. — 5th ed.
p. cm.
Includes bibliographical references and index.
ISBN 0-397-55004-9
1. Nursing. 2. Nurse and patient. I. Nowlis, Elizabeth Ann. II. Title.
[DNLM: 1. Nursing Care. 2. Nursing. 3. Nurse-Patient Relations. WY 100 E47n 1994]
RT41.E4 1994
610.73—dc20
DNLM/DLC
for Library of Congress 93-11761
CIP

Any procedure or practice described in this book should be applied by the healthcare practitioner under appropriate supervision in accordance with professional standards of care used with regard to the unique circumstances that apply in each practice situation. Care has been taken to confirm the accuracy of information presented and to describe generally accepted practices. However, the authors, editors, and publisher cannot accept any responsibility for errors or omissions or for any consequences from application of the information in this book and make no warranty express or implied, with respect to the contents of the book.

Every effort has been made to ensure drug selections and dosages are in accordance with current recommendations and practice. Because of ongoing research, changes in government regulations and the constant flow of information on drug therapy, reactions and interactions, the reader is cautioned to check the package insert for each drug for indications, dosages, warnings and precautions, particularly if the drug is new or infrequently used.

Oversize
RT
41
.E4
1994

Reviewers

Martha Carlson, BSN, MEd, MSN

Certified Family Nurse Practitioner
Parkland College Associate Degree Nursing Program
Champaign, IL

Cecelia Estrada, RN, BSN, MA

Program Coordinator, Vocational Nursing Program
Santa Rosa Junior College
Santa Rosa, CA

Donna J. Sauls, RN, MS

Nursing Instructor
Cooke County College
Gainsville, TX

Kim Sherer, RN, MN

Chair, Nursing Division
Northern Oklahoma College
Tonkawa, OK

Audrey R. Toscano, RN, MS

Assistant Professor, Nursing
Fulton-Montgomery Community College
Johnstown, NY

WILLIAM F. MAAG LIBRARY
YOUNGSTOWN STATE UNIVERSITY

Preface

Nursing: A Human Needs Approach, Fifth Edition, is the central text in a complete package of books for courses in the fundamentals of nursing. *Nursing: A Human Needs Approach,* Fifth Edition, presents the theory and rationale that underlie nursing practice and is intended for the lecture portion of the course. It is coordinated with two softcover volumes, Ellis/Nowlis/Bentz: *Modules for Basic Nursing Skills,* Fifth Edition, Volumes 1 and 2, that teach skilled nursing tasks in a thorough, step-by-step, self-instructional format. The Modules are designed for use in the clinical practice laboratory portion of fundamentals of nursing courses. Our separation of nursing principles and concepts and nursing skills into convenient, independent volumes was one of the most popular features of the previous editions of our package, and we are pleased to continue it in the fifth edition. We also offer a separate *Instructor's Manual/Test Bank,* containing more than 800 class-tested multiple-choice test items covering the contents of this volume. The *Instructor's Manual/Test Bank* is a specially designed book, with test items arranged in a format that enables instructors to select and order them in the way that is most applicable.

The Human Needs Approach

We have retained the human needs approach to nursing that users of previous editions found so valuable. The human needs approach provides a clear framework that enables the student to develop an understanding of the person who becomes a client/patient. This basic framework adapts easily to a variety of conceptual frameworks. It is compatible with the human response patterns formulated by the North American Nursing Diagnosis Association (NANDA) and forms a solid foundation for developing skill in using the nursing process.

You will note that we have used the terms client, patient, and patient/client throughout the text. The individual who is in a hospital is still referred to and thinks of him- or herself as a patient. The person in a community setting is more likely to be referred to as a client. Much of what beginning nursing students will learn has applicability in both settings. We have continued to emphasize the centrality of respect for the dignity of the individual in whatever setting the nurse practices.

Organization

In developing this revision, our major goal was to make the text more useful to both the student and the instructor. In keeping up with current trends in the nursing profession, we have expanded the material on the nursing process. In this edition we have added a new unit—Special Needs—to which we have moved the chapters on Coping With Chronic Illness and Coping With Loss. Also in this unit are three new chapters: Diagnostic Testing, Pharmacotherapeutics, and The Experience of Surgery, which are intended to make topics more easily accessible to the student and to make our text more complete. The other major change in organization is the moving of the unit on Physiological Needs to a position that precedes the unit on Psychosocial Needs.

UNIT ONE: Introduction to Nursing. Unit One consists of three chapters that introduce the student to the health care setting. Those students with prior backgrounds in health care may be able to cover some of this material rapidly. But many students entering nursing have had no health-related experience. It is our belief that on the very first contact with a patient, students must see themselves in the role of the nurse. Furthermore, we believe that the patient has a right to expect the practitioner, whatever his or her role, to fit into the total plan for care in a meaningful way. To do this, the student needs an understanding of the total health care situation.

Chapter 1, The Profession of Nursing, includes information related to nursing history as well as information on the current status of nursing. A brief introduction to nursing theory in the form of an emphasis on nursing as encompassing study of the person, health, environment, and nursing care has been included. The major nursing theorists are presented and special emphasis is given to the definitions of nursing. Chapter 2, The Health Care System, includes a broad look at the entire health care system. Chapter 3 remains Legal and Ethical Issues.

Unit Two: Health and Illness. Unit Two continues to provide the basis for the human needs framework. Chapter 4 has been divided into 2 chapters, so that the discussion of homeostasis could be expanded to include more anatomy and physiology and so that the content on homeostatic regulation that used to be included with sensory perception and cognition could be added.

Unit Three: The Nursing Process. The nursing process is presented in Unit Three and is integrated throughout the entire text. Coverage has been expanded to provide the beginning student with more guidance in using the nursing process in all areas of practice. Furthermore, in each chapter where it is appropriate, the nursing process is the major organizing framework. The use of nursing diagnoses and examples of nursing care plans serve as learning aids for the beginning student. An alphabetical listing of the Nursing Diagnoses developed by NANDA is found inside the front cover for easy, quick reference. To further facilitate the use of nursing diagnoses, the student can turn to Appendix A, which contains definitions of the nursing diagnoses approved by NANDA through 1992. In Chapter 10, the NANDA taxonomy of Nursing Diagnoses has been added to facilitate the student's understanding of the conceptual framework for the NANDA list.

Unit Four: The Essentials of Nursing Practice. Unit Four includes four chapters that discuss the use of communication in nursing practice. Chapter 13, Basic Communication Skills, provides the foundation for the communication process. Chapter 14, Working With Groups, Chapter 15, Coordinating Care, and Chapter 16, Health Teaching, focus on different uses for communication skills, all of which are necessary to professional nursing practice.

Unit Five: Human Needs Through the Life Span. Unit Five is divided into four chapters. Chapter 17, General Concepts of Growth and Development, sets the stage for understanding the needs of individuals at different stages in the life span. Chapter 18 deals with Infancy and Adolescence and Chapter 19 deals with Adulthood. Special emphasis is placed on Chapter 20, Special Needs of the Older Adult, because the elderly compose the largest percentage of those who become clients in the health care system.

Unit Six: Physiological Needs. Unit Six is the longest unit and begins with the most basic need, that for Safety in the Environment. In this chapter all aspects of safety for both patient and nurse are emphasized. Information on universal blood and body fluid precautions as recommended by the CDC, as well as basic information on how the AIDS virus is transmitted, is included. Information on regulation of body functions has been moved from this unit to the chapter on Homeostasis (Chapter 4), including the discussion of body temperature regulation.

Unit Seven: Psychosocial Needs. In Unit Seven psychosocial needs are presented as positive needs. The need to identify oneself as part of a social group is presented in Chapter 33, Social, Cultural, and Ethnic Identity. Chapter 34, Mental Health, covers those needs related to love and belonging and the ability to cope with daily living. Chapter 35, Self-Concept, explores the various aspects of self-concept including personal identity, role function, and body image. Chapter 36, Values and Beliefs, presents such concerns as the work ethic *vs.* the leisure ethic and individuality *vs.* community, as well as discussing the more traditional religious beliefs. In Chapter 37, Human Sexuality is presented. Material on safer sexual practices in an era of AIDS has been added.

Unit Eight: Special Needs. New for this edition, this unit is intended to bring together discussion of various nursing responsibilities that were scattered throughout the last edition and that have become over time part of the fabric of nursing. The nurse's responsibilities in working collaboratively with the physician in administering medication and making sure that diagnostic tests are carried out correctly are discussed in the first two chapters. The nursing care of those experiencing surgery, chronic illness, or death are the topics of the other three chapters in this unit.

Nursing Process

Nursing Process forms a solid base for the clinical nursing chapters. This is evident within each of these chapters in the form of Sample Nursing Care Plans, Nursing Care Studies, and incorporation of the five Nursing Process steps as major headings in the text.

- **Sample Nursing Care Plans** in the clinical nursing chapters provide examples of how the nursing diagnoses discussed in the chapter can be implemented in nursing care. These displays feature a nursing diagnosis, supporting data, desired patient outcomes, and nursing actions and rationales.
- **Nursing Care Studies** at the end of many chapters present clinical situations that show nursing theory applied to real situations and highlight critical thinking in action.
- **Nursing Process Format.** A strong Nursing Process format in all the clinical nursing care chapters provides a solid theoretical underpinning and helps teach the student how to apply the Nursing Process to clinical nursing practice. The nursing care for the problems and disorders discussed in these chapters are presented using the five nursing process steps as specially designed, recurring headings, which can be easily located by the student from chapter to chapter.

Key Features

To provide students with a fundamentals text that makes the mastery of concepts and principles as easy as possible, we have made use of features that make information readily available to the student both in terms of learning and in terms of reviewing. The following paragraphs describe those features.

- **Flexibility.** In structuring the organization of this revision, we have tried to use a conceptual framework that not only speaks to the setting in which nursing is practiced and to the person who becomes a patient/client, but also presents an understanding of health and illness and a framework of nursing practice that includes a definition of nursing, the roles of the nurse, and a methodology for action. We recognize, however, that some instructors will want to reorder topics to fit their own programs, so we have written the text in as flexible a manner as possible. Two alternative sequences are suggested in the *Instructor's Manual/Test Bank,* but other variations also are possible.
- **Readability.** We have sought to make *Nursing: A Human Needs Approach,* Fifth Edition a book that beginning students can and will read. We have used simple, straightforward language and have taken care to define technical and professional terms.
- **Practical Applications.** Nursing Care Studies and Sample Nursing Care Plans continue to be an integral part of this text. Nursing Care Studies at the end of most chapters give students the opportunity to apply their knowledge within the context of concrete situations. The situations presented in Nursing Care Studies are ones that might face a beginning nursing student. Sample nursing care plans serve as examples for students who will soon be writing their own care plans for their own patients. They teach students a valuable practical skill that they will use throughout their careers. The Nursing Care Plans also aid students in understanding nursing diagnoses by presenting possible solutions to problems related to specific nursing diagnoses and the rationales for those actions.
- **Structured Heading Format.** A structured heading format is used that breaks the discussion into clear manageable segments and that, in the clinical nursing chapters, provides the student with an orderly way to find the discussions on anatomy, physiology, disorders, and nursing process.

Pedagogical Features

Nursing: A Human Needs Approach, Fifth Edition, is set up to be easy for students to study and to use as a reference. Each chapter contains the following features:

- **Objectives** at the beginning of each chapter are intended to guide students in their study. The nature of the objectives varies with the subject under consideration: some are presented in very specific behavioral terms, and others are more general.
- **A Comprehensive Chapter Outline** gives students an overview of each chapter.
- **A List of Study Terms** are placed at the beginning of the chapter for this edition, where the student can use them to identify the most important concepts in the chapter.
- **Key Points** highlight and summarize the important points in each chapter (replacing chapter summaries in previous edition).
- **Study Questions** that relate to the chapter objectives are provided. These questions are designed to give students an opportunity to selectively test their mastery of the information covered in the chapter.
- **Critical Thinking Activities** along with the rationale for nursing actions and the Care Studies help the student to develop critical thinking skills.
- **Boldface Terms** in text make the definitions of the study terms readily accessible to the student.
- **Many Illustrations** complement and enhance the text discussion.
- **Tables and Displays** within the chapter summarize and emphasize important information.
- **Relevant Sections** in *Modules for Basic Nursing Skills,* Fifth Edition, are listed at the ends of chapters for the convenience of instructors and students.
- **References and Readings** suitable for beginning students are listed for each chapter. The references include certain more advanced publications that have become classic in nursing, but we have tried to avoid listing publications that are not available in the usual nursing library.
- **Appendices** are included on definitions of nursing diagnoses, common abbreviations, abbreviations of medical conditions, combining forms, and voluntary associations.
- **A Comprehensive Glossary** includes all the study terms, plus other definitions. For each study term, the chapter where the term is defined appears in parentheses following the term.

Recurring Displays

Four kinds of recurring displayed material appear in this text in a special displayed format:

- **Nursing Diagnosis Displays.** Within the clinical nursing chapters, these displays relate to the human need under discussion. NANDA-approved nursing diagnoses form the basis of these displays, which help to reinforce the language of nursing.
- **Potential Complications Displays.** These displays underscore the collaborative nature of nursing in

many situations and help the student to recognize the kinds of situations in which they will work with other health care professionals in meeting the needs of their patients.

• **Nursing Issues and Trends.** These displays are designed to bring to the attention of the student the topics of importance in health care settings today and to foster interest and concern for the larger issues relating to the roles and responsibilities involved in nursing.

• **Nursing Research: Implications for Practice.** Current research is featured in these displays and is intended to make the student aware of how this growing knowledge base impacts on the way in which nursing care is delivered.

New for the Fifth Edition

• **Recurring Displays.** New recurring displays that enhance the student's understanding of the nurse's role in the care setting include

Nursing Issues and Trends
Nursing Research
Potential Complications

• **Pedagogy.** To strengthen the pedagogy in this edition we have added

Key Points: To facilitate study.
Critical Thinking Exercises: To encourage students to apply an analytic process to the work they do.

• **Three New Chapters.** In response to the suggestions of reviewers and faculty, we have added three new chapters to strengthen the knowledge base as well as the content on the basic concepts and principles that underlie nursing practice. These chapters are

Diagnostic Testing
Pharmacotherapeutics
The Experience of Surgery

• **Stronger Human Needs Framework.** Homeostasis and Human Needs are two separate chapters in this edition, reflecting a stronger human needs framework and the importance of homeostasis in the function of all body systems.

Interface with Modules for Basic Nursing Skills, Fifth Edition

The separate *Modules for Basic Nursing Skills, fifth edition,* focus on the student's practice and mastery of nursing skills and procedures. Each module contains step-by-step instructions and carefully chosen photographs and illustrations, along with a main objective, a rationale, a list of prerequisites, a set of learning activities, a vocabulary list, a performance checklist, and a quiz. The two volumes are three-hole punched with perforated pages so students can tear out pages and hand them in or keep the modules in notebooks, and faculty can re-organize them to suit their needs.

Ancillaries

The teaching–learning package for this newest edition of *Nursing: A Human Needs Approach* includes the **Instructor's Manual, Computerized Testbank, Study Guide, and Overhead Transparencies.**

JRE
EAN

Acknowledgments

Over the years that we have been teaching and writing within the nursing field, we have received assistance, support, and encouragement from many individuals.

Our first thanks go to the students who have challenged us, grown with us, and gone on to be contributing members of the nursing profession. Their responses and feedback have greatly influenced the direction, style, and content of this text.

Secondly, we want to thank our professional nursing colleagues, both those within nursing education and those within nursing service. Of particular note are the reviewers listed separately. Our colleagues continually assist us in remaining current in practice and provide input that enriches the content.

The many people at J.B. Lippincott have been simultaneously our critics, our champions, our colleagues, and our friends. Without them and their vision, this book would never have come to fruition. In particular we wish to thank Donna Hilton our sponsoring editor, Marian Bellus our developmental editor, and Amy Jirsa our project editor.

Our families have endlessly applauded our efforts, remained patient, and complained only minimally about the tremendous inroads on our time that writing demands. We would not be the same people or the same nurses without the kind of personal caring and responses that they provide for us. Thank you seems inadequate to express what we feel for them. They know they are central to our lives.

Janice Ellis and Elizabeth Nowlis

Contents in Brief

Expanded Contents

Sample Nursing Care Plans

Nursing Care Studies

Nursing Research: Implications for Practice

Nursing Issues and Trends

Nursing Diagnoses

Potential Complications

Introduction to Nursing

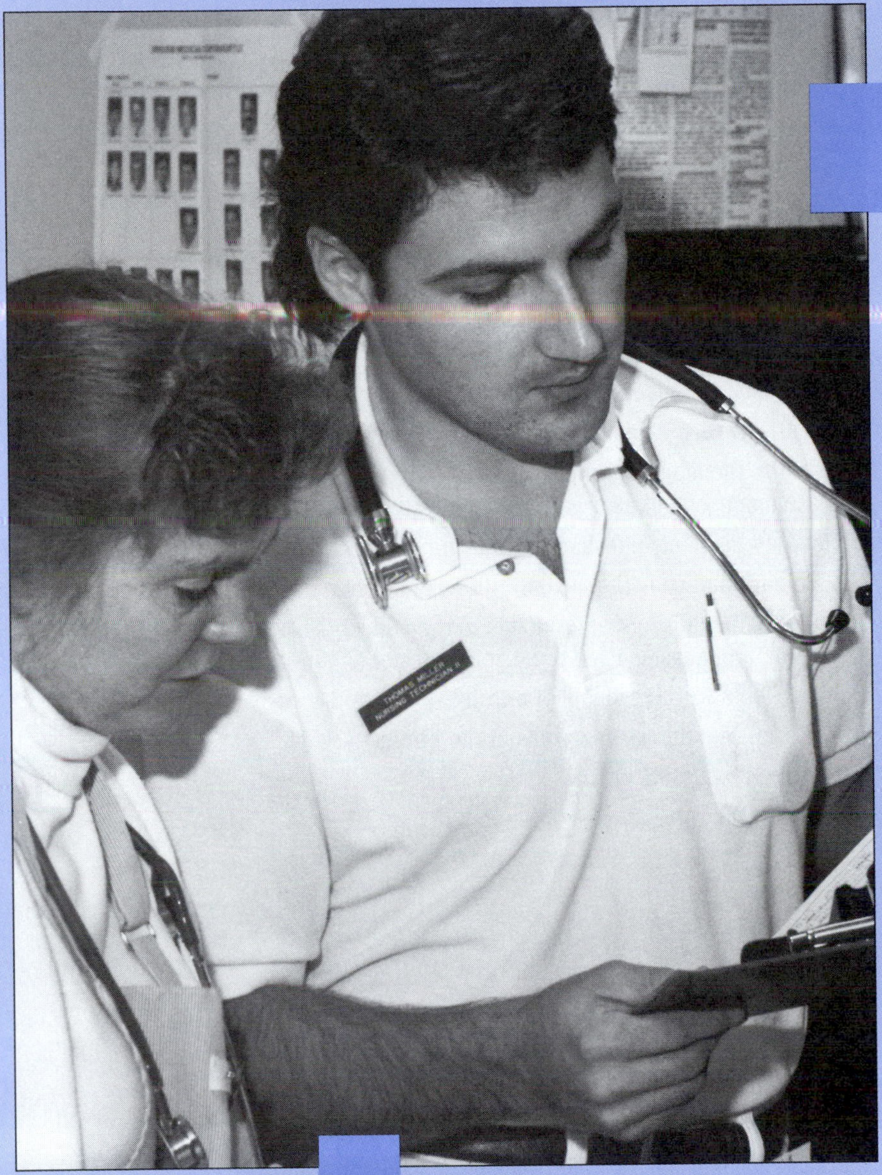

I

The Profession of Nursing

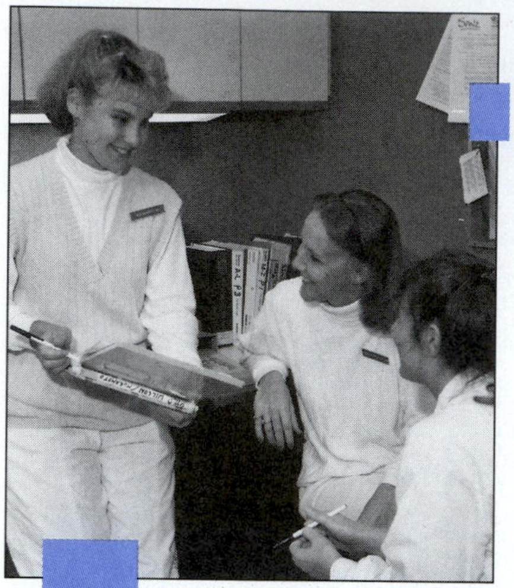

1

Objectives

After completing this chapter, you should be able to:

1. Outline the historical background of nursing.
2. Identify the contribution of significant individuals in nursing.
3. Discuss the "differentiated practice" issue.
4. Differentiate among the various pathways to nursing careers.
5. Identify a variety of employment settings where nursing is practiced.
6. Identify the major characteristics of functional, team, primary nursing, and case management as organizational systems for nursing.
7. Identify the central focuses of four major nursing organizations.
8. Compare and contrast the definitions of nursing used by different groups.
9. Identify the different approaches to the concepts of person, environment, health, and nursing used by various nursing theorists.
10. Describe a working model of nursing.
11. Differentiate the various roles of the nurse.
12. Define the nursing process.
13. Discuss the role of decision-making in nursing.

Study Terms

accountability
adaptation
advocate
associate degree program
associate nurse
authority
baccalaureate program
basic needs
case management
certification
conceptual model
continuing education
continuing education unit (CEU)
diploma program
entry into practice
functional nursing
independent role
ladder concept
mandatory licensure
nurse practitioner
nursing process
permissive licensure
primary nurse
primary nursing
registered nurse
scope of practice
team nursing
theory
total patient care

Ellis, Nowlis: Nursing: A Human Needs Approach, 5th ed. © 1994, J.B. Lippincott Company

Outline

Historical Background

The Folk Image of Nursing: The Nurse as Mother
The Religious Image of Nursing: The Nurse as God's Worker
The Renaissance Image of Nursing: The Nurse as Servant
The Emergence of Modern Nursing
Nursing in the United States
The History of Nursing Licensure

Employment Opportunities for Nurses

Hospital-Based Practice
Long-Term Care Facilities
Home Health Care
School Nursing
Occupational Health Nursing
Ambulatory Care Centers
Independent Practice
Temporary Nurse Agencies
Other Employment Settings

Pathways to Nursing Careers

Nursing Assistants
Practical Nursing
Registered Nursing
Graduate Education in Nursing
The Ladder Concept
Continuing Education
Specialized Fields of Nursing and Certification

Scope of Practice in Nursing

Entry Into Practice
Differentiated Practice

Systems of Care Delivery in Nursing

Functional Nursing
Team Nursing
Total Patient Care and Primary Nursing
Case Management
The Role of the Nursing Student in the System of Care Delivery

Nursing Organizations

American and Canadian Nurses Associations
Student Nurses' Associations
International Council of Nurses
National League for Nursing
Other Nursing Organizations

The Definition of Nursing

International Council of Nurses Definition
American Nurses Association Definition
National Council of State Boards of Nursing Definition
Definitions in State Licensing Laws

Theories of Nursing

Rogers' Science of Unitary Man
Peplau's Interpersonal Relations Model
Johnson's Behavioral Systems Model
Orem's Self-Care Model
Roy's Adaptation Model
Neuman's Systems Model
Watson's Theory of Human Caring
Henderson's Basic Needs/Activities

Developing a Working Model of Nursing

The Role of the Nurse

The Social Versus the Professional Role
The Independent Role Versus the Collaborative Role

The Nursing Process

The Art of Nursing

Decision-Making in Nursing

Who Makes Decisions
Accountability and Authority

As you begin the new venture of preparing to become a nurse, you will find that nursing students today are a highly diverse group. Among you are recent high school graduates and experienced individuals embarking on new careers. Your educational attainments may vary from a general equivalency diploma (GED) acquired through independent study to a baccalaureate degree in another discipline. Your employment experience is also widely varied: some of you have probably had no previous health-related employment, whereas others have worked for years as practical nurses or members of medical corps. This rich variety of backgrounds adds depth and breadth to nursing (Fig. 1-1). You can contribute to the education of others by sharing your background, knowledge, and experiences with them; and you can learn from those around you.

As an introduction, let us look at the long history of nursing. Although nursing as an educated profession is of relatively recent origin, nursing as a vocation is at least as old as recorded history.

Historical Background

Nursing has a history as long as that of humankind. Human beings have always faced the challenge of fostering health and caring for the ill and dependent. Those who were especially skilled in this area stood out and,

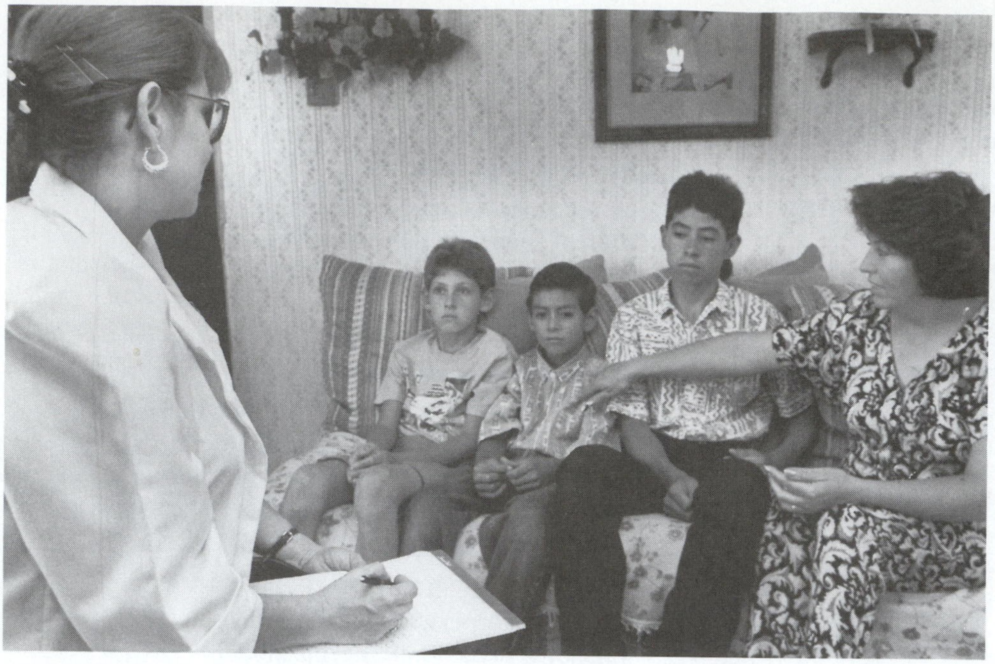

Figure 1-1. Nurses today are as diverse in their work settings and roles as in their backgrounds.

in some instances, passed their skills along to others. Uprichard (1973) described the early history of nursing using three images: the folk image, the religious image, and the Renaissance image.

The Folk Image of Nursing: The Nurse as Mother

The early development of nursing was rarely documented, so we must speculate about its character from what we know of early civilizations. The nurse was generally a member of the family or, if not, then a member of the community who demonstrated special skill in caring for others. Nursing in this perspective was seen largely as a feminine role—an extension of mothering. Indeed, the word itself may have been derived from the same root as the words nourish and nurture. This view of nursing was prevalent in the earliest historical records and is still present in primitive cultures.

There is more documentation of medical care in early civilizations than of nursing care. Records show that in ancient Egypt laws were enacted regarding sanitation and medical schools. Evidence shows that Egyptian physicians performed many types of surgery with success.

The first hospitals may have been built in India. These hospitals were staffed by men, but the families of patients probably performed most of what we would consider today to be nursing care. The men on the staff served as assistants to the physicians.

The Religious Image of Nursing: The Nurse as God's Worker

In the Bible, a woman named Phoebe is identified as the first *deaconess*, a word meaning servant or helper. Deaconesses cared for widows, orphans, and the sick. Olympias, a woman of Constantinople, set up a hospital to care for the sick. In Rome, Marcella established a monastery for those in need of care. Fabiola, who was converted to Christianity by Marcella, established hospitals for the sick poor. In the Middle Ages, the traditional role of religious groups in caring for the ill was continued by various orders of monks and nuns. When the Crusades attempted to regain Jerusalem from Muslim control, the Knights Hospitalers, an order of religious workers who cared for the injured and fought to protect them, marched with the armies. During this time, unfortunately, the knowledge of hygiene and sanitation gained by Greek, Roman, Egyptian, and other ancient civilizations was forgotten. There was no growth or development in knowledge regarding care of the sick.

Throughout the Middle Ages and into the Reformation, religious orders ran almost all of the hospitals and provided most of the nursing care in Europe. With the advent of the Reformation and the presence of Protestant religious groups, the nature of these orders changed. Women might join for a limited period of time, rather than devoting an entire lifetime to service. They were again referred to as deaconesses, the term used in the early church. For example, a church order of deaconesses was organized by Pastor Theodor Fleidner in Kaiserswerth, Germany called the Sisters of Mercy of the Church of England. Another order established St. John's House, an Anglican hospital in London. The Protestant nursing groups were comprised totally of women, and only one nursing order made up of men, the Brothers Hospitalers of St. John, remained in the Catholic church. The Muslim religion has a similar tradition of service to others in the name of God. Rofiada al Islamiah, one of the wives of Muhammad who cared for the sick and injured, is considered the mother of nursing in the Mideastern Muslim countries (Meleis, 1985).

The Renaissance Image of Nursing: The Nurse as Servant

The Renaissance saw the decline of monastic orders and a rise in individualism and materialism. There was a radical change from the image of the selfless nurse that had developed in the early Christian period and the Middle Ages. Care of the ill was delegated to servants and those unable to find any other means of support. The hospitals of this time were plagued by pestilence and filled with death; those who worked in them were seen as corrupt and unsavory.

The Emergence of Modern Nursing

To some extent, the three early images of the nurse were held simultaneously for hundreds of years. Then, in the 19th century, one woman changed the course of nursing: Florence Nightingale. Although born to wealth and a family well placed in Victorian English society, Florence Nightingale had a firm belief in Christian ideals that made her disdainful of a life of luxury. She believed her true calling was to minister to the sick. As an intelligent and well-educated woman, she recognized that optimum care of the sick required education. She persevered against family and social opposition and initiated personal study and research into sanitation and health. She studied with Pastor Fleidner at Kaiserswerth, where she stayed for 3 months. Her first appointment, in 1853, at the age of 33, was to reorganize the care for the sick at a hospital established for "Gentlewomen in Distressed Circumstances."

Nightingale's success in her first post led Britain's secretary of war to recruit her for a far more arduous reorganization. Britain was then engaged in a major war in the Crimea; reports were coming back that more men died of wounds in the hospitals than on the battlefield. Funds were raised and nurses recruited for Florence Nightingale's Crimean campaign. When she arrived at the front, Nightingale found that conditions in the military hospitals were abominable. The absence of sewers and laundry facilities, the lack of supplies, the poor food, and the disorganized medical services contributed to a death rate of more than 50% among the wounded. Nightingale insisted on retaining control of all of her supplies, funds, and personnel. Her efforts and those of her staff reduced the death rate among the wounded to under 3%. She eventually completely reformed the military's approach to the health care of the British soldier.

Nightingale returned to England in poor health and for the rest of her life (she lived to age 90) lived as a semi-invalid. This, however, did not stop her from continuing her work. She wrote extensively about hospital sanitation and supported measures to enhance the health of the British soldier. In 1860, she created a school of nursing, which was the model for most nursing education in England. The school was organized around three components: 1) a trained matron with undisputed authority over all members of the staff, 2) a planned course of theoretical and practical training, and 3) a home attached to the hospital in which carefully selected students were placed in the care of "sisters" responsible for their moral and spiritual training. (The English term "sisters" used for secular nurses reflects nursing's religious history.) Nightingale established educational standards for the students—she concerned herself not just with health care needs but with human needs.

Her school prepared nurses for hospital care (where they were called "ward sisters") and for supervisory and teaching positions. Nightingale also set up a program for preparing "district" nurses, the public health/visiting nurses of England. She wrote that these district nurses needed additional education because they would be working more independently than the hospital staff members.

Nightingale's strong statements about the role of nurses and their need for lifelong education are still quoted widely today. Perhaps she, more than anyone else, can be credited with establishing nursing as a profession (Fig. 1-2).

Nursing in the United States

The history of nursing in the United States is similar to that of nursing in Europe, although it is much shorter. In the United States, nursing was undertaken at its best by members of religious orders or benevolent societies, and at its worst by untrained attendants in secular hospitals. The secular hospitals often had a workhouse atmosphere, sometimes housing the poor and insane and serving as orphanages and even houses of correction. In the United States, as in Britain, war provided the impetus to improve nursing practice and upgrade training.

During the Civil War, a desperate need arose for

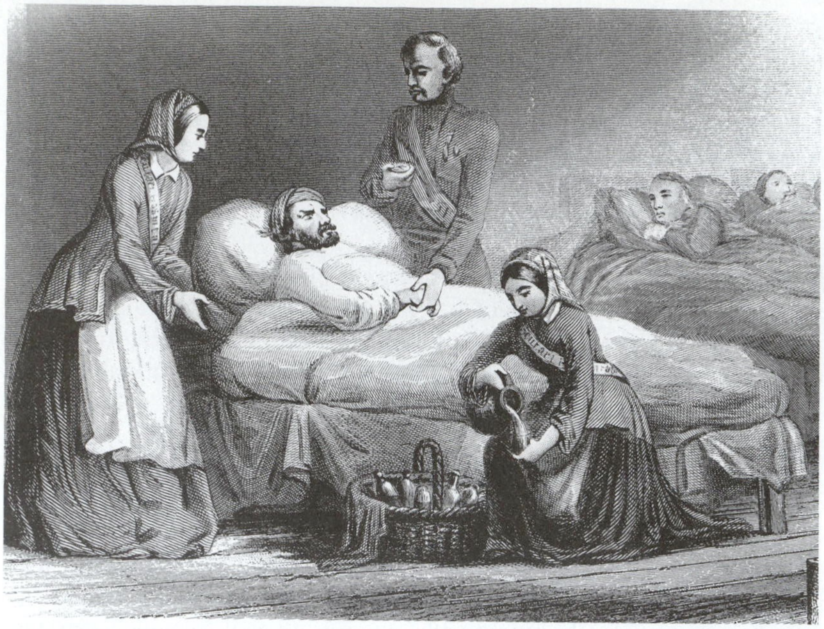

Figure 1-2. Florence Nightingale's work in the 19th century helped to establish nursing as a profession.

nursing care both for battlefield casualties and for soldiers who became ill with fevers and illnesses that were exacerbated by unsanitary living conditions and inadequate diets. Many women, even entire religious orders, offered to serve as nurses. Unfortunately, these individuals were untrained.

A volunteer organization, the United States Sanitation Commission, recruited women, initiated short but intensive training programs, and provided literature on the care of the sick and injured to the government and to groups in the South. One member of the commission, Dorothea Dix, was appointed Superintendent of Women Nurses for the Union Army, the highest position held by a woman in the military even though she was not a nurse.

Some of the outstanding individuals caring for the sick and wounded during that long war were Mary Ann Bickerdyke, who fought to get incompetent and drunken surgeons removed from duty; Clara Barton, who later was instrumental in founding the American Red Cross; Harriet Tubman, an African American woman who before the war had led slaves to freedom; and Sojourner Truth, an African American activist who had spoken out against slavery and for women's rights. Undoubtedly hundreds of dedicated but now forgotten women also contributed to the well-being of the sick and injured in that bloody conflict.

In 1872, what many consider the first school of nursing opened at the New England Hospital for Women and Children. (Other records suggest that the Women's Hospital of Philadelphia provided a training program a few years earlier.) One of the first graduates of New England Hospital was Linda Richards, who became a leader in early nursing. Mary Mahoney, the first African American trained nurse, also graduated from that school. Although some Nightingale schools were started, the majority of nursing schools established in the United States did not follow the model of independence that was characteristic of the Nightingale schools, and programs of study varied greatly in length, from a few months to several years.

Most of these programs remained subservient to hospital administrations, with a focus on learning through practice. During the 1880s and early 1890s hospitals with as few as 20 beds opened their own nursing schools to provide for the care of their patients. Although major cities had excellent hospital schools, many of the smaller schools lacked standards and exploited students. An influential nursing leader of that period was Isabel Hampton Robb. She was a vocal proponent of the 3-year nursing program and the 8-hour workday for nurses. She was also active in founding the Nurses' Associated Alumnae of the United States and Canada, which was a forerunner of both the American and Canadian Nurses Associations, and in the movement to provide for nursing licensure. Robb also wrote the first nursing textbook.

Another important nurse of that era was Lillian Wald, who was instrumental in establishing a visiting nurse service for the poor in the New York City slums. This early beginning of community health nursing established nursing in the minds of many people as a selfless and caring vocation.

By the turn of the century, nursing education had become standardized in the 3-year hospital school. In 1919, the University of Minnesota adapted its 3-year hospital program and established the first baccalaureate program in nursing. Such collegiate programs, however, remained very much in the minority until after World War II. Most baccalaureate programs consisted of a 3-year nursing curriculum followed by 2 years of college work. Only gradually did the baccalaureate program change to the now traditional 4-year academic program.

During World War II, more nurses were needed than were being prepared. Therefore, the government established the Cadet Nurse Corps. Students joined this branch of the armed services, and the government paid for their education. The curriculum was streamlined and shortened to graduate more nurses more quickly. Even after the war, the nursing shortage persisted. The fact that nurses had been educated more rapidly through the Cadet Nurse Corps supported Mildred Montag's contention that a well-planned program that used carefully directed care experiences could provide adequate nursing education in 2 years.

The associate degree nursing program was developed by Montag from pilot projects started in 1952 in seven junior colleges and one hospital school of nursing. Although Montag envisioned this program as complete in itself, and separate from baccalaureate education, many changes have occurred since that time. Efforts are now being made to provide access to baccalaureate education for nurses with associate degrees who wish to continue their education.

Many other changes have occurred in nursing in the last 30 years. Nurses have moved into more independent roles as care providers. They have assumed responsibility for increasingly complex health care technology. They have established specialty areas of practice and methods of promoting advanced knowledge and skill. Nursing continues to be a growing and changing field. It provides a challenge to many within it, and we hope it will provide you with purpose and direction.

The History of Nursing Licensure

Nurses started to organize in the late 1890s and began pressing for licensure. They felt that licensing standards would be the best way to ensure the public of safe care by adequately trained nurses. In 1901, New Zealand became the first country to provide for this licensure. Two years later, the first laws permitting the licensure of nurses in the United States were passed in North Carolina, New Jersey, and New York. When individuals are allowed to be licensed if they meet certain standards, it is referred to as **permissive licensure**. The first law *requiring* licensing of those who wished to practice nursing was enacted in 1938 in New York. When everyone who wishes to practice must meet the standards and be licensed, it is referred to as **mandatory licensure**. Each state, territory, province (in Canada), or nation has individual laws regulating the practice of nursing and establishing the licensing procedure. State boards of nursing within the United States cooperate and nurses' organizations have supported measures for standardized licensing requirements to facilitate the movement of nurses. Because a nursing licensure is primarily to safeguard the public, each governmental body that controls licensing places some restrictions on who may be licensed. These restrictions usually relate to commission of felony crimes, certain drug-related offenses, and indicators of lack of mental competence. The specific governmental licensing authority should be contacted to determine what restrictions exist.

Not until 1950 was there enough uniformity for nurses in all states and territories to take the same licensing examination. That examination, called the State Board Test Pool Examination, provided for tests in each of five areas: medical nursing, surgical nursing, obstetric nursing, pediatric nursing, and psychiatric nursing. Although the tests were constantly updated in content, their format remained the same until 1983, when the National Council of State Boards changed it to reflect a uniform approach to the whole field of nursing. This new test, called the NCLEX-RN (National Council Licensing Examination for Registered Nurses), provides for a single examination, given in several sections but scored as a unit. Beginning in 1989 the actual score of any individual taking the examination was not reported, only the statement *Pass* or *Fail.* The questions are based on a nursing process approach (see Unit 3) and cover knowledge essential for basic safe practice. These examinations are given in February and July, on the same days everywhere in the nation. Eligibility to take the examination is determined by the licensure laws of each jurisdiction. Some time in the mid to late 1990s the test will be converted to a computerized format. When this occurs, tests will be administered at varying times because individuals will not receive the same questions. There will be a pool of questions and the computer will score as the individual answers questions and then present appropriate additional questions. Testing will end when the person has answered enough questions to give a clear determination of passing or failing. See Chapter 4 for further information on nursing licensure.

Employment Opportunities for Nurses

Although the majority of nurses are employed by hospitals, nurses are now also working in other settings. New

WILLIAM F. MAAG LIBRARY
YOUNGSTOWN STATE UNIVERSITY

graduates are most often employed in settings where supervision and consultation are available.

Hospital-Based Practice

Within hospitals, nurses provide the care that society most commonly thinks of as nursing. They tend people of all ages during illness and through surgery and help families experiencing childbirth. The hospital setting gives increasing opportunities to nurses with specialized education in critical care, emergency care, and other specialty areas. Hospitals also employ nurses as managers, staff educators, and clinical specialists. A master's degree in nursing is usually required for the latter positions. Some large hospitals now employ nurse researchers who have doctoral degrees and the expertise to design and carry out nursing research projects. Even within the hospital, nursing is a diversified occupation.

Long-Term Care Facilities

Increasing numbers of frail elderly clients, persons with acquired immunodeficiency syndrome (AIDS), those with severe head injuries, and others who need ongoing care reside in long-term care facilities. Nurses in these settings often are expected to supervise other caregivers and exercise a high degree of independent judgment. Working in long-term care requires that nurses manage not only a health care environment but a living environment as well.

Home Health Care

Many individuals with illness or disability are able to remain in their own homes with the supervision, teaching, and assistance provided by home health nurses. Care may be provided for a limited time after an acute illness or it may be needed on an ongoing basis. Nursing in this setting requires a high degree of autonomy as well as creative abilities to adapt technical skills to various home situations. The home health nurse must be able to teach clients and their families how to care for themselves and to be active participants in their own health care.

School Nursing

Many school districts hire nurses to oversee health screening and health promotion activities for school-age children (Fig. 1-3). These nurses may on occasion treat an illness or emergency, but their focus is on promoting health, screening for deficits needing treatment, and providing support to school staff in working with children with disabilities or chronic illnesses. With increasing societal concerns about the welfare of children, some schools have established clinics that deliver a broad spectrum of medical and health services in the school setting. Nurses are often the major provider of services in these clinics.

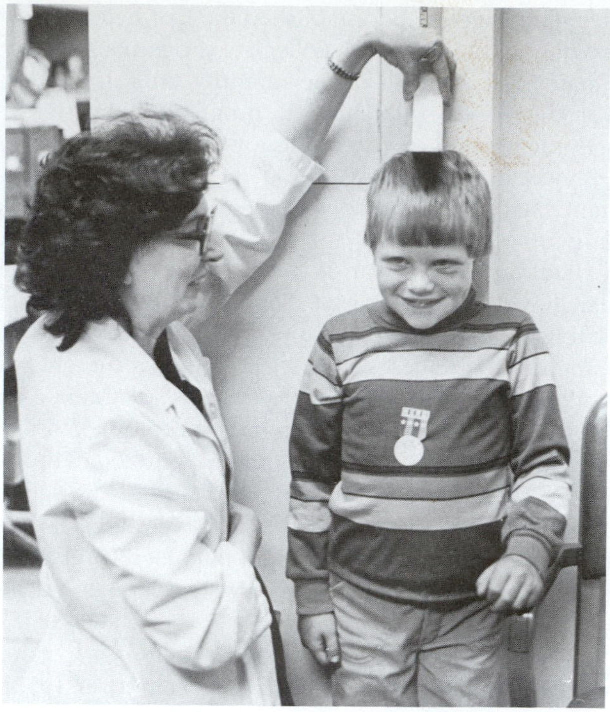

Figure 1-3. Overseeing health promotion activities for children is one responsibility of the school nurse.

Occupational Health Nursing

The workplace provides employment opportunities for nurses to help adults in health promotion activities. Assisting in maintaining a healthy and safe working environment, encouraging appropriate screening, and serving as a resource for health promotion activities provide an ongoing challenge. Occupational health nurses may also care for on-the-job injuries and illnesses that occur at work. With increasing costs of health care, the role of the occupational health nurse in some settings has broadened to include management of individual worker's cases to ensure that overall health care is being delivered in the most appropriate and economical manner.

Ambulatory Care Centers

Ambulatory care centers include doctors' offices, community-based clinics, and commercial walk-in care centers. These centers focus on the treatment of commonly occurring illnesses and accidents and on screening for health problems. Nurses in these agencies focus on teaching self-care to clients and their families as well as on meeting the demands of the current health problem. Ambulatory surgery centers care for individuals before, during, and immediately after surgical procedures. The patient/clients return home as soon as they are able. Therefore, teaching of self-care is a major responsibility of nurses in these centers.

Independent Practice

A small, but growing, number of nurses are in independent practice. Some of them have nurse practitioner education and function as nurse midwives, nurse anesthetists, or mental health nurses. Still others are in general nursing practice assisting individuals in developing plans for their own care, teaching, screening, and providing some direct care services. Nurse-managed care focuses on promoting health and supporting self-directed efforts at managing health problems.

Temporary Nurse Agencies

These agencies employ nurses to work in many different settings on an "on-call" basis. An agency nurse may work in a hospital or in a long-term care setting. Typically the facility contacts the agency for additional nurses when its own staff is not adequate to meet demands. Some agencies can provide full-time work for nurses on their rosters. Others focus on nurses who want part-time employment. Some temporary agencies specialize in providing opportunities for nurses to work in distant places or to accompany individuals who have health problems while they travel.

Other Employment Settings

Many businesses are beginning to recognize that a nursing background provides the expertise necessary to market health care equipment, audit health care records, or work in other health-related positions. An increasing number of nurses are performing these jobs.

Pathways to Nursing Careers

There are many different levels of care providers within the area of nursing and many different settings in which nursing is practiced. In addition, educational pathways to these levels may differ. You must understand the field of nursing education as a whole, as well as your own current position in it.

Nursing Assistants

Nursing assistants, also known as nurses' aides, nursing technicians, or orderlies, are employed in many settings. Nursing assistants are typically restricted to performing specific tasks that require little background knowledge, such as helping to bathe, feed, and walk patients. In facilities with a shortage of licensed personnel, nursing assistants may be taught more complex skills. Because nursing assistants lack a theoretical understanding of the potential consequences of nursing procedures, this poses potential safety concerns. The federal government requires that nursing assistants in nursing homes have a specified number of hours of classroom and clinical training. Requirements for nursing assistants in acute care facilities are less standardized. In some states, these nursing assistants need no special education. The facility that hires the individual provides orientation and education, which may range from informal to highly structured. Instruction continues on the job. In other states, nursing assistants for both nursing homes and hospitals are required to complete a specified educational program, typically at a vocational school, community college, or health care facility. The course of study rarely exceeds 8 weeks.

A few states allow nursing students to be employed in assistive positions within nursing, based on their nursing education. The regulations governing this role for students vary widely. If your state has such a program, you will want to clearly understand the limits of what you are allowed to do as an employed nursing student and to guard against performing in ways that are outside the provisions of the law. Do not confuse this role as an employee with the provisions of the law that allow you to practice within your nursing program as a student. Your school of nursing is responsible for instructing you in your legal role as a student when practicing within the program.

Practical Nursing

Practical, or vocational, nursing focuses on direct patient care. Educational preparation typically lasts one calendar year and takes place in a high school, vocational school, or community college. In North Dakota, an associate degree in practical nursing from a 2-year college is required to become a practical nurse; this is the only state with such a requirement. The academic and science requirements have usually been less rigorous than in programs preparing registered nurses; the focus of such preparation is intensive clinical experience. Practical nurses are expected to work under the supervision of a registered nurse or a physician, although supervision may be more remote in long-term care than in acute care facilities. The title Licensed Practical Nurse (LPN) or Licensed Vocational Nurse (LVN) is earned by passing a state licensing examination.

Registered Nursing

There are three routes to becoming a **registered nurse**. The registered nurse is a graduate of a nursing education program that is approved by the state; he or she also has passed a qualifying examination. Although each route has a slightly different focus, all three prepare graduates for the state examination for licensure as a registered nurse. Every school of nursing must be approved by the state board of nursing or its equivalent. Some are also accredited by the National League for Nursing (NLN). NLN accreditation is voluntary and aimed at ensuring that uniform standards of excellence are met.

Diploma Programs

Diploma programs conducted by hospital schools of nursing are the oldest type of nursing education. Most of the students' clinical experience takes place in the sponsoring hospital. Relative to other programs, more time is spent in clinical practice, and graduates are generally expected to have acquired more clinical proficiency. Many such programs arrange for all science and social science subjects to be taught at a nearby college or university. The graduate receives a diploma on completion of the program, which lasts $2\frac{1}{2}$ or 3 years. In a few programs, the student receives an associate degree in nursing from an affiliated college as well as a diploma from the hospital school. Other diploma programs are affiliating with 4-year colleges to develop baccalaureate programs. Some states, such as North Dakota and the far western states, no longer have diploma programs. Graduates of diploma programs are eligible to take the licensing examination for registered nursing in all states except North Dakota.

Associate Degree Programs

The newest type of preparation for nursing, the **associate degree program**, is conducted by community and junior colleges. Clinical facilities are obtained by contract with hospitals and other health care providers in the community. The general goal of associate degree programs, which last 2 years, is to prepare students for entry-level positions in direct care. The graduate receives an associate degree in nursing and is eligible to take the examination for registered nurse licensure in all states except North Dakota.

Baccalaureate Programs

In 4-year **baccalaureate programs** in nursing, offered by colleges and universities, students receive more instruction in basic sciences, social sciences, and humanities than do students in other types of programs. Nursing theory is taught in greater depth and community health nursing, leadership skills, and elementary research procedures are also included. Graduates of baccalaureate programs are prepared to enter graduate programs in nursing and are eligible to take the registered nurse licensing examination in all states.

Graduate Education in Nursing

Both master's degrees and doctorates can be earned in nursing. Most master's degree programs require a baccalaureate degree with an upper division major in nursing, and many graduate schools require that the candidate's basic nursing program be accredited by the NLN. A minimum of a master's degree with a major in a clinical specialty, such as maternal-child care, is required for a teacher of nursing. A master's degree in a functional area such as nursing administration may be required for many supervisory positions. Specialty positions may also require a master's degree. The doctoral degree in nursing may be oriented toward clinical care or research. Some nurses pursue doctorates in such associated fields as physiology or education.

The Ladder Concept

Many practicing nurses find that they want further education or a more advanced degree. Pursuing this ambition is not always easy; however, efforts are being made to provide for a systematic progression from one degree level to another. In the **ladder concept** (Fig. 1-4), the steps in such a progression are visualized as a ladder. In some geographic areas, educational institutions have developed **articulation** between various levels of nursing education, which means that the individual who graduates from one level is prepared to move directly into the next level with no loss of educational credit and no repetition of educational content.

The nurse who wishes to obtain a higher degree should inquire about the details of various programs. Some colleges and universities allow credit for previous experience if the applicant passes an examination; oth-

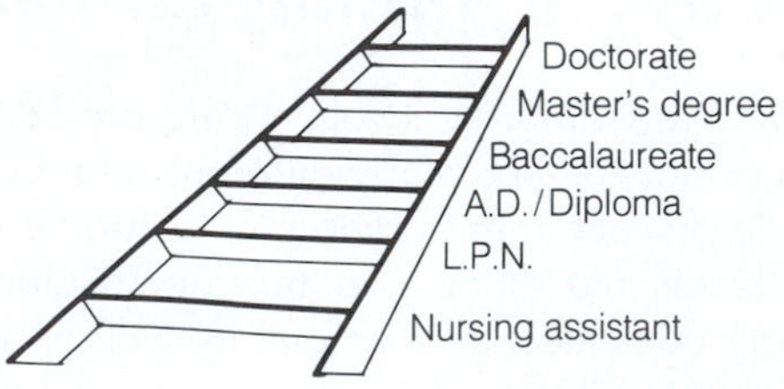

Figure 1-4. The ladder concept.

ers allow the student to construct an independent study program to meet individual needs. Some external degree programs in nursing award degrees to candidates who can demonstrate the desired level of competence, regardless of how they achieve such competence and without requiring specific courses or college attendance.

The program's accreditation and the status and standards of the accrediting bodies must be verified. Nurses should also keep in mind that a baccalaureate degree in business or health administration or another related field provides different career opportunities from a baccalaureate degree with a nursing major.

Continuing Education

The term **continuing education** is applied to any education that maintains and upgrades skills but is not a part of a formal degree program. Ever since the days of Florence Nightingale, experts have emphasized the importance to nurses of lifelong learning so that they may continue to provide high-quality nursing care. Continuing education for nurses is provided by many colleges and universities. In addition, professional organizations, private educational organizations, and employers all serve as continuing education providers. To facilitate comparison of the requirements of continuing education programs, the **continuing education unit (CEU)** is often used as a measure; one CEU represents an hour of instruction. When continuing education is provided by colleges and universities, either CEUs or college credit may be awarded. In some states, continuing education is required for maintaining a license. The requirements, which are not uniform, range from 15 hours every year to 15 hours every 2 years (Ellis & Hartley, 1992). Just as you investigated a basic nursing program, you should investigate continuing education offerings to see if the content will meet your needs and if the faculty has the necessary expertise to teach the course offerings.

Specialized Fields of Nursing and Certification

Nurses may specialize in a variety of ways. Some hospital practice specialties, such as coronary care, require formal postgraduate courses. Such courses admit any registered nurse regardless of the type of initial nursing education. Postgraduate specialty classes in such areas as coronary care are often offered as part of a clinical agency's education program or through the continuing education division of a college.

Education as a **nurse practitioner** leads to more independent nursing practice. The nurse practitioner sees outpatients for health supervision and management of minor illnesses and chronic conditions; there are pediatric nurse practitioners, family nurse practitioners, women's health care specialists, and others. Some nurse practitioner programs admit any registered nurse; others admit only registered nurses with baccalaureate degrees. Some programs award a certificate of completion and others award master's degrees. The educational program typically lasts 1 or 2 years. Standards are not yet uniform, although the trend is toward postbaccalaureate master's level programs.

Certification is professional recognition of specialized expertise as a nurse practitioner or in a field of nursing such coronary care. The American Nurses Association (ANA) in cooperation with some specialty nursing organizations has established the American Nurses Credentialing Center that provides for certification in a wide variety of specialties. Other nursing specialty organizations have established independent mechanisms for certification in their particular specialty. The candidate for certification provides evidence of the required education and clinical competence and then takes an examination in the specialty. Advancement and salary increase may follow certification.

Scope of Practice in Nursing

Scope of practice refers to the breadth of opportunity to function. The scope of practice for a nurse includes the type of client, the setting in which the nurse is prepared to practice, and the specific activities the nurse is prepared to perform. Although many employing agencies do not differentiate between the scope of practice for nurses prepared at the baccalaureate level and those at the associate degree level, nursing educators and leaders of nursing organizations have identified differences in scope of practice based on education. Each program is designed to prepare individuals to practice within its defined scope of practice. Perhaps the most universally used definitions and descriptions of scope of practice are those developed by the three councils of the NLN, which consist of representatives of the three types of programs: associate degree, diploma, and baccalaureate (Displays 1-1, 1-2, and 1-3). The state or provincial nurse practice act is the legal determinant of scope of practice. Nursing associations and health care institutions may also develop statements regarding scope of practice.

Entry Into Practice

There has been vigorous discussion about whether the differences in scope of practice between the graduates of the diploma, associate degree, and baccalaureate programs in nursing should be reflected in differences in licensure. This has been termed the **entry into practice** issue. Since 1968, the ANA has held that nursing

Display 1–1

Educational Outcomes of Associate Degree Programs: Roles and Competencies

The goal of associate degree nursing programs is preparation of registered nurses to provide direct client care. The three roles of the associate degree graduate are Provider of Care, Manager of Care, and Member within the Discipline of Nursing.

Role as Provider of Care

Characteristics
Critical thinking
Clinical competence
Accountability
Commitment to the value of caring

Nursing Process as a Basis for Decision-Making
Assessment
Diagnosis
Planning
Implementation
Evaluation

Settings
Acute care
Long-term care

Knowledge Base
Nursing concepts, principles, processes, skills
Understanding of health and health deviations
Nutrition, pharmacology, human development
Communication, teaching–learning principles
Current technology
Humanities; biologic, social and behavioral sciences

Role as Manager of Care

Characteristics
Collaboration
Organization
Delegation
Accountability
Advocacy
Respect for other health care workers

Skills
Delegation
Consultation
Evaluation

Settings
Policies and procedures are specified
Guidance is available

Knowledge Base
Principles of client care management
Principles of communication and delegation
Legal parameters of nursing practice
Roles and responsibilities of members of the health care team

Role as a Member Within the Discipline of Nursing

Characteristics
Commitment to professional growth
Continuous learning
Self-development

Contributes Through the Following
Participation on committees
Attendance at conferences
Membership in nursing organizations

Knowledge Base
Ethical standards
Legal framework for practice
Importance of nursing research
Rules and regulations governing practice
Roles of professional organizations
Political, economic, and societal forces affecting practice
Lines of authority and communication within the work setting

Information compiled from *Educational Outcomes of Associate Degree Nursing Programs: Roles and Competencies,* Council of Associate Degree Programs, National League for Nursing, New York, Pub. No. 23-2348, 1990.

education should be offered by institutions of higher learning and not service institutions. The ANA also took the position that there should be two levels of nursing, professional and technical, and that the minimum educational requirement for the professional level should be the baccalaureate degree. In 1978, the ANA reaffirmed its support for two levels of nursing practice but did not recommend titles; the future minimum entry requirements specified were the associate degree for the first level and the baccalaureate degree for the second level. In 1986, the ANA took a position supporting the titles Registered Nurse and Associate Nurse for these two levels.

In 1986, North Dakota became the first state to alter its regulations for the nursing licensure examination to require a baccalaureate degree for the registered nurse license and an associate degree for the practical nurse license. Similar changes were proposed in other states,

Display 1–2
Role and Competencies of Graduates of Diploma Programs in Nursing*

Role:

The graduate of the diploma program in nursing is:
- Eligible to seek licensure as a registered nurse
- Able to function as a beginning practitioner in acute, intermediate, ambulatory, and long term health care settings

Functions within professional nursing practice as:
- Provider, manager, leader, teacher, advocate

Competencies:

- Provides nursing care to individuals, families, and groups
- Provides for promotion, maintenance, and restoration of health
- Supports and comforts the suffering and dying
- Utilizes management skills
- Assumes leadership role
- Teaches individuals, families, and groups
- Functions as an advocate for the consumer and the health care system
- Practices based on theoretical knowledge, ethical principles, and legal standards
- Accepts responsibility and accountability for professional practice
- Utilizes opportunities for professional development
- Participates in health-related community services
- Utilizes critical thinking

Compiled from *Role and Competencies of Graduates of Diploma Programs in Nursing,* 2nd Ed., Council of Diploma Programs, National League for Nursing, New York, Pub. No. 16-1735, 1989.

Display 1–3
*Characteristics of Baccalaureate Education in Nursing**

Baccalaureate education prepares generalists in nursing and provides:

- Knowledge of theory
- Competence in the practice of nursing
- Appreciation of professional nursing's historical present, and potential impact on society
- Foundation for continued professional development
- Foundation for graduate study

Liberal education from scientific and humanities disciplines is foundational for:

- Critical thinking
- Decision-making
- Independent judgment
- Understanding and respecting people, various cultures, and environments.

"Graduates are able to:
- Provide professional nursing care including health promotion and maintenance, illness care, restoration, rehabilitation, health counseling, and education.
- Synthesize theoretical and empirical knowledge from nursing, scientific, and humanistic disciplines with practice.
- Use the nursing process to care for individuals, families, groups, and communities.
- Accept responsibility and accountability for the evaluation of the effectiveness of their own nursing practice.
- Enhance the quality of nursing and health practices within practice settings through the use of leadership skills and knowledge of the political system.
- Evaluate research for the applicability of its findings to nursing practice.
- Participate with other health care providers and members of the general public in promoting the health and well-being of people.
- Incorporate professional values as well as ethical, moral, and legal aspects of nursing into nursing practice.
- Participate in the implementation of nursing roles designed to meet emerging health needs of the general public in a changing society."

From *Characteristics of Baccalaureate Education in Nursing,* Division of Baccalaureate and Higher Degree Programs, National League for Nursing, New York, Pub. No. 15-1758, 1987.

but were not adopted due to widespread opposition. Almost all those who proposed changes in the law advocated that nurses who were already licensed at the time of such a change should continue to practice with the same license and that changes in requirements should pertain only to those who graduate after the new law takes effect. This was the procedure in North Dakota.

A change in licensure requirements in any state will be affected by a number of issues, including: 1) the numbers of applicants to nursing schools; 2) the nursing manpower supply; 3) the geographic distribution of nurses; 4) the increased cost of further education; 5) the availability of articulation between one level of nursing education and another; 6) restrictions on mobility if some states change their licensure requirements and others do not; and 7) disagreement among nurses on the best direction for change. Because decisions being made now will shape your future and the future of nursing, it is particularly important to remain informed and let your views be known.

Differentiated Practice

As the nursing shortage became more pronounced in the late 1980s, there were fewer advocates of licensing change and more who spoke in favor of differentiating the scope of practice of individuals with differing preparation through careful job description and selection. As agencies establish *differentiated practice*, the background of the individual is examined and matched with the job requirements.

Currently, employment opportunities for graduates of the various types of programs may or may not differ, depending on such factors as local nursing needs, the type of education an individual educational program provides, and individual ability. Graduates of all three types of programs are hired for entry-level staff positions in hospitals, nursing homes, and ambulatory care settings.

Systems of Care Delivery in Nursing

Many different methods of assigning accountability and authority for patient/client care exist in the field of nursing. When you go to a new health care facility, you must learn its system to function effectively. Although each facility creates its own approach, a few basic systems are in use; understanding them will help you to understand a particular facility.

Functional Nursing

In a functional method of assignment, each nursing staff member is assigned specific tasks to perform rather than specific patients to care for. In this situation, one person might take all the temperatures, someone else would pass all the medications, and still another person would give baths. This method is efficient for accomplishing tasks; however, it does not make any one person accountable for the overall care planning for an individual patient. Care is more likely to be routine and not individualized; the patient may feel unimportant and unknown.

Functional nursing is still used for certain aspects of patient care in which a high degree of technical skill is needed. An example of this is in intravenous therapy. The "IV nurse" is responsible for choosing equipment, starting intravenous fluid lines, and maintaining the functioning of the intravenous lines. This particular job requires a high degree of technical skill that can best be maintained by performing it frequently. Fewer complications develop with intravenous therapy when highly skilled persons are responsible for it.

Functional nursing might also be used in emergency situations when the main concern is accomplishing tasks necessary for the fulfillment of basic human needs. For example, if there were a severe blizzard and only a few staff members were able to get to work, the focus would be on meeting the basic needs of patients for toileting, food, and essential medications. Everyone would recognize that the emergency had made attention to higher needs such as learning about one's health problem impossible and that comprehensive, long-term planning of care would have to wait until the emergency was over.

Team Nursing

Team nursing was devised as a way to provide greater accountability for care and to allow the expertise of the registered nurse to be spread among more patients. It has been especially welcomed when shortages of registered nurses exist. A registered nurse usually acts as the team leader. Other members of the team might be practical nurses, nursing students, or nursing assistants. Persons within the team are assigned specific tasks or pa-

Nursing Issues and Trends: *Differentiated Practice*

With registered nurses being educated at both associate degree and baccalaureate levels, nursing has been challenged to identify the special characteristics of the graduates of each type of program. Most individual programs have identified expected outcomes for their particular graduates. Through differentiated practice some employers are setting different expectations for graduates from each program. Not all nurses have been comfortable with this practice. They are concerned that this may limit opportunities based on individual ability.

tients appropriate to their levels of education and expertise. The team leader has overall responsibility for the work of the team. The heart of team nursing is the team conference, in which the team members meet to discuss and plan care (Fig. 1-5). High-quality care can result if conferences are held regularly, but they tend to be omitted because of the difficulty of finding adequate time for meetings. Another concern is the tremendous load carried by the team leader. Often this nurse is expected to plan and manage care for numerous patients.

Emergency and trauma teams provide a different example of the use of the team in health care. The central concern in an emergency is that lifesaving or life-preserving tasks be accomplished quickly and skillfully. One person, usually a physician, has overall responsibility, and every other person present, including the nurse, has specific functional assignments. The group works together as a team, but during the emergency itself, each person is expected to act independently. For example, the nurse may establish intravenous lines, prepare medications, and monitor vital signs while the physician is examining the patient. A respiratory therapist may set up ventilating equipment and be prepared to ventilate the patient as soon as the physician directs. After the emergency, the team may meet to assess its functioning and to work out improved methods of delivering high-quality care.

Total Patient Care and Primary Nursing

The original method for assigning nursing care was the *case method* in which one nurse cared for one patient. This nurse often worked 24 hours a day, 7 days a week,

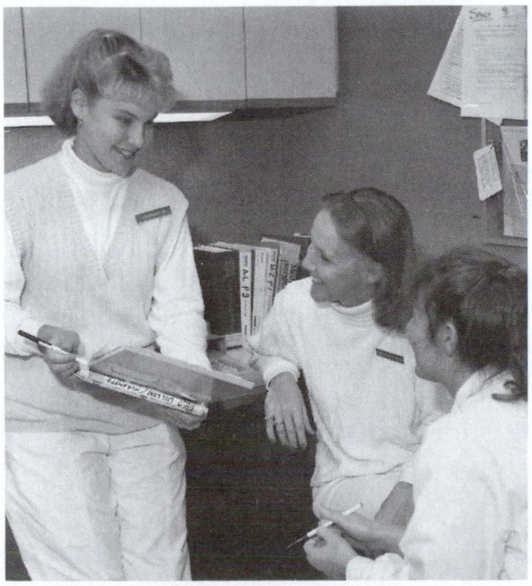

Figure 1-5. Team nursing. Members of a nursing team are assigned specific tasks appropriate to their own levels of education and expertise.

and was responsible for all aspects of the patient's care, including preparing meals. Although difficult for the nurse, this approach provided optimum care for the patient. The nurse knew everything about the patient, and the patient knew the nurse. This system was modified as private nurses began to work fewer hours; several nurses would care in rotation for the same patient. Some private duty nurses still use the case method. While on duty, the nurse is responsible for all the care needed by the patient. When the nurse is off duty, another nurse is totally responsible for the patient. In some hospitals today, nurses are assigned to the total care of a group of patients. This modification of the case method is often called **total patient care** assignment.

Primary nursing is a recent innovation that builds on the total patient care concept. In **primary nursing**, one nurse, termed the **primary nurse**, is assigned overall responsibility for a patient. This nurse is accountable for obtaining a complete baseline assessment of the patient and writing the nursing care plan. During the times while he or she is working, the nurse provides all the direct care needed by that patient. When the nurse is not working, other nurses care for the patient; however, the primary nurse remains responsible for the patient. The primary nurse may even be consulted at home if a question arises as to appropriate care. In many facilities using primary nursing, another nurse caring for the patient may be assigned as the **associate nurse**. The responsibilities of the associate nurse vary. In some places, the associate nurse assumes the responsibility for adjusting the plan of care when the primary nurse is not working. The primary nurse would then not be consulted at home if a change in care were needed. In other facilities, the associate nurse adjusts the plan of care only if an emergency or unexpected change in the patient's condition occurs.

The advantage of primary nursing is the fixing of responsibility and accountability for patient care. Because the patient knows whom to consult regarding problems and concerns and the nurse is able to know the patient well, high-quality care results. Increasingly, research data show that this intense care by a registered nurse results in shorter hospital stays, fewer complications, and increased satisfaction for the patient.

One disadvantage of primary nursing is the need to have enough registered nurses available to ensure that the case load for each nurse remains at a manageable level. There are also problems associated with instituting a change in role and function in a facility that has had another system for care delivery. In a facility with primary nursing, nursing assistants do not provide direct patient care; they only do nonpatient care tasks, such as organizing equipment and supplies and taking messages and specimens to other departments. This results in a need for more registered nurses and fewer nursing assistants in a facility. Also, the role of licensed practical nurses in primary nursing is not consistent. Some facilities believe that they have no role. In other facilities, they care for the patients when the primary nurse is not working, but are responsible only for carrying out the plan of care prepared by the primary nurse; they do not alter or adjust the plan.

Case Management

Case management is not an entire system of care delivery, but one method of coordinating all the care that an individual client receives. A variety of approaches to case management have been adopted, but the common thread is that one person, usually a registered nurse, takes responsibility for the entire course of care from first contact with the agency through and sometimes after discharge. Based on predetermined standards for care and critical timelines, the case manager organizes the delivery of care, evaluates the client's response during the process, and plans for any modifications to the standard plan that is needed. The value to the client is a smooth progression of care and fewer complications. The value to the system is a lower cost for providing that care.

The Role of the Nursing Student in the System of Care Delivery

In most educational programs, the nursing student is assigned to total care of one or two patients regardless of the system of care delivery used by the facility. The extent of the student's responsibilities is based on ability and level in the educational program. It becomes your responsibility, with the help of your instructor, to fit your role into the system being used. The major requirement is that you clearly and directly communicate with the nursing staff so that everyone understands your areas of accountability. You might be assigned to care for Martha Wilson. As a beginning student, you might be giving all care related to hygiene, activity, rest, and nutrition, but might not yet have learned to perform procedures related to elimination. In a team nursing system, most of your communication may be with the team leader, but you would also need to talk with the person assigned to direct care of Mrs. Wilson. In a primary nursing system, you would communicate with the primary nurse regarding the care you provide. In a functional system, you might need to talk with several different people who had been assigned to various aspects of Martha Wilson's care. Adequate communication with others will create good relationships and make your learning experiences more positive.

Nursing Organizations

Within the field of nursing, numerous organizations can help you remain informed about current issues in nursing. The largest are the American Nurses Association in the United States, the Canadian Nurses Association (CNA), and the National League for Nursing. In addition, many other organizations are related to specialized fields of nursing or specific areas of employment.

American and Canadian Nurses Associations

The ANA is the official professional association for registered nurses in the United States. The CNA fulfills that role in Canada. These two organizations were formed in 1911 from an organization called the Nurses Associated Alumnae of the United States and Canada. The original purpose of the organization was to promote high professional standards and to work toward nursing licensure laws as a means of ensuring the public of those standards.

Since that time, they have broadened their scope of activity and today work in many different areas. One major goal is to influence national legislative and governmental actions in relation to health care in general and nursing in particular. The organizations follow actions being taken, provide expert testimony to decision-making bodies, and disseminate information to members. Another goal is to serve as a forum for setting standards for nursing practice and supporting efforts to maintain those standards throughout their nations.

The ANA is structured as a federation of state and territorial nursing organizations. Individuals join at the state level. Every 2 years delegates are sent by each state and territory to a convention. General policy and direction are provided through the representatives at the convention. A board of directors and many commissions, councils, and committees are responsible for the day-to-day functioning. There is also a large paid staff. The *American Journal of Nursing* is the official publication of the ANA, although the editorial board of the magazine is entirely independent. The ANA also publishes many documents relevant to nursing practice.

The CNA is also a federation with individual membership at the provincial level. In addition to the same activities undertaken by the ANA, the CNA is responsible for the nursing licensure examination in Canada. Its official magazine is *Canadian Nurse.*

Student Nurses' Associations

The National Student Nurses Association (NSNA) is the student counterpart of the ANA. It holds its convention yearly. The NSNA focuses on professional concerns similar to those addressed by the ANA and in addition supports special programs to recruit minority students into nursing. Each state has a constituent organization of the NSNA. Many individual organizations are located at schools of nursing. The official publication of the NSNA is *Image*. The Canadian University Student Nurses Association is a counterpart to the NSNA in Canada. It also has provincial and local chapters.

International Council of Nurses

The International Council of Nurses (ICN) is a federation of national nursing organizations with headquarters in Switzerland. The ICN promotes nursing at the international level and maintains communication among nurses in different countries. Every 4 years the ICN forms a congress, which is attended by delegates from throughout the world. The congress establishes general policy and direction for the ICN. The organization is governed by a board comprised of the presidents of the member organizations.

National League for Nursing

The NLN is an organization open to any individual or organization interested in promoting high-quality nursing. Constituent groups are organized by state or geographic region in most areas of the country. In those areas without constituent leagues, individuals join the national organization directly. The NLN supports the development of effective nursing education through a voluntary national accrediting program based on criteria designed to identify a high-quality educational program. The NLN also supports many studies and publications related to nursing education. As part of its testing program, the NLN has developed tests that can be used for admission assessment and tests of proficiency that can be used to evaluate student attainment. *Nursing and Health Care* is the official publication of the NLN.

Other Nursing Organizations

Many nursing organizations are related to specialty areas in nursing practice. These groups focus on continuing education and the establishment of standards for specialty practice. Many have developed mechanisms for certifying nurses as specialists in their area of practice. The Association of Operating Room Nurses (AORN), Association of Women's Health, Obstetrical, and Neonatal Nursing (AWHONN; formerly called NAACOG, the Nurses' Association of the American College of Obstetricians and Gynecologists), and the American Association of Nurse Anesthetists (AANA) are just a few of the major organizations of this type.

Some nursing groups have been organized to promote scholarship and leadership in nursing. The *American Academy of Nursing* is composed of those who are invited to join in recognition of their contribution to the field of nursing. Members are termed "fellows" and use the initials FAAN (Fellow of the American Academy of Nursing). *Sigma Theta Tau* is a national nursing honorary organization that invites leaders in the community, in the senior classes of baccalaureate nursing programs, or in graduate programs to become members. Sigma Theta Tau supports research in nursing. Some organizations within nursing are organized around certain social or cultural concerns. The *National Black Nurses Association*, the *American Indian Nurses Organization*, and the *Assembly of Men in Nursing* are examples of these. Other organizations focus on specific goals, such as the *National Organization for the Advancement of Associate Degree Nursing* (NOAADN), which supports continued registered nurse licensure for associate degree graduates and supports excellence in associate degree nursing programs.

The Definition of Nursing

Given the wide differences among the places where nurses practice and in the clients with whom they work, it is probably not surprising that no single definition of nursing is accepted as best by all nurses. We present several definitions of nursing, each of which might be useful in a particular situation.

International Council of Nurses Definition

In 1973, the ICN adopted a definition of nursing written by Virginia Henderson. It states, "The unique function of the nurse is to assist the individual, sick or well, in the performance of those activities contributing to health or its recovery (or to peaceful death) that he would perform unaided if he had the necessary strength, will or knowledge" (Henderson, 1966, p. 15). One major strength of this definition is that it clearly identifies a realm of health care that belongs uniquely to nursing: assisting individuals with aspects of life that they would ordinarily perform unaided. This definition emphasizes that nursing is primarily related to daily living and helps to distinguish nursing from other health care occupations that provide direct care, such as physical therapy.

Henderson's definition does not focus on curing patients of illness but on caring for them in such a way as to enhance their lives. It embraces health as well as illness. It emphasizes the importance of supporting patients and their families when the patients' lives must end as well as when health can be restored. This definition encompasses the full range of an individual's needs—physical, psychological, social, and spiritual—and stresses that nursing involves caring for the whole person. Above all, it underscores the independence and autonomy of the patient/client.

American Nurses Association Definition

In *Scope for Nursing Practice: A Social Policy Statement*, the ANA defined nursing as the "diagnosis and treatment of human responses to actual or potential health problems." Human responses were identified as:

> 1. Reactions of individuals and groups to actual problems (health-restoring responses), such as the impact of illness—effects on the self, family, and related self-care needs; and
> 2. Concerns of individuals and groups about potential problems (health-supporting responses), such as monitoring and teaching in populations or communities at risk in which educative needs for information, skill development, health-oriented attitudes, and related behavioral change arise (ANA, 1981).

The ANA Model Nurse Practice Act provides a format for the legal definition of nursing:

> The performance for compensation of professional services requiring substantial specialized knowledge of the biological, physical, behavioral, psychological, and sociological sciences and nursing theory as the basis for assessment, diagnosis, planning, intervention, and evaluation in the promotion and maintenance of health; the case finding and management of illness, injury, or infirmity; the restoration of optimum function; or the achievement of a dignified death.
> Nursing practice includes but is not limited to administration, teaching, counseling, supervision, delegation, and evaluation of practice and execution of the medical regimen (ANA, 1980).

This definition recognizes that nursing is based on sound knowledge, that it involves a consistent methodology, that it involves more than direct care, and that it is involved with persons who are ill, those for whom prevention is the focus, and those who are dying. The final clause leaves the definition open ended to allow for change and growth.

National Council of State Boards of Nursing Definition

The National Council of State Boards of Nursing Model Nursing Practice Act defines nursing as "assisting individuals or groups to maintain or attain optimal health throughout the life process by assessing their health status, establishing a diagnosis, planning and implementing a strategy of care to accomplish defined goals, and evaluating responses to care and treatment" (National Council of State Boards of Nursing, 1982).

Definitions in State Licensing Laws

None of the states or territories uses the exact wording of the Model Nurse Practice Act or the Council of State Boards definition. The definition found in each state law is the result of the entire legislative process of hearings, committee meetings, and floor debate before final voting. During this process, the proposed law usually undergoes changes and compromises. Some concepts, however, are usually found in all of these laws: a reference to performing services for compensation, the importance of the knowledge base, and the use of a nursing process approach.

All but six of the state statutes refer to the execution of the medical regimen, and ten include a reference to treating human responses to actual or potential health problems. Twenty-four laws include a statement that additional acts may be identified by the health care community as appropriate to nursing practice. This type of generalization allows the profession to grow and change without coming into conflict with the law.

It will be important for you to read the laws governing the practice of nursing where you reside and to make sure that you understand the provisions contained in that law (LeBar, 1984).

Theories of Nursing

A **theory** is comprised of a group of concepts, their definitions, and statements regarding the interrelationships between those concepts developed for the purpose of explaining, predicting, or controlling the phenomena under consideration. The accuracy and value of any theory must be supported by careful research. A **conceptual model** is a group of concepts and general statements of relationship that are not supported by research.

Although some writers argue that the current formulations in nursing are not sufficiently supported by research to be called theories and should instead be designated as conceptual models, it seems to the authors that this argument is not useful. Whether called conceptual models or theories, these formulations are being used as guides for nursing practice and research and have value for the development of nursing as a science.

We present a general overview of some of the most common nursing theories in current use (Table 1-1). This is not a complete description of each theoretical model, but will introduce you to the language used and alert you to alternative ways of looking at the same subject. If your nursing program is using a particular theory as a central focus, you will need to study that theory more extensively, using the references at the end of the chapter.

All of the nursing theories speak to the concepts of *person, health, environment,* and *nursing.* These four concepts and their interrelationships are central to the domain of nursing. As you study this text, consider how the material in it relates to these four concepts and their relationships. Additional information on theories of nursing is found in Chapters 5 and 8.

Rogers' Science of Unitary Man

Martha Rogers' model (Rogers, 1970) emphasizes that the environment within which the person exists is a space–time continuum that is four dimensional (it has height, width, depth, and time). She identifies the person as a unified, organized energy field with a unique pattern that is continually exchanging matter and energy with the environment. Furthermore, the person is a unitary whole that cannot be understood in terms of its parts. The development of the person is unidirectional (in one direction) toward increasing complexity and innovation. The categories used by the North American Nursing Diagnosis Association for organizing nursing diagnoses (see Chapter 10) have much in common with Rogers' description of the unitary person. Rogers does not view health and illness as separate states, but she also does not view them as poles at either end of a continuum. Health for the individual represents increasing innovation in patterning. Nursing is aimed at the repatterning of the person and the environment to allow optimal development.

Peplau's Interpersonal Relations Model

Hildegarde Peplau (1952) views the person as striving to reach equilibrium (although that is never achieved except in death) and maintains that this striving creates tensions and needs. The condition of health implies that the person is moving in the direction of being creative, constructive, and living in community with others. When immediate needs are met, more mature needs will arise, allowing for growth. Nursing assists individuals to meet their needs through interpersonal relationships. Peplau's environmental focus is on significant persons who interrelate.

Table 1–1. Similarities and Differences of Conceptualization in Six Selected Nursing Models

	Person				
	Goal	*Composition*	**Health**	**Environment**	**Nursing**
Peplau	Equilibrium	System with physiologic, psychological, and social components	Meeting needs	Significant others	Therapeutic interpersonal process
Johnson	Balance	Behavioral system with seven subsystems	Equilibrium	External inputs	External force to restore stability
Orem	Constancy	Whole with physical, psychological, interpersonal, social aspects	Meeting self-care needs	External forces	Actions to limit self-care deficits
Roy	Equilibrium	System with biopsychosocial components	Adaptation	External conditions	Manipulation of stimuli to foster coping
Neuman	Balance	Composite of physiologic, psychological, sociocultural, developmental variables	Equilibrium	Internal and external stressors	Reduction of stressors
Rogers	Increased complexity of pattern	Indivisible energy field	Increasing innovativeness of patterning	Contiguous, continuously interacting energy field	Repatterning to facilitate potential

Leddy, S. and Pepper, J. M. *Conceptual Bases of Professional Nursing*, p. 148. Philadelphia: J. B. Lippincott, 1985.

Johnson's Behavioral Systems Model

Dorothy Johnson describes a person as a behavioral system composed of interrelated subsystems. Health exists, she says, when the system has achieved a dynamic equilibrium. Her definition of environment encompasses everything that provides input to the person. Nursing is needed when the system is in disequilibrium; the goal of nursing is to assist in restoring equilibrium and system stability (Johnson, 1980).

Orem's Self-Care Model

In Dorothea Orem's model (Orem, 1952), the human being is a unity that can be viewed as functioning biologically, symbolically, and socially. The person has universal self-care requisites (needs) and self-care requisites associated with individual development. In addition, the person may have therapeutic self-care requisites resulting from deviations from health. Health is defined here as a state of wholeness and integrity in which the individual is capable of self-care and is related to normal structure and function. The environment encompasses all factors external to the person. When the person is not capable of self-care, a state that Orem calls having a self-care deficit, nursing either assists the person to return to a condition in which self-care is possible or provides the care needed.

Roy's Adaptation Model

The person in Sister Callista Roy's model (Roy, 1984) is described as a biopsychosocial being, a unified system seeking equilibrium. Health is a state of equilibrium reached through **adaptation** to the stressors in life. (See Chapter 6 for a discussion of stress and stressors.) Health and illness are on a continuum in Roy's model, with death at one end and peak health at the other. The environment encompasses external conditions and influences that affect the person, either contributing to the stress or assisting in the adaptation process. Nursing is directed at supporting and fostering adaptation in all spheres of life. This may be accomplished by directing actions toward any of four modes (methods) of adaptation: physiologic, self-conceptual, role function, and interdependence relations.

Neuman's Systems Model

In Betty Neuman's model (Neuman, 1982), the person is viewed as an open system (*ie*, one that receives input from and has output into the environment). The environment consists of both internal and external forces, which surround the person at any time. Neuman describes health as a state in which all parts and subparts of the person are in harmony with the whole. If the person's total needs are met, the individual is in a state of optimal wellness. Forces that tend to disrupt the individual are labeled "stressors," and the person possesses defenses against the disturbances they cause. Nursing is concerned with all of the variables that affect the person's response to stressors and may involve blocking stressors or strengthening defenses against them.

Watson's Theory of Human Caring

Jean Watson described nursing as the science of human caring. She states that caring involves an interpersonal process that includes values, will, commitment, knowledge, actions, and accountability for consequences. She sees human caring in nursing as far more than an emotion, but rather as a response to the total person: body, mind, and soul. The caring person is responsive to others as unique individuals and uses knowledge of health–illness, person–environment interactions, the caring process, and self as a basis for taking action. The caring person assists another in meeting human needs through providing a supportive, protective, or corrective environment.

Henderson's Basic Needs/Activities

Virginia Henderson's definition of nursing (Henderson, 1966) was adopted by the ICN. Henderson viewed the person as having biologic, psychological, sociologic, and spiritual components. These are reflected in her list of 14 activities of the person (Display 1-4). She states that body and mind are inseparable and that each person is unique. She does not emphasize any particular concept of the environment. She defines health as a state in which a person is able to engage independently in the 14 activities. Nursing focuses on helping the person to accomplish these activities or providing the conditions under which the individual can accomplish them.

Developing a Working Model of Nursing

Because no one theoretical or conceptual approach to nursing is supported by all nurses, each school of nursing adopts or devises one that will guide its curriculum development and be used by students in providing nursing care, and this is termed a working model. As you grow in your own knowledge and experience, you will adopt the theory or blending of theories that is most useful to you in your work. Nursing theories (and the

Display 1–4
The Nature of Nursing

The unique function of the nurse is to assist the individual, sick or well, in the performance of those activities contributing to health or its recovery (or to peaceful death) that he would perform unaided if he had the necessary strength, will, or knowledge. And to do this in such a way as to help him gain independence as rapidly as possible.

. . . The nurse is the authority on basic nursing care—by basic nursing care I mean helping the patient with the following activities or providing conditions under which he can perform them unaided:

1. Breathe normally.
2. Eat and drink adequately.
3. Eliminate body wastes.
4. Move and maintain desirable postures.
5. Sleep and rest.
6. Select suitable clothes—dress and undress.
7. Maintain body temperature within normal range by adjusting clothing and modifying the environment.
8. Keep the body clean and well groomed and protect the integument.
9. Avoid dangers in the environment and avoid injuring others.
10. Communicate with others in expressing emotions, needs, fears, or opinions.
11. Worship according to one's faith.
12. Work in such a way that there is a sense of accomplishment.
13. Play or participate in various forms of recreation.
14. Learn, discover, or satisfy the curiosity that leads to normal development and health and use of the available health facilities.

From Henderson. The Nature of Nursing, pp. 15–16. New York: Macmillan, 1966, and Basic Principles of Nursing Care, rev. 1969. International Council of Nurses, Geneva, pp. 4, 12–13. Reprinted with permission.

working models derived from them) have four components, and these components include how the person is viewed, what health means, the relationship of the environment to the individual, and how nursing is viewed.

In this text, our working model of nursing will use the definition conceived by Virginia Henderson, in which the individual is viewed as having biologic, psychological, sociologic, and spiritual components.

The *person* is approached as a total person, with needs that are both universal and specific to that individual. Although the person responds as a totality, it is useful for learning purposes to consider the various needs separately. These needs are presented in Units 5, 6, and 7. Throughout the text we will be giving examples of how these needs are interrelated and the ways in which they affect one another. Adaptation is presented as a process used in meeting needs (see Chapter 6).

Health is viewed as a state in which the individual is in dynamic equilibrium with the environment and within the self. This state is called *homeostasis*; it allows for growth and development. Illness may disrupt health, but some aspects of health coexist with illness. Health and illness are presented in detail in Chapter 7.

The *environment* involves other people (the interpersonal environment), inanimate objects (the physical environment), and forces external to the person (the sociocultural environment). The physical environment is the focus of Chapter 21, which reflects on the need for safety. Chapters 13 and 14 focus on the interpersonal environment and the nurse's role within it. The sociocultural environment is the focus of Chapter 33. Various aspects of the environment are discussed in relation to individual needs throughout the text.

In this text, the individual will be the major focus of *nursing*, although nursing also encompasses families and communities. The nursing process is the methodology through which nursing is provided to the client or patient. This is a problem-solving approach to patient care.

The Role of the Nurse

Analysis of the *role* of the nurse can be approached from many different perspectives. Perhaps the most basic one involves comparing the social role of an individual in a personal relationship with the professional role of a nurse in a relationship with a patient/client. Another way of viewing the nurse's role involves recognizing the many different components found in the professional role. A final aspect is the role of the nurse in interpersonal relationships within the health care setting.

The Social Versus the Professional Role

A positive *professional role* bears many similarities to a positive *social role*. At their best, both are based on honesty, which engenders the trust basic to any sound relationship. In both the professional and the social roles, one should respect the rights and autonomy of others. Both people in a relationship are responsible for that relationship and its outcomes.

There are, however, major differences between the

professional role and the social role (Fig. 1-6). Social relationships may have a variety of purposes, which change as the participants develop and change in relation to one another. Some social relationships have no particular explicit purpose. The professional relationship, however, is purposeful and goal directed. The participants focus on the goal of the relationship—which is often explicitly stated—and direct their efforts toward accomplishing it.

In social relationships, it is assumed that the needs of all participants are equally important. The focus of a professional relationship with a patient/client, however, is the *client's* needs and concerns. Let us examine what this means in a practical way. A nurse who is experiencing stress or a personal crisis might need to talk about such problems with a sympathetic and supportive person. It would be inappropriate, however, to expect the patient/client to meet that need. A person assumes the role of patient/client because of existing stresses and needs, and it would be inappropriate to introduce more. This does not mean that personal stresses and difficulties do not affect the nurse's functioning; this would be an unrealistic expectation. It means that the nurse should address such difficulties outside the nurse–patient relationship by seeking out a friend, colleague, or counselor. The nursing relationship focuses on the needs of the patient/client.

The professional is also expected to bring to the relationship expertise and knowledge beneficial to the patient/client. The patient/client expects the nurse to meet needs the patient/client is unable to provide for independently.

Finally, the professional relationship is time limited; the participants expect that it will end when the goal has been reached. The social role, on the other hand, tends to be open ended; termination of the relationship is not foreseen at the outset.

The nurse's professional role has a wide variety of components. Some of these are based in communication skills, others relate to providing care, and others are managerial in nature. The role also encompasses acting as an advocate for the client in the complex health care system and supporting the profession of nursing.

The Nurse as Communicator

The nurse uses communication as a tool in establishing an interpersonal relationship with clients and families. Within this context, the nurse establishes trust and alters communication in ways that are most helpful and supportive to the client and family. Communication is used to interview clients and gain the information needed to provide optimum health care. In some settings, such as psychiatric nursing, this is the principal form that nursing takes.

Communication is used to maintain the open sharing of information among those participating in the overall health care plan. It appears in written form in medical records and in nursing care plans. It also includes information given orally to other nurses, other health care professionals, individuals, and groups of individuals.

Communication is also the basis for the teaching function of the nurse. Nurses teach ways to maintain and enhance health as well as ways to cope with illness and its consequences. Teaching is individualized to the particular situation of the client and family and is based on knowledge of both the individual and the health care problems.

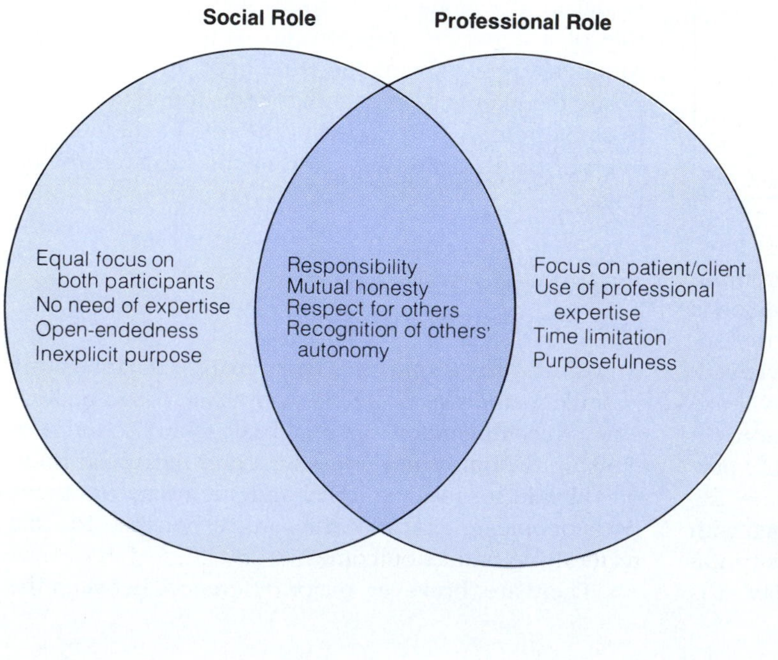

Figure 1-6. The social versus the professional role.

The Nurse as Provider of Care

In providing care, the nurse is responsible for all aspects of the nursing process (see Chapters 8–12). This process includes the skills necessary for assessing the client/patient, identifying the nursing diagnoses, planning for care, implementing the care planned, and evaluating that care. A full description of skills necessary for basic nursing care are found in *Modules for Basic Nursing Skills,* volumes I and II. Some of the care provided is part of the independent function of the nurse. Other care is part of the physician's medical treatment plan (*eg,* giving medications).

The Nurse as Manager of Care

Management of care includes setting priorities for one client and among clients. It may include arranging for consultations with other health care professionals and directing the care of nursing assistants or other nurses. Managing care might also include working within an institution to set up policies and procedures for nursing care. In this text we will focus on managing the care of one client.

The Nurse as Client/Patient Advocate

In the complex health care system of today, the individual often feels overwhelmed. Systems and organizations are designed for their own effective functioning and do not always respond to the needs of the patient/client. As a person functioning as part of the system, who therefore understands it, the nurse is often able to act as an **advocate** for the patient/client. In this role, the nurse helps the individual to seek out the kind of care needed, to ask for modification when appropriate, and to exercise his or her own rights regarding health care. An advocate assists individuals in speaking out for themselves and speaks out for those who cannot do so independently.

The Nurse as Member of the Profession

The nursing profession itself has responsibilities to society for providing safe and effective care. As a member of the profession, with the privilege to practice accorded by a license from the state, each nurse has responsibilities, which include maintaining standards of practice, assisting with the development of the profession, and participating in efforts to monitor the profession. Most responsibilities are carried out through participation in committees within the work setting and through participation in nursing organizations.

The Independent Role Versus the Collaborative Role

Much of the discussion thus far has focused on the **independent role** of the nurse. Within the realm that is uniquely nursing, the nurse is accountable for the patient's care. No one else provides nursing, and if the nurse does not, the patient's well-being is in jeopardy. Both the law and the ethical standards of nursing make nurses responsible for their practice. The nurse makes independent decisions regarding what care is needed, how it should be provided, and who should provide it. This does not mean that the nurse does not consult with others to seek input as necessary, but that ultimate accountability lies with the nurse.

This accountability emphasizes the unique contribution of the nurse to the health care of the individual; however, the nurse also must work with the physician in carrying out the medical plan for care. The duty to cooperate is an important responsibility. Some people call this cooperative aspect of nursing the dependent function of the nurse, to differentiate it from the independent function that is uniquely nursing. Others do not like to use the term dependent to describe any segment of nursing because it may lead people to assume that this area of function does not require depth of knowledge and decision-making ability. *Collaborative,* working together, is the most accurate word to understand this area of nursing responsibility. In the *collaborative role,* in addition to nurse-prescribed interventions, the nurse acts to ensure that information essential to the physician in diagnosing and treating illness is communicated and that specific aspects of the medical plan of care, such as giving medications and treatments, are implemented.

These two aspects of nursing are both important. However, which function is emphasized will depend on the specific patient/client situation. For example, in a long-term care setting, the majority of the nursing time and effort may be focused on the nurse's independent function of trying to identify problems in meeting the basic needs for daily living, whereas during an emergency in an intensive care unit, the nurse may focus most attention on implementing the physician's plan for treating the medical crisis. The nurse may have to decide which function is more important in a given situation, but from the perspective of the overall nursing process, both roles are necessary and neither should be neglected.

The Nursing Process

In whatever setting the nurse practices, the methodology, or approach, to nursing is the same. This methodology, called the **nursing process**, is a problem-solving approach to patient care. Its basic components are *assessment, diagnosis, planning, implementation,* and *evaluation.* Some writers subdivide these basic steps into additional steps, which results in a seemingly different process. In reality these different lists of steps are different ways of looking at the same process, not different processes. Because the standards for nursing practice developed by the ANA and the majority of nursing literature use the five basic steps, we use that structure in this text.

Assessment encompasses all the activities used to gather information. It includes interviewing, observing, the physical examination, and reviewing any pertinent records.

Then the nurse must sort that information and make decisions about the nature of the individual's problems or concerns. The result is a statement of the patient's problem that is termed the *nursing diagnosis.* This step is called *nursing diagnosis* or *analysis.*

Planning encompasses the activities that are used to determine the appropriate course of action. Doris Carnevali and colleagues (1984) state that plans fall into four categories: assisting the person to continue with self-care through instruction and direction, providing independent nursing care, referring the person to a physician or other care provider, and continuing to provide nursing care prescribed as part of a medical regimen. Outcome criteria to be used in evaluation are established during the planning step.

Implementation is carrying out the plans made and involves direct care skills. Information on carrying out direct care skills will be found in *Modules for Basic Nursing Skills,* volumes I and II. Another aspect of implementation is the use of communication and teaching skills with patients. Implementation may also involve using communication skills with others on the health care team and working with groups of people.

Evaluation of the outcomes of nursing care is an essential part of the nursing process. The criteria for specific desired outcomes are established during planning, then the outcomes evaluated later. Evaluation is used to determine the success of actions and to redirect the nursing process.

Unit 3 discusses in detail the use of the nursing process.

The Art of Nursing

Nursing is both a science and an art. The nursing process is part of the science of nursing. The science of nursing is much easier to describe than is the art, but it is no more important. The art is embodied in the manner in which individual nurses practice. It is a product of the individual nurse's personality as well as the knowledge the individual nurse has.

Martin Buber, in his treatise entitled *I and Thou* (1958), focused on the importance of being authentically oneself in a relationship. He stated that only as we are truly ourselves in a relationship can we discover who we really are. He said further that our being authentic opens the path for the other individual to be authentic and discover himself or herself within the relationship. If nursing exists to assist others in their move toward maximum health and if health is associated with achieving one's maximum potential, then the health of both nurse and client is enhanced by an authentic relationship.

Individual nurses demonstrate the art of nursing more effectively than it can ever be described on paper. As you begin your practice, look for examples of nursing art in action and seek ways to develop in yourself the art as well as the science of nursing.

Decision-Making in Nursing

Who Makes Decisions

Whenever a decision needs to be made in health care, the first consideration is who should make that decision. This is sometimes referred to as *locus of decision-making.* The answer depends on the patient/client involved and the nature of the decision to be made. If at all possible, the decision-making responsibility should rest with the person who will be most affected by the outcome; in the care setting, this is usually the patient/client. For patients/clients to make good decisions, they must have enough information. The legal issue of providing adequate information to the patient/client is discussed in Chapter 3. When the individual patient/client is unable to make personal decisions because of youth, mental incompetence, or the severity of the illness, decisions are made by an appropriate guardian.

On many occasions in health care, it is appropriate for the patient/client and the health care provider to share decision-making. This is especially true when the decision requires an ethical or legal commitment on the part of the health care provider or when the expertise of the health care provider is essential in coming to an appropriate decision. In this instance, the health care provider talks with the patient/client and together they come to a decision.

Other decisions are made by the health care provider alone. Decisions that fall into this category are those that require only professional judgment (such as when a medication must be scheduled) or those that revolve around the provider's tasks. Sometimes the health care provider must make decisions for the patient/client because the latter is incapacitated. This might be true for the unconscious patient or the infant.

When making decisions of this kind, you should consider the patient/client's point of view.

Determining where decision-making responsibility should lie can be difficult. After learning of the importance of individual autonomy, a student may turn over all decision-making to the patient/client. Doing this may result in clients feeling very ill at ease because they expect health care workers to assist with making decisions. Having to shoulder the entire burden of decision-making may also further confuse a somewhat disoriented elderly person. On the other hand, some students become so involved with their new knowledge that they assume that all of the health care decisions should rest with the person having the greatest professional knowledge. When decisions need to be made, it is wise to consult with an instructor or more experienced nurse to verify where the responsibility for decision-making should lie.

Accountability and Authority

Much is being written in health care about **accountability**, which refers to responsibility for the outcomes related to decisions and actions. An accountable person strives to be well prepared to make sound decisions and act appropriately. The accountable person evaluates the outcomes of decisions and actions and accepts responsibility for those outcomes. The accountable person also tries to alleviate any problems created by his or her actions. **Authority** refers to having the power to carry out the actions necessary to achieve the desired outcome. Nurses sometimes find themselves being asked to be accountable for outcomes when they do not have the necessary authority to affect the situation. When you are asked to be accountable for outcomes, it is important to establish clearly that you have the authority to affect actions.

As a student, you will be expected to be accountable for your own decisions and actions. It is critical that you clearly evaluate yourself, know your own abilities and limits, and operate within them. Although you may be a novice, the patient/client is entitled to the same high standard of care whether it is being delivered by a student or by a registered nurse. When you meet a new situation, it is your responsibility to consult with your instructor and obtain supervision when needed. You will need to understand clearly when you have authority for decision-making and when final authority rests elsewhere. Often you will be asked to make a decision yourself, but then to check with someone else before actually carrying out your decision. This process will help you become more skilled and at the same time will protect patient/clients.

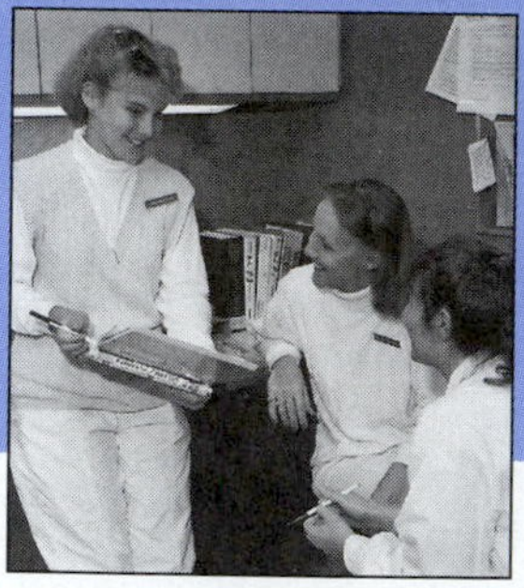

Key Points

- The history of nursing provides insight into how nursing has evolved to what it is today.
- Nursing as we know it today grew out of the work of Florence Nightingale in establishing nursing schools and began its professional development in the United States with the establishment of educational systems and licensure. Currently, controversy surrounds the type and amount of education required for entry-level professional practice.
- The settings in which nurses practice continue to grow and diversify, including hospitals, long-term care facilities, schools, home health agencies, occupational settings, and ambulatory care centers.
- Nursing organizations provide nurses a means by which they can work together on professional issues. Some of these organizations have written definitions of nursing that provide guidelines in practice. The definitions incorporated into licensing laws in each jurisdiction form the legal framework within which the nurse must practice.
- Theories of nursing provide framework for nursing education and practice. The four major concepts central to these theories are the person, health, the environment, and nursing. These concepts form the basis for a working model of nursing for this text.
- The professional role of the nurse includes that of communicator, provider of care, manager of care, patient/client advocate, and member of a profession. In carrying out these roles, the nurse may be operating independently or collaboratively with other health care professionals.
- The nursing process involves assessment, diagnosis, planning, intervention, and evaluation. Throughout this text the nursing process will be emphasized as a valuable tool.
- The approach to the patient/client is a problem-solving one. Within this context, however, decision-making is not always the responsibility of the nurse alone. Sometimes the decision-making lies entirely with the client, and other times the nurse and client share decision-making.
- Accepting responsibility and being accountable are essential characteristics of the registered nurse.

Study Questions

1. What are the three general images of nursing seen in early nursing history?
2. What are the major contributions that Florence Nightingale made to nursing?
3. What is the definition of nursing written by Virginia Henderson?
4. Explain the steps in the nursing process.
5. How does the social role differ from the professional role?
6. How do the independent role and the collaborative role of the nurse compare?
7. In what situations does the nurse make decisions for the patient?
8. Describe the difference between the nurse's role in functional nursing and the nurse's role in primary nursing.
9. What are the advantages of team nursing?
10. What are the differences among the three types of programs that prepare registered nurses?
11. Define the ladder concept.
12. Identify the four major concepts that are central to all theories of nursing.
13. List and describe the steps in the nursing process.

Critical Thinking Activities

1. Obtain the Nurse Practice Act for your state and read the definition of nursing. Compare and contrast it with the model definitions written by the ANA and National Council of State Boards of Nursing.
2. In the library, look up a definition of nursing written by one of the theorists named. Compare and contrast this definition with that adopted by the ICN.
3. Think of a situation in which you were a client dealing with a professional. Analyze the situation and describe behaviors by the professional that tended to define the relationship as professional and not social.
4. Research the ways in which an associate degree graduate could obtain a baccalaureate degree in nursing in your community or area. Evaluate the programs in terms of accessibility, cost, and flexibility for adult learners.
5. Research the avenues for continuing education for nurses, other than degree programs, that are avail-

able in your community. Evaluate the providers relative to credentials of instructors, acceditation of offerings, and cost.

6. Find a description of a problem-solving process in a field other than nursing and compare the steps of the two processes.

References and Readings

American Nurses Association. *Scope for Nursing Practice: A Social Policy Statement.* Kansas City, Mo.: ANA, 1981.

———. *Model Nurse Practice Act.* Kansas City, Mo.: ANA, 1980.

———. "First position paper on education for nursing." *American Journal of Nursing* 65 (December 1965): 106–111.

Barritt, E. R. "Florence Nightingale's Values and Modern Nursing Education." *Nursing Forum* 12, 1 (January 1973): 6, 47.

Beitz, J. M. "Survival Skills for the RN Student." *Nursing '89.* 19, 10 (October 1989): 66–69.

Buber, M. *I and Thou* Translated by Ronald Gregor Smith. New York: Charles Scribner's Sons, 1958.

Carnegie, M. E. *The Path We Tread: Blacks in Nursing 1854–1984.* Philadelphia: J. B. Lippincott, 1986.

Carnevali, D. L.; Mitchell, P. H.; Woods, N. F.; and Tanner, C. A. *Diagnostic Reasoning in Nursing.* Philadelphia: J. B. Lippincott, 1984.

Christy, T. "Entry into Practice: A Recurring Issue in Nursing History." *American Journal of Nursing* 80, 3 (March 1980): 485–488.

———. "Equal Rights for Women: Voices from the Past." *American Journal of Nursing* 71, 2 (February 1971): 288–293.

———. "First Fifty Years." *American Journal of Nursing* 71, 9 (September 1971): 1778–1784.

Donahue, M. P. "The Past in the Present: The Unquestionable Relevance of Historical Analysis to the Resolution of Increasingly Critical Problems Affecting Nursing." *Journal of Professional Nursing* 6, 1 (January-February, 1990): 9.

Ellis, J. R., and Hartley, C. L. *Nursing in Today's World: Challenges, Issues, and Trends.* 4th ed. Philadelphia: J. B. Lippincott, 1992.

Fiedman, E. "Troubled Past of an 'Invisible' Profession: Nursing in the United States." *Journal of the American Medical Association* 264, 22 (December 12, 1990): 2851–2852, 2854–2855, 2858.

Franzoi, S. L. "A Picture of Competence." *American Journal of Nursing 88,* 8, 109–112.

Geissler, E. M. Nurturance Flows Two Ways. *American Journal of Nursing* 90, 4 (April 1990): 72–74.

Gordon, M. *Nursing Diagnosis: Process and Application.* 2nd ed. New York: McGraw-Hill, 1987.

Gordon, S. "Fear of Caring: The Feminist Paradox." *American Journal of Nursing* 91, 2 (February 1991): 44–48.

Gropper, E. I. "Florence Nightingale: Nursing's First Environmental Theorist." *Nursing Forum* 25, 3 (1990): 30–33.

Grubbs, J. "The Johnson Behavioral System Model." In *Conceptual Models for Nursing Practice,* edited by C. Riehl and C. Roy, 2nd ed. Norwalk, Conn.: Appleton-Century-Crofts, 1980.

Henderson, V. *The Nature of Nursing.* New York: Macmillan, 1966.

Johnson, D. "The Behavioral System Model for Nursing." In *Conceptual Models for Nursing Practice,* edited by C. Riehl and C. Roy, 2nd ed. Norwalk, Conn.: Appleton-Century-Crofts, 1980.

Kalisch, P. A., and Kalisch, B. J. "Nurses on Prime-Time Television." *American Journal of Nursing* 82 (February 1982): 264–266.

———. "The Image of the Nurse in Motion Pictures." *American Journal of Nursing* 82 (April 1982): 605–607.

———. "The Image of Nurses in Novels." *American Journal of Nursing* 82 (August 1982): 1220–1224.

Kim, M. J., and Moritz, D. A., ed. *Classification of Nursing Diagnosis.* New York: McGraw-Hill, 1982.

King, I. *Toward a Theory for Nursing.* New York: John Wiley and Sons, 1971.

Kippenbrock, T. A. "I Wish I'd Been There: A Sense of Nursing History." *Nursing and Health Care* 12, 4 (April 1991): 208–212.

LeBar, C. *Statutory Definitions of Nursing Practice and Their Conformity to Certain ANA Principles.* Kansas City, Mo.: American Nurses Association, 1984.

Malone, R. E. "The Challenge of Third World Nursing." *American Journal of Nursing* 90, 7 (July 1990): 32–37.

Meleis, A. I. *Theoretical Nursing: Development and Progress.* Philadelphia: J. B. Lippincott, 1985.

National Council of State Boards of Nursing, Inc. *Model Nursing Practice Act.* Chicago: NCSBN, 1982.

———. "North Dakota Rule Changes Require Associate, Baccalaureate Education." *Issues* 7(2): 1–3, 1986.

Neuman, B. *The Neuman Systems Model: Application to Nursing Education and Practice.* Norwalk, Conn.: Appleton-Century-Crofts, 1982.

Orem, D. E. *Nursing: Concepts of Practice.* 4th ed. New York: McGraw-Hill, 1991.

Orlando, I. J. *The Discipline and Teaching of Nursing Process (An Evaluative Study).* New York: G. P. Putnam's Sons, 1972.

Pavelka, M. "Definition of Nursing Practice." *Issues* 3, 2 (Summer 1982): 48–50.

Peplau, H. *Interpersonal Relations in Nursing.* New York: G. P. Putnam's Sons, 1952.

Perkins, J. L., Bennett, D. N., and Dorman, R. "Why Men Choose Nursing." *Image* 14: 1 (January 1993) 34–38.

Pooyan, A., Eberhardt, B. J., and Szigeti, E. "Work-Related Variables and Turnover Intention Among Registered Nurses." *Nursing and Health Care* 11, 5 (May 1990): 255–258.

Roberts, M. M. *American Nursing: History and Interpretation.* New York: Macmillan, 1954.

Rogers, M. *An Introduction to the Theoretical Basis of Nursing.* Philadelphia: F. A. Davis, 1970.

Roy, Sr. C. *Introduction to Nursing: An Adaptation Model.* Englewood Cliffs, N.J.: Prentice-Hall, 1984.

Uprichard, M. "Ferment in Nursing." In *The Challenge of Nursing,* edited by M. Auld and E. Birnum. St. Louis: C. V. Mosby, 1973.

Watson, J. *Nursing: Human Science and Human Care—A Theory of Nursing.* New York: National League for Nursing, 1988.

Welch, M. "Florence Nightingale: The Social Construction of a Victorian Feminist." *Western Journal of Nursing Research* 12, 3 (June 1990): 404–407.

The Health Care System

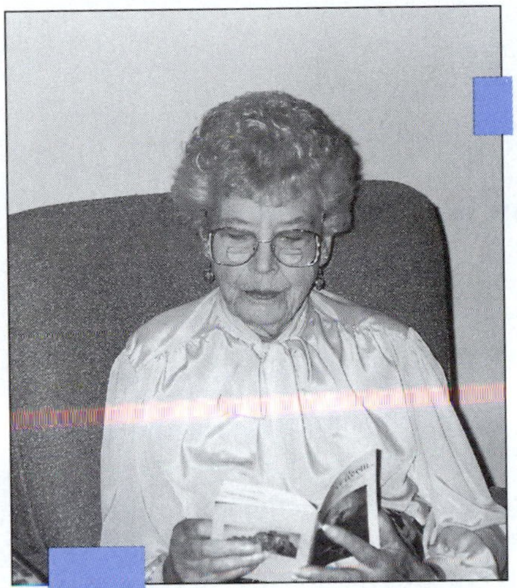

2

Objectives

After completing this chapter, you should be able to:

1. Discuss what is meant by health care as a system.
2. Identify the major components of the health care system.
3. Identify the role of accreditation in health care facilities.
4. Discuss the various ways in which health care is funded.
5. Explain the role of diagnosis-related groups (DRGs) in funding health care in the United States.
6. Identify several major societal trends that affect health care.
7. Explain the different types of health care workers.
8. Differentiate between independent and collaborative functioning.
9. Discuss problems in the delivery of health care and approaches to solving those problems.

Study Terms

accreditation
burnout
community mental health agencies
contraindications
cost containment
collaborative functioning
health care team
health maintenance organization (HMO)
home health agency
hospice
independent functioning
long-term care
Medicaid
medically indigent
Medicare
nurse practitioner
nursing home
nursing orders
open system
preferred provider organization (PPO)
primary health care
prospective reimbursement
quality assurance
quality management
rehabilitation
retrospective reimbursement
secondary health care
sheltered care
tertiary health care
third-party payer
utilization review

Outline

Health Care as a System

Major Components of the Health Care System

World Health Organization
Government Agencies
Third-Party Payers
Health Maintenance Organizations
Preferred Provider Organizations
Primary Health Care Providers
Institutional Providers of Health Care
Voluntary Associations
Health Promotion Organizations

Accreditation of Health Care Facilities

Ellis, Nowlis: Nursing: A Human Needs Approach, 5th ed. © 1994, J.B. Lippincott Company

Funding of Health Care

Sources of Health Care Funds

Methods of Reimbursing for Health Care Costs

Nursing Concerns Related to Reimbursement

Cost Containment

Quality Assurance

Societal Trends Affecting the Health Care System

Increasingly Sophisticated Technology

Changes in Health Care Worker Supply

Changes in Health Care Institutions

Increased Numbers of Elders in the Population

Health Care Reform

Individuals in Health Care

Specific Health Care Occupations

Differences in Preparation for Health Care Roles

Credentials for Practice

Functioning Within the Health Care Team

Problems in the Delivery of Health Care

Depersonalization of Care

Loss of Privacy

Communication Barriers

Need for Continuing Education

Overlapping Responsibilities

Burnout

The Student's Role in Problems of Health Care Delivery

Since World War II, health care has experienced extraordinary growth in size and complexity. Although advances in health care are almost invariably welcomed, concern runs high about how health care is delivered and about the high cost of such care. To help you better understand the vast system you are entering, let us take a look at its components and how they function.

Health Care as a System

The delivery of health care may be usefully viewed as a *system.* It is composed of interrelated parts that act together to form the whole. A familiar analogy is a school system, whose components may be roughly defined as buildings; personnel who teach, clean, administer, and perform other tasks; a school board, elected to set policy; the curriculum; and supplies. Lacking any of these components, the schools would be unable to perform their overall task of educating children.

The extent of a system depends partly on how it is defined. We can look at the health care system of an entire nation or narrow our investigation to a particular locality. Whatever the case, any system may be analyzed in terms of input and output.

Input consists of all the information and material entering the system. Input may or may not be used by the system. Input into the health care system includes patients entering the system, money used to support the system, and new ideas about health and health care.

Output is whatever is produced by the system. The output of a health care system is primarily people whose health care needs have been met. It also includes those who have left the system with health care needs unmet. Other important outputs are the development of new technology, provision of new health care workers, and information regarding health care for the community.

If a system is to operate correctly, continuous *evaluation* is a necessity. Evaluation must focus on not only the system's output, but also the means used to produce that output. Evaluation should consider measurable characteristics of a system such as efficiency, economy, and successful procedures performed and more abstract matters such as personal satisfaction.

The health care system is an **open system**, that is, there is continuing interaction between the system itself and the environment outside the system. New patients, new practitioners, new technology, and new dollars enter the system continually. The approaches and attitudes of those within the system and the influence of organizations and government agencies are also inputs to the system. The flow of output is constant as well. The system never remains stagnant.

Major Components of the Health Care System

There are many different components of the health care system. Governmental agencies, voluntary associations, health care workers, and businesses all make an impact on health care.

World Health Organization

The World Health Organization (WHO) is an arm of the United Nations, established in 1945 for the purpose of promoting health throughout the world. In carrying out its mission, WHO provides assistance to nations that request help in such areas as sanitation, immunization programs, preventive health care, and care of those with health problems. WHO teams, composed of a doctor, a nurse, a sanitary engineer, and other needed personnel, go to an area to teach health professionals and community members. The team also provides some basic health care. WHO provides data regarding communicable diseases and health-related problems on a worldwide basis. It also publishes material related to health. The headquarters for WHO is in Geneva, Switzerland.

Government Agencies

Government at all levels is deeply involved in health care. The following is by no means an exhaustive list of all of the ways in which the government is involved in health care, but it illustrates the breadth of that involvement. At the local level a health department inspects the sanitation of places selling or serving food, oversees the management of communicable disease in the community, and provides standards for clean water and sewage disposal. Air pollution standards may also be monitored. This type of public health activity has been instrumental in significantly improving the health of individuals. In developing countries the lack of resources to support this activity remains a major concern and barrier to health. Some local communities support hospitals and clinics to provide care for those who are without financial resources. The cost of operation of such facilities and the question of who should be cared for and to what extent are serious economic issues in most communities.

At the state or provincial level rests licensing of individual health care providers and institutions. The state or province may also provide educational opportunities for health careers and approve educational programs in private institutions. State and provincial health departments usually develop policies for managing communicable illness. These may include the operation of laboratories that focus on the diagnosis of such diseases. Some states have an agency that must approve the opening of any new health care facility or the acquisition of major equipment to prevent duplication of costly services. The state may also operate health facilities such as psychiatric hospitals, acute care hospitals, and long-term care facilities. Environmental hazards may be controlled at the state level. In Canada, the provinces each operate a health insurance system that finances health care for all residents of that province. In the United States, the states provide part of the funding for health care for individuals receiving public assistance. Because of concerns regarding cost and access to health care, some states are discussing state-managed health care programs.

In the United States, the federal government provides direct care to some people through Veterans' Administration (VA) hospitals, Native American health care facilities, Public Health Service hospitals, and military hospitals. Indirectly, the federal government pays for care to many others through Medicare (the Social Security program for health care reimbursement to those on Social Security retirement or disability benefits and those in renal failure who need dialysis) and Medicaid (the program for assistance to the indigent, administered by the states). In addition, the federal government provides money for research at both its own National Institutes of Health (NIH) and other institutions through research awards. The federal government exercises control through regulations governing conditions under which reimbursement will be made. For example, the federal government regulated the training of nursing assistants in nursing homes by limiting reimbursement for Medicare and Medicaid patients to those nursing homes that met the training standard. Other governmental agencies affect health care through such activities as monitoring and controlling environmental hazards.

Thus, the United States government is deeply involved in health care. Health care providers must stay informed about government activity that relates to health care and become active participants in decision-making of government bodies. In general, your input through nursing organizations and other political groups has a much more profound effect on health care than individual action might have.

Third-Party Payers

Many people have some outside source that pays all or part of their health care costs. This outside source is often referred to as a **third-party payer**. Some government agencies fund medical programs and thus may be considered third-party payers. Insurance companies are third-party payers and some employers independently fund care through their own health plans.

In response to rising costs and consumer demands, third-party payers have moved from being passive payers to active participants in the health care field. Many payers (both insurance companies and government) now request second opinions before costly surgery is done; they conduct **utilization reviews**, in which they look at patient records to determine whether facilities and treatments were used appropriately; and they support health education projects aimed at decreasing preventable illnesses. A more controversial approach has been to increase premiums for those whose lifestyle or behavior, such as smoking, puts them at higher risk for health problems.

Health Maintenance Organizations

Health maintenance organizations (HMOs) provide full health care services to their members for a fixed prepaid fee. Because the income of the HMO is fixed and all needed care is provided without additional cost to the client, an incentive exists to contain costs. Thus, HMOs emphasize illness prevention and early treatment before costly hospital treatment is required. Some HMOs own hospitals; others contract for inpatient care with hospitals in the community. Although a few HMOs have been in existence since the 1930s, they have recently surged in number as a result of federal legislation creating special incentives for the founding of new HMOs.

Preferred Provider Organizations

Preferred providers are individuals, groups, or organizations that have contracted to provide certain types of care for a group of employees or subscribers to a health care insurance plan. Typically, the preferred providers have agreed to accept fees that are slightly lower than the prevailing community fees. The insurance company or employer will not require the individual to pay a deductible amount if the preferred providers are used. The preferred providers make their profit through controlling costs and having an increased caseload.

Primary Health Care Providers

Primary health care is the level at which a person first contacts the health care system. Routine checkups, including well-child examinations, and care for episodes of illness form the basis of primary health care. *Physicians, dentists,* and *psychiatrists* have all traditionally provided primary care. Primary health care is also provided by *nurse practitioners,* who are nurses with advanced education and clinical expertise in a broad range of diagnostic and curative services as well as the supportive and educational services ambulatory patients need. *Physician's assistants,* who have completed a specialized program of study at a university, work with individual physicians and provide basic health-screening examinations and care for routine health problems. They may also prescribe some medications. Primary health care providers may function independently on a fee-for-service basis, or they may be employed by an institution that provides health care.

Institutional Providers of Health Care

Acute Care Hospitals

Of the many types of institutions and organizations that provide health care, the best known is the *acute care* hospital. The community hospital that provides care beyond what the primary care provider does is called *secondary health care.* These community hospitals provide care for health needs such as childbirth and common surgeries and illnesses. A third level of care is *tertiary health care.* Tertiary health care institutions provide specialized services such as a burn unit, trauma center, or cancer treatment facility for a larger geographic area. The most specialized facilities, those that pursue research and extensive teaching, are usually associated with large universities or medical centers. Each type of hospital has a place in the overall system, and all employ nurses in both direct care and administration.

Long-Term Care Facilities

Long-term care facilities provide care for weeks, months, and even years. A single institution may provide several types of long-term care, each in a different unit. Other institutions provide only one type of long-term care.

Sheltered care is offered for those who have reached their maximum level of functioning but still require supportive services. Sheltered care often is increasingly provided in small group homes within the community for those with mild to moderate mental or physical handicaps. Sheltered care may also be provided in larger institutions such as state institutions for the mentally retarded.

Nursing homes provide a living center where skilled nursing resources are provided. Some individuals, such as frail elderly persons, who reside in nursing homes are not expected to improve but to remain in need of total continued care. Nursing homes also care for people who have been hospitalized and are not yet able to manage independent living. Within the nursing home they regain strength and skill to return home. In the nursing home, the focus is on total quality of life, not simply on health care.

Rehabilitation is the process of assisting individuals with a disabling condition to return to optimum independence and health (Fig. 2-1). Rehabilitation services may be offered in one unit or wing of a larger acute care hospital or nursing home. Other rehabilitation centers are independent institutions. A multidisciplinary group, including physicians, nurses, physical and occupational therapists, and other appropriate individuals, designs a program for each individual. The patient/client, family, and other support persons are included in the planning process as much as possible.

Home Health Agencies

Home health agencies provide a wide variety of services that support individuals in their own homes. The current emphasis in acute care is on discharging patients as soon as possible. The result is that individuals return home still needing supportive services to regain health. Other individuals need home care on an ongoing basis to be able to remain at home rather than in an institution such as a nursing home.

The largest part of home health service is usually

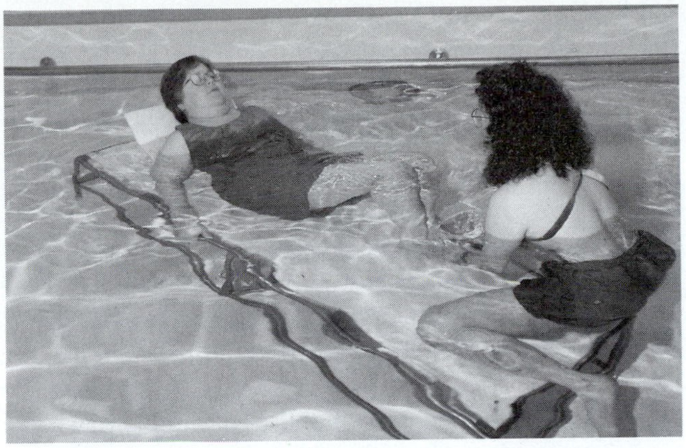

Figure 2-1. Rehabilitation centers seek to restore function and autonomy.

nursing. Registered nurses provide ongoing assessment and skilled care. Licensed practical nurses may provide some kinds of ongoing direct care. Those who need help with personal care, such as bathing, may be cared for by a nursing assistant. Most agencies also have home health aides who provide simple meal preparation, grocery shopping, and house cleaning. In addition to nursing, physical therapy, occupational therapy, and respiratory therapy may be provided in the home.

Providing care in the home requires adaptation to situations in which equipment and supplies may differ from those in institutions. Home care also involves teaching people to care for themselves or for family members and providing the support to help them do this successfully.

Community Mental Health Agencies

Community mental health agencies provide supervision and treatment for those with mental or emotional illnesses. The aim is to assist those individuals to remain in their own communities. One serious concern for many communities is the inadequacy of funding to meet the needs of those who require mental health care. This has been one factor in mentally ill persons becoming homeless.

Hospices

Hospices are organizations that provide care and support to dying individuals and their families and caregivers. Although hospices may differ in their organization, most provide a variety of home health services. They may also provide for hospitalization for symptom management and for *respite care* to relieve at-home caregivers for a period of time. A hospice usually has volunteers who provide personal support as well as professionals. Bereavement counseling for families and caregivers is also a part of hospice services. The essence of hospice care is providing personal dignity and choices so that the individual can die as he or she wishes to die.

Voluntary Associations

The United States has a long tradition of private support for health-related causes through *voluntary organizations* focusing on specific diseases or groups of diseases. These nonprofit organizations raise funds through public contributions and corporate and foundation grants to support research, specialized professional education, public education, and sometimes direct patient services. People with a particular illness may derive valuable psychological support from meeting their counterparts. These organizations often sponsor support groups for both patients and family members. As a nurse you may decide to refer patients and their families to appropriate voluntary organizations (see Appendix E).

Health Promotion Organizations

Health promotion includes activities aimed at achieving a higher level of health and well-being. The emphasis on improving health and well-being has resulted in many new types of organizations. Health clubs may be simply places where indoor racquet sports and exercise equipment are available, but many also provide classes on nutrition, exercise techniques, and stress reduction. Other health promotion resources include private practitioners who teach methods of stress reduction and weight reduction clinics. Some employers provide a variety of health promotion activities for employees. They may provide health education, exercise facilities, and even monetary incentives for weight control, smoking cessation, and exercise programs.

Accreditation of Health Care Facilities

Accreditation is a process of granting approval to a facility that meets certain standards. The standards set by any accrediting agency are designed to promote excellence in care. These standards apply to physical facilities, personnel, policies, and procedures. An accreditation team visits the facility, reviews compliance with standards, and writes a report. Accreditation may be granted or renewed or may be denied. Usually recommendations are written to point out areas for performance improvement. Standards set by accreditation bodies have had profound effects on institutions.

The National League for Nursing (NLN) operates a division titled the Community Health Accreditation Program (CHAP) that accredits home health agencies. The NLN board that operates the CHAP program includes nurses, other home care professionals, and consumer representatives. The focus of CHAP has been recognition of high-quality services and assurance to the public that the agency meets these standards. Accreditation of home care services by this organization is accepted by all federal government programs as evidence of appropriate standards and therefore no additional accreditation is required.

The Joint Commission for the Accreditation of Healthcare Organizations (JCAHO) was initiated for the purpose of accrediting hospitals. It now accredits hospices and home health agencies as well. The JCAHO board is composed of representatives from the American College of Surgeons, the American Society of Internal Medicine, and the American Medical Association. For many years the American Nurses Association advocated for a seat on the board for a representative of nursing. This was accomplished beginning in 1993. Another recent change for the JCAHO was the addition of a consumer representative. The federal government accepts JCAHO accreditation of hospitals and does not require other accreditation.

Funding of Health Care

The cost of health care is a major concern throughout the world. No economy can support uncontrolled health care cost escalation. The inflation in the economy over the past 20 years coupled with new advances in health care technology have caused costs for health care to rise much faster than the average costs in society as a whole. Major efforts are now being made to control health care costs.

Sources of Health Care Funds

Funds for payment of health care come through various channels, although each source ultimately derives its income from money earned by individual citizens. This is a basic concept: there is no health care that does not cost individuals. The cost for one individual may be spread across a large group through insurance premiums or taxes, but as costs rise, the cost to the individual also rises.

In all the developed countries of the world except the United States and South Africa, a national plan for health care is provided by governmental mandate. These plans sometimes are totally tax driven and managed by an agency of the government. Other plans provide for a combination of private insurance and governmental support.

In the United States, specific health care programs are operated by the federal government, but no current plan covers all residents. Each of the federal health care funding programs in the United States is aimed at a specific group. Each year proposals are made before the Congress regarding the enactment of a some type of national health insurance. Each proposal is slightly different, and you might familiarize yourself with current proposals being made.

Private Health Insurance

Private health insurance companies pay for a large share of the cost of acute hospital care in the United States. The basis of insurance is that risk is spread over many individuals so that the burden of cost is lessened for each. Consequently, a large number of people pay more for insurance than they would for their own health care if they paid for it directly because they have remained well. For those suffering major illnesses, the insurance pays more for their health care than they have paid for their insurance.

An insurance policy frequently requires that the individual pay some portion of the health care costs before the insurance begins paying. This amount is referred to as the deductible. The higher the deductible amount, the lower is the insurance premium. Insurance policies also have upper limits on the total amount they will pay for a given episode of illness. Certain health problems may be specifically excluded from coverage. For example, some policies will not pay for any treatment considered to be experimental in nature.

Insurance provided to groups such as employees or students of a particular school costs less than insurance purchased as a private individual because the groups have a large proportion of well individuals. Some people cannot purchase individual insurance policies because of existing health problems that make the risk of their having a serious illness greater. Those who are unemployed, self-employed, or employed by a small firm do not usually have group insurance available to them.

Governmental Funding of Health Care

The United States government makes an extremely large expenditure for health care. The following outlines the major programs the government supports.

United States Public Health Service. The United States Public Health Service plays a broad role in overseeing health care in the United States. Through funding research, setting standards for drugs, preventing communicable disease, and cooperating with international agencies, it promotes health. In addition, the Public Health Service operates hospitals and clinics that provide care for merchant seamen, the Coast Guard, and military dependents and retirees, although the amount of direct care given is being gradually reduced and patients/clients are being redirected into the community.

Medicare. **Medicare** is a program administered by the Social Security Administration that provides health care for those over age 65, dependents on Social Security, and those in renal failure. Part A of Medicare, which pays for hospitalization, is automatically provided to anyone receiving Social Security retirement benefits. Part B, which pays for physicians' fees, is voluntary and paid for through a deduction from the Social Security check. Medicare is like insurance in that it pays only specified amounts for specified health problems (Fig. 2-2). A deductible is required before Medicare begins paying. Those who can afford it usually purchase supplemental private health insurance to pay for some of the expenses that Medicare does not cover.

Medicaid. **Medicaid** is a federally funded program administered by the various states to provide health care for those on public assistance or who meet other low-income standards. Each state sets its own standards for Medicaid. Medicaid tends to pay for acute illness, but not for health maintenance. Low-income individuals who are employed are not usually eligible for Medicaid nor are those who are temporarily unemployed. The state of Oregon has negotiated with the federal government for a radically new approach to Medicaid. The state is trying to structure a plan for minimum health care services that will be available to all low-income people. To do this, difficult decisions are being made as to what constitutes minimum care, what procedures should and should not be covered, and how individual decisions will be made.

Military Hospitals and Clinics. The health care of military personnel and all of their dependents is provided by the military service. Most of the physicians and nurses are military officers, and many of the personnel are members of the military. All care, both preventive and for illness, is provided without charge. Funds are appropriated by Congress as part of the military budget.

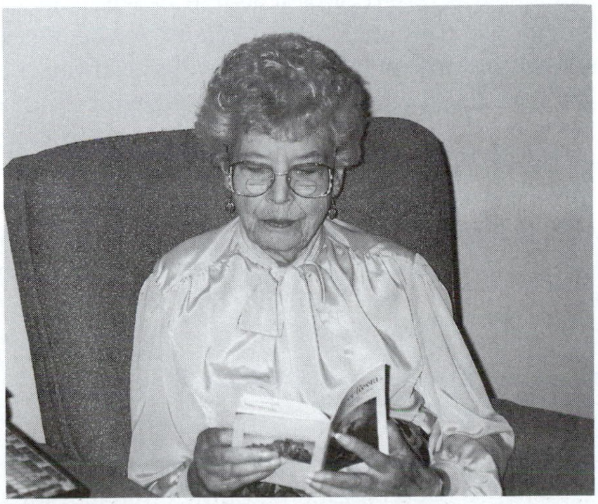

Figure 2-2. Medicare is a federally funded program for those receiving Social Security benefits that pays specified amounts for specified health services.

Under certain circumstances military personnel and their dependents receive health care from agencies within the community. This care is paid for through the Civilian Health and Medical Program of the Uniformed Services (CHAMPUS), which is also funded through the military budget.

Indian Health Service. The Indian Health Service (IHS) is operated by the Department of the Interior to provide care for Native Americans living on reservations. Historically, a great deal of criticism has been leveled at the inadequate funding of health care through the IHS and the inadequacy of the health care provided. The Native Americans living on reservations have had a much higher incidence of many communicable diseases, a higher infant mortality rate, and in general a shorter life expectancy than the general population. In the last 10 years, Native Americans on reservations have become increasingly involved in administering all reservation activities. Changes have been made in health care programs, and improvement is being identified.

Other Federal Programs. A few other federal programs provide limited funds for certain special projects. These projects have become fewer in number and have had a lower level of funding in recent years. This means that not all those eligible for assistance can receive it. An example is the Women, Infants, and Children (WIC) program. It provides nutritional supplementation and health maintenance care for a limited number of low-income pregnant women, nursing mothers, and infants.

State and Local Government Programs. State and local government programs provide services that affect the health of the community at large. Immunizations may be provided free or at cost. Care may be provided for patients with communicable diseases such as tuberculosis and sexually transmitted diseases. Well-child clinics may be provided. Free or low-cost lunches and breakfasts may be provided for children from low-income families.

Each state has some form of workers' compensation that pays for care required from a job-related illness or injury. This program may provide complete rehabilitation, vocational counseling, and job retraining when necessary. Workers' compensation usually provides workers with some form of income for living expenses while they are unable to work because of job-related illness or injury.

Charity

Free or low-cost care may be provided by private charitable groups. In the past, these were the primary sources of care for those in low-income groups, but government programs have replaced much of what was formerly provided through charity. The Shriners' hospitals for crippled children and special hospitals for children with leukemia and other forms of cancer are notable examples of charitable health care services still functioning. Many charitable groups help by continuing to provide care when insurance and other funding is expended. Some hospitals provide free or low-cost care to those who apply for help. Some voluntary organizations provide special care or limited assistance for those with certain disease conditions.

Personal Payment

Even individuals with insurance usually must pay some of their health care costs directly. Over-the-counter medications and prescriptions may need to be purchased or payments made for physicians' services or dental care. Those without insurance or those with major medical costs may face health care costs that overwhelm personal resources.

Health Maintenance Organizations

Often, HMOs are grouped with insurance plans. They do have many similarities in that both spread risk over a large group. The difference is that the HMO is both the provider of care and the payer for care. In this context, HMOs have been leaders in promoting cost containment in health care. The individual pays a monthly fee to the HMO and receives all care, both health maintenance and illness care, from the organization. There is a strong incentive in HMOs to emphasize preventive care and early treatment to avoid major costly crises.

Methods of Reimbursing for Health Care Costs

In the past, all third-party payers paid for care after it had been delivered, a method called **retrospective reimbursement**. In this system, the payer determined what percentage or amount it would pay for a specific procedure or each day of care and paid that amount when billed, after the procedure was completed or the patient discharged. The more procedures that were done or the longer the stay, the more money was paid. Although this worked for many years, it has been extremely costly. Some experts in health care finance believe that this system does not provide adequate incentives to health care providers to try to decrease costs by decreasing unnecessary procedures and days of stay.

In 1983, the federal government began initiating a new **prospective reimbursement** system for payment through Medicare and Medicaid. In this system, a standard fee is established for a group of medical diagnoses called a diagnosis-related group (DRG).

There are 467 DRGs, each with its set reimbursement fee. The set fee for each DRG is based on statistical studies regarding costs. A fee does not increase if the hospital stay is longer than average nor is the fee reduced if the stay is shorter than average. However, in situations, (called outliers) in which the patient's hospital stay is *significantly* longer than the average, extra payment is permitted. If the patient has an additional medical diagnosis that would affect the outcome of the care, such as heart failure in the person with a fractured hip, this is designated a comorbidity and the reimbursement amount is increased. Clearly, detailed and accurate medical records are essential for any health care organization to receive the maximum reimbursement. There are also methods by which a health care provider can apply for greater-than-average reimbursement based on educational and research programs, the type of patients usually served, and other such factors.

Prospective reimbursement was designed to give health care providers an incentive to shorten hospital stays and decrease the costs of providing care. Because this method of payment does result in cost savings, private third-party payers (such as insurance companies) are switching to their own prospective reimbursement plans.

Medicare also pays for a limited period of nursing home care or home care after hospitalization when that care is skilled, not custodial, in nature. In the restructuring of Medicare after 1983, regulations for reimbursement were tightened to limit the costs to the Social Security system. This restructuring has resulted in increasing problems for those agencies seeking reimbursement. Records are reviewed very carefully to determine that visits or care provided meet the criteria for skilled care.

The individual patient pays a deductible for each hospital stay. The deductible amount was increased when Medicare was reorganized. The restructuring also increased the amount of the individual patient's deductible for Part B (physician-related services) and raised the monthly premium for Part B. The overall Medicare reimbursement was based on a schedule of what Medicare had determined were "reasonable fees" for health care. Many private care providers charges have always been larger than the fee established by Medicare. Thus, the individual paid not only the deductible but also the difference between what Medicare determined was a "reasonable fee" and the actual fee. Medicare was further revised in 1990 and private care providers were prohibited from billing in excess of the deductible. This provision of the law has not been enforced, however.

Nursing Concerns Related to Reimbursement

Because nursing is the largest single health care occupation, there has been considerable concern regarding the effect of reimbursement plans on nursing practice. One concern is that overriding attention to lowering costs may not be compatible with providing high-quality care.

For example, the future well-being of a patient/client may depend on the individual's achieving a certain level of self-care skills. This in turn may require an extra day's stay in a care facility. Because there will be no increased reimbursement for the extra day and the extra day will not make a difference in the outcome for this hospital stay, will it become impossible to provide the time needed for patient teaching?

Another concern has been in regard to staffing patterns for nursing care. One way to save money in a health care facility would be to reduce the total number of staff and to change the ratio of relatively more costly staff (registered nurses) to less costly staff (nursing assistants). Most evidence indicates that these changes would be counterproductive because the result would be a lower level of care, which would produce more complications and longer-than-average lengths of stay. However, some business managers still believe that, in their facilities, the registered nurses would just work harder under the new staffing conditions to ensure that patients were well cared for; thus, the new ratios would save money for the facility. Although in the near term some savings might be realized by changes in staff composition, the long-term effects of increased workloads on staff stress and morale are bound to have an undesirable effect on the quality of care.

Some nurses have expressed concern over the way the DRGs were determined. DRGs revolve around medical diagnosis and may not reflect the differences in level of nursing care required by the patient. Also, some facilities have a disproportionate number of high-risk patients with complex conditions, so that their average care costs may be greater than the national average.

Failure of the system to provide direct reimbursement for services directly provided by nurses has also been a concern. For example, a nurse practitioner will not be paid directly but must bill through a physician to be reimbursed in most instances. Historically, public health nurses did a great deal of case finding and they initiated care of families (Zerwekh, 1992). Regulations now require that nurses have referrals from physicians to provide nursing care. This may be interfering with good care as well as being counterproductive to cost savings.

Cost Containment

Because the cost of health care has risen at a rate greater than the general inflation rate, concern over health care costs is widespread. Many decisions being made revolve around **cost containment**, the effort to slow the rate at which costs are rising. Third-party payers, government agencies, and consumer groups have all become advocates of cost-containment efforts.

Regardless of the method of reimbursement, it is important for those in health care to make every attempt to contain costs. In a health care facility, supplies may be conserved or care planned so that the cost involved is the minimum cost consistent with good care. For example, if disposable waterproof pads are being used under a patient who cannot control urination, it is important to use only the number necessary to protect the bed. Using several layers will only result in more wrinkles under the patient and will not provide more protection because each pad is waterproof. Another cost-containment measure is the careful scheduling of diagnostic tests so that those that would interfere with other testing are performed last; this way the patient does not have to spend a day simply waiting for a test to be performed.

As a student, you will be asked to use sterile supplies carefully and correctly so that supplies are not wasted. When choosing supplies and equipment, you should use the size, number, and type appropriate to the particular procedure and not large sizes when small will do, a box of items when one is needed, or sterile equipment when simple cleanliness is all that is required. As you become more responsible for planning care for patients, you will become aware that well-written plans can save the time of other staff members who care for the same patient. You will initiate teaching that

Nursing Issues and Trends: *Cost Control in Health Care*

Because health care costs have risen so dramatically in the last 20 years, concern for cost control assumes a major role in all settings. Cost-control efforts have resulted in very short stays in acute care hospitals with rapid discharge to long-term care or to the home. Some patients express distress that their individual situation is not adequately addressed by early discharge. They may be weak, easily fatigued, and may still have skilled care needs. Finding an appropriate balance between the need of the system for cost control and the need of the individual for care presents a major challenge to the nurse.

may make earlier discharge possible. You can effectively contribute to cost containment in many ways while maintaining quality of care.

Quality Assurance

Quality assurance includes all the evaluation programs in health care agencies. Such programs provide mechanisms for setting standards for care, monitoring care to identify whether those standards are being met, and setting up plans to remedy problems or provide for improvement. Accrediting bodies require systematic evaluation of health services. The federal government also requires that physicians and hospitals receiving payment from Medicare have such programs in place. Nurses are very much involved in the quality assurance programs. Through committees they may help to set standards for nursing care. They may participate in monitoring activities and make suggestions for ways to correct problems or improve care. Although standards for medical care are set by physicians, nurses often serve as surveyors to examine patient records and collect data with regard to medical services. Increasing numbers of institutions are striving to provide high-quality care by a process called **quality management**. The focus of quality management is to not simply evaluate after actions, but to examine situations before taking action and directly plan for ways to increase quality.

Societal Trends Affecting the Health Care System

Increasingly Sophisticated Technology

Each week brings announcements of new research and development in the area of health care. From organ transplantation to sophisticated magnetic resonance imaging for diagnosis, each new technology creates many questions and problems. High cost raises concerns about access to care and questions regarding who will pay for the necessary equipment and care. The question of which health care facility will have the equipment or perform the procedures involves concerns about prestige, income, quality of care, and unnecessary duplication of services. In most jurisdictions, restrictions are placed on institutional purchase of equipment through the requirement of a certificate of need, which is granted through a health planning agency of the government. This procedure is designed to prevent costly duplication of equipment that might be underused. The federal government has now designated, for the purposes of reimbursement, specific institutions as approved centers for heart transplants. Thus, the proliferation of these services is effectively limited. Similar mechanisms are being considered for the practical management of other new technology.

Changes in Health Care Worker Supply

Societal changes in health care demands and the increasing sophistication of the health care provided require more well-prepared health care workers. The shortage of nurses that became apparent to everyone in 1987 had been predicted earlier by nursing leaders who studied the trends in nurse use and nursing education.

As nurses are employed in a greater variety of settings, as the number of individuals requiring long-term care increases, and as acute care becomes more technologically advanced, the demand for registered nurses grows. The American Nurses Association and the National League for Nursing are cooperating in efforts to recruit qualified students into nursing and have been urging the federal government to provide support to nursing education. Another factor that has been cited as contributing to the nursing shortage problem is the number of nurses who leave nursing because of the high level of stress and the demands of the field. Some employers are seeking ways to reduce stress to retain nurses.

The increased complexity of acute care initially resulted in fewer positions for licensed practical nurses and the elimination of nursing assistant positions. The number of schools preparing practical nurses also decreased, and the total number of graduates of these programs declined. As the shortage of registered nurses persisted, more acute care hospitals began to hire nursing assistants. When nursing assistants provide truly assistive tasks to registered nurses, this may help to alleviate the shortage. However, when these individuals are used beyond their educational background, quality of care begins to suffer.

The supply-and-demand cycle for nursing continues to change and as the health care system adapts, the shortage of nurses is alleviated in some areas although it continues in others. Shortages continue to be most acute in the inner cities and underserved rural areas.

Changes in Health Care Institutions

The increased complexity of the health care system is creating pressure on the institutions providing care. Increasing economic pressures require a more sophisticated approach to business management. In addition, competition for clients, especially for those areas of health care that tend to be profitable, has increased.

A pattern has developed of closing small independent health care institutions, with more care being provided by large, multifaceted health care corporations. These large health care institutions have been able to remain financially stable because of their diversity and economies of size. A concern has been expressed that this may decrease local control and accountability and decrease accessibility of care, particularly in rural areas.

Increased Numbers of Elders in the Population

The age group over 70 is the fastest growing category in the United States, a fact that has had immense impact on health care. Older people tend to have more chronic illnesses and require more health care than younger people do. As persons age, they may need more community support services to maintain their independence; some eventually need full-time care. The costs of this care are covered only in part by Medicare and supplemental health insurance. Many elderly persons spend large sums of money each month on prescription drugs, physicians' fees, and health care supplies. Others suffer from inadequate care because their incomes are too low to cover these additional costs. Health care providers have sometimes been slow to recognize that elderly people have some unique needs and that care must be adapted for them. Developing systems of care delivery that effectively meet the needs of elders and finding appropriate ways to fund that care are challenges to the whole society.

Health Care Reform

Health care reform continues to dominate the list of political issues. With rapidly rising costs, changes in demand, and an economic downturn, the issue cannot be ignored. Both at the state and national levels many proposals are being presented. Some states have made significant changes in their systems. A national task force will develop proposals for congressional action.

Some of the topics currently being debated are:

- Is health care a right or a privilege?
- If health care is a right, what level of health care is owed the recipient?
- Should preventive care be included?
- Should only emergency needs be met?
- Should costly procedures such as organ transplants be provided?
- What current governmental programs could be eliminated to free money for health care?
- Should taxes be increased to provide additional health care?

These are difficult questions because funds used for health care must be raised somehow.

Those who are not able to pay for health care or for health insurance are considered *medically indigent.* The group includes not only the unemployed but also those who are employed in jobs with low wages and no benefits. In the past, when people in these groups had emergent health care needs, they were cared for in state, county, or city hospitals or in private hospitals that absorbed the cost of their care. As health care becomes more expensive and government bodies have more demands on their funds, these resources are being exhausted. Formerly, private hospitals supported charitable care by charging higher fees to those who could pay. Private hospitals are now being prevented from supporting charitable care in this way by the reimbursement policies of insurance companies, Medicare, and Medicaid. Thus, a crisis has arisen.

Individuals in Health Care

Specific Health Care Occupations

The increasing complexity of health care makes it impossible for an individual working independently to provide total care to a patient. This circumstance has given rise to an ever-growing number of health care occupations, each with a specific area of expertise and responsibility. Any individual who has a direct or indirect impact on the patient's care is considered a member of the **health care team** in the broadest sense of the term. And the patient, too, must be a central member of this team if the team is to accomplish its goal of optimum health care.

Some of the professionals who compose the health care team, such as doctors and nurses, are well known. Others—such as orthotics technicians, who make braces and prosthetic appliances—are familiar only to specialists. Many of the professionals in newer and less well-known occupations administer new diagnostic or treatment techniques or assist more extensively prepared professionals. Nursing and its role is discussed in Chapter 1. Here we will discuss other health care occupations.

Physician

In a hospital you may encounter a wide variety of physicians, with different levels of education and in different health care roles. The private physician is one who is in practice in the community. The physician admitting a patient to the hospital is frequently referred to as the *attending physician.* The attending physician visits the patient daily and oversees care, although other physicians may be consulted.

Consulting physicians, or consultants, are usually in a specialty practice and are asked to see the patient and provide advice to the attending physician. A consulting physician may assume care for a specific problem. For example, a primary physician may admit a patient with a suspected heart problem. A cardiologist, who is a specialist in diseases of the heart, may then be called in as a consultant. The cardiologist may ultimately assume responsibility for all care related to the heart condition. In some cases the consultant reviews the case, indicates whether specialty care is warranted, and has no further role.

The *house staff* is composed of physicians who are part of an educational program and are salaried by the institution. House staff function at many levels; all are licensed physicians. *Residents* are house staff physicians who have enrolled in a program for specialty practice such as surgery or obstetrics. Residency programs for family practice provide experiences in many different areas of medicine. Residents are often referred to by the year of their progress in the specialty. An R1 is in the first year of residency; an R3 is in the third year. *Fellows* are more experienced physicians who are studying a subspecialty, such as bone marrow transplant, or who are engaged in research projects. The policies regarding their involvement in care are established by the hospital.

In a hospital with a large population of low-income individuals without personal physicians, the house staff doctor may be the primary physician for the patient. In a private hospital in which the majority of patients are admitted by private community physicians, the house staff may serve a more supportive and assisting role, working with the community physician in care. House staff usually provide 24-hour medical coverage and are available for emergencies.

Dietitian

The *dietitian,* or nutritionist, is responsible for planning the menus to meet the dietary needs of all the patients. In addition, the dietitian meets with individual patients for nutritional assessment and then plans individualized diets and provides patient teaching for specialty dietary needs. The staff dietitian is consulted when special nutritional problems arise.

Physical Therapist

The *physical therapist* (PT) assists patients in returning to maximal independence and function in mobility through exercise and physical treatments (Fig. 2-3). Some exercises and treatments are done at the patient's bedside; other exercises may be done in the physical therapy department. Physical therapy treatments can be uncomfortable and exhausting for patients, and the nurse should communicate with the PT to learn the exact nature of the treatment and what the patient will be experiencing.

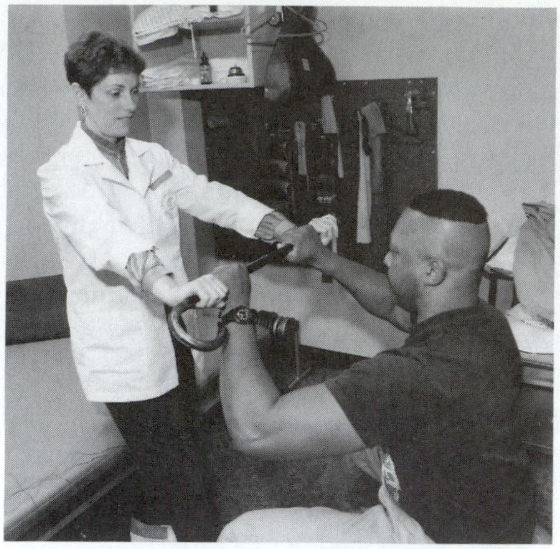

Figure 2-3. The physical therapist is one member of the health care team.

Occupational Therapist

The *occupational therapist* (OT) works with activities of daily living and fine motor skills. Rather than assign a patient/client specific exercises, the OT will often suggest activities that provide the needed motor function. The OT makes splints and other assistive devices to help the person accomplish activities of daily living such as eating and dressing. The OT may also provide activities appropriate for the diversion of the ill person. An OT in a psychiatric setting provides activities that assist the individual in coping with problems and developing more positive feelings about the self.

Respiratory Care Therapist

The *respiratory care therapist* (RCT) provides specialized treatments to support optimum respiratory function. The RCT (sometimes called a *pulmonary therapist*) is usually responsible for the maintenance of respiratory equipment such as oxygen delivery devices and respirators. Most RCTs are educated in associate degree programs, but some have baccalaureate preparation. They become certified through their national association. Some states license RCTs.

Pharmacist

The *pharmacist* is responsible for dispensing all medications. The pharmacist also serves as the primary resource person regarding medications. In some hospitals, pharmacists are based in a central pharmacy; in others, pharmacists are based on patient care units and play a more active role as consultants for both nurses and doctors regarding drug therapy. In the community, pharmacists play a primary role in education regarding medications.

Social Worker

The *social worker* focuses on the family and the patient in the community. This worker may help arrange community resources for care, help find sources for funding health care for the individual, and provide personal support to the patient and family.

Other Health Care Workers

Display 2-1 lists a number of health care occupations you may encounter. You may find that some of these occupations are not represented in your locality. Some may have different titles, and certain of these occupations may have overlapping functions. Nevertheless, you should understand these occupations and their areas of responsibility. If you are unfamiliar with some, look them up in a medical dictionary. As you meet fellow workers in the health care setting, you may want to inquire about their roles on the health team.

Differences in Preparation for Health Care Roles

Educational preparation for health care careers differs greatly. The longest preparation is typically that of the physician who chooses a specialty or subspecialty. Each move into a more specialized level of practice increases the length of the physician's preparation. In contrast, preparation for some health careers consists entirely of on-the-job training, such as that received by some nursing assistants. Educational preparation may also vary within a single occupational group. Nursing, as we have seen, provides three pathways to registration: a diploma, associate degree, or baccalaureate degree. However, nursing education programs are subject to approval by state Boards of Nursing, which tend to have a standardizing effect.

Some health care workers with identical titles may have had vastly different amounts of preparation because there are as yet no laws governing their training. One such field is respiratory care therapy: some RCTs have formal educational backgrounds of considerable depth, whereas others have received only on-the-job training.

Recognition of such differences is important when you are responsible for delegating tasks or sharing them with others. A licensed practical nurse (LPN) can be expected to observe a patient more knowledgeably than would an orderly. If a patient is in need of close observation and your team consists of an LPN and an orderly, you would delegate this task to the LPN. It is also necessary to know the range and limits of others' expertise. For instance, an RCT with a thorough background in respiratory physiology might help you to understand a particular patient's problem, whereas an RCT with on-the-job training would be unable to do so. During your orientation to a new facility, you might inquire about the educational backgrounds of staff members with whose occupations you are unfamiliar.

Credentials for Practice

Just as educational preparation differs, so do the *credentials* necessary for practice. The standards for licensure as a nurse are relatively uniform throughout the country and certify minimum ability to practice safely. Licensure is *mandatory* in most places. Medicine, dentistry, and some other health care occupations have similar standards.

For other categories of workers, licensure is not mandatory but *permissive*. This means that one may be licensed but may also practice without licensure. In some states, licensure of practical (vocational) nurses falls into this category.

Some professional organizations provide *certification* for practitioners of their specialty. Competence is determined by tests and other criteria, and certification is completely controlled by the profession itself. Physicians are certified as specialists in this fashion. Nurses are being certified in specialized fields by the same kind of mechanism.

In the United States, laws governing health care occupations are made at the state level. The resulting local variations may limit the mobility of individuals in certain occupations.

All these variables make it difficult for the beginning nurse to know "who's who." It is, of course, far more difficult for patients, who usually turn to a familiar figure for interpretation and guidance as they move through the modern health care system. The nurse is often that familiar figure and thus must be capable of interpreting the roles of other members of the health care team to the public.

Functioning Within the Health Care Team

An individual member of a health care team may, at different times, function independently or collaboratively. Each mode of functioning has its place and needs

Display 2–1

Some Health Care Occupations

Child Care

Child life coordinator
Pediatrician
Pediatric nurse practitioner

Dental Care

Dentist
Dental hygienist
Dental assistant
Dental laboratory technician

Drug Therapy

Pharmacist
Pharmacy technician
Pharmacologist

Eye Care

Ophthalmologist
Optometrist
Oculist

Laboratory Testing

Pathologist
Cytologist
Medical technologist
Medical laboratory technician
Certified labortory assistant
EEG (electroencephalographic) technician
ECG (electrocardiographic) technician

Nursing

Registered nurse
Licensed practical (vocational) nurse
Nursing assistant (aide or orderly)

Medicine

Physician (many specialties, some listed in specific categories)
Resident
Intern
Extern
Physician's assistant

Mental Health

Psychiatrist
Psychologist
Psychiatric social worker
Mental health technician

Physical Medicine and Rehabilitation

Physiatrist
Physical therapy technician
Registered physical therapist
Registered occupational therapist
Occupational therapy technician

Radiation and Radiology

Radiologist
X-ray technician
Radioisotope technician

Recordkeeping

Medical records administrator
Medical records technician
Medical records transcriptionist

Respiratory Care

Respiratory care therapist
Respiratory care technician

Social Work

Medical social worker
Caseworker
Community liaison worker

Speech and Hearing

Otolaryngologist
Audiologist
Speech therapist

Surgery

Surgeon
Operating room nurse
Surgical technician
Anesthesiologist
Nurse anesthetist

to be understood in light of the efforts of the team as a whole.

Independent Functioning

An individual functions independently when working within his or her own area of expertise. Within that sphere, the person ascertains what needs to be done and initiates action. Others may or may not be consulted, but the final decision is the individual's. Throughout this text, we will point out areas in which it is appropriate for registered nurses to function independently.

A type of nursing in which **independent functioning** is the dominant model is *primary nursing care*. In this situation, one nurse has complete responsibility for the patient's nursing care—supportive care, hygiene, and all other nursing needs—while on duty and, in addition, plans for ongoing care. Of course, the nurse in such a setting works cooperatively with other personnel and performs some collaborative functions related to the physician's medical plan of care, but the primary nurse is fully and exclusively responsible for all nursing functions. The primary nursing approach minimizes communication problems, enhances continuity of care, and helps patients feel that they are being seen as whole people. The major drawbacks to primary nursing care are its high cost and the shortage of registered nurses in some areas of the country.

Independent functioning may take a different form for nurses with specialized educational preparation. Those with backgrounds in such areas as coronary care and anesthesia function independently in ways beyond the scope of the general staff nurse. They make judgments that were once considered the physician's responsibility. Nurse practitioners in such fields as pediatrics, obstetrics, and family practice also exercise expanded independence justified by their superior education and skill.

Collaborative Functioning

In Chapter 1, we mentioned **collaborative functioning**. This phrasing indicates that two or more individuals must be involved for effective action to occur. Collaborative functioning is required, for example, when the team approach is used to manage certain long-term health problems, such as rehabilitation after spinal cord injury. The physician, the nurse, the occupational and physical therapists, and others involved in the patient's care meet to discuss the patient's problems and determine overall priorities and goals. Increasingly, the patient and the family also participate in such efforts. After general priorities and goals have been established by the team, its individual members may work together on some problems and independently on others. This method of making decisions is time consuming but can result in care of exceptionally high quality.

Another example of collaborative functioning is the writing of a "prescription" or "orders" for care. The person with the most extensive preparation or experience in a given area of health care makes decisions for care that will be carried out by others. This practice makes the expertise of one individual available when that person is not present. In the past, health team personnel functioned in response to the physician's orders. Today various other people may also make decisions for others to carry out. The nurse in charge of a patient's care may write **nursing orders** to be carried out by other nurses and by nursing assistants. The physical therapist may write a *prescription* for the patient's exercises, to be carried out by the assistant or by nursing personnel. The person who carries out such orders is functioning in a collaborative role.

It must be clearly understood that relying on orders from another does not relieve an individual of responsibility for his or her own actions. The person who writes the order is responsible for his or her own decision-making process and the orders written. The person who carries out that order is responsible also. He or she must understand the directions clearly, recognize potential **contraindications** to that action, perform the task skillfully, and evaluate the results. The person carrying out the task can be held legally liable for damage resulting from lack of skill, performance of an action when clear contraindications are present, or failure to stop when an unexpected or adverse result occurs. As you can see, carrying out the orders written by someone else does not absolve anyone of responsibility.

Nurses probably function collaboratively most frequently when they engage in *team nursing*. Team nursing is an effort to make the most effective use of various types of personnel and to provide the most effective nursing care through joint decision-making. The team leader is usually a registered nurse with the background and ability to organize and plan care for a group of patients. Members of the team may be other registered nurses, licensed practical nurses, student nurses, and nursing assistants.

The core of the team nursing concept is team planning of care. At a daily *team conference* (Fig. 2-4), care is planned and problems are considered. Of course, some aspects of care are best dealt with by a single individual, for the sake of both efficient use of time and the patient's needs, and need not be considered by the entire team. Conferences usually focus on difficult problems or the overall direction and guidance of the patient's care. Specific aspects of care are then assigned to different team members for implementation. Herein lies one drawback of team nursing: because different team members perform different tasks, the patient en-

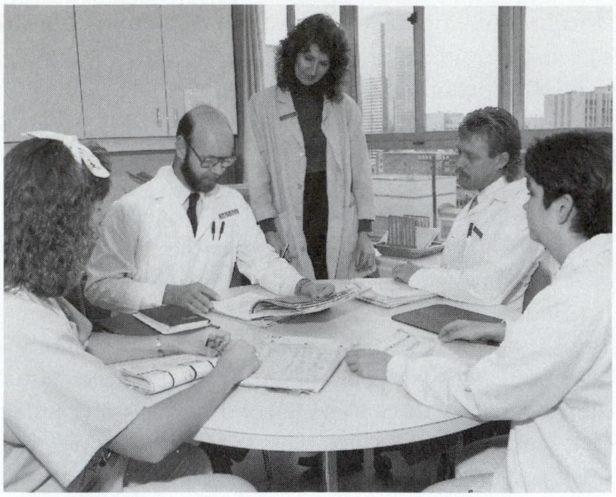

Figure 2-4. An interdisciplinary team conference.

counters many individuals in the course of care and may not know where to turn with a given question or request. Communication is the solution to this problem.

Problems in the Delivery of Health Care

A coordinated health care team in which each person functions optimally is the ideal toward which we should all be striving. However, many problems stand in the way of its realization. We shall discuss some of these problems here, and you may encounter others in your particular work setting.

Depersonalization of Care

The health care system is very large with many components. It is easy for each health care provider to look at a narrow segment of the person and to treat everyone alike without regard to individual personalities. The larger the system, the more easily this depersonalization happens. The individual begins to feel unimportant and as if no one truly cares what happens. This feeling affects the individual adversely in a variety of ways: the person may be less likely to seek health care appropriately; having sought health care, the person may be less likely to carry through with recommended treatments, medications, and care; the person may have more emotional problems related to health, and this may slow recovery.

Loss of Privacy

With an increasingly complex health care system and growing computerization of records, concern is mounting about the loss of individual privacy. Insurance companies require copies of records to verify care and review costs. Governmental agencies require reports regarding certain diseases. Governmental funding agencies review records to evaluate care and control costs. These situations allow more people to have access to private medical records and to have information about individuals. This loss of privacy concerns many people. To combat the loss of privacy, more effort is being made to restrict access to records, to check carefully for proper authorization before information is shared, and to question whether some types of information need to be shared.

Communication Barriers

One of the most complex problems in health care is communication. As more people become involved in a particular patient's care, communication among them becomes both more important and more difficult. Communication can and does break down. The result is fragmented care, which causes patients to believe that no one sees them as whole individuals and that some of their needs are neither recognized nor met.

Need for Continuing Education

As health care has grown more complex, certain occupational groups (including nurses) have had to upgrade their skills and relinquish tasks requiring less skill. This circumstance has sometimes been perceived as threatening. Appropriate continuing education may be costly or may be difficult to access. All nurses must value lifelong learning and systems are needed to make that possible.

Overlapping Responsibilities

Another problem in the delivery of health care is that the advent of new health care occupations sometimes causes responsibilities to overlap. Such overlap arouses feelings of competition and occasional antagonism.

Burnout

In addition to the shortage of nurses, a maldistribution of health care workers exists, that is, larger numbers of health care workers are present in urban and affluent areas and too few in rural and impoverished ones. There are also specific fields of nursing with special needs, such as critical care nursing and care of elderly persons. When there are not enough well-prepared people for the needs of the clients, those who are there may feel pressured and overworked. They may feel unable to give the kind of care they wish to give. This frustration may lead to **burnout**, a condition of personal stress characterized by fatigue, feelings of depression and hopelessness, and decreased problem-solving ability. This problem may be lessened through a variety of approaches. They include caring for one's own general health, using stress reduction techniques, and changing one's job focus within the nursing profession. These are outlined in Chapter 6.

The Student's Role in Problems of Health Care Delivery

In the face of all these problems, what can you do as a nursing student—and later as a practicing nurse—to progress toward the ideal of a functioning, coordinated health care team that meets the needs of the health care consumer? You can act effectively both as a nurse and as a concerned citizen.

You can work to view the patient as a whole person. By recognizing individual differences and altering care to meet individual needs, you can help the person to feel cared about and satisfied with care. You can protect the patient's privacy through the careful use of records and concern for confidentiality in what you say and what you write.

If insufficiently prepared individuals have been given responsibilities that exceed their competence, you can be active in promoting on-the-job educational opportunities for them and in lobbying the power structure to upgrade its hiring criteria.

If individuals with overlapping areas of responsibility are competing, you can promote and participate in negotiations to establish policies—or even laws—that protect workers' rights but maintain a high level of care. You can demonstrate your readiness to compromise with others when appropriate and emphasize your commitment to the goal of optimal patient care.

You can keep abreast of current practice through reading, continuing education, and attention to your patients so that you are able to meet and adapt to change. You can strive to make your communication with other members of the health care team more complete and more direct. You can ask questions and encourage the establishment of routines and procedures that improve communication. Through such actions, you will be making the health care team more effective.

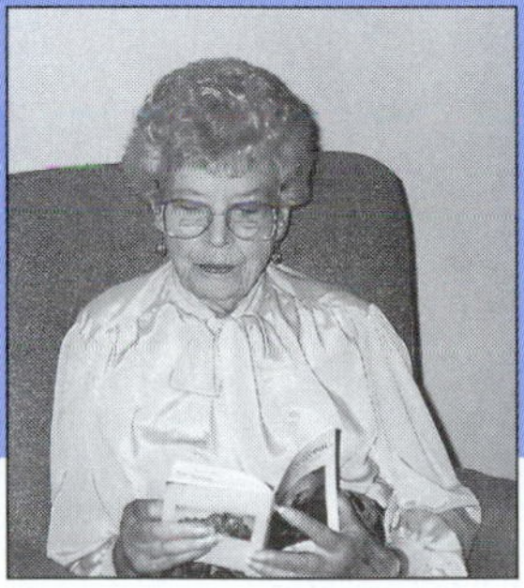

Key Points

- Health care can be conceived of as an open system with constant input and output for which constant evaluation is essential for the system to function at its best.
- Both governmental agencies and private sector organizations are a part of the system with primary health care providers, institutional providers, community health agencies, and voluntary organizations all supplying entry into the system.
- Funding of health care has become a major concern because of inflation and increasingly sophisticated technology. Cost containment is a goal of many programs in health care; every individual in the system can contribute to this end.
- The many different members of the health care team have differing educational preparation, credentialing systems, and specialized functions. The nurse has the responsibility to know the role that each person plays and be able to convey this information to the patient.
- Familiarity with the responsibilities of the many health care occupations helps the nurse to work more effectively with others. The nurse is often in a key position to assist with the coordination of care.
- Even student nurses can contribute to effective function of the health care team, by the way they provide care to the patient and by the way they interact with other members of the health care team.

Study Questions

1. Explain how health care can be described as a system.
2. What is a third-party payer?
3. Differentiate an insurance plan from a health maintenance organization.
4. Outline the various ways in which the government is involved in funding of health care.
5. List sources for health care funding other than the government.
6. Explain how prospective reimbursement differs from retrospective reimbursement.

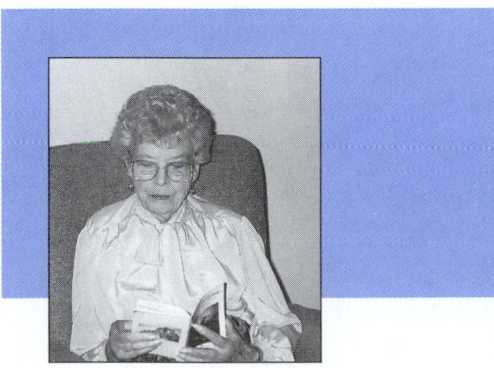

7. Identify situations in which members of the health care team would function independently or collaboratively.
8. List several problems involved in health care delivery and identify an action that a nursing student could take to assist in resolving or preventing each problem.

Critical Thinking Activities

1. Identify a community-based health resource or agency and find out the services provided, the qualifications of the care providers, the method by which clients can obtain this service, and the cost to the client. Suggest situations in which a patient/client might use this resource.
2. Choose a health care occupation about which you know very little. Research the educational preparation needed and the customary responsibilities of the position. Identify situations in which a nurse would interface with individuals in this occupation. Make sure everyone in your class chooses a different occupation. Then hold a conference in which information is shared.
3. Identify the nearest comprehensive health care facility that conducts major research and provides education as well as serves patients with unusual, difficult, or complex care needs. Describe possible patient situations that would require transfer to this facility.

References and Readings

Califano, J. A. "Guiding the Forces of the Health Care Revolution." *Nursing and Health Care* 8, 7 (September 1987): 401–404.

Dougherty, S. "Primary Nursing: It Takes Teamwork." *Nursing '89* 19, 6 (June 1989): 32W–32Z.

Feutz, S. A. "How to Cope with Under Staffing." *Nursing '91* 21, 8 (August 1991): 54–55.

Fralic, M. F., Kowalski, P. M., and Llewellyn, F. A. "The Staff Nurse as Quality Monitor." *American Journal of Nursing* 91, 4 (April 1991): 40–42.

Healthy America: Practitioners for 2005. Durham, N.C.: Pew Health Professions Commission and Duke University Medical Center, 1991.

Malone, R. E. "The Challenge of Third World Nursing." *American Journal of Nursing* 90, 7 (July 1990): 32–37.

Manning, G. "Hospital-based Skilled Nursing Facilities to the Rescue." *American Journal of Nursing* 91, 6 (June 1991): 58–60.

Pillar, B., Jacox, A. K., and Redman, B. K. "Technology: Its Assessment and Nursing." *Nursing Outlook* 38, 1 (January/February 1990): 16–19.

"Occupational Health Groups Seek Licensure in 26 States." *American Nurse* 17, 5 (May 1985): 1, 20.

Zerwekh, J. V. "Public Health Nursing Legacy: Historical Practical Wisdom." *Nursing and Health Care* 13, 2 (February 1992): 84–91.

Ethical and Legal Concerns in Nursing

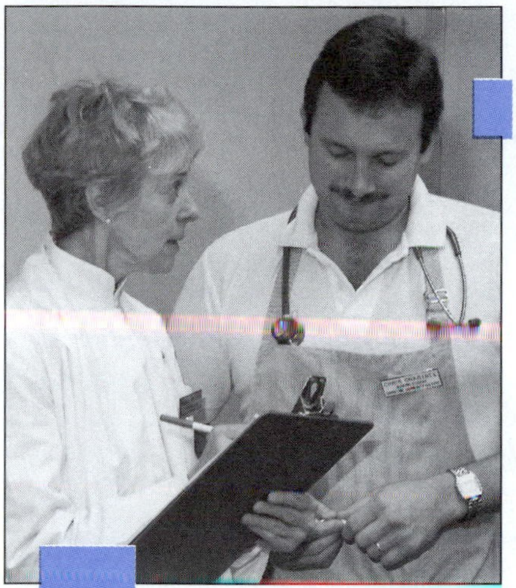

3

Objectives

After completing this chapter, you should be able to:

1. Explain the difference between ethical decision-making based on the consequences (teleologic approach) and based on duty (deontologic approach).
2. Describe bioethics, medical ethics, and nursing ethics.
3. Discuss four contemporary ethical issues in health care.
4. Explain the focus of the Code for Nurses.
5. Discuss the role of the law in nursing licensure.
6. Explain the function of the state Board of Nursing.
7. Differentiate between common law and statutory law.
8. Discuss consumer rights as a component of health care.
9. List some common legal concerns for nurses.
10. Identify ways in which nurses can protect themselves from legal action pertaining to negligence and informed consent.

Study Terms

administrative law
advance directives
allocation of resources
artificial insemination
assault
battery
bioethics
common law
confidentiality
consent
deontologic decision-making
emancipated minor
ethics
false imprisonment
Good Samaritan law
informed consent
liability insurance
libel
licensure by endorsement
malpractice
mandatory continuing education
negligence
Nurse Practice Act
paternalism
patient autonomy
placebo
reasonably prudent nurse
reciprocity
slander
statutory law
surrogate mothering
teleologic decision-making
tort
utilitarianism

Ellis, Nowlis: Nursing: A Human Needs Approach, 5th ed. © 1994, J.B. Lippincott Company

Outline

Ethics and the law are different issues although they often have an impact on one another. **Ethics** "is a direct, focused interest in positive human values and their meaning, and an interest in making our values more real and effective through our choices" (dePender and Ikeda-Chandler, 1990, p. 18). The law, "in its generic sense, is a body of rules of action or conduct prescribed by controlling authority, and having binding legal force." A law is "that which must be obeyed and followed by citizens subject to sanctions or legal consequences" (*Black's Law Dictionary*, 1983, p. 457). Often the law is an expression of the ethical position of a society. For example, recent reinterpretation or refinement of the law has offered protection to special, particularly vulnerable groups. To implement this, many state laws now declare that abusing either a child or an elder is a crime. At other times, the law may be at variance with the ethical position of one or more individuals in a society.

Ethical and legal issues are of increasing concern to society as a whole. The phenomenal advance of medical technology with implications for nurses, changes in the ways we live, and the diversity of our values and beliefs all interact to daily create new questions. The legal and ethical concerns we discuss here are of concern not only to nurses and other health care workers but to private individuals as well.

The health care worker who pilfers or takes from the facility items that are not individually considered costly (*eg*, pencils) may not view this action as unethical or illegal. Yet, the cumulative replacement costs for small items is a growing concern for health care agencies. People who knowingly take small items are deluded into not considering the action one of "stealing." The fact that legal action probably would not occur does not make such action ethical.

Because nursing is so intimately involved with ethical decision-making as well as with the constraints and protection of the law, each of us in nursing has a special obligation to be informed and thoughtful about the positions we choose to support. Aside from nursing, at some time in your life, you will be directly involved in ethical/legal decision-making in which you will be required to examine your innermost personal values.

Each of us subscribes to a personal system of moral belief by which we judge whether particular actions are right or wrong. We establish these ethical systems or codes early in our lives and they become important determinants of our later behavior toward others. Groups of individuals, such as nurses, who engage in a common activity or occupation often share codes of ethics as well. These codes are, for the most part, thoughtfully written and worth careful scrutiny. They do not, however, reduce the responsibility of the individual to be the final judge of moral behavior; Munson (1988) points out that "principles in codes and oaths are not self-justifying. We can always ask about each of them." Like other professional codes, codes for nurses provide a public statement of ethical responsibility.

Ethical Decision-Making

Because the actions of nurses can have a profound effect on the well-being of others, a great many ethical issues are involved in nursing practice. Some of these issues are specific to nursing and are a consequence of nursing's care provider function; others are common to all thoughtful people in a modern society. For us to make intelligent choices regarding these issues, we need to examine closely our personal moral belief systems and to be aware of the bases of our ethical decision-making.

Ethical theory speaks of several approaches to decision-making. Socrates warned that decisions on ethics should not be made on feelings alone but on "hard facts and reasoning." In 1863, John Stuart Mill stated that ethical decision-making should focus on creating the "greatest good" for the most people, a philosophy he called **utilitarianism**. A variety of ethical theorists have written diverse opinions on this complicated subject. Let us consider two of the possible approaches to ethical decision-making: the *teleologic approach* and the *deontologic approach*.

Teleologic decision-making is based on the premise that an ethical decision is right if the consequences of an action derived from that decision are favorable and "do not harm." The term "teleologic" derives from the Greek word *telos*, meaning goal. Nursing practice is greatly influenced by the teleologic approach to decision-making. A common example is the decision to give large doses of pain medication to the suffering, terminally ill patient even though the medications may shorten the patient's life somewhat. The teleologic ethicist might argue that the consequence of the action (relief of pain) far outweighs the possibility of hastening death. Of course, even within the teleologic framework, there is the problem of determining what is beneficial.

Deontologic decision-making defines ethics, as the Greek word *deon* suggests, in terms of "duty" rather than consequences. To do one's duty is to do good and be ethical. Duty is determined by the individual's belief system. For one person, the highest duty may be toward a religious belief, or God; for another, the highest duty may be toward a government. A nurse operating under a deontologic code might choose to medicate the terminally ill patient only lightly because sustaining life at all costs has long been a duty of nursing. Hastening death would be viewed as a violation of duty and therefore, unethical. The basic issue in this framework is determining what constitutes one's value system.

In an attempt to reconcile these two positions, many ethicists have proposed different philosophical bases for ethical decision-making. Both as a student and as a practicing nurse, you will have to make a number of significant decisions regarding your own position with respect to issues of professional and personal ethics. You can base your choices on any of a number of possible premises and approaches. Some of the decisions you make may conflict with those of your colleagues. Just be sure that your decisions are thoughtful ones and that they focus on a concern for the well-being of others.

Bioethical Issues

Bioethics is a broad term that, by definition, refers to ethics arising from biologic functioning. Emanating from this definition has come the field of *medical ethics*, a field of study that addresses moral problems that have surfaced because of modern health care technology or new research and knowledge of disease states. The rapidly expanding issues surrounding the development and use of high technology in health care and its vast cost have raised ethical questions regarding appropriate use within treatment settings. More recently, the area of *nursing ethics* is gaining increasing attention. Nursing literature has given needed focus to the question of the nurse's participation and interest in maintaining ethical behavior that may be at variance with the medical community. Nurses closely interface with the physician and others on the health care team and may find themselves in confrontations. Although this may be uncomfortable for each person involved, understanding that ethically caring about the patient/client and the family may be a healthy and productive activity for everyone concerned.

Many health care agencies have established ethics committees. A variety of people, such as consulting ethicists, administrators, physicians, nurses, pastors, and consumers, serve on these important committees. These individuals examine and guide decisions on human rights, quality of life, allocation of medical resources, and other issues of an ethical nature in health care.

Nursing Issues and Trends: *Nursing Participation in Ethical Decisions*

Ethical decisions in relation to health care are frequently made by families and doctors without input from nurses who are caring for patients. This situation places enormous stress on the nurse who spends entire days in close contact with the patient and is immersed in the situation. Frequently the decisions made require the participation of the nurses. Increasingly, nurses are asking that decisions that will include their actions be made in a collaborative environment in which they can be involved. Ethics committees with nursing membership are one avenue for nurses to be involved in policy decisions. Interdisciplinary team conferences that include family members and all members of the health care team provide an environment that promotes collaboration in the individual situation.

Reproductive Issues

The current study and research in reproduction has raised a variety of ethical matters. Several questions revolve around the use of **artificial insemination**, which is the implanting of sperm into a female by a technical process rather than through intercourse. The issue is no longer limited to the use of insemination for procreation purposes with committed couples. A great deal of controversy surrounds **surrogate mothering**, a situation in which the natural mother cannot provide an adequate and functional uterus. Her ova can be fertilized in a laboratory by her husband's sperm, and the resulting embryo can then be transferred to another woman's uterus for implantation and eventual birth. Some argue that this is ethical because the surrogate is simply offering the uterus as a harbor for growth until the child can be born. Even more questionable are instances in which the sperm of a man are instilled for fertilization into a woman who is not his mate so that the child is born of a natural father and a surrogate mother. Because a monetary arrangement usually is made, some ethicists consider "mothering for hire" unethical.

Even more issues are raised by gene manipulation to alter basic tissue composition. The possibilities and risks of both surrogate mothering and gene manipulation are still largely speculative. Because of the possible risks, Congress continues to hear bills asking for the halting of research in these areas. At present, however, the legislation that has passed has been more advisory than restrictive in nature.

Another ethical issue in the area of genetics is whether persons who have been identified as carriers of particular genetic traits should have to undergo genetic counseling or not be allowed to have natural children. Does regulation take away the inalienable rights of these individuals to act according to their own consciences, or is protecting society from becoming the caretaker of persons who will not be able to function fully on their own in life a more important consideration?

Abortion and Infant Death

The issues of abortion and infant death have a direct impact on nursing. Whether one should take steps to promote life in an infant known to be genetically defective has become a major question. Some nurses consider elective abortion ethically defensible; in good conscience, they participate in the procedure itself and in the care of the patient. Others who consider the procedure unethical refuse in good conscience to participate in any phase of care. Still others decline to participate in the abortion but consider it ethical to care for the patient after the procedure. Each position involves an individual ethical decision that should be respected and honored, even if one disagrees. Because these issues involve fetuses and infants, they are particularly sensitive ones that bring forth strong emotions. In 1973, the United States Supreme Court decision of *Roe vs. Wade* made it legal for a physician to terminate a woman's pregnancy in the first 3 months with her approval. The rights of fathers are now under ethical scrutiny in many states. States' rights have redefined the law so that some allow abortions to be performed during trimesters other than the first if maternal health is in danger. In other states, licensure of those allowed to perform abortions is regulated. This continues to be a controversial issue, with strong feelings on both sides. Nurses can refuse to participate in the abortion procedure if doing so is counter to their ethical stance. In any event, this is a divisive ethical issue that will continue for some time to come. Abortion will continue to be an issue for nurses in the coming century.

A new ethical issue in this area is that of the

"harvesting" of fetal cells. By this, we mean that research is underway concerning the transplanting of organ cells from a dead fetus into a person who has a disease in hopes that the fetal cells might proliferate (grow) and provide improved organ function. A limited number of experiments have used fetal cells from the pancreas in the hope that this will help persons with diabetes and cells from the brain in the hope that they may produce neurohormones in persons with Parkinson's disease. A major concern of ethicists is that babies could be conceived and aborted for the express purpose of cell harvest and, in some cases, for payment of money. It is clear that this emerging issue will stimulate ethical debate because it will affect everyone and, in particular, the health care professional.

You may work in settings where these questions arise. To function comfortably as a nurse, you will need to consider your own beliefs and make your own ethical decisions. Building your own system of ethics can be a lifelong process.

Sterilization

Sterilization is another ethical issue because the surgical ligation of a woman's fallopian tubes or the performance of a vasectomy on a man renders these individuals incapable of conceiving children. Some religions consider this unethical in that it interferes with natural law. Many persons, however, acknowledge that adults have the right to make their own decisions about this matter.

A more controversial issue is sterilization of individuals who cannot make such decisions for themselves, such as those certified to be mentally incompetent. The argument for preventing pregnancy is that these people, because of their mental limitations, could neither care for a child nor be suitable parents.

An extreme position of some private citizens and those in the judicial system is that repeated male sexual offenders, particularly those who prey on children, should be forced by law to undergo orchiectomy (removal of the testicles) to decrease or remove the libido. These situations bring forth questions of human rights versus the protection of others.

Allocation of Resources

Allocation of resources refers to the decisions made regarding the distribution of dollars and other resources, such as personnel, equipment, and facilities.

One aspect of allocation of resources is the availability of donor organs that have saved many lives but have also raised some significant bioethical concerns. Because the need for replacement organs is far greater than the supply, who decides which patient gets a chance at life and which one does not? How is such a decision made and who should pay for the expensive procedures involved in implanting and maintaining donated organs? Should only those who can afford them be eligible for lifesaving transplants? Should government, hospitals, or insurance companies absorb the cost?

Another issue is that of the ethical use of critical care units with their associated high cost and use of highly educated health care staff. Studies done some years ago revealed that only a small portion of these patients survived 3 years after discharge. A computer that interprets inputed data regarding the medical status of an intensive care patient on life support and compares this information with hundreds of catalogued histories of similar patients so that survival chances can be electronically predicted is being used experimentally. Certainly, relying on computerized survival forecasts is unsettling, but physicians envision the possibility of combining this mechanical guidance with medical judgment to use medical technology more appropriately.

Confidentiality

Confidentiality is protection of the patient's privacy in both written and oral communication. The patient's diagnosis, problems, and condition should be discussed only with those who need such information to provide or improve the person's care. The patient has a right to decide what information will be shared. In establishing a relationship with a patient, therefore, you should explain that you may share what you are told with others on the health care team who are involved in some aspect of the patient's care. The person can then decide what is to be shared.

You should consider carefully which portion of the patient's remarks are relevant to care, and thus should be shared, and which should be kept confidential. For instance, a woman might confide that she had had a child as an unmarried 14-year-old. If she were an obstetric patient, such information could be important to her care and ought to be shared. If she were being treated for pneumonia or bronchitis, however, such information would not be pertinent. If you are in doubt about the relevance of information a patient has given you, consult your instructor or an experienced nurse who respects confidentiality before you share the information more broadly.

Sometimes information about a patient is shared for teaching purposes. In such cases, the identity of the patient is concealed. If you are writing a paper on the care of a particular patient, you must take care to conceal the patient's identity by using only initials. In the interests of privacy and confidentiality, patient information should not be discussed in public places where others may overhear. Even when names are not used, personal characteristics may be mentioned, and rumors—false or true—may result.

Confidentiality of written records is preserved by allowing access to the records only to those who need such information to enhance the patient's welfare. In general, the policy requires that the patient's written permission must be secured before the record can be viewed by anyone uninvolved in care. Even within the health care team, however, some people are simply curious. Reading a patient's record simply to satisfy curiosity is considered unethical.

Truth Telling

Is it ever ethical to withhold the truth from a patient? Some also question whether it is appropriate to give placebos without the patient's knowledge. A **placebo** is a pill or capsule that appears identical to a medication but does not contain any active ingredients. Should a physician always tell patients of their conditions, even when this information may lead to great mental anguish? How might a nurse help in these situations? Questions about *truth telling* are difficult ones for those of us in health care delivery.

A related issue is that of **informed consent,** which has both ethical and legal considerations (see later discussion). The ethical issue is determining the meaning of the term "informed." In how much depth should patients be told information that they may later view as harmful? For example, being told about all the dreadful details of open heart surgery may make a patient decide against having the procedure.

Paternalism

Paternalism is the process by which others make decisions for people without including them in the decision. Although well intentioned, taking the decision-making power away from an individual can be unethical. Because an important part of the nursing role is that of identifying patients' problems and carrying out interventions, nurses can, without meaning to, remove the responsibility from the individual and function in a paternalistic mode. Is this behavior by nurses unethical? Should you as a nurse, allow patient participation and if not, have you deprived the patient of rightful power?

Paternalism and its impact can also be an issue for health care. Regulations requiring that fluoride be added to drinking water to decrease the incidence of caries and that children be vaccinated are examples of paternalism in health care (Fig. 3-1).

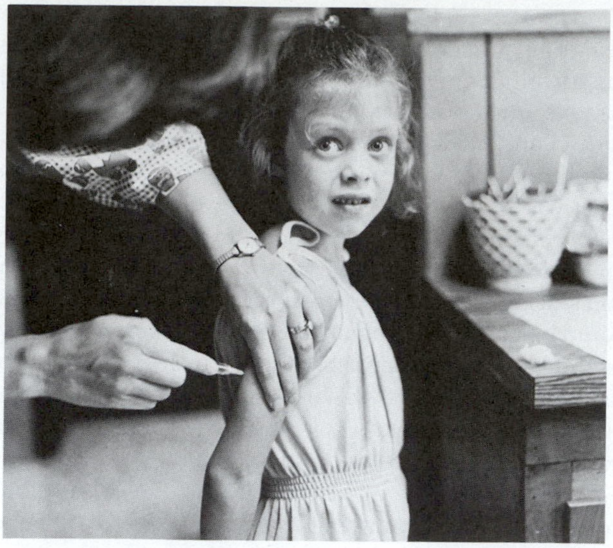

Figure 3-1. Mandatory immunization of children is an example of paternalism in health care.

Paternalistic actions raise complex ethical problems. Many of the actions just mentioned are intended to protect the individual and society but how far should this go? Is taking away the opportunity for individual decision-making on these issues ethical? The health care system is constantly confronted with such questions.

Ethical Concerns Surrounding AIDS

No other issue has aroused individual and collective emotions more in the last 15 years than has the acquired immunodeficiency syndrome (AIDS) epidemic. Early on, those infected were primarily gay men and intravenous drug abusers. These lifestyles caused a minority of persons to question the appropriateness of using great amounts of money and resources to assuage the epidemic. As an increasing number of heterosexuals, teens, women, and infants have become infected, early opponents of medical intervention for these people are rethinking their position.

If predictions regarding rising rates of human immunodeficiency virus (HIV) and AIDS prove accurate, the magnitude of need could deplete medical resources in many countries throughout the world. The cost of maintaining a person who develops AIDS has been estimated at over $85,000 from diagnosis to death (Goldsmith, 1991, p. 1055). What about the resulting reduction in other health programs? The dilemma is an ethical one, in which some think the expenditure unreasonable and disproportionate, whereas others strongly see the issue as a humanitarian obligation.

Other important, related issues concern the ethical right to privacy so that employment, housing, and medical insurance will not be denied. Other international issues are also relevant, such as travel and immigration restrictions. Concerns surrounding the rights of individuals throughout the world to be protected from becoming infected versus the rights of persons infected with the AIDS virus to maximize life are being debated.

Debated questions regarding containment of the epidemic and the care of victims move to the forefront. Who should be tested for infection? Some think everyone should be tested; others feel health care workers, including nurses, should be tested. The American Nurses Association (ANA) has made a public statement against mandatory testing of nurses. Not only is the cost of testing programs an issue, but from an ethical viewpoint, the rights of individuals not to be tested and protection of confidentiality must also be considered. A professional issue is that of possible termination of employment if a nurse tests positive for the AIDS virus.

Truth telling is also an issue. Should the infected person, family members, or sexual partners be told about the presence of infection? What about the rights of the individual who prefers not to know or the rights of one who may become infected through not knowing?

Many neverending issues have become apparent because of this disturbing epidemic. Should intensive care units be used for AIDS patients? Should surgeons be placed at risk performing surgery on persons with HIV infection or, conversely, risk transmitting the virus to patients if the surgeon is HIV infected? Can nurses refuse to care for persons with AIDS? Most health care facilities and programs in nursing maintain a policy that a mission of nursing is to care for all individuals, regardless of disease or contagion.

End of Life Issues

Perhaps no other ethical topic is as important to nurses as that of end of life issues. When the quality of life has deteriorated to the point where no meaningful survival is possible, should life be prolonged? Who decides when a patient is no longer competent to make such decisions? These questions center on the right of the individual to decline extraordinary means of medical intervention that can extend a life whose quality to that person is unacceptable. Also debated is the issue of whether a person can direct the withholding of water and food in an effort to end one's life. This sensitive issue involves both ethical and legal considerations. Does a legal right imply a moral right to self-determination (Salladay and McDonnell, 1992)? To allow individuals more power in this decision, the majority of states have some provision for "advance directives." This means that the person who is mentally competent can make a legal judgment before or during a serious illness directing that extraordinary measures not be used if quality of life has decreased and there is no reasonable chance for recovery. Advance directives include what were formerly known as "Living Wills" and Durable Powers of Attorney for Health Care (Schwarz, 1992). We will discuss this in much more detail in Chapter 41.

Other Bioethical Issues

Numerous other issues involve medical ethics, nursing ethics, or bioethics. It is outside the scope of this text to discuss all of them. We might mention, however, three other ethical issues worthy of thought by nurses who have the welfare of patients in mind.

One concern is the *ethical care of the elderly client.* With the growing number of elders in our society, all nurses should be concerned about the ethical care of the older person. Numerous articles have been written about neglect in hygiene heeds, which leads to decubitus ulcers, and social isolation, which results in low self-esteem. The inappropriate use of medications has also been cited in some settings—oversedation to control agitated behavior and underuse of pain-controlling agents. Although an individual nurse may not be involved in the abuse of any patient, the responsibility to report such a situation is ethically correct.

A second ethical consideration is **patient autonomy**, that is, respecting the patient's right to refuse treatment. This acknowledges the fact that the patient is a vital member of the health care team and should be allowed and encouraged to aid in the decision-making. This area was discussed in Chapter 1.

Lastly, let us consider the area of *medical experimentation.* Munson writes that "there is something 'experimental' . . . about every individual treatment, beginning with the diagnosis itself," but that the patient "has the right to expect the doctor does nothing to him just in order to learn" (Munson, 1988, p. 261). Nurses should also consider their ethical behavior when learning from the patient or conducting research. Confined populations, such as those in prisons or in government hospitals, have long been used for experimental programs because they constitute a controlled group in the statistical sense. This practice raises the ethical question of possible coercion. Certain rewards may be offered to a prisoner in return for participation in a research program. Is such action unethical or is it justified if it furthers needed research? Agencies and "human rights" committees have been established to protect individuals from becoming victims, but reporting an abuse should become the ethical responsibility of any nurse.

Organizations Concerned with Medical Ethics

Several organizations, both domestic and international, monitor the ethical implications of scientific advancements. In addition, professional organizations have committees that promote ethical practice.

The Hastings Center (Briarcliff Manor, NY) is a private, nonprofit organization that conducts educational and research programs in medicine, the life sciences, and the professions. The United States Senate Committee on Ethics is an arm of the Senate whose mission is to propose legislation, when appropriate, to address ethical issues in our country. The International Society for Assessment of Science and Technology at The Hague (Netherlands) encourages scientists throughout the world to engage in a cooperative effort of ethical evaluation of scientific and technologic endeavors. An international organization called the International Association of Ethicists consists of a selected number of the world's most prominent ethicists. This group has been vocal concerning the ethical infringement on human rights.

Because of increasing interest in ethical issues, many subgroups have been formed to address special interest areas. These groups are both national and local; they consider ethical behavior in such areas as education, religion, business, health care, and service agencies.

Reaching decisions that are ethical, either in a personal or professional sense, is not easy. Furthermore, "ethical decision making cannot be avoided in nursing" (Ellis and Hartley, 1992, p. 200). At times, we need to change our decisions as circumstances change or as we gather more information. In reality, we bring to the decision-making process all that we are as individuals—our past, present, and future; family, community, and spirituality also play a role. Perhaps, as Wright (1987) suggests, a commitment to caring is the real foundation of ethics.

Display 3–1
ANA Code for Nurses

1. The nurse provides services with respect for human dignity and the uniqueness of the client unrestricted by considerations of social or economic status, personal attributes, or the nature of health problems.
2. The nurse safeguards the client's rights to privacy by judiciously protecting information of a cofidential nature.
3. The nurse acts to safeguard the client and the public when health care and safety are affected by the imcompetent, unethical, or illegal practice of any person.
4. The nurse assumes responsibility and accountability for individual nursing judgments and actions.
5. The nurse maintains competence in nursing.
6. The nurse exercises informed judgment and uses individual competence and qualifications as criteria in seeking consultation, accepting responsibilities, and delegating nursing activities to others.
7. The nurse participates in activities that contribute to the ongoing development of the profession's body of knowledge.
8. The nurse participates in the profession's efforts to implement and improve standards of nursing.
9. The nurse participates in the profession's efforts to establish and maintain conditions of employment conducive to high quality nursing care.
10. The nurse participates in the profession's efforts to protect the public from misinformation and misrepresentation and to maintain the integrity of nursing.
11. The nurse collaborates with members of the health professions and other citizens in promoting community and national efforts to meet the health needs of the public.

Source: American Nurses Association, 1976. ANA Publication Code No. G56R25M 4/77. Reprinted with permission.

The Code for Nurses

The ANA Code for Nurses is the general standard for professional behavior of practicing nurses in the United States (Display 3-1). This code has not been revised since 1976. A similar code exists for Canadian nurses called the Canadian Nurses Association Code of Ethics for Nursing. Both of these codes continue to be viable documents for guiding the ethical behavior of nurses. Copies of these codes and their interpretation are available from the respective associations.

The International Council of Nurses (ICN) in Geneva, Switzerland, also has a code for nurses. Using five distinct sections, it reflects many of the values set forth by the ANA code; either may serve as a useful directive for the ethical behavior of nurses throughout the world. As individuals in a profession that influences the lives of others, nurses are obligated to thoughtfully examine their own decisions on ethical questions. However, nursing is a profession with explicit ethical principles and every nurse must adhere to them in matters that reflect on the profession as a whole. Any individual who finds it impossible to comply with the ethical standards of the nursing profession would do well to reconsider a career as a nurse. Because you will be guided by your own religious and philosophical beliefs, it would be wise to reflect and clarify your position on the issues discussed in this chapter before you encounter them in a clinical situation.

Consumers' Rights in Health Care

The rights of health care consumers are attracting increasing attention in conjunction with the growth of consumer protection in other areas of life. In 1959, the National League for Nursing (NLN) was the first organization to formulate a protection statement for patients. Unfortunately, this was not widely circulated at the time. Then, in 1973, the American Hospital Association (AHA) published *A Patient's Bill of Rights* (Display 3-2). Because of the AHA's size and membership and because of growing public interest in consumer issues, this document elicited widespread discussion. The document affirms the patient's right to receive respectful care and needed services; to have a communicative patient–physician relationship; and to be informed of experimentation, medical care costs, and hospital policies. The document also addresses confidentiality. The bill also implicitly gives patients the right to refuse treatment—an emerging legal issue of the 1990s. For example, suppose your patient refuses to be transported to the x-ray department for another film, believing that this is unnecessary. You might encourage the patient to discuss the reasons for refusing the x-ray examination with the physician, but at the same time, recognize that it is the patient's right to refuse. How much this bill has changed the care received by patients is unclear, but medical care facilities in this country have encouraged its distribution to consumers of health care.

Nurses' organizations, including state and provincial groups, have also published consumer protection documents. In each of these, the role of the nurse is specifically mentioned. One example is The Health Care Consumer Bill of Rights, written and circulated by the Washington State Nurses Association in 1980 (Display 3-3).

Personal Behavior

Behavior at work is also a matter of ethics. What you do as a student nurse reflects not only on you but on your program and other student nurses. There is, however, considerable difference of opinion as to what constitutes correct and incorrect behavior. A useful guideline to consider is whether specific behavior will enhance or impair your ability to work effectively with the patient. For example, provocative behavior, whether the student is a male or female, is unethical because it would greatly inhibit the ability to care for the person as a patient.

A serious, related problem is that of the chemically impaired nurse who uses alcohol or drugs inappropriately or illegally. If you are aware of such a problem, you cannot ethically ignore it. Safety for the patient and concern for the nurse are both issues. You should share your knowledge of the existence of the problem with the person who is abusing and with your immediate supervisor so that help can be obtained.

Boards of nursing and individual agencies and facilities have policies regarding this growing problem. A minor infraction may result in a recommendation that the nurse enter a chemical abuse treatment program. Nurses who commit a more serious infraction such as being unable to maintain sobriety or taking drugs from the facility and falsifying records may forfeit their licenses. Selling substances for profit usually results in criminal action being taken.

Accepting Attitudes

A nonjudgmental attitude reflecting acceptance of the patient as a person, regardless of your opinion of the person's lifestyle, is an obligation of the health care professional. In the extreme, a person wounded by the police because of violence in the streets and the policeman in the incident deserve the same quality of care. The person who develops lung cancer as a result of long-term heavy smoking or the victim of AIDS who has a history of risk factors is equally deserving of quality of care. You have an ethical obligation to withdraw your care from any patient about whom you cannot be objective and caring.

The Translation of Ethics into Law

When ethical issues become a concern for a community or society as a whole, a law may be written and passed that seeks to translate ethics into what the majority considers to be acceptable behavior. This transformation of ethical standards into law is one of the ways society attempts to guard against abuses that could victimize the defenseless. Its origin goes back to earliest times when people began living together in communities, and it became clear that certain rules had to be made. For the well-being of all the members, during periods of danger and uncertainty, certain standards of behavior were essential. In tribal times, these rules were unwritten and often enforced by a tribal council. When tribes became more rigidly structured and increased in size, eventually

Display 3–2
A Patient's Bill of Rights

Introduction

Effective health care requires collaboration between patients and physicians and other health care professionals. Open and honest communication, respect for personal and professional values, and sensitivity to differences are integral to optimal patient care. As the setting for the provision of health services, hospitals must provide a foundation for understanding and respecting the rights and responsibilities of patients, their families, physicians, and other caregivers. Hospitals must ensure a health care ethic that respects the role of patients in decision making about treatment choices and other aspects of their care. Hospitals must be sensitive to cultural, racial, linguistic, religious, age, gender, and other differences as well as the needs of persons with disabilities.

The American Hospital Association presents *A Patient's Bill of Rights* with the expectation that it will contribute to more effective patient care and be supported by the hospital on behalf of the institution, its medical staff, employees, and patients. The American Hospital Association encourages health care institutions to tailor this bill of rights to their patient community by translating and/or simplifying the language of this bill of rights as may be necessary to ensure that patients and their families understand their rights and responsibilities.

Bill of Rights*

1. The patient has the right to considerate and respectful care.
2. The patient has the right to and is encouraged to obtain from physicians and other direct caregivers relevant, current, and understandable information concerning diagnosis, treatment, and prognosis.

   Except in emergencies when the patient lacks decision-making capacity and the need for treatment is urgent, the patient is entitled to the opportunity to discuss and request information related to the specific procedures and/or treatments, the risks involved, the possible length of recuperation, and the medically reasonable alternatives and their accompanying risks and benefits.

   Patients have the right to know the identity of physicians, nurses, and others involved in their care, as well as when those involved are students, residents, or other trainees. The patient also has the right to know the immediate and long-term financial implications of treatment choices, insofar as they are known.
3. The patient has the right to make decisions about the plan of care prior to and during the course of treatment and to refuse a recommended treatment or plan of care to the extent permitted by law and hospital policy and to be informed of the medical consequences of this action. In case of such refusal, the patient is entitled to other appropriate care and services that the hospital provides or transfer to another hospital. The hospital should notify patients of any policy that might affect patient choice within the institution.
4. The patient has the right to have an advance directive (such as a living will, health care proxy, or durable power of attorney for health care) concerning treatment or designating a surrogate decision maker with the expectation that the hospital will honor the intent of that directive to the extent permitted by law and hospital policy.

   Health care institutions must advise patients of their rights under state law and hospital policy to make informed medical choices, ask if the patient has an advance directive, and include that information in patient records. The patient has the right to timely information about hospital policy that may limit its ability to implement fully a legally valid advance directive.
5. The patient has the right to every consideration of privacy. Case discussion, consultation, examination, and treatment should be conducted so as to protect each patient's privacy.
6. The patient has the right to expect that all communications and records pertaining to his/her care will be treated as confidential by the hospital, except in cases such as suspected abuse and public health hazards when reporting is permitted or required by law. The patient has the right to expect that the hospital will emphasize the confidentiality of this information when it releases it to any other parties entitled to review information in these records.
7. The patient has the right to review the records pertaining to his/her medical care and to have the information explained or interpreted as necessary, except when restricted by law.
8. The patient has the right to expect that, within its capacity and policies, a hospital will make reasonable response to the request of a patient for appropriate and medically indicated care and services.

**These rights can be exercised on the patient's behalf by a designated surrogate or proxy decision maker if the patient lacks decision-making capacity, is legally incompetent, or is a minor.*

Display 3–2 ***(continued)***
A Patient's Bill of Rights

The hospital must provide evaluation, service, and/or referral as indicated by the urgency of the case. When medically appropriate and legally permissible, or when a patient has so requested, a patient may be transferred to another facility. The institution to which the patient is to be transferred must first have accepted the patient for transfer. The patient must also have the benefit of complete information and explanation concerning the need for, risks, benefits, and alternatives to such a transfer.

9. The patient has the right to ask and be informed of the existence of business relationships among the hospital, educational institutions, other health care providers, or payers that may influence the patient's treatment and care.
10. The patient has the right to consent to or decline to participate in proposed research studies or human experimentation affecting care and treatment or requiring direct patient involvement, and to have those studies fully explained prior to consent. A patient who declines to participate in research or experimentation is entitled to the most effective care that the hospital can otherwise provide.
11. The patient has the right to expect reasonable continuity of care when appropriate and to be informed by physicians and other caregivers of available and realistic patient care options when hospital care is no longer appropriate.
12. The patient has the right to be informed of hospital policies and practices that relate to patient care, treatment, and responsibilities. The patient has the right to be informed of available resources for resolving disputes, grievances, and conflicts, such as ethics committees, patient representatives, or other mechanisms available in the institution. The patient has the right to be informed of the hospital's charges for services and available payment methods.

The collaborative nature of health care requires that patients, or their families/surrogates, participate in their care. The effectiveness of care and patient satisfaction with the course of treatment depend, in part, on the patient fulfilling certain responsibilities. Patients are responsible for providing information about past illnesses, hospitalizations, medication, and other matters related to health status. To participate effectively in decision making, patients must be encouraged to take responsibility for requesting additional information or clarification about their health status or treatment when they do not fully understand information and instructions. Patients are also responsible for ensuring that the health care institution has a copy of their written advance directive if they have one. Patients are responsible for informing their physicians and other caregivers if they anticipate problems in following prescribed treatment.

Patients should also be aware of the hospital's obligation to be reasonably efficient and equitable in providing care to other patients and the community. The hospital's rules and regulations are designed to help the hospital meet this obligation. Patients and their families are responsible for making reasonable accommodations to the needs of the hospital, other patients, medical staff, and hospital employees. Patients are responsible for providing necessary information for insurance claims and for working with the hospital to make payment arrangements, when necessary.

A person's health depends on much more than health care services. Patients are responsible for recognizing the impact of their life-style on their personal health.

Conclusion

Hospitals have many functions to perform, including the enhancement of health status, health promotion, and the prevention and treatment of injury and disease; the immediate and ongoing care and rehabilitation of patients; the education of health professionals, patients, and the community; and research. All these activities must be conducted with an overriding concern for the values and dignity of patients.

A Patient's Bill of Rights was first adopted by the American Hospital Association in 1973. This revision was approved by the AHA Board of Trustees on October 21, 1992.
©1992 by the American Hospital Association, 840 North Lake Shore Drive, Chicago, Illinois 60611. Printed in the U.S.A. All rights reserved. Catalog no. 157759.

forming the nations we know today, the rules of earlier times became formal laws. Over time, two main sources of laws came into existence: statutory laws and common laws. In our present world, nurses have the responsibility to be knowledgeable about all legislation but, in particular, about laws that define ethical behavior.

Statutory Law

The first and more powerful type of law is **statutory law** (enacted law), which is law voted in by a governmental legislative body. In the United States, this body may be the state legislature or a county or city council.

Display 3–3
Health Care Consumer Bill of Rights

Consistent with the WSNA purpose to foster high standards of nursing practice, the following beliefs have been adopted as the Health Care Consumer Bill of Rights. The Association recognizes, however, that societal forces exist over which the individual has no control.

Health care consumers have the right to:

1. Health services that respect the dignity and worth without regard to nationality, race, religious philosophy, color, status, age, sex or affectional preference.
2. Equal access to health services designed to provide high level wellness/illness care.
3. A health care program that is consistent with their own value systems, including consultation with alternative health care providers.
4. Information and knowledge about their health status and care to the extent requested.
5. Accept or refuse health care intervention after being informed of the potential and probable consequences.
6. Choose behaviors that impact negatively or positively on their level of wellness.
7. Information relative to mechanisms that may be used if they believe appropriate health care has not been provided.
8. Expect that health care providers will speak on their behalf when health care or safety is affected by incompetent, unethical, or illegal conduct of any person.
9. Privacy by having information of a confidential nature judiciously protected.
10. Determine the extent to which the family is to be included in their health care program.
11. Die with dignity and in a way consistent with their personal values.
12. A reasonable estimate of the costs of care.
13. Prior knowledge if the provider proposes to engage in or perform experimentation affecting their care or treatment. (The consumer has the right to refuse to participate in such research projects without jeopardizing access to health care.)

Adopted by the Washington State Nurses Association Board of Directors, July 1980.

Published collections of such laws are called codes. Many laws relating to the health care system have been passed under federal jurisdiction and were discussed in Chapter 2. Many state and provincial level laws affect nursing practice. Laws concerning abortion rights, advance directives for end of life issues, school attendance, immunization, and provision of housing for the disadvantaged are all state laws that have implication for nurses. Nurse practice acts are also important examples of enacted state laws.

Common Law

The second type of law is **common law**, the collective term for common knowledge, customary procedure, and judicial decisions. Using these last three sources, a judge interprets the law and issues a decision. The roots of common law in this country and in Canada are planted in England. Common law is applied in a number of decisions involving nursing. A judicial decision on a case involving an applicant denied admission to a particular nursing program would become the law in that situation. Another example is a case in which the court must determine what is prudent nursing practice in a given situation. A number of nurses might testify as to correct practice and current nursing journals might be consulted. On the basis of this evidence about customary procedure, a common law decision is made.

The Courts

In the United States, the courts are one part of our national government, along with the executive branch and the legislative branch. Although courts do not initiate law, they interpret existing laws in the process of deciding disputes (the judicial process). If there is a jury, a single judge usually hears a case. When a jury is not called, more than one judge may enter into the decision. The United States Supreme Court, as the name suggests, ranks above state and lower courts.

Administrative Law

Because of lack of time and energy, it is sometimes difficult to administer statutes. The legislature may delegate power to an administrative department of the government. The rules and regulations established by this administrative body become **administrative law**, which is then part of statutory law (Creighton, 1986, p. 3). Agencies or boards assume responsibility for writing the rules used to enforce laws that apply to their purposes and mission. The courts have traditionally upheld the power of administrative law because they view those agencies so empowered to be expert in their areas of interest. An example for nurses is that of the state nursing boards.

Crimes and Torts

A distinction needs to be made between a crime and a tort. A *crime* is a violation of law that threatens the society as a whole, and punishment is sought by the state.

An example pertinent to nursing is a violation of the narcotic laws. Punishment may be imprisonment, a fine, or some form of restitution.

A **tort** is a civil action in which one or more persons is seeking compensation because of the wrongful act of another. Torts are often instances in which a private individual is injured but society is not threatened. Negligence is a tort. If guilt is found, the remedy may involve compensating the wronged party monetarily or by a required action.

When crimes are committed, "there is a heavy burden on the prosecution to prove its case beyond a reasonable doubt, whereas in civil actions, the plaintiffs have only to show a preponderance of evidence in their favor" (Creighton, 1986, p. 227). Occasionally, then, evidence may be insufficient to convict under the criminal laws, but it could be adequate in a civil or tort action to convict the offender. Most legal cases in which nurses are involved are civil actions in which an individual is suing.

The Role of Policy and Procedure

The policies of a health care facility or a school of nursing are established to guide action in various situations. Such policies are based in part on the legal requirements of the locality. Courts often accept hospital policy as evidence of common usage and therefore as the common law. For this and other reasons, you need to learn (or at least know where to find) the policies of your school of nursing and those of the facilities where you practice.

Specific Legal Concerns

A number of legal concepts and terms are of particular interest to nursing, and it is wise to be familiar with them. To augment those we will discuss here, you may want to consult a text on the legal aspects of nursing or do some reading in the current literature.

Negligence and Malpractice

Negligence is the legal term for an act that resulted in harm to another person or the omission of an act that would have prevented such harm. To be found negligent, one must have failed to act as a "reasonably prudent person" would have acted in a similar situation and the act or failure to act must have caused harm.

Malpractice is a narrower term referring to negligence on the part of a professional person. In the case of a nurse or other professional, the standard of the reasonably prudent person is made specific to the profession. That is, your standard of action even as a student is held to be the **reasonably prudent nurse**. An understanding of this principle is important.

Whenever you perform a nursing procedure, you are subject to the standard of the reasonably prudent practicing nurse. You may be slower or less dexterous, but the outcome for the patient must be the same as would be provided by a practicing nurse. This principle ensures safety and a high standard of care for the patient. It is clear that a patient should not be harmed in any way from receiving care from a student. Malpractice is a civil wrong and is punished by a monetary fine rather than a jail sentence. It is assumed that the harm caused by malpractice was not intentional.

Informed Consent

A decision to accept treatment is called **consent**. Every patient/client has a legal right to be informed about his or her condition and the potential benefits and hazards of a proposed treatment. This information is the basis on which the patient can decide whether to accept the proposed plan of care. A patient's decision to accept a proposed treatment based on a clear understanding of the benefits and hazards of that treatment is called **informed consent**. Consent must be both informed and freely given and can be legally withdrawn at any time. In other words, the patient can change his or her mind. This is a legal issue as well as an ethical one.

Consent may be either oral or written. In practice, consent for minor, noninvasive, and temporary treatments is typically oral. Most nursing care measures fall into this category. Consents for major, invasive, and potentially harmful procedures—surgery, radiation, and certain diagnostic tests—are obtained in writing.

It is the physician's responsibility to obtain consent and to provide appropriate information regarding medical treatment (Ellis and Hartley, 1992, p. 180). Some hospitals have forms that give the patient the options for a "full or complete disclosure" of information or "partial disclosure." Not all patients wish to know details of potential complications, for this knowledge might cause undue psychological distress. If such a disclosure form is used, the information given by the physician and the appended signature should be congruent with the option chosen.

Many large hospitals have designated persons available who can witness legal documents such as consent forms. Often, this is done in the admitting department before the patient is transferred to the unit. However, a nurse is sometimes asked to witness a patient/client's signature on a medical or surgical consent form. Doing so does not transfer to the nurse the legal responsibility for providing information about medical treatment and ascertaining that the consent is informed. The nurse is attesting that the person named in the document did indeed sign it freely. The nurse should make certain that the form being used is the appropriate one and is filled out correctly. The physician remains legally responsible for ensuring that the consent is informed.

The nurse is responsible for obtaining consent for nursing measures. When you give a patient information to obtain consent, you must make sure he or she understands the information before you proceed.

Age and Consent

Every adult is assumed to be capable of giving personal consent unless a court or other legal authority has determined otherwise. Advanced age is by no means a sufficient justification for assuming a patient is unable to give consent.

The legal age of consent is 18 years in most jurisdictions, but there are several exceptions. An **emancipated minor**—an underage person who is financially independent and does not live in the parent's home—is usually permitted to give consent. This is often the case in instances relating to reproduction and pregnancy, birth control, and venereal disease. You will need to learn the legal requirements for consent in your state or province.

Growing concern for human rights has led to the inclusion of children in decision-making about their own care as soon as they seem able to understand. Of course, parental consent must still be obtained, but it is also highly desirable to elicit the consent of the child. Children are typically included in decision-making by the age of 7 or 8 years.

Consent for the Incapacitated

Alternatives are available to obtain consent when the individual is temporarily incapable of giving personal consent. In an emergency when an immediate threat to life exists, two physicians are required to concur that an emergency exists and that the patient is unable to give consent. Consent is then usually requested from the next of kin. If this proves impossible, the staff will abide by the facility's policy on such situations, which provides for maximum legal protection of the health care providers and needed care for the patient.

Situations often arise with the extremely ill elder who either temporarily or permanently does not have decision-making capacity. The most useful solution is that the client has revealed appropriate decisions with a family member or close friend before becoming impaired and who has then been granted a Durable Power of Attorney for Health Care. This person then legally "speaks" for the incapacitated in making decisions. If such a person does not exist, the policy of the health care agency should be consulted.

Assault and Battery

Assault is threatening bodily harm (or making a person feel threatened); **battery** is touching or harming a person without consent. This charge may seem entirely irrelevant to health care, but performing certain treatment procedures without informed consent may constitute battery in the eyes of the law. The concept of assault has

Nursing Research: *Implications for Practice*

Wilson, D. M. "Ethical Concerns in a Long-Term Tube Feeding Study." *Image* 24, 3 (Fall 1992): 195–199.

Ten patients, with an average age of 54 years who had been tube fed for 6 months or longer, were studied. These individuals were residents of a long-term care facility. The investigation process focused primarily on five questions:

1. Who should make the decision to tube feed?
2. How should tube feeding decisions be made?
3. What are valid reasons for initiating and continuing tube feeding?
4. Is it permissible to withdraw tube feeding once it is initiated?
5. Is tube feeding an effective and appropriate life-supporting technology?

The study concluded that even though tube feeding is effective in sustaining life over a long period, persons involved in decision-making should weigh the "burdens and the benefits of the procedure." The physician was the predominant decision-maker, and only minimal consultation occurred with the nursing staff or family members. Although the investigator believes that the patient should be consulted, only two of the residents in the study were responsive. With the increase in the aging population and the success of new interventions in treating acute illness, the use of tube feeding will increase. The author suggests more definitive policies regarding the initiation of tube feeding, including the active participation of the patient and family whenever possible.

been expanded to include psychological assault. However unintentional an act may be, this can be interpreted as instilling "fear" in a patient. A patient can hold a nurse accountable for psychological assault in a court of law.

Instances of both child and elder abuse that constitute legal definitions of battery have been reported increasingly, both within institutions and in the home. The unfortunate trend of elder abuse appears to be on the rise and should be of particular concern for nurses in both the acute care and chronic care settings (Kimsey, Tarbox, and Bragg, 1981, p. 465).

False Imprisonment

Confining a person without consent and without due process is considered **false imprisonment**. Using restraints without having followed appropriate procedures and documented the circumstances is defined as false imprisonment. The major method for protecting oneself against legal action when restraints are imperative is to document the procedure carefully in writing, with the reasons for the action. A physician's order should also be obtained promptly. In this instance and many others, clear documentation is your best defense against unwarranted legal action.

Refusing to discharge a person, who judges himself or herself competent, from a health care facility can also be considered false imprisonment. Most facilities have a procedure for this occurrence, which instructs consultation with the physician in an attempt to dissuade the person from leaving. Some hospitals request that the patient sign an AMA (against medical advice) form to relieve the nurse, physician, and hospital of any liability should the patient be harmed or bring forth allegations of false imprisonment. Many hospitals have discontinued using such a form but ask that the nurse, after notifying the physician and talking with a patient who is insistent, document the person's leaving in the patient's record.

Narcotics Control

In many institutions, nurses are responsible for both administering and accounting for narcotics and other controlled substances, responsibilities with important legal ramifications. The hospital establishes policies and explicit procedures for discharging this responsibility. Altering or falsifying narcotic records is a crime. If you discover an error, you have a duty to report it. Established procedure usually entails notifying the unit supervisor and pharmacy personnel as well as filling out a report. By following such procedures carefully, you protect yourself against legal action and possible loss of licensure.

Libel and Slander

Libel is a damaging written statement that defames a person's character or makes the person an object of ridicule. **Slander** is an oral statement to the same effect. Statements may be considered to be libel or slander even when they are true. You should be careful about what you write in a patient's record or say about a patient to others. Such statements should be factual and free of opinions and attitudes that might damage a person's reputation. If a nurse reports to other staff members that he or she believes a patient is "faking" pain, and as a result, pain medication is withheld and staff members ignore the patient, the nurse's remarks could be considered slander. If the nurse had instead presented the facts of the situation and discussed the patient's care in a manner that resulted in more individualized attention to the patient's real needs, no damage would have occurred to the patient and slander could not be charged. Slander may also be charged if staff members make indiscreet comments about a patient in a public area of the hospital. In general, statements about the patient should be made only to those involved in care.

Invasion of Privacy

Every individual has a right to privacy, including personal information and one's belongings. Looking in a patient's suitcase, purse, or wallet or trying to obtain personal information without that person's knowledge is an *invasion of privacy*. Consent must be obtained before one looks through a person's personal effects. When you need information about a patient, be straightforward and honest with the person about what you need to know and the use to which the information will be put. Giving out information about a patient, including diagnosis, without permission is also an invasion of privacy.

Wills

A seriously ill hospitalized individual sometimes decides to prepare or amend a will. Such a legal change or amendment is called a codicil. Most institutions have persons on the staff who can objectively witness the signing of a will. This is often done by an employee in the business or admitting office. It is unwise for a student or even a staff nurse to witness a will. In fact, some hospitals do not allow any employee or student to witness a will. Witnessing a will can be a far different matter from witnessing consent forms for the performance of a procedure. The patient's condition at the time of signing a will is one of the complicating matters. Because wills can involve not only disposition of property

To My Family, My Physician, My Lawyer and All Others Whom It May Concern

Death is as much a reality as birth, growth, and aging—it is the one certainty of life. In anticipation of decisions that may have to be made about my own dying and as an expression of my right to refuse treatment, I ______________________ (print name), being of sound mind, make this statement of my wishes and instructions concerning treatment.

By means of this document, which I intend to be legally binding, I direct my physician and other care providers, my family, and any surrogate designated by me or appointed by a court, to carry out my wishes. If I become unable, by reason of physical or mental incapacity, to make decisions about my medical care, let this document provide the guidance and authority needed to make any and all such decisions.

If I am permanently unconscious or there is no reasonable expectation of my recovery from a seriously incapacitating or lethal illness or condition, I do not wish to be kept alive by artificial means. I request that I be given all care necessary to keep me comfortable and free of pain, even if pain-relieving medications may hasten my death, and I direct that no life-sustaining treatment be provided except as I or my surrogate specifically authorize.

This request may appear to place a heavy responsibility upon you, but by making this decision according to my strong convictions, I intend to ease that burden. I am acting after careful consideration and with understanding of the consequences of your carrying out my wishes. *List optional specific provisions in the space below.*

(Continued)

Figure 3-2. Sample advance directive. (Reprinted by permission of Choice in Dying, formerly Concern for Dying/Society for the Right to Die, 200 Varick Street, New York, NY 10014)

but often have an impact on the dynamics of a family at a time of crisis, they are contested perhaps more than any other legal document. Unfortunately, on occasion, legal action has been taken by families accusing the nurse of witnessing an invalid will to receive funds or at the very least, coercing the patient into what the family considers to be an unfair settlement of property. It is prudent for nurses not to take on such responsibilities but to delegate them to persons who have a legal background or have been designated by the health care agency to perform this service.

Advance Directives for Health Care

A companion issue to defining death is the question of determining when life-support measures should be started and when they should be discontinued. For many years there has been a debate over the legalities and ethics of placing individuals on ventilators, of instituting resuscitation, and of continuing life-prolonging therapies.

In October 1990, the United States Congress passed two sections of the Omnibus Reconciliation Act which was to become known as the Patient Self-Determination Act. Under this law, any health care facility that receives funds from Medicare or Medicaid is required to discuss advance directives with all inpatients (Paridy, 1991, p. 13). Not only is this act important in focusing attention on the legality of end of life issues, but it provides increasing patient autonomy. ". . . This new law seems to be increasing communication between the health care provider and the patient regarding his or her wishes" (Omery, 1991, p. 123).

"Forty-one states and the District of Columbia have enacted legislation that acknowledges advance directives. Advances in medical knowledge and the development of life sustaining technologies have changed the very nature of death" (Schwarz, 1992, p. 920). To make their personal wishes known, some individuals write directives under the *natural death act* of their state. These were originally called "living wills" and were not legally binding. In an **advance directive**, the individual prepares a "directive to physicians" that identifies exactly what the person does not want done in regard to life support. The law carefully states how this document must be written. Usually it cannot be witnessed by close relatives or anyone who would gain from the person's death. It is not necessary to have an attorney prepare the document, but the document must be prepared before serious illness or injury occurs. Copies of the docu-

Durable Power of Attorney for Health Care Decisions (Cross out if you do not wish to use this section)

To effect my wishes, I designate ______________________________, residing at ____

(Phone #) ________________, (or if he or she shall for any reason fail to act, ____ (print name)
(Phone #) ________________, residing at ______________________)
as my health care surrogate—that is, my attorney-in-fact regarding any and all health care decisions to be made for me, including the decision to refuse life-sustaining treatment—if I am unable to make such decisions myself. This power shall remain effective during and not be affected by my subsequent illness, disability or incapacity. My surrogate shall have authority to interpret my Living Will, and shall make decisions about my health care as specified in my instructions or, when my wishes are not clear, as the surrogate believes to be in my best interests. I release and agree to hold harmless my health care surrogate from any and all claims whatsoever arising from decisions made in good faith in the exercise of this power.

I sign this document knowingly, voluntarily, and after careful deliberation, this ______ day of __________, 19____.

____
(signature)

Address ______________________
____

I do hereby certify that the within document was executed and acknowledged before me by the principal this ______ day of __________, 19____.

____
Notary Public

Witness ______________________
Printed Name ______________________
Address ______________________
____

Witness ______________________
Printed Name ______________________
Address ______________________
____

Copies of this document have been given to:

(Optional) My Living Will is registered with Concern for Dying (No.——) Distributed by Choice in Dying, 200 Varick Street, New York, NY 10014 (212)366–5540

Figure 3-2. (Continued)

ment then are given to the physician, to next of kin, and to others as appropriate. This directive may be rescinded or altered at any time. Only adults who are fully capable of reasoning can legally prepare such a document (Fig. 3-2).

Definition of Death

Defining death is both a legal and an ethical issue. The growing feasibility of organ transplants has promoted a definition that recognizes that death can occur before all bodily tissues are dead. Life-support devices raise serious ethical questions about the maintenance of lives that could not otherwise continue. When should life-support measures be removed? To answer these questions, many states have enacted laws defining death.

In 1968, a committee at Harvard Medical School examined the definition of "brain death." Although other groups have also examined this issue, the Harvard definition has become the basis for many legal statutes relating to brain death. This definition involves two types of evidence. The first is clinical signs. Three categories of clinical signs are to be examined. The first is "unreceptivity and unresponsivity," a condition in which the person shows no response of any kind to stimuli. The second clinical sign of brain death is "no movement or breathing." The movement must have been absent for at least an hour. There must be no spontaneous respirations for three full minutes after the respirator is turned off. The third category is the "absence of cephalic reflexes." A list of the specific reflexes to be checked is included in the Harvard definition.

The second type of evidence of brain death involves tests to be carried out. An electroencephalograph (EEG) recording obtained through use of standard procedures must show no brain activity for at least 30 minutes. Another test looks for blood flow in the brain; absence of blood flow in the brain indicating that the cortex of the brain is no longer functioning must be demonstrated by specific scanning techniques. The third type of test measures the oxygen consumed by the brain; if the brain is completely inactive it will use almost no oxygen. Use of this type of definition of death allows medical staff to plan for organ removal while the organs are still viable, but at the same time, protects the individual.

Nurse Practice Acts

Throughout the United States and in most other countries, there is a legal basis for nursing practice. Each United States state or Canadian provincial legislature has enacted an official statute called the **Nurse Practice Act**, which defines nursing, specifies educational standards, assigns the authority to regulate schools of nursing, governs who can practice nursing, and establishes a Board of Nursing.

Nurse practice acts have incorporated the important concept of accountability. Nurses must assume responsibility for their own actions when delivering care to clients. This means that nurses should know their reasonable scope of practice and should not extend their role into areas in which they are either unprepared or unsure. With the increasing shortage of nurses, accountability may become a major problem. Accountability is only one aspect of the movement to refine nurse practice acts to clarify standards of practice. Nursing students are equally accountable under the law and should never exceed their knowledge base, relying on the needed supervision of their instructors and staff when performing patient care. Because provisions of nurse practice acts vary among the states and provinces, you should carefully read the code for your area.

Definition of Nursing

In the eyes of the law, nursing entails a specific body of actions and expertise. The law also delineates specific areas of practice for nurses as compared with physicians. These are discussed in Chapter 2.

Boards of Nursing

Each state and province has an administrative body responsible for carrying out the provisions of the Nurse Practice Act. In the United States, it is usually the state Board of Nursing. In some states the Board of Nursing is part of a larger department that deals with all professional licensing. The responsibility of the Board of Nursing is to develop the specific regulations that will be used to implement the Nurse Practice Act. This responsibility includes overseeing nursing education, arranging for licensure examinations, licensing nurses who transfer from another legal jurisdiction, and revoking the licenses of nurses who do not maintain the standards set by the state. Information on the current *licensure law* in any given state may be obtained by writing directly to the state Board of Nursing. The addresses of the state boards are published in the January and August issues of the *American Journal of Nursing*, the official publication of the ANA.

The Boards of Nursing of all of the states and territories are organized into a National Council of State Boards of Nursing. This national group contracts with a testing agency to prepare and administer the National Council Licensing Examination for RNs (N-CLEX). This national group also serves as a forum for discussion of areas of common concern by representatives from the state boards.

Obtaining a Registered Nurse License

To obtain a license as a registered nurse, an individual must graduate from a nursing program approved by the state Board of Nursing and pass the N-CLEX. Nursing is fortunate to have a uniform licensing system throughout the entire United States. The same examination is given each year in every state on the same two dates, one in February and one in July. This may change when computerized testing services become available, which is projected to occur in the 1990s. Applicants using a computerized examination will answer only enough questions to indicate either success or failure. At this point, the testing procedure will stop. At present, each state accepts the score of 1600 as a passing grade on the examination. The pass/fail score is reported to the individual and to the program of nursing.

After initial licensure in one state, it is relatively easy to secure a license in another state, a process is called **licensure by endorsement** or **reciprocity**. Licensure by endorsement is granted on the basis of the candidate's initial educational program and original licensing examination. Some states also require evidence of having practiced nursing since the original licensure or evidence of continuing education. For the newcomer who has not met these requirements, states usually have established methods of meeting the standards.

Revoking a Nursing License

A license may not be renewed at the end of the licensing period if the nurse fails to send in the renewal request, pay the required fee, or complete whatever continuing education may be required by a particular state.

A license that is not renewed is considered lapsed. To obtain a license again, the individual would have to comply with the directions of the Board of Nursing.

When a license is revoked, it is removed for cause. The causes for which a nursing license may be revoked are defined by law. Conviction for a felony crime, evidence of obtaining and selling drugs, or actions that might have brought harm to a patient are examples of causes that are included in the law. To revoke a license, the Board of Nursing must hold a hearing, a legal proceeding in which formal testimony is heard. The nurse may have legal counsel and may appeal a decision by the board to a higher court.

Continuing Education

Some states have added provisions to their licensing laws requiring nurses to pursue continuing education as a prerequisite to renewing their licenses. This is called **mandatory continuing education**. Most leaders in health care believe that because of rapid change in health care and the resultant need for providers to expand their knowledge, continuing education is beneficial. The legal requirement has proven difficult and expensive to monitor, causing some states to discontinue this as a prerequisite to licensure renewal.

In states where continuing education is not mandatory, nurses are urged to pursue voluntary continuing education to keep their practice current. One need not enroll in a degree program to undertake continuing education. Courses are offered by colleges and universities, employers (*in-service* or *staff education*), and private agencies.

Personal Legal Responsibility

Nurses are always legally responsible for their own actions. This means that they can be held accountable by a court if actions they take do not meet the standards for the nursing profession. Although courts recognize that no one is without error and that mistakes do occur, a nurse causing a problem for a patient can be required to pay for care or provide a monetary settlement to offset the pain and difficulty experienced even if the error was inadvertent.

Preventing Legal Action

The best protection against legal action is providing the very best care of which you are capable. Remember again that, as a student nurse, you are held to the same level of responsibility as an RN. To practice safely, you must know your own abilities and limitations, you must seek assistance appropriately, and you must never move ahead independently into new areas without making sure that you have the necessary knowledge and skills (Fig. 3-3).

Expressing awareness of the patient as an individual and establishing good communication is another important aspect of preventing legal action. Legal action often springs from feelings of alienation and anger rather than from the actual facts of the situation. Listen to patients' concerns and express a caring attitude.

The maintenance of complete, clear, and accurate patient records is an important defense against any legal action. These records document the care provided and the problems encountered. Records you make can be helpful to the entire health care team and to the facility if legal action is brought. You will be learning to use patient records correctly as you progress in your nursing education.

A formal form called an incident report or quality assurance form is used by the institution to document safety and legal concerns. It has been recommended that a report should be completed when *any* unusual situation occurs with a patient, family, or visitor or between yourself and another staff member. This record of what happened may be helpful later if any legal or disciplinary action is proposed. These reports are filed by the hospital or agency but do not become part of the patient's record.

Professional Liability Insurance

Most registered nurses and student nurses find it highly desirable and prudent to carry professional **liability insurance**, which pays attorneys' fees, court costs, and any judgment ordered in a law suit. Such insurance is available through the ANA for its members, through the

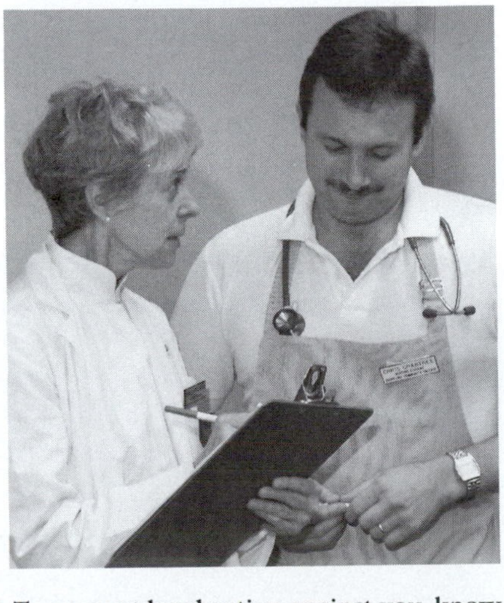

Figure 3-3. To prevent legal action against you, know your limitations as a student and seek assistance appropriately.

National Student Nurses' Association for its members, and from private insurance companies. Some schools of nursing carry group policies for their students. The cost of such insurance coverage is modest. Hospitals provide liability coverage for their employees and nursing staff in a variety of ways, but they do not commonly cover the practice of nursing students. It would be prudent for you to explore whether any coverage is available to you in the program in which you are enrolled or in the hospital in which you are receiving your clinical experience. You may want to consult your instructor regarding insurance so that you can purchase your own insurance plan, if necessary.

If you are buying your own liability insurance, be aware of the two types of coverage: claims-made and occurrence. A claims-made policy must be in effect on the date when you receive a notice of a lawsuit being filed. This means that if you have not kept up your policy by paying premiums and a suit is brought before the time of limitation has run out, you will not be covered. Occurrence policies cover you legally if, at the time of occurrence, you had paid your insurance premiums; then there is retroactive coverage. These are two important distinctions to consider.

Some insurance companies that provide malpractice insurance require different premiums from various areas of nursing practice that they claim have differing risks of liability. For example, a nurse in a physician's office may pay a premium below that of a nurse in critical care or a nurse practitioner.

Good Samaritan Laws

Almost every state and province has what is called a **Good Samaritan law**, which provides immunity to nurses and physicians who render care in an emergency situation outside the health care facility. The most common situation is that of assisting at the scene of an accident or natural disaster. The intent of this protective law is that care be rendered in a prudent and skillful manner but if the care is not successful, the care provider will not be held liable. In a few states, such as Vermont, it is considered contrary to the law *not* to render aid if one is trained to do so.

The Nurse as Witness

An expert witness, including a nurse, is an "individual willing to testify in court who by education and experience has acquired sufficient knowledge of a particular subject or activity—not within the ken or realm of an ordinary person" (Northrop and Kelly, 1987). An attorney in the proceedings requests the expert witness (nurse) to testify; the nurse is usually paid for the required time. It must be a personal choice whether to participate as such a witness. Some nurses practice as consultants to attorneys before trial and are also available as expert witnesses when the need arises. Usually, the expert nurse/witness is testifying as to what is prudent or customary within the profession. This role can be helpful to society and also personally rewarding, regardless of how stressful (Groff, 1985, p. 250).

On occasion, a nurse will be *subpoenaed* as a witness. A subpoenaed witness will be asked to testify regarding the specific facts of a particular case. The nurse who is subpoenaed must appear or risk a contempt citation. The nurse must be reminded that "one of the obligations or duties of a citizen is to aid the administration of justice and to appear in court" (Creighton, 1986, p. 184). When a nurse is witnessing on behalf of or against another nurse, the situation can become extremely sensitive.

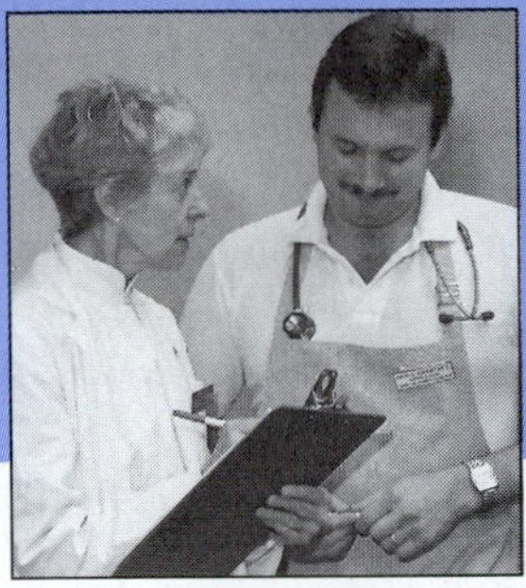

Key Points

- Ethical and legal concerns are an important part of becoming a nurse.
- The nurse is faced with many bioethical questions that require examination and reexamination of personal moral beliefs.
- To provide guidance on ethical matters, specific groups and organizations have developed codes to help nurses and other health care professionals in making their decisions.
- Legal aspects of nursing practice are governed by statutory law, that is, law enacted formally by a legislative body, and common law, that is, law based on precedent or common practice.
- Malpractice involves caring for persons in such a way as to cause harm. This is an issue that affects all those working in the health care setting.
- Other legal issues that affect health care workers are assault and battery, false imprisonment, narcotics control, libel and slander, and invasion of privacy.
- End of life issues deal with such matters as the establishment of a legal definition of death and advance directives to protect patients from inappropriate resuscitative measures when meaningful survival is not possible.
- The law defines nursing as a specific body of actions and expertise and empowers Boards of Nursing to mandate policy.
- Licensure is obtained through accredited education and the demonstration of proficiency by an examination. Continuing education, whether related to licensure or voluntary, is an important professional responsibility.

Study Questions

1. What are three reasons for using the law to uphold ethical behavior?
2. What is the function of Boards of Nursing? How do they help the patient/client?
3. Give an example from nursing practice of a problem that would fall under the jurisdiction of common law and one that would fall under the jurisdiction of statutory law.
4. How do consumer's rights protect the patient/client?
5. What legal problems could arise from assisting a patient to a shower?
6. What is the difference between claims-made and occurrence malpractice insurance?
7. Discuss the advantages and disadvantages of participating in a liability insurance program, both as a student and as a staff nurse.
8. What information is requested on an incident form from your facility?
9. What is the policy of your clinical facility regarding access to patient records? Who has access to current records; to records from previous hospitalizations?
10. How has your facility responded to the Patient Self-Determination Act?

Critical Thinking Activities

1. Suppose a patient told you something in confidence that, for safety reasons, must be divulged. Give the rationale for revealing the information based on a teleologic and a deontologic approach.
2. Explain why you think it is important to have a code for nurses and identify two parts of the code that directly affect the way you care for patients.
3. After examining the policy manual of your facility, identify three sections pertaining to ethics. Share these with those in a small group, giving the rationale for including these sections.
4. Bring to class one current article from a non-professional periodical or newspaper on an ethical issue in health care. Analyze the issue and identify any ethical issues that are in conflict.
5. Keep a brief journal of your clinical experience for a week, relating the thoughts you have concerning ethical issues. Share it with your instructor only if you so choose.
6. Compare the American Hospital Association's Patient's Bill of Rights with the Health Consumer Bill of Rights.
7. Evaluate the various policies of malpractice insurance available to students and staff nurses.
8. Obtain a copy of your state's Nurse Practice Act from the library. Compare and contrast the definition of nursing with that used in your program of nursing.

References and Readings

American Nurses Association Committee on Ethics. "Withdrawing or Withholding Food and Fluid." *American Journal of Nursing* 88, 6 (June 1988): 797–805.

Anderson, B. J., Ayers, N., and Harvey, A. B. "Serving Justice: Giving a Deposition." *American Journal of Nursing* 91, 3 (March 1991): 32–35.

Barritt, E. R. "Florence Nightingale's Values and Modern Nursing Education." *Nursing Forum* 12, 1 (January 1973): 6–47.

Bell, T. "The Right to Know. . .detained patients. . .informed of Their Rights." *Nursing Times* 87, 27 (July 1991): 3–9.

Bergerson, S. R. "Charting with a Jury in Mind." *Nursing '88* 18, 4 (April 1988): 51–56.

Betta, P. A. "Documenting to Stay Out of the Courtroom." *Imprint* 38, 2 (April-May 1991): 39–40.

Black's Law Dictionary. 5th edition. St. Paul: West Publishers, 1983.

"Blowing the Whistle on Incompetence." Anonymous. *Nursing '89,* 19, 7 (July 1989): 47–50.

Cahill, J. (Ed.). *Nurse's Handbook of Law and Ethics.* Springhouse, PA: Springhouse Corp., 1992.

Calfee, B. E. "Protecting Yourself from Allegations of Nursing Negligence." *Nursing '91* 21, 12 (December 1991): 34–37.

Chervenak, F. A., and McCullough, L. B. "Justified Limits on Refusing Intervention." *Hastings Center Report* 21, 2 (March-April 1991): 12–17.

Creighton, H. *Law Every Nurse Should Know.* 5th edition. Philadelphia: W. B. Saunders, 1986.

Cushing, M. "How a Suit Starts." *American Journal of Nursing* 85, 6 (June 1985): 55–56.

———. "Demystifying Informed Consent." *American Journal of Nursing* 84, 4 (April 1984): 437–438.

Daly, B. J. "Development of a Special Care Unit for Chronically Critically Ill Patients." *Heart and Lung: Journal of Critical Care* 20, 1 (January 1991): 45–51.

dePender, W., and Ikeda-Chandler, W. *Clinical Ethics: An Invitation to Helping Professionals.* New York: Praeger Publishers, 1990.

Donovan, N. M. "Confidentiality vs. Duty to Warn." *Nursing and Health Care* 12, 8 (August 1991): 432–436.

Dunning, S. E. "Caught in the Cross Fire." Nursing '92. 22, 11 (November 1992): 49–51.

Elliott, C. "Where Ethics comes from and What to Do About It" *Hastings Center Report.* 22, 4 (July–August 1992): 28–35.

Ellis, J. R., and Hartley, C. L. *Nursing in Today's World: Challenges, Issues, and Trends.* 4th edition. Philadelphia: J. B. Lippincott, 1992.

Fleetwood, J. "Solving Bioethical Dilemmas: A Practical Approach." *Nursing '89* 19, 3 (March 1989): 62–64.

Fowler, M. D. M., and Levine-Ariff, J. *Ethics at the Bedside.* Philadelphia: J. B. Lippincott, 1987.

Freitas, L. "Historical Roots and Future Perspectives Related to Nursing Ethics." *Journal of Professional Nursing* 6, 4 (July-August 1990): 197–205.

Gilbert, D. A. "The Ethics of Mandatory Elder Abuse Reporting Statutes." *Advances in Nursing Science* 8, 2 (January 1986): 51.

Goldsmith, M. "Costs in Dollars and Lives Continue to Rise." *Journal of the American Medical Association* 266 (August 28, 1991): 1055–1057.

Grant, A. B. "Exploring an Ethical Dilemma." *Nursing '92.* 22, 12 (December 1992): 52–54.

Groff, B. "Anatomy of a Malpractice Trial." *American Journal of Nursing* 85, 3 (March 1985): 248–250.

Horner, J., and Miehl, J. L. "The Deontological Decision-Making Model as a Bioethical Tool." *Journal of Association of Operating Room Nurses* 54, 2 (August 1991): 208–209.

Johnson, L. G. "Preparing for a Deposition." *Nursing '90* 20, 7 (July 1990): 44–47.

Kelly, M. "The Omnibus Budget Reconciliation Act of 1987: A Policy Analysis." *Nursing Clinics of North America* 24, 3 (September 1989): 791–794.

Kimsey, L. R., Tarbox, A. R., and Bragg, D. F. "Abuse of the Elderly: The Hidden Agenda." *Journal of the American Geriatric Society* (October 29, 1981): 465–472.

Klop, R., van Wijmen, F. C. B., and Philipsen, H. "Patients' Rights and the Admission and Discharge Process." *Journal of Advanced Nursing* 16, 4 (April 1991): 408–412.

Light, K., and Connelly, R. "Is the ANA Guilty of Paternalism in Its Guidelines on Withdrawing or Withholding Food and Fluid?" *Nursing Forum* 24 (March-April 1989): 19–23.

Mandell, M. "Practical Ways to Survive a Law Suit." *Nursing '92* 22, 8 (August 1992): 56–57.

Miedema, F. "A Practical Approach to Ethical Decisions." *American Journal of Nursing* 91, 12 (December 1991): 20–25.

Mitchell, M. K. "Perspectives in Nursing 1989–1991. Lifting the Veil of Secrecy. . .the Consumer has a Right to Information." NLN Publication 1990 #41-2281, 155–158.

Munson, R. *Intervention and Reflection: Basic Issues in Medical Ethics.* 3rd edition. Belmont, Cal.: Wadsworth Publishing, 1988.

Nagy, M. "The OBRA Regulations: Their Impact upon Nursing Practice." *Chart* 87, 3 (March 1990): 4.

Nelson, J. L. "Taking Families Seriously." *Hastings Center Report.* 22, 4 (July–August 1992): 6–12.

Northrop, C. E. "How Good Samaritan Laws do—and don't—Protect You." *Nursing '90* 20, 2 (February 1990): 50–51.

Northrop, C. E., and Kelly, M. E. *Legal Issues in Nursing.* St. Louis: C. V. Mosby, 1987.

"OBRA Message is Clear: Quality or Bust. . .Omnibus Budget Reconciliation Act." *Nursing and Health Care* 9, 3 (March 1988): 123–124.

Omery, A. "The New Patient Self-Determination Act: Increasing Emphasis on Patient Autonomy." *Dimensions of Critical Care Nursing* 10, 3 (May-June 1991): 123–125.

Paridy, N. E. "New Act Makes Directives Part of Hospital Policy." *Health Care Strategic Management* 10, 3 (May 1991): 13–15.

Partridge, K. B. "Nursing Values in a Changing Society." *Nursing Outlook* 26 (June 1978): 356–360.

Rabb, J. D. "Implications of Moral and Ethical Issues for Nurses." *Nursing Forum* 15, 2 (February 1976): 168–179.

Report of the Ad Hoc Committee of the Harvard Medical School to Examine the Definition of Brain Death. A Definition of Irreversible Coma. *Journal of the American Medical Association* 205, 6 (August 1968): 85–86.

Robinow, J. "Where You Stand in the Eyes of the Law." *Nursing '89* 19, 2 (February 1989): 34–42.

Salladay, S. A., and McDonnell, M. M. "Facing Ethical Conflicts." *Nursing '92* 22, 2 (February 1992): 44–47.

Schwarz, J. K. "Living Wills and Health Care Proxies: Nurse Practice Implications." *Nursing and Health Care* 13, 2 (February 1992): 92–96.

Sisney, K. F. "The Relationship Between Social Support and Depression in Recovering Chemically Dependent Nurses." *Image* 25, 2 (Summer b1993): 107–112.

Stepp, J. "OBRA Provides Guidelines for Quality Assurance Programs." *Provider* 16, 3 (March 1990): 34.

Sweeney, M. L. "Your Role in Informed Consent." *RN* 54, 8 (August 1991): 55–60.

Trinkoff, A. M., Eaton, W. W., and Anthony, J. C. "The Prevalence of Substance Abuse Among Registered Nurses." *Nursing Research*. 40, 3 (May–June 1991): 172–175.

Weeks, L. C., Gleason, R., and Reiser, S. "How Can a Hospital Ethics Committee Help?" 89, 5 *American Journal of Nursing* (May 1989): 651–654.

Wilson, D. M. "Ethical Concerns in a Long-Term Tube Feeding Study." *Image* 24, 3 (Fall 1992): 195–199.

Wright, R. *Human Values in Health Care: The Practice of Ethics.* New York: McGraw-Hill, 1987.

Health and Illness

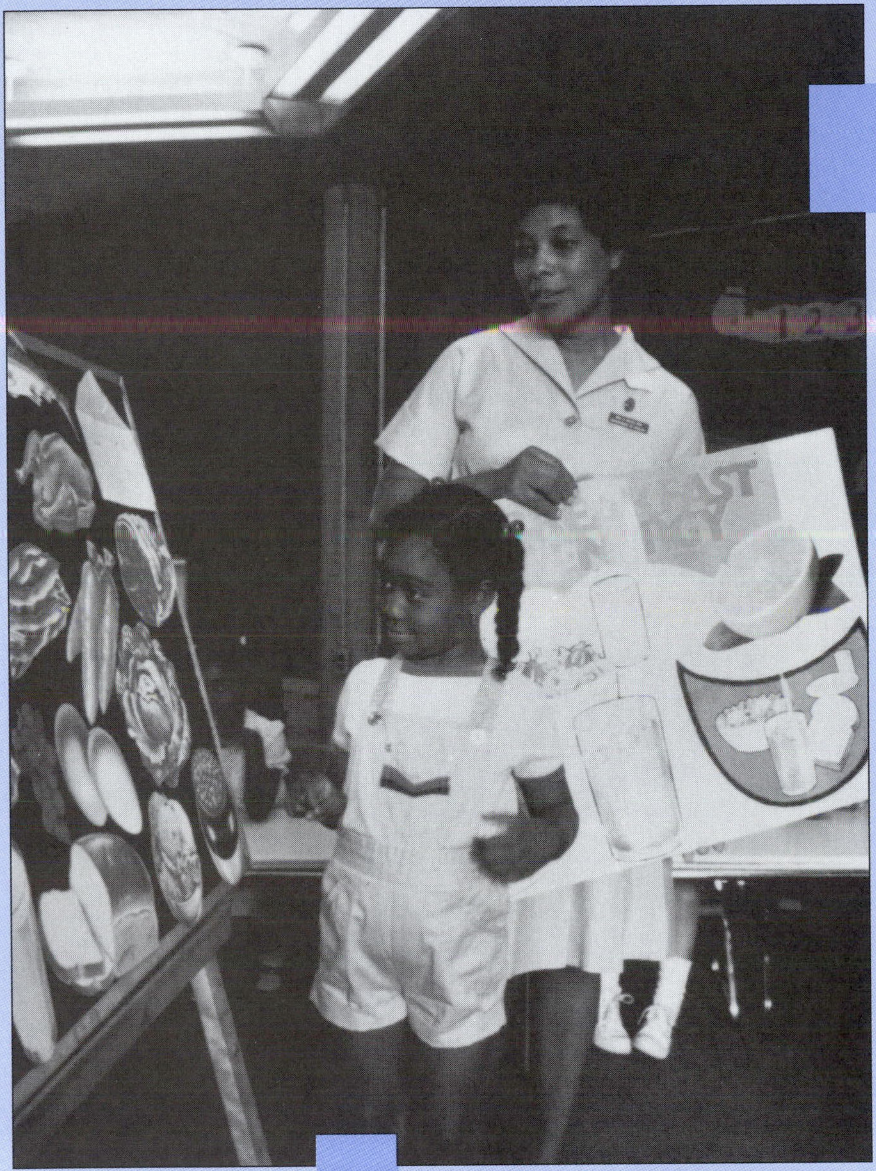

II

Homeostasis

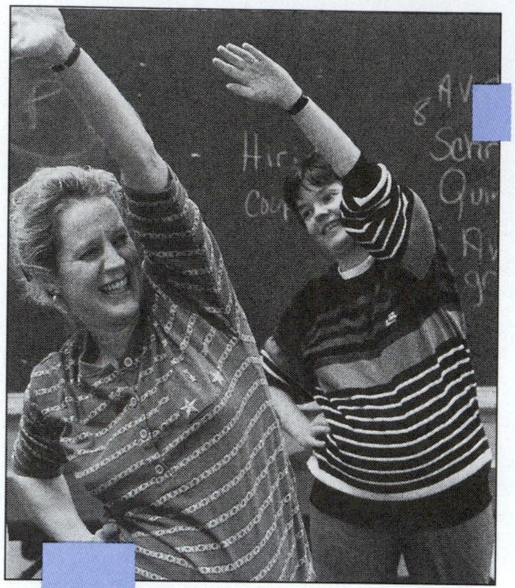

4

Objectives

After completing this chapter, you should be able to:

1. Compare the definitions of homeostasis and homeodynamics.
2. Discuss these concepts as they relate to nursing care.
3. Define an adaptive force.
4. Describe several internal and external physiologic and psychological adaptive forces.
5. Explain how the nurse can serve as an adaptive force.

Study Terms

adaptive force
autonomic nervous system
conduction
convection
endocrine system
equilibrium
evaporation
heat loss
holistic nursing
homeodynamics
kinesis
neuroendocrine system
parasympathetic system
physiologic homeostasis
psychological homeostasis
radiation
stressor
sympathetic system

Outline

Ellis, Nowlis: NURSING: A HUMAN NEEDS APPROACH, 5th ed. © 1994 J.B. Lippincott Company

W. B. Cannon, an endocrinologist, coined the term homeostasis in 1926 to describe the ability of primarily physiologic processes of the body to maintain a steady state. More recently, the term has been applied to psychological processes as well. For our purposes, **homeostasis** is the tendency of all living tissue to restore and maintain itself in a condition of balance or **equilibrium**.

In *Nature and Human Nature*, Frank (1951) speaks of homeostasis as an orchestra, each organ sensitively responding to the rest to create stability. "The internal environment is like the external environment—it is continually changing, maintaining a dynamic equilibrium by larger or smaller fluctuations and sometimes by violent alterations as it continues to oscillate between the limits of living existence."

As time passed, researchers and writers attended more and more to the high level of bodily energy and activity required to maintain a steady state. Langley (1965) focused primarily on the bodily systems and the intricate interactions among them necessary to maintain homeostasis and thus maintain equilibrium. Dubos (1965), building on Cannon's earlier work, emphasized the ability to adapt to an ever-changing internal and external environment as the key to survival for human beings. Although the word homeostasis may appear to imply stillness, homeostasis is actually a dynamic state of balance maintained by the body's constant shifting and adaptation to threat.

To better reflect the quality of change and energy of the process, the word **homeodynamics** came into use. Rogers (1970) preferred this newer term and expanded its definition to include five important concepts.

1. Human beings are *holistic*, each part influencing the whole. (This premise is the one on which holistic health is founded; it is discussed in Chapter 7.)
2. As human beings, we are constantly interacting with those around us and with the environment in which we live.
3. Underlying this interaction is a natural *life continuum* (see Chapter 17); it is sequential and cannot be reversed. This is the recognition of the progression of life as we know it.
4. Because of the internal processes and external interaction, human beings undergo many changes that cause reorganization and integration.
5. The reorganization and integration are by no means solely physical. Human beings have the innate capacity for imagination, abstract thought, and appreciation of beauty, and the sentiment to love and care for each other.

The shift in perspective from the more specific, physiologic definition of homeostasis to the more inclusive one of homeodynamics appears to fit much more clearly the philosophy of nursing. We will use the term homeostasis in this text, however, with the understanding that it applies to both physiologic and psychological equilibrium.

Physiologic Homeostasis

The body's capacity to regulate internal processes so that the vital functions of respiration, circulation, and metabolism are maintained in a relative state of balance is termed **physiologic homeostasis**. For example, changes in heart rate, blood pressure, body pressure, body temperature, fluid and electrolyte balance, blood glucose concentration, and blood oxygen level are all measurable indicators of the body's ability to adapt to changing conditions both internally from disease or externally from the environment. Adaptation to changing needs is vital to organism survival, and homeostatic control is the body's means of adapting to those needs.

Although the cardiovascular, renal, respiratory, gastrointestinal, and musculoskeletal systems are all important in maintaining homeostasis, it is the complex interactions of the brain and the nervous and endocrine systems, commonly called the **neuroendocrine system**, that form the basis for homeostatic control. Neuroendocrine response consists of the activities of the autonomic nervous system and the endocrine systems. The main mechanism by which they are able to achieve their interrelated functions is feedback control, the process by which the chemical product of one system has a stimulatory or inhibitory effect on another system. The self-regulatory nature of these mechanisms is a feature of vital importance to the organism in terms of the body's ability to monitor itself at all times, even during sleep. The regulatory activities of the nervous system generally are more rapid in nature, whereas those of the endocrine system are mainly those of the slower-acting hormones.

Autonomic Nervous System

The **autonomic nervous system** is the part of the nervous system that controls smooth muscles not under voluntary control, such as the heart. Without our conscious control, it provides homeostatic regulation of other smooth muscles such as those of the blood vessels and digestive tract. It is subdivided into the parasympathetic system and the sympathetic system. The **parasympathetic system** provides a steady state during normal conditions and the resting state and is involved in the ongoing processes of digestion and elimination. Maintenance of normal heart rate and blood pressure, secretion of digestive enzymes, and peristaltic motion are examples of responses of the parasympathetic system. The **sympathetic system** comes into play during a state of emergency when the body must respond quickly. Its purpose during such times is to provide the body with the ability to expend a quick burst of energy—a fight-or-flight response. Such responses as increased heartbeat, blood glucose level, and increased mental alertness are examples of sympathetic responses. The functions of the sympathetic and parasympathetic systems are complementary, the effects of one opposing the effects of the other.

Two parts of the brain that play an active role in the functioning of the autonomic nervous system are the medulla oblongata and the hypothalamus, whose functions are discussed below.

The *medulla oblongata*, the lower portion of the brain stem, is continuous with the spinal cord. In addition to housing the nerve centers for both motor and sensory nerves, it is the control center for heart rate, blood pressure, and respiration. It responds to signals from the sympathetic and parasympathetic nervous system in the regulation of these vital functions. A network of cells called the reticular formation within this area of the brain monitors physiologic status through its connections with the sensory and motor pathways and the level of central nervous system activity, that is, wakefulness, attentiveness, and sleep.

The *hypothalamus*, located at the base of the brain, has various regulatory functions, including general regulation of water balance, body temperature, sleep, thirst, and hunger, as well as the development of secondary sex characteristics.

Endocrine System

The **endocrine system** is a regulatory system that maintains homeostasis by producing *hormones* that act as couriers, linking one body system to another (Fig. 4-1). We are holistic persons in large part because of the interrelationships among these essential organs.

The glands of the endocrine system are scattered throughout the body. The various glands secrete hormones directly into the blood to maintain the balance necessary to preserve or to attempt to correct imbalances in homeostasis. Making up this system are the pancreas, gonads, adrenals, pituitary, thyroid, parathyroid, and thymus. Together, they regulate the other systems of the body that have both physiologic and psychological functions. Because you will be studying this complex system in more detail in later courses, we will discuss its important role in regulation only in general terms.

Together, the glands of the endocrine system affect the various stages in physical, intellectual, and emotional growth, including the onset of puberty (see Chapters 17–20). Reproduction is also regulated by the hormones of the endocrine system, and your experiences in maternal and family nursing will help you further in understanding their effects in this area. Metabolism and

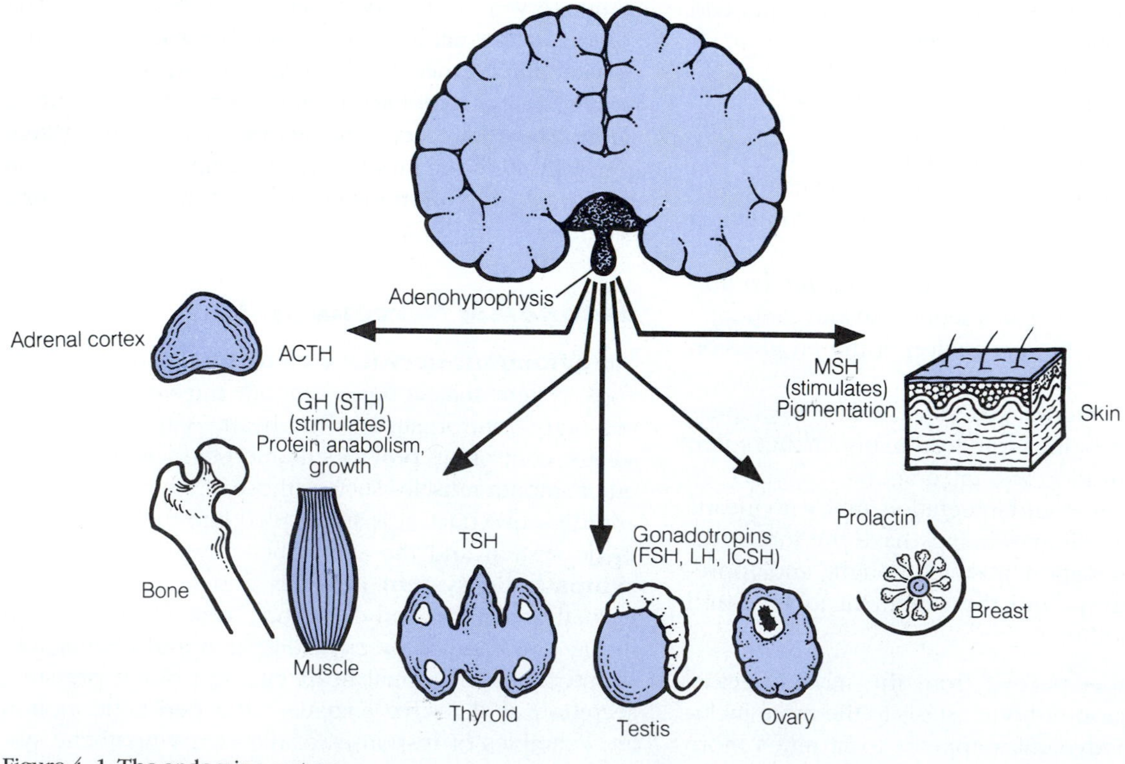

Figure 4-1. The endocrine system.

regulation of the vital systems of the body are also controlled through endocrine processes.

Regulation by the Neuroendocrine System: Body Temperature

Although the nervous system regulates respiration and heart action as well as body temperature, in this chapter we focus on regulation of body temperature. Because of the complexity of the processes involved in regulation of respiration and heart action, these subjects are presented in separate chapters.

Body temperature is systemically controlled by a small structure within the anterior portion of the brain called the hypothalamus. In a way, the hypothalamus is the thermostat of the body. It receives sensory input and responds with alterations that protect the body from changes occurring in the external environment and within the body due to illness. Through this mechanism, the hypothalamus attempts to balance heat production and heat loss.

Heat is produced by metabolism and is therefore a by-product of all activities and processes within the body. The specific dynamic action of foods is the energy expended in the process of digestion and absorption. Because heat is always produced in this process, eating can produce an almost immediate increase in feelings of warmth. Muscular activity also produces considerable heat. Shivering is an involuntary muscular activity that has the effect of increasing the body temperature. Infections and inflammations increase tissue metabolism and thus increase tissue heat.

Heat loss occurs through four processes: radiation, conduction, convection, and evaporation. **Radiation**, the loss of heat to another object without contact, occurs constantly. **Conduction** is loss of heat through direct contact with another object. **Convection** is heat transfer caused by moving air, which carries heat away from the body surface to be replaced by cooler air. **Evaporation** also has a cooling effect because the conversion of liquid to a gas requires heat energy. Evaporation of moisture occurs constantly from the surface cells and more extensively through the secretion of perspiration from glands beneath the skin.

Heat loss is increased by the dilation of peripheral vessels, which transfer heat from the body core to the surface, where heat loss can occur more readily. Increased perspiration also hastens heat loss by providing for more evaporation. The process of heat loss can be enhanced by using fans or a breeze to increase convection or by applying moisture to the body to bring about evaporative cooling. An automatic cooling blanket increases conduction of heat from the body by circulating cool water through tubing within the blanket. Such a blanket is usually equipped with a rectal thermometer and a means of regulating the temperature of the blanket.

Heat loss is minimized by the contraction of muscles in the hair follicles, causing "goose pimples," which in turn raise hairs on the body surface to provide an insulating layer and decrease convection. This process is most effective in individuals with large amounts of body hair. Vasoconstriction of the body surface decreases all forms of heat loss and preserves the heat of the body core.

The human body's temperature must be maintained within narrow limits for the optimal functioning of its various physiologic processes. The normal temperature range is only 97°F (36.1°C) to 100.4°F (38°C). The "normal" body temperature is considered to be 98.6°F (37°C) when measured orally. Axillary temperature (temperature measured under the arm) is normally 1°F (0.6°C) lower, and rectal temperature is 1°F (0.6°C) higher than oral measurement. Some researchers believe, however, that imprecise measuring techniques account for these differences.

Because it is subject to a 24-hour cycle called its *circadian rhythm*, body temperature is highest from 4:00 to 8:00 PM and lowest in the early hours of the morning. Women also experience a temperature change associated with the menstrual cycle: the body temperature increases 0.5 to 1°F at the time of ovulation and decreases again at the time of menstruation.

Nursing Research: *Implications for Practice*

Caruso, C.C. and Hadley, B.J. and Shuka, R. and Frame, P. and Khoury, J. "Cooling Effects and Comfort of Four Cooling Blanket Temperatures in Humans with Fever." *Nursing Research.* 41,2 (March–April): 68–72.

Eighty-nine persons with fever were randomly assigned, with physician approval, to one of four cooling blanket temperatures. The subjects were evenly distributed as to sex, race, cause of fever, and initial body temperature. The subjects were monitored throughout and after the procedure. Body temperature was reduced by all four cooling blanket settings. Significantly, patients were more comfortable and shivered less at warmer temperatures.

Normal temperatures vary among individuals. Elderly persons often have relatively low normal temperatures, probably a function of their slower metabolisms. Normal temperatures in infants and young children may be a full degree higher than those in adults. For this reason, a single temperature reading provides only general information unless it is considered along with other data on the patient.

Adverse conditions such as extremely hot or cold weather and the body's own immune response can cause life-threatening conditions such as hypothermia and fever. These topics are discussed in greater depth in Chapter 21.

Psychological Homeostasis

Psychological homeostasis can be defined as a state of mental well-being. This implies the ability of the human being to maintain a state of equilibrium in the face of the stressors experienced by the individual from day to day, an adaptability to circumstances. To maintain or reestablish a state of mental well-being, an individual's basic psychological needs must be met, needs such as those for love and belonging, which are discussed in Chapter 5 as they relate to nursing. It is stressors that interfere with a person's ability to meet needs and as a consequence threaten homeostasis. Chapter 6 discusses how stressors affect physical and psychological homeostasis in both positive and negative ways.

Adaptive Forces

Key to the notion of homeostasis is the influence of adaptive forces. As can be seen in Chapter 5, many nursing theories involve adaptation. For our purposes, an **adaptive force** is any force, internal or external, that tends to maintain or restore physiologic or psychological homeostasis.

Those forces that are adaptive, however, can become stressors. A **stressor** is any stimulus or agent that poses a real or perceived threat to the person. For example, a medication meant to be an adaptive force can cause an allergic reaction and cause the body to be out of homeostatic balance.

Internal Adaptive Forces

Internal adaptive forces are sometimes referred to as compensatory mechanisms, that is, physical or psychological mechanisms capable of causing shifts toward greater homeostatic balance.

Vital signs are one reflection of the internal physiologic adaptive process. For example, when body temperature is elevated, respiratory rate increases in an effort to ventilate and cool the body. Body fluids and chemical balance in the blood can similarly undergo alterations to compensate for disturbances. The senses also perform as adaptive forces. For instance, sightless people develop heightened senses of hearing and **kinesis** (awareness of one's body in relation to space). Virtually all body tissues possess some capacity to help correct imbalance in another organ or body part.

Many internal adaptive forces are psychological in nature. Some are coping mechanisms, such as the ability to reason and solve problems. For example, a young man paralyzed in an accident may return to school where he can acquire not only knowledge but also increase his self-esteem, self-confidence, and a degree of self-actualization. Mental ability thus compensates in a healthy manner for physical disability.

Various psychological *defense mechanisms* are internal adaptive forces—some more functional than others—that people use to protect themselves from feelings of shame or anxiety or loss of self-esteem. These are used in daily life in response to the external environment as a way of coping. Two examples with which you may be familiar are denial and rationalization. Defense mechanisms are considered in detail in Chapter 6.

External Adaptive Forces

External adaptive forces can also be both physiologic and psychological. Food, water, oxygen, and medications are examples of external physiologic adaptive forces. Giving aspirin to a patient with an elevated temperature is an application of an external physiologic force. Meanwhile, the patient's internal physiologic adaptive forces, such as increased respiratory rate and perspiration, are helping to lower body temperature. Providing a safe and therapeutic environment for the patient also involves the application or use of adaptive forces, such as control of room temperature, lighting, sounds, and odors. A call light placed within reach of the immobilized patient is a crucial external adaptive force. An example of a primarily psychological external adaptive force is a caring person who sits quietly and listens to the patient. Groups that provide a safe environment for belonging and personal growth may in themselves be an adaptive force. These may be religious or neighborhood groups. Therapy and counseling programs also belong to this category. Norman Cousins (1980) said that Dr. Albert Schweitzer explained the success of an African witch doctor this way: "The witch doctor succeeds for the same reason all the rest of us succeed. Each patient carries his own doctor inside him . . . . We are at our best when we give the doctor who resides within each patient a chance to work."

The Nurse as an Adaptive Force

An adaptive force tends to maintain or restore homeostasis. Clearly, nursing care is the application of adaptive forces to promote the patient's recovery. For example, nurses bathe the patient to combat bacteria, administer drugs to bring about a variety of bodily changes, hydrate the patient to prevent fluid loss, teach health measures to the patient to prevent further illness, and communicate with the patient to offset stress and loneliness. In addition, nurses can become adaptive forces by their own approaches to patients.

The nurse as an adaptive force is a role that carries with it both satisfaction and responsibilities. It is a role that is honored, trusted, and genuine. Nurses are enablers, empowering persons to live their lives focused toward health. When illness does arise, the adaptive force of the nurse is altered to aid the individual in regaining health or moving to a peaceful death.

Homeostasis and Nursing

We have emphasized the basic concept of homeostasis not just because of its physiologic importance but also because it encompasses an important theoretical concept of health. Homeostasis and health are integral to nursing, and each chapter on nursing care incorporates both concepts.

Cannon and Frank focused on the way the organs and structures in the body interact continually to maintain homeostasis. The anatomy and physiology of homeostasis in this context is that of the body's organs and internal structure. As we move through the text, the anatomy and physiology aspects of each system will be outlined so that you will understand more clearly how that system fits into human homeostatic activity.

We can use the Cannon–Frank definition of homeostasis to describe one aspect of your role as a nurse. As a nurse, you will formulate health care plans that maximize the functioning of organs in the various bodily systems. When problems arise, your nursing actions will assist the patient in correcting those problems. For example, if the person is having difficulty breathing because pneumonia has affected the lungs, you might put the head of the bed in a higher position or give the oxygen that has been ordered. Your knowledge of homeostasis as it involves the organs of the body will allow you to help patients regain a physiologic state of relative homeostasis.

Another aspect of nursing can best be described by going back to the description of homeodynamics. The idea that human beings are holistic is basic to nursing and provides the conceptual framework for many nursing programs. In **holistic nursing**, nurses view patients as total persons, with physiologic, psychosocial, and spiritual traits, needs, and problems. Because human beings interact with those around them and with the environment, nurses must consider the patient's family and home when giving care, recognizing that the patient is part of a family or community. Nurses' perspectives are enhanced by the fact that nurses are witnesses to all aspects of the natural life continuum. They are present at the wondrous moment of birth and the mystical moment of death. They care daily for patients with differing levels of homeostasis and at different stages of the life span. What nurses see is that individuals, throughout

Nursing Issues and Trends: *Learning Techniques to Maintain Homeostasis from Other Cultures*

Humans have attempted to use a variety of methods throughout history to maintain homeostasis. Herbs, meditation, and religion have all played a large part in some areas of the world. Traditional medicine as practiced in the West has also attempted to attain a balance of the external and internal environments. Global communication has more recently portrayed the benefits of the ancient Oriental practice of "tai chi" as an effective means of achieving physical and emotional homeostasis. Tai chi involves performing rhythmic body movements. The purpose is to position the person in a posture of physical and mental accord or balance which is believed to ensure homeostasis. Even the young and the very old may engage in tai chi. The relaxed faces and graceful movements of tai chi are testament to the value of this exercise. Care providers should develop appreciation for the contributions of a variety of nontraditional means of maintaining homeostasis.

life, undergo many changes for which adjustments must be made. Applying this concept, nurses can encourage and assist patients in integrating the changes so often caused by illness so that functioning can continue. This integration and growth that results are all part of homeodynamics. Being part of that process gives nurses the opportunity to create hope as well as provide care, both of which are needed for balanced lives.

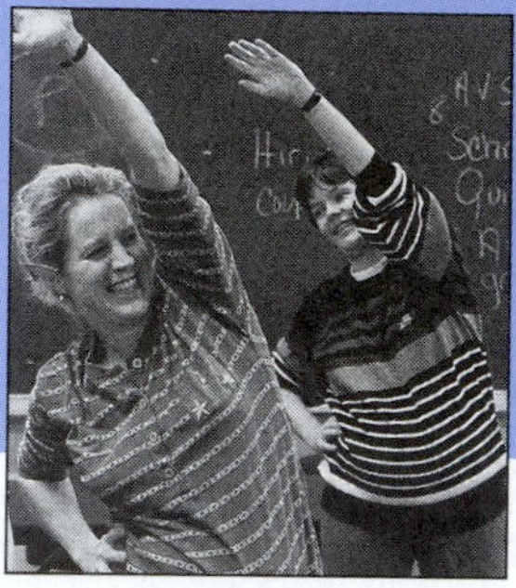

Key Points

- Homeostasis is a basic concept in nursing. It refers to the interplay of the various bodily systems, as well as the continual interaction among the individual, other people, and the physical environment.
- The term homeodynamics is preferred by Rogers and others because it more clearly reflects the description given for homeostasis and because it can be used to provide holistic care.
- Internal and external adaptive forces help to maintain or restore homeostasis. The nurse serves as an adaptive force for patients by providing care that answers needs and helps to maintain homeostasis.

Study Questions

1. How does homeostasis relate to health?
2. How do the body systems interact with one another to maintain homeostasis?
3. What are some internal adaptive forces?
4. Name some external adaptive forces.
5. What are some major ways a nurse can serve as an adaptive force?

Critical Thinking Activities

1. Analyze your own current health status in relation to the maintenance of homeostasis.
2. Select a patient for whom you have been caring and analyze the patient's status as it relates to homeostasis.
3. Using your knowledge of anatomy and physiology, explain the response of the respiratory system to maintain homeostasis with levels of increased activity.
4. Give the rationale for actions the nurse can take as an adaptive force to minimize the effects of social isolation for the elderly patient.

References and Readings

Beecher, H. K. "The Powerful Placebo." *Journal of the American Medical Association* 159 24 (December 1955): 1602–1606.

Cannon, W. B. "Some General Features of Endocrine Influence on Metabolism." *American Journal of Medical Science* 171 (1926): 1–20.

Cousins, N. *Anatomy of an Illness.* New York: W. W. Norton, 1980.

Dubos, R. *Man Adapting.* New Haven: Yale University Press, 1965.

Evans, P. J. "Thinking of Maslow." *Nursing Times* 76 (January 24, 1980): 163–165.

Frank, L. K. *Nature and Human Nature.* New Brunswick, N.J.: Rutgers University Press, 1951.

Guyton, A. C. *Human Physiology and Mechanisms of Disease.* 5th edition. Philadelphia: W. B. Saunders, 1992.

Langley, L. L. *Homeostasis.* New York: Reinhold Book Corporation, 1965.

Munson, R. *Intervention and Reflection: Basic Issues in Medical Ethics.* 3rd edition. Belmont, Cal.: Wadsworth, 1988.

Rogers, M. E. *An Introduction to the Theoretical Base of Nursing.* Philadelphia: F. A. Davis, 1970.

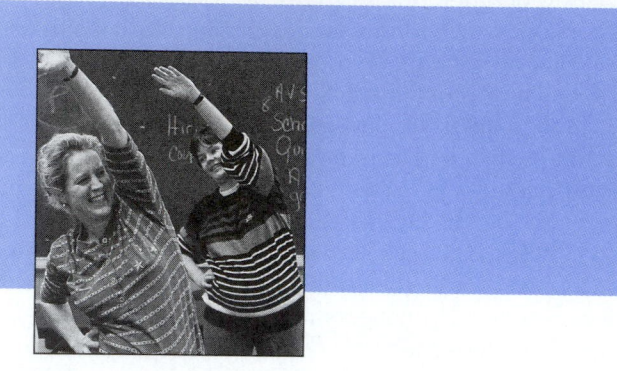

Human Needs

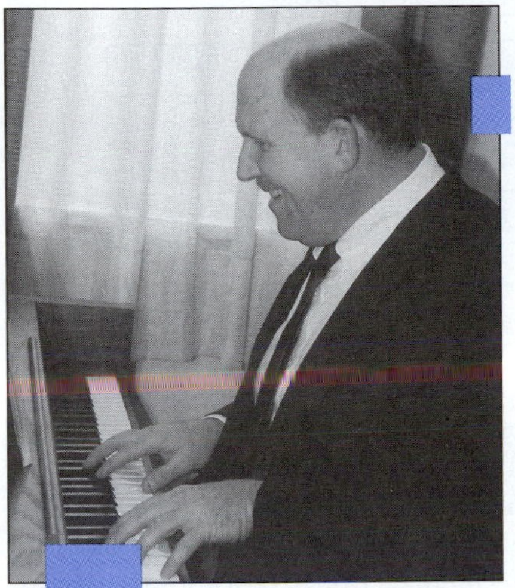

5

Objectives

After completing this chapter, you should be able to:

1. List, in ascending order, Maslow's hierarchy of needs.
2. Explain how Maslow's hierarchy of needs guides the setting of priorities in nursing care.
3. Discuss the importance of the human needs concept to theories of nursing.
4. Define a human need.
5. Discuss why safety needs are so important for the individual.
6. Name and discuss some of the physiologic and psychological needs of the individual.
7. Distinguish between a need, a deficit, and a problem.
8. List some of nurses' particular needs.

Study Terms

deficit
hierarchy of needs
life span
need
physiologic needs
problem
psychosocial needs
self-actualization

Outline

Ellis, Nowlis: Nursing: A Human Needs Approach, 5th ed. © 1994 J.B. Lippincott Company

Recognizing the holistic nature of the human being, we have now expanded the concept of homeostasis to include the psychological, social, and spiritual needs. A theory of human needs developed by Maslow (1943) remains important to us as nurses, even though some limitations are apparent when the theory is applied to the nursing role. First, let us look at the work of Maslow and then explore some of the conceptual models of nursing that were presented in Chapter 1, with an emphasis on the belief of each regarding human needs. For our purposes, we will consider the work of Rogers (1970), Peplau (1952), Johnson (1968), Orem (1971), Roy (1984), Neuman (1982), and Henderson (1966). In so doing, we understand that many other theories regarding the nursing role have contributed remarkably to the concept of nursing as a helping profession.

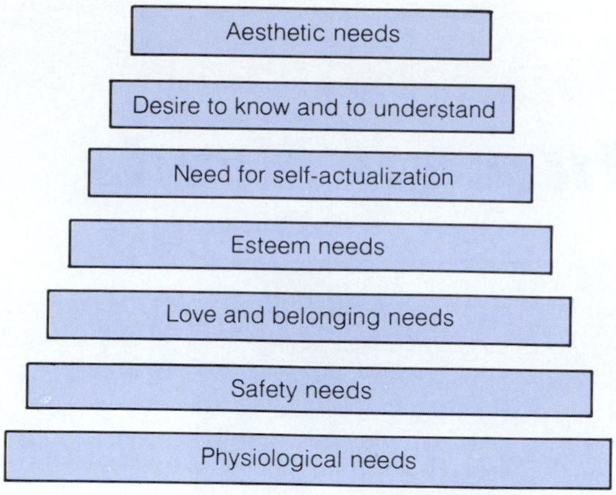

Figure 5-1. Maslow's hierarchy of needs.

Maslow's Theory of Needs

Maslow developed a construct called the **hierarchy of needs**. According to Torres (1986, p. 56), Maslow believed that there were "similarities of the unified organism/human who is constantly motivated to meet changing needs." Maslow's motivational theory contains a directional pattern that is tied neither to the age or life span of human beings nor the influence of the environment.

When establishing the hierarchy, Maslow arranged human needs into seven groups. He then ranked the groups in an ascending order with physiologic needs first (Fig. 5-1). His theory is helpful in developing an understanding of the person by focusing on the possibility of growth as each individual satisfies physiologic needs and is *motivated* to fulfill higher and more individually rewarding needs.

An important application for nurses is to remember that physiologic needs must be met for survival. Only when these needs have been met is a person motivated to fulfill such higher needs as esteem, self-actualization, knowledge, and aesthetic attainment. For example, a patient experiencing severe difficulty in breathing invariably shows little interest in health teaching. The basic need for oxygen is foremost, and not until it is met can the patient pay attention to learning. The nurse is integral to meeting patients' needs and helping them to meet their own needs.

Physiologic Needs

Physiologic needs are the physical needs inherent in all human beings; among them are the needs for oxygen, food, fluids, sleep, and procreation to ensure the continuation of human existence. Physiologic needs are sometimes referred to as basic needs. The effects of their denial are both obvious and measurable. Physiologic needs must be met at least minimally for life to continue. Below the level of subsistence, death occurs. However, even physiologic needs are variable and somewhat subject to mental control. For example, starving prisoners of war survived against all odds by remembering passages of literature or working mathematics problems; they were, in effect, satisfying intellectual and aesthetic needs in place of a physiologic need. More commonly, people experiencing stress overeat not because the need for food is greater at a particular time but because food serves as a "reward" and partial substitute for emotional safety.

Safety Needs

According to Maslow, the need for *safety* is one level above basic physiologic needs. Safety is both physiologic and psychological. The infant experiences safety when held securely and lovingly in the arms of a parent. A playpen, too, can convey physical safety and limits; for a time, most young children play contentedly within such confinement. Only gradually does the child feel safe enough to venture out and explore further; even then a perceived threat, such as the greeting of a stranger, can send the child running back to the safety of the parent.

Safety remains important to adults. We need not only a safe physical environment, a shelter, but also the feeling of psychological safety. Individuals also need to feel that their community is safe. Studies of communities threatened by street violence and disasters, such as hazardous waste contamination, earthquakes, or fires, have found that both psychological disruption and family discord result from threats to community safety. To feel psychologically safe, most of us need relatively structured lives and definite social expectations for our own

Nursing Issues and Trends: The Need to Feel Safe

All humans, since the beginning of time, have shared the basic need to feel both physically and psychologically safe. Street crime, domestic violence, and internal wars have interfered with this most primary need. Any of these leads to high levels of anxiety which can affect health. We can respond to violent societal changes in two ways. First, as individuals living in an unsafe world, we can use our collective power to make a statement that threatening others is never acceptable. Secondly, we must provide care for victims of threatened or actual violent acts with understanding and sympathy. Nurses have an unusual challenge in becoming active in this cause.

behavior and that of others. We need freedom from separation, quarreling, disorder, and the sense of loss. To feel safe, we need regular contact with people we trust and with whom we feel close. These people function as a system of support.

Love and Belonging Needs

The security we gain from *love and belonging* enhances the feeling of safety (Fig. 5-2). We also learn about ourselves from the responses of those around us. We learn which aspects of our behavior are acceptable or unacceptable. Our feeling of structure and security is reinforced when we know where we stand in relation to others and who we are to them. This reflection of ourselves in the eyes of others—as well as our ability to share in the lives of others—is the essence of belongingness. We all need mutually meaningful relationships with other people.

The love of which Maslow speaks is not, by definition, sexual. For some people it may be not just love of a single person, but devotion to a group or even a cause. For an infant or young child, on the other hand, the need for love from a mother figure is at the more elementary or physiologic level. Spitz's classic observational study (1945) of two groups of infants and children demonstrates this fact. Each group received the same high-quality physical care, but one group was talked to, held, and caressed, whereas the other group received little demonstrative affection. Not only did the children who received little love develop signs and symptoms of lassitude, withdrawal, physical ailments, and delayed development, but their mortality rate was significantly higher than the other group.

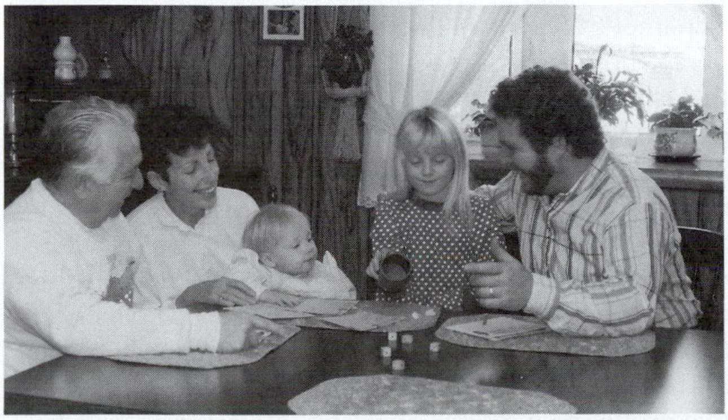

Figure 5-2. The need for love and belonging is a basic human need.

Adults who are similarly neglected are often able to sublimate or transfer the fulfillment of their love needs to a pet, an artistic endeavor, or a charitable pursuit. The need for love may exist on more than one level.

Esteem Needs

Self-esteem is derived largely from feeling that we are valued by those around us. We feel good about ourselves when the people who are important to us express acceptance and approval. But self-esteem also comes from within; it is related to our assessments of our own adequacy, our performance and capacity in the various arenas of our lives, both personal and professional. Self-approval (*ie*, liking oneself) is essential.

Some people who achieve great *esteem* in the eyes of others lack self-esteem and try to compensate by frantically pursuing wider public recognition. Most people gain and maintain self-esteem by performing their jobs competently and contributing to the well-being of their families, professions, and communities. Some unfortunate people spend their lives in self-doubt and sadness.

The Need for Self-Actualization

Maslow calls **self-actualization** "being true to oneself." More precisely, it is the effort to fulfill one's potential; to do in life, with joy, what one both wants and is suited to do (Fig. 5-3). As Maslow writes, "The farmer plants

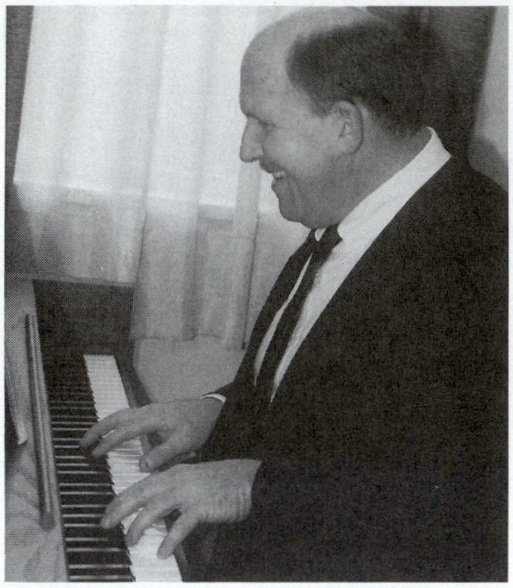

Figure 5-3. Self-actualization: to do in life, with joy, what one both wants and is suited to do.

and tends his crops, the nurse nurses." But to be truly self-actualized, a person must grow: the farmer takes pride in the increasing ability to grow plants, and the nurse sharpens his or her skills and experiences through growing empathy with the patient. Self-actualization, then, is not confined to what one chooses to *do* in life; it also includes what one *feels*. Philosophy, morality, and religion, honestly explored, can enhance self-actualization. Although few individuals ever achieve full self-actualization, reaching for one's potential enriches life.

The Need to Know and Understand

The striving for knowledge is an outgrowth of self-actualization. Motivated by curiosity, people seek answers to the secrets of their world. Perhaps it is this need that led us to our great advances in technology and the exploration of outer space. Opportunities for learning are more abundant today than ever before: the media expose us to masses of information, continuing education is available even in small communities, and written self-help programs are readily accessible. It is becoming increasingly common for adults to pursue new horizons by returning to school or learning new skills. The *need to know and understand* is not necessarily related to the gratification of immediate goals; it may be its own reward.

Aesthetic Needs

The highest level in Maslow's hierarchy is the level of *aesthetic needs*. Highly developed in the artist who creates beauty on paper or canvas, the aesthetic need can also be satisfied by appreciation of others' artistic efforts and by the cultivation of beauty and form in the details of daily life. Sometimes, when talking in general terms, we must be cautious. For example, an economically disadvantaged family that finds it difficult to acquire sufficient food or adequate housing may have an increased need for aesthetics to offset its deprivation. Throughout their lifetimes, people constantly move through the various levels, often in response to the external world. Much of what we consider "routine" nursing care consists of meeting needs to *prevent* problems from occurring.

The Hierarchy of Needs in Setting Priorities

One of the important values of Maslow's theory is that it can be used to identify priorities when planning care for patients. In identifying what is of primary importance to the patient and adding our expertise, we can design a plan of care that is the most effective in fulfilling that person's needs. For example, oxygenation is often the most important because it is a basic need. When the person can breathe more easily, that person may consider pain most important and priorities for care appropriately shift so that comfort is provided. The nurse must have skills in identifying priorities and yet remain flexible when caring for patients.

Once patient needs have been identified, priorities can be assigned to them. This is the process of determining which need is the most important for a patient at a particular time. The priorities may change as the patient's status changes.

The guiding principle in establishing priorities for care is that you must first help the patient meet physiologic needs. When a patient is short of breath, it is not appropriate to discuss the importance of keeping an accurate record of intake and output. If a patient is in obvious pain, it would similarly be wise to delay teaching about a therapeutic diet. Helping patients fulfill their basic needs first makes it possible for you to assist in the fulfillment of their higher needs. For example, the patient whose basic needs have been met and who is in the state of recovery is ready to be consulted about plans for long-term care and the prevention of recurring illness.

You may also prevent problems by foreseeing when the fulfillment of essential needs may be threatened. Recognizing the need for full oxygenation or lung expansion after surgery, you can teach the patient the techniques of coughing and deep breathing the evening before the scheduled surgery to avoid such postoperative problems.

Nurses should be a vocal part of society and serve as advocates for those needing health care. Nurses should know that the government and the health care system are also continually setting priorities, both in programs and in allocation of funds and staff. Sometimes the basic needs of which Maslow wrote become a top national priority, such as funding the school lunch programs and providing food stamps so that people can attain proper nutrition. These programs sometimes take priority over programs for the chronic mentally ill. In 1965, health care of elderly persons became a national priority. In response, national health insurance (Medicare) for elderly persons brought about more comprehensive health care for elders, often preventing catastrophic illness in this age group. If immunization programs are a top state priority, those at risk for communicable disease may escape illness. There are many other areas, both national and international, that need priority setting in providing for basic need fulfillment for individuals. Many older adults view Medicare coverage of prescription drugs as a priority although the government is only now beginning to address this issue.

Human Needs and Theories of Nursing

In Chapter 1 we described the nursing models formulated by several of the leading theorists: Rogers, Peplau, Johnson, Neuman, and Henderson. Each of the theorists recognizes that all individuals have primary and secondary needs that must be met to attain an acceptable quality of life.

The manner in which needs are met distinguishes one theorist from another. Many stress the interaction with the external environment, whereas others stress attaining a balance that is both external and internal. Regardless of the views of the individual theorist, implicit in a definition of nursing is consideration of our own needs and the needs of patients/clients. The nurse acts as a facilitator whose skills are used to meet identified needs. We should understand that theories regarding the nursing role have contributed remarkably to the concept of nursing as a helping profession. Historically, earlier theories focused on the nurse's giving direct attention to solving dilemmas for the person and thereby meeting the patient's needs. In the 1960s and afterward, many of the theorists saw the patient as a system interacting with aspects of the environment. Because of this view, more recent theories of nursing have tailored Rogers' original four themes more specifically to the art of nursing by using language that incorporates person, health, environment (an earlier theme), and nursing. These later concepts greatly change the view of the nurse as primarily a person solving problems for others to meet their needs to that of a skilled individual assisting others to meet their own needs within the construct of a wider world. (For additional references regarding the writing of these authors, refer to the references at the end of Chapter 1.)

Regardless of framework, each theory is useful to us in relationship to human needs and should not be disregarded. In a much broader sense, you may seriously consider each nursing theory as you formulate your own philosophy of nursing practice.

Rogers' Science of Unitary Man

With the use of the space–time continuum, Rogers (1970) viewed the person as an organized energy field, which she called holistic or *unitary man*. This unitary man is in constant interchange with environment energy and matter. Rogers holds to a homeodynamic principle as she views the directional ongoing complexities of man and the environment's mutual energies.

Under the Rogerian theory, needs would arise when the exchange of energy is unequal or the equation out of balance. Because a person is viewed as being on a continuum in life from conception to death, a need could also arise when this ongoing development is interrupted. Although Rogers does not directly address illness, one might assume that illness with its accompanying needs may also occur when energy sources are depleted.

Peplau's Interpersonal Relations Model

Peplau (1981) incorporates many of the principles held by Maslow in that she believes that human beings are oriented to move toward growth and the fulfillment of a higher needs level. Like Maslow, Peplau recognizes that needs can be both physiologic and psychological in origin. As a spokesperson for nursing, she sees the nurse strongly in the relationship role. Within that role, nurses function in many capacities to assist patients to meet their needs: teacher, consultant, adviser, and, as a more recent term suggests, manager of care.

Johnson's Behavioral Systems Model

Johnson's beginning premise (1968) is that the person is a behavioral system and has, as Rogers also believes, dynamic *equilibrium*. Johnson also incorporates some of Rogers' theory in giving importance to the interaction with the environment. She views the individual as a total system and feels that when this system is influenced by events so that equilibrium is disturbed, needs emerge that can cause problems. One important aspect of Johnson's theory is interpersonal behavior. Patients who are ill may have dependency needs that may cause interpersonal problems that have an impact on equilibrium.

Orem's Self-Care Model

Orem (1971) uses ability to provide one's self-care independently as the maxim of health. The three theoretical parts of nursing theory are self-care, self-care deficits, and nursing systems. The self-care deficits are clearly the patient's needs, and Orem relies on the nursing systems to assist the individual in meeting these needs. Orem's model reflects the current definition of nursing diagnoses in that much of the language centers around deficits. Nursing interventions are identified whose purpose is to minimize or correct that person's deficits in independent functioning.

Roy's Adaptation Model

Once again, the individual is viewed as holistic in that all human beings have biopsychosocial characteristics. Rather than emphasizing environment, Roy (1984) believes that the person continuously interacts with both internal and external stresses. This process necessitates adaptation, which can be seen as successfully meeting needs, and when this does not occur, problems arise and illness is possible. Roy builds into her theory a complex of subsystems that, for our purposes, is not relevant. She views the nurse as helping the patient/client in the process of adaptation in such a way that needs are fulfilled and problems resolved.

Neuman's Systems Model

Environment and adaptation are both important to Neuman (1982) as she describes human beings as *systems* that interact reciprocally with the environment. When stress is exerted on the person, a variety of "variables" come into play to act as "buffers." These protective elements may be elements of the physiologic, psychological, or social makeup of the person. These variables may be age, support systems, or living conditions. In meeting the patient/client's needs, the nurse focuses on reduction of stressors. Problems arise when these protective responses are inadequate or those usually present are depleted or break down. Neuman shows a strong belief in assessment as a tool in the prevention of undue stress being placed on the individual.

Henderson's Basic Nursing Care Components

Henderson, a prolific writer of nursing theory, emphasizes the role of the nurse in meeting human needs. She uses the terms health, illness, and death, but not environment (1966). The nurse is assigned the role of providing for or substituting actions that, in health, the patient/client would perform. Using a list of 14 activities, she views the person who can independently perform these as being in a state of health. These 14 activities represent basic needs of the person. Specific problems emerge as the individual becomes incapable of engaging in these activities. (See Display on the nature of nursing in Chapter 1.)

Needs and the Nursing Process

The organization of this text reflects both a way of categorizing human needs and the approach to meeting those needs that makes up nursing practice. This approach, the nursing process, is discussed in detail in Chapters 8 through 12. You will use the nursing process as a framework for identifying the needs of patients and for determining the interventions that help the patient to meet those needs.

Identifying Needs, Problems, and Deficits

When you use the nursing process, you will identify patient needs, deficits, and problems. To do this, you must be able to distinguish among the three, all of which are different. We have defined **need** as that which is necessary or required for optimum functioning. The word **deficit** is derived from Latin and means lacking. Many people have a physical or even a psychological deficit. Each person has a need for safety in the environment. Being able to use the senses to perceive danger is important to meeting this need. Suppose a person has a sensory deficit in the left hand caused by a physical condition and is unable to feel light touch. If the person is right handed and has no motor loss, he or she may make adjustments to the deficit and not perceive it as a problem. If, however, this individual is not able to adjust to the lost sensation and is in danger of injury, a problem exists.

A **problem** is present when a need is not met. Let us say that the water pitcher is inadvertently placed beyond the reach of a frail elderly patient. The patient's need is for fluid. After a time, the patient will feel thirst, demonstrating a fluid *deficit.* The *problem* is that the water is not accessible. Lack of water in turn creates such other problems for the patient as dry mouth, flaky skin, and general discomfort. Or consider the nurse who reports to work in the afternoon, forgetting to wear a jacket and then shivers all the way home in the evening. Here, the *need* is for body warmth; there is a heat *deficit*; the *problem* is inadequate clothing. In planning care, clearly differentiating needs, deficits, and problems will help to more explicitly define goals and nursing actions.

Changing Needs Throughout the Life Span

People in all phases of the **life span** have similar needs. However, because of the differences in their developmental level, the nursing process may have to be modified for each to best meet these needs. For example, the infant and elderly person both have a need for safety in the environment, but the assessments and interventions used may be different to accomplish the goals. With each of the human needs presented below, it is essential that you consider the variations appropriate for each stage of the life span. The need to develop fully throughout the life span (see Chapters 17–20) is paramount over all other needs. This need is both physical and psychological. Physical growth can be directly affected if one is not nurtured socially and psychologically. The need to progress through the continuum of life in homeostatic balance is a universal one.

Meeting Physiologic Needs

An awareness of the various needs of the individual and where they fall in the hierarchy of needs is helpful in the use of nursing process.

Making sure physiologic needs are met requires awareness, knowledge, and skill (Fig. 5-4). The nurse can monitor some physiologic needs visually (*eg*, sleep and rest); others can only be tracked with special equipment (*eg*, fluid and electrolyte balance). The physiologic requirements of the healthy human being are both obvious (oxygenation) and not so obvious (activity). Meeting some of them is primarily the nurse's responsibility, whereas other needs are managed by other members of the health care team.

The safety needs of patients, which include both physical and psychological safety requirements, are essential for the patient's sense of well-being (see Chapter 21). Meeting a patient's need for physical safety means constantly monitoring the health care environment for any safety hazards. Concern for the patient's physical safety also requires that all medical equipment be functioning well and that thought and care go into the administration of all drugs and medications. To be in an environment that is safe and free of harm is a basic need. An important part of this is to be free of infection. An invasion of any of the body systems by microorganisms can threaten life. Within the hospital setting, this need is intensified by the increased danger of contamination. The duty to provide an infection-free environment falls primarily on the nurse, who is with the patient more than any other person on the health care team. The use of aseptic practices and barriers to ward off or contain infection and the monitoring of the environment for potential hazards that may jeopardize safety help to fulfill this need (see Chapter 21 of this text and Module 3 in Ellis, Nowlis, and Bentz, *Modules for Nursing Skills*, Volume I.)

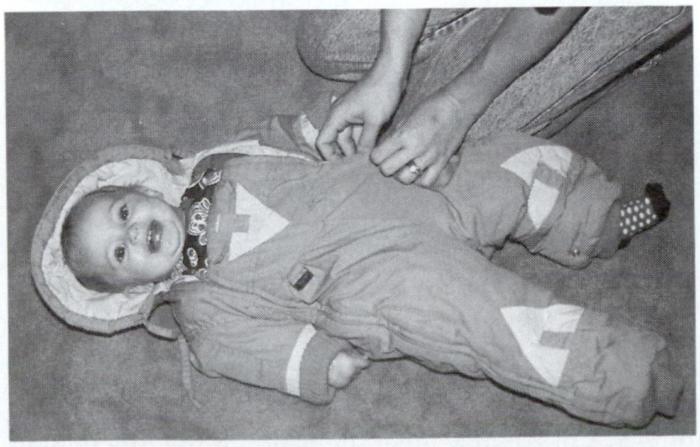

Figure 5-4. Clothing to provide warmth fulfills a physiologic need.

Tied closely to the need to be free of infection is the need for the patient to have intact skin that can protect the body from infection (see Chapter 22). Adequate hygiene can prevent the rapid growth of microorganisms that can endanger health; it can also help to satisfy the patient's need for comfort. Ill patients often must rely on the nurse for their personal hygiene. Bathing, clean garments, and an uncluttered environment also give a patient a sense of comfort.

From birth, activity is an essential part of development and life (see Chapter 23). Patients continue to have a basic need for activity even when their abilities are altered or diminished by illness. Activity maintains muscle tone. An adequate activity level also positively affects other systems; heart action increases in rate, the lungs expand more fully, and elimination is facilitated. In addition, activity gives the patient a sense of vitality. Numerous studies have been done linking exercise to improved health status and psychological well-being. To meet this basic need, the nurse should prepare and implement a plan to provide the maximum amount of activity appropriate for a specific patient.

As important as the need for activity is the body's basic need for rest and sleep (see Chapter 24). When the body rests, muscles have time both to get rid of wastes and to take nourishment to function effectively. The other systems of the body rest as well; circulation slows, respirations are quieter, and the mind becomes less stressed. Sleep, which is different from rest, is basic to survival. Human beings cannot live without periods of sleep to renew vital functioning. Patients who are dealing with physical and emotional deficits must have extra sleep to meet their other needs, such as the need for activity and emotional stability. Nurses can help provide time for patients to get essential sleep by carefully considering this need in the plan of care.

The need for the body to receive adequate nutrients is also physiologic (see Chapter 25). Although human beings can survive longer without food than without water, both are required to maintain life. Much of the body is made up of water; one important function of all body fluid is to transport nutrients. Food provides the substances needed for energy, healing, and general organ function. Patients recovering from an illness have an increased need for both water and food. Assessing, correcting, and providing fluid intake is often a fundamental aspect of care planning.

Adequate elimination of excess water and waste products from the metabolism of food within the body is necessary for proper functioning of the various systems (see Chapters 26 and 27) because it ensures that excess fluid and wastes are not retained in body tissues. When a patient has an elimination problem, the nurse assists in its reduction. When a patient is unable to care for elimination needs, the nurse must assist the patient in carrying out this function.

All human beings have an immediate and constant need for oxygen (see Chapter 28). Lack of oxygen affects all systems. Some body tissues die within minutes without proper oxygenation. All patients are continuously monitored by the nurse to ensure that each has an adequate airway through which to receive oxygen as well as a concentration of oxygen in the blood sufficient to sustain all functions of the body at the highest level.

Also self-evident is the basic need for effective circulation, both to carry nutrients to tissues and to carry off waste products from those same tissues (see Chapter 29). This need cannot be ignored because it directly affects all other body systems. By using a variety of nursing interventions, nurses support and improve the patient's circulation.

Fluid and electrolyte needs revolve around the intracellular and extracellular balance provided by chemicals in a fluid environment (see Chapter 30). The balance is fragile, and thus these needs of the internal body must be constantly met to sustain life.

Cognition and sensory perception needs are orchestrated primarily by the nervous system (see Chapter 31). Their fulfillment allows the patient to respond to other needs such as the need to think and to use the senses. Because sensation and perception are vital to all other systems, nurses must be sure to integrate these needs into their plan of care.

Persons have a need to be free of pain and in a state of comfort (see Chapter 32). Although pain can be a warning system and therefore protective, relentless pain, which prevents the fulfillment of other needs, should be eliminated whenever possible. Listening to patients and accepting their analysis of pain with sensitivity is a first step in providing a pain-free state. If pain cannot be eliminated, it can usually be reduced in intensity so that other needs can take precedence.

Meeting Psychosocial Needs

In this text we will also focus on **psychosocial needs**, which include the need for social, cultural, and ethnic identity; mental health; and a system of values and beliefs. Meeting these needs requires psychosocial skills on the part of the nurse, and those skills are among the first ones you will need to acquire to interact effectively with your colleagues on the health care team and with your patients/clients (Fig. 5-5).

Meeting the psychological needs of patients requires personal integrity as much as technical skill. Chapter 3 addressed ways in which paying careful attention to ethical issues can help to meet the psychological safety needs of the patient. The maintenance of confidentiality assures patients that no embarrassing or harmful information will be divulged without their permission. Being honest with patients promotes trust, which makes them feel safe in their interactions with the nurse. The competence you exhibit when planning, organizing, and implementing care (see Chapter 11) is also reassuring, as is the confidence you display.

Another need of people is to attain social, cultural, and ethnic identity (see Chapter 33). This gives us a sense of belonging because it links us with a significant past and present and allows us to be different. It encourages a feeling of being part of a group of persons who have similar backgrounds. Being recognized as having a particular social, cultural, or ethnic identity is a prerequisite to sharing that identity with others in a constructive way.

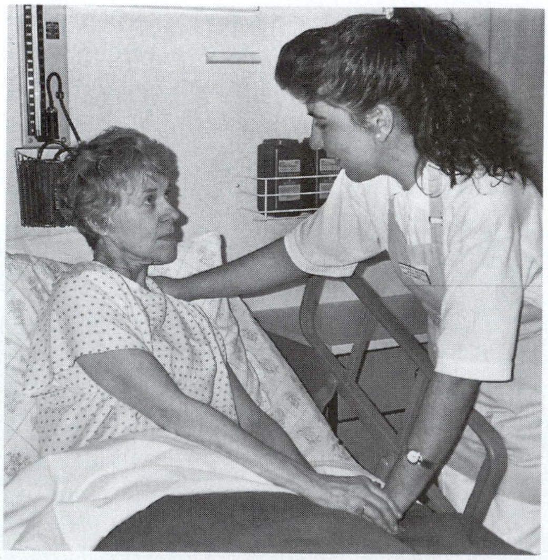

Figure 5-5. A nurse may meet the need for full functioning through interacting with patients.

We all have a need to be mentally healthy, to feel that we are psychologically in control. Mental health (see Chapter 34) implies feeling good about oneself. Illness can substantially interfere with this because the patient role often requires a person to be passive or dependent, which can lead to diminished self-esteem. Within the hospital setting, small but meaningful ways can be found to support self-esteem and to help offset anxiety and depression. Maintaining privacy, including the patient in decision-making, and recognizing the patient as a sensitive, feeling person, all help build a patient's self-esteem. The manner of offering care should say, "You are an important person as well as a patient to me."

The need to have a self-determining set of values and beliefs is basic to all human beings (see Chapter 36). Exploring one's own particular values and beliefs is an important part of affirming one's identity and attaining self-esteem. Patients may have an increased need to strengthen their values and belief systems when illness threatens their well-being and, in many instances, their lives.

The need for sexual identity is also basic to human beings (see Chapter 37). Not everyone has the same need to be sexually active, but people certainly need to feel either feminine or masculine and to express those feelings in ways appropriate for them.

Meeting Special Needs

A variety of special needs surface in our lives and the lives of our patients and require unique attention. They are particularly relevant to the completeness of this text.

Communication (see Chapter 13) is a basic need of all people. For patients who, through illness, have lost the ability to communicate verbally, other ways of communicating must be found. Although our communication is professional, at times it also serves social needs as well as we interact with the patient. Communication is involved in satisfying a deep psychological need of patients to understand what is occurring and what might take place. Reasonable explanations are especially important when the patient is anxious about why the body is not functioning properly. Clarifying and answering the patient's questions may quiet unnecessary fears. The nurse's health teaching role (see Chapter 16) answers the patient's need to know and understand. One of the basic factors of health teaching is patient receptiveness or desire to learn. Health teaching often focuses on the preventive goal of attempting to ensure that other problems do not arise.

At other times in our lives special needs emerge. One of these times occurs when the patient has to undergo a diagnostic test or be given medications that have physical and psychological significance (see Chapter 38). Having tests may be perceived by the patient as an expectation by others on the health care team that there is "something wrong" with the body. This can cause understandable fear and anxiety so the patient needs to be well informed and adequately prepared. Because of the inherent dangers in administering medications, the nurse should recognize that strict safety principles must be observed at all times to provide the need for safety (see Chapter 39). Psychological ramifications must be considered. Including the patient in both the knowledge and actions of the many drugs now used therapeutically allays a degree of fear and can maximize the patient's physiologic therapeutic response.

Surgery is another major stressor that produces special human needs (see Chapter 40). Whether the surgery is to be performed on an outpatient basis or in the acute care setting, the realization that there is loss of control during the perioperative period is, of itself, extremely frightening for patients. The nurse's role is one of supporting the physiologic and psychological strengths of the patient as surgery is performed and the person moves toward recovery or necessary adaptations to life.

To be able to come to terms with losses in life and with one's own death is also a basic but special need (see Chapter 41). In some cases it is possible to find opportunity in pending death. It is not uncommon to see a terminally ill patient seeking self-actualization. This is not to be construed as a frantic final attempt to find some meaning in a life soon to be extinguished. One's last days can be a time of growth, of exploration of self, of relating to family and friends in a new way, and of seeing clearly the world around in all its excitement. Granted, many do not find the physical strength to pursue such adventures. On a less intense level, illness causes many patients to find strengths in themselves never before defined. The nurse can provide restful times and encouragement to patients who do, indeed, grow with physical and mental adversity.

Special needs are particularly evident at times of bereavement; patients' families and those significant to them are also important to the nurse's caring role. There is a need to be psychologically healed when something or someone of significance is gone from our lives. There is a sense of needing the support of others and needing to reconnect or become involved in what has previously been worthwhile. Personal growth and reaffirmation can develop when loss occurs and needs arise.

Chronic illness can cause a multitude of problems, resulting in ongoing and special human needs. Fear of progression and unknown effects on one's life are major concerns. There may also be family role needs as well as financial adjustments. Identifying needs unique to the patient and support strengths is an essential role for the nurse in these situations (see Chapter 42).

The Nurse's Own Needs

Nurses also have needs. The most effective nurses are holistically well balanced individuals who are able to identify their own needs and seek healthy ways of fulfilling them.

Physiologic needs must be met before the nurse can effectively give care to others. The nurse on the unit who has a severe headache or is worried about circumstances at home, for example, is unlikely to contribute fully to the care of patients.

Nurses have a need to feel safe. With procedures to protect themselves against infection and unsafe working environments, nurses have minimized several safety problems. By establishing reciprocal, open communication with others on the health care team as well as with patients, nurses gain psychological safety. The team members' honesty with one another builds trust, which in turn, is passed on to patients.

Nurses' love and belonging needs are appropriately satisfied by caring family and friends. One important aspect of this level of need, however, is the satisfaction of belonging to a respected profession—nursing—and being accepted as a member of the health care team. This acceptance as a member of a group and the sense that one is competent in performing the tasks of nursing generate a feeling of self-esteem. More than many other professions, nursing allows its practitioners to see clearly just how important they are to others who need their assistance.

The need for self-actualization is individual, but it is a strong component for nurses who believe in realizing life to the fullest. The need for professional and personal growth is a concept central to being a nurse.

The strong emphasis on increasing knowledge for nurses, through in-service and continuing education programs, is evidence of the need to know and understand. Many nurses progress to higher education to attain degrees that allow them to move up professionally. But not all knowledge has to be confined to nursing. Many nurses find intellectual excitement in reading or attending classes relative to other aspects of their lives.

It is the fortunate nurse who gives attention to the aesthetics of life. Art, music, and beauty can help to offset some of the rigorous and sad aspects of nursing. Nurses would do well to consciously cultivate aesthetics to experience the enjoyment they can create.

Nurses should be reflective about their needs and how those needs can be satisfied. People close to them, and particularly patients, should never be victimized because of frustrations or inadequate mechanisms for coping with needs. The holistic approach is essential for both nurses and patients.

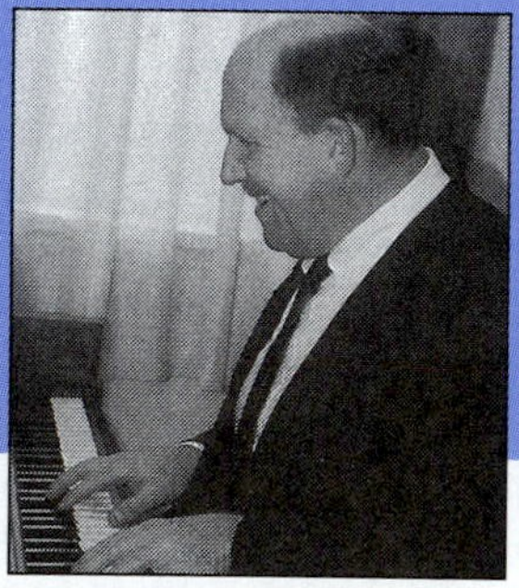

Key Points

- Understanding the concepts of needs, deficits, and problems is vital to planning patient care. A deficit can produce a need, and a problem can prevent a need from being met.
- To maintain homeostasis, human needs must be met adequately. Maslow's hierarchy of human needs can guide the nurse in setting priorities for nursing care.
- The most effective care is that which is prioritized using the nursing process. Maslow's hierarchy is helpful in directing care that is individualized to specific needs.
- Nursing theorists have added to our understanding of the whole person and the individual's needs.
- Many universal physiologic and psychosocial needs are apparent as well as special ones.
- Part of nursing is to ensure the safety of each patient in every situation and to recognize the serious consequences of failure to observe safety precautions.
- Physiologic needs include the need to be free of infection and the need for comfort, activity, sleep, rest, proper nutrition, elimination, oxygenation, circulation, fluid and electrolyte balance, and appropriate interaction with the environment.
- Basic psychosocial needs include those for a social, cultural or ethnic, and sexual identity; the need for mental health; and the need to have a system of values and beliefs.
- Patients have other special physiologic and psychosocial needs that are important for the quality of life, including the need to communicate, the need to have fear minimized, and the need to come to acceptance of our own death and the death of others and losses in life.

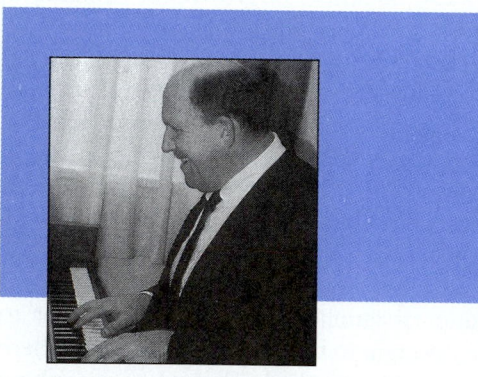

- Chronic illness carries with it a variety of special needs.
- Nurses have needs and the most effective nurses are those who acknowledge their needs and grow both professionally and personally.

Study Questions

1. Give an example of a patient for whom you are giving care and explain how the patient's illness might alter the order within Maslow's hierarchy of needs.
2. Discuss ways in which the environment of the health care facility can interfere with the fulfillment of the patient's psychosocial needs.
3. How can health care facilities more successfully meet patients' psychosocial needs?
4. In what ways do nurses respond to patients' physiologic needs?
5. A patient complains to you about having dry skin. What is the need and what is the problem; explain your answer.
6. What do you believe are some of the needs of nurses?
7. What actions could you take to meet your personal needs at the present time?

Critical Thinking Activities

1. Select a patient in the clinical area as an example. What specific deficits do you see as preventing that person's needs from being fulfilled?
2. Identify what you see as your primary and secondary needs. Compare these with Maslow's hierarchy of needs. Are they in the same or a different order?
3. In a clinical or discussion group, have each member select a different age and outline the primary needs of a person at that age. Compare and contrast what each member has identified. Compare the group's views with Maslow's.

References and Readings

Byrne-Coker, E., Fradley, T., Harris, J., Tomarchio, D., Chan, V., and Caron, C. "Implementing Nursing Diagnoses within the Context of King's Conceptual Framework." *Nursing Diagnosis* 1, 3 (July-September 1990): 107–114.

Diamond, L. K. "Empowerment through Self-Healing." *Revolution: The Journal of Nurse Empowerment.* 2, 2 (Summer, 1992): 116–121.

Hanchett, E. S. "Nursing Models and Community as Client. . . Public Health/Community Health Nursing." *Nursing Sciences Quarterly* 3, 2 (Summer 1990): 67–72.

Headricks, M. M. "Needs Assessment: Sense or Nonsense?" *Journal of Continuing Education in Nursing* 14, 5 (September-October 1983): 13–15.

Hektor, L. M. "Martha Rogers: A Life History." *Nursing Science Quarterly* 2, 2 (Summer 1989): 63–73.

Henderson, V. *The Nature of Nursing*. New York: Macmillan, 1966.

Holzapfel, S. K. "The Importance of Personal Possessions in the Lives of the Institutionalized Elderly." *Journal of Gerontological Nursing* 8 (March 1992): 156–158.

King, I. M. "Health as the Goal for Nursing." *Nursing Science Quarterly* 3, 3 (Fall 1990): 123–128.

Kyle, B. A. S., and Pitzer, S. A. "A Self-Care Approach to Today's Challenges." *Nursing Management* 21, 3 (March 1990): 37–39.

Laschinger, H. K., and Duff, V. "Attitudes of Practicing Nurses Towards Theory-Based Nursing Practice." *Canadian Journal of Nursing Administration* 4, 1 (March-April 1991): 6–10.

Little, C. "Health for All by the Year 2000: "Where is it Now?" *Nursing and Health Care.* 13, 4 (April 1992): 198–203.

Macnee, C. L. "Perceived Well-being of Persons Quitting Smoking." *Nursing Research.* 40, 4 (July/Aug 1991): 200–203.

Maslow, A. H."A Theory of Human Motivation." *Psychological Review* 50 (1943).

Maslow, A. H. *Motivation and Personality.* 2nd edition. New York: Harper & Row, 1970.

Neuman, B. *The Neuman Systems Model: Application to Nursing Education and Practice.* Norwalk, Co.: Appleton-Century-Crofts, 1982.

Orem, D. E. *Nursing: Concepts of Practice.* New York: McGraw-Hill, 1971.

Peplau, H. E. *Interpersonal Relations in Nursing.* New York: G. P. Putnam's Sons, 1952.

Rogers, M. E. *An Introduction to the Theoretical Base of Nursing.* Philadelphia: F. A. Davis, 1970.

Roy, Sr. C. *Introduction to Nursing: An Adaptation Model.* 2nd Ed. Englewood Hills, N.J.: Prentice-Hall, 1984.

Spence-Laschinger, H. K. and McWilliam, C. L. "Health Care in Canada: The Presumption of Care." *Nursing and Health Care.* 13, 4 (April 1992): 204–207.

Spitz, R. "Hospitalism: Inquiry into Genesis of Psychiatric Conditions in Early Childhood." *Psychoanalytic Study of the Child* 1 (1945).

Torres, G. *Theoretical Foundations of Nursing.* Norwalk, Conn.: Appleton-Century-Crofts, 1986.

Wu, R. *Behavior and Illness.* Englewood Cliffs, N.J.: Prentice-Hall, 1973.

Stress, Adaptation, and Coping

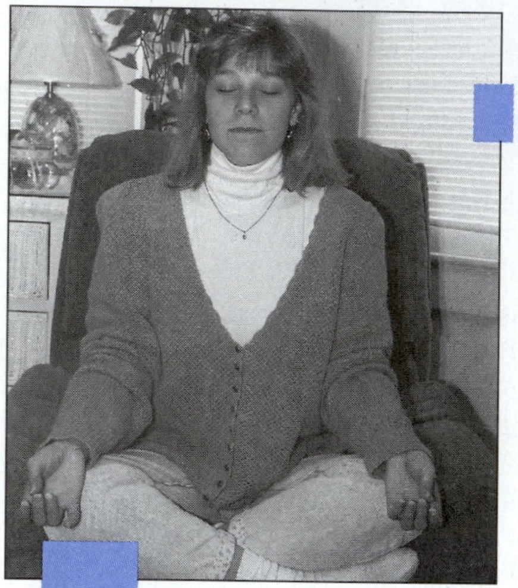

6

Objectives

After completing this chapter, you should be able to:

1. Explain the differences between stress and stressor.
2. Discuss how adaptation and coping relate to health.
3. Outline the factors that affect the impact of stressors.
4. Explain the general adaptation syndrome (GAS).
5. Outline the physical, cognitive, emotional, and behavioral signs and symptoms of stress.
6. Define active, passive, and natural immunity and describe how each is acquired.
7. Identify the major task of the macrophage cells.
8. Explain how cell-mediated immunity, complement, and interferons participate in adaptation.
9. List the cardinal signs of inflammation.
10. Outline what happens in the inflammation process.
11. List the factors that affect healing.
12. Explain the differences and similarities among soft-tissue, bone, and nerve healing.
13. Summarize the relationship between stress and illness.
14. Discuss a variety of ways of coping with stress.

Study Terms

active immunity
adaptation
antibody
antibody mediated immunity
antigens
autogenic training
behavior modification
biofeedback
cardinal signs of inflammation
cell-mediated immunity
coping
coping mechanisms
defense mechanisms
distress
eustress
first intention healing
general adaptation syndrome (GAS)
humoral immunity
immune response
local adaptation syndrome (LAS)
natural immunity
negative feedback
passive immunity
progressive relaxation
regeneration
relaxation response
second intention healing
self-hypnosis
stage of exhaustion
stage of resistance
stress
stressor
support system

Ellis, Nowlis: Nursing: A Human Needs Approach, 5th ed. © 1994 J.B. Lippincott Company

Outline

The terms *stress* and *coping* are widespread in the popular literature as well as in health-related publications. This frequency reflects a growing awareness of the importance of these concepts in understanding health and illness.

A **stressor** is any agent or stimulus that poses a real or potential threat to homeostasis. A stressor disturbs homeostasis when it interferes with a person's ability to meet needs. Although the view persists that all stressors are harmful, minor stressors may not actually interfere with needs and may even contribute to the ability of the person to cope with major stressors that may later be encountered (Selye, 1976).

Stress is the internal state of the person as he or she responds to the stressor. It is a complex set of reactions that help to prepare the person's reaction to the stressor (Selye, 1973). A successful response to the stressor is termed **adaptation**. Adaptation would be any way the body tries to assist the individual to meet needs and maintain homeostasis.

Just as there are many different types of stressors, there are many modes of adaptation. One of them is **coping**, the process by which a person solves problems, makes decisions, and relieves tension created by stress. Coping involves both unconscious behaviors that relieve tension and choices of actions designed to promote adaptation. Understanding these processes will assist you in supporting individuals and families experiencing stress as they move toward greater homeostasis.

Origins of Stressors

Stressors are found in all aspects of life. They may originate within as well as outside us. They may be physiologic or physical in nature, or they may be social and psychological (Display 6-1). Their common feature is their potential to disturb homeostasis.

Some stressors are *internal physiologic factors*. For example, the accumulated waste products of fat metabolism can become a stressor: they are acid in nature and pose a threat to the body's acid–base balance (see Chapter 30). Drugs, disease-causing organisms within the body, and hormonal and metabolic changes may likewise function as stressors.

External physical factors may also be stressors. Extreme heat or cold, loud noises, bright lights, and trauma are all physical causes of stress. Although people differ in their ability to withstand physical and physiologic stressors, all these factors can cause predictable stress in all individuals and, if extreme enough, may even threaten survival.

Much less predictable are internal psychological stressors and external social stressors. *Internal psychological stressors* are thoughts and feelings that produce stress. Low self-esteem, loneliness, and hopelessness, for example, can create stress. Even though such feelings may not be based on realistic perceptions, they can pose a threat to a person's integrity.

Display 6–1
The Origins of Stressors

External Physical
Internal Physiologic
External Social
Internal Psychological

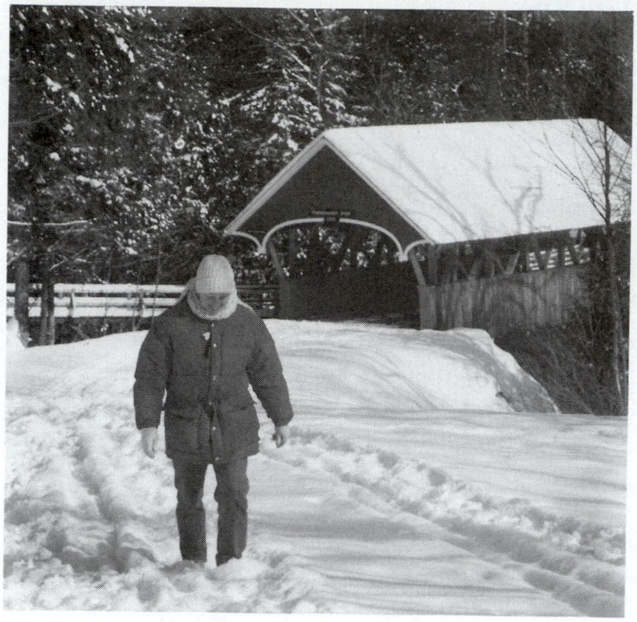
Figure 6-1. Extreme cold causes the body severe stress.

External social stressors are threatening stimuli arising from interactions with other people. Conflict and pressure to perform are common external social stressors. For example, a critical and demanding employer, a spouse who shirks responsibility, or a rebellious child could threaten a person's stability. Psychological and social stressors are almost always intertwined. Feelings change as a result of interactions with other people, and relationships are altered by our perceptions of ourselves. Change itself is one of the most common social stressors; changes in one's job, home life, responsibilities, relationships, and circumstances require adjustments and can thus produce stress.

Factors Affecting the Impact of Stressors

Not all stressors have equal impact on an individual's homeostatic balance. The factors that must be considered when evaluating the potential effect of a stressor are its magnitude or strength, its duration, the person's prior experience with the stressor, its perceived significance to the individual, and the presence of additional stressors.

Magnitude

A stimulus may be extremely weak or strong; this is what we call its relative magnitude. For example, cold is a stressor, but different degrees of cold arouse different amounts of stress within an individual (Fig. 6-1). The greater the cold, the greater the stress. Magnitude also affects the extent to which the stressor affects the whole person. A skin rash over a small area may be a small stressor. Enlarge that same rash to cover major body surfaces, and it becomes a major stressor. Burns and other injuries are also graded in the same way.

Holmes and Rahe (1967) tried to quantify the magnitude of common social and psychological stressors by assigning them "stress points" on a scale of 1 to 100 (Table 6-1). Although this scale is the result of many years of research into stress, it is best used as a general guide to a given stressor's magnitude rather than as an absolute scale applicable to any individual. Others have expanded on this concept and proposed stress scales for specific groups, such as a stress scale for nurses (Kinzel, 1982).

Duration

The duration of a stressor is another important factor in its effect. The longer the stressor acts on the person, the more difficult it will be for the body to meet basic needs and maintain homeostasis. Again cold serves as a good example. It is easy to understand that someone could quickly run to a car without wearing a coat when the temperature was 35°F. Although that person would feel cold, the body could meet the need for temperature regulation through increased heat production, and the cold would not pose a serious threat to homeostasis. However, if the person were exposed to this temperature overnight without proper clothing, the ability of the body to adapt could be seriously compromised, and the person might not survive. The body would be unable to meet the need for an appropriate temperature.

Similarly, the duration of psychological stressors is important. A working environment in which there was an occasional burst of anger might not cause undue stress. That same anger repeated frequently throughout each day would have a different effect on the individual.

Cumulation

Stress is also cumulative, that is, separate stressors added to each other have a greater effect than does any one of them singly. The stress resulting from two differ-

Table 6–1. The Social Readjustment Rating Scale

Life Event	Mean Value	Life Event	Mean Value
1. Death of spouse	100	22. Change in responsibilities at work	29
2. Divorce	73	23. Son or daughter leaves home	29
3. Marital separation	65	24. Trouble with in-laws	29
4. Jail term	63	25. Outstanding personal achievement	28
5. Death of close family member	63	26. Spouse begins or stops working	26
6. Personal injury or illness	53	27. Beginning or end of school	26
7. Marriage	50	28. Change in living conditions	25
8. Fired at work	47	29. Revision of personal habits	24
9. Marital reconciliation	45	30. Trouble with boss	23
10. Retirement	45	31. Change in work hours or conditions	20
11. Change in health of family member	44	32. Change in residence	20
12. Pregnancy	40	33. Change in schools	20
13. Sex difficulties	39	34. Change in recreation	19
14. Gain of new family member	39	35. Change in church activities	19
15. Business readjustment	39	36. Change in social acitvities	18
16. Change in financial state	38	37. Mortgage or loan less than $10,000 (e.g., car)*	17
17. Death of close friend	37	38. Change in sleeping habits	16
18. Change to different line of work	36	39. Change in number of family get-togethers	15
19. Change in number of arguments with spouse	35	40. Change in eating habits	15
20. Mortgage over $10,000 (e.g., house or business)*	31	41. Vacation	13
21. Foreclosure of mortgage or loan	30	42. Christmas	12
		43. Minor violation of the law	11

Reprinted with permission from *Journal of Psychosomatic Research* 11, T. H. Holmes and R. H. Rahe, "The Social Readjustment Rating Scale," Copyright 1967, Pergamon Press, Ltd., pp. 213–218.
*These dollar amounts were established in 1967. Today's figures might be expected to differ.

ent items in Table 6-1 is thus additive. Holmes and Rahe add together the points associated with the various stressors operating in an individual's life to arrive at a figure representing total stress. It does not matter, they say, whether total stress is a result of many minor factors or one major event; the effect on the person is the same.

Perception

Individual perception plays a critical role in the impact of any stressor, but it is particularly important in social or psychological stressors. Individual sensitivity makes it possible for predictions about the effects of stressors to be wrong.

Lazarus and Folkman (1984) use the term *cognitive appraisal* to refer to the process that occurs within the person when a stressor is confronted and then categorized according to its significance. It is an evaluative process that focuses on meaning and significance. If someone perceives a particular stimulus as stressful, that stimulus will function as a stressor for that individual regardless of how others may view it. For example, one person may view having guests in the home as a pleasant and comfortable event. Another might perceive the same occasion as creating a great deal of stress. The second individual might worry that guests might criticize the home or the arrangements or that the occasion would reveal the person's social inadequacies.

Cognitive appraisal is also important in physiologic stress. Siegel (1986) has written of the difference in quality of life, response to treatment, and longevity that can be seen in individuals who respond to cancer with hope and confidence versus those whose appraisal leads them to despair and defeat. He underscored that all healing must be done by the body itself and that an attitude of hope sets the stage for healing. He emphasized that if a given illness shows only a 20% recovery rate, it is not promoting false hope to encourage a person to believe that they can be within that 20%.

Prior Experience

Prior experience affects both physical and psychological reactions to a stimulus. An example is contact with the virus that causes chickenpox. Once an individual has been exposed to that virus, the body's defense system

Nursing Issues and Trends: *Are We Blaming the Victim?*

As we identify the role of stress in illness and the potential for enhancing healing and well-being through personal action, the concern has been raised that the end result may be blaming the patient for illness or failure to heal. How much of the **cause** of any illness is related to stress? Is there a difference between stress making a problem worse and stress causing the problem? What factors cause illness that are beyond the control of the individual? Can we as health professionals help people to feel more in control of their own lives and health, and still not feel guilt when all does not go well? New knowledge presents us with new challenges!

has developed the ability to counteract it; in another encounter, that same virus is easily destroyed and does not cause as much stress in the person.

Psychological stressors exhibit an analogous relationship. One's expectations about whether a situation will be stressful often arise from earlier encounters with similar situations. If those situations produced stress, then the individual may ascribe stress to every similar situation. By contrast, if a stimulus has been associated with previous unstressful experiences, one is more likely to approach it as unstressful. For example, the individual who has successfully dealt with a major loss in life will usually be able to cope more successfully with another loss. However, if the loss was not successfully managed, a new loss might be an even greater stressor.

In health care, the nature of a person's previous contact with the health care system is an important factor in the amount of stress experienced in the system now. One individual may perceive hospitalization as a major stressor because it is associated with the terminal illness of a family member. Another person may have contacted a hospital only in a situation in which the hospital was seen as a refuge and relief from responsibilities. This individual might not perceive hospitalization as a stressor.

Stress: The General Adaptation Syndrome

Hans Selye, a Canadian physician and endocrinologist, was one of the first researchers to define and describe stress (Selye, 1973). According to Selye, whenever a person confronts a major threat, the body responds in a predictable way. This response is the same no matter what the nature of the threat. Selye labeled the body's response to threat the **general adaptation syndrome** (GAS). This term emphasizes that the response is both generalized and *adaptive*—that is, aimed at neutralizing the threat and restoring the body to homeostasis. Stress, then, is the state in which the body is prepared to act to preserve itself.

Selye and other writers have pointed out that stress is both a normal and an essential part of human life. If it lacked the ability to respond, the body would be overwhelmed by threats. Selye (1978) has also suggested that without threat and accompanying opportunities to respond, development would be inhibited. Stress that is helpful and valuable in this way Selye calls **eustress**.

Distress, on the other hand, is stress so extreme or prolonged (or both) as to deplete the body's reserves, induce exhaustion, and contribute to illness and even death. To understand how such outcomes could occur, let us examine what happens during stress.

The GAS is the collective response to threat of the many body systems that help prepare the body for action. The GAS is a neuroendocrine response that arises through the *autonomic nervous system*—the branch of the nervous system that governs such involuntary functions as glandular secretion, heart action, and the activity of smooth muscle in the gastrointestinal tract and the blood vessels. The autonomic nervous system has two components, the *sympathetic nervous system* and the *parasympathetic nervous system*. It is the sympathetic nervous system that responds to stress.

The primary endocrine glands involved in the stress response are the pituitary, the adrenals, and the thyroid. The *pituitary* is a small gland located at the base of the brain. The anterior portion of the pituitary, often called "the master gland," secretes several hormones that affect the functioning of other endocrine glands. The posterior portion of the pituitary functions separately. It releases antidiuretic hormone (ADH), which causes the kidneys to retain water in the body.

The *adrenal glands* are located on top of the kidneys. They are composed of two sections, the center, or *medulla*, and the outer layer, or *cortex*. The hormones secreted by the cortex, called adrenocorticosteroids, are the most critical in the stress response. Adrenaline (also called epinephrine) secreted by the medulla also plays a role in stress.

The *thyroid gland* is located on the anterior side of the trachea. The thyroid hormone, thyroxine, has a major effect on the body's basic *metabolism* (the physical and chemical processes that produce energy). The thyroid gland may have particular significance in long-term stress.

Stages of the General Adaptation Syndrome

The GAS has three distinct stages: 1) the alarm reaction, 2) resistance, and 3) exhaustion. The physiologic processes are complex. Figure 6-2 illustrates the neuroendocrine response in the GAS.

The Alarm Reaction

The *alarm reaction* activates the neuroendocrine response: the sensory nerves receive an external stimulus and relay it to the brain. The brain, in turn, identifies the stimulus as a threat. In the medulla of the brain are located the centers of the autonomic nervous system. These centers stimulate the sympathetic nervous system to respond. The response generated in this way is often called the flight-or-fight response because it prepares the body for both kinds of action.

The respiratory rate increases. The heart beats more rapidly and the peripheral blood vessels constrict (causing a rise in blood pressure). The adrenal medulla is stimulated to secrete the catecholamines (epinephrine and norepinephrine), which further increase heart rate and respirations and cause additional *vasoconstriction* (decrease in the diameter of blood vessels) and higher

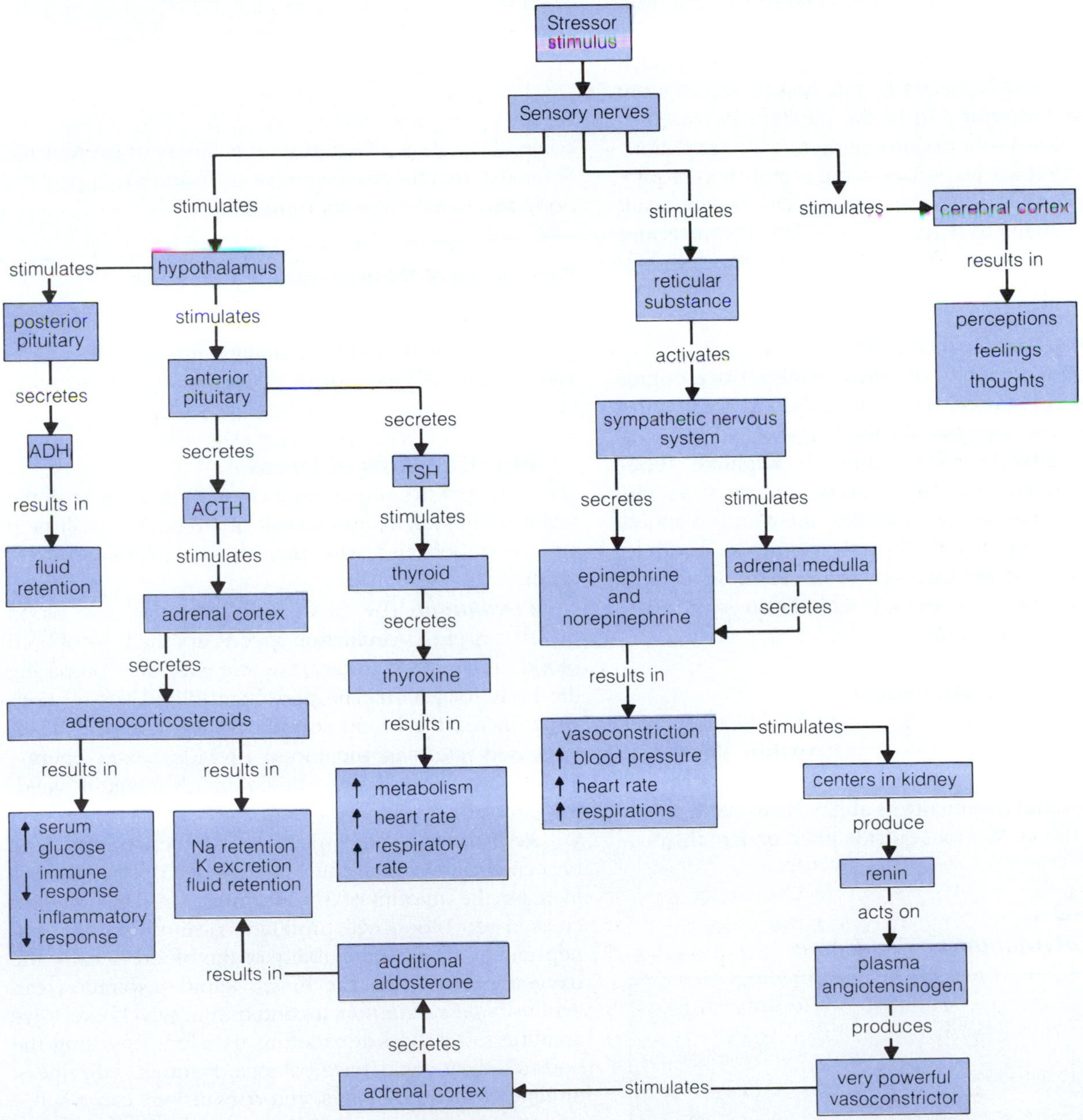

Figure 6-2. Physiologic processes of the general adaptation syndrome (GAS).

blood pressure. The kidneys are stimulated to release a hormone (renin) that raises blood pressure even further.

Simultaneously, the stimulation of the central nervous system causes a response in the hypothalamus (one of the structures of the brain). The hypothalamus activates the anterior pituitary gland, which in turn stimulates the adrenals through adrenocorticotropic hormones (ACTH) and the thyroid through thyroid-stimulating hormone (TSH).

The adrenal cortex increases its production of the adrenocorticosteroids (aldosterone and glucocorticoids), hormones that help to increase glucose content in the blood and to retain sodium and water in the body. These adrenocorticosteroids also depress the immune system, the body's ability to wall off organisms through inflammation, and therefore the increase in those hormones increases the risk of infection. The thyroid secretes an additional thyroid hormone, thyroxine, which increases the body's metabolic rate and produces more energy. The posterior part of the pituitary increases its release of ADH, further contributing to water retention.

These complex responses occur rapidly and require the body to use considerable energy. The overall result is enhanced ability to defend against outside threats and enhanced functioning as a result of optimum oxygenation and circulation (Display 6-2).

The Stage of Resistance

The body's adaptation to the stressor takes place during the **stage of resistance**. Having mobilized its abilities, the body neutralizes or destroys the threat. Production of hormones starts decreasing through **negative feedback**. In other words, as the levels of hormones rise and there is no further stressor stimulus, the glands respond by decreasing production. Thus, the hormones return to prestress levels. When the body is successful in its fight against the threat, the GAS ends with the stage of resistance as homeostasis is restored.

The Stage of Exhaustion

If the stage of resistance is not successful, the body may enter a third stage, the **stage of exhaustion**. This stage, a prolonged state of preparedness, depletes the body's energy stores and eventually its ability to maintain resistance to the threat. Without outside intervention, the outcome of the stage of exhaustion is illness or even death. Some external mechanism must be found to support the body and make adaptation possible.

Display 6–2
The General Adaptation Syndrome

Stage 1: Alarm reaction
Stage 2: Resistance
Stage 3: Exhaustion

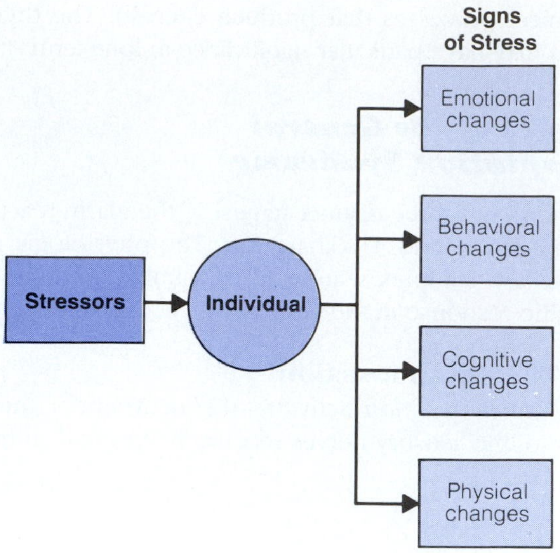

Figure 6-3. Stress causes multiple changes.

Signs and Symptoms of Stress

Stress is manifested in a variety of ways—physical, cognitive, emotional, and behavioral. Knowing these signs and symptoms will enable you to recognize stress in yourself and others (Fig. 6-3; Display 6-3).

Physical Signs of Stress

Let us review the physiologic changes that occur in the major body systems as a result of stress. This will help you to understand why the physical signs of stress occur.

Circulation. The heart rate increases and blood pressure rises. As circulation speeds up, the flow of both blood and oxygen to tissues increases, thus preparing the body for action. The peripheral blood vessels constrict, increasing blood supply to the brain and heart. Increased sugar in the blood provides extra energy. Fluid is retained. (This would be an advantage if bleeding occurred.)

Respiration. The respiratory rate increases and the bronchial passages in the lungs dilate. Both processes increase the amount of air exchanged in the lungs. Increased red blood cell production, stimulated by epinephrine, enhances the ability of the blood to carry the oxygen provided by the lungs. Rapid respiration can lead to *hyperventilation*, a condition in which excessive amounts of carbon dioxide are exhaled, upsetting the body's delicate acid–base balance. Faintness, dizziness, tingling of the extremities, and convulsions can result.

Digestion. Because of decreased production of di-

Display 6–3
Common Signs and Symptoms of Stress

Physical Signs

Circulation	Heart rate increased Blood pressure increased Peripheral vessel constriction Fluid retention
Respiration	Increcreased rate Increased depth
Digestion	Decreased secretions Decreased peristalsis Abdominal distention Nausea and vomiting Heartburn
Elimination	Frequency of urination Gas and constipation Diarrhea
Muscle tension	Headaches Clenching of jaw Grinding of teeth Backache
Metabolism	Increased blood sugar Decreased healing Decreased inflammation Fat mobilized

Cognitive Changes

Mild stress	Increased alertness Attention to detail Increased problem-solving ability Increased learning
Moderate stress	Narrowing of focus Decreased learning Decreased problem-solving ability
Severe stress	Tunnel vision Vacillating between decisions Impulsive decision making Clinging to ideas
Emotions	Tenseness Anxiety Irritability Inappropriately directed anger Decreased self-esteem Malaise Suspicion
Behavior	Tasks not completed Errors common Change in activity level Talk about self Rapid speech Scattered thoughts in speech Aggression with little provocation Purposeless or random activity

gestive enzymes and decreased *peristalsis* (muscular contractions that aid digestion), stress can result in anorexia, abdominal distention, nausea, and vomiting. Nutritional needs increase, however, making special attention to diet desirable. Possibly because the lining of the stomach becomes less resistant to acid stomach secretions, heartburn and even ulcers are common.

Elimination. Although urine production may decrease, frequency of urination may increase because of autonomic nervous system stimulation of the bladder. When peristalsis decreases, gas and constipation may result. In some cases, however, defecation increases in frequency to the point of diarrhea.

Muscle tension. Muscle tension in the head, back, and neck is a common symptom of stress. Tension headaches may result from the tensing of scalp and neck muscles. Some people grind their teeth because of tension of the jaw muscles. Backaches are common. At times, muscle tension is clearly visible; even when pain and discomfort are absent, muscle tension can sometimes be identified by palpating the muscle.

Metabolism. Many metabolic changes occur in stress. The increased production of glucose by the liver results in increased blood sugar concentration. The type of protein produced in the liver is changed, and this alteration slows healing. Calcium is mobilized from the bone, an effect that is not noticed in short-term stress but becomes significant when stress is prolonged. Fat is mobilized to provide more energy. Within cells, the membranes that contain inflammation-enhancing enzymes are stabilized, thus preventing the release of these enzymes and curbing inflammation.

Cognitive Changes Caused by Stress

Cognitive changes are those changes that involve thinking. Mild stress typically increases mental alertness and the ability to learn, to attend to details, and to solve problems, at least for a while. Energy, ability, and productivity are all likely to increase: the person feels "up."

As stress increases or persists, however, the thinking processes function less effectively. Learning becomes more difficult, and even simple instructions may be forgotten. Those about to undergo surgery, for example, often fail to remember instructions and information they have just received about preparation for surgery.

Severe or chronic stress undermines problem-solving ability. The severely stressed person is less able to remember information that would be helpful in problem solving, and his or her thinking may become so narrowly focused (a condition often called "tunnel vision") that pertinent ideas are not connected. Such a person's ability to weigh alternatives and make sound decisions is deficient. Vacillating among different positions is common, as is impulsive, ill-considered decision-making. However irrationally arrived at, the person may cling to a choice in the face of conflicting arguments in an effort to minimize feelings of uneasiness.

Stress also typically decreases the number of problems a person can deal with at one time. One problem may be approached successfully, but additional problems are likely to seem overwhelming.

Emotional Responses to Stress

In addition to changes in cognitive ability, unpleasant emotions also accompany high levels of stress. The most common feeling is tenseness or anxiety—the nonspecific feeling that something is wrong. When asked the source of these feelings, the person may not know; alternatively, the person may invoke one or several unconvincing explanations. As a result of this inner turmoil, irritability and anger may be directed at anyone with whom the person comes in contact. When you work with a person who is undergoing stress, it is helpful to remember that anger expressed is not usually a response to your behavior or personality but a response to the situation.

Stress typically undermines self-esteem and trust in one's own abilities. Loss of self-esteem is in turn often accompanied by self-centeredness and diminished ability to concern oneself with others' feelings and needs. All experiences tend to be interpreted as uniquely significant to oneself. For example, a person under stress might suspect that routine questions and procedures signify that the illness is more serious than he or she has been told. Such a person might also make unreasonable demands on family members.

As stress persists, malaise—a general lack of energy and ability to initiate action—may set in. A person may feel purposeless and adrift. Some people become depressed.

Behavioral Signs of Stress

People's behavior changes under stress in response to the foregoing physiologic, cognitive, and emotional changes. Tasks may be left undone or incomplete. Errors become more common. Some people become less active; others take on more tasks in an effort to alleviate the feelings they are experiencing. In both cases, actual accomplishment is diminished. Urging a person under severe stress to accept new responsibilities (such as self-care) may precipitate further problems. The focus of conversation tends to be the self. Speech may become more rapid. Conversation may be disjointed because of a tendency to lose one's train of thought and introduce scattered ideas.

Outbursts of anger accompanied by shouting, door-slamming, and other aggressive behavior may occur with relatively little provocation. Random, purposeless movement, such as pacing, jangling keys, and fiddling with one's hair and clothing, is common.

Adaptive Processes

The body adapts to daily stressors in many ways in addition to the GAS. At any time, various processes that meet basic needs are taking place within the body. These are called adaptive processes and are essential to the maintenance of homeostasis. Most of these processes are also controlled by the neuroendocrine system by means of feedback mechanisms, such as the ones discussed for stress, through which signals are sent to the neuroendocrine system, which responds by decreasing or stopping the adaptive process. In this way, a relatively steady state is maintained.

The kidneys are an important part of the constant adaptive process. They are able to conserve or excrete water and various body chemicals. The lungs are also important in that respirations can increase and/or decrease in both rate and depth depending on the needs of the body. The temperature-regulating mechanisms control dilation of vessels near the surface of the body so that heat may be conserved by constricting surface vessels or dissipated by dilating surface vessels. Increasing the circulation of blood close to the surface where heat may escape is another means by which temperature is regulated. As we discuss the various body systems throughout this book, we will try to help you understand how adaptation is facilitated in each system.

In addition to this constant nonspecific adaptation, the body has specific processes aimed at adaptation. These include the immune responses, the local adaptation syndrome, the macrophage system, and mechanisms for tissue healing and repair.

The Immune Responses

The **immune responses** are specific cell responses to specific types of stressors. The immune system is a complex combination of cells distributed throughout the body. Basically three types of cells in this system are responsible for the immune process. The *macrophage* is responsible for ingesting the foreign substance that enters the body, digesting it, and presenting portions of it to the lymphocytes for further action against it. There are two types of lymphocytes: the *T lymphocytes* that provide for *cellular immunity* and the *B lymphocytes* that form antibodies for *antibody-mediated* (**humoral**) **immunity**.

Macrophage Cells

The *macrophage cells*, formerly called the reticuloendothelial system, are in a network of tissues throughout the body—especially in the blood, general connective tissue, spleen, bone marrow, lymph nodes, mucosal tissue, and liver (where such cells are called Kupffer's cells). The function of this group of cells is the destruction of invading microorganisms in a process known as *phagocytosis*. Bacteria enter the body constantly through the lungs, through the mouth, through the bowel wall, and in many other ways. It is the macrophage system that continually destroys these invaders so that they do not cause a problem. In addition to initially destroying some invaders, the action of macrophages serves as one step in more extensive immune responses when they are necessary.

Cell-Mediated Immunity

Cell-mediated immunity is controlled by the T lymphocytes and the macrophages and acts against cancer cells, viruses, and foreign tissue. Two categories of T lymphocytes, *regulatory T cells* and *effector T cells*, are important in this process.

There are two types of regulatory T cells. The first type supports the action of the B lymphocytes and they are called *T helper cells*. These are the cells that are initially invaded by the human immunodeficiency virus (HIV). Those T cells that depress action of B lymphocytes are called *T suppressor cells*. The *effector T* cells produce and release lymphokines, which are important in causing the breakdown of the targeted foreign cells. Lymphokines also help to bring macrophages to these targeted cells. This process is responsible for destruction of new malignant cells and for the rejection of foreign tissue such as transplants. One type of effector T cell is called a *killer T cell*, which is able to cause death of the targeted cell.

Antibody-Mediated Immunity

The B lymphocytes develop into plasma cells, which can produce specific substances, known as **antibodies** or *immunoglobulins*, that are active against specific invading agents called **antigens**. These immunoglobulins are divided into five classes or groups. Each class is made by a different group of B lymphocytes and varies according to the type of antigen against which it acts. There are three methods by which the body develops antibody-mediated immunity: active immunity, passive immunity, and natural immunity (Table 6-2).

Active immunity. When certain types of antigens invade the body, the B lymphocytes initiate a process in which specific antibodies to that antigen are produced. It takes several days to 2 weeks for the body to produce a sufficient quantity of the antibody to completely destroy the antigen. However, this exposure provides the B lymphocytes with the "pattern" for making the antibody against this specific antigen. If the same antigen again invades the body, this antibody will be produced in large amounts quickly, thereby preventing illness. This process, which protects the body from subsequent episodes of certain viral diseases such as mumps and measles, is called **active immunity**.

Until the 19th century, the only active immunity that existed was that which occurred naturally: an invading antigen was destroyed after setting in motion the capacity for rapid antibody production, thus creating an immunity. Medical science has since developed a variety of ways to induce active immunity in individuals with-

Table 6–2. Types of Immunity

	Method by Which Acquired		
How Acquired	*Active (body produces own antibodies)*	*Passive (body receives antibodies from external source)*	*Natural*
Naturally acquired	Development of natural antibody in the course of certain viral and bacterial illnesses	Receipt of a specific antibody through the placenta or in mother's milk	Inborn genetic characteristic
Artificially acquired	Introduction of a specific antigen	Introduction of a specific antibody	

out their having active disease. Attenuated (non–disease-producing) virus may be introduced orally (such as poliomyelitis vaccine), by injection (such as diphtheria immunization), or by scratching or pricking the skin (such as smallpox vaccination).

All three methods provide for an artificially acquired active immunity that lasts all one's life. "Boosters" are necessary in the case of some conditions, such as tetanus, to reinvigorate the body's ability to produce antibodies. Active immunization is one of the cornerstones for maintaining general public health and protecting the community from epidemic infections.

Passive immunity. Immunity acquired through antibodies not produced by one's own body is called **passive immunity** because the body is not active in the process. An infant's acquisition of passive immunity through the placenta before birth and the mother's milk when breast-fed, is an example of natural acquisition. A person may also acquire passive immunity through an injection that contains antibodies, such as gamma (γ) globulin. This is called artificial acquisition. Passive immunity is effective for only a limited time. The body soon destroys the antibodies that were ingested or injected and, because it has not developed the ability to produce these antibodies, no residual immunity remains.

Providing passive immunity is important when it is known that a person is exposed to a disease and that the body will take a long time to produce sufficient antibodies. In that situation, providing the antibodies from an outside source will protect the individual from the effects of the disease. For example, if a person who is not immunized against tetanus is exposed to tetanus infection through a wound, the tetanus antibody can be given and tetanus infection can be prevented.

Antibodies for passive immunity are most commonly contained in antiserum or immune serum produced in cells from other species (such as egg or horse serum). Because these antisera are foreign proteins in the body, they have the potential to serve as strong antigens, producing a severe and potentially fatal allergic reaction called anaphylactic shock. Therefore, their use is limited to situations of critical need, and active immunization is encouraged whenever possible. In the case of a few diseases, human gamma globulin (which is one of the antibodies produced by the B lymphocytes) may be used to produce passive immunity. The human antibodies do not cause the widespread allergic reactions caused by antisera from other species. The use of gamma globulin is limited to prevention of diseases that are common in people because the donated blood from which the human gamma globulin is obtained must contain the appropriate antibody.

Natural immunity. Some antigens are not capable of producing illness in some organisms. This phenomenon is called **natural immunity**. The simplest type of natural immunity is that of entire species; certain viruses invade one species and not another. For example, there is a type of distemper that only cats acquire and another type that only dogs acquire. Human beings do not get either type. However, disease acquisition is a complex process and many factors may be interacting to produce any particular disease; therefore, the extent of natural immunity is difficult to determine.

The Complement System

The complement system is composed of a specific group of proteins that are always present in the circulating blood. These proteins attach themselves to foreign cells and facilitate the other immune processes. They attract the macrophages and help to stimulate the release of histamines and other cell chemicals that are active in inflammation. They help to destroy the cell membrane of the invader and modify it, making it more vulnerable to macrophage attack. Finally, they help to adhere the immune cells to the antigen and adhere both to the vessels wall where the immune process can be completed.

Interferons

Interferons are a group of proteins produced by cells. They act on the gene to prevent the cells from replicating the virus that invades the cell. Interferons are not specific to the invading virus, as an antibody is, but act on all viruses. Interferon from animals is not effective in human beings; therefore, until recently it was difficult to study interferons because the only source was human leukocytes. Recent research in which the genetic material in bacteria has been altered and recombined (recombinant DNA research) offers promise of greater knowledge about the use of interferons. Other areas of research include methods to increase the body's production of its own interferon.

Local Adaptation Syndrome

The body has several means of responding to localized threats, such as a bacterial invasion. These responses limit the effects of a physiologic stressor and establish the preconditions for restoration of homeostasis to the affected body part. Selye (1956) termed these processes the **local adaptation syndrome** (LAS) to differentiate them from generalized responses to stressors. According to Selye, the LAS is also characterized by the three stages of alarm, resistance, and exhaustion. When the stage of exhaustion is reached in the LAS, general body responses are called on.

The Inflammatory Response

The inflammatory response is a type of LAS in which the body produces localized tissue changes that confine the injurious agent and prepare the area for destruction of the agent and subsequent healing.

Inflammation has many different causes. Infection by a microorganism is one. Others include dead tissue, wounds, and trauma to tissue. The common element is the process the body institutes to repair the tissue. The ending *-itis* is used to designate an inflammatory condition, as in arthritis (inflammation of a joint) and iritis (inflammation of the iris of the eye). You will learn that some conditions designated *-itis* are always caused by infection (such as appendicitis), whereas others (such as tendinitis) rarely involve infection. Therefore, it is important that you explore each term individually and not make an assumption about the cause from the suffix alone.

Signs of inflammation. The immediately apparent signs of inflammation are redness and heat from increased blood supply, swelling from the movement of fluid from vascular spaces to the interstitial spaces, pain, and decreased function (Display 6-4). These five signs are often called the **cardinal signs of inflammation**. You have probably observed these signs many times in such varied locations as a sprained ankle and the area around a large cut. You may also have experienced the effects of an inflammation in an internal organ you cannot see. For example, you may have had an irritated, inflamed stomach, the signs of which were pain and decreased function in the form of nausea, the accumulation of gas, and belching. The redness and swelling were no doubt present, but not visible without a special examination. The temperature of the tissue cannot be ascertained.

Mediators of inflammation. A *mediator* is a body chemical that causes other substances or tissues to react. A variety of body chemicals serve as mediators of inflammation. *Histamine*, one of the major mediators, affects the blood vessels in the area of the injury, causing them to become more permeable, so that large molecules of protein and white blood cells can leave the circulatory system and move into the tissue more easily. *Prostaglandins*, another group of mediators, act on blood vessels, causing them to dilate; they also cause contraction of muscles, which may result in pain. Other actions of prostaglandins are currently being studied. *Plasma kinins* also cause blood vessels to dilate, act on smooth muscle, and stimulate nerve endings, causing pain. Other mediators have been identified and are being explored; this entire area of physiology is receiving considerable attention from researchers.

White Blood Cell Responses in Inflammation

White blood cells, *leukocytes*, are active in coping with the injurious agent. As the vessels dilate, the blood flow slows. The fluid portion of the blood moves out through the more permeable vessel walls. This movement causes the white blood cells to move toward the vessel walls (a process called *margination*), form a cobblestone-like layer along the wall (a process called *pavementing*), and leave the vessel in large numbers (a process called *emigration*). The white cells move purposefully toward the injurious agent in a process called *chemotaxis*. Chemotaxis can be affected by the nature of the injurious agent, the chemicals released, and the effect of the plasma protein called complement.

The bone marrow responds by releasing increased numbers of white blood cells in a process called *leukocytosis*. There are three major groups of white cells: granulocytes, monocytes, and lymphocytes. The granulocytes are divided into polymorphonuclear neutrophils, eosinophils, and basophils. Each type of white blood cell has specific functions in the inflammatory process, and each type may be present in proportions that differ depending on the nature of the injurious agent and how long the inflammatory process has been present. A white blood cell count may be done to measure the total number of white cells. A differential blood count, often called a "dif," provides both the total number of white blood cells and the percentage of each different type. This differential count may aid in determining the source of the inflammation and whether it is an acute or chronic condition.

Vascular and Fluid Changes

Initially the small arteries serving the area of injury dilate (vasodilation), increasing the blood supply, and any small capillaries that were not full then fill with blood. The blood vessels become more permeable, allowing fluid and proteins to leave the vessel and move into the interstitial spaces. This fluid is called an *exudate* and is responsible for swelling. Each of the five different types of exudate has a different content.

Serous exudate is fluid with a low protein content.

Display 6–4
Cardinal Signs of Inflammation

1. Redness
2. Heat
3. Swelling
4. Pain
5. Decreased function

It usually is the first fluid to appear in the inflamed area. The fluid in a blister and the secretion from the nose during hay fever are both serous exudate. *Fibrinous exudate* contains the compound fibrinogen and forms a thick mesh, as the fibers in a blood clot (the fibrin network). Fibrinous exudate causes the growth of scar tissue and adhesions where it remains; however, it is effective in controlling the spread of infection. *Membranous exudate* develops on a mucous membrane surface and forms a cohesive membrane. This may be seen in the bowel in pseudomembranous colitis, which may occur as a toxic response to certain drugs and in a membranous exudate formed on the throat in diphtheria that sometimes interferes with breathing. *Purulent exudate* contains white blood cells, protein, and debris from bacterial and tissue destruction. It occurs in the presence of certain pus-forming (pyogenic) bacteria. Infected skin wounds contain purulent exudate. *Hemorrhagic exudate*, also called *sanguineous exudate*, contains red blood cells and occurs when a vessel has been damaged or when capillaries become so permeable that red blood cells can migrate through them. Exudates may also be combinations of the above types. For example, serosanguineous exudate is a combination of serous exudate and hemorrhagic exudate.

Resolution of Inflammation

Resolution occurs when the leukocytes have completely destroyed the injurious agent. The stimulus to the inflammatory process is ended, the fluid that caused swelling is reabsorbed, the capillaries return to normal permeability, and vasodilation ceases. The fibrin network is reabsorbed, and normal structure and function are restored. The tissue that was inflamed is left exactly as it was before the inflammation started. This is the ideal ending of inflammation.

Supporting Resolution of Inflammation

In the initial stage of the inflammatory process, the use of cold packs causes vasoconstriction, which tends to decrease swelling. This process helps minimize pain and loss of function. When capillary permeability has returned to normal (in approximately 24–48 hours), heat is used to increase circulation, which in turn promotes resolution of the inflammation. Anti-inflammatory drugs may be prescribed by the physician to decrease the inflammatory response.

Chronic Inflammation

Acute inflammation, like a sprained ankle, is usually rapidly controlled, but certain types of inflammation, such as rheumatoid arthritis, are not resolved for weeks, months, or even years. These chronic inflammations appear to involve an immune response rather than simply a local response. The same kinds of exudates do not develop in chronic inflammation; rather, vascular structures and fibroblasts (cells that create connective tissue) increase in number. There is more chance for tissue damage that will result in deformity. In other cases of chronic inflammation, small (1- to 2-mm) lesions called granulomas form. These form around small foreign bodies (such as a splinter) and some microorganisms (such as the tuberculosis bacillus). They may remain in place for years or until some additional stimulus causes the inflammation to become acute again.

Tissue Healing and Repair

Whenever tissue has been damaged by trauma, microorganisms, or the inflammatory process itself, a repair process is initiated. If possible, the body heals the tissue itself, providing new cells of the same type to replace damaged ones. This process is called **regeneration**. Sometimes the body is unable to replace the cells with the same tissue, and scar tissue is used to complete the repair process. Scar tissue repairs the structure of the tissue but does not replace the cellular function. This may not be a concern if the tissue is primarily supportive in nature but may be a serious problem if the cells replaced had important functions.

Regeneration occurs with ease in skin and mucous membranes unless the area of injury is large or deep. Some tissues, such as those in the liver and the kidney, regenerate well if the underlying structure was not damaged by the inflammation. If the structure was damaged, the new cells regenerate in a haphazard pattern and are not functional. Bone tissue regenerates well, recovering complete function in most instances. Regeneration is limited in muscle tissue and does not occur at all in the heart muscle. Muscle that has been severely damaged and replaced with scar tissue may be less able to contract and in addition may be more susceptible to injury from strain. Neurons (nerve cells) do not ordinarily seem to regenerate at all after early childhood, although the processes (the projecting strands) of the nerve cell body may regrow if the body of the nerve cell is intact. Experiments are being conducted concerning techniques for encouraging nerve regeneration.

Factors Affecting Healing

The speed and completeness of the healing are affected by many different factors (Display 6-5). Some of these can be manipulated to enhance healing; others must be accepted as unchangeable.

Nutritional status can greatly change the rate of healing. To build new tissue, the body must have all the components available. Protein, vitamins C and A, iron, and zinc are particularly important. There must also be

Display 6–5
Factors Affecting Healing

Age
Nurtitional status
Oxygen supply
Circulation
Hormone status
Rest
Foreign material present
Necrotic tissue present
Infection present
Tissue separation or movement

enough calories to provide the extra energy needed for the healing process. Nutrition is one factor that can be altered to facilitate healing. This subject will be discussed more completely in Chapter 25.

Oxygen is essential for the body's metabolic processes to proceed effectively. When an individual has a lung disorder that interferes with adequate oxygenation of the blood, healing will be delayed. Extra oxygen may be provided, but this is not effective if the lungs are not capable of gas exchange. Some work is being tried using hyperbaric oxygen, which is oxygen under high pressure, to increase the oxygen supply in tissues. This technique appears to enhance healing in some situations.

Circulation to the affected area must be adequate for the necessary nutritional components and the oxygen to arrive where they are needed. The adequacy of circulation is of particular concern with elderly persons because they often have compromised circulation caused by disease processes. Circulation may also be a problem in a lower extremity or in an area where the blood vessels were damaged.

Hormones in the body can influence the rate of healing. Some hormones, such as the male androgens, are anabolic, that is, they promote the production of tissue. Other hormones, such as the adrenocorticosteroids, which are secreted in stress and are given to people for many disease states, slow healing.

Age is an important factor in the speed and completeness of healing (Fig. 6-4). The younger the individual, the faster the healing process. In the young person the body cells are still growing and replicating rapidly, and the entire metabolic and hormonal pattern is structured to support growth. Therefore, when healing is necessary, this pattern supports rapid, thorough healing. As an individual ages, the pattern changes, and tissue repair is slower. For example, a fractured femur in a newborn may heal completely in 3 weeks, but in a person 70 years of age it may take 6 months.

Rest is necessary for the body to use its energy stores for the healing process. The need for rest is a major concern when a large area requires healing. For example, after surgery, a person may need to plan for rest periods during the day as well as for adequate sleep at night to allow the body to repair itself. Those who do not get sufficient rest may find their healing delayed.

Foreign material present in the tissue can impede healing. Until the foreign material is removed, the stim-

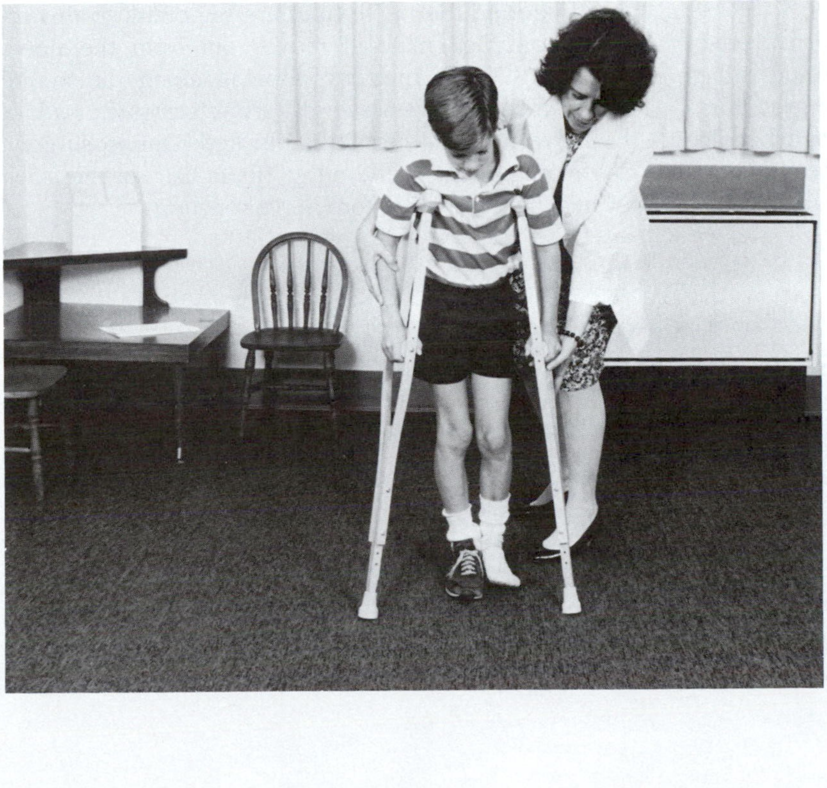

Figure 6–4. Age is an important factor affecting healing.

ulus for a continuing inflammatory response is present and exudate continues to form. *Necrotic* (dead and decaying) *tissue* can act in the same way to prevent healing. In most cases the body is able to break down necrotic tissue through enzyme action and then remove the products, but when large amounts of necrotic tissue are present, the body is unable to do this adequately. Necrotic tissue may then need to be removed surgically to allow tissue to heal. This procedure is called *debridement.* Infection in a wound also continues tissue destruction and the stimulus for inflammation. Until the infection is controlled, either by the action of the body's own defenses or by the use of medication, the wound will not heal.

Tissue separation or movement will interfere with healing by requiring that large areas be filled with tissue and by constantly breaking down the new tissue being formed. In soft tissues this causes only a moderate problem because the tissue is flexible. In rigid tissue such as bone, movement may completely destroy the ability to heal, leaving a broken bone permanently separated.

Soft-Tissue Healing

Three types of soft-tissue healing occur. **First intention healing** results when the edges of the tissue are touching. A blood clot holds the edges together as connective tissue cells move out and close the gap (Figure 6-5). Healing occurs all along the surface at the same time, and the result is little or no scarring. In tissue where there is tension, sutures may be needed to hold the edges together until the tissue is strong enough to do so. Surgical wounds are examples of wounds that heal by first intention.

Second intention healing occurs when the edges of tissue are not touching and granulation tissue (which becomes scar tissue) must gradually fill the gap. Burns on the skin and surgical wounds that have become infected heal by second intention. During the inflammatory process, the macrophages invade the area and remove microorganisms and cellular debris. Then fibroblasts, which are connective tissue cells, and vascular endothelial cells begin to enter the area. By the third to the fifth day, small blood vessels are forming in the area, and soft pink granulation tissue is visible in the bottom of the wound. This tissue is fragile because of the new cells it contains. Gradually, granulation tissue is built up from the bottom of the wound. As tissue development progresses, more connective tissue is formed, and the blood vessels begin to degenerate. The connective tissue fibers contract and form the dense tissue that is the scar. Scars tend to continue to contract, and this contraction may contribute to functional and cosmetic problems on the skin surface. In internal tissues, the contracting scar may put traction on organs such as the bowel, causing pain and dysfunction. Internal scars of this type are called *adhesions.*

Bone Healing

The first stage of bone healing is like soft-tissue healing. A blood clot occurs between the ends of the bone, and a type of granulation tissue called *procallus* then forms. Next, osteoblasts, which are bone-forming cells, enter the area and form a cartilaginous tissue called *callus,* which is similar to bone but does not have the calcium salts in it. Then the tissue is remodeled and calcium salts are laid down, resulting in strong bone.

Nerve Healing

Although cells of nerves do not regenerate, the peripheral nerve fibers do. The Schwann cells that form the sheath around the nerve fiber are important to this regeneration. Cell material moves out from the nerve stump at 1 or 2 mm/day, moving along the neural sheath. If connective tissue scar grows across the path of the nerve fiber, its growth is blocked. During surgery, careful alignment of the nerve fibers can set the stage for healing that will restore nerve function.

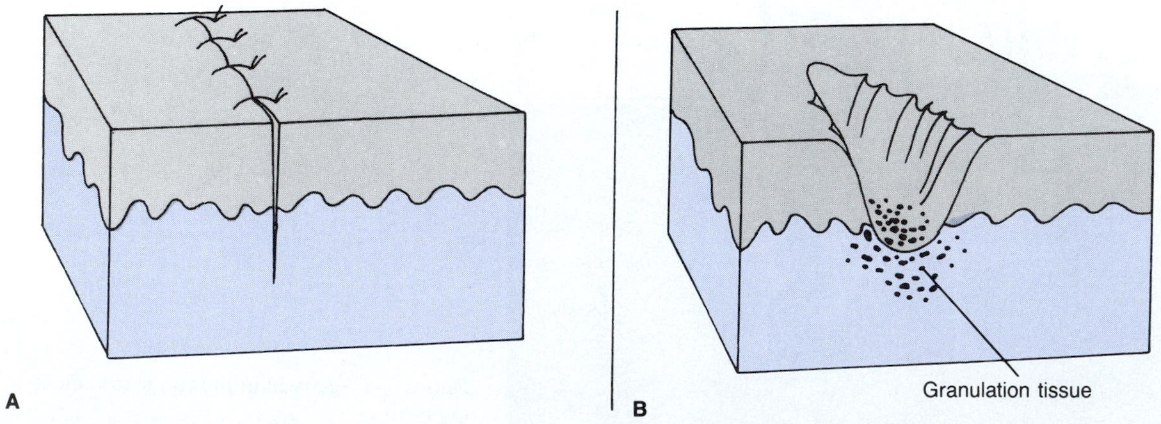

Figure 6-5. Soft-tissue healing.

Stress and Illness

The role of excessive stress in illness is receiving growing attention from researchers. It is widely believed that constant stress depletes the body's resources, making it more susceptible to additional stressors that may act on it. This hypothesis helps explain why an individual may develop a cold in one instance but not another when exposed to two identical viruses. Holmes and Rahe (1967) state that the likelihood of physical illness increases with an increase in total stress points. Their research has led them to conclude that individuals who score higher than 300 points on their scale have a 90% chance of becoming ill within a year. A score of 150 to 300 points means a 50% chance of becoming ill, and a score of fewer than 150 points indicates a 10% to 20% chance of illness. Such illness may be major or minor, and of course, its exact nature cannot be predicted. Thus, Holmes and Rahe advocate efforts to limit the number of stress-producing changes in one's life at a given time.

Aspects of the stress response itself may also develop into chronic conditions. An example is increased blood pressure. Unremitting stress may produce chronic high blood pressure, which in turn may bring about potentially dangerous illness.

Prolonged stress can also cause body organs or systems to break down. Stress ulcers in the stomach and inflammation in the colon are examples. Although researchers have tried to link specific stressors to specific illnesses, such efforts have not yet met with success. It may be that the specific illness an individual develops is more dependent on basic genetic makeup and physiology than on the nature of the stressor.

When new stressors are superimposed on existing illness, they may interfere with the body's ability to cope with that illness, which may then become more severe or overwhelming. A constant state of stress may also arouse unpleasant emotions, such as anxiety or depression. If these feelings become severe enough to impair the individual's ability to function, they may require treatment.

Conversely, reducing the number or magnitude of stressors may increase the body's ability to cope with existing illness. A stable and supportive emotional life enhances one's ability to cope with physical illness, just as sound physical health enables one to cope better with emotional stressors.

Coping with Stress

Coping is a process by which a person continues to participate in daily life and meet role responsibilities in the face of stressors. At its most basic, coping is getting up in the morning and putting both feet on the floor and acting despite whatever distressing feelings are present. In some situations of severe stress, this may be initially all that can be expected. For example, those whose homes were destroyed in a tornado, who found shelter for their families, notified relatives, and participated in cleanup efforts were coping effectively although they were experiencing overwhelming emotions. However, the most effective long-term coping techniques relieve the tension created by stress and help the individual to solve problems and make decisions.

In addition to deliberately chosen actions, some coping processes are automatic or unconscious; these are termed **coping mechanisms** or **defense mechanisms**. They effectively help to lessen feelings of tension and therefore can be valuable to the individual for providing a short period of relief from overwhelming feelings and perhaps allowing energy to be restored. These mechanisms have limitations, however, because they do not lead to resolution of the problem that is creating the feelings of distress or tension. These coping mechanisms—regression, rationalization, repression, suppression, denial, compensation, sublimation, substitution, projection, displacement, identification, reaction formation, conversion, restitution, and fantasy—will be discussed more completely in Chapter 34.

Still another important way to cope with stress is the deliberate use of strategies that relieve the tension and therefore may make constructive action or problem solving more possible. These strategies are usually referred to as stress management strategies. They are necessary for everybody, but especially for those who work in high stress occupations such as nursing and for those who already face a severe illness. As you read this section, you might review your own stress management strategies, evaluate their effectiveness, and determine whether you need to expand your repertoire.

Each individual—nurse, client, anyone else—needs some individual mode for stress management. Some of the techniques available can have exceptionally positive effects but only with considerable time and persistence. All require the individual to be an active participant, not a passive recipient, of treatment. **Behavior modification** techniques—the reinforcement of desired behavior—appear to be especially well suited to teaching responses that must become semiautomatic to be effective, such as relaxing instead of tensing one's back muscles when angry. Some people may find a given technique helpful for moderate stress, but less so for severe stress.

Eliminating Stressors

The best way of managing stress may be to eliminate the stressor from one's life. Physical causes of stress are commonly handled this way. You protect yourself from the cold, for example, by wearing adequate clothing. You avoid foods to which you are allergic, and you come in out of the rain. But it is usually much more difficult to eliminate psychosocial stressors from our lives. Sometimes this is the result of ambivalence: if a certain situation causes stress but also has the potential to elicit pleasure or growth, one may be unwilling to abandon it. Sometimes it is impossible to eliminate stress. For example, a particular job might be severely stressful but, for a variety of reasons, essential. Willingness to examine the stressors in one's life openly and honestly can be productive. People under stress often fail to recognize the alternatives available to them. It may be possible, for example, to find a less stressful job, give up an expensive club membership, or stop socializing with a difficult neighbor. Alternatively, one can often eliminate several minor stressors, thus freeing resources to cope with a major stressor that cannot be avoided.

Increasing Resistance to Stress

Maintaining a high level of general health is important for maintaining adaptation and coping with stress. Remember that each individual is a whole person in whom one process cannot be separated from all others. Sound nutrition, which provides the body with the nutrients needed for energy, development, and repair, is essential. The components of meeting nutritional needs will be discussed in detail in Chapter 25. Regular activity that conditions muscles and the cardiovascular and respiratory systems is another essential component of good health. This will be discussed in Chapters 23 and 29. Adequate rest and sleep are also essential for health and are discussed in Chapter 24.

A healthful lifestyle also includes adopting safety measures such as wearing seat belts in automobiles and helmets when bicycling. Avoiding health-damaging habits such as smoking, taking drugs, and drinking excessive alcohol is important to health maintenance. Seeking appropriate health care such as immunizations, physical examinations, and screening tests are additional ways to promote health. All of these actions can assist an individual to cope effectively.

It is also possible to become more resistant psychosocially to stress. People who cope effectively with small problems and stressors as they arise develop skills that will prove useful when stress is high. Treating small problems as challenges to learn coping skills can set the stage for handling stress in the future.

One productive way to help others cope with stress is to encourage them to review successful coping methods they have used in the past. Doing so can promote sound problem solving in the current situation. Stress seems to be more easily tolerated if one feels in control of the situation. The sense of control is achieved by making conscious choices and decisions and undermined by allowing others to direct one's life.

Basic Life Skills

Psychosocial stress can arise from an inability to manage the day-to-day tasks of adult life, such as organizing one's time, budgeting finances, communicating assertively, and sharing one's feelings with others. Individuals may handle such daily tasks well but have trouble making sound, well timed decisions about major changes in their lives. Some people need help identifying the skills they lack and deciding where to seek assistance. Learning to manage ordinary tasks well tends to enhance self-image as well as reduce stress. Classes in *basic life skills* are widely available and nurses may refer clients to these resources.

Physical Activity

In addition to helping the body resist stressors more effectively, physical activity helps prevent the cyclic neurohormone patterns that keep the GAS activated when stress occurs. Purposeful physical discharge of accumulated tension acts as negative feedback, preventing the stress response from persisting beyond its usefulness. If you are tense just before a test, for example, you might benefit more from jogging around the block than from sitting and worrying. Vigorous exercise expends nervous energy and enables you to focus more usefully on the test itself (Fig. 6-6).

Humor

Humor is commonly used as a coping strategy. Successful coping humor tends to be that which promotes an alternative appraisal of the situation at hand and enhances feelings of mastery. For example, a middle-aged person may cope with the problem of decreasing close vision by joking that it improves the appearance of others by putting them in "soft focus." Humor may also provide a temporary psychological escape from a difficult situation.

Laughter physiologically relieves tension, leaving a more relaxed feeling in its wake. During laughter the respiratory rate and depth increase; there is an increase in endorphins (neurohormones that relieve pain and increase feelings of well-being); and immune system response is enhanced. According to Berk and Tan (1989) serum cortisol levels decrease with laughter and mirthful laughter increases spontaneous lymphocyte production and natural killer T cell activity. Immunoglobulins, especially IgA, increase as individuals use humor to cope

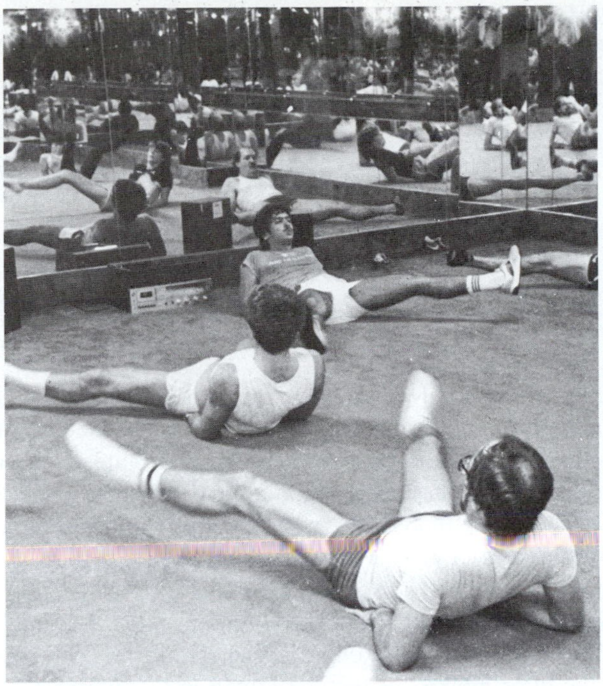

Figure 6-6. Physical activity is an effective method for decreasing stress.

with stress (Lefcourt, 1988; Dillon, 1985) and when individuals are in a positive mood (Stone, 1987).

Norman Cousins (1974) used laughter as part of his personal strategy for fighting a serious autoimmune disease. He chronicled the illness and his recovery in *Anatomy of An Illness.* Hospitals with "in-house" television channels used for patient education may also add cartoons and comedy shows to these channels to provide hospitalized patients with access to the benefits of humor. Health care workers may use humor as a way to cope with their own stress while working.

To use humor effectively for clients, you must establish your professional competence and a trusting relationship first. When you have established that relationship, you can then try limited, light humor to see how the individual responds. Some individuals are not comfortable with humor from health care professionals. If this is true, then you should not use humor. Effective humor does not offend people; therefore, you should avoid all sexual, religious, or ethnic comments. Many individuals welcome the atmosphere that carefully chosen humor creates.

Spiritual Resources

For many individuals, their spiritual beliefs are an important part of their coping strategy. In a study of elderly persons, Manfredi and Pickett (1987) identified that prayer was one of the two most common coping strategies used to respond to the major stressors of loss and conflict. Values, beliefs, and supporting spiritual resources are discussed more completely in Chapter 36.

Maintaining Support Systems

An individual's **support system** is composed of the people who offer emotional and practical support. The members of one's support system may include family members, friends, neighbors, coworkers, and anyone with whom one has a caring relationship. A sound support system is important in stress management. Human beings live in community with each other, and concerned and caring people can serve as the solid foundations in one another's lives. Sharing difficulties and concerns often makes them seem less overwhelming and helps identify ways of overcoming them. Occasionally one needs to transfer responsibilities and tasks to someone else temporarily to lighten one's load. The concern of others also promotes feelings of self-worth, important in coping successfully with stress. When clients need additional social support, they may be referred to support groups such as those operated by the American Cancer Society for people with cancer and their families. When a group includes others who have experienced the stressor with which you are coping, it offers a particularly valuable resource. Throughout this text we will provide you with names of organized support groups to whom you might refer an individual client. Appendix E provides a brief list of support resources you might find useful to clients.

Biofeedback

Biofeedback is a means of monitoring a biologic process, such as temperature or blood flow, by machine and using feedback from the machine to learn to alter that process. Biofeedback may be used in stress management to provide information on circulatory or vascular responses to stressors. By identifying and learning to control an undesirable response, such as rising blood pressure, one may be able to minimize the detrimental effects of stress. Learning to use biofeedback is time-consuming, and refresher courses may be necessary to maintain the skill.

Therapeutic Massage

A variety of approaches to massage are used to relieve muscle tension and promote relaxation. In some states massage therapists must have completed a brief educational program and be licensed to practice. Those who use therapeutic massage often report the relief of backaches and headaches related to stress. Massage promotes a general feeling of well-being, releases endorphins (neurochemicals that decrease pain), and enhances circulation.

The Relaxation Response

The **relaxation response**, a state characterized by decreased sympathetic nervous system activity, decreased muscle tone, pupil constriction, decreased blood pressure, decreased heart rate, and decreased respirations, can also counteract the effects of stress (Benson et al., 1974). An overview is presented in Display 6-6.

Four conditions must be present to initiate the relaxation response: 1) an environment with minimal stimuli; 2) minimal muscular activity and decreased muscle tone; 3) a mental device to help shift one's thoughts away from the source of stress; and 4) a mentally passive attitude (Benson et al., 1974).

Many different approaches are used to teach people to invoke the relaxation response at will. Most of the following techniques are subject to ongoing research.

Progressive Relaxation

Progressive relaxation is a method of ending muscle tension associated with stress. It was first described in 1938 by Jacobson. The first step is to help the person identify tight muscles and evidence of tension. Then the individual is taught to relax these muscles voluntarily. One way of doing so is to alternately tighten and relax specific muscles, beginning with the feet and gradually moving upward until the whole body is relaxed. After learning to relax progressively, some people learn to invoke relaxation of the entire body at will. This response can then be used in situations of stress.

Meditation

Although *meditation* has been practiced for hundreds of years in various Christian mystic and Far Eastern traditions, it has received widespread popular attention in this country only in the last 25 years. The meditation method most widespread in the United States is transcendental meditation, the conceptual structure and vocabulary of which are drawn from Hindu religious thought and religious terminology. Many Americans, however, pursue transcendental meditation as an aid to life enrichment and stress management rather than as a religious experience. Religious beliefs are not essential to the effectiveness of these meditation techniques.

Meditation invokes the relaxation response by helping one structure one's thoughts and actions to shut out stimuli. Meditation is practiced in a quiet, private, pleasant place. The position of the body is one that tends to promote relaxation and decrease muscle tension (Fig. 6-7). Repetition of a word or phrase is used as a mental device to focus one's attention.

Meditation produces definite changes in the brain wave pattern measured on an electroencephalograph. Sympathetic nervous system activity also appears to be diminished. People who regularly practice meditation report that they feel an increased sense of well-being and are calmer, less nervous, and able to function more effectively. Meditation requires a significant investment of time, both to learn and to practice (Wallace and Benson, 1972).

Display 6–6
The Relaxation Response

1. Decreased sympathetic nervous system activity
2. Minimal muscular activity
3. Decreased blood pressure
4. Decreased heart rate
5. Decreased respiratory rate

Nursing Research: *Implications for Practice*

Pruitt, R.H. *Effectiveness and Cost Efficiency of Interventions in Health Promotion.* Dissertation. University of Maryland at Baltimore, 1989.

The effectiveness and cost efficiency of a stress management health promotion program in a group of U.S. Army employees was studied. These individuals attended a stress management class taught by a nurse and then practiced relaxation on a daily basis. A control group did not attend the health promotion program. The individuals in the program showed significant differences in their stress-related physical symptoms and significantly lower systolic blood pressure. The researcher also analyzed the results from a cost perspective and concluded that this health promotion program was cost effective.

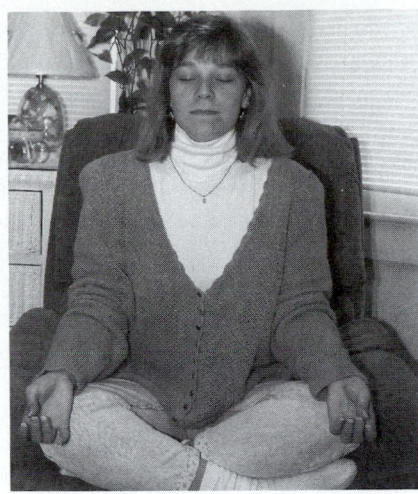

Figure 6-7. The relaxation response can be induced in a variety of ways.

Autogenic Training

Autogenic training is a set of exercises designed to help one focus on physical sensations and autonomic body processes. The exercises teach systematic concentration on heaviness of the limbs, warmth in limbs, calm regular heartbeat, slow deep breathing, warmth in the abdomen, and coolness of the forehead (Schultz and Luthe, 1959). Through this technique psychosocial stressors are shut out and the relaxation response invoked.

Self-Hypnosis

Self-hypnosis—inducing a hypnotic state in oneself at will—is sometimes taught as a stress management technique. A hypnotic state is a form of relaxation response in which external stimuli can be completely shut out. Some individuals are successful at this technique, which requires a professional instructor and an investment of time to master. Others are not able to use self-hypnosis even with extensive instruction.

Guided Imagery

Guided imagery is a process in which a person is helped to create a mental image that is positive to shut out other stimuli. The person chooses the image (such as an ocean beach or a peaceful meadow) and then is helped to focus on that image through a quiet, soothing, monologue from another person. As the person focuses more and more completely on the image, he or she can block out unpleasant stimuli such as pain or nausea.

Psychotherapy and Counseling

Mental health professionals use a variety of psychotherapeutic techniques to help individuals learn to manage stress. When you study the care of clients with mental health problems, you will learn about types of therapeutic intervention. Unfortunately, segments of society still stigmatize those who seek counseling help and this may affect the willingness of clients to take advantage of these services.

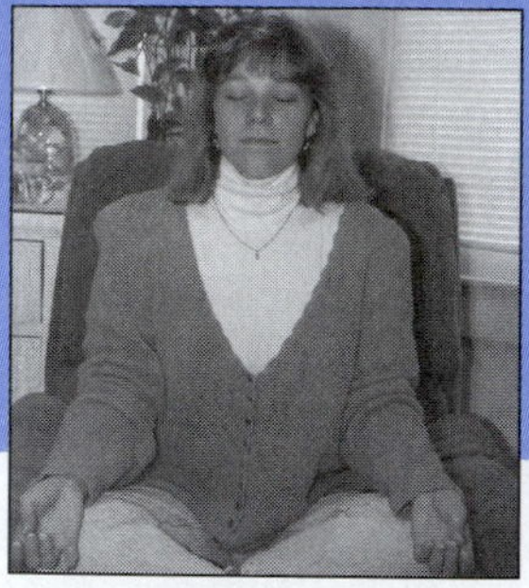

Key Points

- A stressor is a stimulus that poses a real or perceived threat to homeostasis and may interfere with meeting basic needs.
- Stress is an internal response of the individual to a stressor.
- A person responds to stressors through adaptive processes that are designed to meet the person's basic needs and prevent a disturbance of homeostasis.
- Stressors may be internal, external, physical, or psychological. Their impact is affected by the perception of the individual, the magnitude of the stressor, the duration of the stressor, the number of stressors occurring at one time, and prior experiences with the particular stressor.
- The general adaptation syndrome (GAS) is a physiologic response of the body to any type of threat. It consists of three major stages, and its purpose is to make the person more able to resist the threat.
- Stress that does not disturb homeostasis and that prepares the person to meet greater stressors has been termed eustress. Stress that is extreme and prolonged and interferes with homeostasis is called distress.
- Physical signs of stress include changes in circulation, respiration, digestion, elimination, muscle tension, and metabolism. Cognitive changes include changes in thinking patterns.
- Tenseness and anxiety often accompany stress as well as changes in behavior and less effective overall functioning.
- Certain types of stressors result in an immune response. Humoral immunity may be either actively or passively acquired and prevents the development of certain infectious diseases. Cell-mediated immunity is controlled by lymphocytes and macrophages. It causes the breakdown of unwanted cells. Complement facilitates the success of the various immune processes.
- Interferons protect cells from viruses that invade them and are a subject of special research seeking to identify ways they might be used to combat disease.
- Inflammation is a type of local adaptive process that produces localized tissue changes that can help to contain and resolve disease processes. The cardinal signs of inflammation are redness, heat, swelling, pain, and decreased function.
- Exudate is the fluid responsible for swelling, and it may be serous, fibrinous, membranous, purulent, or hemorrhagic in nature.
- Macrophage cells help to protect the body against microorganisms that enter through mucous membranes or open wounds and help to initiate the inflammatory process.
- Both cold and heat are used to assist in the resolution of inflammation. Inflammation may become chronic and create permanent tissue damage.
- Regeneration is the process by which damaged cells are replaced with identical functional cells. The healing process is affected by nutritional status, oxygen supply, circulation, hormones, age, rest, the presence of foreign or necrotic material, infection, and tissue separation.
- Soft tissue may heal by first intention and by second intention.
- Bone heals by a process of callus formation.
- Nerve cells do not regenerate, but peripheral nerve fibers can regenerate if scar tissue does not block the pathway.
- Coping with stress is important in maintaining health. Methods of stress management include physical activity, the relaxation response, increased attention to basic life skills, support systems, biofeedback, and psychotherapy and counseling.

Study Questions

1. How is adaptation related to stressors?
2. How do stressors differ?
3. What causes the general adaptation syndrome?
4. List physical, cognitive, emotional, and behavioral signs and symptoms of stress.
5. What is the relaxation response?
6. Name at least three ways in which the relaxation response can be initiated.
7. Describe three additional methods of reducing stress.
8. What type of immunity occurs when you have chickenpox?
9. What causes the swelling of inflammation?
10. List factors that affect healing.

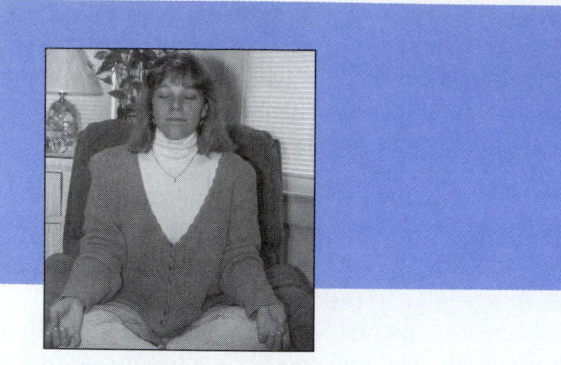

Critical Thinking Activities

1. Using the Social Readjustment Rating Scale developed by Holmes and Rahe, evaluate your current life and assign life change points to yourself. According to Holmes and Rahe, how likely are you to experience an illness? What steps could you take to reduce your own stress?
2. Through an interview, determine a patient's/client's total life change points. Identify the person's medical diagnosis. How might life stress affect this person's illness?
3. Investigate a specific stress management technique that is taught in your community. Write a brief report that includes information on the time required, the cost, the number of people completing the training, your analysis of the effectiveness of this strategy.
4. Identify a situation in which you felt a great deal of stress (such as your first day in the nursing program). List all the objective signs of stress that you exhibited at that time. Compare your own responses to stress with those outlined in the chapter.
5. Reflect on the way in which you use humor in your own life. Identify situations in which you have used humor as a coping technique.

References and Readings

Bellert, J. L. "Humor: A Therapeutic Approach in Oncology Nursing." *Cancer Nursing* 12, 2 (April 1989): 65–70.

Berk, L., and Tan, S. "Eustress of Mirthful Laughter Modifies Natural Killer Cell Activity." *American Journal of Medical Sciences* (December 1989): 298 (6): 390–396.

Benson, H., Beary, J. F., and Canol, M. P. "The Relaxation Response." *Psychiatry,* 37 (February 1974): 37–46.

Cohen, F., and Lazarus, R. S. "Coping and Adaptation in Health and Illness." *Handbook of Health, Health Care, and Health Professions.* New York: Free Press, 1983.

Cousins, N. *Head First: The Biology of Hope.* New York: Dutton, 1989.

———. *Anatomy of an Illness.* New York: W. W. Norton, 1980.

Delongis, A., Cogne, J. C., Dakof, G., Folkman, S., and Lazarus, S. "The Relationship of Daily Hassles, Uplifts, and Major Life Events to Health Status." *Health Psychology* 1 (1982): 119–136.

Dillon, K. "Positive Emotional States and Enhancement of the Immune System." *International Journal of Psychiatry in Medicine,* 15, 1 (January 1985): 13–18.

Folkman, S., and Lazarus, R. S. "An Analysis of Coping in a Middle-Aged Community Sample." *Journal of Health and Social Behavior* 21 (1980): 219–239.

Golemeir, D., and Schwartz, C. G. "Meditation as an Intervention in Stress Reactivity." *Journal of Consulting and Clinical Psychiatry* 44 (March 1976): 456–466.

Holmes, T. H., and Rahe, R. H. "The Social Readjustment Rating Scale." *Journal of Psychosomatic Research* 11 (1967): 213–218.

Howard, K., and Scott, R. A. "A Proposed Framework for the Analysis of Stress in the Human Organism." *Behavioral Science* 10 (1965): 141–160.

Jacobson, E. *Progressive Relaxation.* Chicago: University of Chicago Press, 1938.

Kinzel, S. L. "What's Your Stress Level?" *Nursing Life* 2 (2): 54–55, March–April 1982.

Lazarus, R. S., and Folkman, S. *Stress, Appraisal, and Coping.* New York: Springer, 1984.

Lefcourt, H. M. "Humor and Immune System Functioning." *International Journal of Humor Research* 18, 1 (January 1988): 93.

Leff, E. W., and Leff, H. Z. "If You're Having Another Bad Day." *American Journal of Nursing* 87, 10 (October 1987): 1362–1363.

Lerman, C., Rimer, B. Blumberg, B. Cristinzio, S., Enstrom, P. F., MacElwee, N., O'Connor, K., and Seay, J. "Effects of Coping Style and Relaxation on Cancer Chemotherapy Side Effects and Emotional Responses." *Cancer Nursing* 13, 5 (October 1990): 308–315.

Macinick, C. G., and Macinick, J. W. "Strategies for Burnout Prevention in the Mental Health Setting." *International Nursing Review* 37, 2 (March-April 1990): 247–249.

Manfredi, C., and Pickett, M. "Perceived Stressful Situations and Coping Strategies Utilized by the Elderly." *Journal of Community Health Nursing* 4, 2 (February 1987): 99–110.

Ploeg, J., and Faux, S. "The Relationship Between Social Support, Lifestyle Behaviours, Coping, and Health in the Elderly." *Canadian Journal of Nursing Research* 21, 2 (Summer 1989): 53–65.

Porth, C. *Pathophysiology: Concepts of Altered Health States.* 3rd edition. Philadelphia: J. B. Lippincott, 1990.

Rich, V. L., and Rich, A. R. "Personality, Hardiness, and Burnout in Female Staff Nurses." *Image* 19, 2 (Summer 1987): 63–66.

Schultz, J., and Luthe, W. *Autogenic Training.* New York: Grune & Stratton, 1959.

Selye, H. Interviewed by Lawrence Cherry. "On the Real Benefits of Eustress." *Psychology Today,* 11 (March 1978): 60–61.

———. *Stress Without Distress.* Philadelphia: J. B. Lippincott, 1956.

Selye, H. "A Code for Coping with Stress." *AORN Journal* 25 (January 1977):35–42.

———. "Evolution of the Stress Concept." *American Science* 61 (November-December 1973): 692–699.

———. *The Stress of Life.* New York: McGraw-Hill, 1956.

Siegel, B. S. *Love, Medicine, and Miracles.* New York: Harper & Row, 1986.

Simon, J. M. "Humor and Its Relationship to Perceived Health,

Life Satisfaction, and Morale in Older Adults." *Issues in Mental Health Nursing* 11, 1 (Winter 1990): 17–31.

———. "Humor Techniques for Oncology Nurses." *Oncology Nursing Forum* 16, 5 (September-October 1989): 667–670.

Stone, A. "Evidence That IgA Antibody is Associated With Daily Mood." 52, 5 (May 1987):, 1–9.

Tamez, E. G., Moore, M. J., and Brown, P. L. "Relaxation Training as a Nursing Intervention Versus Pro Re Nata Medication." *Nursing Research* 27 (May-June 1978): 160–165.

Wallace, A. "An Active Role for Patients in Stress Management." *Professional Nurse* 5, 2 (November 1989): 65–66, 68–69, 72.

Wallace, R. K. "Physiological Effects of Transcendental Meditation." *Science* 167 (March 27, 1970): 1751–1754.

Wallace, R. K., and Benson, H. "The Physiology of Meditation." *Scientific American* 226 (October 1972): 84–90.

Basic Concepts of Health and Illness

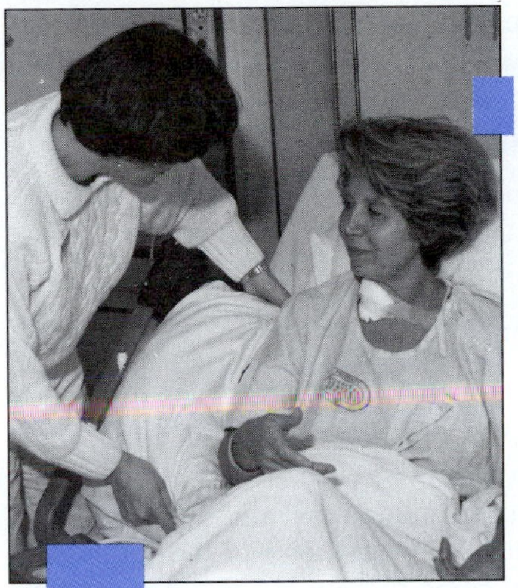

7

Objectives

After completing this chapter, you should be able to:

1. Discuss two definitions of health.
2. Differentiate between illness and disease.
3. Explain how illness and health can coexist.
4. Explain how health and illness can be perceptual and subjective.
5. Name community programs that focus on health promotion and preventive health care.
6. Distinguish between acute and chronic illness.
7. Name and briefly discuss the five stages of illness.
8. List the major causes and the risk factors of illness.
9. Discuss the common patient responses to illness.
10. Define restoration of health (healing).
11. Explain what is meant by "nontraditional healing."
12. Discuss the importance of rehabilitation throughout illness.

Study Terms

acute illness
acupuncture
anxiety
biofeedback
chronic illness
dependence
depression
fear
guilt
health promotion
health maintenance
high-level wellness
host
hostility
imagery
intervention
malingering
nontraditional healing
pathogens
preventive health care
regression
rehabilitation
self-care
stressors

Outline

Ellis, Nowlis: Nursing: A Human Needs Approach, 5th ed. © 1994 J.B. Lippincott Company

The concepts of health and illness are fundamental to an understanding of the well or ill person and the nurse's role. In nursing, medical, and social science literature, many definitions of health and illness are offered. Understanding and thinking about them may change the way we provide care. Is health just feeling well? Who decides if a person is healthy? Is a person healthy only if all body systems are functioning optimally? On the other hand, is illness a state of not feeling well? Who determines if an illness is present and if only one body system is not functioning, is the person considered ill?

Do you consider yourself healthy right now? What might happen that would make you regard yourself as ill? As we shall see in this chapter, there are several answers to each of these questions. A look at both past and present views of health and illness will prove useful to us as nurses.

Historical Views of Health and Illness

Before medical advances permitted a better understanding of the causes of illness, *health* was often looked on as a fortunate happenstance and *illness* as an unexplained event. In some cultures, staying healthy was believed to require adherence to a complicated set of rituals, including avoiding some foods, eating plenty of others, staying out of drafts, wearing warm clothes, and thinking "good" thoughts. Early in the history of our country, youngsters were often routinely "dosed" with laxatives to prevent constipation, rubbed with liniments to prevent lung congestion, and buttoned or even sewed into heavy winter underwear to prevent chilling.

Still earlier civilizations viewed illness as an unavoidable natural phenomenon. People incurred bouts of illness on a regular basis. Their beliefs about illness were based not on scientific knowledge but on a need for some explanation for what they were experiencing. Illness was held by some to be punishment or retribution for a misdeed or bad thought. Many people believed that thinking "ill" of another could have punitive power and induce illness in that person—hence the custom of sticking pins into an effigy. Some of these beliefs persist today.

During the devastating epidemics of bubonic plague in Europe in the 14th century, many of those who had touched the bodies of the dead became ill themselves. This experience gave widespread support to the "myth of contagion"—the idea that contact with the dead human body would cause a person to die. It is from the roots of the word "contact" that contagious is derived. Later, as the causes of diseases became clearer, people who were ill were thought of as "just not strong enough" to overcome their illness.

In earlier times, healing was also defined largely in terms of functioning: if you felt well enough to resume working, you had been healed. Most healing methods, such as the prescribing of special foods and herbs, had not been developed scientifically. A few such remedies were effective. Foxglove, for example, was used to alleviate fatigue, water retention, and fast pulse, which were not yet recognized as symptoms of heart disease. It contains digitalis, which is still used today in treating heart disease. Similarly, isolation of patients, which was formerly enforced to promote rest, is now recognized to be an effective way to prevent the spread of organisms. But in most matters relating to health, illness, and healing, scientific advances have significantly changed our ideas.

Early medical and nursing practice was illness oriented. Physicians and nurses helped ill persons to improve or recover. Except for participating in "well baby checks," nurses followed the medical definition of health as absence of disease. Little in the nursing literature concerned health or health maintenance. As the field of nursing expanded, new definitions were needed to include preventive health measures and to encompass a broader view of healing. The need to heal is now seen as a basic one, whether it is the need to heal physically, to survive psychosocial trauma, or to find spiritual recovery. The healing process is viewed as a "holistic" one, which means that the total person is involved.

Definitions of Health

Many theorists have defined health. Not only are there different definitions of the state of health but also different views on assigning responsibility for maintaining health. Earlier definitions have been replaced as health care has changed. Baronowski (1981) lists four reasons to define health.

1. Health may best be promoted by activities other than medical care. This reason distances health from the more narrow meaning that only medical intervention can regain or maintain one's health.
2. Knowledge about health enhances our knowledge of human beings and the role of health. This suggests that if we understand what health is, we can begin to recognize behaviors that promote wellness.
3. By defining health, we can define and mobilize appropriate professional guidance to promote health in individuals.
4. A definition of health can serve as the basis for comparative cost–benefit studies of the treatment of disease and health promotion.

By defining health, we can focus on those groups in our society that will benefit most from programs in health promotion and we can set priorities for maximizing the well-being of more of our citizens. Let us explore some definitions of health.

Medical Model

Belloc and Breslow (1972) proposed a medical model definition of health as the state of being free of signs or symptoms of disease. This definition suggests that illness is the presence of signs or symptoms of disease, a topic we will discuss presently. The medical model definition has limited meaning for nursing. If health is simply the absence of the symptoms of disease, nursing care for a patient with diabetes, for example, would focus on minimizing signs and symptoms of the illness, a rather limited plan of care. The medical model does have some application, however, as nurses assess for signs and symptoms as part of the nursing process (discussed in Unit 3). This model also has limitations with regard to the increasing focus on prevention of disease.

Role Performance Model

Parsons (1958) formulated the role performance model, which classifies health as the ability to perform all those roles for which one has been socialized. For example, a young woman may perform the roles of mother, wife, student, and worker. This definition is relevant to nursing. Nurses often assess patients/clients for deficits. To assess a role performance deficit, a nurse would determine what the patient is unable to do because of the illness. The activities in question may be activities of daily living (ADLs) or something more profound. For example, a nurse might want to look at how the illness interferes with the person's work or how it interferes with personal relationships. Is the illness detracting from the value and quality of life?

World Health Organization

The definition of health adopted by the World Health Organization (WHO) in 1947 characterized health as "the state of complete physical, mental, and social well-being and not merely the absence of disease or infirmity." The word complete is somewhat misleading in that it suggests an absolute standard. In actuality, few people who are perceived by themselves and others as healthy have achieved a state of complete and perpetual well-being. This definition was also much too abstract for nursing. It has some meaning as a goal statement but lacks practical applicability.

In 1981, WHO began an ambitious project that took a more pragmatic approach to improving world health. After gathering data from member countries, WHO planned to implement an international network of assistance in health matters that would answer more closely the individual needs of the countries involved. The purpose, as stated in the proposal, was to "work together to attain the goal of a level of health for all the people of the world by the year 2000 that would permit them to lead a socially and economically productive life." In 1991, the attorney general of WHO stated that "the monitoring of progress toward the goal of health for all has shown that at best it has been slow . . . it is becoming clear that we need to improve our understanding of the close relationship between health, the economy and development" (Little, 1992). The third edition of this document, written in 1992, stated that at any one time, 20% of the world's population was not healthy. This fact has rekindled the effort of the organization to mobilize programs that will interface with local health representatives in an effort to improve health and reach the previous goal.

High-Level Wellness

A more inclusive definition of health—actually more of a description than a definition—is Dunn's (1961) concept of **high-level wellness**. Emphasizing the relationship between wellness and the family, community, environment, and society, Dunn discusses the individual's inner and outer worlds and the need for a balance of energy between them. In other words, health involves more than the self.

For nurses, Dunn's definition is more practical than the original WHO definition because Dunn's description links wellness to specific factors that nurses can consider when planning care. Nursing becomes more holistic (involving the total person) when the patient's internal and external environment are taken into account. Dunn is clearly referring to a state of homeostasis much like that defined in Chapter 4—the tendency of all living tissue to restore and maintain itself in a *condition* of balance and equilibrium.

Health-Illness Coexistence

Lamberton (1983) proposed a particularly interesting definition of health in which health and illness are viewed as coexistent, that is, present at the same time and interacting. Shortridge and McLain (1983) apply the Lamberton model to nursing action by distinguishing among interventions "for each degree of health state: promotion of high-level wellness; maintenance of wellness; prevention of potential disruption in health; treatment of actual alterations in health; and restoration for resolving alterations in health" (p. 74). We will discuss later the ways in which nurses help patients toward a state of health.

Tillich (1961) used the term "unhealthy health." This follows his definition of health as a multidimensional unity in human beings; although health may be present in one or more human dimensions, it may not be present in others. For example, a person may have a leg fracture, but after treatment and casting, may feel relaxed, well, and able to carry out the responsibilities of life. Only one dimension, that of mobility, has been altered.

Needs Fulfillment Model

This text is based on the premise that human beings have certain needs and nursing can assist people in meeting those needs. A useful and applicable definition of health springing from this foundation would be needs focused, defining health as a state in which needs are being sufficiently met to allow an individual to function successfully in life with the ability to achieve the highest possible potential. It must be recognized that different people hold different beliefs about what, for themselves, constitutes being healthy. Although the fulfillment of basic needs is crucial to everyone, psychosocial needs may vary significantly in degree and type from one individual to another. To feel truly healthy, the athlete, for example, may require a high degree of muscle coordination and strength not essential to most of us. The artist, in contrast, may regard a high and sustained sense of creativity as essential to a feeling of health. Needs also vary with age. Many illnesses are associated with certain ages. For instance, upper respiratory infections are common during the early school age years, and cardiovascular disease is common during the mature years. The needs fulfillment model is a dynamic approach to health, allowing persons to seek increasing satisfaction in their performance and goals of life. This text is based on this model because this approach will allow you to share in planning care so that you and the patient share perceived needs and appropriate ways to fulfill them. Maslow's hierarchy of needs has relevance for us when we address patients' needs for it helps us prioritize in such a way so that basic needs are considered first and then, the person can move to higher psychosocial levels. For example, a woman who has had a breast surgically removed successfully may choose to join a community organization that helps others facing the same experience. This woman who has survived illness can now gain satisfaction from becoming a role model in helping others.

Other Definitions of Health

Several theorists have used the person's ability to make adaptations as a foundation for a definition of health. Dubos (1959), Dunn (see previous discussion), and more recently, Sister Callista Roy (1984) defined health as "man's ability to respond positively, or to adapt" to changes in the environment. According to Roy, whether such a change is "a direct assault that causes injury or a subtle variation in psychological nature, man has mechanisms to cope with the changing world."

Although the various definitions of health differ in perspective, each definition incorporates in some manner the concept of the wellness–illness continuum (Fig. 7-1). This concept is based on the principle that, throughout life, there are gradients of health status. The points on the continuum, of course, are not sequential. For example, not all persons experience a period of serious illness just before death. Some may be in a physical and psychological state of high-level wellness, only to suffer a sudden heart attack that results in death. However, the wellness–illness continuum provides nurses with a general, useful concept of health status.

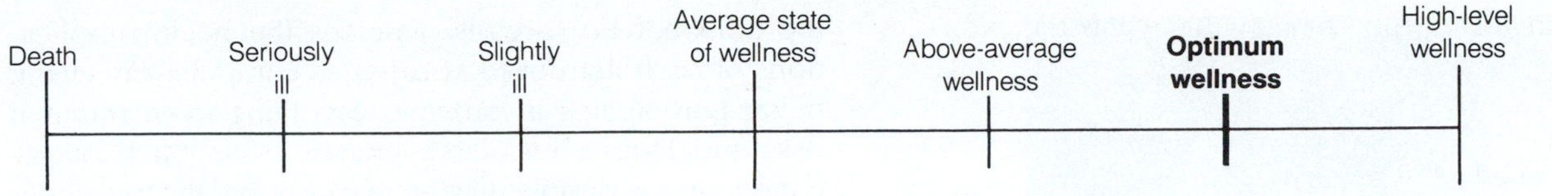

Figure 7-1. The Wellness-illness continuum.

Health as Perceptual and Subjective

Most of the definitions of health just presented acknowledge that health has a subjective component. This aspect of perception and subjectivity gives nurses great potential for assisting patients. The concept also has implications for health promotion and maintenance, subjects that will be discussed later in this chapter.

Balog (1982) suggests that health care provides a perceptual confirmation of a patient's health or illness. We give patients a view they may not have perceived of their health or lack of it, and we also communicate this view to others on the health care team.

Perceptions of health may affect all patients for whom we care, and we can often improve perceptual status by performing basic nursing actions. Suppose, for example, that you enter the room of a patient who looks pale, unkempt, weak, and sad. You know from your assessment data that the patient has been very ill but you proceed to give care that includes understanding and good hygiene, with an emphasis on improving appearance and providing for the patient's general comfort. Later, as you place the patient in a wheelchair in the sun near the window, the patient remarks, "My, I certainly feel much better now." The patient's disease is still evident; the patient, by some of the definitions we have examined, is not in a state of health. However, the patient *feels* healthier (Fig. 7-2).

Subjective feelings of health are always changing. You might feel particularly well on arising in the morning, with an unusually high sense of well-being, only to experience an upsetting confrontation with a classmate soon after arriving at school. Suddenly, you do not feel well at all and realize how external factors have affected your earlier feelings of good health. Yet most such people have a sense of well-being and regard themselves as healthy. Similarly, many people with chronic conditions and diseases, such as multiple sclerosis or rheumatoid arthritis, attain a high level of adjustment and would describe themselves as basically healthy. However, the onset of a common cold might prompt these same individuals to describe themselves as ill.

An interesting phenomenon is that of "the worried well." Because so much has been written in the media about disease, outlining risks and symptoms and offering frightening statistics on incidence, some persons have perceptions that are overly fearful regarding illness. Many become so worried that they imagine they actually have certain illnesses and seek out physicians for confirmation of their suspicions.

Health Promotion and Health Maintenance

Health promotion involves a person's becoming informed and taking actions that will promote a state of health. **Health maintenance** is the act of incorporating these health promotion actions into the lifestyle, leading to maintaining one's health on a continuing basis.

In 1992, the U.S. Department of Health and Human

Nursing Research: *Implications for Practice*

Miller, M. P. "Factors Promoting Wellness in the Aged Person: An Ethnographic Study." *Advances in Nursing Science* 13, 4 (June 1991): 38–51.

Using an interview technique, the investigator studied the perceptions and interpretation of wellness of a selected number of aged persons using as criteria outside involvement, quality of relationships, and degree of health-seeking activities. The study revealed that those who maintained an interest in life and the community, enthusiasm for learning, and participation in health maintenance activities had a more positive self-assessment of their wellness status than did those who did not. This research has implications for those who care for older clients. Health care professionals should include these domains in their care, encouraging clients to participate in any activities that promote a concept of wellness.

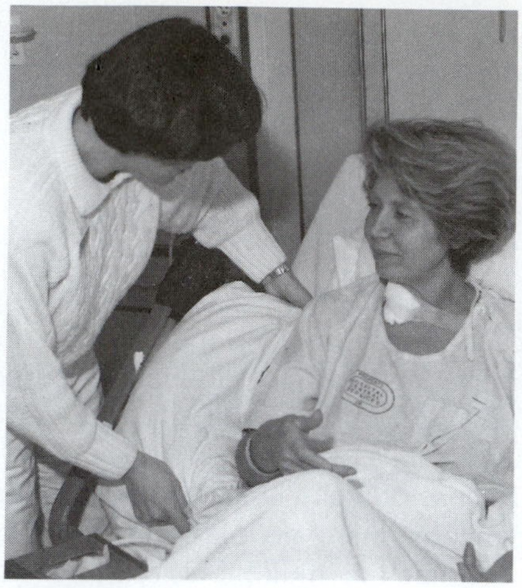

Figure 7-2. Providing for a patient's comfort can sometimes make the patient feel healthier, even when disease is still present.

Services presented a document outlining a national strategy for improving the health of this country over the coming decade. This document focuses on health promotion as well as disease prevention. We will discuss this important document more fully in sections of this chapter.

Society is presently motivated toward both health promotion and health maintenance. A look at any bookstore health section will quickly reveal how important the topic of health promotion has been since the early 1980s. The size of such a collection of books is far larger than that on almost any other subject—the range is endless. Look, for example, at the number of books available on diet or exercise. It is certainly encouraging that more people than ever before are seeing value in regular exercise and learning the benefits it provides for the cardiovascular and respiratory systems. Eating "healthy" is also a major area of interest receiving increasing popular attention. Low-salt meals are now available in many restaurants, and investigations continue as to whether decreasing sugar intake and lowering the level of additives in food products enhances health. Vitamins top the list of nonprescription medications sold in this country.

People are also becoming more interested in mental health maintenance. It is reasonable to assume that not only does good physical health contribute to sound mental health, but having a restful mind contributes to physical well-being. Many people find self-help groups useful. Groups that meditate or use relaxation techniques are common. Classes and seminars on raising self-esteem, becoming more assertive, finding one's identity, and parenting are on the increase as people place value on maintaining their psychological health. Behavior often reveals a great deal about the approach to health maintenance. At one end of the spectrum is the person who carefully assesses the health implications of each item of food eaten, is compulsively clean, never participates in activities involving even minimal risk, and lives a restricted, unvaried life. Such overly conscientious people may be inappropriately apprehensive; some suffer from extreme death anxiety and need counseling. What might appear initially as an earnestly conscientious degree of health maintenance is, in reality, neurotic or irrational behavior. At the other end of the spectrum, you may know someone who consistently refuses to make any effort at health maintenance despite the person's full knowledge of the dangers of smoking, drinking and overeating, and ignoring the signs of illness.

Most people fall somewhere between the two extremes. It is widely recognized that an individual can have some control over his or her health by pursuing proper exercise, diet, hygiene, psychological growth, and stress reduction.

There are two important and interesting aspects to health promotion and health maintenance. The first is that people have to accept that there is or may be a problem before they undertake actions to correct or prevent it. This has been called the health belief model by many theorists. The second factor involved in health promotion and health maintenance and related to the first is that of cultural and ethnic diversity.

Health Belief Model

One of the most powerful aspects of health promotion and maintenance is that of the person's perceptions, which have been discussed. This has been known as the health belief model, which says that people do not make genuine changes toward health unless they perceive there is a problem. The first perceptual level is that of *perceived susceptibility.* This is a time of active learning and self-assessment. The question may be asked, "Do I have a problem?" The second stage is *perceived severity.* If I have determined that I have a problem, how much is it interfering with my life physically or emotionally? The related question is urgency; does something have to be done about it now or can help with the problem be delayed? Third, *perceived benefit* is a motivational stage; will seeking help bring about positive changes and if so, to what extent? Fourth and last, *perceived barriers* are resources, skills, and support available. This model incorporates the idea of empowerment or inclusion of the individual in both assessing health status and weighing options for action.

Ethnic and Cultural Identity

Ethnic identity also influences our perceptions of health and the need for promotion and maintenance. Many of our responses to illness are learned from the group with which we identify. Using the major social, cultural, and ethnic groups of our society as a background, Chapter 33 explores perceptions of health and illness, as well as healing practices.

The subjective nature of health is even more evident when we consider other cultures. In some countries, for example, worms in the intestinal tract are common throughout the general population. Because this condition is so prevalent, people in these countries may not make changes to prevent infestation. If this condition occurred to people in a more developed country, alleviating the problem would be a top priority.

Definitions of Illness

Let us clarify the distinction between the words disease and illness. A *disease* is a physical or psychological defect and its results may be predictable. An *illness* is an individual event and is unique each time it occurs. The distinction is important for "healing professionals" because dealing with an illness requires different skills than treating a disease (dePender and Ikeda-Chandler, 1992, p. 28).

In defining *illness,* it makes sense to build on the several definitions of health. If health is the absence of signs and symptoms of disease, then illness, according to the medical definition, is the presence of those signs and symptoms. There are difficulties inherent in this definition. What is disease? If you feel healthy and have no signs or symptoms of high blood pressure, are you ill? According to the definition that equates illness with signs and symptoms of disease, you are ill. This definition arouses considerable disagreement. If, however, you expand the definition of illness to include the presence of any disease whether or not there are signs and symptoms, you will find other problems.

Illness With Evidence

Closely related to the disease theory is the theory of "illness with evidence," which defines illness in a specific medical sense. This rather narrow view states that there must be demonstrable evidence of an organic nature for someone to be considered ill, that is, a person who does not feel well but has no objective signs of organic disease is not ill. This places the definition of illness entirely within the scope of health care professionals.

Role Performance

Building on Parsons's role performance model, illness can be defined as a state in which individuals cannot fulfill the roles society expects of them. "Calling in sick" is one type of social confirmation that the person is ill. Among the unemployed, illness is not as evident to the rest of society. For example, the woman or man who maintains the home and does not work outside it may have more difficulty convincing others that she or he is ill. If one feels too ill to perform one's usual tasks, denial of illness can be prolonged until the illness progresses to the point of requiring medical assistance.

The role the person plays and the expectations that go with it also make a difference in the definition of illness. Partly because of the bias of ageism, if an elderly person is feeling "under the weather" (ill), the rest of the family may not be very concerned because this person may not have the variety of daily tasks that other members of the family have and more illness may be expected among the aged. However, if a mother or father is too ill to perform all the tasks assigned to the parent role, the rest of the family becomes very anxious.

Lack of Needs Fulfillment

Within the human needs framework of this book, illness is defined as a state in which someone's needs are not sufficiently met to allow the individual to have a sense of physical and psychosocial well-being. This is directly related to homeostasis in that imbalance elicits needs. As needs are addressed and fulfilled, the state of homeostasis for an individual improves.

Most often, the deprivation involves basic needs. But disruption in the fulfillment of the higher level psychosocial needs can also make the individual ill and unable to function. The inability to cope is indicative that needs are not being met (see Chapter 34).

Acute and Chronic Illness

An **acute illness** is characterized by sudden onset, and its pace or progression is rapid and steady. An acute illness does not necessarily require medical attention. It may or may not threaten survival, but numerous acute illnesses can, without expedient intervention, lead to death. However, treatment for an acute illness is usually short term, and there are usually no residual effects. An acute illness with which we are all familiar is the common cold with infection of the upper respiratory tract.

As defined by the U.S. Department of Health, Education and Welfare (1976), a **chronic illness** is one that persists for 3 months or longer, requires medical management, and is characterized by the presence of signs and symptoms. The onset of a chronic illness is slow as is the recovery period (see Chapter 42). A person can have the same illness in both acute and chronic forms at different times. For example, the elderly person who falls and fractures a hip becomes acutely ill with the sudden onset of incapacitation. After stabilization of the fracture, this same person may enter a time of chronic illness because the healing process of elderly persons is slow. Some chronic illnesses can have an acute episode and then resume their original chronic course. With such illnesses, the intermittent acute phases are called *exacerbations*, and the return to the chronic state with abatement of symptoms is termed a *remission*. Some examples of chronic diseases are multiple sclerosis, diabetes, arthritis, and emphysema.

Stages of Illness

Whether an illness is acute or chronic, the sick individual experiences stages of the illness. These stages are not unlike the stages of dying or bereavement described by numerous researchers. People do not necessarily move sequentially through such stages but may revert to earlier positions from time to time. The similarities between the stages of illness and the various stages of loss derive from the fact that illness may represent a loss of body function that alters lifestyle and affects self-identity and self-esteem. The stages of illness may vary depending on the individual and on the severity and length of the illness (Display 7-1).

Disbelief and Denial

The first stage in an illness may be a feeling of some surprise or even frank disbelief that signs and symptoms are occurring. Denial may bring a strong belief that the problems will "all go away." It may be fairly easy at first to attribute the symptoms to something besides an illness. For example, the full feeling in the head that often precedes a cold may be attributed to a "slight allergy" that will quickly go away. Disbelief and denial may be engendered by fear, which encourages the hope that whatever discomfort or other symptoms are being experienced will resolve themselves on their own and disappear.

Irritability and Anger

The second stage of illness involves a feeling of irritability or anger. The irritability arises from a sense that the body or mind is not acting as expected and is interfering with life to some degree. This irritability may grow into a more defined feeling of anger. The anger, if directed inward, can lead to guilt. This phenomenon is demonstrated by patients who say, "If I had only rested more (taken my vitamins; dressed more warmly; not smoked), perhaps I would not be feeling this way." Fear may also increase during this second stage.

Display 7–1
Stages of Illness

Stage 1	Disbelief and denial
Stage 2	Irritability and anger
Stage 3	Attempting to gain control
Stage 4	Depression and despair
Stage 5	Acceptance and participation

Attempting to Gain Control

During the third stage of an illness, an individual attempts to gain some control over the state of illness through self-diagnosis, applying what seem to be appropriate remedies. Taking the proverbial two aspirin tablets to see if the "catch" in the knee will go away is a good example. During this stage, denial no longer works and fear increases so if self-diagnosis and interventions fail, the person usually seeks professional help.

Depression

The most common stage of illness is **depression**, which is a sad, dejected state, sometimes including feelings of hopelessness. Studies show that even such an innocuous illness as the common cold produces some depression, caused by the illness's interference with daily living combined with a general lack of well-being. Depression induced by illness can vary in length and intensity. The patient who is ill for a short period of time may suffer only a mild depression or fleeting moments of sadness. For example, a person with an uncomplicated pneumonia that is responding to treatment may feel depressed occasionally, mainly because of the interruption of the routine of daily life. On the other hand, a patient who has an orthopedic condition, such as a broken hip that requires a long period of immobility for healing, may develop a state of depression that, although it does have "highs and lows," persists throughout convalescence.

The patient with a lifelong chronic illness may plunge into a sudden, deep depression on hearing the diagnosis. After subsiding somewhat, this depression may become as chronic as the disease itself. The chronically ill patient may "fight" depression throughout life, enjoying long periods of time when the depression lifts or disappears, only to become depressed again with exacerbations of the condition.

The more seriously ill become aware of the possibility that they may not recover sufficiently to regain the previous quality of life, a possibility that sometimes evokes more fear than the prospect of death. The patient with a terminal illness may or may not develop depression initially but is likely to become depressed when hope begins to fade. Later, a patient facing the end of life can understandably enter a stage of profound depression. Patients may openly weep, only minimally communicate, refuse to eat, and either have difficulty sleeping or appear to sleep much of the time. There are also terminally ill persons who move through depression to a state of comfort, needing to relate to those who are important to them.

Acceptance and Participation

Accepting the reality of the illness and gaining control of it through participation in decisions regarding management of the illness is a positive stage of revitalization for the ill person. The knowledge that "something is being done and I am a part of it" alleviates some of the depression. Even those who are terminally ill have many options at this stage (see Chapter 41).

Persons at Risk for Illness

Research has been useful in identifying persons who may be at increased risk for illness. Those who totally ignore preventive health practices knowingly or unknowingly place themselves at risk for illness. However, in groups of people living under similar conditions, it is hard to predict which individuals will become ill. Regardless of the same exposure to disease agents, some become ill while others remain healthy. A variety of factors, such as age, life events, and the person's perception of health and illness enter into consideration (Fig. 7-3). Psychological stress has been widely investigated as a contributing factor to illness. Though it remains impossible to measure the damage stress causes a given individual or the quantity of stress that must be imposed to produce illness, some studies show a direct relationship between stress and the onset of illness. Cumulative loss, especially the kind that produces feelings of abandonment, as well as other stress can place persons at risk for illness. The concept that accumulated stress can cause illness has implications for nurses. Reale (1987) suggests, "Evaluating stressful changes in your patient's life may shed light on the cause of his illness" (p. 53). This is further explored in Chapter 34.

Specific Causes of Illness

Our understanding of the sources of illness has expanded explosively over the past several decades. Unscientific generalities have been replaced in some instances by specific knowledge of causes. As some diseases that bring about illness become extinct, others never previously known to exist are being identified.

Invasion of Body Defenses by Pathogens

Pathogens are disease-producing microorganisms. Many such microorganisms are always present in the human body but in numbers insufficient to cause illness. If these pathogens multiply enough to threaten homeostasis, illness occurs. In this context, it is essential for nurses to understand the notion of "necessary but not sufficient." For a certain disease to occur, the pathogen that causes it must be present. However, the mere presence of the pathogen may not be sufficient to bring on the illness. For example, it is necessary for the tubercle bacillus to be present for a person to develop tuberculosis. However, the organism alone may not be sufficient to produce the illness. If the **host** (the person who is carrying the organism) is debilitated or has an impaired immune system, however, this combination and the presence of the bacillus could be sufficient for tuberculosis to occur.

Immune System Disturbances

The *immune system* normally protects the body by attacking and subduing invading pathogens and foreign substances. A disease such as acquired immunodeficiency syndrome (AIDS) destroys an essential part of the immune system, allowing pathogens that would not ordinarily be invasive to cause "opportunistic infections." This means that the impaired immune system has given certain pathogens the "opportunity" to infect the individual.

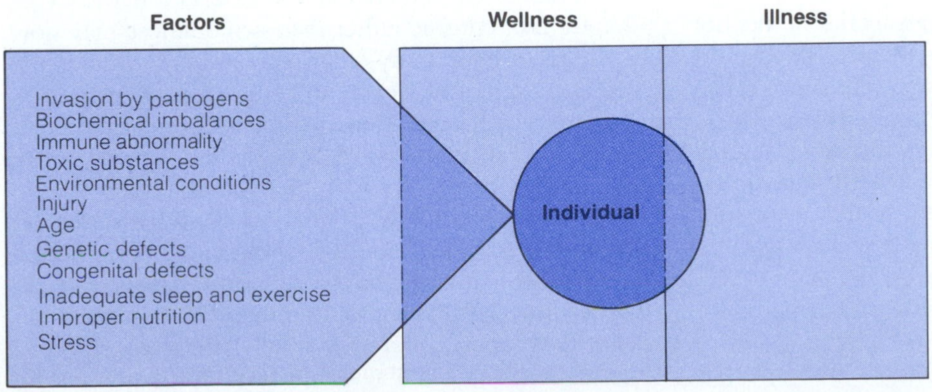

Figure 7-3. Single or multiple factors that can cause illness.

At other times, the immune system can become "confused" and attack parts of the body itself, causing cellular destruction and illness. Many illnesses have currently been described as being what is termed *autoimmune.* Many chronic illnesses appear to be autoimmune although in some cases, proof remains elusive.

A depressed immune system leading to illness can be caused by some drugs, including those used to combat cancer, which cause a decrease in the numbers of white blood cells that are important components of the body's immune system, or defense against pathogens. In other people, the immune response can be reduced by age, stress, alcohol, or the use of illicit drugs such as cocaine. Regardless of the reason for a decrease in the immune system, nurses should understand that susceptibility to disease increases and the patient is at a high risk for illness.

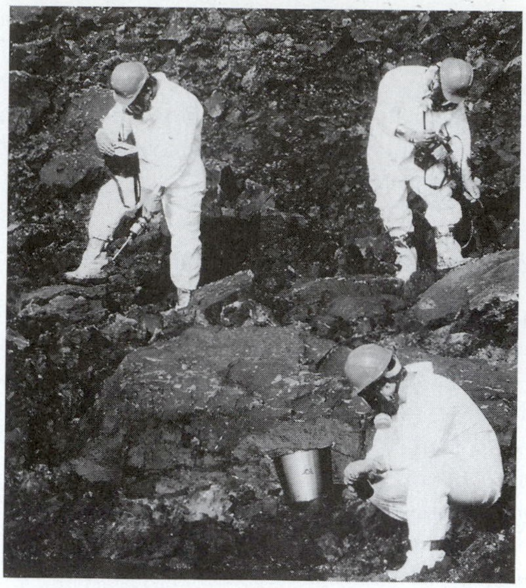

Figure 7-4. Workers must protect themselves against potential toxic effects of chemicals.

Biochemical Imbalances of the Body

Imbalances of the body's chemical structure and hormones can cause illness. These essential body chemicals have a wide variety of purposes and actions. Within the body, a delicate balance exists between fluid in the tissues and the chemicals called *electrolytes.* Through a complex process, these tiny particles regulate the intracellular and extracellular fluid balance. The more important electrolytes to consider are sodium, potassium, calcium, bicarbonate, and chloride. Another important electrolyte balance within the body is that of acid and base. Whenever a chemical mechanism is sufficiently out of balance (the normal range is narrow), illness can occur. Such an imbalance might occur if an individual had an inadequate intake of fluids for a lengthy period of time. Breathing deeply for a prolonged period can also cause an acid–base imbalance. Fluid and electrolytes will be discussed in greater detail in Chapter 30.

Toxic Substances

Toxic substances act as poisons in the body, causing serious tissue damage. Infections can cause serious illness because bacteria excrete toxins. Some substances are toxic only in large amounts over an extended period of time or in conjunction with other substances or conditions. For example, long-term high intake of alcohol can cause diseases of the liver, pancreas, brain, and other organs. The indiscriminate use of drugs can cause serious physiologic and psychological illness. Toxic substances may be absorbed through the skin, inhaled, or ingested orally. For example, some pesticides can be absorbed through the skin or inhaled so that these substances should be avoided or if used, special clothing and masks must be worn (Fig. 7-4).

Injury

Although *injury* is rarely termed illness, injured people *are* ill if illness is defined as interference with functioning and the presence of signs or symptoms. Serious injury or *trauma* is an assault on the body's integrity equivalent in severity to serious medical illness. Responses to injury are similar to responses to illness.

Injury can cause exacerbation of a chronic illness because it is an added stressor. For example, if a person has chronic asthma and sustains an injury, the injury may cause breathing to become compromised, leading to an asthma attack. Directly or indirectly, then, injury can be a cause of illness.

Age

Many people expect illness to accompany aging. **Infirmity**, or general weakening of body systems, is often associated with advanced age. However, gerontologists—those who study the aging process—emphasize that, although elderly persons are at high risk of illness, perhaps because of a decrease in the immune system, health is an attainable goal for most elderly persons.

Because of a remarkable increase in longevity (see Chapter 20), chronic rather than acute illness may now be the pattern for many older persons. According to the U.S. Department of Health and Human Services (1978), 50 years ago chronic diseases, such as arthritis and heart conditions, accounted for 30% of all illnesses; today such diseases represent more than 50%.

Infants, particularly premature newborns, are also susceptible to illness because of their age. For a period of time, the infant has immune response factors from the mother, but the infant's own immune system must undergo development before it is fully effective in protecting the body against illness. Immature body systems are also not adept at adjusting to environmental changes, such as variations in temperature, which could place these youngsters at risk.

Young children have more respiratory illness than do older persons because of exposure to multiple organisms within the school environment, the child's shorter structure of the otonasopharyngeal passages, which allows organisms to gain entry, and the fact that children often do not practice consistent and effective personal hygiene. Other contagious illnesses are also prevalent in children despite immunization.

Genetic and Congenital Defects

Genetic defects are inherited conditions caused by errors in genetic makeup and present at birth. One of the most common is trisomy 21, which results in a group of symptoms formerly known as Down syndrome. Although people suffering from genetic defects vary greatly in their capacity for near-normal function, their death rate from illness and injury is higher than average, probably because of accompanying physical and psychological conditions that undermine the ability to adapt to disease.

Some congenital defects may be considered illnesses. These defects are not inherited but are present at birth and cause major body impairment. One example of a congenital defect is spina bifida or incomplete closure of the spinal canal. One individual may also have more than one congenital defect.

Multiple Causes of Illness

As we have seen, many different factors can cause illness (see Fig. 7-3). It is not uncommon, furthermore, for illness to be brought on by a combination of such factors. A person who does not become ill in response to one such factor may fall ill when a second is imposed. A person paralyzed for years by a stroke (cerebrovascular accident or CVA) may not feel ill until pathogens introduced into the respiratory tract cause pneumonia. Because the stroke-induced immobility increased susceptibility to the pathogens in the respiratory tract, the stroke and the respiratory infection together caused illness. Stress may also be a factor in such a situation.

Factors that may Reinforce Illness

Illness may elicit perceptions and attitudes that interfere with recovery. For example, illness may in some circumstances prove rewarding for the patient. The dependence it engenders can be used manipulatively. "Don't you see I'm ill? How can you leave me?" is a plea that can realign relationships in a negative way. It is hard to show anger, regardless of how justified, toward an ill person. Illness also excuses the patient from having to perform tasks or fulfill obligations. Because people tend to protect the ill from added stress, even the details of everyday life can be temporarily ignored by someone who is sick.

A patient who has accumulated a great deal of paid sick leave at work may unconsciously prolong an illness out of lack of motivation to recover. **Malingering** is the conscious exaggeration of symptoms by the patient to gain rewards of some type. For example, a patient may feign pain to elicit attention.

If you are tempted to assign a patient's behaviors or motives to dependence or malingering, you must consider carefully whether such an assessment is accurate. Judgmental reactions can seriously interfere with your relationship to the patient and the effectiveness of care. Even if such a conclusion is justified, the patient still needs sympathetic care. Good care includes an effort to identify why the patient is behaving in a particular way.

The Illness Role

We play many roles in life. Illness, like other roles, focuses on expectations for behavior. Parsons (1958) assigned four concepts to the illness role: 1) ill people are exempt from fulfilling social responsibilities; 2) ill people are not responsible for being sick; 3) ill people should "want to get well"; 4) ill people should seek competent help.

These assumptions are difficult for many people. Some feel guilt because of not being able to fulfill their usual role in society. Although it is irrational to feel this way, ill people sometimes do feel responsible for their illness. For others, the benefits from being ill occasionally outweigh the desire to get well. The term competent help is relative, and participants in nontraditional medical treatment may feel added guilt if their recovery does not happen.

There are many other concerns for the person who is in the illness role. Of necessity, patients must conform to the routine of the hospital. For instance, the time schedule patients must follow in a hospital may be different from their normal ones. The patient who habitually awakens at 7:30 AM, for example, may be dismayed to find that the night nurse appears at 6:00 AM to administer early morning care. In general, patients are people who, before becoming patients, were able to live by a routine and style that suited them. Hospitalization interrupts this routine and invades privacy. People who find pleasure in being sexually active miss the intimacy sacrificed in this new patient role. The most attractive patient room is not nearly as personalized as even the most modest home. Some facilities refer to the ill as "clients" and a few call them "customers," but it is questionable if these terms offset the discomfort of adjusting

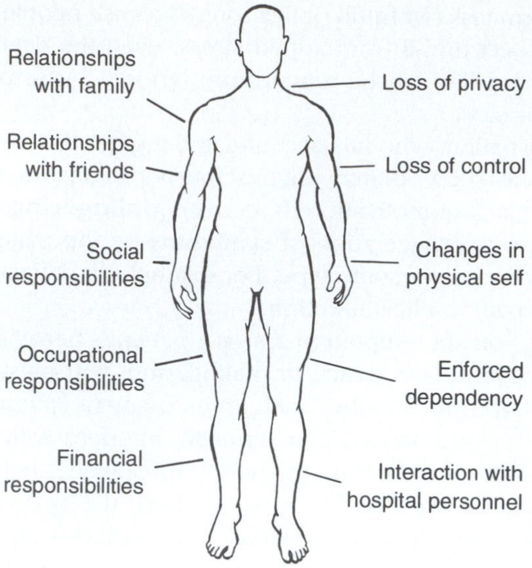

Figure 7-5. Stressors for the ill person.

to being ill and, at the same time, in a strange new environment.

Patients have traditionally been expected to behave passively and dependently. "Good" patients accepted treatment and care with a minimum of questions and adapted uncomplainingly to the routine of the hospital or institution. However, the era of the docile patient is past. That the role of the patient is undergoing change is aptly symbolized by the widespread adoption in health care facilities of the Patient's Bill of Rights (see Chapter 3). More and more, patients and their families perceive themselves as consumers of health care, and they correctly insist on their right to quality care. Providers, in turn, are encouraging patients to take an active part in making decisions about their own care. To participate in such decision-making, the patient must be fully informed. Many *stressors* affect the patient role. Responsibilities outside the hospital, intense interaction with all the personnel within the health care setting, and the strain of undergoing a variety of treatments to regain health place patients under considerable stress (Fig. 7-5).

Common Responses to Illness

Responses to illness may or may not be related to the stage of an illness. For example, the person who is depressed may also be anxious. The individual who has a severe cold may respond with guilt for having to be absent from work. It is essential that nurses do not expect certain responses. In any situation in which the body is not functioning properly, there may be fear for survival.

Every person responds to the threat of illness in a unique way. Individuals develop specific patterns of responding to threats and the occurrence of illness tends to elicit these responses. A person who usually responds to threats with hostility will probably react this way to illness.

Illness may impose necessary changes on an individual's lifestyle. These changes may affect the person's home, job, or family.

Dependence is the inability to function satisfactorily without the aid of someone else. Dependence is inherent in the role of the patient and may be threatening to people who perceive dependence as loss of control. To offset the feeling of threat, many health care professionals are encouraging patients to become even more active in their plans for care. As health care workers, we must take some of the responsibility for assuming that patients should be passive participants. One deterrent, justified or unjustified, is that assertiveness on the part of patients elicits negative responses from health care workers, which forces the patients back into the more traditional passive role. However, more self-care and participation are welcome developments for those who become ill and need advocacy from nurses.

Guilt is a feeling of remorse at having done something wrong. A patient who is the primary wage earner in the family may feel guilty for depriving the family of income. A long-term illness may lower the family's standard of living and possibly cause resentment among other family members. Inability to perform household tasks or fulfill social commitments can also arouse guilt, as can the ill person's inability to provide emotional support or sexual gratification to a loved one.

Anxiety is an ill-defined and disturbing feeling of apprehension. It may take the form of a vague feeling that things are generally not right and that something unknown but unpleasant is going to happen. Lack of understanding of one's illness and its treatment can cause a high level of anxiety, as can simply being ill or being hospitalized and away from one's family. **Fear** is the feeling aroused by danger or threat. Although more acute than anxiety, fear may be easier to deal with because it is usually more clearly defined. Fear of pain is common, as is fear of the outcome of illness, injury, or surgery. Sometimes fear that an important relationship will change or end because of one's illness can cause psychological suffering. Fear of disability is even more severe than fear of death for some patients.

Depression can be an expected result of the person's responses to illness such as dependence, guilt, anxiety, and fear. The person may ask, "Why do I feel this way?" This is particularly true if the person has led a healthy life and suddenly finds that the ability to perform daily activities of life have been hampered. This depression is situational and hopefully disappears on recovery. If the person has a protracted or long illness, some degree of depression may persist.

Regression is reacting to anxiety by reverting to

immature behavior. An ill child who long ago gave up bottle-feeding may, for example, demand a bottle at mealtime. Similarly, a sick adult may become whiny or overreact to inconsequential matters. Irritability can be a form of regression.

The threat posed by illness typically causes patients to become preoccupied with themselves and their health. As the seriousness of an illness increases, even less attention is paid to the outside world or the concerns of others. Sometimes *self-centeredness* leads to demanding behavior and unreasonable requests for attention.

Hostility may be a response to overwhelming anxiety. Patients may occasionally be verbally abusive of the nursing staff. The patient may unconsciously view the nurse as a safer target for pent-up hostility than a family member or other person highly significant to the patient. Such misplaced hostility is difficult for the nurse to manage.

Patient hostility raises the question of nurses' rights. The nurse should not be a convenient target of abuse from a patient or a family member. If abuse is excessive, the nurse might ask the supervisor, physician, or a staff counselor to intervene. Remember that you have the right to remove yourself physically from proximity to a patient whose behavior is combative and unsafe.

Prevention of Illness

Efforts to prevent illness and injury appear to have particular merit in a world with limited resources for the care of people who are ill. Not only does preventing illness avoid the anguish suffered by those who are afflicted but it is cost effective to spend scarce dollars on prevention rather than on expensive treatment. Membership in health maintenance organizations has currently increased because of the economic benefit of keeping people well. Because we truly live in a global community, a focus on **preventive health care** throughout the world is essential. Central to preventive health care is risk reduction. Identifying risks for illness and educating people to reduce taking such risks is the key to prevention. The following are major programs in preventive services.

Immunization has brought about the virtual eradication of such diseases as polio and smallpox in this country. However, there has been a rise in some infectious diseases such as measles and influenza. The Centers for Disease Control and Prevention (CDC) reports that 80% to 90% of the deaths resulting from influenza occur in people over age 65. The resurgence of measles has brought about an active immunization program including school admission laws in many states that mandate immunization before the child is allowed to enter school. Dissemination of information and provision of access to services form the basis of a successful immunization program.

A growing concern is the steady rise in persons infected with the human immunodeficiency virus (HIV). The CDC has proposed a new definition of persons with AIDS in which all adults and adolescents who are HIV positive and who have T helper cell counts (CD4) of less than 200/mm^3 of blood would be added to the AIDS classification. These cells are an integral part of the immune system and if there is no other obvious cause for their reduction, they become "markers" for the presence of AIDS. The purpose behind the new definition is that treatment to prolong the length and quality of life, delaying illness, can be started earlier if persons carrying the virus can be identified. It is estimated that the new definition would double the number of people already reported (Chang, Katz, and Hernandez, 1992, p. 973). This devastating disease is far too complex to discuss in depth here, but more education in safer sex practices and eliminating drug injection abuse are essential in reducing risks for AIDS.

Another factor in preventive health care is to educate women to seek prenatal services early in their pregnancy. National statistics report that one of every four pregnant women does not seek prenatal care during the first trimester. This leads to failure to identify risk factors related to low birth weight and increased infant mortality. Specific risk factors of concern are low socioeconomic status, younger or older maternal age, poor nutrition, smoking, alcoholism, and illicit drug use.

Public awareness and education regarding chronic and life-threatening disease are also preventive health measures. Excessive exposure to direct sunlight can cause skin cancers and increase the development of cataracts. Although some cancers as well as diabetes and neuromuscular disorders cannot be prevented, both the incidence and complications of many of these illnesses can be reduced. For example, moderate- to high-fiber diets have been linked to the reduction of colon cancer; weight control is important when controlling complications of diabetes and activity as tolerated is important in reducing the incapacitation for those with neuromuscular disease.

Adequate rest, proper nutrition, and stress reduction are each important in preventing illness. Nurses can be role models in risk reduction in a variety of areas of life.

Government Policies that Protect People from Illness

A variety of services and information are available regarding living in a safer environment. Both in the United States and Canada, strict policies ensure that food and drugs are safe for the consumer. Regular inspection of food outlets and health standards for food handlers have made the food we purchase safer. The drug agencies outlined in Chapter 39 regulate research and the safe control and dispensing of prescription and nonprescription drugs.

Studies of environmental hazards have also greatly increased in number during the last few years. The conclusions of some of these studies have had such important implications regarding health care that all levels of government have mandated a wide variety of programs and regulations to improve or maintain the quality of the environment and the workplace.

A major factor in illness is that of smoking. The governments of both the United States and Canada have been assertive in encouraging smoking cessation and also in protecting the nonsmoking public. The American Lung Association has released accumulated evidence that what is referred to as "secondhand smoking" or "involuntary smoking" is hazardous. As early as 1979, Tagar reported that the children of heavy smokers had a greater incidence of lung function abnormalities than did the children of nonsmokers (Tager et al., 1979, p. 24). Most hospitals completely or partially ban smoking by patients, visitors, and staff within the facility.

Aside from smoke, there are other *carcinogenic* (cancer-causing) substances in the air, as well as in some of the foods we eat, the clothing we wear, and the products we use. Some of the information regarding environmental hazards is suggestive rather than conclusive. For example, large amounts of certain compounds have produced abnormal cells and illness in animals, but not in human beings. Despite continuing vigorous investigation by scientists and monitoring by those in the health care system, persons still become ill from exposure to unidentified substances in our environment.

Citizens groups have, on occasion, been effective in bringing about needed changes. Nurses, in particular, have responsibilities concerning health hazards in society in general and also in the health care setting. Research aimed at identifying dangers for health care personnel is continuing. (Consult Module 3 in *Modules for Basic Nursing Skills.*)

Restoration of Health

To heal is to restore health or eliminate illness. What brings about restoration? During the 18th and 19th centuries, seriously ill or wounded patients went to hospitals to be cured by the physician. The person was not expected to have an active part in this process. The role of the nurse was to assist the physician and provide routine physical care. Fortunately, all this has drastically changed. *Healing* appears to involve many factors other than direct intervention by the physician.

Nursing Intervention

Patients who receive selected drugs, undergo procedures, and receive direct nursing skills are being helped to heal (see Chapter 15). Much of nursing care assists the patient in the healing process. Providing adequate nutrition, exercise, and sleep and reducing exposure to microorganisms by providing an aseptic environment are nursing tasks that promote healing (Fig. 7-6). Psychological intervention is also important. Physicians and nurses who have built a strong trust relationship with their patients can influence healing. Because of this trust, patients expect a positive outcome. Therapeutic communication, listening, and touch are all important to healing.

Self-Care

An area being increasingly discussed is that of **self-care**, which refers to the patient's active involvement in bringing about healing. A large part of this position that patients should be active participants is that it allows control. This idea also implies changing the role of nursing in the practice of healing. Nurses need to encourage the patient's greater participation in the healing process and view it as an opportunity to change the nursing role. Nurses can provide motivation, structure and education, actions which promote and hasten healing.

Nontraditional Healing

In keeping with the holistic approach to health maintenance, **nontraditional healing** methods imply that "all possible avenues of healing must be used (or considered for use) and that no single healing be used to the

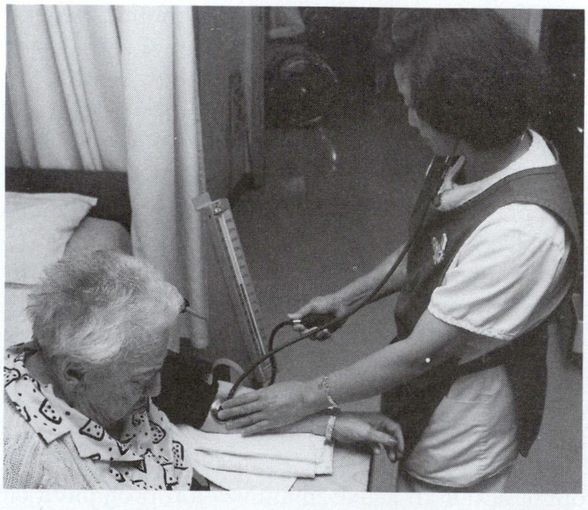

Figure 7-6. Physiologic intervention involves using direct nursing skills.

Nursing Issues and Trends: *Recognition of the Value of Nontraditional Medicine*

The National Institutes of Health of the federal government have formed a committee to study methods for healing that have been called "non-traditional". Healing is at best an imprecise "art". Nontraditional remedies used for healing have varied greatly among different cultures and belief systems. Some in the medical community have actively discouraged the use of nontraditional approaches to healing. It is encouraging that the government is taking part in a serious investigation of healing methods that have for too long been dismissed by western, technological medicine. Traditional and nontraditional methods may work in concert to improve the condition of those who are ill. As health care providers, we can use this opportunity to learn a great deal as patients search for methods which will restore and heal the body and mind.

exclusion of others" (Grant, 1978). It may be reasonable for us to begin to think of healing in subjective terms. Sometimes healing takes place without scientific explanation so that it is viewed as nontraditional. There are documented instances of people who have recovered or healed when medical standards indicate that they should not have. Nurses should be receptive to each person's feelings about healing. Meditation, relaxation, and imaging have long been used to promote healing of the mind and body. **Imagery** is a complex healing technique that basically consists of helping people to visualize the inner workings of their bodies in relationship to their illness and the treatment regimen. Several other techniques have proven useful to individuals in our society. **Acupuncture** is a healing method in which very thin needles are applied to various pressure points to relieve discomfort in other parts of the body. Long practiced in the Far East, acupuncture is gaining acceptance in the United States and Canada. **Biofeedback**, which is a means of providing information on specific body processes through the use of electronic devices, is also widely accepted. Some people find therapeutic touch, manipulation of certain body parts or pressure points, or faith healing additional adjuncts to healing.

There are other exciting pathways to healing. In writing of the crippling illness he suffered, Norman Cousins (1981) said that the value of humor was one of the "natural recuperative mechanisms of the body" (*Anatomy of an Illness*, p. 15). Quoting Hippocrates, Cousins wrote, "the human body is the physician of its own illness."

Rehabilitation

Rehabilitation is a process of education, actions, and treatments that results in maximizing function for the disabled person. Rehabilitation was once seen as appropriate only for the young or for those with obvious potential for improvement. Health professionals typically undertook efforts too late, in the belief that the rehabilitation period began only when the effects of the illness or injury had reached a plateau. This practice unfortunately delayed and sometimes even prevented the person from regaining useful abilities. Because a strong component of rehabilitation is attitude, delay is harmful not only to physical progress, but also to the person's mental well-being.

Rehabilitation should begin as soon as there is evidence of illness or disability. Johnson (1980) wrote, "Rehabilitation is a dynamic process that restores an individual to the highest possible level of function. Emphasis is placed on the individual's remaining abilities rather than on disabilities" (p. 221).

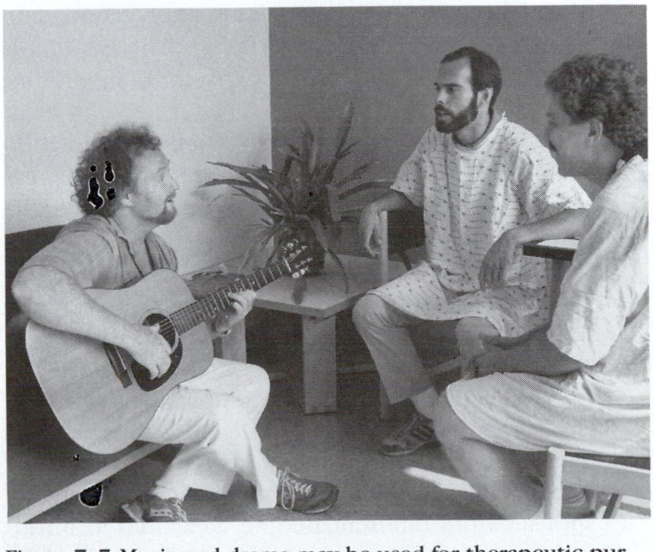

Figure 7-7. Music and drama may be used for therapeutic purposes during rehabilitation.

Rehabilitation is a concerted effort by the patient, as a motivated, active participant and by the health care team. Nowhere is it more important that the patient be a primary member of the health care team than in rehabilitation. The health care team may be much larger than one caring for an individual who recovers without disability. Members of the team may include psychologists, physical therapists, recreational and occupational therapists, and in some instances, music and drama therapists who practice specialties using music and drama for therapeutic purposes (Fig. 7-7).

Rehabilitation is a part of *all* nursing. This important premise implies that each integral part of nursing care for every patient must have as its goal the restitution of the highest possible quality of life for that individual.

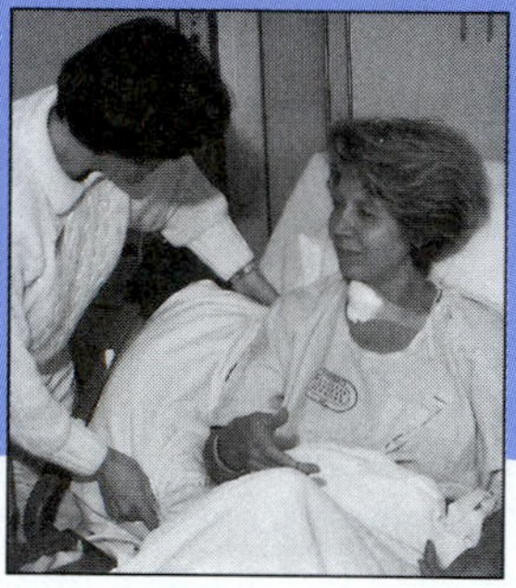

Key Points

- Definitions of health and illness can be both perceptual and subjective in nature. In a human needs framework, health can be thought of as a state in which needs are being sufficiently met to allow adequate functioning of the individual.
- The recent popular emphasis on health promotion and health maintenance is an indication that people want to help control their own health status.
- Acute illness occurs suddenly and progresses rapidly, often requiring expedient intervention, and may result in disability or death. Chronic illness has a slower onset and persists for 3 months or longer.
- The five stages of illness are: disbelief or denial, irritability or anger, attempts to cure the illness through self-treatment to gain some control over the situation, feelings of depression or despair, and finally acceptance.
- The causes of illness include invasion of body defenses by pathogens, immunopathology, biochemical imbalances, exposure to toxic substances or hazardous environmental conditions, injury, age-related conditions, and genetic and congenital defects.
- The patient role is complex, eliciting different responses from different people. Reactions to illness include discomfort with the dependent role, feelings of guilt about not meeting employment or social obligations, anxiety, fear, regression, self-centeredness, hostility, and depression.
- Nurses need to understand the reactions brought on by the crisis of illness so that they can respond appropriately.
- In many new concepts regarding the restoration of health (healing), the importance of maintaining a hopeful and positive attitude is stressed.
- Restoration of health includes rehabilitation, an ongoing program in which nurses play an important part, until physical and psychological functions are regained.

Study Questions

1. Give two examples of how earlier cultures viewed health.
2. Using a needs fulfillment definition of health and illness, how would you describe your state of health if you were ill with the flu?
3. What health programs are available within your community (*eg*, health clubs, YMCA, YWCA, weight reduction centers) and how important are they to you?
4. Define acute and chronic illness and identify ways in which one is different from the other.
5. Name the five stages of illness and describe feelings associated with each stage, again using the example of flu.
6. List four environmental conditions that are risk factors for illness?
7. How can the age of a patient be a risk factor for illness?
8. Of the many common responses to illness involved in the patient role, which do you see as most important for nurses?
9. How do you see yourself responding to some of the feelings of the patient that are a consequence of illness?
10. What does the term nontraditional healing mean?
11. Compare traditional and nontraditional concepts of healing.

12. Why are nurses particularly susceptible to be coming the "worried well"?
13. Name two ways you can personally reduce the risk of illness.

Critical Thinking Activities

1. Write out your beliefs about health maintenance. Discuss these in a small group.
2. Think about the last time you were ill. List your behavioral responses to illness. How were these responses helpful or not helpful to you in resolving your health problem? Discuss this in a small group setting.
3. Investigate a nontraditional health care provider. How does the care provided differ from traditional health care? In what ways are they the same? Give a brief report on what you have learned.
4. Find an article in a current periodical regarding a nontraditional healing practice or philosophy. Identify the most important parts of the article for a small group discussion.
5. Interview a patient/client in a health care facility. Review the patient's plan of care. Compare your interaction with the patient and the plan of care regarding the patient's health status.

References and Readings

Balog, J. E. "The Concepts of Health and Disease: A Relativistic Perspective." *Health Values: Achieving High Level Wellness* 6, 5 (September-October 1982): 7–13.

Baronowski, T. "Toward the Definition of Concepts of Health and Disease, Wellness and Illness." *Health Values: Achieving High Level Wellness* 5, 6 (November-December 1981): 246–256.

Belloc, M. B., and Breslow, L. "Relationship of Physical Health Status and Health Practices." *Preventive Medicine* 1, 3 (August 1972): 409–421.

Benson, A. M., and Williams, N. J. "Wellness Begins with the Nursing Student." *American Journal of Nursing* 88, 12 (December 1988): 1711.

Chang, S., Katz, M., and Hernandez, S. "The New AIDS Case Definition." *Journal of the American Medical Association* 267, 7 (February 19, 1992): 973–975.

Cousins, N. *Anatomy of an Illness.* New York: Bantam Books, 1981.

Crow, S. "Calling in Sick." *Nursing '90* 20, 3 (March 1990): 63–64.

dePender, W., and Ikeda-Chandler, W. *Clinical Ethics: An Invitation to Healing Professionals.* New York: Praeger Publishers, 1992.

Diamond, L. K. "Empowerment Through Self-Healing." *Revolution: The Journal of Nurse Empowerment.* 2, 2 (Summer, 1992): 116–121.

Dossey, B. "Awakening the Inner Healer." *American Journal of Nursing* 91, 8 (August 1991): 30–33.

Dubos, R. *The Mirage of Health.* New York: Harper & Row, 1959.

Dunn, H. *High-Level Wellness.* Arlington, Va.: R. W. Beatty, 1961.

Grant, L. *The Holistic Revolution.* Pasadena, Cal.: Ward Ritchie Press, 1978.

Johnson, J. H. "Symposium on Rehabilitation Nursing." *Nursing Research* 15, 2 (June 1980): 221.

Lamberton, M. M. "Health and Illness: A Co-Existence Hypothesis." *Nurse Practitioner* 8, 2 (February 1983): 47–52.

Levin, L. S. "Patient Education and Self Care." *Nursing Outlook* 26, 3 (March 1978): 170–175.

Lillis, P. P., and Prophit, P. "Keeping Hope Alive." *Nursing '91* 21, 12 (December 1991): 65–66.

Little, C. "Health for All by the Year 2000: Where is it Now?" *Nursing and Health Care* 13, 4 (April 1992): 198–201.

Macnee, C. L. "Perceived Well-being of Persons Quitting Smoking." *Nursing Research.* 40, 4 (July/Aug 1991): 200–203.

McNall, M. C. "Healing We Cannot Explain." *American Journal of Nursing* 89, 9 (September 1989): 1162–1163.

Mengel, T. E. "We Couldn't Come to Terms with Hank Until He Signed a Contract." *Nursing '92* 22, 1 (January 1992): 50–52.

Meyer, C. "Rehab: Primary Nursing as It Was Meant to Be." *American Journal of Nursing* 92, 2 (February 1992): 59–66.

Newman, B. M. "Health as a Continuum Based on the Newman Systems Model." *Nursing Science Quarterly* 3, 3 (Fall 1990): 129–135.

Norris, C. M. "The Work of Getting Well." *American Journal of Nursing* 90, 7 (July 1990): 47–50.

Parse, R. R. "Mysteries of Health and Healing: Two Perspectives." *Nursing Science Quarterly* 4, 3 (Fall 1991): 93.

Parsons, T. "Definitions of Health and Illness in the Light of American Values and Social Structure." In *Patients, Physicians and Illness,* edited by E. G. Jaco. New York: The Free Press, 1958.

Pender, N. J. "Predicting Health-Promoting Lifestyles in the Workplace." *Nursing Research* 39, 6 (November-December 1990): 326–332.

Popkess-Vawter, S. "Wellness: Nursing Diagnoses To Be or Not To Be." *Nursing Diagnosis* 2, 1 (January-March 1991): 19–25.

Reale, J. "Life Changes: Can They Cause Disease?" *Nursing '87* 17, 7 (July 1987): 52–55.

Robertson, J. F. "Promoting Health Among the Institutionalized Elderly." *Journal of Gerontological Nursing* 17, 6 (June 1991): 15–19.

Roy, Sr. C. *Introduction to Nursing: An Adaptation Model.* 2nd edition. Englewood Cliffs, N.J.: Prentice-Hall, 1984.

Shortridge, L. M., and McLain, B. R. "Levels of Intervention for a Coexistence Model." *Nurse-Practitioner* 8, 3 (March 1983): 74–79.

Shugars, D. A., O'Neil, E. H., and Bader, J. D. (Eds.). *Healthy America: Practitioners for 2005.* Durham, N.C.: The Pew Health Professions Commission, 1991.

Spence-Laschinger, H. K. and McWilliam, C. L. "Health Care in Canada: The Presumption of Care." *Nursing and Health Care.* 13, 4 (April 1992): 204–207.

Tager, I. B., Weiss, S. T., Rosener, B., and Speizer, F. E. "Effect of Parental Cigarette Smoking on the Pulmonary Function of Children." *American Journal of Epidemiology* 110 (February 1979): 15–25.

Tillich, P. "The Meaning of Health." *Perspectives in Biology and Medicine* (Autumn 1961): 92–100.

U. S. Department of Health and Human Services. *Healthy People 2000: National Health Promotion and Disease Prevention Objectives.* Bethesda, Md.: Public Health Service Publication No. 91-50213, 1992.

The Nursing Process

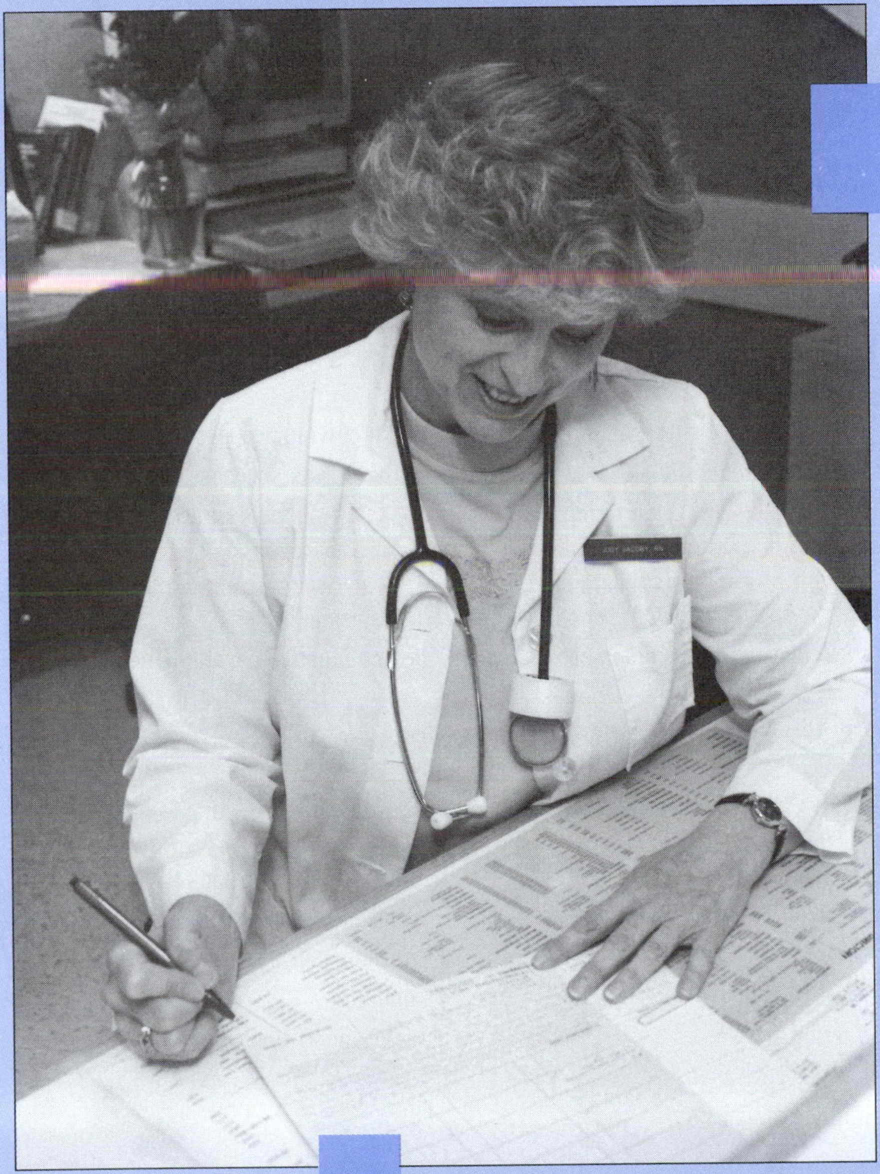

III

Overview of the Nursing Process

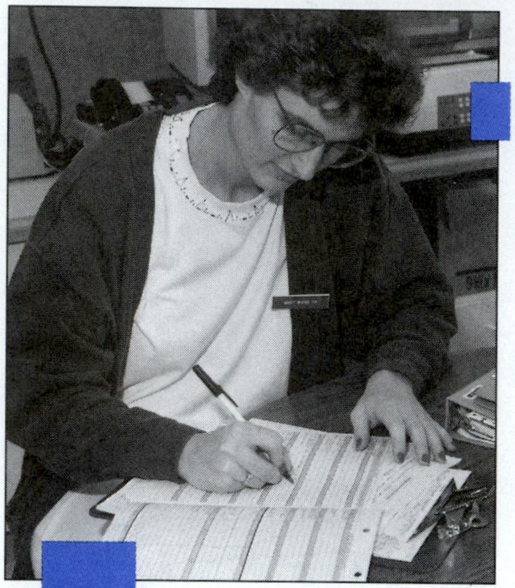

8

Objectives

After completing this chapter, you should be able to:

1. List and define the steps of the nursing process.
2. Explain the development of the five-step nursing process.
3. Compare the steps of the nursing process to the steps in the traditional scientific process.
4. Compare the nursing process to a problem-solving process.
5. Discuss the role of the patient/client in the nursing process.
6. Discuss how the nursing process serves as a framework for evaluation of nursing practice.
7. Discuss the relationship of the American Nurses Association (ANA) *Standards of Clinical Nursing Practice* to the nursing process.
8. Identify four common errors that the novice must be careful to avoid when using the nursing process.
9. Discuss your views of the art of nursing.

Study Terms

assessment
audit
concurrent review
critical thinking
desired outcomes
evaluation
goal
implementation
intuition
NANDA
novice
nursing art
nursing care plans
nursing diagnosis
nursing intervention
nursing observations
nursing process
planning
retrospective review

Outline

Purposes of the Nursing Process
A Background View of the Nursing Process
The Nursing Process as a Problem-Solving Process
Steps in the Nursing Process
The Ongoing Dynamic Nature of the Nursing Process
The Scientific Method Compared to the Nursing Process
Critical Thinking and the Nursing Process
Intuition and the Nursing Process
Documenting the Nursing Process
The Client as Partner in the Nursing Process
Evaluating Nursing Care
Standards for Evaluating Nursing
From Novice to Expert

Ellis, Nowlis: Nursing: A Human Needs Approach, 5th ed. © 1994 J.B. Lippincott Company

Nursing is performed in a wide variety of settings, from the community to the acute care facility. The nurse uses similar approaches to nursing care in all of these settings. This common approach to patient care has been named "the nursing process." The **nursing process** is a variation of the general problem-solving process adapted to the nursing situation. It is the process through which the nurse determines what needs to be done, plans how to do it appropriately, provides care, and then evaluates care.

Purposes of the Nursing Process

The use of the nursing process is not an end in itself. Its primary purpose is to provide for the maintenance or restoration of the client's health, in the broadest sense possible. The process is successful or unsuccessful only measured by the outcome for the client. It is important to keep this in mind as you evaluate your own use of the nursing process. A perfectly organized written plan, reflecting all the correct steps of the process, is not successful if it has not contributed in a positive way toward the well-being of the client.

Second, the nursing process provides a structure to help the nurse organize both the intellectual tasks and the physical skills involved in nursing practice. Nursing is a complex field, and this structure creates order and ensures that important components are not omitted.

Third, the nursing process assists the nurse in examining his or her own practice and evaluating it. Not only can the individual use this as a self-evaluation tool, but entire departments of nursing may use the process to evaluate the nursing care being delivered in a particular agency or facility.

A Background View of the Nursing Process

People looking from the outside at the practice of nursing sometimes erroneously describe nursing in terms of visible tasks performed. This view fails to recognize that a complex intellectual process was needed to determine what actions should be taken and whether changes had to be made in what was being done. Beginning in the 1960s, to help students understand this intellectual process, nursing educators began trying to identify its components. The result was several different descriptions of that process. Some described three steps in the nursing process (Johnson, 1959; Orlando, 1961; Wiedenbach, 1963), some had four (WICHE, 1967; Yura and Walsh, 1983; Little and Carnevali, 1969), and some listed five (Knowles, 1969; Freeman, 1970; Gebbie and Lavin, 1970).

The steps described often reflected which aspects of nursing practice were most important to the particular educator. For example, Orlando emphasized the interpersonal process between the nurse and the client; therefore, her steps were 1) behavior of the client, 2) reaction of the nurse, and 3) nursing action. Other authors included the behaviors of the client and reaction to the nurse as information to be gathered, but focused more extensively on what Orlando had grouped under "nursing action."

Knowles' (1969) approach—1) discover, 2) delve, 3) decide, 4) do, and 5) discriminate—appears to have been chosen partly to provide a device for those trying to remember the process as she described it. When the details of her descriptions are read, all of the components described in other terms by other authors can be found within her steps.

In the 1960s and early 1970s there was discussion within the health care field about whether the term "diagnosis" should be used by any groups other than physicians. The differences of opinion became especially marked when proposed changes in the nursing licensure laws included the term as a nursing function. Physicians stated that diagnosis referred to the diagnosis of disease, which was clearly a medical task. Nurses maintained that "diagnosis" is used in many nonmedical fields to refer to the identification of a problem within the context of each field. Thus, engineers may diagnose problems with bridges, attorneys may diagnose a legal difficulty, and nurses can and should make a nursing diagnosis. This latter view finally prevailed, and the term *nursing diagnosis* gained wide acceptance.

Through the 1970s and early 1980s descriptions of the nursing process began to consist of four or five similarly described steps. The five steps were 1) assessment, 2) nursing diagnosis, 3) planning, 4) intervention or implementation, and 5) evaluation. If the description consisted of four steps, the first was called assessment, which was then subdivided into two sections matching the first two steps of the five-step process. Step 1a was data collection and step 1b was statement of the problem or, later, nursing diagnosis. The other steps bore the same titles used in the five-step processes.

The **North American Nursing Diagnosis Association (NANDA)** (originally called the National Group for the Classification of Nursing Diagnoses) was established to provide a forum in which nurses could come to agreement on terminology and definitions to be used in regard to nursing diagnosis. As the work of this organization became better known and more nurses were emphasizing the intellectual skills involved in diagnostic reasoning, the five-step process grew in popularity be-

Nursing Issues and Trends: *Limitations of Nursing Process*

In order to facilitate understanding, the nursing process is usually presented as a series of steps. This implies to many people that the nursing process should be approached in a straight-line fashion. Some nursing leaders are distressed with this approach and worry that it tends to constrain our creativity. The complexity of nursing requires critical thinking and interpersonal interaction. Knowing comes not only from objective fact but also from personal relationships and even intuition. How can we combine a purposeful, ordered approach to nursing practice with the creativity necessary to provide optimum care?

cause of its emphasis on nursing diagnosis. In 1982, the National Council of State Boards implemented a new nursing licensure examination, based on a five-step nursing process. The steps were entitled 1) assessing, 2) analyzing (or diagnosing), 3) planning, 4) implementing, and 5) evaluating (Fig. 8-1).

Because many health care experts have placed more emphasis on evaluating services based on outcomes in the client or patient, some have suggested that the nursing process be reformulated so that stating desired patient outcomes is a separate step. This is seen in the ANA's *Standards For Clinical Nursing Practice* (1991). However, it is still most common to consider the formulation of desired patient outcomes as part of the planning process.

Here we will present the nursing process in a five-step format. We do not imply that other organizations are incorrect, but rather that at this time this format reflects the emphasis most often used within the nursing profession.

The Nursing Process as a Problem-Solving Process

You may have used a problem-solving approach on other concerns in your life without really thinking about it. The nursing process is only an extension and enhancement of skills you may already possess. The difference in nursing is that you will be asked to apply this process in a thoughtful and organized manner.

For example, your usual pattern of exercise might have included swimming three times a week. Since you started your nursing program, you have been skipping that activity. Yesterday you noted that you felt tired even though you hadn't done "that much." You reviewed your usual pattern of exercise, your current schedule, and demands placed on you by a combination of job, school, and family. You decided that the real problem was that you were not exercising enough. You determined that your goal was to maintain health while going to school and that this required some form of exercise. You looked at your options and decided that the best way to exercise was to walk to and from the farthest parking lot each day. This would be about 20 minutes twice a day. Although not as much as you preferred, you determined that this would meet your minimum needs and fit effectively into your schedule. As the week progressed and you carried out your plan, you remarked to a classmate, "It is a pain at times, but I really do feel better since I put some regular exercise back in my life!"

Now reread the above description outlining the steps. There are various ways of analyzing the process, and different people might specify different numbers of steps. The following analysis of the process has proven consistently helpful to beginning nursing students and practicing nurses.

First, having identified cues that a problem was present, you gathered information to identify clearly the real nature of the problem. The major initial cue was your unaccustomed fatigue. Additional important information was the comparison of your previous regular exercise pattern and your current routine. This was accom-

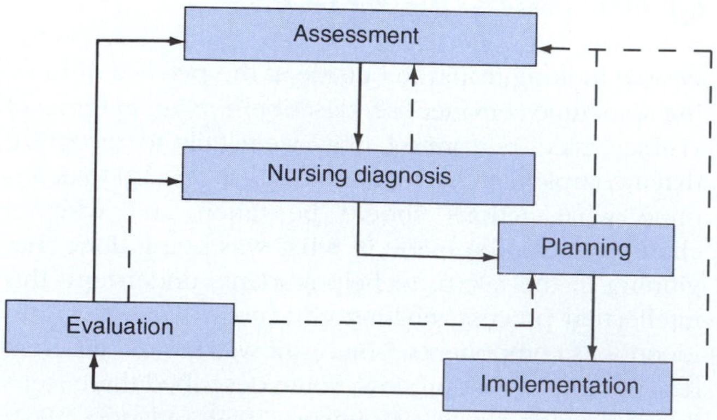

Figure 8-1. The nursing process.

panied by your understanding of the role of exercise in health.

Second, you identified that you were not including sufficient exercise in your current schedule. The clear identification of the real problem and its causes was your second step.

Third, you planned appropriate actions to help resolve your problem. In planning these actions you considered the time frame, the types of exercise you could do, and exactly what your goal was. In this case, you planned a new approach to exercise.

Fourth, the planned actions were carried out. Each day you walked to and from the parking lot. Last, you evaluated the effect of walking on your feelings of well-being and decided that it really did help although you found it inconvenient at times.

These steps are the same ones you will use in the nursing process. The initial step, in which you collected information, is called *assessment.* The second step in which the exact nature of the problem is identified is called *nursing diagnosis.* The third step, in which you identified desired outcomes and planned specific actions to be taken, is called *planning.* The fourth step, in which you carried out the plan, is called *implementation.* The fifth step, in which you reviewed the entire process, is called *evaluation.* From this beginning, let us now examine the nursing process.

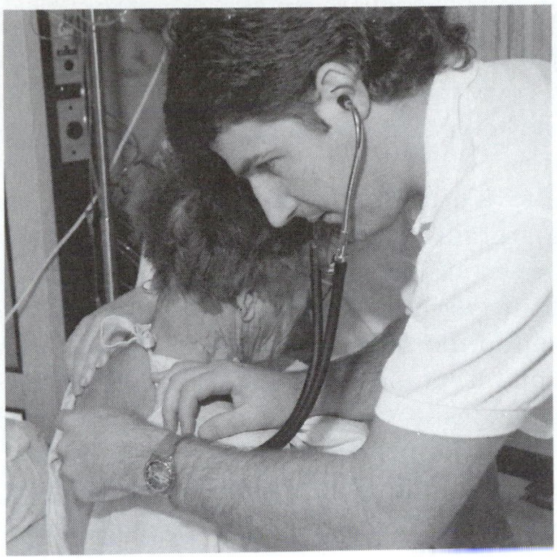

Figure 8-2. Information can be gathered by direct examination of the patient.

Steps in the Nursing Process

Step one, **assessment**, is the process of gathering information in regard to the client. Such information includes data obtained from records and gathered from clients and families through interviews, observation, and physical examination (Fig. 8-2). Deciding what data are needed for a particular client requires a sound background in nursing theory and the basic biologic and social sciences. As a student, you will need to consult texts and experts to determine what information is essential. What method to use for obtaining data is another important decision. Some data must be obtained by direct observation of the client; other facts are best obtained from an interview with the client. Finally, assessment requires skill in deciding what data will be needed. In Chapter 9, this will be discussed in greater detail. For example, John Smith, age 72, enters the hospital for care of a possible mild stroke. The nurse will interview both him and his wife and give Mr. Smith a physical examination. This is the basic assessment.

The term **nursing diagnosis**, step two, refers both to the intellectual process of sorting, classifying, and making decisions about the data collected and to the summary that will be the end result of this process. A variety of individuals and groups have formulated definitions of nursing diagnosis. A commonly used definition states that a nursing diagnosis is a statement of a "human response to an actual or potential health problem" (American Nurses Association, 1981) that can be helped by nursing intervention (see Chapter 10). Nursing diagnosis reflects the unique knowledge base of nursing. For Mr. Smith described above, the nurse might identify the nursing diagnosis "High Risk for Injury: Falls related to dizziness, unsteady gait, and left leg weakness" (see Appendix A).

Step three, **planning**, is the process of determining **desired outcomes** or **goals**, deciding what data should continue to be collected, determining appropriate nursing actions, and setting priorities for those actions. In planning for Mr. Smith, the nurse determines that the number one desired outcome or goal is "No falls or injury during hospitalization." A secondary goal might be that "Mr. and Mrs. Smith state the safety precautions for which Mr. Smith will assume responsibility." The nurse will then outline nursing actions to be taken to achieve these goals: 1) patient to be up only with assistance; 2) keep side rails up; 3) keep call light control within reach; 4) observe for steadiness, gait, and strength when assisting patient; and 5) discuss with Mr. and Mrs. Smith the importance of calling for assistance and the reasons for the restrictions. The nurse put the actions in the order of their importance to accomplishing the goals. As you can see, planning is a time-consuming step in the nursing process.

Step four, **implementation**, is the actual carrying out of the nursing care plan. The nurse caring for Mr. Smith will carry out the actions planned earlier. The designation **nursing intervention** is sometimes used for those nursing actions that may succeed in preventing or alleviating the problem. **Nursing observations** refer to the collection of data on an ongoing basis. Both are *nursing actions*, and both may be part of the nursing care plan (Fig. 8-3). In this case, the first three nursing actions could be considered nursing interventions because they might prevent falls. The fourth nursing action was a nursing observation to collect further information relative to the originally identified problem. The fifth nursing action was an intervention designed to accomplish the second goal that had been set. Specific technical skills needed for carrying out the nursing care plan are found in the *Modules for Basic Nursing Skills*, Volumes I and II. Communication skills necessary for such nursing actions as teaching the patient and family will be discussed in the text.

Step five of the nursing process, **evaluation**, is the process of determining the actual patient outcomes, reviewing the process used, and determining future actions. In determining whether you have met the established goals, you will compare the actual outcome with the originally stated desired outcome. In addition to evaluating for the achievement of outcomes, you will review the nursing process to determine whether any part of it needs to be altered. You might, for example, decide that you need to gather more data or data of a different type. Based on how effective the interventions were, you will determine whether the actions previously planned should be continued or adapted or whether different nursing interventions must be planned. Evaluation for Mr. Smith would require the nurse to discuss the safety measures with Mr. and Mrs. Smith and to determine whether they clearly understood how they could help to maintain safety. Final evaluation would come at the time of discharge, when it would be possible to identify whether falls had occurred during the entire hospitalization.

This, then is a brief outline of the problem-solving nursing process:

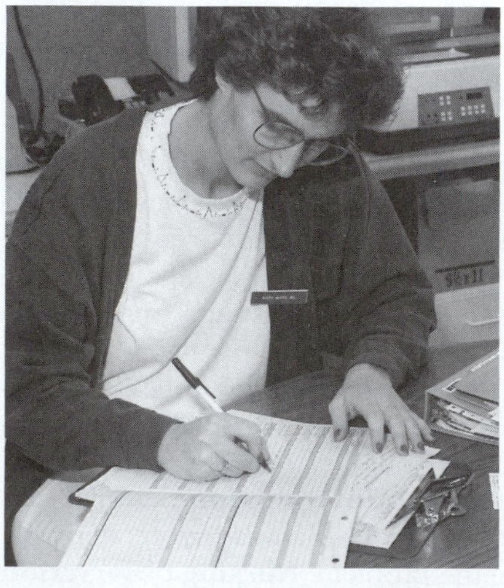

Figure 8-3. Nursing care plans commonly include nursing diagnoses, desired outcomes, and nursing actions.

1. Assessment
2. Nursing diagnosis
3. Planning
   a. Determination of desired patient outcomes/goals
   b. Identification of appropriate nursing actions
   c. Setting of priorities
4. Implementation of the plan
5. Evaluation
   a. Determination of actual patient outcomes
   b. Comparison of actual outcomes to desired outcomes/goals
   c. Review of the nursing process
   d. Determination of further actions needed

The Ongoing Dynamic Nature of the Nursing Process

It is important not to deduce from this explanation that the nursing process always appears in a logical, step-by-step linear pattern. Although the step-by-step pattern is a useful learning device, the reality is that the nurse in practice may carry out two steps simultaneously and move back and forth between steps as the situation requires. The process may follow a path that often might be described as winding, zigzag, or circular rather than straight.

For example, one piece of information might lead to an immediate decision to act. No formal nursing diagnosis might be formulated, the plan might never be written up, and the action might occur immediately. Viewed from the outside, this situation might look as if no planning or diagnosis had been done, only assessment and action.

In another situation, implementation of one plan might be taking place with evaluation occurring simultaneously, and then alternative actions might immediately be tried when the first action was unsuccessful in resolving the problem. Although a later analysis might reveal that additional planning took place within the mind of the nurse, the observer would think that actions had been consecutive, with no intermediate planning step.

At yet another time, one might see a nurse enter a patient's room to implement a previously devised plan. That nurse might then collect new data, immediately begin revising the statement of the nursing diagnosis, and proceed to plan anew. Thus, in this situation, the entire original process was never completed before the cycle began again.

The fluid nature of the nursing process in action requires the nurse to exercise a high level of skill based on a broad foundation of knowledge. The process must be a framework from which to build, not a rigid structure that confines or inhibits nursing creativity. The five steps describe basic aspects of the process, but their order is not meant as a rigid prescription. Figure 8-1 diagrams the nursing process. The standard order of the steps is indicated by solid lines; dotted lines show the other directions in which the process might go.

The Scientific Method Compared to the Nursing Process

You may have studied the traditional scientific method as part of a science course and noted that the nursing process resembles it in some ways. Although the steps are similar, the goals of the two processes are different. The purpose of the scientific process is the acquisition of knowledge. The purpose of the nursing process is the provision of care to a patient. Therefore, some of the careful constraints of the *scientific process*, such as lengthy searching of the literature before any plan is devised, may be unrealistic in the setting where a real problem must be solved quickly to reduce the suffering of an individual.

The steps of the scientific process include identification of the problem, data collection, formulation of a hypothesis, selection of a method for testing the hypothesis, testing it, interpreting the results, and evaluating the hypothesis. We will discuss how these steps relate to the steps of the nursing process.

In the nursing process as in the scientific one, there may be a preliminary identification of a broad problem area or concern. However, in nursing sometimes you start with no major area of concern, but rather from the more general standpoint of concern for the person's current health status. An example in the nursing process might be identifying that a patient looks slightly flushed and wondering if this might be significant. In the scientific process a more specific question begins the process. For example, a nurse researcher noted how much time nurses spend taking temperatures but could not find any research about the process of measuring a person's temperature. The nurse researcher then asked the specific question "How long must a glass thermometer remain in the mouth to obtain an accurate oral temperature?"

The data collection step in science is similar to the assessment step in the nursing process. In each, you try to gain all pertinent information about the problem area. Thus, in nursing, you may be gathering pertinent information about the person's health status. In the scientific process, a complete review of the professional literature relevant to the question is done at this time.

The formulation of a hypothesis in the scientific method involves analysis of the literature to identify relationships among concepts and make a clear statement that explains the facts. In our example, the nurse researcher might have noted that many nurses left thermometers in place for 3 minutes. Based on this information, the hypothesis might be "Leaving a glass thermometer in the mouth for 3 minutes provides an accurate measure of body temperature." A hypothesis is a tentative statement that must be tested before being accepted as an accurate reflection of the facts. In the nursing process, analysis of the data leads to the formulation of a statement of a nursing diagnosis. This diagnosis identifies the nature of the problem being experienced by the patient as well as the factors that contributed to the existence of that problem. Although a nursing diagnosis may be changed and revised, it is less tentative than is a scientific hypothesis.

The next step in both processes involves planning. In the scientific process, one plans a way to test the hypothesis to determine if it is correct. In the nursing process, one plans interventions that will resolve the nursing diagnosis, ongoing assessment that is needed, and the outcomes that will be used to evaluate the success of the plan. In our temperature example, the nurse researcher would plan a way to compare a variety of temperature taking strategies and times and a way to collect these data. In addition, the researcher would plan a method to analyze and evaluate the information obtained.

Implementation follows planning in both sequences. In the scientific method, the hypothesis is tested by carrying out the planned activities and gathering the data. In the nursing process, the planned nursing interventions and ongoing assessment are provided for the client.

The final step of the nursing process is evaluation of whether the desired patient outcomes were accomplished. Additionally, the nurse reviews the entire nursing process and determines whether the nursing diagnosis is accurate and whether plans need to be revised. In the scientific method, the data collected are interpreted and compared to the hypothesis to determine whether the hypothesis is supported by the data. This step involves evaluation of the original hypothesis. At the same time, the researcher evaluates the entire research project and identifies whether there were any weaknesses or limitations in the study and then makes suggestions for further research.

Critical Thinking and the Nursing Process

Much of higher education is engaged in a discussion of the importance of critical thinking and of how the skills of critical thinking can be enhanced (Paul, 1990; Ennis, 1985; Lipman, 1988). **Critical thinking** is "the art of thinking while you are thinking so as to make your thinking more clear, precise, accurate, relevant, consistent, and fair" (Paul, 1990, p. 32). Paul further describes critical thinking as characterized by logicalness, depth, completeness, specificity, significance, and adequacy. Clearly, critical thinking is an essential component of every aspect of the nursing process.

Critical thinking engages the individual in analysis of information. Analysis involves questioning the origin of data, from whom it was received and when it originated, to identify the biases present in the data itself. Analysis incorporates questions about the underlying meaning of data. Another important aspect of analysis is considering the significance of data for the future when planning.

Furthermore, critical thinking requires that the individual synthesize material from multiple sources to attain a unified view of the situation. The person who thinks critically is never satisfied with only one viewpoint, but rather recognizes that the best understanding of any situation is created from many viewpoints and ideas. Through using multiple sources, patterns that have significance can be discerned. Multiple sources of information can be synthesized into an individualized plan for action.

Critical thinking also involves examining all information from an evaluative viewpoint. The naive person accepts all input without question, which may create errors in decision-making. Questioning "What is the source of this information?" "Is this information accurate?" "Is it relevant?" "Is it adequate for decision-making?" "What are the biases reflected in the information?" are marks of critical thinking.

Through critical thinking, you can enhance your skills within the nursing process. Data are gathered with constant questioning. As you identify the nursing diagnosis, you are considering a wide variety of information and patterns. Planning requires a critical approach of evaluating the wide variety of nursing actions available, examining each in relationship to the particular situation, and selecting those most likely to be successful. As you carry out any nursing plan, you will be simultaneously evaluating the patient's response and your own practice. You will be considering the relevance of additional data. Evaluation of outcomes will be a consistent focus of your care and direct you as you consider your next steps.

Intuition and the Nursing Process

In more recent years, some nurses have begun to study the role of intuition in nurses' decision-making (Rew and Barrow, 1989). Questions arise as to what intuition is and how this fits in with the idea of the nursing process. **Intuition** for the purpose of this discussion is a sense of something that is not evident or deducible from the evidence available.

In many settings nurses speak of "knowing" that something is happening to a patient, but they are unable to identify the objective evidence that leads to this conclusion. The more this phenomenon is studied, the more apparent it becomes that experts in any field develop a heightened sensitivity that sometimes results in this type of intuitive knowledge. Whether this is based on rational evidence that has not yet come to conscious awareness or whether expert nurses become responsive to additional aspects of the person is not clear. What is clear, is that experts do and should pay attention to these intuitive cues. They may not base immediate action on intuition but may use it as an indicator of the need for closer monitoring, a more rigorous examination of the data, and for collection of new types of data.

Although you are a beginner in the field of nursing, you can consult with expert nurses. Listen to their statements regarding intuitive knowing. Identify the effects of their intuition on care they provide. The use of intuition is one aspect of the **art of nursing.**

Documenting the Nursing Process

Each health care facility has a standard format for documenting the nursing process as it is used for an individual patient. Many agencies use a document called a **nursing care plan** or *plan of care* that includes statements of nursing diagnoses, desired outcomes/goals, and nursing actions. Sometimes the assessment information used to identify a particular nursing diagnosis is included on the care plan. In most agencies, the assessment and evaluation steps are documented in the patient record or chart. In other agencies all steps of the nursing process are documented in the patient record and no separate nursing care plan is kept.

Throughout this text we will give you examples of nursing care plan entries to help you understand the process. In these examples, we will state a nursing diagnosis with the assessment data that supports it and then outline desired outcomes and list nursing actions with rationale. This format was chosen to help you learn the steps and to see how they fit together as whole.

As a student, you may be required to prepare a detailed nursing process paper. You may be asked to include all steps of the nursing process as well as your underlying rationale for actions, documentation of resources used in planning, and other information that will help your instructor to evaluate your nursing knowledge and your skill in applying that knowledge. This type of paper is a tool to assist you in learning to use the nursing process effectively and therefore is much more extensive than the working care plan used for delivering patient care.

The Client as Partner in the Nursing Process

Philosophically, the field of nursing has moved toward a greater emphasis on partnership with the health care client. This direction recognizes that the health of individuals and families is more important to them than to anyone else, that individuals and families have the right to self-determination, and that maximum effectiveness of any plan is achieved only when goals are shared by all those involved.

Although we speak of the "nursing" process, it is carried out on behalf of the client, and therefore the client is included at each step. Information is collected from and about the client. However, the validity or accuracy of the data must be checked with the client whenever possible (Fig. 8-4). When goals are formulated and plans for action are made, the client should have an opportunity to share in determining those goals and developing those plans. This is true not only because it is the client's right, but also because the plan will be more successful when the client participates. The client is asked to evaluate care not only so that the care may be improved, but also so that care may be improved for other clients with similar problems.

The nursing theory of Orem (1980) places a major focus on the nurse's role in supporting self-care. That emphasis has helped many nurses to examine their own practice and adapt it to give the client a larger role in care.

Another aspect of including the client in the nursing process is the necessity for the nurse to accept a client's personal goals even when those are not what the nurse would choose. One dramatic example is the client who has a bone marrow disorder that will be fatal unless treated by bone marrow transplant. However, the transplant has been given only a 50% chance of success for this client and will certainly cause severe illness and suffering during the period of treatment. The client may choose to not have this treatment but rather to die at home among loved ones. The nurse needs to support this decision, helping the client structure health care and a lifestyle that meets personal goals through hospice care. On the other hand, the client may choose to have the transplant and to struggle against all odds for longer life. The nurse supports this decision, helping the client to maintain maximum function and relationships within the constraints of this major treatment process.

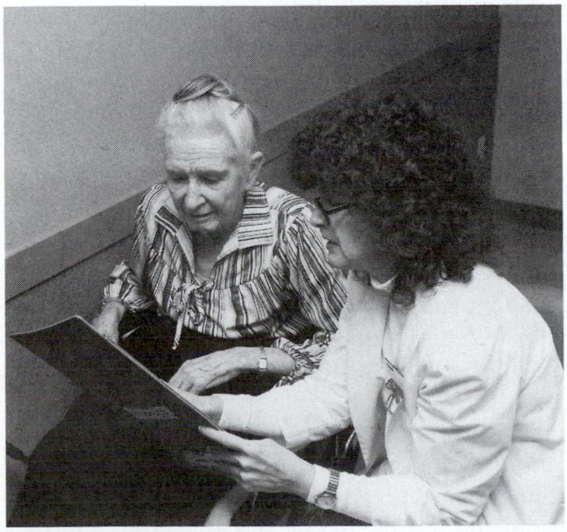

Figure 8-4. Validity of data should be checked with the client whenever possible.

Most instances of including clients in the decision-making process are much less dramatic but no less important. The person who is included in planning for postoperative care and who understands and agrees with the goals of that care will participate much more effectively. This same principle holds true at every level.

Evaluating Nursing Care

In Chapter 1 we explained that quality assurance programs designed to evaluate both the processes and outcomes of care are in place in almost all agencies that provide health care. Process criteria for nursing care are usually based on the steps of the nursing process.

Assessment criteria might identify what is to be included for a particular category of client and how soon after admission an initial assessment should be performed. For example, the criteria for a patient entering for surgery might state that the admission nursing assessment must be completed before the individual goes to the operating room, except in the case of an emergency admission.

Criteria related to nursing diagnosis might include the expectation that initial nursing diagnoses be identified and recorded within the first 24 hours after admission. Another criterion might specify the format in which nursing diagnoses are to be written.

Planning criteria might set the expectation that a plan of nursing care be written for each identified nursing diagnosis. Further criteria might list the necessary components of a correctly written plan.

Criteria for implementation might require that completion of nursing actions prescribed in the plan be documented in the patient's record. Further, the criteria might specify that the documentation include the date, time, and the name of the nurse implementing the plan.

Evaluation criteria might specify that measures for determining the effectiveness of the plan have been included in the written plan. Further documentation indicating that the patient was evaluated by these outcome measures might be required.

You will note that these examples all refer to examining the records to see whether the process was carried out correctly. In most instances, records are reviewed for quality assurance evaluations because records are the most economical method of review in terms of staff time. A review of records is called an **audit**. Audits are the most common method of ensuring quality of care.

However, some quality assurance evaluations are made by having observers visit the unit and note whether they see the criteria being met. This is useful but expensive because the observers must be knowledgeable and each observation is time consuming.

A **concurrent review** is an audit done while the patient is still hospitalized. The advantage of a concurrent review is that there is still an opportunity to effect change and improve care if the review reveals a concern. Concurrent reviews are often difficult to arrange when hospital stays are short.

A **retrospective review** is an audit done after the patient has been discharged from the facility. Retrospective reviews provide an opportunity to review records of several different patients with similar problems and identify general trends in care. Future patients who have the problem studied will benefit from the results of a retrospective review, but the patients whose records are reviewed will not benefit directly because they will already have been discharged.

Evaluating outcomes of care is becoming more widespread. One method of outcome evaluation involves examining whether the individual outcomes established for the client were attained. When doing an overall review regarding the attainment of outcomes, general outcome criteria for a large group of clients may first be established. These outcome criteria address global concerns such as the absence of complications, the length of stay, and ability to manage self-care. Often a level of attainment is specified, such as "90% of patients with this problem will be discharged on or before the fourth hospital day." The process of establishing these general outcome standards is extremely valuable for those providing care. As individuals study the records of many patients, patterns begin to emerge. Expectations are clarified. Thus, care for all patients is improved.

Standards for Evaluating Nursing

The ANA has developed standards for use as guidelines in evaluating nursing. The *ANA Standards of Clinical Nursing Practice* (American Nurses Association, 1991) are divided into two major sections. The first section titled Standards of Care is based on a nursing process approach to care. The six standards represent a six-step approach to the nursing process: assessment, diagnosis, outcome identification, planning, implementation, and evaluation (Display 8-1). Each standard has measurement criteria that can be used to determine whether the standard has been met.

The second section of the document includes Standards of Professional Performance. These standards are written in regard to quality of care, performance appraisal, education, collegiality, ethics, collaboration, research, and resource use. Again, measurement criteria have been developed for use in evaluating whether the standard has been met.

Display 8–1
ANA Standards of Care

Standard I.
Assessment: The nurse collects client health data.

Standard II.
Diagnosis: The nurse analyzes the assessment data in determining diagnoses.

Standard III.
Outcome Identification: The nurse identifies expected outcomes individualized to the client.

Standard IV.
Planning: The nurse develops a plan of care that prescribes interventions to attain expected outcomes.

Standard V.
Implementation: The nurse implements the interventions identified in the plan of care.

Standard VI.
The nurse evaluates the client's progress toward attainment of outcomes.

Source: American Nurses Association Congress for Nursing Practice, Washington, DC, 1991.

In addition to the ANA's general standards, specific standards have been developed for many specialty areas by groups of nurses who work in those specialties. Other standards that affect nursing have been developed by other organizations. The Joint Commission for the Accreditation of Healthcare Organizations (JCAHO) includes criteria for evaluating nursing practice in its standards for accrediting hospitals and other health care agencies. These criteria usually use the terminology of the nursing process.

The state licensing examination (NCLEX-RN) uses the nursing process as a framework for structuring questions. Many employers base their patient care planning system on the steps of the nursing process; as a beginning nurse you must be able to function within such a system. Thus, by the time you come to the end of your educational program, it is essential that you be thoroughly familiar with the nursing process.

If only to comply with standards, then, you need to learn to apply the nursing process. There is, however, an even more compelling reason to do so: the nursing process works! You will find that it lends structure to your thought processes, serves as a framework on which to organize information, and guides you to effective action.

From Novice to Expert

Benner (1984) describes the 1980 Dreyfus model, which outlined five levels of proficiency: novice, advanced beginner, competent, proficient, and expert. This model has particular application to nursing because nursing is a discipline in which the acquisition and development of skill is critical.

According to Benner, the *expert* is able to bring together a wide range of experiences and theory, quickly identify pertinent information, and discard what does not apply. This action leads to rapid and refined assessment of situations as a whole and the ability to intervene effectively without considering a range of wasteful options. As a novice, you must be careful not to make the erroneous assumption that because expert nurses act rapidly, the nursing process is not being used. Expert nurses more visibly demonstrate the use of the nursing process when they are faced with a new or unique challenge in patient care.

At the other end of the spectrum of experience and beginning with fewer ideas, the **novice** must guard against prematurely fixing on a narrow view of the situation and thus failing to explore the many alternatives available for nursing action. As a beginner, you may need to move more painstakingly and in a more ordered way through the nursing process than would an expert. You will not possess the knowledge base and experience to adapt quickly what you are doing and move to a different step in the process. The beginner in any field must operate in a different manner from the expert who has a broad background of experience on which to draw. You will need to rely on the judgment and advice of experienced staff nurses and nursing instructors to guide your decision-making.

You must refrain from moving immediately into action without careful planning, goal setting, and thinking of objectives, as well as frequent consultation. When you move too quickly into action, you may have failed to understand the underlying problem clearly or to consider the possible consequences of your actions. Lack of planning could lead to incorrect decisions about what actions are most appropriate.

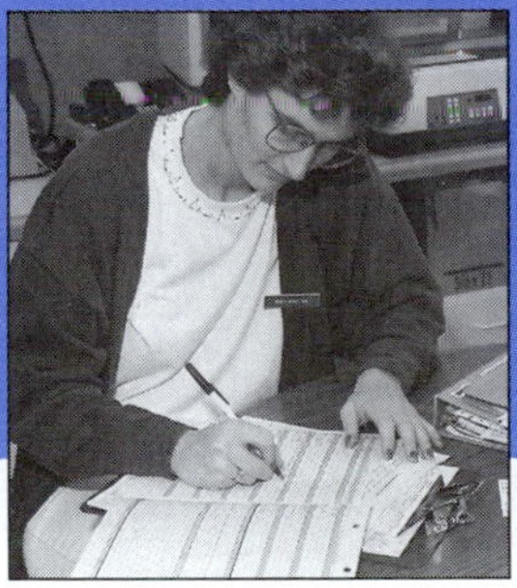

Key Points

- The primary purpose of the nursing process is to provide for the maintenance or restoration of health. It provides a framework for organizing practice and evaluating that practice.
- The nursing process consists of the following steps: assessment, nursing diagnosis, planning, implementation, and evaluation.
- Assessment involves gathering data. Diagnosis requires the analysis of that data to describe the client's problem and its etiology concisely. Planning refers to the careful identification of the desired outcomes and the nursing actions appropriate for achieving those outcomes. Evaluation is an ongoing process that focuses primarily on identifying whether outcomes have been achieved and secondarily on whether the process itself was carried out appropriately for the particular client.
- There are many similarities between the nursing process and the traditional scientific method.
- Intuition may be used by expert nurses as an indicator of the need for increased acuity in assessment of the patient.
- The client is a partner in all of health care and needs especially to be included in the nursing process. Data are collected from the client and, whenever possible, the client validates the accuracy of all data collected. The care plan must be one that is acceptable to the client; therefore, the client's participation is important.
- A variety of standards based on the nursing process has been designed to evaluate nursing practice.
- The nursing process provides a sound basis for moving from novice to expert nurse.
- The judgment and advice of experienced nurses can be invaluable to the beginning nurse.

Study Questions

1. What are the steps of the nursing process?
2. In what ways does the four-step process differ from the five-step process?
3. How are the steps of the nursing process similar to the steps of the traditional scientific process?
4. In what ways might the client be involved in the nursing process?
5. What are the ANA *Standards of Clinical Nursing Practice*? How do they relate to the nursing process?

Critical Thinking Activities

1. Select a particular nursing theorist named in Chapter 1. Investigate what that nursing theorist has written in regard to the nursing process. How does this theorist's viewpoint compare with the one in the text?
2. Obtain a copy of the nursing care plan used in a clinical facility. Identify the steps of the nursing process that are a part of that nursing care plan. If some steps are not included, learn where they would be documented. Evaluate the way the nursing process is documented.
3. If your nursing program assigns a nursing process paper, compare the steps with those given in the text. How does it differ? Analyze this paper to determine what aspects of the nursing process are being emphasized at your level?
4. Interview a registered nurse in regard to his or her use of the nursing process. Ask for that individual's evaluation of its value in practice.

References and Readings

American Nurses Association. *Scope for Nursing Practice: A Social Policy Statement*. Kansas City, MO: ANA, 1980.

American Nurses Association. *Standards of Clinical Nursing Practice.* Kansas City, Mo.: ANA, 1991.

Bailey, J. T., and Hendricks, D. E. "Decisions Made Easy." *Nursing '90* 20, 1 (1990): 120–122.

Benner, P. *From Novice to Expert: Excellence and Power in Clinical Nursing Practice.* Menlo Park, Cal.: Addison-Wesley, 1984.

Benner, P., and Tanner, C. "Clinical Judgment: How Expert Nurses Use Intuition." *American Journal of Nursing* 87, 1 (1987): 23–31.

Buber, M. *I and Thou.* Translated by R. G. Smith. New York: Charles Scribner's Sons, 1958.

Carboni, J. T. "A Rogerian Theoretical Tapestry." *Nursing Science Quarterly* 4, 3 (Fall 1991): 130–136.

Carpenito, L. J. *Nursing Diagnosis: Application to Clinical Practice.* 4th edition. Philadelphia: J. B. Lippincott, 1992.

Ennis, R. H. *Goals for a Critical-Thinking/Reasoning Project.* Champaign, Ill.: University of Illinois, 1985.

Gebbie, K., and Lavin, M. A. "Classification of Nursing Diagnosis." *American Journal of Nursing* 75, 2 (1975): 250.

Iyer, P. W., Tapitch, P. J., and Bernocchi-Losey, D. *Nursing Process and Nursing Diagnosis.* 2nd edition. Philadelphia: W. B. Saunders, 1991.

Johnson, D. "A Philosophy of Nursing." *Nursing Outlook* 7, 2 (1959): 198.

King, I. M. "Health as the Goal for Nursing." *Nursing Science Quarterly* 3, 3 (Fall 1990): 123–128.

Knowles, L. "Decision Making in Nursing: A Necessity for Doing." *ANA Clinical Sessions 1966.* New York: Appleton-Century-Crofts, 1967.

Kyle, B. A. S., and Pitzer, S. A. "A Self-care Approach to Today's Challenges." *Nursing Management* 21, 3 (March 1990): 37–39.

Laschinger, H. K., and Duff, V. "Attitudes of Practicing Nurses Towards Theory-based Nursing Practice." *Canadian Journal of Nursing Administration* 4, 1 (March-April 1991): 6–10.

Lipman, M. "Critical Thinking and the Use of Criteria." *Inquiry: Newsletter of the Institute for Critical Thinking,* Montclair State College (March 1988): 3-8.

Little, D. E., and Carnevali, D. L. *Nursing Care Planning*. Philadelphia: J. B. Lippincott, 1969.

Miers, M. "Developing Skills in Decision-Making." *Nursing Times* 86, 30 (1990): 32–33.

Orem, D. *Nursing: Concepts of Practice.* New York: McGraw-Hill, 1980.

Orlando, I. *The Dynamic Nurse-Patient Relationship.* New York: G. Putnam and Sons, 1961.

Passmore, J. "On Teaching To Be Critical." In Peters, R. S. (ed.): *The Concept of Education.* London: Routledge & Kegan, 1967, pp. 192–211.

Paul, R. W. *Critical Thinking.* Rohnert Park, Cal.: Sonoma State University, 1990.

Rew, L., & Barrown, E. "Nurses' Intuition: Can It Co-Exist With the Nursing Process?" *AORN Journal* 50 (1989): 353–358.

Wiedenbach, E. "The Helping Art of Nursing." *American Journal of Nursing* 63, 1 (1963): 64.

Yura, H., and Walsh, M. *The Nursing Process: Assessment, Planning, Implementing, and Evaluation.* 4th edition. New York: Appleton-Century-Crofts, 1983.

Assessment

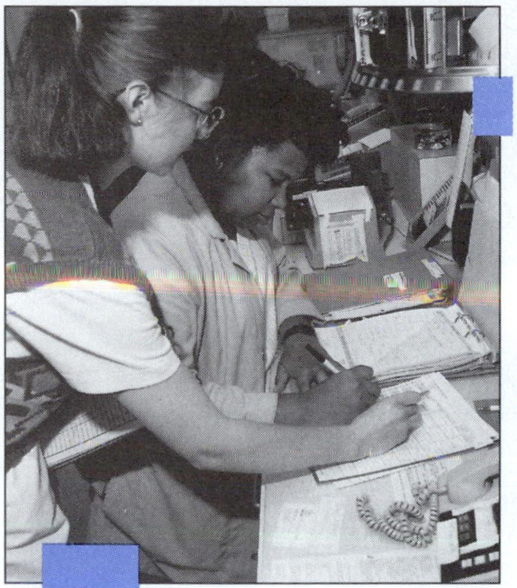

9

Objectives

After completing this chapter, you should be able to:

1. Define assessment.
2. Explain two major purposes of assessment.
3. Identify and explain one organizing framework for assessment.
4. List the sources of assessment data.
5. Identify the data that can be gathered through general observation.
6. Differentiate between structured and unstructured interviews.
7. Differentiate between objective and subjective data.
8. Outline the physical examination process.
9. List data available from records.
10. Describe two different ways you might gather data from colleagues.
11. Differentiate between the requirements of an initial assessment and those of an ongoing assessment.

Study Terms

activities of daily living
developmental self-care requisites
health deviation self-care requisites
interview
modes of adaptation
objective data
observation
pattern
self-care requisites
structured interview
subjective data
universal self-care requisites
unstructured interview

Outline

Assessment is the process of gathering data to provide effective nursing care. The American Nurses Association (ANA) *Standards of Clinical Nursing Practice* (1991) refer to it as "a systematic, dynamic process." It includes gathering information in regard to physical, psychological, sociocultural, spiritual, and developmental aspects of the client.

A nurse has many responsibilities in regard to assessment. The nurse must determine what information is needed in a specific situation. An extensive theoretical background is needed to determine what information should be sought. Determining the priority for gathering this information is another significant nursing responsibility. Some information will be needed immediately and some may be gathered later without compromising care. Additionally, the nurse is responsible for mastering the skills needed for effective assessment. These include the skills of interviewing and physical examination as well as many others. *Modules for Basic Nursing Skills*, Volume I, gives detailed information on assessment skills.

As you learn more and more about health-related problems, you will learn what information is most important in differing situations and you will learn additional advanced skills. In this chapter we provide an overview of data collection. More detailed information about what data would be needed before dealing with a particular human need will be found in the chapter that discusses that specific need. Specialized nursing texts such as those for medical–surgical and maternity nursing will provide greater detail about the assessment needed for individual health care problems.

Gathering information includes obtaining data from patients themselves or their families through interview, observation, and physical examination. It also includes gathering relevant data from the patient's record and from other members of the health care team who have cared for the patient. Further information may be needed from nursing theory in texts and articles. You may also get information from nursing experts, such as your instructor, an experienced nurse, or a clinical nursing specialist (Fig. 9-1).

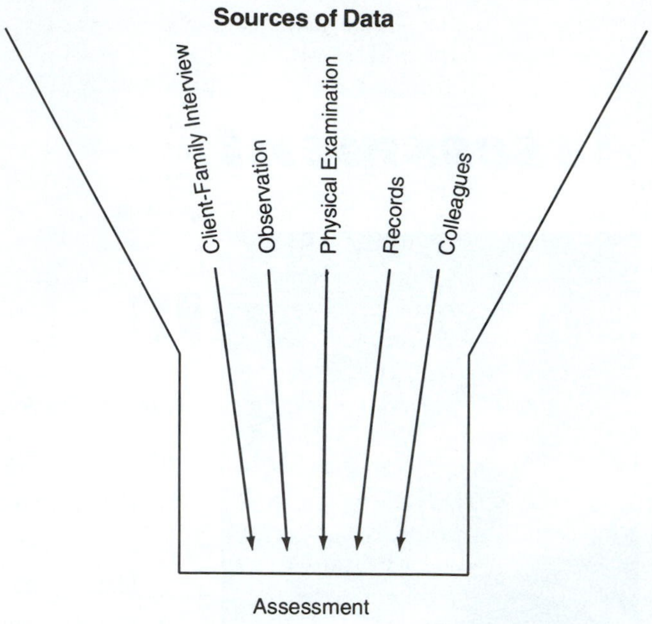

Figure 9-1. Assessment is composed of data from many sources.

Purposes of Assessment

Data are collected to identify the client's problems, formulate nursing diagnoses, plan appropriate actions, and evaluate the effectiveness of health care. For the hospitalized person, continuing data collection serves as the foundation of sound care. Those in home care conduct periodic assessments to guide the client, family, and care providers.

New data may reveal new or modified nursing diagnoses at any time. During the implementation of a plan for nursing care, *data collection* will help you to determine the patient's immediate responses to nursing action and to identify which nursing actions are inappropriate. It may be necessary to halt a plan immediately to safeguard a person, for example, when dizziness might lead to a fall. Data also are collected to evaluate the patient's progress toward desired outcomes. Nurses assist with evaluating progress, lack of progress, or even regression in relation to medical diagnoses as well as in relation to nursing diagnoses.

Accurate and appropriate assessment is a legal as well as a professional responsibility of nurses. Courts have held that failure to make appropriate assessments or to recognize the significance of data gathered is malpractice when a problem was not recognized nor appropriate actions taken resulting in harm to the patient.

Organizing the Assessment Process

As you observe and listen attentively to what the patient tells you, you must constantly relate the resulting information to your knowledge of such basic sciences as anatomy, physiology, pathophysiology, sociology, and psychology. You will also increasingly relate your observations to your knowledge of human needs, nursing theory, and nursing practice and gradually become better able to discern when needs are unmet and basic homeostasis is disturbed. Organizing your data as you collect the information helps you later as you begin to try to discern patterns and trends. When your data are organized, you will find it easier to interpret their meaning.

Numerous systems and tools for data collection have been devised to help nurses remember what data to collect and to organize the information obtained. For many years some nurses used the "21 Nursing Problems" of Abdellah and colleagues (1961) as a guide to assessment. From this list, for example, the nurse would take each possible problem, such as inability to eat and drink normally, and collect data to identify whether or not that problem was present.

Another approach to assessment focuses on the normal healthy individual. Its aim is to collect data on all healthy aspects of the person to identify any deviations from that healthy state. Most currently used systems start from this approach. One of the earliest of these was Henderson's list of **activities of daily living**, which contained her classic statement of "The Nature of Nursing" (1966; see Display 1-4) that identified those things the healthy person would do for the self if able.

The theoretical framework that you use for a basis for your practice will provide your orientation to assessment. Although the assessment will eventually involve the entire person whatever the system used, the system chosen will give special emphasis or a sense of importance to some particular aspect of the data.

Gordon's Functional Health Patterns

Gordon (1987) has developed an assessment framework based on the *functional health patterns.* She states that functional patterns represent patient strengths, and dysfunctional patterns represent areas of nursing diagnoses. A **pattern** is defined as a "sequence of behavior across time" (p. 92). Eleven functional health patterns are presented in Display 9-1.

Roy's Modes of Adaptation

Roy (1984) presents an adaptation model of nursing. She identifies adaptation as occurring within four of what she calls **modes of adaptation**: *physiologic mode, self-concept mode, role function mode,* and *interdependence mode.* Display 9-2 presents her organization of the modes of adaptation. Within each mode, the nurse looks for data that represent three types of stimuli. Focal stimuli are those situations or conditions immediately confronting the individual that can lead to failure to adapt. Contextual stimuli are all other contributing factors in the environment. Residual stimuli are those attitudes, traits, and cultural determinants that may possibly be affecting the present situation, but the effects of which are difficult to validate.

Display 9–1
Gordon's Functional Health Patterns

Health perception/health management
Nutritional/metabolic
Elimination
Activity/exercise
Cognitive/perceptual
Sleep/rest
Self-perception/self-concept
Role/relationship
Sexuality/reproductive
Coping/stress tolerance
Value/belief

Source: Gordon, M. *Nursing Diagnosis: Process and Application.* 2nd edition. New York: McGraw-Hill, 1987.

Orem's Self-Care Model

Orem (1991) focuses on those conditions and processes needed to support effective self-care, that is, **self-care requisites**. Assessment, then, would focus on identifying whether these self-care requisites are available to the individual. She divides self-care requisites into three groups: **universal self-care requisites**, those that are the same for all people; **developmental self-care requisites**, which are based on the person's age and developmental level; and **health deviation self-care requisites**, which are individual needs based on the presence of pathology in the person. Display 9-3 outlines Orem's self-care requisites.

Neuman's Systems Model

Neuman (1982) presents a model of nursing that focuses on the *stressors* influencing the client and the strengths of the client to resist those stressors. Stressors and strengths, as perceived both by the patient and by the caregiver, are explored. Display 9-4 outlines this approach.

Basic Needs as an Assessment Framework

The framework of the person we present here is organized around human needs. We believe that this organization is clearly helpful and understandable to the beginning student and that it can be adapted to the nursing model being applied. The two major categories

Display 9–2
Modes of Adaptation in Roy's Adaptation Model

Physiologic Mode

Oxygenation
Nutrition
Elimination
Activity and rest
Skin integrity
The senses
Fluid and electrolytes
Neurological function
Endocrine function

Self-concept Mode

The physical self
  Body sensations
  Body image
The personal self
  Self-consistency
  Self-ideal/self-expectancy
  Moral-ethical-spiritual self

Role Function Mode

Primary role
  Age/sex/developmental level
Secondary role
  Relatively permanent achieved positions requiring performance (wife, father, son, sister)
Tertiary role
  Temporary, freely chosen (employee, student)

Interdependence Mode

Support systems
Receptive/contributive behaviors

Source: Roy, Sr. C. *Introduction to Nursing: An Adaptation Model,* 2nd edition. Englewood Cliffs, N.J.: Prentice-Hall, 1984.

are the patient's *physical* and *psychosocial needs.* Display 9-5 outlines human needs as presented in this text. In *Modules for Basic Nursing Skills,* Volume I, Module 5, you will find a format for organizing your data based on human needs. Module 5 presents a detailed discussion of the data pertinent to each of the basic needs.

Sources of Data

No matter what conceptual model of data collection you use, the sources of data are the same. There are basically five: 1) *observation,* 2) client/family *interview,* 3) *physical examination,* 4) *records,* and 5) *colleagues.*

Observation

Observation is the process of obtaining data through visual means. Observation reveals **objective data**, that is, data that could be confirmed by another observer. General observation begins when you enter the room and starts with a focus on the patient. Observations should describe the physical appearance or the behavior of the person. Emotions cannot be observed and are not considered objective data. However, behavior that might indicate what a person is feeling can be observed. These behaviors would be the objective data. After noting them, you would interview the client to obtain subjective data regarding the presence of particular feelings.

Most written assessments begin with general descriptive statements of the patient's appearance. Such statements often become so routine that abbreviations are used to indicate these general observations. For example, you may see an initial assessment that states, "WD, WN, BM," meaning: well developed, well nourished black male. These generalized statements contain conclusions as well as objective data. That the client is a black male could be easily verified. However, the statement, "well developed" is open to interpretation in various ways. You should make your observations as factual as possible and reserve opinions and conclusions for the diagnostic process that will follow the collection of data.

Appropriate descriptive statements would describe posture as erect, slightly stooped, or with pronounced deviation to the left, for example. If the patient is in bed, the position in bed is important. Facial expression might be described as animated, flat, or smiling. Behavior might be described as sitting quietly, in continual movement, or slow ponderous movements. Behaviors that indicate feelings, mood, or pain can be described. All of these are examples of objective descriptions. Observa-

Display 9–3
Orem's Self-Care Model Assessment

Universal Self-care Requisites

Air, water, food
Elimination processes
Solitude and social interaction
Prevention of hazards to human life and functioning
Normalcy (state of being normal according to scientific theories and cultural and societal values)

Developmental Self-care Requisites

Maintenance of conditions to support life processes including developmental stages
Prevention of adverse effects on development of conditions such as loss

Health Deviation Self-care Requisites

Seeking appropriate medical assistance for pathology
Attending to the effects of pathology
Carrying out prescribed measures effectively
Caring for or regulating uncomfortable or deleterious effects of prescribed medical measures
Accepting self in relationship to a state of health in need of health care and modifying the self-concept
Altering one's lifestyle to promote personal development while living with the effects of pathology and medical measures

Source: Orem, D. *Nursing: Concepts of Practice,* 2nd edition. New York: McGraw-Hill, 1984.

tions would also include observing all body excretions such urine, stool, vomitus, and sputum.

From your initial observation of the patient, you should expand your observation to include the patient's immediate environment. If this person is in bed, what type of bed? Are side rails in place? What special medical equipment is there for care? Is all of that equipment in current use? Any equipment in current use should be checked to be certain that it is functioning. You may discover an electrical device, which has been unplugged, and is therefore not working or other such problems through careful observation. If the equipment is not in current use, is it for use at a later time or was it formerly used and never removed from the setting? Is there a call light within reach? Are items the patient needs, such as water glass or tissues, placed conveniently? Part of your responsibility will be to manage this environment, and this initial assessment will aid you in establishing a supportive setting for care.

Expand your observation to include the entire room. Consider lighting. If the patient wishes to read, is the light adequate? Is there glare from a window in the patient's eyes? Is the temperature comfortable? Are safety hazards present, such as water spilled on the floor or an obstacle between the patient and the bathroom door? Are supplies for care stored in the room? All of these will be important as you plan for care.

Client/Family Interview

After you have made a general observation of the patient and the environment, you have a basis from which to begin an interview. An **interview** is a conversation between two individuals in which one individual seeks information and the other provides it (Fig. 9-2). In a nursing setting, you will be seeking information from the patient or family or both.

Interviews are often characterized as structured or as unstructured. A **structured** (or formal) **interview** is one in which the questions are predetermined and the interviewer carefully raises each question in turn. An **unstructured** (or informal) **interview** is one in which the interviewer formulates new questions based on the responses of the person being interviewed. Thus, the

Display 9–4
Neuman's Systems Model of Assessment

Stressors and Strengths

Stressors perceived by the patient
Strengths perceived by the patient
Stressors perceived by the caregiver
Strengths perceived by the caregiver

Factors to Be Considered

Intrapersonal Factors
Physical (mobility, oxygenation, etc.)
Psychosociocultural (attitudes, values, expectations, behavior patterns, nature of coping patterns)
Developmental (age, degree of normalcy, present developmental process)

Interpersonal Factors
Resources and relationships of family, friends, or caregivers

Extrapersonal Factors
Resources and relationship of community facilities, finances, or employment

Source: Neuman, B. *The Neuman Systems Model.* Norwalk, Conn.: Appleton-Century Crofts. 1982.

Display 9–5
Human Needs as Assessment Categories

Physical Needs

Safety
Skin integrity and hygiene
Mobility and activity
Sleep and rest
Nutrition
Bowel elimination
Urinary elimination
Oxygenation
Circulation
Fluid and electrolyte balance
Regulation/sensation/perception

Psychosocial Needs

Social, cultural, and ethnic identity
Mental health/coping
Self-concept
Values and beliefs
Sexuality

unstructured interview may move in unpredictable directions.

Nursing interviews typically combine structured and unstructured aspects. The *nursing history form* developed by a particular health care agency is a carefully planned document designed to ensure that essential information is sought (Fig. 9-3). However, the specific questions the nurse would use to elicit that information may not be listed. In addition, the nurse is expected to perceive cues in the client's or family's statements that should be explored further to gain a comprehensive view of the unique individual. Thus, the interview may proceed in an unstructured manner although it was initially designed with a specific structure.

Information elicited in an interview with the client is termed **subjective data**, which means that the data originated with the subject (the patient/client). Subjective data should be clearly identified as such in any written record. In some records this is done by writing, "Client states . . ." In other records the letter "S" precedes all statements of subjective data. A nursing history form consisting of questions to be asked is accepted as being composed of subjective data. When recording subjective data, you must guard against inserting your own opinions or conclusions. For example, if the person appears to be upset or anxious, this fact should not be recorded as subjective data until the person actually says that he or she is feeling upset or anxious. Table 9-1 illustrates the differences between subjective and objective data.

When the client is unable to respond in an interview either because the client is a small child or because the client is too ill, a family member is interviewed. In this context, family is a broad term and includes those persons the client regards as significant support persons. Care must be taken to accurately record the origin of the information.

Many nursing interviews are totally unstructured in nature. While providing care, the nurse may question the patient in regard to certain health problems, about the patient's knowledge of care requirements, or about feelings being experienced. These interviews may be brief, encompassing only a few questions. For example, when a patient has had surgery, the nurse might ask a few pertinent questions about pain to determine whether nursing intervention for pain was needed. In another instance, an unstructured interview might be lengthy as a nurse explores with a patient the plans that have been made for care after discharge from the hospital.

Effective interviewing is a complex skill. It involves active listening, observing behavior and facial expressions, and formulating appropriate replies and questions. Perceptions of feelings, beliefs, or attitudes must always be *validated*, that is, verified with the client, to ensure that they are accurate. The skills involved in interviewing are presented in Chapter 13. Display 9-6 presents a brief example of an unstructured interview.

Physical Examination

After you have spoken with the patient, you are ready to collect data through a physical examination of the patient (Fig. 9-4). In some settings, nurses are responsible for performing complete diagnostic physical examinations, which is an advanced skill found in complete texts on physical assessment (Bates, 1991). However, all nurses must be able to do basic physical examinations, which is what we will discuss here. During the physical examination, you will use the four techniques of inspection, palpation, auscultation, and percussion to gather data.

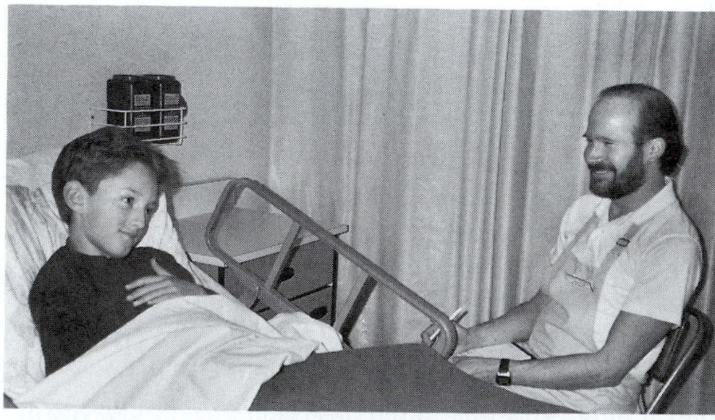

Figure 9–2. Effective interviewing includes listening, observing, and making appropriate responses.

NURSING ADMISSION DATA

	Medications (Prescription and over-the-counter)								Disposition of meds:
T: 98 4/5	Medication and strength	dose	freq.	time last dose	Medications and strength	dose	freq.	time last dose	☒ did not bring
P: 66	1. Lanoxin	.1mg	qd	This a.m.	6.				☐ patient has
R: 18	2. Maalox	2Tsp.	prn	Yes-ter-day	7.				☐ family has
BP: 142/84	3.				8.				☐ retained to ID
Wt (Kg): 73.6	4.				9.				☐ other
Ht: 5'8"	5.				10.				

Date: 4/18/94 Time: 12:50 Signature: N. Nifelt RN

NURSING DATA BASE

☐ OUTPATIENT ☒ INPATIENT ☐ EXPEDITE PATIENT

PATIENT'S STATEMENT OF REASON FOR HOSPITALIZATION AND ANTICIPATED LENGTH OF STAY:
Ankles are swollen – heart "acting up"

INFORMATION GATHERED FROM:
☐ PATIENT ☐ OTHER ____ (Relationship)

LANGUAGE / SPEECH
LANGUAGE DIFFICULTIES: YES/(NO)
Describe:
SPEECH DIFFICULTIES: YES/(NO)
Describe:

COMFORT
PAIN: (YES)/NO Location: chest
Duration: comes and goes Type: Ache
Intensity: 0 1 (2) 3 4 5 (NONE, MILD, MODERATE, SEVERE) Onset: 3 days ago
Relieved By: Resting
Aggravated by: climbing the stairs

EENT
HEARING DEFICIT: (YES)/NO
Describe: A "little" hard-of-hearing
VISION DEFICIT: (YES)/NO
Describe: wears eye glasses
MOUTH/THROAT/TEETH/ PROBLEM: YES/(NO)
Describe:

NEUROLOSENSORY
LEVEL OF CONSCIOUSNESS: (Alert)/Lethargic/Restless/Agitated/Semi-Coma/Coma
PUPIL STATUS (when indicated):
ORIENTATION: Person/Place/Time/Situation — yes yes yes yes
SENSORY DISABILITY: YES/(NO)
Describe:
CMS Parameter Flow Sheet started: YES/(NO)
NEURO Parameter Flow Sheet started: YES/(NO)

RESPIRATORY
QUALITY: Normal/Labored/Shallow/SOB/(SOB with exertion)/(Orthopnea)/Other:
COUGH: Absent/Non-productive/Productive
Describe (cough, sputum, etc.):
LUNG SOUNDS: slight crackles in both lower lobes
RESPIRATORY AIDS (oxygen, nebulizers, inhalers, etc.): YES/NO
HISTORY OF TOBACCO USE: YES/(NO)
Describe:

CARDIOVASCULAR
SKIN COLOR: (Normal)/Cyanotic/Dusky/Jaundiced
SKIN TEMPERATURE: Warm/(Cold)/Hot/Diaphoretic
HEART RHYTHM: Regular/(Irregular)
PERIPHERAL PULSES (when indicated): pedal pulses
POSTURAL BP (when indicated): ____ LYING ____ SITTING ____ STANDING
EDEMA: (YES)/NO
Describe: 1+ to 3 inches above lateral malleolus
VENOUS ACCESS: YES/(NO) Type:

SKIN
CONDITION: (Normal)/Dry/Bruises/Abrasions/Open wounds/Ulcers/Rash/Scars
Description/Location:
HISTORY OF PRESSURE SORES/SKIN BREAKDOWN: (YES)/NO
Describe: Had leg ulcer 1 yr. ago – healed

ROOM NO.: 815W NAME: Jorgenson, Sven

GI / GU
ABDOMEN: (Non-tender)/Tender/Firm/Distended
BOWEL TONES: (Present)/Absent/Hypoactive/Hyperactive
BOWELS: Usual pattern: daily
LAST BM: yesterday
LAXATIVES/ENEMAS: YES/NO No
(No difficulty)/Diarrhea/Blood in stool/Constipation/Impaction/Incontinence
Other:
URINARY: No difficulty/Frequency/Urgency/Pain/Burning/(Nocturia)/Catheter/Incontinence/Foul-smelling urine
Other:

GYN
LAST MENSTRUAL PERIOD: N/A
DISCHARGE/BLEEDING/PAIN: YES/NO
Describe:
CONTRACEPTIVES: YES/NO Type:

NUTRITION
WEIGHT CHANGE: (Gain)/Loss 4 Kg
Length of time:
NUTRITIONAL STATUS: (Adequate)/Malnourished
INTAKE INHIBITED: YES/(NO) Nausea/Vomiting/Chewing or Swallowing difficulties/Other:
SPECIAL DIET: (YES)/NO Type: Low Salt
Dislikes:
MEAL PATTERN: Small breakfast

SUBSTANCE USE
ALCOHOL: YES/(NO)
RECREATIONAL DRUGS: YES/(NO)
Type/Amount/Frequency:
Time of last drink/other:

MOBILITY SAFETY
USUAL ACTIVITY LEVEL: "Just stay home"
ALTERED NOW: (YES)/NO
Describe: sedentary
LIMITATIONS IN MOVEMENT: YES/(NO)
Contractures/Paralysis/Amputation/Weakness/Gait/Balance/Cast/Pain
MOBILITY AIDS: YES/(NO)
Cane/Crutches/Walker/Prosthesis/Brace/Wheelchair
HISTORY OF FALLS: YES/(NO)
Describe:

PSYCHOSOCIAL
RECENT STRESS/LOSS: YES/(NO)
Describe:
AFFECT: Within normal limits/Angry/(Anxious)/Depressed/Flat/Hostile
COPING STYLE: Usual manner of handling stress:
SIGNIFICANT SUPPORT PEOPLE: Son and daughter-in-law

EDUCATION
LIMITED KNOWLEDGE: (YES)/NO (Diagnosis)/Therapy/Procedure
Describe: Does not understand angina
Information requested related to:
BARRIERS (limitations) TO LEARNING: YES/(NO)
Physical/Psycologica/Cognitive/Sensory/Language
Describe:
FAMILY/SIGNIFICANT OTHER AVAILABLE AND ABLE TO LEARN: (YES)/NO
Describe: Son

DISCHARGE
PRIOR TO ADMISSION, PATIENT LIVED: (Alone)/With family/With friends/ECF(name):
PATIENT'S PLANS FOR CARE AFTER DISCHARGE: Go home to own apartment
OBSTACLES IN LIVING ENVIRONMENT: (YES)/NO
Describe: stairs to front door – 1 flight
CARE PROVIDER: YES/NO Describe:
NEED FOR DISCHARGE CARE REFERRAL SERVICES/EQUIPMENT: (YES)/NO
Describe: Home making assistance

Date: 4/18/94 Time: 13:30 Signature: N. Nifelt RN

*SEE ADDITIONAL INFORMATION ON BACK OF FORM

Figure 9-3. Nursing history interview.

Table 9–1. Subjective versus Objective Data

Subjective data (symptoms)	Objective data (signs)
Heart palpitations	Rapid pulse—104 beats per min
Feeling of warmth	Elevated temperature—105°F
Dizziness	Stumbling gait
Burning on urination	Cloudy urine
Nausea	Emesis—brown, liquid, 100 ml
Apprehension	Trembling
Pain	Wincing on movement

Some of the important skills you will need for physical examination are measuring blood pressure, temperature, pulse, and respiration (see Modules 16 and 17). You will need skill in listening to lungs and bowels (auscultation); examining the skin; checking wounds, dressings, drainage tubings, and intravenous infusions (inspection); examining the abdomen by touch (palpation); tapping to identify differences in sound conduction (percussion); and the like (see Module 13). In some instances you will need the skill to perform common laboratory tests such those for occult (hidden) blood in stool or glucose level in the blood (see Module 20).

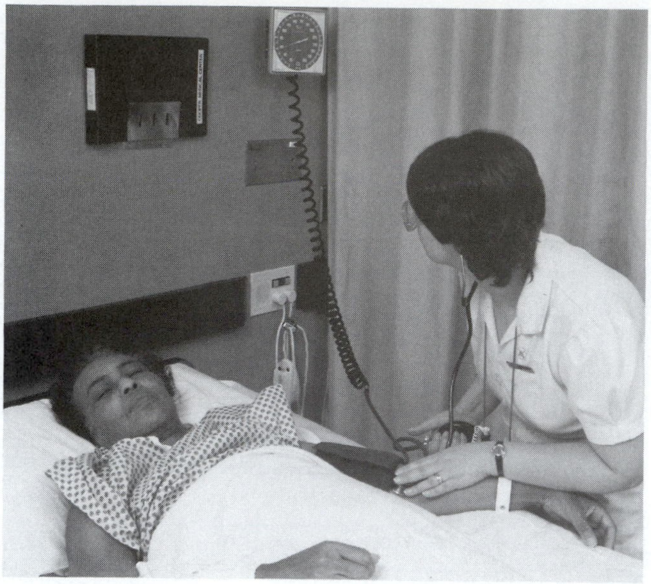

Figure 9–4. The physical examination is an important source of assessment data.

Display 9–6
A Brief Unstructured Interview with a Postoperative Patient

NURSE:	You look uncomfortable. Are you having pain in your incision? (*Note: The nurse is validating her impression.*)
PATIENT:	Well, it's not too bad. I guess I can stand it.
NURSE:	On a scale of zero to ten, with zero being no pain and ten being the worst pain you have had, how would you rate your current pain? (*Note: The nurse is attempting to gain more specific subjective data.*)
PATIENT:	If you look at it like that . . . well, maybe a six.
NURSE:	In that case, I believe you should have the pain medication prescribed by your doctor. The medication will allow you to rest more comfortably and also to move around, which is important to your getting well. Would that be all right with you? (*Note: The nurse is explaining her proposed plan for care and seeking the client's participation in the plan.*)
PATIENT:	OK. I *am* pretty uncomfortable.

Most nurses use a standardized approach for physical assessment, which ensures that all data are gathered. Commonly, the vital signs (blood pressure, temperature, pulse, and respiration) are measured first. Then a head-to-toe approach is used for the rest of the examination. In this approach, you would first examine the head including the eyes, nose, mouth, and ears. From there you would progress to the neck. You would then examine each arm and hand in turn. Next you would examine the chest, including auscultating the lungs and the heart. After examining the chest, from the anterior, you would ask the client to turn or move so you can examine the posterior chest. You would auscultate the lungs from the back and also observe the skin. After helping the patient to return to a supine position, you would examine the abdomen. The genital area is examined if there is reason to believe that a health problem exists in this area. For example, if the patient has a urinary drainage catheter or a dressing in the genital area, it would be essential to inspect it. The legs and feet are examined last.

Other nurses prefer to use a body systems approach to physical examination. In this approach, the nurse will try to gather all information regarding the skin at one time. All information about the gastrointestinal system, including the stomach, the abdomen, and the bowel is gathered. In a similar manner, each body system is assessed.

The time spent on an area of the body varies depending on the patient's health problem. For example, examination of the head would receive more attention in the person with a facial fracture and examination of the abdomen would receive more attention in the person with appendicitis. As you begin to care for patients, your instructor will assist you in determining what areas need greater attention. You may be asked to do a limited portion of the overall patient assessment, gradually adding more detail as you acquire more skill. When this is the case, you must communicate with other members of the health care team to ensure that a complete assessment is done for all patients for whom you care even if you are unable to do it independently.

Records

The patient's written record or chart contains laboratory data and assessments by other members of the health care team such as other nurses, the physician, or the physical therapist. This information will become increasingly important to you as you learn to interpret its significance (Fig. 9-5). In some instances you will be able to thoroughly review a record before meeting the patient. Sometimes, you will only have time to check for the most important information from the record before meeting the patient. In other instances you will be establishing the initial record.

Other written records may be of potential value to you. These may include a card index used for quick reference to current physician's orders and plans for care; the nursing care plan, containing the specific nursing directions for care; and any other checklists and forms maintained by the nursing staff (see Module 6).

Colleagues

Communicating with colleagues about a client is an important way to expand your data base. Most care facilities have some type of "report" when nurses from one shift communicate information to those on the next shift. As a student you may find that the nurses with whom you work are a source of key information to help you provide appropriate care. Nursing care conferences may be held, in which care for an individual or a group of patients is discussed. Such conferences may be formal or informal. Communication with colleagues is discussed more extensively in Chapter 15.

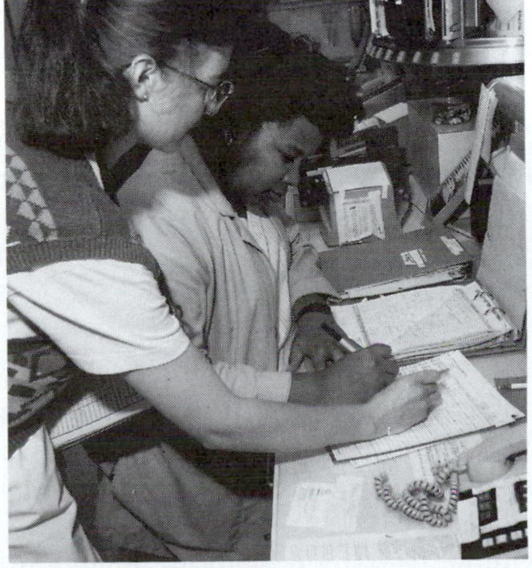

Figure 9-5. Important information can be learned by reading the patient's record or chart.

Formal interdisciplinary conferences are characteristic of rehabilitation settings, hospice care, and long-term care facilities. Because the client is more stable and will be in the care setting for some time, there is an opportunity to plan for formal gatherings of various members of the health care team to share information and to plan together. In many of these settings, the patient and family are encouraged to participate in the conference if at all possible. In the conference, colleagues share perceptions, validate what they have seen, and attempt to gain new insights into what the patient is experiencing. In Chapter 14, we will explore more fully the skill of working with colleagues in groups.

In acute care settings, contacts with colleagues in other health care disciplines are more likely to be informal and unscheduled. Patients' conditions change rapidly, and often there is no opportunity to plan a formal meeting. Instead the nurse may consult the nutritionist regarding nutritional concerns, may confer with the physician during the physician's daily visit, or arrange to meet the physical therapist at the bedside to discuss transfer techniques. The patient can be included in these informal conferences if they take place at the bedside. An important point is that a bedside conference should always include the patient as an active participant, taking care to make sure that the patient understands the conversation. A conference that takes place over the bed without including the patient devalues the person, is disrespectful of individual needs, and may create anxiety. If the patient is not able to participate, such as the patient who is unconscious or confused, members of the health care team should still talk as if the person could understand because it is impossible to determine when a person still has listening ability even though the individual does not have the ability to respond.

Initial Assessment Versus Continuing Assessment

Initial assessment of a patient is comprehensive. It includes the complete nursing history, general observations, a physical examination, a review of the patient's records, and consultation with colleagues. After this assessment, the nurse usually identifies areas that need continued assessment and sets up a plan for ongoing monitoring. Continuing assessment must include aspects that relate to the patient's current health problems and to any further problems that may arise from them. The determination of appropriate actions for continuing assessment is both a professional and legal responsibility for the nurse. Although the nurse will be alert to cues that indicate a problem beginning in a new area, the effective use of time demands that the nurse set priorities for routine assessment.

As a beginning student, you will often be asked to make a comprehensive assessment of a patient even when a registered nurse has already completed such an assessment and identified the data to be collected for continuing assessment. One reason for this is that you need to develop assessment skills and doing so requires practice. The opportunity to assess a patient and then to compare your assessment with that of an experienced nurse is an invaluable method of enhancing your own skill.

A second reason for you to conduct a complete assessment also relates to the fact that you are a novice. It is common for a novice to focus on those areas that have been pointed out as important. You might miss cues that would lead the experienced nurse to expand assessment beyond what was planned. If you missed these cues while caring for a patient, important problems might be missed. The requirement that you always perform a comprehensive assessment ensures the patient an extra margin of vigilance in the provision of high-quality nursing care.

Standards Regarding Data Collection

The ANA's *Standards of Clinical Nursing Practice* (see Display 8-1) indicate that the collection of data is the responsibility of the nurse and should be systematic and ongoing. We have discussed the reasons for systematic data collection. Ongoing data collection is important because changes occur in the individual, necessitating changes in the responses of the nurse. The standards also specify that the data will be documented in a retrievable form. If data are not correctly recorded, in the proper manner and in the proper place, they will not be available for others to use. Communication of routine information may be done through the record, but verbal communication of some data may be essential to prompt response to patient problems. Chapter 15 and Module 6 provide information on how to correctly communicate data.

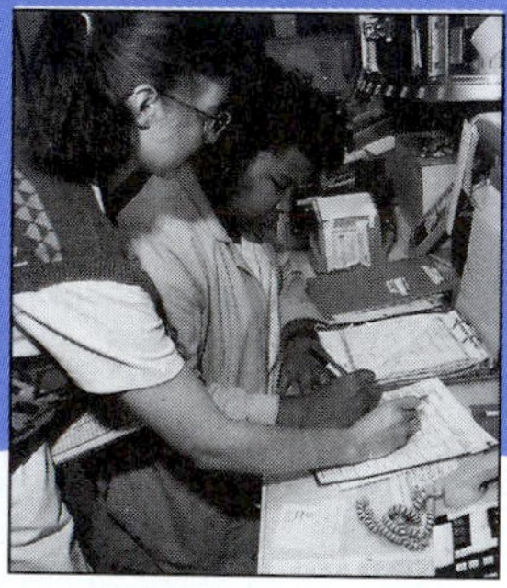

Key Points

- Assessment is the process of gathering data in regard to the patient. It enables the nurse to identify the client's problems, formulate the nursing diagnoses, and identify when a nursing action is inappropriate and the nursing intervention should be halted. It also provides a basis for evaluating the effectiveness of nursing action.
- Accurate and appropriate assessment is a legal responsibility of the nurse.
- The organizing systems for data collection include Henderson's activities of daily living, Gordon's functional health patterns, Roy's modes of adaptation, Orem's self-care requisites, and Neuman's systems approach. The basic needs approach is the focus of this text, and it can be adapted to other nursing models.
- Data are collected through general observation, client/family interviews, physical examination, the study of records, and consultation with colleagues. All of these data collection methods require special skills.
- Subjective data are data that originate with the client. Objective data are observable and verifiable by another person.
- Initial assessment of a client includes a comprehensive nursing history, obtained through an interview, complete observations, a thorough physical examination, a review of records, and consultation with colleagues.
- Continuing assessment is more limited and reflects

aspects related to the client's current and potential health problems.

- The ANA has formulated standards for data collection indicating that such collection should be systematic and ongoing. Data must be documented in a retrievable form.

Study Questions

1. What is assessment?
2. What are two major purposes of assessment?
3. How does Gordon's assessment framework differ from Neuman's framework?
4. How does Orem's framework for assessment differ from Roy's framework?
5. How is a basic needs framework similar to and different from the other frameworks presented?
6. Describe four sources of assessment data.
7. Describe how you would organize a physical assessment.
8. What is the difference between initial assessment and continuing assessment?

Critical Thinking Activities

1. Review a patient's record for 24 hours. Make two lists of data, one containing subjective data and one containing objective data. Compare and contrast these two sources of data.
2. Obtain a copy of the initial nursing history and admission assessment forms used in your facility. Analyze them for structured and unstructured interview items.
3. Arrange with your instructor to attend a formal patient care conference as an observer. Compare the contributions offered by persons in different fields. How do these contributions reflect their differing education and professional focus?
4. Arrange to confer with an experienced nurse about what is planned for continuing assessment of a particular patient. Compare this information with the data gathered for initial assessment. Try to identify the factors that determined which information would be included in the ongoing assessment.

Relevant Sections in Modules for Basic Nursing Skills

Volume I Module
Assessment 5
Documentation 6
Inspection, Palpation, Auscultation, and Percussion 13
Optional
Admission, Transfer, and Discharge 14
Intake and Output 15
Temperature, Pulse, and Respiration 16
Blood Pressure 17
Collecting Specimens 18
Assisting with Examinations and Procedures 19
Performing Common Laboratory Tests 20

References and Readings

Abdellah, F. G., Beland, I., Martin, A., and Matheny, P. *Patient-Centered Approaches to Nursing.* New York: Macmillan, 1961.

American Nurses Association. *Standards of Clinical Nursing Practice.* Kansas City, Mo.: ANA, 1991.

Bates, B. *A Guide to the Physical Examination.* 5th edition. Philadelphia: J. B. Lippincott, 1991.

Beyea, L. S., and Suddarth, D. S. "Assessing Elders Using the Functional Health Pattern Assessment Model." *Nurse Educator* 14, 3 (1989): 32–37.

Enlow, A. J., and Swisher, S. N. *Interviewing and Patient Care.* New York: Oxford University Press, 1986.

Fuller, J., and Schaller-Ayers, J. *Health Assessment: A Nursing Approach.* Philadelphia: J. B. Lippincott, 1990.

Gordon, M. *Nursing Diagnosis: Process and Application.* 2nd edition. New York: McGraw-Hill, 1987.

Henderson, V. *The Nature of Nursing.* New York: MacMillan, 1966.

Neuman, B. *The Neuman Systems Model.* Norwalk, Conn.: Appleton-Century-Crofts, 1982.

Orem, D. *Nursing: Concepts of Practice.* 4th edition. New York: McGraw-Hill, 1991.

Roy, Sr. C. *Introduction to Nursing: An Adaptation Model.* 2nd edition. Englewood Cliffs, N.J.: Prentice-Hall, 1984.

Nursing Diagnosis

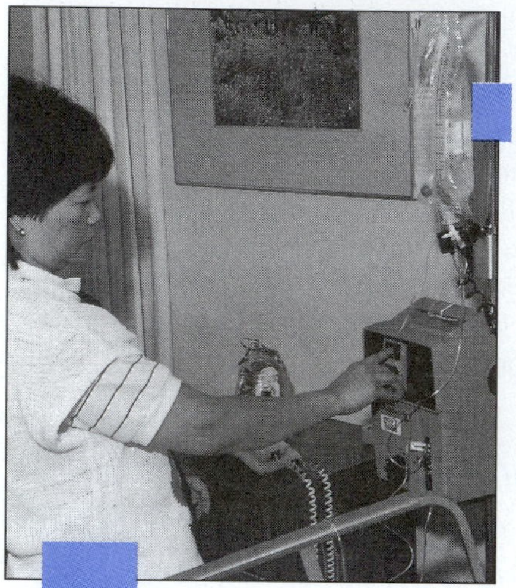

10

Objectives

After completing this chapter, you should be able to:

1. Define nursing diagnosis and differentiate it from medical diagnosis.
2. Differentiate between the process of diagnosis and a statement of diagnosis.
3. Explain the use of defining characteristics in developing a nursing diagnosis.
4. Discuss how knowledge of related factors assists in planning.
5. Name the parts of a complete nursing diagnosis using a two-part statement, and differentiate that statement from a three-part statement.
6. Explain the role of the North American Nursing Diagnosis Association (NANDA) in developing nursing diagnoses.
7. Outline the taxonomy of nursing diagnoses based on the "Human Response Patterns."
8. List the elements of the diagnostic process.

Study Terms

collaborative problem
defining characteristics
diagnostic process
etiology
human response patterns
medical diagnosis
nursing diagnosis
related factors
taxonomy

Outline

Definitions of Nursing Diagnosis
Developing a Standardized System for Nursing Diagnosis
Definition
Defining Characteristics
Related Factors
Risk States as Nursing Diagnoses
Format for Writing Nursing Diagnoses
The Diagnostic Process
Compare Data With Norms
Cluster Data
Interpret Patterns
Identify the Appropriate Nursing Diagnosis
Determine Related Factors
Document the Nursing Diagnosis
Common Errors in Nursing Diagnoses
Nursing Diagnosis and Health
Collaborative Problems

Ellis, Nowlis: Nursing: A Human Needs Approach, 5th ed. © 1994 J.B. Lippincott Company

Nursing diagnosis is both a process and a statement that results from that process. The nursing diagnostic process involves sorting, interpreting, and making a clinical judgment about the data gathered. The **nursing diagnosis** statement provides a concise description of a patient problem that will be amenable to nursing intervention. The American Nurses Association (ANA) *Standards of Clinical Nursing Practice* (1991) states that nursing diagnoses are derived from the assessment data, validated with the client whenever possible, and documented in a manner that facilitates their effective use.

We will discuss many different definitions of nursing diagnosis. All these definitions strive to communicate the fact that a nursing diagnosis is unique to the nursing profession and reflects a unique perspective on the patient. The nursing diagnosis is made by the nurse and treatment is the responsibility of the nurse. You will need to clearly differentiate this from a **medical diagnosis**, which is a statement of a disease state or pathology that is identified by and treated by a physician. Although the nurse works collaboratively with the physician in regard to the disease state, the primary responsibility regarding treatment of the disease state remains with the physician.

Definitions of Nursing Diagnosis

The ANA *Social Policy Statement* (1980) defined nursing as "the diagnosis and treatment of human responses to actual or potential health problems" (p. 9). On the basis of this statement, we would expect a nursing diagnosis to describe a human response and perhaps indicate the health problem to which it is a reaction.

Gordon (1976) defined a nursing diagnosis as *an actual or potential health problem which nurses, by virtue of their education and experience, are capable and licensed to treat.* This definition requires the person making the diagnosis to have mastered the content of nursing education, have nursing experience, and have a knowledge of the licensing laws. It also suggests that nursing diagnoses might change along with changes in nursing education or licensing. Moritz (1982) used a similar definition. She enlarged the one used by Gordon to include that a nursing diagnosis is "a response to an actual or potential health problem which nurses, by virtue of their education and experience, are able, licensed, and legally responsible to treat."

Carnevali and colleagues (1984) indicate that the nursing domain involves the relationship between the patient's daily living status and functional health status. Thus, a diagnostic statement would encompass a description of this relationship. This definition, which is not widely used, is especially helpful to the person who has limited information about what nurses traditionally do and what is included in licensure laws relative to nursing.

Roy (1984) identified three means of categorizing adaptation problems, all of which were appropriate nursing diagnoses. One was the identification of a cluster of assessment data within an adaptive mode and the naming of this cluster. She provided a list of titles to be used to identify these clusters. A second approach was to use as the nursing diagnosis the statement of the behavior identified in the assessment data. This statement would provide a specific basis on which to plan nursing interventions. A third approach was to collect a summary of behaviors from more than one of the adaptive modes and from that form a cluster that would represent one pattern.

Gebbie (1982) defined nursing diagnosis as the judgment or conclusion that occurs as a result of nursing assessment. This puts it into perspective in the nursing process but does not clearly reveal what the substance of a nursing diagnosis would be.

Carpenito (1992) uses the following definition: "A nursing diagnosis is a statement that describes the human response (health state or actual/potential altered interaction pattern) of an individual or group which the nurse can legally identify and for which the nurse can order the definitive interventions to maintain the health state or to reduce, eliminate, or prevent alterations" (p. 5).

The foregoing definitions illustrate the gradual refinement and evolution of the term nursing diagnosis. When the North American Nursing Diagnosis Association (NANDA) was established (see discussion later in this chapter), it attempted to provide a definition that reflected the unique responsibilities of the nurse. The current NANDA definition is as follows: *A nursing diagnosis is a clinical judgment about individual, family or community responses to actual and potential health problems/life processes. Nursing diagnoses provide the basis for selection of nursing interventions to achieve outcomes for which the nurse is accountable (NANDA, 1992)* (Display 10-1).

In the context of a beginning nursing student it is useful to consider nursing diagnoses in terms of whether or not the individual patient or client's basic needs are met or whether threats to meeting these basic needs exist. This will help you to focus your thinking on the areas that are truly nursing responsibilities. According to Henderson's (1966) definition of nursing, you would look for areas in which the client would meet personal needs if he or she had the necessary strength, will, or knowledge to do so. Using Carnevali's viewpoint (1984), you would look for areas in which the

Display 10–1
NANDA Definition of Nursing Diagnosis

> Nursing diagnosis is a clinical judgment about individual, family, or community response to actual or potential health problems/life processes. Nursing diagnoses provide the basis for selection of nursing interventions to achieve outcomes for which the nurse is accountable (1992).

health status was interfering with the patient's daily living. In this context, daily living is a broad concept that covers relating to and performing one's role in life as well as the physical aspects of day-to-day life.

Gordon (1987, p. 15) described four characteristics of a nursing diagnosis, which are shown in Display 10–2.

Display 10-3 summarizes the definitions of nursing diagnosis described here that have contributed to the development of the current NANDA definition.

Developing a Standardized System for Nursing Diagnosis

In 1973 the first national conference on nursing diagnosis was held. The aim was to develop a standardized system for naming nursing diagnoses. Having such a universal system was seen by a group of nursing leaders as essential to the development of nursing as a profession. Without a standardized terminology, it is more difficult to communicate, and both care and research are hampered.

The result of that first meeting was a list of nursing diagnostic statements on which the conference participants agreed. A National Group for the Classification of Nursing Diagnosis was formed. Thereafter a conference was held every 2 years to further develop and refine nursing diagnostic statements. At the fifth national conference a more formal organization was approved; the presence of nurses from outside of the United States was acknowledged; and the *North American Nursing Diagnosis Association* (*NANDA*) was begun.

The nursing diagnoses considered at the conferences are suggested by practicing nurses, both as individuals and as groups, on the basis of their experiences. Diagnoses submitted are reviewed by a committee, published for general review, and reviewed by a task force of clinical experts. The results of all these reviews are considered by the committee, which then recommends for acceptance by the NANDA board a tentative version. Recommendations from the board are presented to the general assembly at the biennial conferences. Comments and suggestions are then returned to the committee, where a final version is developed. This is sent to all of the members of NANDA for a final vote of approval or rejection.

Originally, the NANDA nursing diagnoses were presented only in an alphabetical list, which contained specific statements such as "alteration in elimination: bowel, constipation," and statements that reflected general problem areas, such as "noncompliance." It became obvious that an effective organizing framework for the nursing diagnostic statements was needed to establish greater clarity; therefore, nursing theorists were asked to work together to develop a taxonomy for a classification system. A **taxonomy** is a classification system based on a set of organizing principles.

To help you understand their task, let us consider a familiar taxonomy. The taxonomy in biology is based on the structure and function of living things. Originally, the biologic taxonomy included two major kingdoms, plants and animals, and everything was classified in one of these two groups. Each kingdom was further divided into phyla. Phyla were divided into classes, classes into orders, and so forth down to individual species. Two key features of an effective taxonomy are that all possible items are included and that the categories are defined specifically enough that it is clear to which category an item belongs. As science became more precise and more was understood about biologic function, the biologic taxonomy was revised. The current biologic taxonomy contains five kingdoms: plants, animals, monera, fungi, and protista. The position in the taxon-

Display 10–2
Gordon's Characteristics of a Nursing Diagnosis

1. Conditions described by nursing diagnoses can be accurately identified by nursing assessment.
2. Nursing treatments or methods of risk factor reduction can resolve the condition described by a nursing diagnosis.
3. Because the necessary treatments to resolve nursing diagnoses are within the scope of nursing practice, nurses assume accountability for outcomes.
4. Nursing assumes responsibility for the research required to identify clearly defining characteristics and etiologic factors and to improve methods of treatment and treatment outcomes for conditions described by nursing diagnosis.

Source: Gordon, M. *Nursing Diagnosis: Process and Application*. New York: McGraw-Hill, 1987, p. 15.

Display 10–3
Definitions of Nursing Diagnosis

American Nurses Association (1980) "Human responses to actual or potential health problems."

Gordon (1976) "An actual or potential health problem which nurses, by virtue of their education and experience, are capable and licensed to treat."

Moritz (1982) A response to an actual or potential health problem that nurses by virtue of their education and experience are able, licensed, and legally responsible and accountable to treat.

Carnevali (1982) A statement of a relationship between daily living status and functional health status.

Roy (1982) Three typologies: (1) a name of a cluster of assessment data within an adaptive mode; (2) a statement of the behavior of the client which was identified in the assessment data; (3) a summary of behaviors from more than one adaptive mode in a cluster that represents a pattern.

Gebbie (1982) A judgment or conclusion that occurs as a result of nursing assessment.

Carpenito (1987) A statement that describes the human response (health state or actual/potential altered interaction pattern) of an individual or group that the nurse can legally identify and for which the nurse can order the definitive interventions to maintain the health state or to reduce, eliminate, or prevent alterations.

omy of each living thing had to be reevaluated based on the new system. Although for most living things this was simple, even within such a long established science as biology, differences of opinion exist about the proper placement of some living things in the new system. This may help you to understand why there are disagreements and difficulties associated with establishing a taxonomy of nursing diagnoses.

The theorists and the NANDA committee designed a system for organizing and classifying nursing diagnoses. They titled it "NANDA Nursing Diagnosis Taxonomy I." The designation "I" reflected recognition that the system would be refined and revised. The taxonomy is organized under nine **human response patterns** (called "patterns of unitary humans" in the original text): *exchanging, communicating, relating, valuing, choosing, moving, perceiving, knowing,* and *feeling.* Display 10-4 presents the definitions of each pattern. (These are analogous to the kingdoms in the biologic taxonomy.) They serve as the most general classifications.

Display 10–4
Human Response Patterns

Exchanging	Mutual giving and receiving
Communicating	Sending messages
Relating	Establishing bonds
Valuing	Assigning relative worth
Choosing	Selecting of alternatives
Moving	Activity
Perceiving	Reception of information
Knowing	Meaning associated with information
Feeling	Subjective awareness of information

Source: North American Nursing Diagnosis Association, 1992.

The first level under each pattern provides a category of alterations in the pattern, such as "Alterations in nutrition." Terms such as "altered," "impaired," and "ineffective" are used at this level to show that there is a change, but these terms do not indicate a specific degree of change. Under each alteration category, there is a level containing more specific statements such as "less than body requirements" (which appears under "Altered nutrition"). At each lower level, the statement becomes more specific (Display 10-5).

Display 10–5 presents the NANDA taxonomy as it exists at the time of this writing (NANDA, 1992). You will note that some numbers have no statements. These numbers are nevertheless included to focus attention on the fact that the taxonomy is incomplete in these areas. The statements in parentheses have been suggested but have not yet been through the complete NANDA approval process. They may be accepted in this format or may be altered before being accepted. Every 2 years the NANDA conference meets and additional nursing diagnoses are added to the taxonomy. Appendix A contains an alphabetized list of NANDA-approved nursing diagnoses with their definitions. The inside of the back cover has an alphabetical list of NANDA diagnoses for quick reference.

Clearly there are problems that nurses are diagnosing and treating that are not yet contained in the taxonomy. When the conference approves new diagnoses, NANDA is not stating that this is the first time that nurses have treated these problems, but only identifying agreement on the terminology and classification for that problem. Some specialty nursing groups are examining nursing diagnoses in their own specialties and beginning to

(Text continues on page 161)

Display 10–5
*NANDA Taxonomy I Revised**

Pattern 1: Exchanging: A human response pattern involving mutual giving and receiving.

1.1 [Altered nutrition]
1.1.1. [Cellular]
1.1.2. [Systemic]
1.1.2.1. Altered nutrition: More than body requirements
1.1.2.2. Altered nutrition: Less than body requirements
1.1.2.3. Altered nutrition: Potential for more than body requirements
1.2 [Altered physical regulation]
1.2.1. [Immune]
1.2.1.1. High risk for infection
1.2.2. [Altered body temperature]
1.2.2.1. High risk for altered body temperature
1.2.2.2. Hypothermia
1.2.2.3. Hyperthermia
1.2.2.4. Ineffective thermoregulation
1.2.3. [Altered autonomic response]
1.2.3.1. Dysreflexia
1.3 [Altered elimination]
1.3.1. [Altered bowel elimination]
1.3.1.1. Constipation
1.3.1.1.1. Perceived constipation
1.3.1.1.2. Colonic constipation
1.3.1.2. Diarrhea
1.3.1.3. Bowel Incontinence
1.3.2. Altered urinary elimination
1.3.2.1. [Urinary incontinence]
1.3.2.1.1. Stress incontinence
1.3.2.1.2. Reflex incontinence
1.3.2.1.3. Urge incontinence
1.3.2.1.4. Functional incontinence
1.3.2.1.5. Total incontinence
1.3.2.2. Urinary retention
1.4 [Altered circulation]
1.4.1. [Altered vascular circulation]
1.4.1.1. Altered (specify type) tissue perfusion (Renal, cerebral, cardiopulmonary, gastrointestinal, peripheral)
1.4.1.2. [Altered fluid volume]
1.4.1.2.1. Fluid volume excess
1.4.1.2.2. [?]
1.4.1.2.2.1. Fluid volume deficit
1.4.1.2.2.2. High risk for fluid volume deficit
1.4.2. [Altered cardiac circulation]
1.4.2.1. Decreased cardiac output
1.5 [Altered oxygenation]
1.5.1. [Altered respiration]
1.5.1.1. Impaired gas exchange
1.5.1.2. Ineffective airway clearance
1.5.1.3. Ineffective breathing pattern
1.5.1.3.1. Inability to sustain spontaneous ventilation
1.5.1.3.2. Dysfunctional ventilatory weaning response

Display 10–5 ***(continued)***
*NANDA Taxonomy I Revised**

1.6 [Altered physical integrity]
1.6.1. High risk for injury
1.6.1.1. High risk for suffocation
1.6.1.2. High risk for poisoning
1.6.1.3. High risk for trauma
1.6.1.4. High risk for aspiration
1.6.1.5. High risk for disuse syndrome
1.6.2. Altered protection
1.6.2.1. Impaired tissue integrity
1.6.2.1.1. Altered oral mucous membrane
1.6.2.1.2. [Altered skin integrity]
1.6.2.1.2.1. Impaired skin integrity
1.6.2.1.2.2. High risk for impaired skin integrity

Pattern 2 Communicating: A human response pattern involving sending messages.

2.1 [Altered communication]
2.1.1. [Verbal]
2.1.1.1. Impaired verbal communication
2.1.2. [Nonverbal]

Pattern 3 Relating: A human response pattern involving establishing bonds.

3.1 [Altered socialization]
3.1.1. Impaired social interaction
3.1.2. Social isolation
3.2. [Altered role]
3.2.1. Altered role performance
3.2.1.1. [Parenting role]
3.2.1.1.1. Altered parenting
3.2.1.1.2. High risk for altered parenting
3.2.1.2. [Sexual role]
3.2.1.2.1. Sexual dysfunction
3.2.2. Altered family processes
3.2.2.1. Caregiver role strain
3.2.2.1. High risk for caregiver role strain
3.2.3. [Role conflict]
3.2.3.1. Parental role conflict
3.3. Altered sexuality patterns

Pattern 4 Valuing: A human response pattern involving the assigning of relative worth.

4.1 [Altered spiritual state]
4.1.1. Spiritual distress (Distress of the human spirit)

Pattern 5 Choosing: A human response pattern involving the selection of alternatives.

5.1 [Altered coping]
5.1.1. [Individual coping]
5.1.1.1. Ineffective individual coping
5.1.1.1.1. Impaired adjustment

(continued)

Display 10–5 ***(continued)***
*NANDA Taxonomy I Revised**

5.1.1.1.2. Defensive coping
5.1.1.1.3. Ineffective denial
5.1.2. [Family coping]
5.1.2.1. [Ineffective family coping]
5.1.2.1.1. Ineffective family coping: disabling
5.1.2.1.2. Ineffective family coping: compromised
5.1.3. [Community coping]
5.2. [Altered participation]
5.2.1. Ineffective management of therapeutic regimen (individual)
5.2.1.1. Noncompliance
5.3. [Altered judgment]
5.3.1 [Individual]
5.3.1.1. Decisional conflict (specify)
5.4 Health seeking behavior

Pattern 6 Moving: A human response pattern involving activity.

6.1 [Altered activity]
6.1.1. [Altered physical mobility]
6.1.1.1. Impaired physical mobility
6.1.1.1.1. High risk for peripheral neurovascular dysfunction
6.1.1.2. Activity intolerance
6.1.1.2.1. Fatigue
6.1.1.3. High risk for activity intolerance
6.2. [Altered sleep]
6.2.1. Sleep pattern disturbance
6.3. [Altered recreation]
6.3.1. Diversional activity deficit
6.4. [Altered activities of daily living]
6.4.1. [Home maintenance]
6.4.1.1. Impaired home maintenance management
6.4.2. Altered health maintenance
6.5 [Altered self-care]
6.5.1. Feeding self-care deficit
6.5.1.1. Impaired swallowing
6.5.1.2. Ineffective breastfeeding
6.5.1.2.1. Interrupted breastfeeding
6.5.1.3. Effective breastfeeding
6.5.1.4. Ineffective infant feeding pattern
6.5.2. Bathing/Hygiene self-care deficit
6.5.3. Dressing/Grooming self-care deficit
6.5.4. Toileting self-care deficit
6.6 Altered growth and development
6.7 Relocation stress syndrome

Pattern 7 Perceiving: A human response pattern involving the reception of information.

7.1 [Altered self-concept]
7.1.1. Body image disturbance
7.1.2. Self-esteem disturbance
7.1.2.1. Chronic low self-esteem
7.1.2.2. Situational low self-esteem
7.1.3. Personal identity disturbance

Display 10–5 ***(continued)***

*NANDA Taxonomy I Revised**

7.2. Sensory/Perceptual alterations (specify) (visual, auditory, kinesthetic, gustatory, tactile, olfactory)
  7.2.1. [?]
    7.2.1.1. Unilateral neglect
7.3. [Altered meaningfulness]
  7.3.1. Hopelessness
  7.3.2. Powerlessness

Pattern 8 Knowing: A human response pattern involving the meaning associated with information.

8.1. [Altered knowledge]
  8.1.1. Knowledge deficit (specify)
8.2. [Altered learning]
8.3. Altered thought processes

Pattern 9 Feeling: A human response pattern involving the subjective awareness of information.

9.1 [Altered comfort]
  9.1.1. Pain
    9.1.1.1. Chronic pain
9.2. [?]
  9.2.1. [Grieving]
    9.2.1.1. Dysfunctional grieving
    9.2.1.2. Anticipatory grieving
  9.2.2. High risk for violence: self-directed or directed at others
    9.2.2.1. High risk for self-mutilation
  9.2.3. Post-trauma response
    9.2.3.1. Rape trauma syndrome
      9.2.3.1.1. Rape trauma syndrome: compound reaction
      9.2.3.1.2. Rape trauma syndrome: silent reaction
9.3. [Altered emotional integrity]
  9.3.1. Anxiety
  9.3.2. Fear

*The patterns and numbering system have been developed and approved by NANDA. All nursing diagnoses approved through 1992 are included.

All entries enclosed in brackets are for the purpose of clarifying the structure of the taxonomy and have not been approved as NANDA nursing diagnoses. They may be useful to nurses in understanding the relationships of the concepts and in supporting the development of additional nursing diagnosis statements. Some categories are marked with a question mark to indicate areas where no specific term has been suggested. Modified from NANDA Nursing Diagnosis: Definitions and Classification. Copyright © 1992, North American Nursing Diagnosis Association, St. Louis, Mo.

formulate tentative diagnoses to be added to the taxonomy in the future.

Definition

Each nursing diagnosis approved by NANDA is carefully defined. This definition helps nurses to use the terminology more precisely. Prior to the time when there was agreement on definitions, more than one term might be used to indicate the same problem. This hampered communication in regard to an individual patient and was even more of a problem when trying to gather general information or conduct research in which patients from many different areas of the country were included. There are still areas of disagreement about the precise definitions of some nursing diagnoses. NANDA recognizes that this is a concern but has taken the position that at this time it is more important to continue to expand the taxonomy than to keep refining the definitions of diagnoses already accepted.

When you consider using a nursing diagnosis, you must first carefully review the definition to be certain that the term you intend to use means what you intend to communicate. As you become more experienced in nursing, you will have committed to memory the precise definitions of many nursing diagnoses.

Defining Characteristics

In addition to determining the appropriate label, placement in the classification system, and definition of each nursing diagnosis, NANDA also identifies the defining characteristics of the nursing diagnosis. **Defining characteristics** are those signs and symptoms that indicate that a nursing diagnosis is present. Initially all possible signs and symptoms were simply listed for each nursing diagnosis. In 1989 as the process became more sophisticated, NANDA began dividing the defining characteristics into *critical* (sometimes called major or essential) defining characteristics and *supporting* (sometimes called minor) defining characteristics. Critical characteristics are those that must be present to use the particular nursing diagnosis statement. Supporting characteristics provide additional support that the nursing diagnosis is present but may not be there in all cases. Additionally, supporting characteristics provide guidance for planning nursing interventions. At this time, NANDA has not elected to use its time and efforts to differentiate the defining characteristics for previously approved nursing diagnoses. Just as with the definitions, the organization has felt that expanding the taxonomy is more important than perfecting those parts that are already in place and useful.

Related Factors

Related factors refer to those factors that either caused the nursing diagnosis to be present, contributed to its development, are commonly associated with it, or serve as risk factors for its development. This is also referred to as the **etiology**. Etiology literally means the things from which something originates. It is clear that in most of nursing practice, any individual problem may have more than one etiology. The multiple etiologies of health-related problems are one of the factors that make them difficult to treat. Each etiology may indicate the need for a different approach to treatment. Because the true cause of any nursing diagnosis may be difficult to discern, we recommend you use the term "related factors" rather than etiology.

Risk States as Nursing Diagnoses

NANDA has also developed a systematic approach to situations in which the patient does not yet have a particular nursing diagnosis but is at risk of developing it. Within the assessment data, you may identify that individuals have a number of factors that place them at *high risk* of developing a nursing diagnosis although it is not currently present. In many instances, the nurse is able to prevent the development of a problem through preventive action if the risk factors are recognized. NANDA determined that nurses needed a mechanism for indicating these situations requiring preventive action through the nursing diagnosis taxonomy. Therefore, the "High Risk" title was developed. The nursing diagnosis is stated as *High Risk for . . .* (specify the nursing diagnosis). The related factors include the factors that are placing the individual at high risk. There would be no defining characteristics because the problem is not yet present. In such cases, the focus of the nursing action would be on prevention. This category was originally referred to as *Potential for . . .* but was changed in 1991 to High Risk because that terminology was felt to be more precise. For example, all persons who have surgery may have the potential for some nursing diagnoses, but a limited number actually are at high risk. It is the high risk status that demands nursing intervention.

Format for Writing Nursing Diagnoses

In making use of the NANDA terminology in the writing of nursing diagnoses, the components just described are combined to construct a one-part, two-part, or three-part statement.

The most common format for writing nursing diagnoses is a two-part one. In this format, the initial section is the statement of the nursing diagnosis that has been identified. The statement should be clear and concise, and it should reflect the health problem or response of the client (whether that is the patient or the family). Using the NANDA terminology, this first section would be composed of a specific problem. For example, the specific problem statement might be "constipation." In some of the NANDA categories there is no list of specific problems; instead, there is a general category, followed by "(specify)." For example, the NANDA category "Noncompliance (specify)" might be used for a particular client by stating *Noncompliance: Not adhering to prescribed diabetic diet.* In specifying, the precise individual problem within the category of noncompliance is stated. For convenience, in some settings nurses do not write out the overall category. They simply write the specific problem assuming that all nurses would know the category under which it falls. In this situation you might see the nursing diagnosis stated as *Constipation* or *Not adhering to prescribed diabetic diet.* If you have a choice we recommend that you include the category. This will facilitate your learning of the taxonomy.

The second section of the nursing diagnosis statement contains the related factors. These are the factor or factors that relate to the occurrence of the problem. Factors in the environment, behaviors of the client, existing pathophysiology, maturational factors, factors related to treatments, or a combination of any of these may be part of this statement. In the above example, *Constipation* may be related to lack of fiber in the diet and physical inactivity. Thus, the entire diagnostic statement would be *Constipation related to lack of dietary fiber and physical inactivity.* The inclusion of the related factors as well as the problem statement provides for more precise determination of the appropriate nursing interventions. If the person did not yet have constipation, but the conditions for its development were present, the statement might read *High Risk for Constipation related to lack of dietary fiber and physical inactivity.* In this case you are indicating that the lack of dietary fiber and physical inactivity are placing the patient in a category of "high risk" for developing the problem of constipation.

A three-part format contains the specific NANDA diagnosis, the related factors, and the defining characteristics. This provides a clearer picture of the patient situation and may facilitate planning. In the example above, a three-part statement would be *Constipation related to lack of dietary fiber and physical inactivity, as evidenced by no bowel movement for 3 days, history of hard stools, and discomfort on defecation.*

A one-part statement may be most appropriate for wellness-related nursing diagnoses. A two-part statement is most appropriate for a "high-risk" state because no signs or symptoms are currently present. A three-part statement is especially useful to the novice. Even if this format is not used where you practice, the exercise of clearly identifying the defining characteristics that you relied on in your identification of the problem is valuable in helping you to avoid making assumptions that are not supported by data (Display 10-6).

Display 10–6
Writing Nursing Diagnoses Using the Three-Part (PES) Format*

P Pain (acute)
E related to swollen and inflamed joints
S as evidenced by:
states joints are very painful (rated 7 on a scale of 1 to 10)
Moves slowly
Guards joints carefully

P High risk for altered skin integrity
E related to immobility
S as evidenced by:
is on complete bed rest
does not move about in bed
when turned, bony prominences appear red
is thin (height 5'6", weight 110 lbs.)
states that skin is sore when she lies on it

P Toileting Self-care deficit
E related to stiffness in joints
S as evidenced by:
states cannot bend down onto low toilet seat
unable to clean self after bowel movement because of stiffness
unsteady on feet when up

*Problem, Etiology, Signs and Symptoms
Gordon, 1987

The Diagnostic Process

The process of moving from a broad set of assessment data to specific statements of nursing diagnosis is called the **diagnostic process**. After you have collected your data, you will need to 1) compare data with norms or a state of health; 2) group, or cluster, the information in a way that helps you to discern the patterns that are present; 3) interpret those patterns; 4) identify the appropriate diagnostic statement; and 5) identify the etiology of the problem (Display 10-7). As in most other processes involving reasoning and judgment, the steps do not always occur in a straight, ordered line.

Compare Data With Norms

First you must determine whether a given item of information represents a normal, healthy state or whether it represents a deviation from the norm or suggests that

Display 10–7
The Diagnostic Process

1. Compare data with norms or a state of health.
2. Group or cluster the information in a way that demonstrates the patterns that are present.
3. Interpret the patterns.
4. Formulate a diagnostic statement.
5. Identify the etiology of the problem.

the individual lacks something needed for health. Data that represent a healthy state may be important when planning interventions because it is often possible to build on strengths to assist with resolving problems. Comparing data with norms is often done as the data are collected.

Cluster Data

The second task is clustering (grouping) the data. This requires that you recognize the relationships among the data you have collected and recognize the pattern that is present. As a beginner, you will be asked to recognize simple patterns within assigned areas. For example, you might be asked to study the client's nutritional status. You might identify that the client ate less than one-half of the most recent meal. From the record you learn that the patient has consistently eaten less than one-half of each meal for the 5 days of hospitalization. On interviewing the patient you learn that she does not have any appetite for the food and does not feel like eating when meals are served. The patient's weight is slightly under the normal for her height. All of these items could be clustered together into a pattern regarding nutrition. One of the hallmarks of the expert nurse is the ability to identify clusters of data that relate to each other and form a pattern that might not be readily apparent to the novice.

Interpret Patterns

The third step is to interpret the pattern identified. In this case, you would identify that the patient's weight will not be maintained with the current eating pattern. In addition, the amount currently being eaten does not provide the needed nutrients for an adult woman. Interpreting data requires that you have knowledge of the consequences of certain states, that you recognize directions and trends in data, and that you identify the manner in which an individual patient is responding.

Identify the Appropriate Nursing Diagnosis

The next step is identifying the appropriate the nursing diagnosis (Fig. 10-1). From the NANDA taxonomy you would select the pattern "Exchanging," the subsection on "Altered Nutrition." On the basis of your interpretation, you would select the specific problem "Less than body requirements." In some situations, you will find that there is not yet a standardized statement representing the specific problem you have identified. In such a case, you would need to formulate a brief statement that reveals the specific problem. Consult with your instructor or an experienced nurse to assist you with doing this.

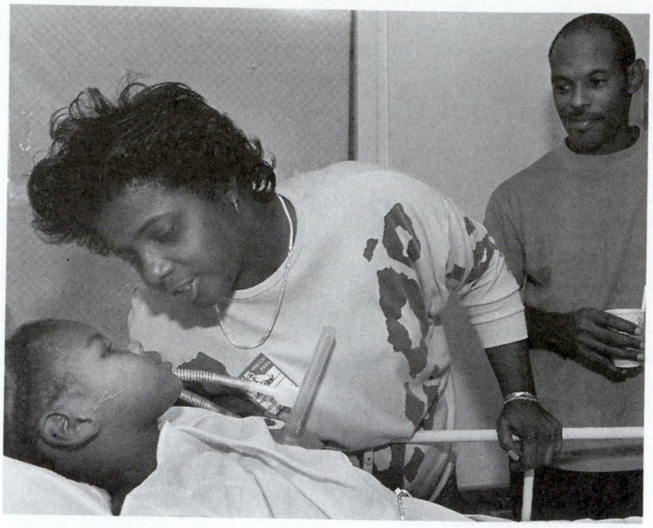

Figure 10-1. Altered Family Processes related to hospitalization of child can be an appropriate nursing diagnosis.

Determine Related Factors

The final step is to analyze the data to determine the related factors. In the nutritional example above, you might have expanded your interview to clarify the patient's perceptions about her loss of appetite. You might then be able to write, "Related to unfamiliarity of food being served and unavailability of usual Vietnamese foods." If you are using a three-part nursing diagnosis statement, you would then add a list of the signs and symptoms you had clustered together.

This brief example shows how you might use a planned diagnostic process. Your diagnostic abilities will grow as you progress in nursing. One mark of the expert nurse is the ability to group data and recognize patterns that do not fall clearly within one area of function. For example, low urinary output, shortness of breath, moist sounds in the lungs, and swollen ankles would be clustered into a pattern by an experienced nurse although two observations relate to breathing, one relates to urinary function, and one relates to the appearance of the lower extremities. The nurse would recognize that this information is related and forms a pattern that reveals the fluid volume status of the person and in fact, indicates excess fluid volume. To formulate the nursing diagnosis the nurse would then consult the NANDA taxonomy, and write the nursing diagnosis as "Fluid volume excess." To complete the statement, the nurse would reexamine the data to identify the factors related to the fluid excess.

Data may be clustered while it is being collected or after it has been collected. One piece of information

Nursing Research: Implications for Practice

Haight, B. K. & Warren, J. "Apathy: Development of a Nursing Diagnosis." *Applied Nursing Research* 4: 4 (186–188) November, 1991.

These researchers used a formal consensus method called a Delphi technique to validate the proposed nursing diagnosis of "apathy." The first group of individuals asked to respond to the mailed questionnaire were 20 elderly people. The second group asked to respond were 40 nurse experts in gerontology or in nursing diagnosis. Three consecutive questionnaires were sent to each subject. Each succeeding questionnaire was developed based on the responses on the previous questionnaire. Information from the study supported the development of a list of major cues and minor cues that would be indicators of this nursing diagnosis. These cues would become defining characteristics if apathy is accepted as a valid nursing diagnosis. The North American Nursing Diagnosis Association relies on the careful research of nurses as decisions are made to add nursing diagnoses to the approved list.

may suggest a pattern and therefore trigger the need to seek other data to verify whether this pattern actually exists. While you are formulating a diagnostic statement, you may reinterpret patterns and alter your initial interpretation of the data. Thus, the process is continuous.

Document the Nursing Diagnosis

Nursing diagnoses must be documented for the patient's record (Joint Commission on Accreditation of Healthcare Organizations, 1990) using whatever format is accepted by the specific agency. Some agencies specify precisely the format that is acceptable. In others, nurses have a wide latitude to use whatever format they deem appropriate. In some facilities, nursing diagnoses are documented in a separate nursing care plan. In other agencies, the patient record contains a problem list that is a combined table of contents and index to the material in the record. Nursing diagnoses are recorded along with the medical diagnoses on this list. All charting is then done in relationship to listed patient problems. This system has the advantage of making it easy to follow the progress of any individual problem over time. Whatever system is used, the important factor is that they are shared with the appropriate staff to be used to focus nursing care.

Common Errors in Nursing Diagnoses

A common error in formulating nursing diagnoses is making someone other than the client the focus of the statement. For example, the statement "husband nonsupportive" may be pertinent data, but it does not give any information about the client's response. There is no direction for the nursing intervention that would resolve this concern. This might be one part of the data necessary to diagnose "Ineffective Individual Coping," but more information is needed. In some settings, more than one family member may be a client. In these settings, nursing diagnoses may be written for each client *and* for the family unit. This is essential in maternity units, where both mother and baby are clients, and in

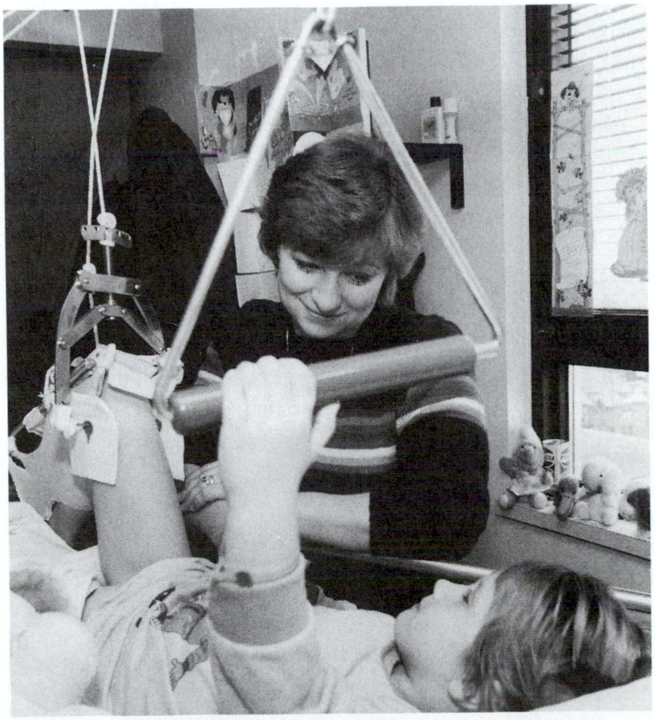

Figure 10–2. Using "fractured tibia" as a nursing diagnosis for this patient would be incorrect; "fractured tibia" is a medical diagnosis.

hospice care, where support of the whole family is of major importance.

Another mistake is stating a need for a service as part of a nursing diagnosis. For example, "needs emotional support" does not give any information about the situation nor the response of the individual, nor does it help to suggest specific nursing intervention. Nonspecific emotional support may inadvertently omit exactly that intervention the client needs to function effectively. The diagnosis "Fear of anesthesia related to mother's adverse response to anesthesia" provides specific information that supports specific intervention.

A single symptom is sometimes used erroneously as a nursing diagnosis. For example, the statement "cough" is important in understanding what the patient is experiencing, but is not adequate to help guide intervention. Is the cough interfering with sleep? Is it raising sputum? Is it creating a sore throat? Is it accompanied by any other signs and symptoms? The cluster of signs and symptoms is needed for the true nature of the problem to be identified accurately and to guide intervention.

Knowing the medical diagnosis is important to understand the client, but it is not the nurse's role to make a medical diagnosis (Fig. 10-2). The nursing diagnoses should describe the patient's *response* to the medical diagnosis. Therefore, "chronic obstructive pulmonary disease with pneumonia," the medical diagnosis, would guide medical intervention. A related nursing diagnosis might be "Ineffective Airway Clearance related to increased secretions."

Another error sometimes seen is reference to equipment used for the patient as if the equipment were the nursing diagnosis (Fig. 10-3). An indwelling urinary catheter has important implications for nursing, but the catheter is not the nursing diagnosis. A patient with a catheter may have a nursing diagnosis of "Total incontinence related to lack of neurologic control." When the diagnosis is written correctly, the focus is on the patient and the problem related to the basic need for elimination.

The common errors made in formulating nursing diagnoses are summarized in Display 10-8.

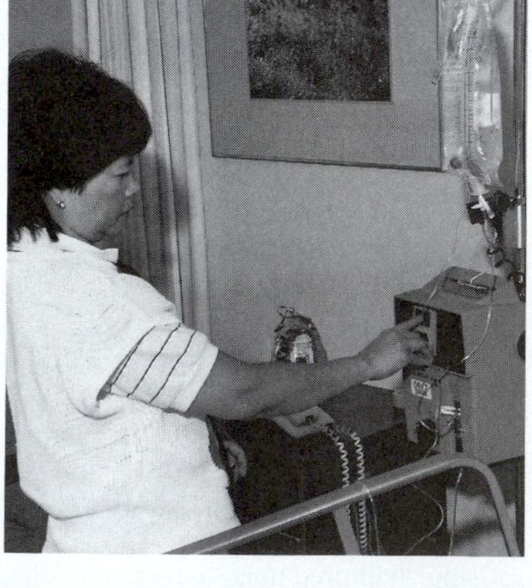

Figure 10-3. Incorrectly referring to a piece of equipment as a nursing diagnosis is a common error beginning students make.

Display 10–8
Common Errors in Nursing Diagnosis

1. Making someone other than the client the focus of the statement
2. Using a need for service as a nursing diagnosis
3. Identifying a single symptom as a nursing diagnosis
4. Using a medical diagnosis as a nursing diagnosis
5. Referring to equipment in use as a nursing diagnosis

Nursing Diagnosis and Health

Some nurses have expressed concern that the NANDA taxonomy focuses on problems and does not recognize healthy states (Gleit and Tatro, 1981). Gordon (1987), however, suggests that a focus on problems is appropriate because the patient has a need for assistance when a problem is present. Nevertheless, many nurses do work with primarily healthy individuals such as new mothers, infants, and school children. How does this kind of nursing fit into a problem orientation?

To address this issue, the current NANDA-approved list of nursing diagnoses contains several nursing diagnoses whose focus is wellness. They include Family Coping: Potential for Growth, Health Seeking Behaviors, and Effective Breastfeeding. Even when the focus for nursing diagnosis is on problems, identification of healthy patterns is important in planning appropriate actions in relationship to health problems.

Display 10–9
Stating a Collaborative Problem

Potential Complication: Gastric bleeding related to peptic ulcer. (Note the nurse assesses for gastric bleeding. If it occurs, the physician will be notified, work collaboratively with the nurse, and prescribe medical treatment for the bleeding.)

Nursing Issues and Trends: *Maintaining a Focus on Wholeness*

With nursing diagnoses that refer to very specific problem situations, the danger exists that we may lose the focus on the whole person that has characterized nursing. The strengths that a person possesses, the life experience he or she brings to any situation, and the social context of the person's life, all have a profound effect on responses to health care problems. How can we understand, use, and respond to these specific concerns and still see the person in a totality? This remains a continuing challenge for nurses.

Collaborative Problems

In addition to independent nursing interventions, nurses often work collaboratively with physicians in the treatment of medical diagnoses. Among the nurse's major responsibilities in these situations are monitoring of changes in the patient's condition and instituting preventive actions.

When such problems arise, the physician is notified so that physician-prescribed treatments can be instituted. Carpenito (1993, pp. 30, 31) defines **collaborative problems** as "certain physiologic complications that nurses monitor to detect onset or changes in status." She suggests that they be recorded in a consistent format as Potential Complication. . . . (followed by specification of what the complication might be). An example is the potential complication of hemorrhage and shock for the person who has just had surgery (see Display 10–9). She further states that "nurses manage collaborative problems using physician-prescribed and nursing-prescribed interventions to minimize the complications of the events."

One may distinguish between a collaborative problem and a nursing diagnosis by asking whether or not the nurse prescribes all the treatments for the problem. If the nurse orders the definitive treatment, then it fits into the nursing diagnosis category. If the nurse must notify a physician and the definitive treatment is prescribed by both the physician and the nurse, then it is a collaborative problem.

Carpenito suggests that nurses be careful to identify priorities for each patient based on that person's individual situation. For some patients the nursing diagnosis will be the priority; for others the potential complication will be the priority.

Identifying collaborative problems requires extensive knowledge of disease states, medical treatments, and the possible adverse responses to each. In each area of nursing there are collaborative problems that occur more frequently and nurses often develop standard protocols for assessment designed to identify collaborative problems. When patients have less common medical diagnoses, the nurse will need to consult references and consult with the physician to clearly establish potential complications and the priorities for assessment.

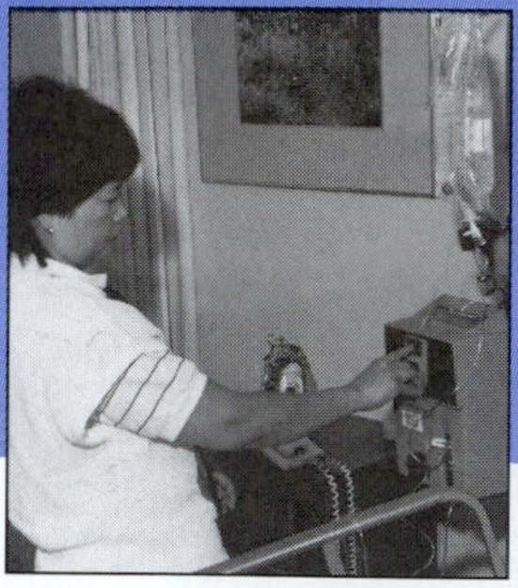

Key Points

- The term nursing diagnosis refers both to an intellectual process and to a statement that is a concise description of a patient's problem.
- Nursing diagnosis is defined by NANDA as "a clinical judgment about individual, family, or community responses to actual or potential health problems/life processes" (1992). This text will focus on whether or not an individual patient/client's basic needs are met or whether threats to meeting these basic needs exist.
- The four characteristics of a nursing diagnosis suggested by Gordon are the following: nursing diagnoses can be identified by nursing assessment, nursing treatments can resolve the condition, nurses are accountable for outcomes, and the nursing profession assumes responsibility for the research related to nursing diagnoses.
- The North American Nursing Diagnosis Association (NANDA) has developed a taxonomy for nursing diagnoses based on nine human response patterns. Under each of these are three levels of statements, each level more specific than the previous one. Each nursing diagnosis has a definition, a list of defining characteristics, and a list of related factors.
- A complete nursing diagnosis usually includes a specific problem and a statement of related factors. The signs and symptoms may also be stated.
- Nursing is concerned with healthy states as well as illness states. Identification of healthy patterns is important in planning appropriate actions in relationship to health problems.
- Collaborative problems are those situations that the nurse monitors and manages by using physician prescribed treatment or nursing prescribed preventive action. The nurse identifies these as potential complications rather than as nursing diagnoses.
- Mastering nursing diagnoses helps to give direction to the nurse's actions and assists in effective communication with colleagues and patients.

Study Questions

1. What is the difference between a medical diagnosis and a nursing diagnosis?
2. Outline and explain the steps of the diagnostic process.
3. Explain each part of a three-part nursing diagnosis statement.
4. What has been the role of NANDA in the development of nursing diagnoses?
5. List the patterns of human response.
6. What is a collaborative problem and how is it different from a nursing diagnosis?

Critical Thinking Activities

1. Using Appendix A, find and write out nursing diagnoses related to the following problems: constipation, patient's inability to do own care, inability to move about freely. Add related factors and signs and symptoms for a hypothetical patient.
2. Exchange lists with another student and critique one another's nursing diagnosis statements.
3. In a clinical facility, examine the nursing care plans. Are nursing diagnoses being used? If not, how are patient problems identified? If so, what format is being used in the facility?
4. Review the NANDA taxonomy. Choose one area of "alteration" under any pattern and prepare a report on that area, outlining the definition and defining characteristics for it. Present your report in a conference.

References and Readings

American Nurses Association. *Standards of Clinical Nursing Practice.* Kansas City, Mo.: ANA, 1991.

American Nurses Association. *Nursing: A Social Policy Statement.* Kansas City, Mo.: ANA, 1980.

Avant, K. C. "The Art and Science of Nursing Diagnosis Development." *Nursing Diagnosis* 1, 2 (1990): 51–55.

Carnevali, D., Mitchell, P., Woods, N., and Tanner, C. *Diagnostic Reasoning in Nursing.* Philadelphia: J. B. Lippincott, 1984.

Carpenito, L. J. *Nursing Diagnosis: Application to Clinical Practice.* 4th edition. Philadelphia: J. B. Lippincott, 1992.

Carroll-Johnson, R. M. (Ed.). *Classification of Nursing Diagnoses: Proceedings of the Ninth Conference.* Philadelphia: J. B. Lippincott, 1992.

Creason, N. S. "How Do We Define Our Diagnoses?" *American Journal of Nursing* 87, 2 (February 1987): 230–231.

Fitzpatrick, J., Ker, M., and Saba, V., "Translating Nursing Diagnosis into ICD Code." *American Journal of Nursing* 89, 4 (1989): 493–495.

Fredette, S. L. "Common Diagnostic Errors." *Nurse Educator* 13, 3 (1988): 31–35.

Gebbie, K. "Toward the Theory Development for Nursing Diagnoses Classification." In *Classification of Nursing Diagnoses*, edited by M. J. Kim and D. A. Moritz. New York: McGraw-Hill, 1982.

Gleit, C., and Tatro, S. "Nursing Diagnoses for Healthy Individuals." *Nursing and Health Care* 2, 2 (February 1981): 456–457.

Gordon, M. *Nursing Diagnosis: Process and Application*. 2nd edition. New York: McGraw-Hill, 1987.

———. "Implementation of Nursing Diagnosis: An Overview." *Nursing Clinics of North America* 22, 4 (December 1985): 875–880.

———. "Nursing Diagnosis and the Diagnostic Process." *American Journal of Nursing* 76 (1976): 1298–1300.

Joint Commission on Accreditation of Healthcare Organizations. *Accreditation Manual for Hospitals*. Chicago: JCAHO, 1990.

Henderson, V. *The Nature of Nursing*. New York: Macmillan, 1966.

Miller, J., Steel, K., and Boisen, A. "The Impact of Nursing Diagnosis in a Long-term Care Setting." *Nursing Clinics of North America* 22, 4 (December 1985): 905–906.

Moritz, D. A. "Nursing Diagnosis in Relationship to Nursing Process." In *Classification of Nursing Diagnoses*, edited by M. J. Kim and D. A. Moritz. New York: McGraw-Hill, 1982.

North American Nursing Diagnosis Association. *Nursing Diagnoses: Definitions and Classification 1992*. St. Louis, MO: NANDA, 1992.

North American Nursing Diagnosis Association. *NANDA Taxonomy I* (rev.). St. Louis: NANDA, 1990.

North American Nursing Diagnosis Association. *Guidelines for Submission*. St. Louis: NANDA, 1990.

Roy, Sr. C. *Introduction to Nursing: An Adaptation Model*. 2nd edition. Englewood Cliffs, N.J.: Prentice-Hall, 1984.

Planning and Implementation

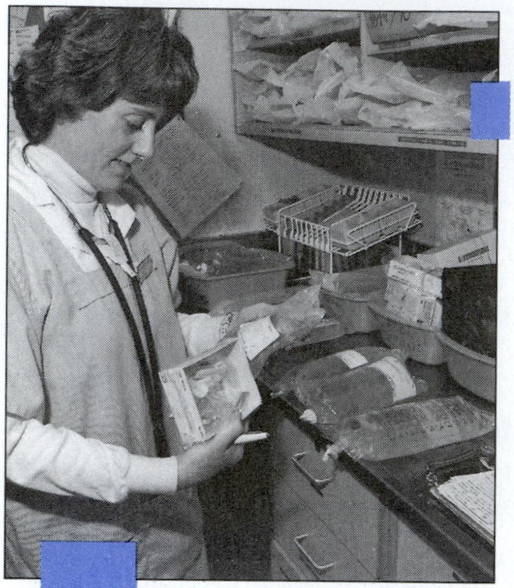

11

Objectives

After completing this chapter, you should be able to:

1. List the contents of a complete plan for nursing care.
2. Discuss how goals and desired outcomes are determined.
3. Discuss how priorities for nursing action are determined.
4. Explain the meaning of "nursing orders."
5. Discuss the types of nursing actions that might be included in a comprehensive plan.
6. Discuss the roles of standardized plans, computerized plans, policies, procedures, protocols, and critical pathways in planning care for an individual.
7. List the factors to be considered in developing technical skill performance.
8. Discuss the impact of patient trust and nursing skill on the effectiveness of nursing actions.
9. Outline the responsibilities of the nurse and the patient in the health care system.
10. Explain how the nurse can safeguard the rights of the patient when implementing care.
11. Outline a nursing process approach to skill performance and collaboration with physician prescribed care.

Study Terms

critical pathways
desired outcome
goal
nursing actions
nursing interventions
nursing orders
patient outcome
objective
outcome
outcome criterion
principle
protocol
rationale

Outline

Planning

Identifying Patient Outcomes
Seeking Information for Planning
Developing a Plan of Action
Setting Priorities
Writing a Plan for Nursing Care
Using Standardized Nursing Care Plans
Incorporating Policies, Protocols, and Critical Pathways in Planning Care

Maintaining Patient Involvement in Planning

Ellis, Nowlis: NURSING: A HUMAN NEEDS APPROACH, 5th ed. © 1994 J.B. Lippincott Company

Nursing care planning is a complex process consisting of several components: setting goals, gathering additional data, developing a plan, setting priorities, and writing the plan. Once the plan is developed, implementing it requires a basic understanding of rights and responsibilities in health care, a wide knowledge base, and the use of both technical and interpersonal communication skills.

Planning

After an assessment has been completed and the nursing diagnoses identified, the nurse is responsible for identifying desired outcomes, planning the appropriate nursing action, and determining when and how the actions should be implemented.

Identifying Patient Outcomes

The first aspect of planning is the identification of patient outcomes or goals. An **outcome** is a "valued health state, condition, or behavior exhibited by the client" (Gordon, 1987, p. 307). Outcomes are projected, that is, a decision is made in advance as to what outcomes are desirable. The terms **desired outcome**, **goal**, **outcome criterion**, and **objective** may each be used in different settings to refer to patient outcomes. To identify appropriate outcomes you must ask, "What is the desired end result for *this* patient in regard to *this* particular nursing diagnosis?" The **patient outcome** serves as a basis for deciding when nursing action is successful, when it can be discontinued, and when it must be altered.

At first glance, the description of a desired patient outcome or goal may be interpreted as a statement of what an optimal healthy state is because that is what you would hope for every patient. In the case of the nursing diagnosis "Bathing Self-care Deficit," the goal or outcome might be stated, "bathes self." However, the goal must be realistic and achievable. "Bathes self" might be an appropriate goal for a patient who is in a rehabilitation program and is expected to be capable of self-care. In a long-term care facility, you might care for a patient with severe brain impairment from a stroke who would not ever be expected to be capable of self-care. For this patient, identifying "bathes self" as the desired outcome would only cause frustration and disappointment because it would never be achieved. An appropriate outcome for this patient would focus on the individual abilities and needs of the patient. The desired outcome might be a state of cleanliness rather than an activity. Thus, we see that outcomes must be individualized—neither so limited as to underestimate the patient's potential nor so complex as to be unobtainable. This is often a difficult balance to achieve.

To be useful, outcomes must be stated in clear, descriptive, and measurable or comparative terms that can be used as criteria for evaluation. In some situations, writing specific outcomes is relatively easy, as in the bathing example above. "Bathes self" is a clearly observable behavior. The addition of a date by which that behavior is expected to be achieved further clarifies the desired outcome and would provide a complete outcome statement (Display 11-1).

In some instances, a more general goal is stated first and then the specific criteria are added. For the nursing diagnosis *High Risk for Fluid Volume Deficit*, a general statement such as "increased fluid intake" might be a general goal, but "increased fluid intake" is too vague a criterion for evaluation. The question arises as to what amount of fluid would represent an increase and how much increase would be necessary before you would agree that the problem has been resolved.

The question of timing is also important in this instance. An amount of fluid that might be adequate for an 8-hour shift is not adequate for 24 hours. Thus, in the case of the fluid outcome, appropriate criteria for evaluation would be added to the statement. It might be written, "Increased fluid intake as evidenced by drinks a minimum of 2,000 ml of fluid during each 24-hour period." Because this quantity could be measured, it would be clear whether or not the desired outcome had been achieved. In instances like that, a desired outcome is written in such a way as to indicate that a change (increase or decrease) in a particular attribute will occur. The record of that attribute might appear on a graph or table, but the desired outcome should still clearly indicate the standards being used for determining success or failure.

Timeliness of outcomes may also be addressed by setting a specific date when the outcome is to be

Display 11–1
Examples of Desired Outcomes and Planned Actions

Nursing Diagnosis

Self-care Deficit:* Feeding related to right-sided paralysis as evidenced by:

1. Cannot use right hand.
2. Indicates has always been right handed.
3. Is eating only a few bites and then turning head away.

Desired Outcomes

1. Feeds self all "finger foods" by 1/19.
2. Food intake includes minimum of 3/4 of each meal served.
3. Feeds self all foods on tray by 2/20.

Planned Actions

1. Record intake from each meal on flow sheet.
2. Arrange tray so that items are convenient to left hand.
3. Sit with patient during meals.
4. Encourage holding finger foods in left hand to eat.
5. After dexterity with finger foods established, assist in using regular utensils to eat. Place plate guard on plate edge to facilitate manipulation of food.

*Approved by the North American Nursing Diagnosis Association

achieved. Whether the outcome is to be accomplished within 24 hours postoperatively or by the time of discharge will make a difference in your further planning.

Note that the desired outcome is worded to make the patient the focus of the statement. This is a desired outcome for the *patient*, not for the nurse or other health care team members. One way of checking a desired outcome statement is to preface it with "For the patient to (be) (have) (do) (say) . . . ." If the statement makes sense when structured in this fashion, you know that you have made the patient the focus of the outcome. In the above example, "For the patient to have an increased fluid intake as evidenced by . . ." is a clear and meaningful statement. If the desired outcome had been written with the nurse as focus, it might have ended with a statement such as "to provide increased fluid intake." The statement "For the patient to provide increased fluid intake" would not make sense because the patient is not providing the fluid. Thinking the wording through shows you that the second statement was not written correctly.

Long-term Versus Short-term Goals

Both long-term and short-term goals are valuable in planning for care (Fig. 11-1). Long-term goals set up expectations for what will be achieved by the time of discharge from a facility or in a specified period of recovery and rehabilitation; they are future oriented. However, long-term goals may contribute to frustration on the part of both the patient and the caregivers if they are not accompanied by short-term or intermediate goals.

A short-term goal might encompass a week, a day, or even one shift. Broken into smaller segments, long-term objectives may seem more manageable and less threatening for both patients and caregivers. Nursing students may feel a greater sense of accomplishment when they set goals for patients that can be reached during the short periods in which they are providing care. They are then able to evaluate the results of their own care rather than only helping to work toward long-term goals, the attainment of which they may not be present to see. For example, a patient with a long-term objective of "2,000 ml of fluid intake each day" might have a short-term objective of "drinks 500 ml of fluid during the 7 AM to 12 noon time period today." This goal would allow the student providing care for the morning to evaluate whether actions taken during that time were successful.

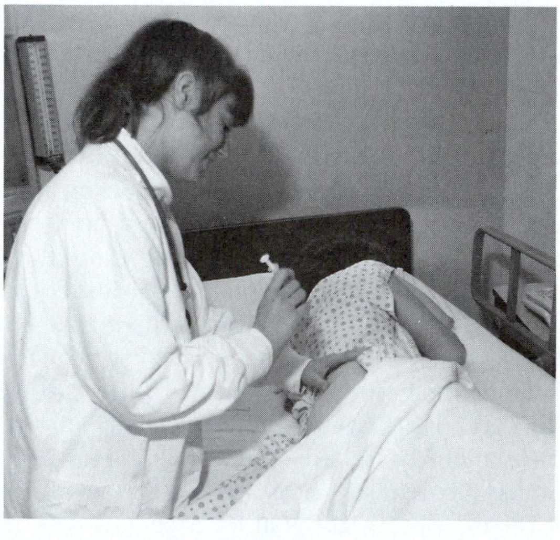

Figure 11-1. Providing comfort from pain may be seen as a short- or long-term goal, depending on the patient's individual situation.

Values and Patient Outcomes

A decision regarding an appropriate outcome or goal is a value-laden decision and must consider the patient's value system and desires, as well as the views of the health care team. This is because the ethical basis of nursing recognizes the right of the patient to care that is compatible with the individual's personal values. In many situations, there is little difference in desired outcomes. This is why standardized outcomes as a part of a critical pathway can be appropriate for most individuals. In the situation of a common surgery, such as an appendectomy, this is often the case.

However, in some cases there is much greater individual variation. Consider the nursing diagnosis "Pain (terminal) related to pressure in spine from metastatic bone tumors." In many instances, the desired outcome might be that the patient express freedom from pain. However, medications used to achieve freedom from pain can cause sedation and clouded thinking. One patient might prefer this to the pain. Another patient might prefer that some pain be present, with less sedation. In such a situation, you would strive to learn the patient's values and try to achieve the outcomes that patient wants.

Overall Goals

Overall goals are sometimes specified for patients with multiple problems. Such goals are often not limited to the nursing diagnosis but instead encompass the patient's overall condition, current status, and the prognosis for the future. Physicians, nurses, and other health care team members usually collaborate with the patient on overall goals, which focus on the expected end of care without setting an exact time for achieving that goal. Examples of overall goals include "a comfortable and pain-free death" or "return to self-care and independent living." Overall goals are never substitutes for the specific desired outcomes written in response to a specific nursing diagnosis but are meant to give general direction to the entire health care process.

Seeking Information for Planning

At this point in the nursing process, you will have collected data that will be useful as you plan nursing action. But before acting, it is essential to obtain more information on the specific problem in question. This information is derived from references and resources. Examples of references include nursing texts, current journals, and the "policy and procedure" book of the facility. Resources might include advanced nurse specialists, the pharmacist, or your nursing instructor. These references and resources will provide the **rationale**, or reason, for your action. Some practitioners use the phrase "facts and principles" when discussing the rationale for nursing action. A nursing **principle** is most often defined as two or more cause-and-effect–related facts that directly suggest a given nursing action. We prefer the term rationale, which is somewhat broader and encompasses a wide variety of facts, principles, and other information that can be considered together as a basis for action. The skilled practitioner may carry much of this knowledge in memory. For the beginning practitioner and the skilled practitioner confronting new or unusual problems, it will be necessary to consult books and periodicals. For example, an experienced nurse faced with "Impaired Skin Integrity" related to immobility would know the nursing actions likely to resolve this problem. As a beginning student, you might need to consult your texts or current periodicals to identify appropriate nursing actions. Nursing requires a disciplined approach to scientific knowledge as a basis for care.

Developing a Plan of Action

The plan for nursing action is a road map to direct you from the current problem to the desired outcomes. When you can clearly view the desired end result, your efforts will have purpose and direction.

In general, nursing actions can be thought of as those that involve technical or psychomotor skills, those that involve communication and interpersonal skills, and those that involve teaching. In addition, the plan may include reporting to other health care team members and documenting information appropriately.

Bulechek and McCloskey (1990) have developed a taxonomy for nursing actions in much the same way a taxonomy has been developed for nursing diagnoses. They identified a complex set of general categories that includes *psychomotor skills, psychosocial interventions, educative interventions, maintenance, surveillance or monitoring, supervision of other health care providers,* and *sociocultural actions.* Although the effort to establish a standardized terminology for nursing interventions is in its infancy, the categories outlined will be helpful in stimulating you to consider all of the possible nursing actions you might need to include in your plan.

In determining the specific actions to be taken, you will weigh all your data to decide what are relevant. You will synthesize what you know about this particular patient with all the theories, facts, and principles you have gathered. You will judge each possible action against the criteria of *appropriateness* (Is this action the correct one for this patient at this time?) and *feasibility* (Can this action be carried out with the resources of time, materials, and staff available?). In addition, you will address the criterion of *acceptability* to the patient (Will this action be acceptable to the patient?). You can

Nursing Research: Implications for Practice

Titler, M.G. "Interventions Related To Surveillance," *Nursing Clinics of North America* 27: (2) 495–515, June, 1992.

Surveillance interventions are the purposeful acquisition of patient data with subsequent interpretation and action by the nurse. This nursing action is also called "monitoring" and requires knowledge and skill. Surveillance occurs after the initial assessment and nursing diagnosis have been determined. In this study 10 surveillance nursing interventions used in critical care settings were described and validated. The general area of surveillance was one category. More specific interventions were: risk identification, vital signs monitoring, neurologic monitoring, fluid monitoring, electrolyte monitoring, acid-base monitoring, invasive hemodynamic monitoring, and intracranial pressure monitoring. The category of shock prevention was included with notes that it included important actions that went beyond collecting data. This study is related to the Iowa Intervention Project which seeks to create a systematic terminology for nursing interventions.

determine this only by sharing your proposed plan with the patient and asking for feedback.

The most effective plan is a specific plan. Therefore, you must determine not only what action should be taken, but also when it should be taken and who should take it. A general directive of "Provide good skin care" does not provide a caregiver with enough information from which to begin. What kind of skin care does this individual need? What areas of skin are in need of attention? How frequently should this care be provided? Who will provide the skin care?

Plans for nursing action should reflect the most current, effective nursing practice. For this to occur, all nurses must remain up-to-date in practice. You must understand the rationale for any action you plan. Although a nursing care plan in a health care facility will not contain the rationale for the actions prescribed, you may, as a student, be asked to provide the rationale for actions you select and to cite references to support that rationale. It is only when you understand the rationale for a particular action that you will be able to determine when to use it.

The actions selected may be referred to as a *nursing prescription* or in some instances as **nursing orders**. They are a prescription in the sense that the nurse prescribes the actions to be used in resolving the patient's problems. They are orders in the sense that the entire nursing team is to follow the directions for care. In a facility with primary nursing, the primary nurse may be responsible and accountable for all plans for nursing care for his or her patients.

A well designed plan of action describes not only the specific actions prescribed, but also how often and when the actions will be carried out. If the patient is cared for by a team, the plan should also specify which member of the team should perform each action. As you progress in your education you may be in a position to delegate planned actions to others on your nursing team. In a facility where total nursing care is performed by one assigned nurse, the provider does not have to be spelled out because it is always the assigned nurse.

For some psychosocial nursing diagnoses it may be appropriate to also include general guidelines for interactions such as "Encourage expression of feelings," "Be non-threatening and calm in all interactions," or "Convey acceptance." These are usually referred to as **nursing approaches.**

For the nursing diagnosis of High Risk for Fluid Volume Deficit mentioned above, in which the desired outcome was "Fluid intake of 2,000 ml in each 24-hour period," the nursing actions might include the following:

1. Explain to patient and wife why fluid intake of 2,000 ml/24 hr is desirable.
2. Offer preferred fluids (ice water, apple juice, or orange juice) every hour between meals.
3. Have patient keep own record of intake at bedside.
4. Provide positive reinforcement when patient drinks fluids.
5. Observe for intake and output balance, urine concentration, and condition of mucous membranes each shift.
6. Record intake and output on flow sheet every shift.

This plan includes teaching the patient about the reason for the desired outcome (number 1), which has the potential for getting the patient to increase fluid intake. Additional actions that will have the potential for achieving the goal of increased fluid intake are numbers 2, 3, and 4. All actions that have the potential for achieving the goal are sometimes identified as *nursing interventions* because they may intervene between the patient and the problem. Next you see a plan for *continuing assessment* (number 5). The final element (number 6) is a plan for *recording* what has been accomplished. These elements are frequently part of a nursing care plan. Although all elements may not be necessary for every nursing diagnosis, considering them all as you plan will help you remember to include all important aspects of the plan.

Setting Priorities

Setting priorities involves deciding which of several nursing diagnoses is the most important and also which planned action should be performed first. When more than one patient is being cared for, setting priorities among the different patients is also important. Setting priorities is necessary because time constraints may make it impossible to accomplish all the desired tasks.

One basis for making decisions about priorities is Maslow's hierarchy of needs (1970). In his framework, the problems related to the basic physiologic needs come before psychosocial needs (Fig. 11-2). This hierarchy of needs does not differentiate among the physiologic needs. Although Maslow's view is useful in some settings, taken alone it fails to recognize individual differences.

Another approach to setting priorities is to see what is the most life-threatening problem. Using this framework, the need for oxygen is a more immediate need than the need for fluid. Similarly the need for fluid would take priority over the need for food. In this approach, psychosocial problems would almost always have lower priority.

A third approach is to consult with the patient and learn what the patient is most concerned about. Many years ago Peplau wrote that "immediate needs must be met before more mature needs can arise" (1956, p. 79). What she spoke of as needs are what we refer to as problems. Her view was that patients' own perceptions of their most immediate needs were the most accurate and that when these were cared for, the patient would be better able to address concerns such as learning and developing interpersonal relationships.

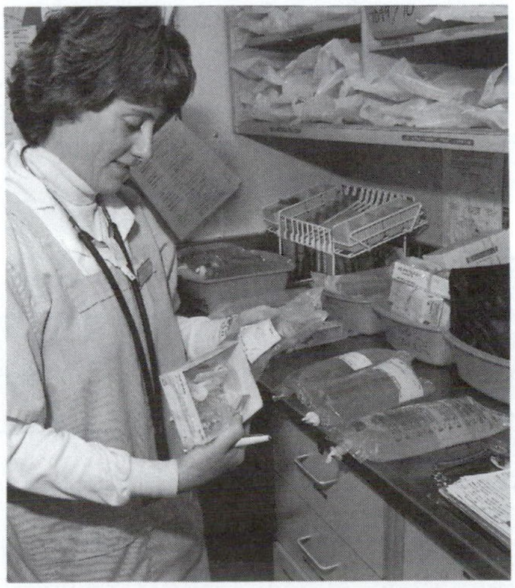

Figure 11-2. In most cases, basic physiologic needs are the first priority. Here the nurse plans for meeting fluid needs.

No one approach to setting priorities is correct in every situation. For the person in a life-threatening situation, looking at those areas critical to life is appropriate. For the majority of patients, however, the question is not survival but much less straightforward. For the terminally ill patient, the most important priority may be relating to family even though there are many physiologic needs. For the person about to be discharged to home, teaching about self-care and management of health problems at home may be much more important than changing a dressing one last time. In trying to determine which of several actions has the highest priority, you might ask yourself which has the greatest potential for achieving the desired outcomes.

The relationship of timing to other care needs also affects priorities. If the patient is going to surgery, nursing actions that relate to preparing him or her for surgery will take priority over those that relate to other matters.

Another way to look at priorities is to ask yourself the question "If I could work on only one of these problems, which would I choose?" Using this method, you would try to identify whether any of the problems had life-threatening potential and work with those first, moving from the most serious problems to the least serious. This may be difficult for you as a beginner because you will be caring for patients who do not have life-threatening problems, and it is often difficult to determine the appropriate priorities among several similar problems.

Time is also a consideration when setting priorities. Both the patient and the caregiver have limitations on the time available. You may have to determine which actions you have time to perform and which the patient has time to do. Be careful that time does not become a primary guide when you determine actions to be taken because this might interfere with effective care.

In the last analysis, setting priorities is particular to the individual patient. Examine the alternatives. Identify the patient's wishes. Consider the demands of time and setting. Weigh the support for the various possible priorities. Then make your decision based on the best rationale you know. Consult with more experienced nurses when you have doubts. Gradually you will become more skilled at setting priorities in a variety of situations.

Writing a Plan for Nursing Care

Each facility has its own approach to writing a plan for nursing care. The written nursing plan is designed to facilitate the provision of effective nursing care by establishing a common approach to problems and communicating this approach to all who are involved in care. The Joint Commission for the Accreditation of Healthcare Organizations (JCAHO) requires that there be a method of documenting that all the steps of the nursing process have occurred but leaves the exact nature of this documentation to the individual agency (1990).

Many agencies choose to have a specific document titled a "Nursing Care Plan." Sections of these plans that are always present are the statement of the problem, or nursing diagnosis, the desired outcomes, and the list of nursing actions to be taken (Fig. 11-3). In some facilities the major signs and symptoms present are included with the nursing diagnosis to facilitate clear understanding of the problem. The nurse who initiates the written nursing care plan usually dates and signs or initials the written record. Whenever the nursing care plan is revised, irrelevant sections are marked out according to the routine in the facility, and new sections are added, dated, and signed. When a problem is resolved, the date of resolution is added and the actions no longer needed are crossed out.

A nursing care plan may contain other care information in addition to the nursing diagnoses and related material. Treatments, procedures, the patient's activity level, and diet ordered by the physician may be noted. There may be a section to record the diagnostic and laboratory tests that have been performed. If other health care workers such as respiratory, physical, or occupational therapists are involved in care, their activities may be included for information. The nursing care plan may be used as the basis for giving a report from one shift to the next to ensure continuity of care.

PATIENT CARE PLAN

Date Signature	Problems Nursing Diagnoses	Expected Outcomes Discharge Criteria	Nursing Actions	Date
6/20/94	Acute pain	1) States no pain	1) Elevate ankle on	6/20/94
R. Redford	related to	2) Moves easily	pillow	
	fractured ankle	without wincing	2) Apply ice to	6/20/94
			ankle continuously	
	States ankle		3) Give prescribed	6/20/94
	painful		pain med. q4h for	
	Winces when moves		24 hrs. then q4h PRN	
6/20/94	Ineffective	1) Coughs and	1) Teach to use	
R. Redford	airway clearance	deep breathes	incentive spirometer	
	related to	effectively	2) Supervise in	
	excessive	2) Lungs clear	deep breathing	
	secretions	on auscultation	and coughing	
			q2h while	
	Crackles and		awake	
	bubbles in		3) Encourage to	
	lower lungs		change position	
			frequently	

Figure 11-3. An example of an individualized nursing care plan.

At one time nursing care plans were temporary documents that were destroyed when the patient was discharged. In current practice, the nursing care plan is recognized as an important part of the patient's health care record and is retained along with the rest of the record. One disadvantage to this approach is that some individuals are reluctant to make alterations to a document. If nursing care plans are not altered and adapted as the patient's condition changes, they lose their value as guides for effective nursing care and a means of communication among the nursing staff.

Some agencies keep all patient-related information in documents in the individual patient record or chart. In these agencies there would be no separate document called a "nursing care plan," but all of the elements of the plan for nursing care would be documented in the chart in some way. Still other agencies maintain nursing plans of care in a computerized record. In these systems it may be possible to obtain a printout of the most current nursing plans to use during the shift. This printout could be used for keeping notes as well as guiding care and would then be discarded at the end of the shift. The permanent record of the plan remains in the computer.

Nursing care plans written by students as part of their education are commonly much more complex and include all parts of the nursing process and typically require that all assessment data and the rationale for all actions be included. Information regarding medications, laboratory and diagnostic tests, and other members of the health care team involved in care may also be included. The student nursing care plan is designed to facilitate learning and to apply the nursing process to the individual patient situation.

Using Standardized Nursing Care Plans

Some facilities have *standardized nursing care plans* that contain the standard plans of care for patients with the medical diagnoses encountered on each unit. For example, a unit that cares for postoperative patients may have a standardized plan for care outlining the typical nursing diagnoses, desired outcomes, and nursing actions for those patients. These may be referred to as "standards of care" (Fig. 11-4). The nurse who is responsible for care planning reviews the standardized plan, then dates and signs those nursing diagnoses relevant to the particular patient. The desired outcomes and nursing actions are then individualized by specific dates, times, and other characteristics. Additional outcomes or actions may be added, and those not appropriate to the patient are deleted. Nursing diagnoses that do not appear on the standardized plan are entered and the rest of the process is then completed for them.

The purpose of standardized plans is to decrease the time nurses must spend on paperwork and facilitate the preparation of well written care plans. However, these plans are not adequate if they are not individualized because they then do not reflect the needs and problems of the particular patient.

The use of computers for all health care record keeping is growing, and the nursing care plan is no exception. Computerized nursing care plans are based on standardized nursing care plans, which are entered into the memory of a computer. These computerized plans vary in their operating details, but they all have certain common characteristics (Fig. 11-5).

MEDICAL PATIENT CARE STANDARDS

Date Signature	Problems	Expected Outcome & Problem Resolution Date	Nursing Actions	Date	Treatments Special Orders
4/5/93	Alteration of respiratory status	Lungs clear to	1. T.C. D.B. q 2 hrs.		
	Ineffective	auscultation	2. Assess lung sounds q shift		
K. Barthold RN	airway	4/8/93			
	clearance				
	rel. to painful				
	incision				
4/5/93	Alteration of skin integrity		1. Turn q 2 hours		
	High Risk	Skin clear	2. Massage around bony prominences		
K. Barthold RN		without redness	and reddened areas. Assess skin q		
		or open areas	3. Use pull sheet/egg crate/sof-care as needed		
			4. Encourage high protein/carbohydrate		
			foods & juices high in Vitamin C.		
			5. Skin Care.		
			Bath: $\bar{c}$ oil Lotion: $\bar{c}$ massage		
			6. Oral Hygiene:		
			Assessment:		
			Care:		

Figure 11-4. An example of a standardized nursing care plan.

05/14/94 14:05 PAGE 2

CARE PLAN FOR PATIENT: JASON SMITH ROOM/BED #: 229-B
DIAGNOSIS: 276.5 - DEHYDRATION, 250.01 - DIABETES MELLITUS, INSULIN DEP., 008.8 - VIRAL GASTROENTERITIS,
414.0 - ARTERIOSCLER

PROBLEMS	GOALS	EST DATE	APPROACHES	DISC
A-04-A -				
08 FEEDING DEFICIT RELATED TO WEAKNESS ONSET DATE 3/03/94	01 FEED SELF SHORT TERM	06/30/94	01 RECORD RESPONSE TO FEEDING REHAB GOAL: + = MET GOAL; - = REQUIRED ASST FEED SELF	REH
			50 VERBAL CUES TO EAT AND FINISH MEAL	NAC
A-05-A -				
01 DRESSING/GROOMING DEFICIT RELATED TO: IMPAIRED MOBILITY	01 DRESS/UNDRESS SELF SHORT TERM	06/30/94	01 RECORD RESPONSE TO DRESSING REHAB GOAL: + = MET GOAL; - = REQUIRED ASST DRESS/GROOM SELF	REH
04 DRESSING/GROOMING DEFICIT R/T WEAKNESS ONSET DATE 3/03/94			06 REMIND TO DRESS/UNDRESS	NAC
			67 ASSIST PRN	NAC
A-06-A -				
08 TOILETING DEFICIT RELATED TO: IMPAIRED MOBILITY ONSET DATE 3/03/94	05 MAKE NEED FOR TOILETING KNOWN SHORT TERM	06/30/94	11 STANDBY WITH VERBAL CUES FOR TOILETING	NAC
09 TOILETING DEFICIT RELATED TO: WEAKNESS ONSET DATE 3/03/94				
B-10-A -				
01 BOWEL ELIMINATION, ALTERED CONSTIPATION RELATED TO: LACK OF EXERCISE ONSET DATE 03/03/94	01 COMFORTABLE & REGULAR BM SHORT TERM	06/30/94	04 RECORD ON BM FLOW SHEET	NAC
			25 GIVE STOOL SOFTENER AS ORDERED	LN
B-15-A -				

CARE PLAN FOR PATIENT: JASON SMITH ROOM/BED #: 229-B
DIAGNOSIS: 276.5 - DEHYDRATION, 250.01 - DIABETES MELLITUS, INSULIN DEP., 008.8 - VIRAL GASTRONENTERITIS,
414.0 - ARTERIOSCLER

Figure 11-5. An example of a computerized nursing care plan. REH, rehabilitation assistant; NAC, nursing assistant, certified; LN, licensed nurse. Content selected from a resident care plan customized from *Care Planning for Long-term Care,* Bellevue, WA.

The computer contains a file of nursing diagnoses that can be brought to the screen for review. Their defining characteristics may also be listed, to aid in the process. After reviewing the nursing diagnoses given, you may select one as written or enter one that the computer does not present. Even if you use a nursing diagnosis presented by the computer, you can usually alter that statement to individualize it if necessary. The etiology is then entered into the computer to provide a complete nursing diagnosis statement. Some programs ask that you also enter the signs and symptoms.

Desired outcomes are then entered. The computer

may prompt you to enter a target date for attainment of the outcomes if you fail to include a date in your entry.

Once the nursing diagnosis has been established and the desired outcomes entered, the computer may also present a list of possible nursing actions. Again you may select from the list, modify listed suggestions, or enter new nursing actions.

The process is repeated for each nursing diagnosis. When all nursing diagnoses have been completed, you indicate that all of this information should be recorded on the nursing care plan. The nursing care plan is then added into the patient's computerized record and a copy may be printed out for use on the unit.

Computers speed the formulation of nursing care plans and make it easy to revise the plans. Each system is different; therefore, you will need to learn the system in use where you practice. Not all nursing care planning systems contain all the features mentioned. In some facilities, the care plan is recorded on the computer, but all aspects must be entered individually by the nurse. In some systems, it can be difficult to alter the plan suggested by the computer. This complication may make it harder to individualize a plan. In a research study comparing individually written and computer-assisted nursing care plans, the investigator found that the computer-assisted plans more consistently contained all relevant steps of the nursing process and were more likely to be updated than individually written plans (Colbath, 1992).

Incorporating Policies, Protocols, and Critical Pathways in Planning Care

Policies, as discussed in Chapter 1, are designed to give guidelines for appropriate action to the employees of any organization. In general, policies describe the responsibilities of each position. They may also describe the actions to be taken when certain situations are encountered. For example, a policy would state the situations in which a registered nurse could start an intravenous infusion without a physician's order. In addition, the policies would specify that this action was the responsibility of the registered nurse not the licensed practical nurse. Policies may be used as general guidelines when planning care.

Protocols are more detailed and specific than policies and list nursing actions needed in greater detail. For example, a protocol for the person receiving pain medication by intravenous infusion might specify the assessment that must be conducted, the frequency of the assessment, and how that assessment is to be documented. A protocol may even include specific conditions that should be reported to the physician. Protocols are designed to systematize nursing practice in a particular setting. They are commonly developed by a committee or task force of nurses who have expertise in the type of care covered by the protocol. Sometimes a protocol is developed to assist nurses with a totally new type of care. In this instance the nursing committee may consult references and contact other agencies to learn about their protocols before developing one for their own agency.

In many health care facilities, nurses are working to establish what are called critical pathways for care. A **critical pathway** is composed of a sequence of standardized short-term patient outcomes that will lead toward an overall long-term outcome. For example, a critical pathway for all patients having a particular surgery may specify precisely how many hours after surgery that the patient is expected to be able to get out of bed, when the bowel sounds are expected to return, and when the person will be taking adequate oral fluids. The use of critical pathways helps the nurse to examine whether the individual patient is progressing as expected. In addition, the use of critical pathways is thought to hasten progress because everyone has a clear goal in mind and works toward that goal. Thus, there are not delays in the patient's progress from one level of care to another.

In some agencies, a nurse is assigned to the individual patient as a *case manager.* The role of the case manager in this instance is to follow the patient's progress in regard to the critical pathway and determine whether the patient is meeting the expected standard outcomes. If the patient is not progressing as expected, the entire situation is examined to determine what is interfering with the patient's progress. Interventions can be altered rapidly or new interventions initiated to help the patient progress. A major goal of critical pathways as an approach to planning for nursing care is to shorten hospital stays and lessen the costs of health care.

Critical pathways can also be used as a basis for standardized care plans. The critical pathways are established with the desired outcomes. Then nursing actions to achieve those outcomes are included. For example, if the critical pathway states that one short-term goal is "return of bowel sounds 24 hours after surgery," then the critical pathway may indicate that after this short-term outcome is achieved, the nurse begins oral fluids. In the situation in which a patient has had bladder surgery, if the critical pathway has a short-term goal of "urine light pink with no clots within 24 hours," the pathway then prescribes the nursing actions to be taken to assist the patient toward the next short-term outcome. In this instance, the next short-term outcome might be that "The patient is voiding independently within 30 hours after return from surgery." To achieve this, the next prescribed action might be "Remove Foley catheter 24 hours after surgery."

Maintaining Patient Involvement in Planning

It is extremely important that patients be involved in planning for their own care. First, of course, it is their right to know what you propose and to determine whether or not they will consent to your proposed plan. However, a plan will be much more successful if the patient is involved not only in giving consent after the plan is formulated but throughout the planning process in considering alternatives and establishing goals and outcome criteria.

Patients often enter a health care setting with predetermined goals, which may or may not be in accord with those of the health care personnel. It is the nurse's responsibility to find out the patient's goals, communicate to the patient the goals the nurse sees as appropriate, and negotiate with the patient to establish a set of goals toward which all can work together. If staff and patient are working toward separate goals, it may be impossible for any goals to be achieved. The American Nurses Association *Standards of Clinical Nursing Practice* specify that outcomes should be mutually formulated with the patient whenever possible (1991).

When data collection is part of the plan, the patient may be able to assist in that process if he or she understands the purpose and the plan for collecting the data. Many technical skills are taught to patients to facilitate self-care. If patients are consulted while the techniques are being established, these techniques will be more likely to be appropriate for the patient's life setting.

Implementation

Implementation is the step in the nursing process in which care is provided to the patient. All the details of the plan are carried out. *Implementing* a nursing care plan requires communication and interpersonal skills as well as technical skills. Communicating with the patient will be a part of every action. Through communication you will demonstrate support for your patient's rights and respect for the patient as a human being. You will also use communication skills to teach patients. In Chapter 13 basic communication skills will be presented, and in Chapter 16 the skills of health teaching will be discussed.

Respecting Patients' Rights

Part of the foundation for effective nursing action is a recognition of and support for the rights of everyone in the health care system. This includes not only the patient, but also the employees and the students. Claire Fagin (1975) defined a right as "a just claim to anything to which one is entitled such as power or privilege. A right is that which one may properly demand or claim as just, moral, or legal" (p. 84). Most rights stem originally from a moral or ethical viewpoint. Some rights are embodied in law. Most of the statements on rights are not legal documents but guidelines for ethical and just behavior.

In Chapter 3 we discussed some of the legal and ethical aspects of patients' rights. We emphasized that patients continue to have rights whatever their ages or circumstances. As a nurse, you will be safeguarding patients' rights in the way you deliver care. You will also have an obligation to safeguard patients' rights when others are providing care. Patients in care facilities are vulnerable because of their illness, their lack of knowledge, and their dependency; often they are not able to speak for themselves. Although each care provider is responsible for obtaining consent in regard to the care he or she provides, the nurse is often in the position to identify when patients have not understood and contact the appropriate person to provide information to the patient.

The right to self-determination and consent is fun-

Nursing Issues and Trends: *A Taxonomy of Nursing Interventions*

Does nursing need another taxonomy? As the work on the taxonomy of nursing diagnosis has progressed, another group of nurses has begun work on the development of a standardized terminology for nursing interventions. The Iowa Intervention Project, directed by nursing faculty at the University of Iowa, has established a beginning framework in which to investigate terminology that nurses use for their intervention activities. It is their belief that research and development in nursing will be facilitated by a standardized terminology. Perhaps in the future, a nurse will be able to search a data base for a term representing an intervention activity and obtain all relevant references without concern that important information was missed because others were using different language.

damental. The patient has a right to make personal decisions regarding health care. The facility in which you practice should provide policies to guide you in determining who can give consent for care when the patient is unconscious or otherwise unable to give consent. Remember that old age or physical illness alone does not imply incompetence.

At times patients rely on nurses to make decisions for their nursing care and well-being and do not wish to or cannot be asked about each detail of care. The new surgical patient is a good example. The patient is in pain and sedated and probably has no idea what actions might be appropriate at any given time. This surgical patient will rely on the nurse to decide when it is time to turn and breathe deeply. For the patient who is unconscious, the nurse may make all the routine decisions about daily nursing care; the family or guardian will make all major decisions including those that require formal written consent.

At times, it is appropriate for the nurse and the patient to come to a mutual decision regarding care. This is particularly true when a patient is learning self-care in regard to a health problem. After discussing the circumstances and the patient's concerns, they reach a joint decision about actions to be taken and mutual responsibilities.

The patient or guardian cannot be expected to make good decisions without adequate information. Part of a nurse's responsibility is to explain the various possible decisions and the possible consequences of actions taken or not taken so that the consent the patient gives is truly informed. Each member of the health care team is responsible for providing the appropriate information relative to the care being planned: the physician's responsibility is to provide information relevant to decisions about medical care, and the nurse's responsibility is to provide information relevant to the nursing plan of care.

The patient has a right to have information of a confidential nature carefully safeguarded. You will need to keep this in mind when you are preparing papers, discussing a patient with your instructor, or presenting information in a conference. Information can be shared with those who need it to provide care. It is also ethical to share information for the purposes of education if the patient's identity is safeguarded from public exposure. Written papers should never identify the patient by name.

Physical privacy is also an important right. You will safeguard this through the use of screening and draping. In multiple-bed rooms, maintaining physical privacy requires constant attention to detail, such as knocking on closed doors and asking permission before you approach a curtained bedside.

The patient has the right to expect that those providing care are knowledgeable and competent and will provide safe care. When directly providing care for a patient or when directing someone else in care, you are responsible for the outcome. As a student, you must always make sure that you know what your own abilities and limitations are and practice within those. Never hesitate to seek help if you are unsure.

Care that respects the dignity and worth of the person, unrestricted by considerations of nationality, race, creed, color, status, age, or sex, is another important right of the patient. Showing respect for individual dignity should be part of every contact with the patient. Your respect for a patient's dignity is revealed in the way you address the patient, the attention you give to personal concerns, and the quality of care you provide.

The patient has a right to individualized care related to his or her unique needs and lifestyle. To support this right, you must treat each person as a unique and important individual. Thorough assessment to identify special needs and concerns provides the basis for care that supports the patient's individuality.

Being able to care for oneself is important in building one's self-esteem and is critical in resuming functioning as an independent person. To support the development of this ability, you must go beyond providing care to teaching the patient about his or her care needs and coordinating care so that the entire health care team is assisting the patient in the move toward independence.

Patients have the right to evaluate care, and when it has not been of high quality, to obtain changes to improve its quality. Often health care providers become upset and defensive when patients identify deficiencies in care. No person or system is ever perfect, and there is always room for improvement. When a complaint is made, look into the situation and then find ways of improving it. Sometimes you will find that what patients have complained about is not the real basis for concern, but patients have perceived that others are treating them with a lack of dignity or failing to recognize their individual uniqueness. Patients may have difficulty verbalizing this perception and may therefore complain about more concrete matters. (See *Modules for Basic Nursing Skills*, Module 1, for a further discussion of patients' rights.)

Acquiring Knowledge of Patients' Responsibilities

Responsibilities always accompany rights. Patients, health care workers, and students all have responsibilities within the health care system.

Most of the literature on patients' rights also discusses staff responsibilities in relationship to these rights but does not discuss the patient's responsibilities. A notable exception is the work of the Group Health Cooperative of Puget Sound. This health maintenance organization is owned and operated by consumers. Part of the philosophy of the cooperative concerns taking responsibility for one's own health. Some people do not agree with placing responsibilities on the consumer. The person who is ill is under stress and has many sources of anxiety. This situation may seem to require that health care workers assume most decision-making responsibility and allow the patient to assume a dependent role. Although patients must often be dependent to a limited extent, historically most health care has been designed to promote a greater level of dependency in patients than was really necessary. Fostering the autonomy and independence of the patient requires a recognition that responsibilities go with independence. Display 11-2 lists some of the general responsibilities of the health care consumer that have been outlined by Group Health (1977). Placing these responsibilities on the health care consumer is a relatively new concept, springing from the recognition that the patient is an active participant in health care and not a passive recipient. This list of consumer responsibilities should be evaluated in light of the abilities of each individual to participate in health care.

Meeting Nurses' Responsibilities in Implementing Care

Nurses have a history of accepting responsibility well. The responsibilities of the nurse include maintaining an adequate knowledge base in regard to nursing care to be implemented, making appropriate decisions for care, and demonstrating technical proficiency in skills. In addition, the nurse is responsible for maintaining effective communication and the appropriate environment for care.

The nurse has independent responsibility for evaluating and maintaining a personal *knowledge base*. This includes knowledge related to the nursing process; knowledge of health, illness, and its effects; and the knowledge necessary to perform nursing care with skill. You are also responsible for knowing the limits of your own ability and working within those limits. This responsibility continues throughout your career. The primary sources of such knowledge will be textbooks, professional journals, continuing education classes, and expert colleagues.

The nurse is responsible for performing skills with *technical proficiency*. This includes performing safely and efficiently, demonstrating dexterity, and being well organized. The development of technical proficiency is essential to functioning effectively as a nurse. You will need to learn correct techniques and develop the ability to organize your work efficiently. Specific technical skills are presented in *Modules for Basic Nursing Skills*, Volumes I and II. In the modules all skills are presented using a nursing process approach. This approach

Display 11–2
Responsibilities of the Health Care Consumer

- Consumers are expected to treat all employees with courtesy and consideration, just as the consumer has the right to be treated with dignity and respect. Good interpersonal relationships form the basis of sound health care, and these relationships are based on the participation of both parties. The person who is mentally incompetent or in an altered state of awareness because of illness is not responsible for behavior, but other consumers are.
- Consumers are expected to supply complete and accurate medical history information. Without this information, the health care team cannot function effectively. In return, the consumer is guaranteed privacy and the confidentiality of all information shared.
- Consumers are expected to ask questions, especially if they do not understand or cannot follow instructions. Although the health care worker is expected to provide information in an understandable manner, the worker is not infallible. For consumers to exercise the right of informed participation, they have the responsibility to communicate their information needs.
- Consumers have the responsibility to communicate their wishes about treatment. To exercise the right to informed consent meaningfully, the consumer must clearly state if consent is being withheld. If consent is being given, the consumer must follow the procedure for providing consent.
- Consumers affected by a research project have the responsibility to decide whether to participate. This decision cannot be left to others. This decision-making responsibility accompanies the right to be informed about the research nature of any treatment or program.
- Consumers have the right to be informed of policies and regulations affecting safety and health, such as smoking regulations. In return, the consumer has the responsibility to adhere to these policies. For example, smoking is not allowed where oxygen is found. Smoking in such an environment creates a hazard for others and is not acceptable.
- Consumers are expected to discuss the problems they encounter with health care workers. They may discuss the problem with the individual involved; or, if doing so would make them uncomfortable, they may speak to a supervisory person. This expectation places some of the responsibility for correcting problem situations on the consumer. If no one knows a problem exists, no one can work to solve it.

should become a basic part of the way you function in nursing.

As you progress, your work will increase in both speed and dexterity. You will need to practice new skills repeatedly until you can use them with ease. Doing so ensures that you can concentrate on the patient, not the equipment, during the procedure. Practice is also necessary to maintain your proficiency at skills you have already acquired but use only occasionally. You will need to ask for supervision when learning new skills to ensure the safety of the patient.

Technical proficiency allows a procedure to be accomplished quickly, causing the patient less fatigue. Technical proficiency certainly assuages the patient's anxiety and may also minimize discomfort. Technical proficiency increases the patient's trust in your abilities and relieves some of the anxiety experienced by the patient facing procedures.

Most health care settings are complex places with complex equipment. A large number of patients have a lessened ability to safeguard themselves. The combination of these two factors creates a high potential for injury. You must always consider patient safety when carrying out a plan for care.

Delegating Nursing Care

Delegation of tasks to others on the nursing team is also a part of implementation (Fig. 11-6). As a beginning student you will not be delegating work to others, but work may be delegated to you. You can begin understanding the skill of delegation by observing registered nurses at work. Identify what tasks are delegated and to whom. Also try to identify how the nurse follows up to be sure delegated tasks are completed. Delegation is discussed further in Chapter 15.

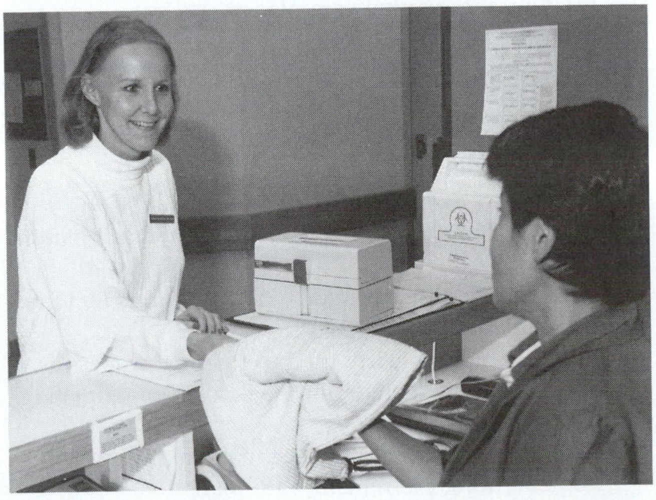

Figure 11-6. Delegation of tasks to others on the nursing team is part of implementation.

Written documentation of the entire nursing process is both a professional and legal responsibility. Information on how to document your care is found in Chapter 15 and also in Module 6.

Using a Nursing Process Approach to Physician-Prescribed Care

The problem-solving approach of the nursing process is appropriate to many situations in nursing. Although nursing diagnosis is directly related to identifying those problems that are nursing's responsibility, the steps of assessment, planning, implementation, and evaluation are relevant to working cooperatively with others on the health care team. Implementing prescriptions or orders of the physician involves far more than merely carrying out tasks. As an educated, independently licensed health care provider, the nurse is always responsible for any care given, whether prescribed by a physician or planned by the nurse. The best safeguard for the patient is a health care team in which all members take responsibility for what is happening, not simply "follow orders."

Assessment is the gathering of data before you act and throughout your contact with the patient. You may be carrying out a procedure prescribed by the physician to relieve a medical problem, but you are still responsible for skillful assessment based on knowledge of the patient, the medical problem, and the procedure.

The condition of a patient is not static and unchanging but rather is a dynamic process. Therefore, you will need to have a clear view of the patient's current condition and status to make good decisions about carrying out medical orders. For example, a physician may order an oral pain medication for a patient. If you observe that the patient is currently nauseated and vomiting, you should not give the medication. In another instance, if the patient was having severe pain unrelieved by the maximum dosage of pain medication that had been ordered by the physician, you would contact the physician in regard to modifying the prescription in some way to more effectively treat the pain.

Planning is necessary before you begin a procedure to ensure that you proceed in an organized manner. You may also wish to facilitate the planning of future procedures by noting helpful ways of doing things. Planning should include setting goals (although they may be simple), as well as identifying the equipment needed and thinking through the procedure.

As part of your planning you need to understand the ordered therapy, its goal for the patient, and how it is to be carried out. Whether it is a medication ordered, a treatment, or an activity plan, you need to understand the basis for it. For example, if a physician orders a medication and you observed that the written dosage is ten times the usual dosage for that medication, you should not simply give the medication; instead, you should call the physician and discuss the order. If the medication ordered is one that must be taken with food, you should schedule the medication to be given with meals. You will often need to use references to review the background knowledge essential for safe practice.

Implementation—performance of the procedure itself—is the only part of the process clearly visible to the patient. Often the entire process will be judged by the patient on the basis of implementation alone.

Finally, when you have completed an ordered procedure, you must always evaluate the effects. Was it effective? What was the patient's response? How could you have performed better? The evaluation step of the nursing process is discussed in detail in the next chapter.

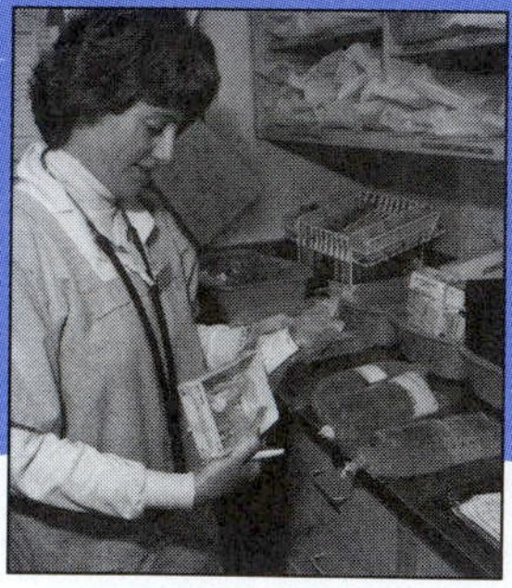

Key Points

- The planning step of the nursing process involves setting goals, gathering additional data, developing a plan, setting priorities, and writing the plan.
- Desired outcomes are identified and clearly stated. The focus of these statements is the patient, and the statements must be in descriptive, measurable, or comparative terms that can be used as criteria for evaluation. Both long-term and short-term goals may be included.
- Patient involvement in nursing care planning results in a plan that is appropriate to the individual and in which the individual is more likely to participate effectively. The patient's values must form the basis for these decisions.
- For patients with multiple problems, goals may include the patient's overall condition, current status, and prognosis for the future.
- Planning may require gathering more information from resources such as nursing texts, current journals, and the policy and procedure book of the facility. These references and resources provide the rationale for your actions.
- Setting priorities requires decisions about the order in which actions should be performed and also about what problem should be addressed first.
- Each facility has its own approach to writing a plan for nursing care. Standardized nursing care plans may be used as a basis for the development of individualized care plans. Computers make the individualization of standard nursing care plans easier. Policies, protocols, and critical pathways may all be used as a basis for standardized planning.
- Implementation of a nursing care plan requires the use of technical and interpersonal skills and should take place within the framework of respect for the rights and responsibilities of all involved. Technical proficiency increases the patient's trust in the nurse's abilities and relieves the patient's anxiety.
- The nurse has independent responsibility for evaluating and maintaining a personal knowledge base, for performing skills with technical proficiency, and for knowing the limits of his or her own ability.
- As an educated, independently licensed health care provider, the nurse is always responsible for any care given, whether prescribed by a physician or planned by the nurse.
- Delegation of tasks and documentation of the nursing process are also important aspects of implementing the nursing care plan.

Study Questions

1. What are the usual components of a nursing care plan?
2. List the characteristics of a correctly written patient outcome.
3. What are the three general types of actions included in a nursing care plan?
4. In what part or parts of the nursing process is it appropriate to include the patient or patient's family?
5. How can the nurse maintain patients' rights while implementing the nursing care plan?
6. Compare and contrast the responsibilities of the patient and of the nurse.

7. What are the components of technical proficiency?
8. How does the nursing process approach apply to carrying out the physician's prescription for care?

Critical Thinking Activities

1. Check the plans for nursing care in the facility where you are a student. What is included in those plans? Compare them with the contents of a plan suggested in the chapter.
2. If the facility where you are a student has standardized nursing care plans, examine them. Check the policy manual to learn how the standardized nursing care plans are used. Evaluate the level of individualization in the standard care plans in use.
3. If the facility where you are a student has computerized nursing care plans, arrange to observe a staff nurse as he or she prepares a nursing care plan from the computer. Ask the nurse what he or she sees as the benefits and problems involved with the use of computerized plans.
4. Select two different nursing diagnoses from the NANDA list and write specific desired outcomes as if for a particular patient.
5. In a group, share your written outcomes with other students. Critique each other's statements and restate correctly when necessary.
6. Choose one NANDA nursing diagnosis. Using the text index, determine where you would find information on appropriate nursing actions for that diagnosis. Write out one nursing action and the rationale for that action as you find it in the text. Share this with other students in a group.
7. Review the nursing diagnoses for a given patient in the facility. Using the various approaches described in the text, identify which diagnosis would take first priority. Discuss your selection of priority with your instructor.

References and Readings

American Nurses Association. *Standards of Clinical Nursing Practice.* Kansas City, Mo.: ANA, 1991.

Bulechek, G. M., and McCloskey, J. C. "Nursing Intervention Taxonomy Development." In *Current Issues in Nursing.* 3rd edition, pp. 23–28, edited by J. C. McCloskey and H. K. Grace. St. Louis: C. V. Mosby, 1990.

Carpenito, L. *Nursing Diagnosis: Application to Clinical Practice.* 4th edition. Philadelphia: J. B. Lippincott, 1992.

Colbath, R. Unpublished master's thesis, Seattle Pacific University, Seattle, WA. 1992.

Fagin, C.M. "Nurse's Rights," American Journal of Nursing 75:1 January 1975: 82–85.

Gordon, M. *Nursing Diagnosis: Process and Application.* 2nd edition. New York: McGraw-Hill, 1987.

Joint Commission on the Accreditation of Healthcare Organizations. *Accreditation Manual for Hospitals.* Chicago: JCAHO, 1990.

Maslow, A. H. *Motivation and Personality.* New York: Harper & Row, 1970.

Matthewman, J. "Combining Care Plans and Kardex." *American Journal of Nursing* 87, 6 (June 1987): 852–854.

Peplau, H. *Interpersonal Relations in Nursing.* New York: G. P. Putnam and Sons, 1956.

Evaluation

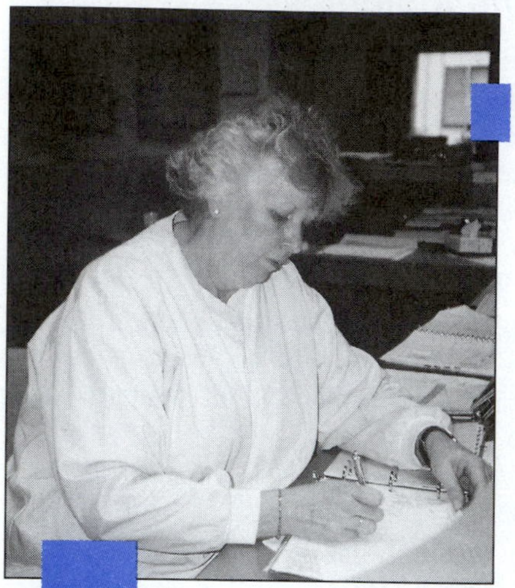

12

Objectives

After completing this chapter, you should be able to:

1. Define evaluation.
2. Discuss the purposes of evaluation.
3. Discuss the differences in evaluation processes used for different purposes.
4. Explain how evaluation could be used to modify the nursing care plan.
5. Identify people in the health care system who have an interest in nursing evaluation.
6. Explain how a nursing student might use evaluation in professional growth.

Study Terms

concurrent review
continuous quality improvement (CQI)
evaluation
peer review organization (PRO)
preadmission/preprocedure review
quality assurance programs
retrospective review
total quality management (TQM)

Outline

Purposes of Evaluation

Evaluation within the Nursing Process

Attainment of Desired Outcomes
Degree of Progress Toward Desired Outcomes
Patient's Evaluation
Discharge Evaluation
Recording the Evaluation

Evaluation of the Entire Nursing Process

Modification of a Plan Based on Evaluation

ANA Standards Regarding Nursing Process

Evaluation Within the Health Care System

Peer Review Organizations
Quality Assurance Programs
Quality Management

Personal Evaluation for Professional Growth

Evaluation is a process of examining and judging something or someone for worth or effectiveness. All aspects of nursing are subject to evaluation. In this chapter we discuss evaluation within the context of the nursing process and within the broader field of the entire health care system.

Purposes of Evaluation

Within the nursing process, evaluation has two major purposes. The first is to determine whether the desired outcomes for the patient have been reached. The second is to examine the entire nursing process to identify whether the assessment was complete, the nursing diagnosis correct, and the planning appropriate, as well as whether the actions taken were responsible for the outcomes and whether they should be continued, discontinued, or revised.

In the context of the wider health care system, evaluation is used to examine the effectiveness of general policies and procedures, the overall responses of clients as a group, the functioning of individual health care practitioners, and the quality of health care delivered.

Evaluation Within the Nursing Process

Evaluation within the nursing process is a nursing responsibility. Just as nurses are responsible and accountable for assessment, planning, and implementation, they are also responsible and accountable for evaluation within the nursing process because it is within the realm of independent nursing function. No one else can properly assume this responsibility. Evaluation includes identifying whether a desired patient outcome was fully met, whether it was partially met, or whether it was not met at all.

To evaluate, you must clearly understand what the desired outcomes are. Then you must collect the data that will allow you to compare the patient's progress with the goal. Both subjective and objective data are important for the purposes of evaluation.

Attainment of Desired Outcomes

Desired outcomes for patients are established during the planning phase of the nursing process. These outcomes are the criteria for evaluation. If the problem and the desired outcome were originally stated precisely and in detail, evaluation is a relatively straightforward task. For example, if the problem was that the patient ate too little to provide for healing and the desired outcome was that the patient eat half the food served on the meal tray, then you would observe the tray to gather objective information about the amount eaten. You could then state either "Yes, the patient did eat half the meal; the problem is solved, and the plan was a success" or "No, the patient ate one-fourth of the meal; therefore, the plan was unsuccessful." This is evaluation at its simplest. The criterion—the standard for judging success or failure—is merely success or failure at attaining the desired outcome.

If the problem and the desired outcome were originally stated in general terms, the first step in evaluation would be to establish criteria. For example, if the desired outcome in the above case was simply that the patient eat more or eat enough, a decision would have to be made about what constituted more or enough. A criterion must be established so that one can determine whether it has been met.

Time lines are also reviewed when evaluating. The idea is to determine whether the desired outcomes were achieved in a timely fashion. If the date and time for attainment of the desired outcome have not yet arrived, your judgment of the success of the plan will consider the fact that additional time to work on outcomes still remains.

Written records facilitate evaluation because care is typically provided by different nursing personnel at different times. If actions and results are recorded, and if there is a record of the desired outcomes and criteria being used to measure results, evaluation can be undertaken by someone other than the nurse who made the plan.

Degree of Progress Toward Desired Outcome

More complex evaluation involves subtler questions and determinations. When there are several desired outcomes for a nursing diagnosis, each one is evaluated. Thus, goals might be partially met if there were three desired outcomes for a nursing diagnosis and only two of the three were accomplished.

Often the degree of progress made toward an individual outcome must be estimated to determine if the outcome is partially met. If the patient has made progress, the nurse must try to determine whether that progress resulted from the action taken or whether the actions have been unsuccessful and any progress is due to other factors. If the action has been responsible for the partial success, the nurse must then consider whether the action should be continued or whether the patient would benefit more from a reconsideration of the plan.

When a desired outcome is not reached at all, the nurse must examine a variety of factors to determine what has interfered with the outcome. You will want to

Nursing Issues and Trends: *Ethical Considerations in Evaluation*

The emphasis in evaluation is increasingly on the outcome or result of any action or project. Results are important in determining success, but the emphasis on outcomes sometimes overlooks the importance of the process used to get there. The ethical position of utilitarianism focuses on the outcomes as opposed to the methods or processes. Is that the preferred ethical position for nurses? Are there ethical considerations that deserve as much emphasis as outcomes? Can outcomes encompass the values regarding the whole person that nursing cherishes? How can nurses assure that their values are part of any evaluation plan in the health care arena?

determine whether the failure was due to a lack of original assessment data, an incorrect identification of the nursing diagnosis, inappropriate outcomes being established, or incorrect actions being planned. It may also be that the nursing care planning was appropriate, but that other factors interfered with success. These factors might include the patient's failure to carry out planned actions, psychological distress in the patient, or the presence of other health problems. A wide variety of social and cultural factors may also interfere with the success of a nursing plan.

Patient's Evaluation

Discussion has focused exclusively on the nurse's evaluation, but the patient's evaluation of care is equally important. Patients need to be encouraged to examine their outcomes and their progress. The patient's opinion of care should be actively sought. If care is producing the desired result but is not being delivered in an acceptable manner, the patient can readily evaluate it.

Discharge Evaluation

At the time of discharge, all nursing diagnoses are reviewed and outcomes are determined. If problems remain unresolved, the nurse has a responsibility to plan for ongoing care. This may include teaching the patient and family to provide care or making a referral to a home health care agency. In some instances, the patient will be moving from the hospital to a long-term care facility. A referral is then written that outlines continuing care needs.

Recording the Evaluation

Evaluation is recorded in the nursing progress notes of the patient's record. When using a narrative format, the problem is stated, and data demonstrating outcomes are written. If the problem was resolved, the simple statement "problem resolved" is included, along with the date of resolution. Actions no longer needed are taken off the care plan in the manner established by the facility.

In a problem-oriented record, the problem is identified, the subject and objective data are recorded, and then the overall final evaluation is recorded. Further information on recording can be found in *Modules for Basic Nursing Skills*, Volume I, Module 6, Documentation.

Evaluation of the Entire Nursing Process

When you examine the entire nursing process, you will ask yourself questions to determine whether you have used the process correctly. For a complete explanation of each of the steps of the process, refer to Chapter 8.

Examine the assessment data you collected. Were your data complete? Did you review all available sources, such as the family and laboratory reports on the chart? Did you collect both subjective and objective data? Were your subjective data clearly identified as originating with the client? Are your objective data written in clear, nonjudgmental terms that could be verified by another observer? Are you lacking data that would have helped you in planning? Have you clearly identified the data that served as the defining characteristics for this diagnosis for this client?

Examine the nursing diagnoses in the light of having completed the entire nursing process. The following questions will assist you. Were there any nursing diagnoses suggested by the data that you failed to identify? Did you select the correct general area of alteration? Did you identify the specific problem accurately? Did you use correct NANDA (North American Nursing Diagnosis Association) terminology? If not, is this a problem for which terminology is not yet standardized? If no standardized terminology exists, did you verify with your instructor or an experienced nurse the clarity of the terminology you used? Did you state the related factors accurately, including all that contributed to the origin or continuation of this diagnosis? Should additional related factors be added to the diagnosis statement to provide better direction for planning?

When you examine your planning, use these questions. Are the desired outcomes appropriate to this client, that is, neither too difficult to be accomplished nor too easy to represent the client's best potential? Are they acceptable to the client? Do they represent true end results, not actions or processes? Are they stated in terms that preserve the focus on the client? Are they objective in nature, that is, observable, measurable, or comparative? Is a date or time for attainment of the objectives included?

Actions are examined in response to these questions. Will the actions designated in the plan alleviate the problem or provide continuous monitoring for the problem? Has patient/family teaching been included, as appropriate? Are the actions under nursing control? Are the actions specific, providing definite tasks to be done? Are they time oriented, including the times and frequency of action? Is there designation of the person who should carry out the action (if necessary in your care setting)? Is the action realistic, given the constraints of the care setting? Have you correctly identified priorities for this patient at this time? If you have stated the rationale for your actions, examine the rationale. Does the statement you have given really provide the underlying scientific reasoning that explains why this particular action will achieve the desired outcome? Is your reference for this rationale available? Displays 12-1 and 12-2 summarize the questions and issues that should be addressed when you evaluate the entire nursing process.

Display 12–1
Guidelines for Evaluation of the Entire Nursing Process

Assessment

1. Data complete?
2. Subjective and objective data included?
3. Subjective data clearly identified as such?
4. Objective data in clear, nonjudgmental terms?
5. Information needed for planning was available?
6. Defining characteristics of nursing diagnoses identified?

Nursing Diagnosis

1. All applicable nursing diagnoses identified?
2. Correct general area of alteration?
3. Specific problem accurate?
4. Correct NANDA terminology used, if available?
5. Terminology verified if no standard available?
6. Related factors accurately reflect what is contributing to problem or its continuation?
7. Are multiple related factors needed in this instance?

Planning

Desired Outcomes/Goals

1. Desired outcomes appropriate to specific client (neither too difficult nor too easy)?
2. Desired outcomes represent end results?
3. Desired outcomes focused on client?
4. Desired outcomes observable?
5. Desired outcomes measurable or comparable?
6. Data for attainment included?

Actions

1. Actions for ongoing monitoring included?
2. Interventions capable of alleviating problem included?
3. Client/family teaching included, as appropriate?
4. Actions are under nursing control?
5. Actions are specific behaviors?
6. Actions realistic within constraints of care setting?
7. Time and frequency included?
8. Person to carry out action included when needed?
9. Priorities identified?

Rationale

1. Explains "why" action will be effective?
2. Reference for rationale available?

Implementation

Communication

1. Correct technique chosen?
2. Technique used effectively?

Skills

1. Correct technique demonstrated?
2. Dexterity demonstrated?
3. Speed of functioning appropriate?

Documentation

1. Documentation done in format prescribed by facility?
2. Documentation included all relevant information?
3. Documentation accurate?

Display 12–2

An Example of Evaluation of Entire Nursing Process Based on Plan in Displays 11-1 and 12-3

Assessment

1. Admission history and physical examination included complete nutritional assessment, height, weight, and handedness.
2. Both subjective data (obtained through asking yes or no questions and having patient respond with head shake) and objective data included.
3. Subjective data identified by stating "indicates."
4. Objective data clear and nonjudgmental.
5. Adequate information for planning was present.
6. Defining characteristics were identified.

Nursing Diagnosis

1. Only one nursing diagnosis identified. Others were present.
2. Specific problem identified.
3. NANDA terminology used throughout.
4. No need to verify non-NANDA terminology.
5. Related factors clear and accurate.
6. Multiple etiologies not provided. Multiple etiologies do not appear appropriate.

Planning

Desired Outcomes/Goals

1. Outcomes appropriate to this patient.
2. Outcomes represent end results—both short-term and long-term included.
3. Outcomes focus on client.
4. Outcomes are observable, objective behaviors.
5. Outcomes can be measured when appropriate or compared with previous behavior.
6. Date for attainment was included.

Actions

1. Continuing monitoring included; however, monitoring of weight should have been included.
2. Interventions were capable of solving problems.
3. No client teaching was specified, although it may be implied in assisting person to eat.
4. Actions specified are within nursing's control.
5. Actions are specific behaviors.
6. Actions are realistic for this care setting.
7. Time and frequency are not specified but actions to be carried out for each meal are implied.
8. Person to carry out action not included. In this facility nurses provide total patient care.
9. Actions were listed in order of priority. Because only one nursing diagnosis was included, no priorities between nursing diagnoses were determined.

Rationale

1. Rationale for actions included.
2. No references given.

Implementation

Communication

1. A structured interview was used for admission. Use of "yes" or "no" questions appropriate for this client.
2. Technique was effective in obtaining needed data.

Display 12–2 ***(continued)***

An Example of Evaluation of Entire Nursing Process Based on Plan in Displays 11-1 and 12-3

Skills

1. Technique for vital signs was in accord with *Modules for Basic Nursing Skills.* No other skills used.
2. Dexterity was demonstrated in taking vital signs.
3. Speed was not a consideration in this plan.

Documentation

1. Entire nursing care plan on correct facility form. Intake and output record complete. Dietary intake noted on appropriate flow sheet.
2. All relevant information included in chart.
3. Information accurate.

SUMMARY: This example of the nursing process demonstrates use of the major steps. The major correction needed is the addition of rationale for actions with references. Further refinement of other steps would improve the specificity of the plan.

Modification of a Plan Based on Evaluation

After you have evaluated both the desired outcomes and your entire nursing process, you will need to decide whether modification is necessary. If you determine that your assessment was incomplete, you will need to reassess the patient. Perhaps your dates for goal accomplishment were unrealistic, or perhaps the patient is able to accomplish more than you originally believed possible. After examining actual outcomes, you may wish to modify the plan to more effectively reach the desired outcomes (Fig. 12-1). To do this, you might have to consult resources and references again. Modification might mean continuing some nursing actions, altering others, or adding completely new actions. Display 12-3 is an example of modifying a plan for nursing action based on evaluation.

ANA Standards Regarding Nursing Process

The American Nurses Association (ANA) *Standards of Clinical Nursing Practice* (1991) address all parts of the nursing process. Specific criteria are listed for evaluating each segment. Attention is drawn to collecting appropriate data in a systematic and ongoing manner. The use of the assessment data to determine nursing diagnoses is emphasized. The standards point out the importance of identifying specific, measurable, attainable outcomes that include a time estimate. Criteria for planning include the importance of individualizing the plan in cooperation with the client and significant others. The standards encourage the inclusion of the patient's participation in planning. Implementation should be consistent with the plan and actions carried out in a safe and appropriate manner. Evaluation should be systematic and ongoing and incorporate both the care provider's and the client's perspectives. The nurse is prompted to use the evaluative data for revision of the nursing care plan. In each area the standards underscore the important role of documentation.

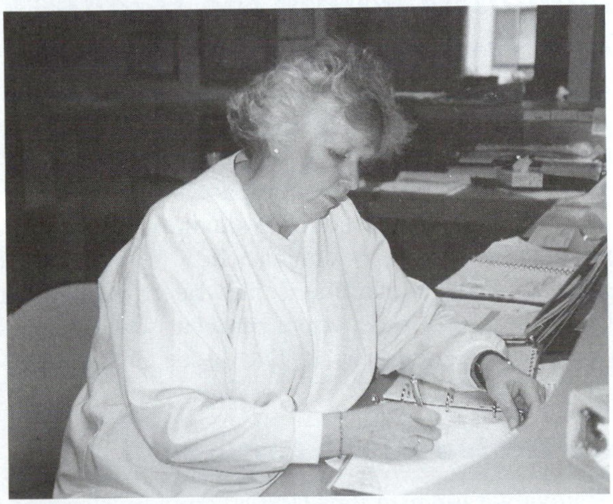

Figure 12-1. Nursing care plans are often modified based on evaluation.

Display 12–3

An Example of Evaluation Regarding Desired Outcomes and Modification of a Nursing Care Plan

Nursing Diagnosis	Desired Outcomes	Evaluation 1/20	Modifications of Plan 1/20
Self-care Deficit:* Feeding related to right-sided paralysis as evidenced by 1. Cannot use right hand 2. Indicates has always been right-handed. 3. Is eating only a few bites and then turning head away.	1. Feeds self all "finger foods" by 1/19. 2. Food intake includes minimum of ¾ of each meal served. 3. Feeds self all foods on tray by 2/20.	1. Now feeds self all "finger foods." 2. Food intake is ¾ of each meal served for ⅔ of meals. Frequently eats only ½ of breakfast. 3. Now holds spoon and feeds self part of meal. Becomes tired before meal is completed and is fed rest of meal.	1. Continue record-keeping as before. 2. Continue tray arrangement as before. 3. Encourage patient to eat in dining room. Sit with her there for meals. 4. Provide finger foods and give recognition for improved ability at holding foods. 5. Continue to use plate guard. 6. Decrease amount served at breakfast and arrange for a midmorning snack to compensate for needed nutrients.

(See Display 11–1 for original plan.)

Evaluation Within the Health Care System

Many elements within the health care system are creating pressure for evaluation. Third-party payers for services, including insurance companies and the federal government, have pressed for evaluation to demonstrate that quality of care is not diminished by cost-containment measures. Cost containment has been implemented through the use of prospective payment schedules based on diagnosis-related groups (DRGs; see Chapter 2).

Peer Review Organizations

Peer Review Organizations (PROs) are a mechanism established by Medicare and Medicaid, two federal health care programs, for evaluating health care services. The programs currently require that each hospital contract with a Utilization and Quality Control Peer Review Organization, commonly called "PROs." Each organization must include a substantial number of physicians and is required to set standards and review care. Groups of physicians organize and apply to be designated a PRO. The Department of Health and Human Services designates these PROs through the awarding of contracts by geographic area. **Preadmission** or **preprocedure reviews** are done to determine whether patients scheduled for admission truly require the performance of a procedure or hospitalization. This is done for such things as elective surgeries. As a result of this type of review, many more surgeries are performed as day surgeries, rather than being done with overnight hospital stays, and diagnostic procedures are performed on an outpatient basis. Preadmission reviews are not required for urgent or emergency conditions. Many health insurance companies are now establishing similar evaluation programs.

Concurrent review is done while patients are hospitalized. Individual patient records are reviewed to determine whether the patient continues to meet the criteria for a hospital stay. A concurrent review is always done when the length of the patient's hospitalization exceeds the standard for that DRG. Careful documentation of the patient's condition is important to demonstrate that continued hospitalization is necessary. Physicians are notified when patients no longer meet these criteria. Concurrent review has resulted in shorter hospital stays because of pressure for earlier discharge.

Retrospective reviews are done after patients are discharged. In retrospective reviews, data about groups as well as individual patients are considered. Appropriateness of treatment plans, infection and mortality rates, and patient outcomes are all considered. Retrospective reviews are used as a basis for suggesting continuing education needs for health care workers. They have also been used to make policy decisions. For example, the Department of Health and Human Services has designated heart transplant centers on the basis of data indicating that greater success is achieved in centers with a larger number of patients and thus more experience with the procedure.

Although the major focus of PROs is evaluation of medical care, many nurses are employed by these organizations to review records against the criteria established by physicians and to carry out the activities of the organizations.

Quality Assurance Programs

Quality assurance programs establish mechanisms for continuous monitoring and evaluation of all aspects of care provided within hospitals. These programs are required for accreditation by the Joint Commission for the Accreditation of Healthcare Organizations (1990). Expert nurses serve on committees to develop the standards that will be used for evaluating nursing services. Once the standards are developed, many individuals may participate in the evaluation process. If records are to be reviewed, medical record employees may carry out the review and summarize the data for consideration by the nursing department. When direct observations or interviews are used to collect data, registered nurses carry out the review. Individual nurses may be asked to participate in reviews, either on their own units or on other units in the facility (Fig. 12-2).

The purpose of these evaluative activities is to identify both areas of excellence and areas where growth or change is needed. Once the information is available, decisions are made as to what the data mean; then action is taken. Commendations for excellent work may be made. Plans may be made for special education events to update the nursing staff when needed. Policies and procedures may be altered.

Quality Management

Quality management (sometimes referred to as **total quality management [TQM]** or **continuous quality improvement [CQI]**) has been introduced to many businesses in the 1990s. The focus of **total quality management** is a "0 defect" program (or product) and continuous improvement. In health care that means not only using evaluative processes to identify problem areas and make needed changes in those areas, but also to identify ways to further improve care, to respond to trends in care that would benefit consumers, and to establish mechanisms to optimize patient and family satisfaction. Some proponents of quality management stress that it must become an overall way of thinking and acting, not simply a set of policies and procedures.

Personal Evaluation for Professional Growth

As a student, you are entering a profession in which self-evaluation will always be essential. Just as you evaluate the nursing process and participate in the overall evaluation of nursing services, you must be committed to self-evaluation.

Students are usually given criteria for their performance. Although an instructor will provide feedback, no instructor will observe everything you do. Therefore, you are in the best position to determine your own progress in relationship to the criteria. If you establish the practice of self-evaluation while you are a student, it will be much easier for you as you progress in your career.

When you are evaluating yourself, consider all the different aspects of functioning. Look at your use of the nursing process, your communication skills, how you work with others, and your technical proficiency. As you identify areas for improvement, set up a plan to seek experiences that will assist your growth. Do give yourself credit for what you do well also because evaluation should not only focus on problems, but should be a source of personal satisfaction regarding your achievements.

CONFIDENTIAL

SWEDISH HOSPITAL MEDICAL CENTER

QUALITY ASSURANCE PHYSICIAN REVIEW

1. Is the documentation in the record clinically pertinent for the following items, specifically:

   a) Does the H&P contain the detail of information appropriate to the reason for admission? YES ☒ NO ☐

   b) Do the Progress Notes give a pertinent report of the patient's course? YES ☒ NO ☐

   c) Are the results of the diagnostic tests documented? YES ☒ NO ☐

   d) Is the therapy rendered documented? YES ☒ NO ☐

   e) Does the chart substantiate the Principal Diagnosis? YES ☒ NO ☐

   f) Is there an adequate Discharge Summary, including condition of patient at discharge? YES ☒ NO ☐

   Comments: ____________________

2. Comments regarding the case: ____________________
   Referred for appropriate P.T. post discharge.

3. To whom should this occurrence be attributed? ____________________

4. SEVERITY:
   0 - No Disability ☐
   1 - Minor Temporary ☐
   2 - Minor Permanent ☐
   3 - Major Temporary ☒
   4 - Major Permanent ☐
   5 - Potential Major or Major Continuing ☐
   6 - Death ☐

5. STANDARD OF CARE: Met ☒ Questioned ☐ Not Met ☐

6. Should this case be referred to the Departmental Q.A. Committee for discussion?
   YES ☐ NO ☒ Other referrals: ____________________

7. Should this case be referred to the Utilization Review Committee?
   YES ☐ NO ☒ Please comment: ____________________

8. Physician Reviewer Initials: JEP Date: 4/24/94

MR-7 rev. 2/89 FC/SHMC SN-6136

CONFIDENTIAL

Figure 12-2. Quality assurance tool.

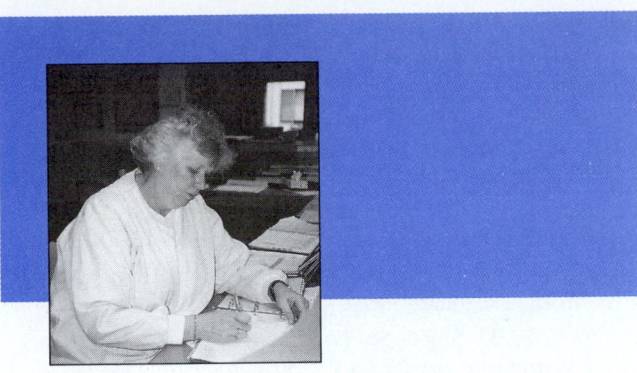

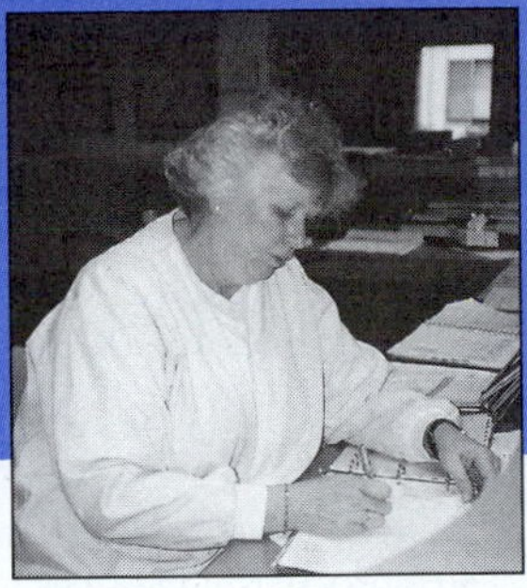

Key Points

- Evaluation is a process of examining and judging something for worth and effectiveness. In nursing, the two major purposes of evaluation are to determine whether desired outcomes have been met and to determine the effectiveness of the entire nursing process.
- Nurses are responsible and accountable for evaluation. When evaluating, the nurse compares the actual outcomes with the desired outcomes as originally stated. Evaluation serves as a basis for revising the nursing care plan. Patients should also be asked to evaluate for themselves their progress toward the desired outcomes.
- At the time of discharge, all nursing diagnoses are reviewed and plans are made for continuing care for problems not yet resolved. All evaluation in regard to desired outcomes is documented on the patient's record.
- The ANA *Standards of Clinical Nursing Practice* address all parts of the nursing process. Specific criteria are listed for evaluating each segment.
- Throughout the entire health care system, peer review organizations are entrusted with the responsibility of evaluating medical care. Nurses evaluate nursing care through quality assurance programs developed within the facility. The purposes of evaluation within the health care system are to recognize excellence, to identify areas needing growth, and to address areas of concern.
- Personal evaluation is also a part of nursing practice. Nursing students are expected to evaluate themselves in relation to criteria set by instructors as well as in relation to criteria they set for themselves. Self-evaluation begins as a student but continues as a career-long responsibility.

Study Questions

1. What are two major purposes of evaluation?
2. What are the criteria for evaluation within the nursing process?
3. What is meant by "determining degree of progress toward a goal"?
4. What is a peer review organization?
5. What is a quality assurance program?
6. How might you use the nursing process in self-evaluation?

Critical Thinking Activities

1. Choose one nursing diagnosis in the Self-care Deficit group. Write desired outcomes that would be appropriate if your patient were each of the following:
   a. An 88-year-old woman who has had a major stroke and is unconscious.
   b. A 50-year-old man who has fractured his femur and is on bed rest, with traction that cannot be removed attached to his leg.
   c. A 3-year-old child who has severe pneumonia.
2. In a group, compare outcomes written by different students. Identify which were the correct components of your outcomes and which areas need improvement.
3. In a small group, discuss the various values that might be present and should be considered when in determining desired outcomes for a person who is terminally ill.
4. In the facility where you are a student, check to see whether a quality assurance program is being conducted. If so, examine the forms being used and answer the following questions:
   a. Is a prospective, concurrent, or retrospective review being conducted?
   b. Is audit of records or direct observation being used as the method for data collection?
   c. Who is expected to do the data collection?
   d. What will be done with the results?
5. Write out personal desired outcomes for yourself in regard to using the nursing process. Arrange a conference to discuss these with your instructor. Save them and review them at the end of the term.

References and Readings

American Nurses Association. *Standards of Clinical Nursing Practice.* Kansas City, Mo.: ANA, 1991.

"ANA Board Acts to Assure Competence of Nurses." *American Nurse* 18, 2 (February 1986): 7.

Curtis, B. J., and Simpson, L. J. "Auditing: A Method for Evaluating Quality of Care." *Journal of Nursing Administration* 15, 10 (October 1985): 14–21.

Ferrell, M. J. "The Relationship of Continuing Education to Self-Reported Changes in Behavior." *Journal of Continuing Education* 19, 1 (January-February 1988): 21–24.

Joint Commission on the Accreditation of Healthcare Organizations. *Accreditation Manual for Hospitals.* Chicago: JCAHO, 1990.

Lang, N. M., and Marek, K. D. "The Classification of Patient Outcomes." *Journal of Professional Nursing* 6, 3 (1990): 158–163.

McLean, P. H. "Professional Growth: Get Ready for Your Next Evaluation." *Nursing '86* 16, 9 (September 1986): 97–98.

Oleske, D. M. "Development and Evaluation of a System for Monitoring the Quality of Oncology Nursing Care in the Home Setting." *Cancer Nursing* 10, 4 (August 1987): 190–198.

Osinski, E. "Developing Patient Outcomes as a Quality Measure of Nursing Care." *Nursing Management* 18, 10 (October 1987): 28–29.

Pasquarello, M. A. "Measuring the Impact of an Acute Stroke Program on Patient Outcomes." *Journal of Neuroscience Nursing* 22, (1990): 76–82.

Pastorino, C. A. "Using Standards of Care in the Practice Setting." *Orthopedic Nursing* 6, 2 (March-April 1987): 23–26.

Royle, J., Montemuro, M., and Roberts, L. "Capitalizing on Staff Enthusiasm to Improve Nursing Process." *Dimensions in Health Services* 63, 4 (May 1986): 16, 18, 20.

Scher, B. B. "Are Checklists Replacing Good Care?" *Nursing '88* 18, 1 (January 1988): 47.

Solomon, S. B. "Sights Set on Quality Care for the Elderly." *Nursing and Health Care* 7, 5 (May 1986): 244–245.

Styles, M. "Together We Can Negotiate Progress, Improve Care." *American Nurse* 18, 7 (July-August 1986): 4, 18.

Communication

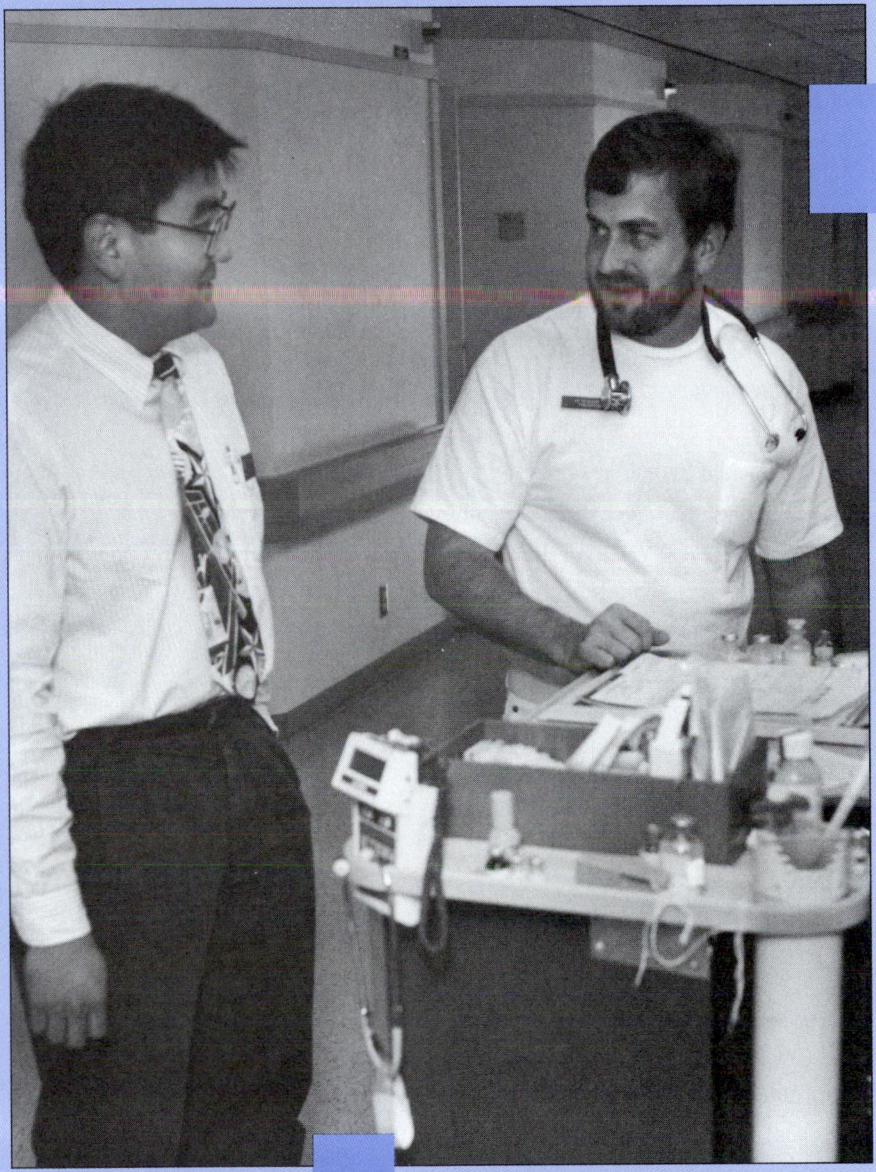

IV

Basic Communication Skills

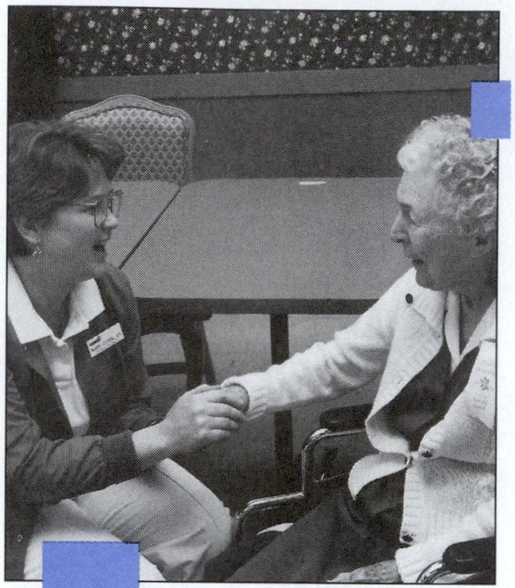

13

Objectives

After completing this chapter, you should be able to:

1. Discuss the role of communication in nursing.
2. Identify the three variables in an interaction.
3. Explain the three phases of an interaction.
4. Discuss a variety of methods of communicating messages.
5. Outline the characteristics of attentive listening.
6. Explain the techniques of verbal communication.
7. Define and describe assertion, submission, and aggression.
8. Discuss a variety of ways in which humor can be appropriately used in nursing.
9. Outline interviewing techniques.
10. List the categories of facilitating responses.
11. List the categories of blocking responses.
12. Discuss how communication relates to the nursing process.

Study Terms

aggression
assertion
attentive listening
belittling
blocking responses
clichés
communication
empathy
exploratory responses
facilitating responses
false reassurance
focusing
general leads
gunnysacking
interaction
interview
leave-taking
nondirective comments
nonverbal communication
opposing responses
pacing
perception
probing
pseudoprofessional comments
reflecting
restating
reviewing
seeking clarification
stereotyped comments
submission
sympathy
therapeutic interaction
trust
validation
voice tone

Ellis, Nowlis: Nursing: A Human Needs Approach, 5th ed. © 1994 J.B. Lippincott Company

Outline

To communicate is, according to the dictionary, "to make known" and "to be connected." This is precisely what **communication** is all about: making oneself and one's ideas, thoughts, and feelings known to another individual and finding out that person's thoughts, ideas, and feelings. Effective communication requires both interest and skill. The skill can be learned; the interest must come from within you.

Many factors affect communication. An individual's cultural background influences the choice of topics communicated, the gestures used, and the entire approach to communicating with others. In Chapter 33 we will explore some of these factors more fully. Developmental level also influences communication. Children use different language and speak at a different level of abstraction from adults. People's beliefs about what should be said and to whom also differ with age level. Chapters 17–20 discuss developmental differences in greater depth.

Communication is critical to every phase of the nursing process. Assessment requires effective communication to gather accurate and comprehensive information about a patient. Planning involves communicating with other members of the health care team and with the patient and family. Explaining your actions to the patient is an ongoing component of direct care. Communication may also be necessary to teach self-care skills or to help the patient cope with emotional problems accompanying illness. Finally, evaluating the effectiveness of nursing care involves communicating with all those who provide care as well as with the patient.

Thus, communication has many different purposes for the nurse. The effectiveness of any given communication is enhanced by the use of skills and techniques appropriate to its purpose. Some skills are valuable in all situations; a few are valuable in one setting or for one purpose but not others. This chapter examines how communication skills and techniques can be incorporated into your nursing care.

The Nature of an Interaction

Interaction is communication between two individuals. The word describes both a particular episode of communication, such as a conversation, and an ongoing relationship. A single interaction may be seen as having three variables: the sender, the message, and the receiver (Fig. 13-1).

Variables in an Interaction

The *sender* is the person trying to communicate. Many factors about the sender affect the interaction. When you are the sender, your skill will facilitate the interaction. When someone else is the sender, your awareness of that person's degree of verbal skill will help you to bridge difficulties in communication.

The *message* is what is being communicated by the interaction. The message may or may not be clear in the mind of the sender. If you are the sender, you should clearly define your message for yourself to communicate it effectively. If the other person is the sender, your awareness that the message may be unclear should prompt you to focus all your attention on understanding it. Sometimes a message is mixed, which means that conflicting ideas or feelings are being communicated simultaneously. When a message is mixed, it may be impossible to make sound decisions without more information.

The *receiver* is the person trying to understand the message. The receiver's skill also contributes to the effectiveness of the interaction. The receiver must listen. Although this sounds simple, it may not be. It is easy for

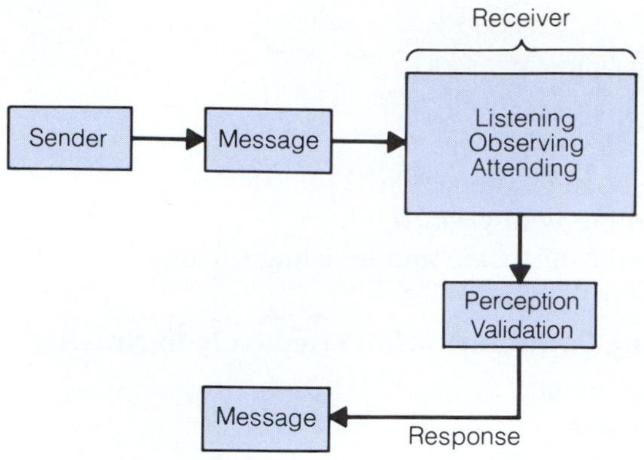

Figure 13-1. The interaction.

the receiver to think about what to say next, rather than listening to the sender. The receiver must also observe; the message is conveyed not only in words but also in the behavior of the sender. The third component of skillful receiving is attending, that is, thinking about the words heard and the behavior observed. To understand the message fully, you need to attend closely to the interaction.

Perception is understanding of and insight into the message on the part of the receiver. Accurate perception of the message is the desired result of the interaction. In addition to the message itself, perception is influenced by the receiver's prior experience, relationship with the sender, and feelings about the interaction. When trust exists between sender and receiver and when previous efforts of communication have been successful, perception is enhanced.

Validation is the process of verifying your understanding of the message communicated by another person. Validation may be accomplished by telling the sender what you understand of the message and asking whether that is correct. You may validate your perception by asking a specific question or by restating what you understood. Until you have validated your understanding of a message, do not assume that you understand it correctly.

Validation may be necessary in the case of factual messages. If a nurse asks you to "take that in to the patient," you should not proceed until you are sure the "that" the nurse is referring to is the same thing you mean by "that." You might validate by asking "You mean, take this breakfast tray?"

Validation is even more important in understanding messages regarding feelings. The words and gestures used to convey feelings are open to different interpretations. When a patient says, "I'm feeling so nervous," don't assume that the patient means the same thing by nervous that you do. The facilitating responses discussed later in the chapter can be used to validate your understanding of a patient's feelings.

Having perceived and validated the message, the receiver becomes a sender and responds to the communication. The interaction is not complete until the receiver responds. The roles of sender and receiver alternate within a single conversation.

Phases of an Interaction

A long-term interaction is not a static phenomenon but a changing, growing process occurring between two people. Experts in the field of communication have subdivided interactions into three phases: the introductory phase, the working phase, and the termination phase (Table 13-1). The length of each phase depends on the interaction and its purpose.

The Introductory Phase

The *introductory phase* of an interaction establishes the relationship between the participants. It may involve the exchange of factual information about both people and the purpose of the interaction. During this phase, the participants determine what the nature of their relationship will be and develop mutual trust. Until trust is well established, only superficial and factual communication can occur. Although the relationship is established during the introductory phase, this relationship will continue to grow and change throughout the lifetime of the interaction. For example, as a student, you introduce yourself to the patient, explain your role in care, and begin your assessment. During this time the patient will be responding, and both of you will be making judgments regarding your expectations of the relationship that will follow.

The Working Phase

The *working phase* of the interaction is the period during which its purposes are accomplished. This phase varies in length depending on those purposes, which might include teaching, therapy, or coordination of care. During the working phase you will continue to interact to accomplish the purposes of care. You may be gathering additional information, teaching about health care, or trying to alleviate the patient's anxiety or distress.

The Termination Phase

The *termination phase* is the end of the interaction. Ideally, the patient knows the purpose of the interaction

Table 13–1. The Phases of an Interaction

Phase	Purpose
1. Introductory	Establishing the relationship
2. Working	Pursuing the relationship's goals
3. Termination	Ending the relationship

and its expected goal and time frame and thus is prepared for termination from the beginning. However, if the relationship is a meaningful one, even an expected and prepared for termination can be difficult. If it is not adequately prepared for, termination can be detrimental to the vulnerable patient or family. It is helpful to review the interaction's purpose and expected end throughout its duration, especially if it lasts a long time. The actual termination should be a summation: the purpose of the interaction is reviewed, and the work, accomplishments, and conclusions summarized. **Leave-taking** is formal recognition that the interaction or relationship is at an end. A short-term interaction may end with a brief farewell and acknowledgment that the interaction is over. If the relationship has been prolonged, bringing it to a smooth conclusion may require several sessions. At the end of your time working with the patient, you will explain that you are leaving, indicate whether or not you will be returning the next day, and perhaps summarize what was accomplished during the period of care.

Methods of Communicating Messages

Meaning is conveyed in a variety of ways, both *verbal* (using words) and *nonverbal* (using gestures and facial expressions). Understanding how these two aspects of communication can be varied to clarify the transmission of an intended message will help you to be a more effective nurse.

Conveying Attitudes

Your underlying *attitude* will usually be communicated to the other person regardless of the techniques you use. Therefore, you might first spend some time considering attitudes that will tend to facilitate the development of a positive relationship. Some individuals lack skill in verbal communication techniques, but nevertheless communicate effectively because of the strongly positive and supportive attitudes they convey.

Honesty and Genuineness

Honesty and genuineness are so closely allied that they are often considered to be the same trait. Honesty is basic truthfulness in your dealings with others. You must first be honest with yourself regarding your own opinions, viewpoints, and values. Failure to be truthful will quickly destroy a trust relationship. If you cannot provide certain information when asked, be direct: state that you are not at liberty to give out the information. Although the person who asked may be angry that the information is being withheld, trust will remain.

Being sincere or genuine is being truly yourself at all times. Although we have many roles in many different situations, we can still be the same basic person in all of those roles. People are reluctant to trust an individual who seems to be a different person in different situations. If you are usually quiet and reserved, not sharing easily, it is inappropriate for you to try to put on a facade of exuberance. You will be uncomfortable, and those around you will perceive that this behavior is not genuine. Genuineness does not mean that you cannot learn new behaviors to function more effectively, but only that you must adapt new behaviors so that you are comfortable with them and so that they genuinely reflect your feelings.

Caring and Concern

Although much has been written in recent years about nursing as an academic field, the underlying purpose of nursing is still the well-being of others—patients or clients and their families. If you do not really care whether they achieve resolution of their health problems and gain the ability to function in more independent and effective ways, you will not be an effective nurse. Patients are not machines to be manipulated, but living, breathing, feeling people. The caring of nursing is based in knowledge and involves both action and simply "being with" another person. Caring is communicated by your interest in their concerns, the tone of voice you use, and many nonverbal behaviors.

Empathy is a part of caring. **Empathy** is sharing the feelings of another, as opposed to **sympathy**, which is feeling sorry for that person. True empathy can come only from similar personal experiences. Therefore, be careful not to claim understanding of another's feelings or situation unless you have experienced something similar. One major strength of the many community self-help groups is that they bring together people who have had similar experiences and can truly empathize with one another (Fig. 13-2). An example is the Compassionate Friends, a group for parents who have had a child die. Although you might be concerned, unless you have lost a child, you cannot really empathize with a parent's feelings as a person in the group can. You can have limited empathy if you have children and can relate the parent's emotions to the strong feelings you currently have toward your children, or if you have experienced the death of someone close to you. When expressing empathy, be sure to acknowledge the limits of your experience.

Feelings of concern and empathy can be draining. They demand a great deal of your energy and strength. Thus, you need to look for ways to renew and restore yourself, either through the support of other care providers or in your private life. Do not ignore your own needs; failure to attend to your own needs can lead to exhaustion and the inability to function.

In some situations you will find it essential to dis-

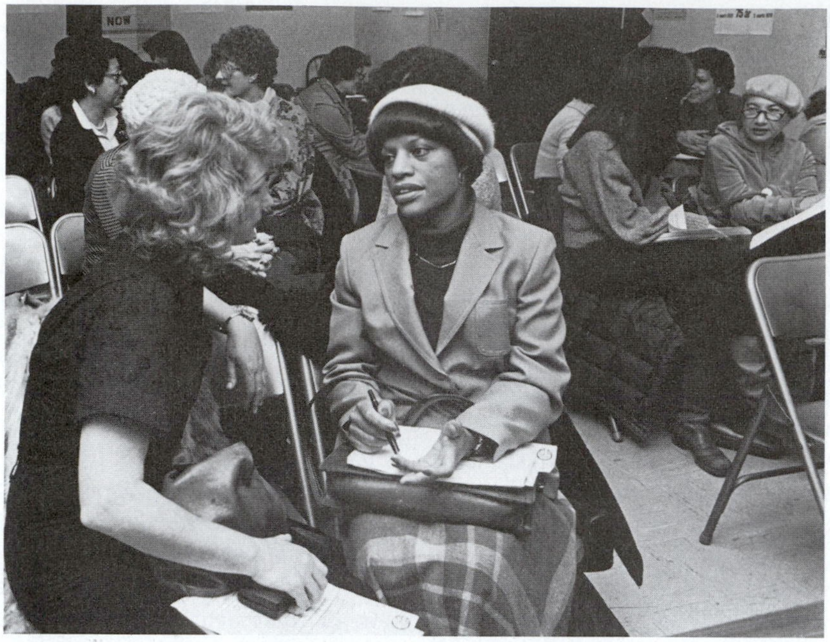

Figure 13-2. Community self-help groups bring together people who have had similar experiences and can empathize with one another's feelings.

tance yourself from patients for your own protection. You, too, are finite, with limits to your strength and resources. Adequate support for an individual with multiple problems may need to come from a variety of people for the care providers not to be overwhelmed with the responsibility. Do not view your need for *distance* as a failure, but strive to recognize it as a realistic response to your own human limitations.

Establishing Trust

Trust is confidence in a person's integrity and ability. Establishing trust between yourself and the patient is essential to effective communication. Throughout this text we will comment on the role of trust and its importance. Trust does not occur automatically but results from the overall pattern of the nurse's behavior in relationship to the patient/client.

You establish trust by being *genuine.* Focusing on the other person promotes trust, as does willingness to treat the other person's concerns as foremost. In nursing, a key to establishing trust is meeting the other person's immediate perceived needs before pursuing your own agenda.

The maintenance of appropriate confidentiality is also critical to trust. If you will be sharing information you acquire from the interaction with others on the health care team, you must make your intention clear at the outset so that the patient does not feel confidentiality was betrayed. Remember that information is only shared for purposes of care or for purposes of education. In the latter instance, the patient's identity is protected.

Truthfulness. *Telling the truth* to the patient is one part of establishing trust. When you are not truthful or are evasive with a patient, you undermine trust not only for yourself but also for the whole health care team. When the patient requests information you are not free to share (*eg,* the medical diagnosis is shared with the patient by the physician who makes that diagnosis), you can be honest and state that the information is not yours to give out and should be sought from the appropriate person. This relieves you of being untruthful or evasive and maintains your trust relationship with the patient.

Sometimes nurses are afraid to be truthful for fear of causing anxiety or distress to the patient. In actuality, anxiety over the unknown or the imagined is often much more distressing than the actual facts would be. In addition, a loss of trust in those on whom one is dependent can produce great anxiety. In health care a decision may be made not to inform a patient about a diagnosis or treatment because it is believed that telling the patient will cause more distress than withholding the information. This type of decision carries potential harm for both the patient and the caregiver. Sissela Bok, an ethicist, has written an excellent treatise on lying (Bok, 1978), in which she writes of lying to the sick and dying. She concludes that trust "requires a stringent adherence to honesty in all but a few carefully delineated cases" and that these exceptional cases should be considered individually. An example might be when a client is suicidal, and caregivers feel that information would increase the chance of suicide. Reasons must be set forth, the alternatives debated, and someone close to the client included in all decision-making.

Following through. Trust is also established by *following through on commitments* made to the client. For example, when you say you will return in 15 minutes, you should be able to be relied on to do that. When you promise to get the patient fresh water, you must do so. These small things build a confidence that you can be relied on for the larger tasks. If you are consistently reliable, then when some inadvertent problem makes it impossible for you to fulfill a particular commitment, the patient will be more able to understand and accept the unusual situation. If, however, you are frequently unreliable, the patient will never develop feelings of trust toward you.

Competence. Competence in carrying out care makes the patient/client more confident in you and enhances trust. Time spent in practice laboratories and preparation before doing procedures will help you to be more self-assured and competent. This competence will, in turn, help you to establish trust with a client.

Listening Attentively

Listening includes not only hearing what someone says, but also understanding the message and remembering it. Listening carefully is as much a skill as speaking correctly. **Attentive listening** is an approach to listening in which the other person becomes the center of your attention. Attentive listening conveys to the other person that what is being said is important and that he or she is significant as a person. You can learn to listen attentively and to increase both what you understand and what you remember of the message the person is trying to convey.

Some of the skills you will need to be a good listener have to do with your nonverbal actions; others have to do with the attitudes you convey.

Barriers to Effective Listening

First, let us consider some of the common barriers to effective listening. One is not valuing what the other person has to say. If you do not value the other person's viewpoint, you will not listen effectively. Another is being distracted by a person's appearance. When a person is attractive, most people are attentive. When a person is unattractive, people tend to be less attentive. Clients are often not at their best, and thus those around them may tend to discount what they have to say.

Another problem involves listening for facts alone. Facts are important, but feelings, values, and opinions are also significant communications. If you prematurely form an opinion about what the person is feeling or thinking, you may fail to accurately receive communication that conveys a different message.

Setting the Stage for Listening

Following the behaviors given below will help you to be a more effective listener (Display 13-1).

Focus on understanding what the other person is saying, not on what your reply will be. You really cannot think of two things simultaneously, and if you are thinking about your reply, you will not pick up all the cues the other person is giving you.

Display 13–1
Attentive Listening Guidelines

Focus on understanding the other person.
Maintain eye contact.
Place yourself at the same level as the other person.
Sit, if at all possible.
Allow the other person enough time to speak.
Respond frequently with general leads.
Respond frequently with nonverbal behaviors such as nods.

Maintain eye contact while the person is talking if at all possible. Looking around, doing other tasks, or shifting your position frequently will give the impression that you are not listening.

Place yourself at the same level as the other person if at all possible. If you look down on the other person, you give the impression of being superior. This will inhibit another person's communication (Fig. 13-3).

Sit down for the conversation, if possible. If you are standing during the conversation, the patient may think you are ready to leave momentarily and may not begin discussing anything that will take more than a few minutes to say.

Allow the person time to speak. Considerable patience may be required, because many individuals in health care facilities are hampered by their illness in their ability to communicate. When a person pauses to find the right word or just to catch a breath, do not take that as a cue to begin speaking. Calmly wait, allowing time for thought, and do not begin speaking yourself

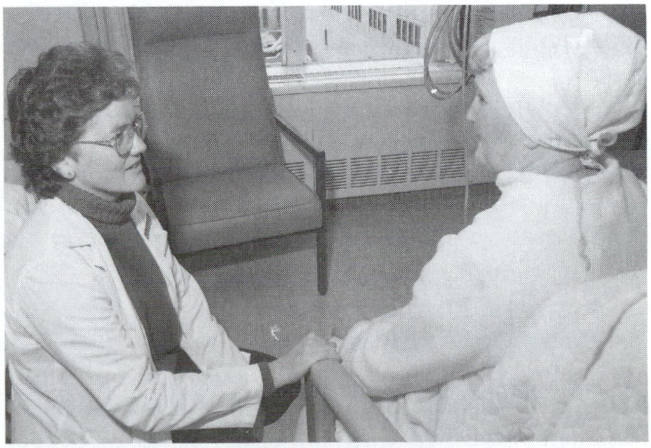

Figure 13-3. Talking at eye level conveys a message of personal interest and equality of relationship.

until you clearly perceive that the other person is finished.

Respond frequently with general leads to communicate that you are being attentive and that you wish the conversation to continue. Responding with such nonverbal cues as nods also indicates your attention and interest.

Increasing Your Understanding

In addition to listening you will need to *understand* what the person is saying. Understanding means that you have processed the information and have accurately identified the message the person is trying to convey. The following are guidelines to help you increase your understanding.

Listen with empathy. Empathy reflects an understanding of the position of the client and an attempt to see things from that point of view.

Leave your own emotions and feelings behind as much as you can. Try to put your own concerns, fears, and problems aside so they do not prevent you from listening.

Listen for what is NOT said. What the person leaves out or avoids may convey important information. When a person avoids a topic or does not respond to questions, it may indicate that the topic is difficult or painful.

Listen to the way things are said as well as what is said. Attitudes and emotional reactions may be the most important content.

Control your own reactions to emotion-laden words that might tend to distract you. If you become upset or distressed over the words, you will be less effective in understanding the person's message.

Understanding Nonverbal Communication

Nonverbal communication reveals feelings and attitudes without using words, often more effectively than words do. Nonverbal behavior can convey meaning independently, or it may enhance or contradict verbal communication. Touch, tone of voice, and facial expressions communicate feelings to an infant before that infant is able to understand the meaning of any spoken word. At the other end of life, a warm touch communicates caring to a person so near death that words are no longer meaningful.

Types of Nonverbal Behavior That Communicate

Almost any type of human behavior can communicate a message. The first step in understanding nonverbal communication is to learn to identify significant behavior (Display 13-2). You will need to practice looking for such behavior in yourself as well as in others. It is as important to be aware of the messages you are sending nonverbally as it is to understand those you receive from others.

Display 13–2
Types of Nonverbal Communication

Position	Eye contact
Gestures	Touch
Distance	Silence
Facial expressions	

Position. The position of your body in relation to that of the patient expresses relative attentiveness and relative power. Directly facing a person usually indicates interest and attention. When the two people's faces are at the same level, communication is encouraged because they tend to feel equally important. If two people are at unequal heights, the lower person usually perceives the higher person as authoritarian.

Gestures. Gestures are expressive movements of the hands and head. Common gestures include pointing and using the hands for emphasis, as well as nodding and shaking the head. Nodding is usually taken as indicating attention, agreement, or approval. Gestures can also spontaneously express such feelings as agitation, elation, despair, worry, and relief.

Physical distance. The physical distance between people communicates the degree of emotional intimacy existing or desired. Many studies have found the message communicated by distance to be related to people's perceptions of the space around their bodies, often termed "territory" or "personal space." The area within which normal body odors can be detected, approximately 12 to 18 inches, is perceived as one's *intimate space.* People often feel invaded and threatened when another person moves abruptly into their intimate space. Because nurses must often do so in the course of caring for patients, it is important to proceed slowly at first, explaining what you plan to do, and asking permission.

Personal distance, between approximately 18 inches and 4 feet, is close enough to permit people to speak quietly and personally, but allows for more independence and seems less threatening than intimate distance. It is a comfortable distance for most people. *Social distance,* from 4 to 12 feet, is more formal. Conversations conducted at this distance can be heard by casual passersby, and people usually choose their words with this in mind. Most people are reluctant to talk about personal matters at this distance.

Public distance, over 12 feet, is appropriate for

speaking to groups rather than individuals. Communication at this distance is often formal, preplanned, and focused on ideas rather than feelings.

Culture deeply affects people's perceptions of appropriate physical distances. People of Central and South American, Southern European, and Middle Eastern background tend to be more comfortable at closer distances than people of Asian, Native American, and Northern European backgrounds.

Facial expressions. Facial expressions are the most accessible aspect of nonverbal communication (Fig. 13-4). The position of the mouth, eyebrows, and eyes expresses feelings overtly. However, it is easy to misinterpret familiar facial expressions. Although smiling usually indicates pleasure and frowning usually expresses displeasure or unhappiness, some people habitually smile when they are nervous or anxious, and others frown when they are concentrating or lost in thought. Assumptions about the patient's mood on the basis of facial expressions are thus risky; always validate your perception.

Eye contact. Eye contact is also subject to different interpretations. In most Western cultures, eye contact is perceived as expressing honesty, straightforwardness, and attentiveness. In some Native American and Asian cultures, however, looking straight into the eyes of a person you do not know well may be considered rude. In situations that require you to wear a mask, such as isolation, eye contact can have a reassuring effect on the patient. If you watch closely you will see that an individual's pupils tend to dilate when the person is interested and alert. Changes in pupil dilation are signals of changes in emotional response and communication.

Touch. Most people associate touch with mothering, comfort, and caring. In fact, touch can express caring when no other mode of communication can bridge a barrier between two people (Fig. 13-5). Touch may be a way of expressing feeling, releasing tension, or simply making contact with another human being. Thus, the nurse may touch the dying patient to express grief; the patient may grasp the nurse's hand for reassurance. People's perceptions of touch depend on past experience, assumptions, and the nature of the situation. Some people associate touch with discipline, rejection, or pain. Mentally disturbed individuals may perceive touch as threatening. It is important to be alert to the meaning and value of touch for both the patient and yourself.

When using touch with patients, do so based on its value and meaning to the patient rather than to you. It may sometimes help to state what you are trying to convey with touch: "It's hard to be alone at a time like this. I'll stay with you during the test." Touch may be inappropriate for mentally ill or agitated people because they are not able to interpret it accurately and may perceive it as threatening. It is also inappropriate if the patient misinterprets it as a sexual gesture.

Silence. Silence also conveys meaning and can enhance communication. Silence at an appropriate moment in a conversation may communicate your willingness to let the other person think about a reply. Silence on the part of a patient may indicate that he or she is digesting information or marshaling personal resources. Sometimes sitting quietly with a patient communicates unconditional acceptance. However, silence makes many people anxious; such anxiety, conveyed by other nonverbal behavior, defeats the purpose of silence. You may be able to overcome anxiety by initially limiting silences to a few minutes and gradually increasing their duration as you become more comfortable. If 5 minutes is the most you can handle without becoming anxious, you might articulate this limit in advance by saying, "I'll stay another 5 minutes with you, and then I'll leave."

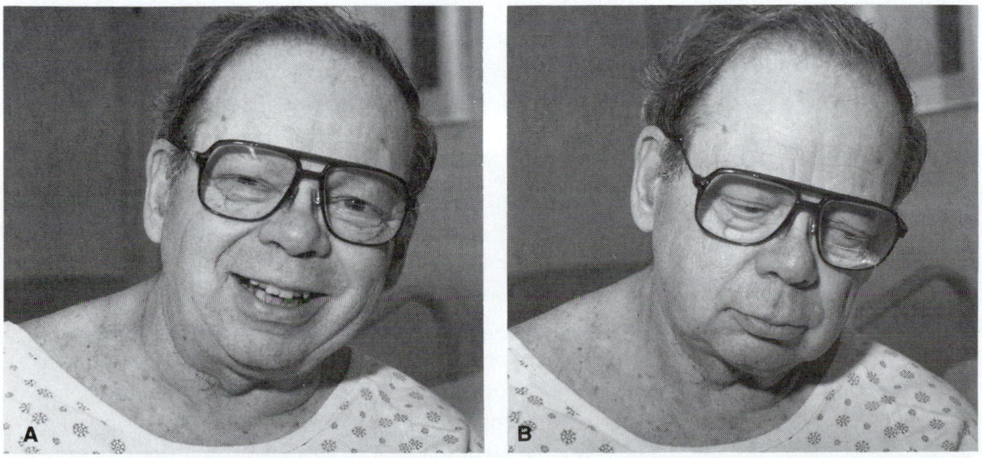

Figure 13-4. Nonverbal communication and the patient: What message is the patient communicating in each photograph?

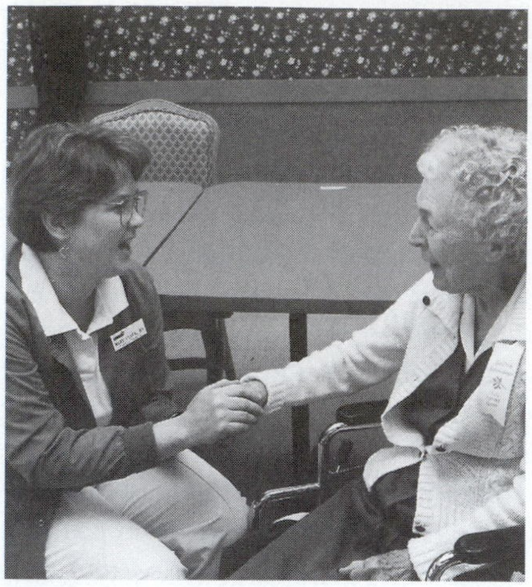

Figure 13-5. Touch is a nonverbal expression of caring.

Interpretation of Nonverbal Behavior

Interpretation of nonverbal behavior ought to be approached systematically. You might begin by consciously noting the usual meanings of common types of nonverbal behavior.

The second step is to broaden your understanding and sharpen your ability to interpret nonverbal behavior by familiarizing yourself with typical nonverbal styles of different cultures. Many (though not all) Southern European, Middle Eastern, Hispanic, and African American people tend to use more vivid nonverbal language than Northern Europeans and Asians. It is easy to interpret behavior erroneously if you use your own background as a reference point for everyone you meet.

The third step is to read as much as you can about nonverbal cues. Many of the publications listed in the references at the end of this chapter make fascinating reading. You might also discuss them with other nurses to broaden your understanding.

The most definitive step, of course, is to validate your perception of a person's behavior by describing what you observed and asking the person whether you interpreted it correctly.

Intervention Based on Nonverbal Communication

Once you are sure you have interpreted a given behavior correctly, you can plan your nursing intervention. If the patient validates your interpretation, you may proceed accordingly. If the person denies your interpretation, you should first consider the possibility that you might be in error. Interpreting nonverbal behavior is by no means simple, and such errors are common. If further observation and objective data reinforce your interpretation, you might want to seek the opinion of another nurse. Then, if your interpretation is seconded, try responding to the nonverbal message you interpreted. For example, a patient admitted for diagnostic studies is tossing and turning, unable to sleep. Approaching the patient, the nurse says, "I notice you're having difficulty sleeping, and you look tense. Are you worried?" The patient replies, "Oh, I'm OK. I'm sure you have lots to do with so many sick patients." The nurse reconsiders the original observation and decides to respond to the nonverbal behavior rather than the patient's statement. The nurse sits down to talk to the patient and helps relieve the patient's anxiety. The patient finally falls asleep. In many instances, responding to the patient's nonverbal behavior is significantly more helpful than responding to a verbal denial of that behavior's message.

Using Verbal Communication

Verbal communication consists of all the words people exchange. Words can be a source of considerable confusion; you can probably recall becoming involved in an argument only to discover that you and your adversary differed only over the meanings of terms, not basic ideas. In addition to the words themselves, pacing and voice tone significantly affect the receiver's perception of verbal messages. Finally, it is important to choose communication techniques capable of accomplishing the purpose you have in mind.

Language Use

Words have different meanings to different people. Expensive, for example, means something different to a welfare recipient than to a surgeon. Similarly, two people who both answer "fine" when asked how they feel may be in different states of mind and health.

Furthermore, people's vocabularies vary a great deal. Technical words and abbreviations are like a foreign language to many patients. As a nursing student, you undoubtedly know how it feels not to understand all the technical terms being used around you.

It is important to consider the patient's educational level, degree of sophistication, and fluency in English when choosing your words. Because it is crucial to communicate with patients even if they speak little or no English, many facilities have developed resource lists of people on the hospital staff or in the community who are willing to serve as translators. If such a list does not exist in your facility, you might promote the development of one.

The use of volunteer translators can, however, create problems. The translator may not know technical terms in either English or the other language, which can lead to incomplete or inaccurate communication. Thus, health care facilities that treat many patients who speak a particular language often employ a professional translator, who acquires familiarity with the health care setting and with technical terminology. If a translator is not available, or to supplement the translator's role, you may want to seek out a book or pamphlet of translations. These books typically have lists of words and phrases in English with their counterparts in the other language.

In general, clarity, brevity, and simplicity are desirable attributes of language. *Clarity* involves choosing words of clear and unmistakable meaning. *Brevity* means presenting your message briefly and without unnecessary digressions to avoid confusion about what is important and what is less so. *Simplicity* involves choosing simple, commonly used words in preference to technical or rarely used terms.

Pacing

Pacing is the rate at which you speak. It is a common error to forget to pause between statements or questions to allow the receiver time to process the message and formulate a response.

When you are anxious or busy, you tend to speak at a rapid pace. You may fail to allow the other person enough time to think and respond, and you may not be clear yourself. Slowing the pace of an interaction can allow you to think more clearly about what you are saying and to listen more effectively. A slower pace makes what you say easier to understand. With children, elderly persons, those who hear poorly, and those who have received drugs that alter alertness, it is especially prudent to slow your pace to enhance their understanding.

Voice Tone

Voice tone refers to the manner of expression used in speaking, and it can change the meaning of words. Something said in a loud voice can mean something entirely different from the same thing said softly. Voice tone also expresses urgency, impatience, sarcasm, condescension, anger, and many other attitudes and emotions; most people are quick to perceive such feelings, although they may not realize they are doing so.

When speaking to a person with a hearing impairment, it is important to speak not only loudly enough but also slowly and clearly. Avoid mumbling. Using lower tones and speaking more slowly will assist the hearing-impaired person to hear more clearly.

Techniques of Verbal Communication

A large repertoire of communication techniques and skill at using them are extremely valuable in nursing. It is also important to recognize and avoid responses that tend to interfere with communication.

Giving Clear Information

Giving clear information is an important communication skill. When you first meet a patient, you should introduce yourself by name and explain your role. This same approach is important when communicating with hospital staff. When giving information, you will want first to make sure you understand what you want to say and then provide that information in simple, easily understood language. Organize your thoughts into a logical progression that the other person can follow. This will help that person to comprehend your message. The beginning of effective communication is learning to express factual material in a clear and understandable manner. For example, when you are caring for a patient and a physician visits the patient, you will need to present a clear and concise verbal report of the patient's condition. You want your information to be well organized, accurate, and easily understood. You will also use this skill when you give a report to the registered nurse after having completed your care.

Asking Questions

It is appropriate to ask a patient questions only if you need the information to assess the patient's problems and plan nursing care. You have an obligation to let the patient know the purpose of your questions and the uses that will be made of the answers. If you will be sharing the information with others on the health care team, you should tell the patient before you ask any questions. If, for example, you will share the information you acquire from an interview with your instructor, you might say, "My instructor will review my interview with me to help me plan your care." If you are recording the answers to your questions on the nursing record, the fact that you are doing so conveys the message that the information will be shared.

When specific information is needed to plan and provide care, you will need to ask specific questions. Such questions are of two types: open ended and closed. Open-ended questions allow for the other person to respond in detail; an example is "What are your plans for managing your care after discharge?" The newspaper reporter's traditional list—who, what, where, when, and how—may be of value to you in posing open-ended questions (Table 13-2). Questions that can be answered with a brief yes or no are called closed questions; an example is "Will you have help when you go home?" By deciding whether or not you want a detailed answer, you can determine when to use each kind of question. In general, open-ended questions are far more useful. Closed questions are essential when the person is unable to speak but capable of nodding or shaking the head. Such questions need to be planned carefully to gain the necessary information without "putting words in the patient's mouth."

Table 13–2. Asking Questions

Type of Question	Example
Closed	"Do you have pain?" "Do you feel tired?" "Will you have help at home?"
Open-ended	
What	"What do you think caused this episode?" "What is your opinion about the best solution?"
Where	"Where were you when you started getting this feeling?" "Where will you stay after discharge?"
When	"When did you first become concerned about this?" "When did the pain begin?"
How	"How do you remember to take your medications?" "How do you usually discipline Johnny?"

Plan your questions to proceed from the general to the specific. Such a progression will help the patient concentrate and will demonstrate that your questions are purposeful. For example:

NURSE: "What are your plans for care after you're discharged?"

PATIENT: "Well, I'm not sure. Guess I haven't thought much about it."

NURSE: "Your physician said you should limit your activity. What is your understanding of what that means?"

PATIENT: "I believe he said something about not doing any housework or cooking."

NURSE: "How will you arrange for meals?"

Facilitating Responses

If you have no specific questions in mind, but wish instead to explore the patient's feelings, worries, or uncertainties, direct questions may be of less value than **facilitating responses**, which are responses that encourage the other person to communicate with you. Although facilitating responses are occasionally considered therapeutic techniques, we believe that the entire interaction, rather than a particular statement or response, is therapeutic. Facilitating responses are tools whose purpose is to encourage and support the other person in communicating and personal problem-solving. Use of facilitating techniques is based on a belief in the other person's integrity, worth, and ability to solve his or her own problems. Only if you believe in the other person's capabilities will you be able to act as a facilitator instead of trying to be the patient's problem-solver (Table 13-3).

Facilitating responses may be subdivided into three categories: nondirective comments, exploratory responses, and aids to decision-making. Though each has a purpose, nondirective comments are generally the most useful.

Nondirective comments encourage the other person to continue talking in the same vein. Comments such as "yes, go on, mm-hmmm" indicate that you are attending to what is being said and demonstrate willingness to continue listening. Such comments are called **general leads**. Another type of nondirective response is **reflecting**, or simply repeating the patient's exact words in the form of a question. The patient says, for example, "I just can't stand staying in bed any longer!" and the nurse replies, "You can't stand staying in bed any longer?" This response allows the patient to hear what he or she is saying and to think about it. Overuse of this technique can, however, make the patient uncomfortable and self-conscious. A third type of nondirective response is **restating** or repeating the other

Table 13–3. Responses That Facilitate Communication

Response	Example
Nondirective Comments	
General leads	"Yes," "Go on," "Mm-hmmm."
Reflecting	PATIENT: "I'm really scared." NURSE: "You're really scared?"
Restating	PATIENT: "I just can't seem to sit still." NURSE: "You're feeling nervous?"
Exploratory Responses	
Placing events in time sequence	"When did that happen?" "Was this before or after . . . ?"
Encouraging comparisons	"Was this similar to . . . ?" "Are there differences this time?"
Focusing	"You said . . . . Could you explain that more fully?" "This seems to be an important point."
Seeking clarification	"What would you say is the main concern?"
Validating	"What I understand from what you said is . . . . Is that correct?"
Aids to Decision-making	
Serving as a resource	"Children under 14 can visit if special arrangements are made."
Pointing out information	"Have you considered . . . ?"
Reviewing	"Now you said the main concerns are . . . ."
Considering consequences	"If you do . . . , what might happen?"
Encouraging formulation of a plan	"What do you think you might do?"

person's statement in different words. This technique helps the other person recognize the message being received. If, for example, the patient says, "I need a stronger sleeping pill," the nurse may reply, "Your present sleeping pill isn't effective?"

Exploratory responses help encourage the other person to examine a situation more completely. Placing events in *time sequence*, for example, might be promoted by asking, "Was that before or after . . . ?" or "What happened next?" **Focusing** the conversation involves identifying an important statement and pursuing it: "You said your brother is helpful. Could you explain more about that?" *Encouraging comparisons* may help the other person weigh and evaluate the significance of something: "Does this feel like . . . ?" **Seeking clarification** is asking for a clearer explanation of something that has been said: "I don't quite understand what you mean. Could you explain more fully?" *Validating*, which we have already mentioned in another context, involves identifying what you believe the other person is trying to say and asking whether you are correct: "Do you mean . . . ?"

Aids to decision-making are responses that encourage the other person to make informed decisions. One way to do so is by serving as a *resource*, providing information or directing the patient to an appropriate source of information. Information giving is appropriate only when the patient has indicated a need for or interest in such information. If such a need is not apparent to the patient, information giving might be construed as interfering or directive. In such a situation, *pointing out information* that might be of help lets the other person know that certain information is available, but allows the person to decide whether to pursue it. **Reviewing** is helping to summarize what has been said, to consider diverse approaches, and to organize ideas. It is sometimes appropriate to encourage the patient to *consider the consequences* of proposed plans of action. When doing so, let the patient imagine and work out all the possible consequences; this process promotes independence and self-direction. The final step is encouraging *formulation of a plan*. This might involve constructing a time frame: "What do you think you might do first?" "What would come next?" You can encourage the patient to be specific in planning by saying, "Can you give me an example of what you plan to say?" or "Would you explain how you will go about that?" It is important to remember that your role is to encourage the patient to formulate a plan; you must neither formulate a plan for the patient nor encourage the person to adopt your plan.

Blocking Responses

Responses that hinder communication, express lack of interest in what the patient has to say, or undermine the patient's sense of adequacy are called **blocking responses**. A single blocking response will not usually destroy the effectiveness of an interaction, but many blocking responses will tend to make communication shallower, less sharing, and less effective at promoting problem-solving.

Stereotyped comments—overused and automatic phrases—are probably the most common blocking responses. People tend to interpret the use of stereotyped comments as indicating lack of interest, condescension, or evasion. **Clichés** like "Things will be better tomorrow" and "Keep a stiff upper lip" are almost always perceived as unfelt and insincere. **Belittling** is the use of clichés to minimize the seriousness of the patient's problem: "Lots of patients here are much sicker than you are!" **False reassurance** is the use of clichés to insist that all is well: "You'll be back on your feet again in no time!"

Introducing an *unrelated topic* into a conversation effectively communicates that you do not want to talk about the previous topic. For example, the patient brings up worries about discharge from the hospital, and you reply, "Well, that's a long way off. I notice you have several new cards here." Usually the patient recognizes your discomfort and abandons the earlier topic.

The various types of **opposing responses** are readily recognizable as blocking. *Rejecting* the patient's statement, such as by saying, "Don't think about that," indicates that you do not want to listen. *Denying* the truth of the patient's statement—"That's ridiculous!"—effectively discourages further sharing of feelings or ideas, as does *challenging* its validity: "How can you possibly know something like that?" *Defending* other staff members or the institution against the patient's complaints puts you in the position of opposing the patient. Responding defensively tells the patient, "I'm on the other team, not on your side." A more appropriate response takes such complaints seriously without necessarily agreeing with them.

Pseudoprofessional comments—remarks that are phrased in the language of psychology but are not professional in context—are becoming more common as people become more familiar with psychological concepts and terminology (Table 13-4). They can be very detrimental to relationships with patients. **Probing**—asking for personal information unrelated to the patient's health care—is inappropriate if you are merely satisfying curiosity; doing so can undermine the patient's trust. Patients should be free to share only what they decide to share. When such information will be used to plan care, the patient ought to be informed of the purpose of the questions. Probing often grows out of a mistaken belief in the value of extensive information for its own sake, without regard to its usefulness in planning care. *Demanding an explanation* for the patient's expressed feelings or behavior can cause the patient extreme discomfort. Although sometimes in-

Table 13–4. Responses That Block Communication

Response	Example	Response	Example
Stereotyped Comments		Defending	PATIENT: "I'm not sure that doctor knows what he's doing." NURSE: "Now, you have a very good doctor. He certainly wouldn't do anything that wasn't in your best interest."
Clichés	"Chin up." "It's for your own good."	*Pseudoprofessional Comments*	
Belittling	PATIENT: "I don't want to live like this." NURSE: "You'll feel differently in the morning."	Probing	"Now, you must tell me everything about your relationship with your son."
False reassurance	"You'll be just fine!" "Nothing to worry about!"	Demanding explanations	"*Why* do you feel that way?"
Introducing an unrelated topic	PATIENT: "Am I going to get better?" NURSE: "Well, the color of that robe sure makes you look better. Blue really is your color."	Interpreting	"Underneath you really feel anger at . . . ."
Opposing		*Personal Opinions*	
Rejecting	PATIENT: "I feel as if I'm never going to get well." NURSE: "Don't think like that; it's depressing."	Agreeing	"That's right. You do need to look at the bright side."
Denying	PATIENT: "I'm not worth bothering about." NURSE: "Of course you are. That's silly."	Disagreeing	"I don't think you understand." "No, you're wrong about that."
Challenging	PATIENT: "Just touching her hand made me well." NURSE: "It isn't possible for that to happen."	Approving	"I'm glad to see you're cheerful today."
		Disapproving	"Now don't be so glum."

tended to promote self-understanding, such a response rarely has that effect because the meaning is outside the patient's awareness. *Interpreting* the patient's comments can be perceived as demeaning or as an invasion of personal rights. In general, only the person who makes the comment has the right to interpret it.

Offering *personal opinions* is a common blocking response. Whether you are *agreeing, disagreeing, approving*, or *disapproving*, the opinion indicates that you believe one viewpoint to be correct and others incorrect. Such a message can have several undesirable effects. A patient struggling uncertainly to make a personal decision may give up and defer to you. A patient who disagrees with your expressed belief or opinion may be reluctant to say so because "You are the professional." If you agree with or approve of an expressed feeling, the patient may later not share less positive feelings in the belief that they will meet with your disapproval. Feelings should never be labeled correct or incorrect, good, or bad; they simply exist.

It is important here to distinguish health teaching (see Chapter 16) from the less formal situations we have been discussing and to distinguish between feelings and behavior. It is appropriate in health teaching to approve of a given behavior you want to promote because the desirability of that behavior is demonstrable and not merely a matter of opinion.

Assertive Communication

To work well with others, you must learn to express yourself clearly and directly. You must learn the differences among assertion, aggression, and submission, and learn to use assertive techniques. **Assertion** can be defined as "asking for what you want, stating your opinion, expressing your feelings in direct and honest ways that show respect for yourself and the people you are communicating with" (Nicarthy, 1981, p. 2). In contrast, **submission** is "giving in to other people's requests, demands or feelings without regard to what you want or how you feel" (Nicarthy, 1981, p. 2). **Aggression** is "standing up for your rights, but expressing yourself in a way that violates the rights of others or shows them no respect" (Nicarthy, 1981, p. 2).

Assertive techniques are most often needed in work with others on the health care team but may also be needed in work with patients. You may find that a patient would be helped by learning to use these techniques in his or her own life. The best way to learn these techniques is to practice them. You may want to role-play situations with another student to practice assertive techniques. When helping a patient to become assertive, you may want to have the patient practice what he or she will say in the given situation.

General Guidelines for Assertive Behavior

Always try to look the other person directly in the eyes while talking. Eye contact tends to focus a person's attention on what is being said and makes you appear more self-confident. In most of Western society, looking directly into someone's eyes while speaking also gives the impression that what is being said is true.

Speak loudly and clearly enough to be easily heard. If you mumble or speak softly, you often give the impression that what you are saying is not really important. Others may just move the conversation on rather than stop to ask you to repeat what you have just said. If you are having difficulty with making assertive statements, you may have difficulty making your statement more than once. By the second try you may think, "Oh, what's the use?" and give up. Sometimes you may need to raise your voice slightly to gain the attention of others in the group. This does not mean that you interrupt or become strident, but that you make yourself heard.

Whenever possible, begin your statement with the personal pronoun I or my. Doing so identifies the message as conveying your own viewpoint or preference. Personal pronouns direct the other person to look beyond his or her own viewpoint and help you to avoid inappropriate generalization.

Use gestures that are sure and outgoing. Gestures such as leaning forward, moving your hand decisively, holding your head up, and standing straight convey confidence in what you are saying. These gestures encourage others to take your statements seriously.

When you have said what you wanted to, stop talking. If you continue to ramble on, you begin to sound less sure of yourself, and what you have said loses its force. What might have been clear in your initial statement may become less clear as it is surrounded by qualifying statements.

Display 13-3 summarizes the general guidelines for assertive behavior.

Display 13–3
General Guidelines for Assertive Behavior

1. Use eye contact.
2. Speak loudly and clearly.
3. Begin statements with I or my.
4. Use sure and outgoing gestures.
5. Stop talking when you are done.

Common Uses for Assertive Communication

Saying No. To learn to say no effectively, you must first examine your own preferences. Some people have spent so long being submissive that they truly do not know what they prefer. Saying no when you want to say no is an important skill. Those who do not learn to say no often find themselves feeling harried, disorganized, and frustrated because they do not control their own lives.

You might begin by saying no to small requests that are not convenient, and then move into being able to say no in major situations in life. It is not necessary to be rude or abrupt to say no, but it is important to be firm. If those around you are not used to your saying no, they may be persistent until they accept that you do mean what you say. For example, suppose you are working with another nursing student. Both you and the other student are busy with your care. You have determined that you will finish just in time to get to a postclinical conference. The other student asks you to make a bed for her so that she can get to the conference on time. A submissive response would be to say yes, and then to try to get the bed done along with your own work, thereby running the risk of being late for class. An aggressive response would be to become angry at the other student for asking for your help. An assertive response would be to say, "I'm sorry; I barely have time to get my own work done before going to conference, so I can't help you." It is not always necessary to explain your reasoning when making an assertive response, but doing so often makes your refusal seem less abrupt. When you are saying no to a colleague, an explanation may make interpersonal relationships more comfortable. If the other person is a stranger (such as a salesperson), you might prefer to say simply, "No, thank you." In some situations explanations just make you seem less firm. The other person sees an explanation as something with which to argue. It is possible to be polite and even gracious in saying no without giving any explanation—for example, "Oh, I'm very sorry, but there's no way I can help you now." In many situations this may be the best action.

Withholding a decision. In some situations you may not want to say yes or no because you do not have enough information or you have not yet made up your mind. It is your right to withhold a decision when you want to. Stating "I have not yet decided" is one approach. If you plan to make a decision, you may say, "I will make a decision tomorrow."

Expressing an unpopular opinion. When everyone else seems to have one viewpoint and you have a different one, it may be important to your feelings of integrity and self-esteem to express your own viewpoint. Doing so is often difficult. First, you might make sure that you truly understand the other people's viewpoint by using facilitating techniques to encourage them to express their views clearly. Demonstrate respect for the other people, even when you do not agree, by not attacking their view as wrong and by acknowledging their right to their own opinions. You might say, "I don't agree with that position myself, but I recognize that others support your view" or "That isn't the way I would approach that problem, but I can recognize that you felt it was best." Express your own opinion as an opinion or an alternative viewpoint, not as the truth. "I have always thought of it from this perspective." "My opinion is almost the exact opposite of what you expressed." If the difference is over a factual matter, acknowledge that you could be wrong and suggest seeking an authoritative source to verify the fact. "I could be wrong, but I didn't really think that was the generic name for that drug. Let's check the formulary." When it becomes clear that you and another person have a difference of opinion that cannot be resolved, be willing to drop the subject and move on to something else. "I don't think we'll ever agree on what the best action would have been, so let's talk about something else." Continuing to push for your viewpoint will increase distance and seldom accomplishes anything positive.

Asking for something. Whether you are asking for an item, a behavior, or an attitude, there are skills to asking. First, be as exact as possible so that the other person knows what you are asking. If you are asking a physician to spend time explaining a procedure to the patient, do not spend all of your time going over information in the hope that the physician will come to the same conclusion you did. Instead, clearly state, "I found that Mr. Mele was very confused about what procedure you are performing tomorrow. Would you please talk with him about it this evening?" Wherever possible, give a reason for your request. Note that terms of politeness, such as please and thank you, are appropriate in assertive communication. When asking for help, do not belittle or criticize yourself for needing help. Doing so gives others the impression that you are not competent, which may not be the case at all. Asking for help is an acceptable behavior. On the other hand, do not use flattery or try to make someone feel guilty to obtain a positive answer to your request. Such tactics detract from your credibility as a responsible person. Making negative comments or implying that you expect the person to refuse also lessens your stature. Give an individual the freedom to make his or her own decisions without prejudging. When an individual refuses a request, it is appropriate to suggest a compromise that might assist you but at the same time decrease the burden on the other person. In fact, offering a trade-off of assistance is often the best way to approach another person. "I need help with turning and moving Mrs. Evans. If you could help me with that, I would be glad to feed Mr. Walesa."

Giving criticism. When you feel that you must express an opinion about someone else's behavior, think carefully about your approach so that you do not alienate the person. Offer criticism only when there is sufficient privacy so that others do not overhear what you have to say. This thoughtfulness demonstrates respect for the other person's dignity. Clearly state your own feelings about the situation: "I am upset when I hear you speak to Mr. Otho like that." Describe the specific behavior you are criticizing: "You said you didn't think he was trying." Avoid using global or encompassing terms like always and never, which imply that you never see the person in a favorable light; using them will create antagonism. Try to focus on one instance of the behavior you are criticizing. Doing so lets the other person know that you will deal with situations as they arise and not save criticisms until you have collected a whole list. Saving up negative comments—sometimes called **gunnysacking** because it is akin to saving criticisms in a gunnysack and dumping them on the unsuspecting person all at one time—is extremely detrimental to interpersonal relationships. First, gunnysacking is not honest; if you do not comment on behavior when it occurs, you imply that it is acceptable. Second, it can be devastating to an individual's self-esteem to be confronted with many criticisms at one time. When you criticize, you should also be prepared to suggest alternative behaviors or changes that will correct the situation.

Accepting criticism. Criticism can be accepted in an assertive manner. First, you need to listen to the criticism without immediately jumping to the defensive. Think about the criticism, repeating it in your own mind if necessary to be sure you understand exactly what is meant. If it seems unclear, ask for an example of the behavior being criticized. Then judge for yourself. Is this criticism fair? If it is fair, do not offer excuses. Instead suggest changes that you can make. If you cannot think of a way to change, ask for suggestions for change. If you believe the criticism is not fair or correct, reply with "I" statements that express your feelings and views, not with statements that attack the other person. Say, "I feel distressed that you think that about me, because I don't see the situation in that light at all."

Display 13-4 summarizes the situations in which assertive communication is useful.

Special Purposes of Communication in Nursing

The appropriateness of the various techniques of verbal and nonverbal communication depends on the purpose

Display 13–4
Situations in Which Assertive Communication Is Useful

1. Saying no.
2. Withholding a decision.
3. Expressing an unpopular opinion.
4. Asking for something.
5. Giving criticism.
6. Accepting criticism.

of the interaction, which may range from socializing to leading a group.

Socializing

Socializing is engaging in ordinary social conversation; its content may include such impersonal topics as the weather and politics and such personal topics as children, family, and occupation.

A facility in which nurses rarely socialize with patients would be perceived as cold and unfriendly. Socializing is pleasant and relaxing and enhances our knowledge of one another. However, the nurse's social conversation with patients has been a cause of concern for many practitioners. The patient's physical well-being is a prime consideration—social conversation should not promote fatigue or interfere with needed rest. Another issue is the patient's privacy—social conversation should not pry into personal and family matters. A third concern is the patient's emotional well-being—it may be that the response to the concerns or feelings the patient expresses should be therapeutic, not social. Finally, social conversation should not become a forum for the nurse's problems and opinions.

As a nurse, you need to assess the situation and decide what the patient needs. If you decide that socializing is appropriate, it is your responsibility to make sure such conversation does not create a problem where none existed, by, for example, causing undue fatigue or probing into personal matters. Socializing should provide a time for patients to discuss topics of interest to them, not an opportunity for you to talk about topics of personal interest to you.

What you reveal about yourself will vary considerably in different situations and with different patients. The crucial guideline is that socializing must not undermine the effectiveness of the professional relationship. A student nurse might feel comfortable sharing personal thoughts with a patient of the same sex. With a patient of the opposite sex, however, such talk might be misconstrued as romantic interest and interfere with future therapeutic interaction. Some nurses feel comfortable revealing their thoughts and feelings to other people; others are more private even in their personal lives. Each nurse must decide how much and what to share in each situation. What is right for one may not be right for another.

Some people question whether nurses and patients should establish long-term friendships that will persist outside the care setting. Again, this is an individual matter. Sometimes such relationships are successful. In other instances, the two people find they have little in common once the professional connection ends. The nurse needs to be aware that a one-sided loss of interest can be painful for the other person. The ex-patient is apt to be more dependent emotionally and thus to be hurt more when the friendship ceases. Again, recognition of the various possible outcomes, critical self-evaluation, and the making of a considered decision constitute the best possible course of action.

Using Humor

Humor can be a valuable tool in making all of life more comfortable. In his book *Anatomy of an Illness*, Norman Cousins (1979) even proposes that humor can be used to enhance an individual's adaptation. However, not all humor is alike, and not all situations are appropriate forums for the use of humor. Let us examine some ways in which you might effectively use humor.

Light humor and an opportunity to smile or laugh will often dissipate tension and embarrassment. For example, passing gas in a loud fashion is not considered socially acceptable behavior. However, after surgery, passing gas is considered a desirable sign that the bowel has resumed functioning. When a patient apologizes or expresses embarrassment about passing gas, a nurse might reply, "Oh, we give medals for that after surgery." This light remark lessens the patient's embarrassment without making it a topic of major concern.

You might use humor directed against yourself as a means of lessening the discomfort felt by those around you when you make a mistake or are clumsy. Do this carefully so that you do not convey the impression that you are not serious about your responsibilities. For example, if you should spill a basin of water on yourself, you might say, "Well, I've heard those old nursing jokes about 'we'll have a bath,' but I didn't really plan to join you in bathing right now."

Humor directed against another individual can be damaging to that person's self-esteem and should not be used without real knowledge of that person and thought about what you are saying. It is possible for humor to mask aggressive comments. If the person making the joke responds to a complaint from the person who is the butt of the joke by implying that the response shows a lack of sense of humor, the jokester may have been expressing aggression. Gentle humor directed at another person can demonstrate friendliness or be a nonthreatening way to point out an inappropriate behavior. For example, if a patient is getting out of bed when the physician has prescribed bed rest, you might jokingly say, "Mr. Simmons, if you don't stay in bed we'll have to do something drastic like tie your toe to the call light."

Humor may defuse strong feelings occurring in an argument between two people. Two nurses may be angrily differing. You might say, "Hey, can this wait until we schedule the boxing ring and order up the gloves from central supply?" This tactic will be acceptable to those involved only if you have previously established a relationship of trust with them.

In some situations humor is inappropriate. When a person has suffered a major loss or is depressed about the seriousness of a health problem, a joke might convey that you do not recognize the gravity of the situation. It makes you appear uncaring and insensitive. In a formal situation, jokes may seem out of place and make others uncomfortable.

Some types of jokes are not appropriate in a professional context. You should avoid jokes that are sexually suggestive, contain innuendo, or involve profanity. Although both you and the patient may engage in such joking in a personal situation, the care setting demands different standards from you. Such jokes might embarrass the patient or might make the patient misconstrue the type of interest you have in him or her.

Interviewing

An **interview** is "a purposeful, goal-directed interaction between two people" (Johnson, 1993, p. 110). The goal in an interview is to establish a relationship and gain information about the patient/client that will assist you in providing effective care. The skill and sensitivity of the interviewer are crucial to the successful outcome of an interview. Research has indicated that spontaneity, warmth, and caring are the most important personal attributes for a successful interviewer (Shapiro, 1979).

In an interview you will be moving from a position of a relative stranger to the client to an interaction in which you are discussing personal and intimate aspects of life. This is considered acceptable in our society because you are seen as a helping professional. An unspoken contract exists that includes your commitment to confidentiality regarding the content of the interview and use of the information only for the client's benefit.

The skills of listening are critical to being a successful interviewer. You will need to listen attentively to hear the factual answers to questions you ask and also to understand the feelings, emotions, and concerns expressed in other ways. In addition, the interviewer is an active participant in the interaction. This means that the interviewer guides the direction of interaction, exploring avenues perceived as significant and helping to keep the interaction focused toward the goal.

The Phases of an Interview

The phases of an interaction are present in an interview. The *introductory phase* includes setting the stage for the interaction. As the interviewer, you are responsible for establishing the best physical environment possible. This may be difficult in a busy acute care setting. It is sometimes hard to arrange for privacy in a multiple-bed room or to avoid interruptions and the presence of others. If you are sensitive to these concerns, you can arrange for the maximum privacy possible and sit close to the patient so that you can both speak quietly, maintaining confidentiality. It is important, too, to ensure that the immediate needs of the client are cared for. If the person has pain, that should be addressed; if elimination needs are present, they should be taken care of so the client will be able to focus on the questions being asked.

As part of the introductory phase, you will introduce yourself and present the goals and purposes of the interview. It is at this time that you assure the patient of the confidentiality of information and explain that confidential means that information will be shared only with those involved in this patient's care. If a patient asks you not to share information with others involved in care, you, as a student, should explain that you cannot make that agreement. You need the guidance and assistance of experienced professionals and should not put yourself in the position of having to make decisions based on information you have pledged not to share.

During the *working phase*, you will ask the questions planned for the interview. An interview may be *structured* or *unstructured*. These two types of interviews were discussed in Chapter 9. Reviewing the structured questions before beginning the interview will help you to focus on the client, rather than the questions.

The use of attentive listening skills to pick up cues to what is important and what areas should be explored more fully is crucial. You will also need to use nondirective comments and leads to encourage the person to express ideas more completely and give more complete descriptions. The skillful interviewer may assist the patient to identify relationships between facts and feelings in a way that would not have been possible without the interviewer's interaction. In addition to gathering information about potential problems and concerns, you will also be seeking knowledge of the client's strengths and resources. These will be important to build on as you plan strategies to assist with resolving problems.

Ending the interview with skill is important to the *termination phase.* You will want to close in such way that the patient/client realizes that additional information would be welcomed at a later time and without making the patient feel shut off or rejected. As you near the end of the interview, you might say to the patient, "We are almost at the end of my questions" or "Just a few more questions and we will be done." This gives the patient time to prepare for the ending of the interview, and if he or she has been deciding whether or not to share some information, indicates that this decision should be made.

The interviewer might briefly summarize the main concerns expressed in the interview. For example, you might say, "It appears that what is most urgent for you right now is getting relief from the constant pain in your foot. We will make that our first priority." This lets the patient know that you have understood and accepted his or her most important concern and will focus on that.

The final closing statement should indicate your appreciation and recognition of the effort the patient has put forth in the interview and an open-ended invitation to share any other information at a later time. Your willingness to listen and the importance you place on what the patient has to say reinforces the impression that you respect and value the person.

Therapeutic Interaction

When a patient experiences unpleasant feelings or has a decision to make or a problem to solve, the nurse can help to minimize anxiety, handle grief, clarify feelings, or solve the problem. Interaction for this purpose is called **therapeutic interaction**.

Therapeutic interaction proceeds systematically, in accordance with the five steps in the nursing process. First, the need for therapeutic interaction must be identified. In your nursing assessment, you will note and evaluate such things as nonverbal cues indicating anxiety, statements of feelings, and signs of grief. The problem confronting the patient should be identified, if it is known.

Second, you will plan your interaction. To do so effectively, you will first set a goal. What is your purpose in interacting with this particular patient? It may be for the patient to exhibit behavior less indicative of anxiety, to state that anxiety has decreased, or to plan action to solve a problem. In most cases, a nondirective approach using facilitating responses proves most helpful. When possible, plan for time to sit down and talk with the patient unhurriedly. This is a particularly appropriate time to review what you know about using nonverbal messages to enhance communication.

Third, you will implement the planned interaction by talking with the patient, encouraging discussion of concerns and feelings. Often this alone enables patients to manage their own feelings. You may also want to encourage a patient's problem-solving efforts. Remember that the patient benefits from the least possible direction on your part.

The last step, of course, is to evaluate the effectiveness of your interaction, examining the results in terms of the planned goal. If the goal was not met, consider the possible explanations. It is often helpful to review your interaction with particular attention to the facilitating or blocking responses you might have made. Try to determine whether such responses may have been responsible for failure to meet your goal. It is important to guard against unrealistic expectations, in terms of both the goal and the effort required to achieve it. Several interactions over a period of days may be more effective than a single interaction.

Working With Groups

Whether you are the leader of a group or a participant in a group, you will find that you will be more effective if you consistently use assertive communication techniques. Others will feel that they know where you stand and can rely on your being direct and honest. This encourages them to behave in a similar manner and leads the entire group toward its goals. In Chapter 14 we will discuss in greater detail working with groups.

Coordinating Care and Initiating Change

All of the areas in which the nurse is responsible for coordinating care for the patient require communication skills. Most of the time you will need to use assertive communication techniques when dealing with colleagues in care. See Chapter 15 for a more extensive discussion of coordinating care.

Health Teaching

Teaching patients, families, and other staff members is a major responsibility of the registered nurse. Because teaching is such a comprehensive task, we have devoted Chapter 16 to health teaching.

Using Communication Effectively in Nursing

Communication skills are basic to effective functioning in nursing. You will use communication with other health care personnel as well as with patients and families. Much of your success will depend on using the right communication techniques for the situation.

Assessment

Whether the situation involves a patient or another staff member, you will want to begin with careful assessment. As part of your assessment, you will need to consider the relationship you already have established. You will also want to consider the other person's current life situation. What cues have you received about feelings and concerns? Assess your own current status. How much energy or strength do you have to give at this time? Identify the unmet needs and problems of those in the situation.

Planning

When you have clearly established the current status, it is time to look toward the future. What outcome do you desire from this interaction? Do you hope to relax the other person? Do you want to bring about change in the person's behavior? Do you wish to encourage the other person in independent problem-solving? Once you have clearly established the goal of your communication, you can plan the type of communication to use. One of the difficulties with effective communication is that events may move so rapidly that you have little time to reflect before you speak. As you be come more skilled at using the various communication techniques, you will also become more skilled at processing assessment and planning information quickly, so that you can move into active communication.

Implementation

Once you have established a plan, move ahead with your communication. Keep in mind that no single reply or single situation is going either to save or destroy an individual. You will make mistakes (everyone does), but you learn from those as well as from situations in which everything goes well. Keep in mind that your positive attitude can make up for technical communication errors.

Evaluation

After an encounter with another person, you will gain more insight if you spend time reflecting on the interaction. The most important consideration is whether or not you met your goal. Then you might want to analyze the interaction itself. Was your assessment thorough, or did you miss information you needed? Were the planned communication techniques appropriate to the

Table 13–5. An Interpersonal Process Recording

Description of the Setting: We were in the patient's room after AM care, patient sitting in the large chair by the window, nurse sitting in a straight chair facing the patient. No other persons were present.

Purpose of the Interaction: For Mr. J. to make plans for care after discharge.

Objective Description of the Interaction (include all statements made and behaviors seen.)	Feelings Occurring During the Interaction	Analysis of Interaction
NURSE: Mr. J., have you thought about your care after you leave the hospital?	I was very nervous. Mr. J. appeared calm.	Used a closed question. An open-ended question would have been better.
PATIENT: No. *(Kept looking out of the window.)*	Seemed abrupt. Was he avoiding the subject? I got more tense.	He did answer my question.
NURSE: When you go home, you will still need to use a walker. How will you manage that at home? *(I leaned forward.)*		Open-ended question. More opportunity for him to respond.
PATIENT: Well, I guess I can get around the apartment.		He did respond more.
NURSE: Um-hmmm. *(I nodded.)*	I began to relax because I felt more in control of myself.	Used a general lead. Was "attentive listening."
PATIENT: *(Made eye contact.)* But I don't see how I can cook a decent meal.		He introduced a concern.

situation? Did you use the techniques correctly? One way of evaluating your own communication patterns is through the use of an "interpersonal process recording." If you write down the various aspects of the interaction and then analyze them, you can share the content of the interaction and your analysis with an instructor or a more skilled nurse to gain feedback for improvement. Table 13-5 is a format for an interpersonal process recording.

Nursing Care Study
A Therapeutic Interaction

Mrs. Shadle is a 75-year-old patient in a long-term care facility for care following the repair of her fractured hip. Mrs. Langley is the registered nurse in charge of the unit. Entering Mrs. Shadle's room on her nursing rounds, Mrs. Langley notes that Mrs. Shadle is sitting in a wheelchair with her hands in her lap, hair uncombed, shoulders down, and head bowed. Mrs. Shadle emits a long sigh and does not look up as the nurse approaches.

NURSE: "You look like you are feeling down."

PATIENT: "Who wouldn't? I'll never leave this awful place."

NURSE: "Never leave this awful place?"

PATIENT: "That's right—I can't ever go home because I can't walk, can't do a thing." *(Tears start to flow down her cheeks.)*

NURSE: *(She sits down beside Mrs. Shadle and takes her hands.)* "Mrs. Shadle, do you mean that you believe you won't be able to walk again?"

PATIENT: "That's right—and I can't be home in this thing." *(She points at the wheelchair.)*

NURSE: "You are going to physical therapy. Can you tell me what you did there yesterday?"

PATIENT: "I stood up between those bars and tried to walk—but I could only go halfway and I got so tired."

NURSE: "Yesterday you went halfway. Do you remember what you were doing in physical therapy last week?"

PATIENT: "That was when I first started going. It took two of them to hold me up."

NURSE: "So last week it took two people to hold you up, and this week you walked half way down the bars."

PATIENT: "I guess that is better, isn't it? But it goes so slowly."

NURSE: "It's a slow process, but it has been steady. What do you suppose you might be doing next week at this time?"

PATIENT: "Maybe I'll be able to walk the whole way." *(Her face brightens.)*

NURSE: "You may even be using a walker so you can walk around the room." *(Mrs. Langley has communicated with the physical therapist and knows that this is the plan.)*

PATIENT: "Really? I might be able to go home if I could use a walker."

NURSE: "Mm-hmm."

PATIENT: "I guess this isn't such a bad place for a while."

NURSE: *(She gives Mrs. Shadle's hand a squeeze and stands up.)* "I'll have Miss Johnson, the nursing assistant, help you comb your hair and clean up to go to physical therapy. I'll be back to check on how

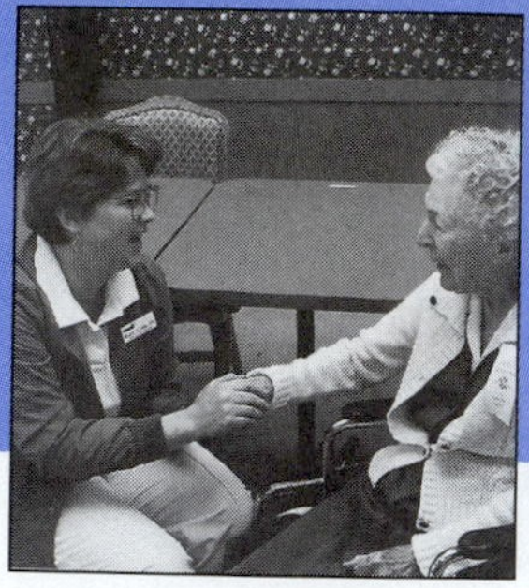

Key Points

- Communication is a process of sharing ideas, thoughts, and feelings with another person. It is essential in relationships with patients, clients, and health care personnel and in every phase of the nursing process.
- An interaction consists of an exchange or series of exchanges between two individuals. The person trying to communicate is the sender. The other person is the receiver. What is being communicated is the message.
- An interaction has three phases: the introductory phase, the working phase, and the termination phase. Each is important to the overall communication that occurs.
- The message in a communication is transmitted both verbally and nonverbally. Feelings and attitudes are often more accurately reflected by the nonverbal behavior than by the verbal content.
- In using verbal communication, language use, pacing, and voice tone need to be considered. The techniques of verbal communication are intended to help the nurse interact more effectively.
- Facilitating responses are those that encourage another person to explore ideas, thoughts, and feelings and to solve problems.
- Blocking responses are those that tend to cut off communication.
- Position, gestures, and physical distance are components of nonverbal communication. Facial expression and eye contact can be used to assess mood, but these perceptions must be validated.
- Attentive listening is a skill that conveys respect and concern and is a way of acknowledging that the other person is significant. Sitting down, allowing time, maintaining eye contact, and focusing on what is being said are all parts of attentive listening.
- Assertive communication is a method that can be used by the nurse to express his or her own preferences and wishes in a clear and direct manner. It is useful in working with other health care workers and is most commonly needed when one is saying no, withholding a decision, asking for something, or giving or accepting criticism.
- Humor has a place in nursing but must be used carefully to not demean or belittle another person or communicate a lack of understanding of a serious situation.
- Communication skills are used in socializing, in interviewing, in therapeutic interaction, in health teaching, and in coordinating care and working with others.
- A nursing process approach is appropriate when communication is used in nursing. This requires the nurse to assess the person and the situation, clearly identifying the problem; plan the communication carefully; carry out the communication using appropriate techniques; and evaluate the effectiveness of the communication, both in terms of outcome and in terms of the nurse's own performance.

Study Questions

1. Describe the three variables in an interaction.
2. What occurs in the introductory phase of an interaction?
3. What are the components of nonverbal interaction?
4. How does physical distance affect individuals in an interaction?
5. How do attitudes affect the message being communicated?
6. Give an example of the use of humor in nursing.
7. What are the differences between the techniques appropriate for socializing and the techniques appropriate for therapeutic communication?
8. Why is agreeing considered a blocking response?
9. In what situations is slower pacing desirable?
10. What behaviors can you use to convey attention when listening?
11. List four major purposes of communication.

Critical Thinking Activities

1. Complete a nursing history on a patient in the clinical facility. Analyze your own interview techniques in relationship to attentive listening, use of open-ended questions, and effectiveness in encouraging the patient to talk.
2. Plan a 5-minute conversation with a given patient. After leaving the patient, write down the entire conversation. Note nonverbal as well as verbal interaction. Identify the type of interaction: socializing, teaching, or other.

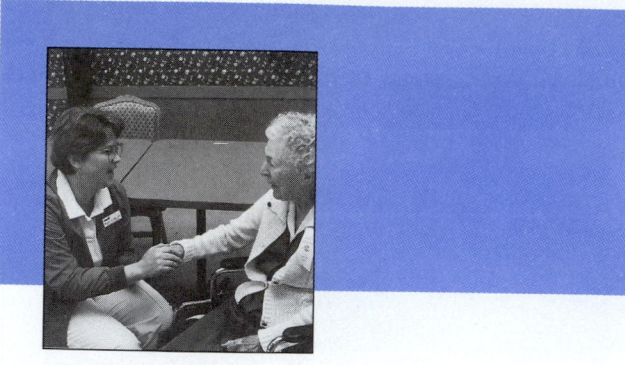

3. a. Plan a conversation in which you will encourage the patient to explore his or her feelings about hospitalization or illness. Review the section on facilitating techniques as you plan.
   b. Carry out the planned interaction.
   c. Record the interaction, noting nonverbal as well as verbal interaction.
   d. Review your interaction in regard to facilitating and/or blocking responses used.
4. With another student, practice using assertion to say no to requests. Practice asking for something. Critique each other's skill in using assertion.
5. While in a clinical facility, be alert for the use of humor with patients. Note these instances. What purpose did they serve? Were they appropriate? Share your notes and ideas with a group of students.

References and Readings

Apse, A., and Stetler, C. B. "Avoiding Terms of Bewilderment." *Nursing '85* 15, 12 (December 1985): 42.

Barnett, K. "A Theoretical Construct of the Concepts of Touch as They Relate to Nursing." *Nursing Research* 21 (March-April 1972): 102–110.

Baugh, C. "Practical Ways to Assert Yourself." *Nursing '89* 19, 3 (March 1989): 57.

Bok, S. *Lying.* New York: Vintage Books, 1978.

Brammer, L. M. *The Helping Relationship: Process and Skills.* Englewood Cliffs, N.J.: Prentice-Hall, 1973.

Burnside, I. M. "Caring for the Aged: Part 5, Touching Is Talking." *American Journal of Nursing* 73 (December 1973): 2060–2063.

Buxman, K. "Make Room for Laughter." *American Journal of Nursing* 91, 12 (December 1991): 46–51.

Buxman, K., and Lemons, C. "Fighting the Fear of Public Speaking." *Nursing '91* 21, 8 (August 1991): 108, 110, 112–114.

Chappelle, M. L. "The Language of Food." *American Journal of Nursing* 72 (July 1972): 1294–1295.

Cochrane, D. A., Oberle, K., Nielsen, S., Sloan-Roseneck, J., Anderson, K., and Finlay, C. "Do They Really Understand Us?" *American Journal of Nursing* 92, 7 (July 1992): 19–20.

Cousins, N. *The Healing Heart.* New York: W. W. Norton, 1983.

———. *Anatomy of an Illness.* New York: W. W. Norton, 1979.

Egolf, D. B., and Chester, S. L. "Speechless Messages." *Nursing Digest* 4 (February 1976): 26–29.

Epstein, C. "Breaking the Barriers to Communication in the Health Care Team." *Nursing '74* 4 (December 1974): 63–68.

Fast, J. *Body Language.* New York: Simon and Schuster, 1970.

Field, W. E., Jr. "Watch Your Message." *American Journal of Nursing* 72 (July 1972): 1278–1280.

Goldsborough, J. "On Being Non-Judgmental." *American Journal of Nursing* 70 (November 1970): 2340.

Gordon, T. *Parent Effectiveness Training.* New York: Wyden, 1970.

Grening, L. "A Formula to Avoid Miscommunicating." *Nursing '90* 20, 9: 122–127.

Hall, E. *The Silent Language.* New York: Doubleday, 1973.

Hein, E. "Listening." *Nursing '75* 5 (March 1975): 93–102.

Herth, K. "Laughter: A Nursing Rx." *American Journal of Nursing* 84 (August 1984): 991–992.

Johnson, B. S. *Psychiatric—Mental Health Nursing.* Philadelphia: J. B. Lippincott, 1993.

Jurgens, A., Meehan, T. C., Wilson, L. H. "Therapeutic Touch as a Nursing Intervention." *Holistic Nursing Practice* 2, 1 (November 1987): 1–13.

Krieger, D. "Therapeutic Touch: The Imprimatur of Nursing." *American Journal of Nursing* 75 (May 1975): 784–787.

Krieger, D. *The Therapeutic Touch: How to Use Your Hands to Help or Heal.* Englewood Cliffs, N.J.: Prentice-Hall, 1979.

Loesch, L. D., and Loesch, N. A. "What Do You Say After You Say Mm-hmmm?" *American Journal of Nursing* 75 (May 1975): 807–809.

Lynch, J. J. "The Simple Act of Touching." *Nursing '78* 8 (June 1978): 32–36.

Nicarthy, G. *Assertion Skills for Young Women: A Manual.* Tucson: The National Female Advocacy Project, New Directions for Young Women, 1981.

Osborn, S. M., and Harris, G. G. *Assertive Training for Women.* Springfield, Ill.: Charles C. Thomas, 1975.

Radulovic, P. O. "Under the Cover of His Charm." *American Journal of Nursing* 73 (October 1973): 1731–1737.

Richardson, B. K. "Seven Ways to Win Your Patient's Trust." *Nursing '87* 17, 3 (March 1987): 44–45.

Robinson, L. "The Crying Patient." *Nursing '72* 2 (February 1972): 16–20.

Robinson, V. "Humor in Nursing." In *Behavioral Concepts and Nursing Interventions*, edited by C. E. Carlson. Philadelphia: J. B. Lippincott, 1970.

Shapiro, M. B. "Assessment, Interviewing for Clinical Psychology." *British Journal of Social and Clinical Psychology* 18 (June 1979): 211–218.

Teasdale, K. "The Concept of Reassurance in Nursing." *Journal of Advanced Nursing* 14 (July 1989): 444–450.

"The Doctor-Nurse Game: A Special Survey Report." *Nursing '91* 21, 6 (June 1991): 60–64.

"Touch: A Symposium." *Nursing Forum* 18, 1 (1979).

Working with Groups

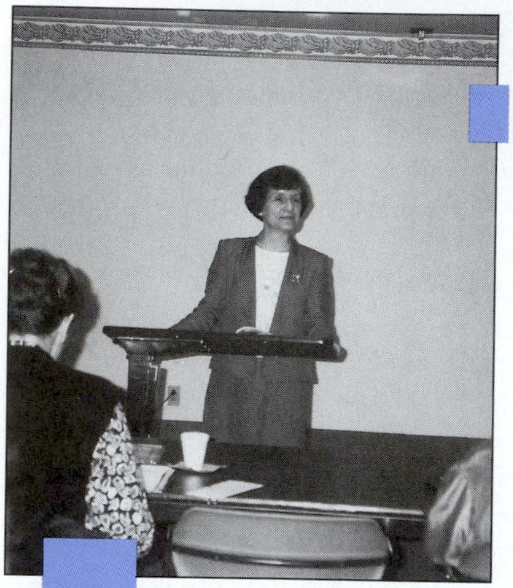

14

Objectives

After completing this chapter, you should be able to:

1. Identify situations in which a nurse would participate in a group.
2. Outline four aspects of group structure.
3. Discuss the various factors involved in group process.
4. Define the three major leadership styles.
5. Identify four or more additional leadership styles that may be used with groups.
6. Name and describe the aspects of the five stages of a group.
7. Identify ways in which a group member can facilitate the functioning of a group.
8. Identify ways in which a group leader can facilitate the functioning of a group.
9. Discuss common problems seen in groups.
10. Outline attributes to be considered when analyzing a group.

Study Terms

accommodation stage
aggregate
authoritarian leadership
autocratic leadership
cohesion
consensus
considerate leadership
democratic leadership
directive leadership
dissolution stage
feedback
formal group
goal
group
group process
influence
informal group
initiating leadership
initiation stage
laissez-faire leadership
motivational leadership
multicratic leadership
negotiation stage
norms
operation stage
orientation stage
participative leadership
power
primary group
relations-oriented leadership
secondary group
semiformal group
task-oriented leadership
termination stage
working stage

Ellis, Nowlis: Nursing: A Human Needs Approach, 5th ed. © 1994 J.B. Lippincott Company

Outline

A **group** is a collection of individuals united in a common goal. Although this goal may not be directly stated or clearly defined, it is the reason the people are associated together. Groups of two are called dyads, and three, triads. A group achieves a goal that cannot be achieved as well by a single individual.

A number of people who happen to gather together without a common goal are merely an **aggregate**. For example, students crossing a campus between classes form an aggregate, but if six of them stop to help someone who is injured, those six become a group.

Groups and Nursing

Nurses function with many different groups in many different ways. For you to work effectively with various groups as a nurse, you must have a firm understanding of the different types of groups that exist and how they function.

The most obvious groups in which you presently participate are groups of students. From the beginning of your education, you have been in small groups of students who were united in pursuit of the goal of successfully completing a course. In these groups, called classes, the chances of success in meeting the goal were greater if all class members met their obligations, such as appearing on time, being quiet when appropriate so that everyone could hear information that was being shared, and so on. Classes are more formal in structure than are many of the groups in which nursing students participate. You may have a group conference with your instructor and peers before or after the clinical experience to discuss patient care and other concerns. Here the environment may be more relaxed, with either the instructor or a student leading the group. However, all participants are encouraged to enter into the discussion. Many students find that group study is useful. A small number of classmates meet to study together before examinations. This group meeting may take place in the home of a group member. There may or may not be a group leader.

As a registered nurse, you will be functioning with many different types of groups of health care workers. Even though you may be giving primary care to one or more patients, you are responsible for communication with and accountability to the group of nurses on your unit. On other units, nurses may be members of a team of only two or three people focused on the care of a number of patients, each member providing the skills appropriate to his or her role. The responsibilities of primary and team nursing are discussed in Chapter 15.

Nursing groups exist within the community. On the local level are special interest groups. These nurses have a common interest or specialty that allows them to share resources and express concerns within their area of interest. Examples of these groups are nurses who work in fields such as the operating room, oncology, or rehabilitation.

Other groups are broader, with regional, state, or national interests. The goals of these groups may vary, but all are concerned in some way with the enhancement of nursing care or the working situation for nurses. It will be important for you to be able to function effectively in these professional groups.

You will also be working with patients and clients in family groups. These family groups are significant in the life of the individual, and your ability to provide high-quality care will often depend on your ability to understand and work with family groups.

In your practice you may find yourself working with groups of patients with common concerns or needs. You may be helping them to discuss their concerns or providing information essential to their future health and independence. If you do not understand the nature of the group, you will be less effective in your teaching.

Regardless of the type, goal, or composition of a group, the **group process** has usefulness for all its members. Among its functions are opportunity to explore the ideas of others within the group and the inclusion of others with whom one can validate decision-making matters. Groups offer the opportunity to explore similarities and differences with other group members as well as providing a relatively safe environment (Fontes, 1987, p. 212).

Types of Groups

Groups can be discussed in terms of two types—primary and secondary.

Primary Groups

A **primary group** is the most important personal group of which an individual is a part. Traditionally, the primary group has been identified as the family. An individual is born into this group or comes into it through an intimate relationship, such as adoption or marriage. The family provides basic sustenance to the young and meets the psychosocial needs of its members. In some societies, the family remains the dominant social group throughout life. In modern Western society, many individuals are separated from their original primary group because of geographic mobility, changes in outlook on life, and conflict with the family. Many of these individuals form new primary groups that provide basic support. These groups may not be related by any formal or legal structure, but they are significant in the lives of those involved in them. When you are working with patients, it will often be important to identify the primary group that forms a support system for the individual.

Secondary Groups

Secondary groups are less intimate groups in which membership tends to be short term rather than lifelong. Some secondary groups are informal. **Informal groups** are characterized by a lack of specific membership, unverbalized goals, and lack of a definite structure. An example of an informal group is a group of friends who gather to go skiing. Some individuals invited to be part of the group may be unable to go, and others may be invited to take their places without formal action. The goal is to go skiing, but other goals of communication, companionship, and relief of boredom may exist without being clearly identified. Although someone may serve as the organizer of the group, there is no formal process by which this person becomes a leader.

Secondary groups may also be formal groups. In **formal groups**, the structure is clearly specified and outlined. The membership rules and processes are also definite. The goals may be written in clear and elaborate terms. An example of a formal group in nursing is the American Nurses Association. This organization has written bylaws that require a formal process for change. Members must meet certain criteria to belong, and the members can be identified by the membership list. The goals of the organization are adopted at formal meetings where voting is conducted in accordance with the group's rules and regulations.

A large number of the secondary groups in which you will function in nursing will be **semiformal groups**. As the name implies, these groups are not as structured as the formal groups, but they do have some clearly structured aspects. The structured aspects may be different for different semiformal groups. A common semiformal group in nursing is the nursing team. The leader is specifically assigned to that role. Members are specifically designated, and they remain in the role of members for the shift. The goals are general, that is, group members wish to provide for optimum care of the patients to whom they are assigned. The manner in which the team members will interact, how decisions will be made, and when the group will meet are not specified. Another semiformal group might be a committee established to consider a problem in the work setting. Individuals might volunteer to serve on the committee. The committee might determine its own chairperson through an election or simply by asking who is willing to serve. The goal is clearly stated, but the process that the committee will use to function is not clearly stated and may be adapted as the committee members see fit. When writers discuss small groups and their functioning, they are frequently referring to semiformal groups.

Group Structure

Structure refers to those fixed dimensions of the group that can be used to identify it. Group structure is important because it affects the way the group functions. Changes in group structure can cause corresponding changes in function.

Size is the most apparent aspect of structure. A small group may consist of only a few people; moderate-sized groups average 20 to 30; and large groups may number 100 people or more. Appropriate size varies with the purpose of the group. Optimum size is determined by the group's tasks and the way its members function. Hare's study and other reports have indicated that as the size of the group increases, individual members have less opportunity to contribute and lead (Hare, 1962). Therefore, membership participation tends to decrease as the size of a group increases (Bass, 1973). In a large group, it takes much longer to gather information and make sure that everyone understands the issues.

Reaching a decision may be more difficult in a larger group. In a small group, it may be possible to get everyone to agree on a decision reached; in a large group, reaching universal agreement is often impossible. In general, the ideal-sized group for decision-making purposes is one that is as small as possible but that has enough different ideas and viewpoints to provide the information needed for a good decision. In most situations in which you find yourself as a nurse, a relatively small group of 3 to 15 individuals will prove most effective.

Membership is another aspect of structure. How individuals become members of the group and who the members are is part of the structure. Members who choose to be part of the group may have a greater sense of commitment than those who are appointed to a group, but this is not always true. Sometimes appointment to a group is seen as an indication of ability or status and is therefore prized. In some groups membership is stable, that is, the same persons continue to be members. This stability facilitates the accomplishment of tasks because everyone knows what has already occurred and is a part of the entire process. In groups in which membership varies, time must be devoted to integrating the new members into the group; otherwise the group will eventually become unable to function.

Meeting times are another aspect of structure. Whether the group meets in the daytime, in the evening, or as part of the work schedule is another facet of its basic structure. In informal groups, meeting times may not be specifically stated. In semiformal groups, meeting times may vary and be decided by the group as it progresses. In formal groups, rules may mandate meeting times. The frequency of meetings is also a consideration. If meetings are far apart, members may need to spend time reviewing past information to progress. If meetings are spaced closely together, individuals may not have time to complete tasks assigned by the group. Again, there is no ideal frequency for meetings; the appropriate intervals will depend on the task of the group and the other obligations the group members have.

Another aspect of structure is the *stability of relationships and roles.* Whether or not the relationships among the individuals in the group remain stable is important. Do the group members continue with the same responsibilities? Is the same person the leader? The task often determines the leader, and a change in this task may necessitate a change in leadership and group participation. For example, if an in-service conference is planned to discuss nursing diagnoses, the leader may be one who has expertise in this area and can effectively facilitate the group's exploration of this topic. If the next in-service conference concerns infection control, a new leader may be designated. The members' interest in these two topics may vary by individual so that relationships change. Changing relationships within the group may produce growth in individuals but may slow the group's attainment of a task-oriented goal.

Group Process

Group process, also called group dynamics, is the way in which a group functions. There are many different aspects of group process: the assigned roles, functional roles, power and influence, norms, decision-making, and cohesion. In any individual group, some aspects may be more important than others. The interaction among the different aspects of group process is significant (Fig. 14-1). Therefore, you should not consider one aspect in isolation from the others.

Roles Within the Group

It is essential that the leader clearly understand what is expected from members of the group. If expectations are not clear, the members may feel role ambiguity, which means that the leader's uncertainty is communicated to the members. When members of a group feel unsure of their leader and, in turn, of precisely what is expected of them, conflict can occur.

In many groups, *formal roles* are delineated. The leadership role is an assigned one, and ambiguity does not occur. The expectations of the leader may differ depending on the leadership style being used in the

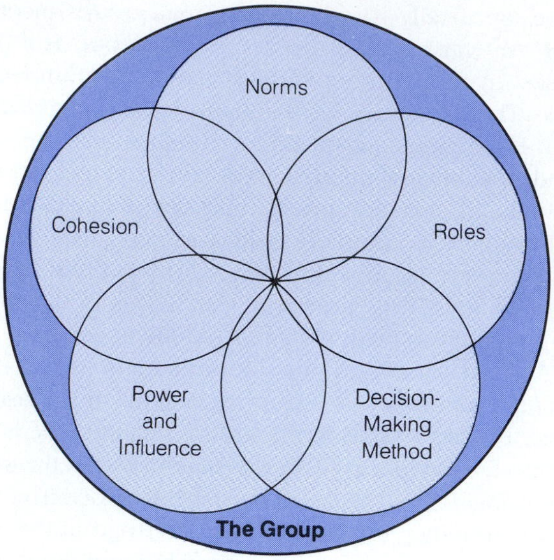

Figure 14-1. Factors within a group that interact to affect the functioning of the group.

group. Individual members within groups may have specific tasks or assignments that define their roles, such as keeping minutes or notes or reports of finances.

Functional roles are the ways in which people behave in the group, regardless of their formal assignment. Functional roles may facilitate the group process or block it. A member may respond in a characteristic way in all of the group activities; for example, one group member might always try to solicit the viewpoint of each person in the group before a decision is made. This behavior may facilitate full participation by everyone. Another individual may always find fault with the ideas of everyone. This role would tend to interfere with group function.

Table 14-1 provides a list of some of the commonly identified functional roles that facilitate group function. These roles are not always present, nor does the same person always fulfill the same role. People do function differently at different times on the basis of their own needs and resources. You will notice that some of the facilitating roles help the group to accomplish its primary task. Other *facilitating behaviors* help to meet the psychosocial needs of the individuals within the group and therefore make the group process move more smoothly.

The list by Smith (1965) is a classic list of functional roles that block group effort (Table 14-2.) Each of these *blocking behaviors* lessens the ability of the group to function effectively and to accomplish its goal. Some of the behaviors, such as debunking, interfere with the contribution of others or make others feel less valuable to the group. Other behaviors, such as seeking recognition, take time the group needs for its primary tasks.

Table 14–1. Facilitating Roles Taken by Group Members

Role	Type of Interaction
Those That Facilitate Group Process	
Diplomat	Takes responsibility for maintaining group harmony.
Humorist	Releases group tension through appropriate use of humor.
Listener	Demonstrates friendliness, warmth, and sympathy by listening to the concerns of others.
Encourager	Actively seeks the participation of others in the group.
Problem identifier	Identifies problems in the group process and brings them to the attention of the group.
Confronter	Assists others in looking at behaviors that are blocking group process.
Those That Facilitate Accomplishment of Goals	
Liaison	Communicates the needs, concerns, and issues of the group to outside authorities.
Specialist	Provides information and access to outside resources.
Focuser	Focuses attention of the group on the goal.
Summarizer	Brings together the ideas and information presented to assist the group in making a decision.
Compromiser	Identifies commonalities and areas of agreement.
Contributor	Gives own ideas, viewpoints, and suggestions so that the group can consider them.
Originator	Presents new ideas and directions for the group.
Worker	Is willing to accept responsibility for tasks that are needed to accomplish the goal.

Power and Influence

Power is the ability to influence the actions of the group. Power may be exercised by individuals within the group or jointly by several persons. Power can shift from one person to another in response to a situation. A person who wishes to affect the actions of the group needs to understand where the power in that group lies. Power may be exerted by making or obstructing group decisions and by furthering or obstructing its actions. Similarly, power can be used to move a group toward or away from its goals.

Power may have a variety of sources. *Legitimate power* comes from expertise or knowledge related to the task or goal of the group or from an appointed authority

Table 14–2. Blocking Roles Taken by Group Members

Role	Type of Interaction
Eager beaver	Is unwilling to take time for decision-making and discussion; wants to act immediately.
Talker	Takes more than a proportionate share of group time.
Brilliant one	Offers ability and ideas, but sees own contributions as invariably the best.
Emotional one	Invariably reacts strongly, either positively or negatively, to others' ideas.
Bored one	Appears uninterested in the group's goal or task.
Silent one	Does not talk or contribute.
Conformist	Always agrees with others; never voices conflicting ideas.
Recognition seeker	Draws attention to self and own contributions.
Playboy/Playgirl	Socializes instead of focusing on the goal.
Suspicious one	Believes that everyone is motivated by self-interest and desire for advancement.
Nonconformist	Will do anything to be different and stand out in the group.
Politician	Opposes the leader and works to acquire power and influence.
Aggressive one	Fights and overrides others to get own ideas accepted.
Debunker	Puts down others' ideas but does not contribute.
Special pleader	Has a vested interest in the outcome and tries to direct the group in a personally beneficial direction.
Blocker	Tries to keep the group from acting.

Adapted from William S. Smith *Group Problem-Solving Through Discussion,* Appendix B. 1965 © by the Bobbs-Merrill Co., Inc. Indianapolis.

such as that of the employer. This power is considered legitimate because it is clearly recognized, is openly acknowledged, and has a purpose in the group. Some power is *coercive,* that is, it comes from being strong and decisive in action, not necessarily from any expertise or knowledge base. Coercive power may cause action to be taken, but may not create action that moves the group effectively toward its goals. Even when coercive power moves the group toward its goals, such power may create unpleasant feelings in other group members.

Influence is the ability to affect the decisions and actions of another individual in the group. Influence is similar to power and the same person often possesses both. Influence over others can affect the group as a whole, if those being influenced share power in the group. If the person being influenced has little power, however, change may not occur in the group as a whole. Influence may be exerted overtly by openly suggesting that another person behave in a certain way. Influence is also exerted covertly by rewarding desired behavior and ignoring undesired behavior.

Norms

Norms are the rules governing behavior within the group. Some groups adopt formal norms, such as adopting the rules presented in the book *Robert's Rules of Order,* for the conduct of official business. Other groups' norms are unstated, and members learn them in the context of the group. Examples of such norms are whether or not it is acceptable to interrupt others when they are speaking and whether or not acceptance by others requires sustained active participation in the group or allows for discontinuous participation. Unstated norms are usually communicated by members' responses to particular instances of behavior. If a certain kind of behavior is accepted, or even rewarded, it will continue and may spread to other members. If it is punished by negative responses or ignored, it will usually decrease in frequency and eventually cease. Groups may change norms by discussing them and deciding to adopt new ones. Norms may also be changed by the behavior of an influential member.

Decision-making

Every group must have some way of coming to decisions if it is to accomplish its goals. There is no one right way to make decisions; rather, the appropriate decision-making method depends on the group and the tasks involved. The most important aspect of any decision-making method is that everyone clearly understands how decisions will formally be made.

Although many processes are used to make decisions formally, other subtle or even hidden influences may sometimes determine decisions. The art of persuasion and its impact on decision-making has been increasingly studied. Members of the group may influence one another toward a particular resolution. The charisma of a leader may be a strong factor in determining the outcome of a decision.

Sometimes the formal process of presenting ideas as motions and *voting* on them proves most acceptable to the members of the group. Whenever this system is used, the group must be prepared to work effectively with those who voted on the minority or losing side of a question. Finding ways to prevent discouragement or loss of commitment on the part of those whose views are not adopted is part of the group's task.

Another means of arriving at decisions is **consensus**: alternatives and compromises are proposed, modified, debated, and discussed until a conclusion is reached that all members of the group support. The process of reaching a consensus can be time consuming. Furthermore, it may fail if some participants in the group are unable or unwilling to compromise. If successful, however, consensus effectively promotes group cohesion and ensures that all members of the group will support its decisions.

A third way of making decisions is through **authoritarian leadership**, that is, a single individual decides among alternatives suggested by the group. Decisions can be made rapidly this way; however, group members tend to feel less investment in decisions they did not help to make. If the members all agree with the decision, however, this lessening of commitment may not occur.

Cohesion

Cohesion is the state that results from loyalty, enthusiasm, and involvement on the part of the group's members. For a high degree of cohesion to exist, the group must be important to the individual members. Such feelings prompt them to maintain the existence of the group. If the level of cohesion is low, members of the group may care little whether the group continues to exist. Cohesion affects individuals' willingness to work toward the aims of the group, as well as their commitment to and satisfaction with the group.

This group satisfaction is also reflected in the feelings each member has for the others. Bass and Stogdill (1981, p. 424) found increased cohesiveness when members of a group regarded each other with esteem. Cohesive groups also display less hostility than do less cohesive groups.

Cohesion is enhanced when the members agree on a group's goals and norms and when they feel they have participated in decision-making. It tends to be highest when all participants in the decision-making process are satisfied with the end result. Cohesion is thus a valuable outcome of meeting the group's psychosocial needs.

Styles of Leadership

There are many styles of group leadership, each of which has strengths and weaknesses. No single leadership style is appropriate for every group. A leadership style is most effective when it is compatible with the purpose of the group and the feelings of the individual members. On occasion, a leadership style may change with either a change in leader or a change in the task. At times, a combination of leadership styles is used so that maximum effectiveness is achieved by the group process.

There are three main styles of leadership: autocratic, democratic, and laissez-faire. Many successful leaders adopt a *multicratic leadership style* in which the type of leadership used is adapted for the situation.

Autocratic Leadership

Autocratic or **authoritarian leadership** is a type of leadership that is centralized and directive (Fig. 14-2). The leader makes decisions for the group and often assigns tasks to individual members. In some instances, the nursing team will function in an authoritarian manner. The team leader decides when the group will meet, assigns tasks, and oversees the work of the group. The autocratic leader's position may be based on experience, education, or influence over others. Most of the power in the group is held by the leader, who also establishes group norms. An autocratic leadership style is efficient and tends to be minimally time consuming, but it has disadvantages. The members of the group may feel little personal satisfaction in the group's accomplishments because typically little time is devoted to meeting personal needs. Cohesion may be lacking if the members do not feel personally committed to or responsible for the group. When decisions are made by an authoritarian leader, the members of the group may feel little commitment to supporting those decisions. Sometimes, although the leader exercises overt power, other group members exert covert influence over him or her. Authoritarian leadership is essential in emergency situations in which someone takes charge and directs everyone's activities toward the resolution of the problem. Any type of group decision-making would be too time consuming in an emergency.

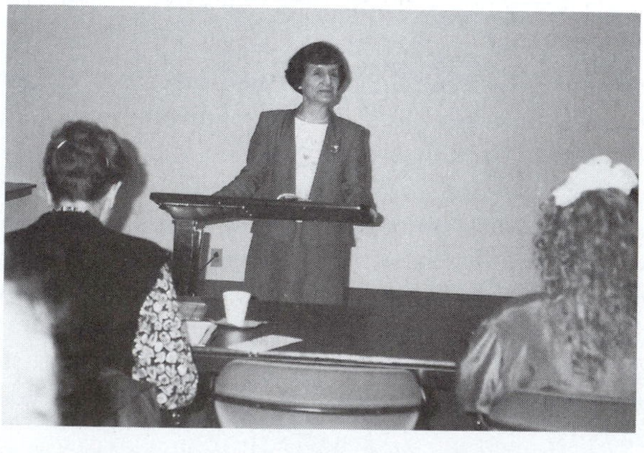

Figure 14-2. Autocratic leadership is leader centered.

Democratic Leadership

In **democratic leadership**, a leader shares decision-making with the other group members through voting or consensus (Fig. 14-3). The leader may be chosen by the group or appointed and subsequently accepted by the group. Democratic leadership tends to be more time consuming than authoritarian leadership, and decisions may be harder to reach. On the other hand, democratic leadership usually elicits a wider variety of ideas and options. Creative solutions to problems are more likely because many individuals are contributing. Group members tend to feel committed to decisions they have shared in making, and thus they are more willing to work actively toward the group's goal. Power and influence may either be widely disseminated throughout the group or concentrated in a few people. Norms are usually based on group decisions, and cohesion tends to be high. The members feel important to and part of the group, which in turn enhances feelings of personal satisfaction.

Democratic leadership is exemplified by a clinical conference group that chooses a different person each time to lead the group's next meeting. The group members together define the purpose of the upcoming meeting and share responsibility for any necessary preparation. At the meeting, the leader is responsible for facilitating the group process so that all members have an opportunity to share their knowledge and expertise on the patient care problem under discussion. All members of the group act together, by voting or by consensus, to choose a course of action.

Laissez-faire Leadership

In **laissez-faire leadership**, the role of the leader does not reside in any particular individual. Leadership may rotate or the group may operate without an acknowledged leader. Lack of an explicit leader can seriously hamper a group's efforts. A leaderless group tends to have difficulty maintaining its focus on the goal and there are few norms. Decision-making is extremely difficult; the group may find itself unable to move in any direction. Such a group's means of decision-making is consensus, which may be difficult to attain with no one to guide the discussion. A laissez-faire group may be comfortable and unthreatening to some participants, who enjoy its freedom and lack of structure, but acutely uncomfortable to others, who usually withdraw from laissez-faire groups.

Some clinical conferences operate as laissez-faire

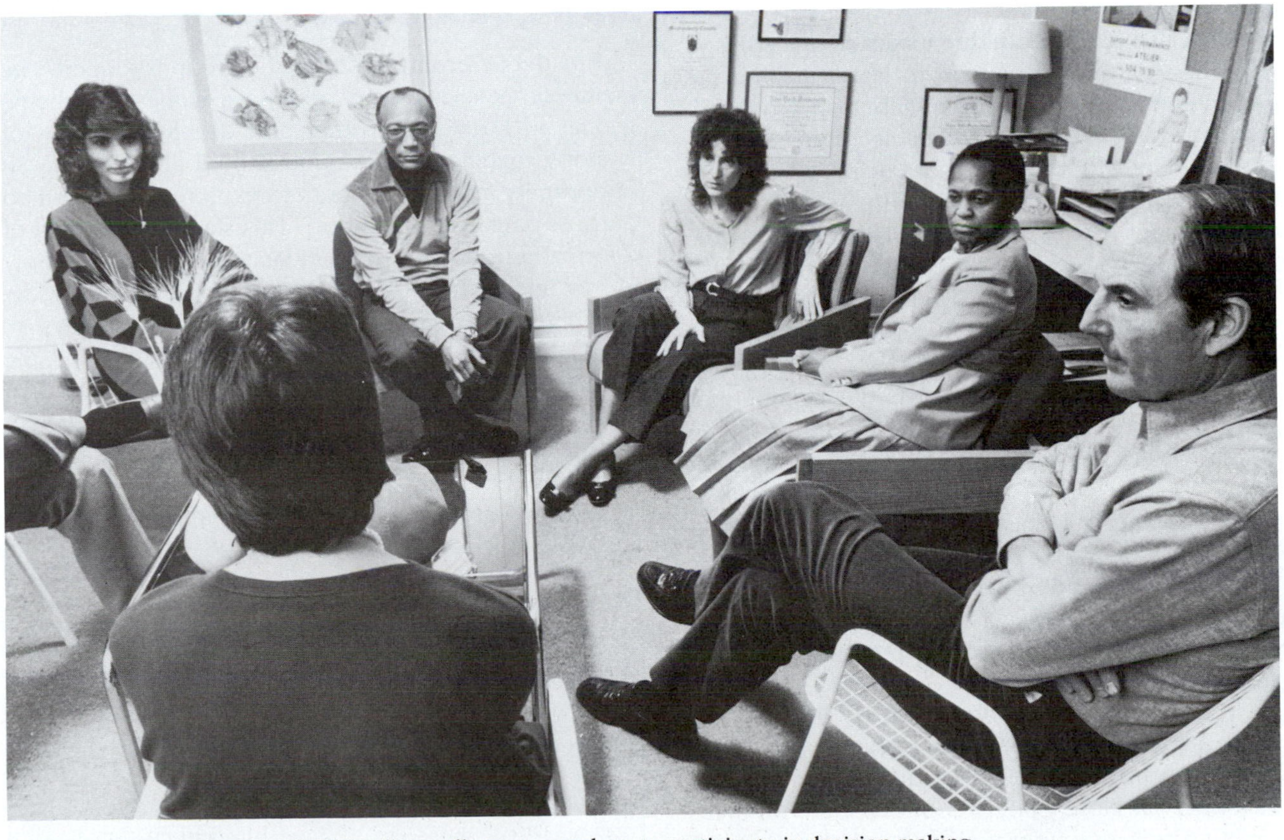

Figure 14–3. Democratic leadership allows all group members to participate in decision-making.

groups. Such a group may be composed entirely of people who welcome lack of structure. Although no one directs the group, everyone shares concerns and ideas. A goal is essential to a laissez-faire group. However, if the group lacks a purposeful focus, one individual with power and influence can easily usurp control of the group. It is also possible for nothing to happen. Without explicit goals, it is difficult for a laissez-faire group to be effective.

Other Leadership Styles

The three main models of leadership style—autocratic, democratic, and laissez-faire—may be combined and referred to as **multicratic leadership**. As the group or goal changes, the leader may alter his or her style to fit the group or task. Some additional leadership styles can be described as considerate, directive, initiating, motivational, participative, relations oriented, and task oriented (Bass and Stogdill, 1981).

In **considerate leadership**, the leader's style includes *consideration* for each group member as a person. This leader may encourage growth in individuals so that they will be able to assume future leadership roles. The behavior of such a leader includes treating others more as equals, providing an environment that puts members at ease, and giving praise for good performance.

In **directive leadership**, the leader designs the approach to solving the task and directs group members to adhere to the plan. Some group members may be comfortable with such direction, whereas others feel decreased involvement when their participation is not a key component. **Initiating leadership** is the type in which the leader may or may not personally direct the group's activity but feels responsible for maintaining standards and setting deadlines for the completion of tasks. Initiating leaders identify their own role and the roles of those within the group.

Participative leadership allows the members of the group to participate actively in all phases of identifying the problem and making decisions about forming solutions. There is power sharing in that the leader is willing to relinquish a degree of power to the group (Bass, 1973).

Motivational leadership involves leaders who have a high degree of skill in interpersonal relations. They believe firmly in the task and persuade others in the group of its importance.

In **relations-oriented leadership**, leaders not only have a concern for their group members as individuals but have a high degree of trust and do not have the need to supervise closely nor to control the group. Completion of tasks is a group victory rather than a personal one for the leader. In contrast to the relations-oriented leader, one who is *task-oriented* finds the task itself of primary importance. The purpose of **task-oriented leadership** is to keep the group cohesive and functional to bring about successful completion of the task. Consideration of each member as a person and cementing interpersonal relations is not a priority.

The Stages of a Group

As in the life of an individual, there are stages in the life of a group. These stages are, however, not absolute. In fact, different stages may occur simultaneously. A group may move backward as well as forward, just as a person may regress. The group's experience at earlier stages will inevitably affect how well the group functions in the later stages. Familiarity with these stages will enable you to work more effectively in a group.

The stages of a group have been characterized in two different ways. These two systems describe the same process, but label it differently. One identifies five stages (Olmstead, 1959) and the other three stages (Cartwright and Zander, 1968). We will describe the five-stage model and explain how it relates to the three-stage model (Display 14-1).

Stage I: Orientation

During the **orientation stage**, the group is formed. The members meet, learn one another's names, and begin getting to know each other and developing ways of working together. This period should also provide an opportunity for the members to explore their common purpose as part of the group. This stage may consist of a formal introduction and orientation, or it may simply be an informal and unstructured opportunity for the members to relate to one another in their own ways.

If there is no opportunity for orientation, the members may always feel isolated from one another. Without an orientation period, trust may never develop, and the members may prove reluctant to take risks in the group. Orientation ought to be seen as essential to an effective group; it is by no means a waste of time

Display 14–1
Two Models of the Stages of a Group

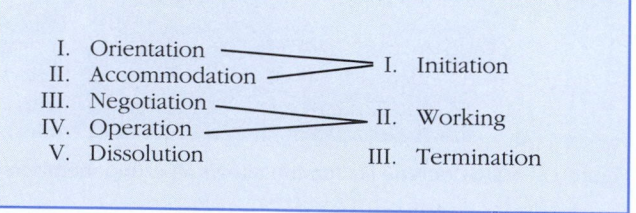

I. Orientation	I. Initiation
II. Accommodation	
III. Negotiation	II. Working
IV. Operation	
V. Dissolution	III. Termination

merely because the group is not yet addressing itself to work.

Orientation will recur whenever a new member joins the group. A new person changes the character of the group and thus requires that the other members change. A group may either try to orient a new member while maintaining the working phase or return temporarily to the orientation stage. If you recognize its importance, you will be able to facilitate orientation and help others to recognize its importance. If membership changes frequently, the group may never be able to move beyond the orientation stage and may thus be unable to accomplish its work.

Stage II: Accommodation

The **accommodation stage** is the beginning of the process of working together. During this period, the members adjust their behavior to work more effectively with others. If, for example, one member has difficulty expressing his or her thoughts, others in the group must learn to give that person time to make a contribution. If the group fails to make such accommodations, some individuals may be shut out of participation. In the long run, the group will suffer from this lack of input. Accommodation may continue to be necessary whenever new situations arise in the group. The three-stage model of group process treats orientation and accommodation as a single stage termed the **initiation stage**.

Stage III: Negotiation

The **negotiation stage** is the stage during which decisions are made. For a group to make decisions, a decision-making system must be adopted. Groups arrive at decisions in a number of ways, and no single approach is correct. Instead, members must find the approach that is most effective for their particular group and its purpose.

Stage IV: Operation

During the **operation stage**, the goal of the group is translated into action on the basis of the decisions made at stage III. This phase is often informally called the group's action time. If, for example, the nursing team has decided that a class needs to be presented on charting, the planning and presenting of that class is the operation stage.

As its work progresses, the group may be required to make further decisions. To do so it must return temporarily to the negotiation stage. The interrelationship between decision and action explains why the three-stage model simply combines negotiation and operation and calls the result the **working stage**.

Some groups make few decisions because their work is clear-cut. Thus, negotiation may be almost nonexistent. In other cases, decision-making is the group's work, and the operation stage is consequently limited.

Stage V: Dissolution

The last stage is identical in the three-stage and five-stage models. Whether it is called the **dissolution stage** or the **termination stage**, it is the process of ending the group—ending one's participation and withdrawing—when its purpose has been accomplished. In some groups, termination occurs at different times for different members. In other groups, termination occurs for all the members at once. If the group has been highly cohesive, termination may be a difficult stage. Some groups find termination so unpleasant that they search for a new purpose to remain together as a group. Nursing students who have worked together for a semester may find their relationship so worthwhile and supportive that they elect to continue as a social group. This effort may be successful if all of them make the transition to the new purpose. If the group's cohesion grew out of its shared purpose and the new purpose is not strong enough to re-create such cohesion, the new group may prove disappointing.

Termination is usually worked through more effectively if sufficient attention is paid to it as a necessary stage in the life of the group. If termination has been planned from the beginning to occur at a given time or at the conclusion of certain work, it may be acknowledged or discussed from time to time so that the members recognize that it is in the nature of the group to end. When the time comes to end the group, the members may want to have a leave-taking in which the function of the group is reviewed and its accomplishments are evaluated. Such an occasion can round out and complete the experience of the group.

Understanding Group Needs

Just as a person has individual needs, a group has collective needs. Meeting the needs of groups is more complex than meeting individuals' needs. For group needs to be met most effectively, the individuals in the group must feel that their individual needs are being met. When such needs are met, the group can function with purpose and direction. When they are not met, the group may become dysfunctional and even disintegrate.

Like individuals, groups have both physical and psychosocial needs (Table 14-3). Like individual needs, group needs form a hierarchy on which the physical needs are the most basic and the psychosocial needs are higher. Like an individual, a group must generally have

Table 14–3. The Needs of a Group

Physical	Psychosocial
Time	Common goal
Space	Action
Size	Sense of accomplishment
Comfort	Personal satisfaction

its basic needs met before it can address its higher level needs, although it is possible for a group to ignore basic physical needs when its higher needs are particularly cherished.

Physical Needs of a Group

A group's physical needs involve time, space, and comfort, which may be characterized as *environment.* Physical needs are as important to a group as they are to an individual. A group needs adequate time together to function. Inadequate time will frustrate the individual members of the group and prevent the group from functioning effectively. Another important consideration is a mutually satisfactory time to meet. If group meetings conflict with other aspects of members' lives, their performance in the group will be impaired, and they may have to withdraw. Meetings ought not to be so prolonged that fatigue sets in, interfering with interest and productivity. For the same reason, it may be more productive to meet early in the day.

The place where a group meets ought to be both adequate in size for the number of participants and constructed in such a way as to allow the group to function. The arrangement of furniture, acoustics, lighting, and privacy all affect the suitability of the space. Familiarity is also an important factor; a familiar location where group members feel safe may enhance interaction. On the other hand, a new locale may distinguish the group from outsiders and thus help its members to focus on the goal. For the group to be physically comfortable, such matters as room temperature, the type of chairs, and distracting noises need to be considered.

Psychosocial Needs of a Group

The psychosocial needs of any group include a common goal, action, a sense of accomplishment, and the personal satisfaction of the individual members. When these psychosocial needs are met, the members will be happier with the group and tend to remain in it, and the group will move more effectively toward its goals.

Every group has some purpose or **goal**, whether or not it is explicitly stated. For example, although some of their other individual goals may vary, the members of a particular college class share the general goal of learning the content of the course.

A group acts in such a way as to move toward its goals. This action may or may not be successful, but a group that is not trying to move toward its goals will soon dissolve. If the students enrolled in a course do not participate actively in it, they fail to constitute a real group. Action is essential to the definition and the continued existence of any group.

A *sense of accomplishment* originates in the members' feeling that the group is making progress toward its goals. Such progress need not be massive or rapid for a sense of accomplishment to develop; the key factor is its significance in the eyes of the group members. This sense of accomplishment is rooted in the work of the group as a whole rather than the contributions of individual members.

Personal satisfaction results when the individual members of a group feel that they are valuable contributors to the group. This process is enhanced when the members feel that the group meets some of their personal needs. The degree to which a group meets personal needs may vary considerably, depending on its purpose. The purpose of some groups is such that individual needs must be submerged in the needs and function of the group. If the members accept this as the way the group will function, its work will not suffer. The members must find their personal satisfaction in accomplishing the goals of the group. If an individual expects the group to meet personal needs, such as a need for recognition, and it fails to do so, he or she may not contribute to the group and may even undermine it. Being clear about the expectations of the group for meeting individual needs and discussing them openly will help to resolve this dilemma.

The major purpose of some groups, such as psychotherapy or counseling groups, is to meet the needs of individual members. In such a group, it is appropriate to expect others to help meet one's personal needs. In other groups, such as nursing teams, the primary goal is to meet others' needs. The personal needs of the nursing staff are met only when they coincide with this primary purpose. In most groups both personal needs and group goals are being sought. For example, a nursing goal is to provide excellent individualized care. An individual nurse's personal need for self-esteem might be met by providing a high standard of care. Thus, group goals and individual needs blend.

Each group needs **feedback**, that is, a system by which to recognize progress, evaluate that progress, and revise actions if the goal is either too slow in being realized or not being attained. Feedback may be given formally by the leader in regular reports or by the appointed leader within the group. Sometimes feedback is offered more informally from members when the group is assembled. When feedback on progress is negative and dissatisfaction is felt among some members, the feedback process may be informal and shared only among a few trusted members. This kind of feedback can be disruptive and can lower group cohesion.

One type of feedback is a planned review of *group content.* The content of the meeting includes the issues presented, topics discussed, and the decisions that take place. An example of content recording is the taking of minutes, which is routine with many groups. Written minutes are shared later with members of the group and act as a useful summary of what took place during a meeting.

Another type of feedback is a planned review of *group process.* Group process includes such aspects as which members talk and which members respond to issues or raise questions. It also includes nonverbal communication of feelings and relationships between members. To formally evaluate group process, one person is identified as a process recorder, records how the group is interacting, and reports to the group at a designated time. The information on process provides a pattern of how the group functions and may be especially useful in developing increased group effectiveness. This is often done by groups of students as a learning exercise, but it can also be done to provide feedback to other kinds of groups. You can also informally evaluate group process for yourself. This may be especially valuable if a group does not function effectively and you would like to identify the problem.

It is only with continual *evaluation* that true group progress can take place. Continual evaluation, based on both objective and subjective group data, can allow one or more of the original goals to be altered or new goals to emerge. Evaluation may set the stage for changing the leadership or the composition of the group. With thoughtful evaluation, members often experience renewed energy and enthusiasm. There is further information on techniques useful for gathering information to evaluate a group under the section below, "Analyzing a Group."

Being an Effective Group Member

It is not widely recognized that participation in a group is enhanced by understanding and skill. An effective participant is valuable to all other group members and contributes significantly to the group's ability to meet its goals (Fig. 14-4). In an effort to enhance your skills as a group member, let us examine some of the characteristics that make for effective group membership.

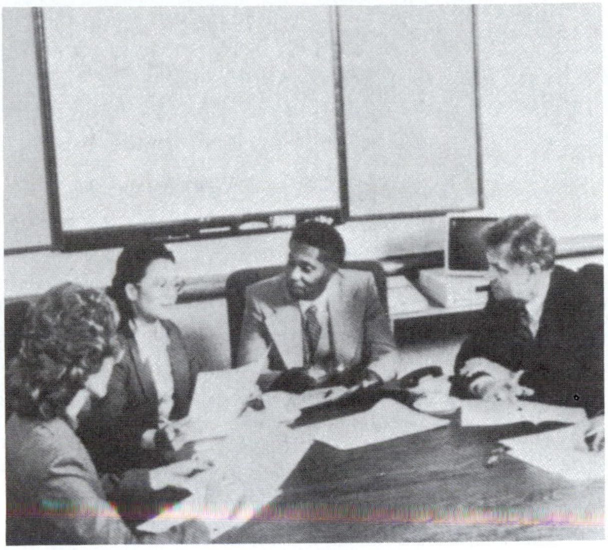

Figure 14-4. Are you an effective group member?

Understanding the Group

Basic understanding of how groups function and of those factors that facilitate or block effective function helps the group member participate actively. When you understand the stages through which a group passes, for example, you can participate enthusiastically in orientation, recognizing its importance to the group's eventual success. Similarly, if you understand that the group's leadership style is democratic, you will recognize that you are expected to play a part in the decision-making process. If the group's initial leadership is autocratic and you find yourself uncomfortable with that style, you will be better able to negotiate for shared responsibility if you understand what the alternatives are. In general, the greater your familiarity with all aspects of group life, the greater your ability to work effectively in a group.

Willingness to Collaborate and Compromise

Because no two individuals can be expected to think identically, groups depend on their members' willingness to pursue collaboration and compromise. Collaboration includes your willingness to work with someone else rather than independently. Compromise includes finding areas in which you are willing to defer to another's preference and areas in which they will defer to yours. It can be enlightening to examine your own approach to groups in which you participate. Do you work cooperatively with others, sharing the workload and the rewards? Do you see yourself as a realistic compromiser, or do you expect others to adjust to and accept your viewpoint? However creative and exceptional your viewpoint, it will not be the most effective alternative unless the group as a whole claims ownership of the idea. This cannot happen if you promote its adoption by running roughshod over the ideas and opinions of others. Your willingness to compromise and collaborate can elicit a similar willingness in others, thus facilitating the work of the group.

Focus on the Goal

Whether a group's goal is the personal growth and satisfaction of its members or an action-oriented outcome, it is highly desirable to keep that goal in mind as you work with the group. If the goal is personal growth, it is clear that time devoted to working on interpersonal relationships within the group is well spent. If the goal is to write a procedure for administering medications, you will direct your efforts to that end and not dissipate the energies of the group pursuing other aims. Although working on interpersonal relationships might become necessary in the latter group, it would not be the central focus.

Concern for Others

Belief in the worth of each individual is a basic ethical principle of the nursing profession (see the Code for Nurses in Chapter 3). One way of acting on this belief is to concern yourself with others in the group. Such concern can be expressed by encouraging others to share their thoughts and ideas, accepting their ideas without "putting down" those people with whom you disagree, and striving for the personal satisfaction of all members of the group, not just your own satisfaction.

Direct and Honest Communication

The functioning of any group is enhanced when the members are direct and honest in their communications. If you are asked for your opinion, state it clearly and briefly. It is false modesty to wait until you are pressured to share your views. If you disagree with a certain position, say so. Disagreement can be expressed without personally attacking others. It is unproductive for the group if you disagree but do not say so and are then reluctant to participate further. Concerns you feel but do not voice can undermine your ability to function and to relate to others in the group. Direct and honest praise of others' ideas and contributions is also valuable. Insincere praise tends to be resented, but sincere praise enhances others' self-esteem and thus the group's potential for success.

Many of the skills and techniques discussed in Chapter 13 will be of value to you as a participant in groups. For example, you might use the skills of questioning to gain more information from those in the group. You might use the facilitating techniques to encourage participation by others, to acknowledge their contributions, and to make them feel wanted. You may find that you need the assertive skills to make your own contribution and to keep others from exerting coercive power. Part of learning to function effectively in a group is learning to assess the situation accurately and to use the appropriate communication skills.

Sharing the Responsibility

If each member accepts responsibility for an appropriate share of the group's tasks, the group's goal is more likely to be accomplished. If one or two people become burdened with all the tasks of the group, they may become resentful and eventually withdraw. There is also a danger that overburdened group members will cause tasks to be left undone or done poorly because of insufficient time and energy.

Being an Effective Leader

When you have the opportunity to be a leader in a group, you have the opportunity to contribute significantly to the accomplishment of the group's goals. An effective leader is able to focus the efforts of the group, identify problems, and assist others in making their most effective contributions.

Understanding the Group

Even more than the member, the leader, to be effective, needs an understanding of the function of groups in general and of the specific group in particular. How do people become members of this group? What are the group's goals? Is the leadership style predetermined or is it the choice of the leader or of the group members? It is important for you to review all the components of group function and to determine how these apply to the group you are planning to lead.

Providing for Physical Needs

The leader needs to take responsibility for the physical needs of the group. This does not mean that the leader must provide for all physical needs. It may be appropriate for the leader to ask others to arrange a meeting room, set up chairs, and do the other necessary tasks. However, the leader should follow through to see that these needs are satisfied. Part of providing for physical needs is planning for the use of time. Is unlimited time available? Are there deadlines that must be met? What time commitment can be expected of the group members?

Facilitating the Stages of the Group

Members of a new group must have an opportunity for *orientation,* that is, get to know one another, review or develop the group goals, and establish working relationships. All this is accomplished more efficiently and effectively if the leader plans ahead for the orienting process. The leader will convene the group and introduce group members to one another. Identifying and clearly stating norms for behavior is also a helpful part of orientation. If the group must observe certain limits, these should be explored. Assisting the group to look beyond the immediate situation to recognize its goals is also important in orientation. Goal recognition helps to give direction and focus to the group.

To enable the group to work together effectively, the leader must assist members with *accommodation* by facilitating the meeting of psychosocial needs. Throughout the life of the group, the leader must remain sensitive to the psychosocial needs of the group members. Giving recognition, asking for participation, and listening carefully all enhance the self-esteem of others. The use of effective communication skills is critical to this task. The life of the group revolves around the quality of the communication that occurs. The communication skills most important in meeting the psychosocial needs of the group were discussed in detail in Chapter 13. The leader must listen with skill, clarify communication, identify individual perceptions, and provide support to the members.

The method to be used for *decision-making* must be explicit so that all members understand their role in relationship to decisions. In some groups one of the first decisions is what decision-making method will prevail; in other groups the decision-making method is prescribed by others. To bring the group to a decision, the leader must recognize when the group needs to make a decision and work to facilitate decision-making. Groups that never come to a decision are never able to meet their goals. The leader can help to explore similarities and differences of opinions, restate the goal, and suggest compromises when appropriate.

Focusing the attention of the group on the need to *take action* is the responsibility of the leader. The leader may ask for specific suggestions or reinforce ideas for action that are presented. One part of the leader's responsibility is involving everyone in the proposed actions. To do this, the leader needs to identify the strengths and weaknesses of the members. Pointing out individual abilities encourages those individuals to participate.

The effective leader helps the members of the group with *termination* by helping them to evaluate their work and conclude their relationships. Summing up what has been done and acknowledging the contributions of individuals are important steps in this process.

Identifying and Correcting Group Problems

Throughout the life of the group, it is necessary for the leader to analyze events and activities in the group and to help it adopt more effective patterns of functioning. Many different kinds of problems can occur. Analyzing the stage of the group, the group process, and the roles of group members can help you to identify problems. Although any member of the group can assist in solving the problems of a group, the leader has a special responsibility in regard to problem resolution. The following are common problems encountered when working with a group.

Lack of Motivation

One reason for a lack of motivation is a lack of clearly spelled out goals. When motivation seems to be lacking, it is often helpful to review the goals of the group. Failure to accomplish tasks that can be clearly seen as leading to the goal also results in decreased motivation. Members begin to think that the group will never accomplish anything and therefore see no reason to work. Moving the group toward decision-making and facilitating the establishment of concrete plans for action also serve to increase motivation within a group. If a single individual within the group seems to lack motivation, it is often helpful to make a specific effort to include that person, solicit ideas from him or her, and find a task that this individual can perform.

Competition

When members of a group are competing against one another for recognition or status, the work of the group may not be hindered if that competition leads individuals to take on specialized functions at which they work hard. If, however, the competition interferes with decision-making, pointing out areas of agreement and common ground and making suggestions for compromise may be useful.

Blocking Behavior

Most group members will exhibit some blocking behaviors at some time in a group. For example, one member may divert the group into social conversation on occasion. Simply refocusing the group on the goal is usually sufficient to prevent this from becoming a problem. Blocking behaviors become problems for the group when an individual persists in a blocking role within the group. Ignoring the behavior in the hope that it will change is seldom effective. When you have identified a blocking behavior, try also to identify the behavior you want the individual to exhibit. Sometimes the most effective response is to confront the individual openly, describe the blocking behavior (do not label the behavior), state why it is counterproductive, and offer a suggestion for a positive contribution the individual might make to the group. For example, "John, you have put down every idea that has been proposed, but you haven't offered any alternatives. That isn't helping us get the job done. Could you try to identify some positive aspect of the suggestions that have been made?" In some instances you might decide that open confrontation would not be productive. You might then find it helpful to interrupt the person and point the group in an appropriate direction. You might state, "We've discussed that aspect for quite a while; let's get back to the question of when we will hold the program. Does anyone have a suggestion?"

The force of the entire group may be used to obtain a change if the leader reflects the group's feelings about what is happening. The leader must be certain that he or she knows the group's feelings before using this technique. "Sue, I sense that the other members of the group are becoming impatient with your unwillingness to make a decision. No solution is ever perfect, but I believe we do have enough information to proceed."

Conflict

Differences of opinion in a group are not necessarily a problem. In fact, they may indicate a high degree of interest in the goal and a high level of commitment to the tasks of the group. However, it is possible for healthy conflict to become heated enough to make others in the group uncomfortable or to interfere with the group's ability to make decisions or take action. This kind of conflict may be dealt with in a straightforward manner in which the behavior is described, its effect on the group is pointed out, and the desired change in behavior is clearly stated. "Juan and Michael, you both seem to feel very strongly about this issue, but your heated discussion is making others uncomfortable, and we don't seem to be getting any closer to agreement. We need to work out some kind of compromise that you both are comfortable with. Would each of you consider what areas of common ground you see?" If the individuals themselves are not able to see areas in which compromise is possible, the leader may make suggestions for compromise. If a conflict between two members seems to stem from a lack of understanding of each other's points of view, the leader might offer to interpret the viewpoints. "Ivan, I think you have missed Ann's main point. It is really similar to what you were saying a while ago. Ann, would you explain what you meant?"

Sometimes the conflict is healthy, and the different viewpoints need to be fully explored. The leader might want to highlight the opposing viewpoints and solicit input from other group members. "Jessie, you believe that we should not use our limited funds for the convention expenses. On the other hand, Rachel, you were saying you believed representation at the convention was important for us. What are the opinions of some of you others?"

Conflict that arises from struggles for prestige or power in the group or from personal attacks by one member on another are more problematic. It is important that the leader not put others down or cause them to feel that they have lost face in the group. Focusing on "I" statements (that is, statements of one's own feelings) and then suggesting another course of action may be helpful. "I feel uncomfortable when you speak like that to Kim. Let's talk about the issue. How can we get a better turnout at our next program?" Sometimes it is helpful for the group to discuss the problem behavior before returning to the task. However, be wary of becoming mired down in personal problems that keep the group from ever being successful at its task. If the goal of the group is to assist with personal behavioral growth, then discussing problem behavior is essential. The leader must exercise judgment in deciding when such a discussion would be helpful. "Maria and Sophie, something seems to be going on between the two of you that is making you both angry. I think we need to clear that up before we go on."

Conflict resolution is a current topic frequently discussed among theorists on group behavior. Many suggest using someone outside the group, called a consultant or facilitator. When conflicts are serious and cannot easily be resolved within the group itself, this method is useful. First, the consultant is an objective person who has no vested interest in particular "sides" of a question. Second, the consultant usually has special expertise and understanding of group process and can use that knowledge to bring factions together and restore cohesiveness. This is most useful when the conflict is an ongoing problem and the group must continue to work together for some time.

Analyzing a Group

To enhance your own understanding of groups and to facilitate the functioning of groups of which you are a part, it is often helpful to analyze a particular group.

You will find it helpful to analyze both the structure and the functioning or process of the group. You will also want to examine the content of group discussions and evaluate the effectiveness of the group in accomplishing its goals.

Identifying Structure

Identifying the structure of a group is the easiest step and therefore should usually be done first. Look at the size, the membership, the meeting times, and how long the group has been functioning together. You might want to identify how often new members join the group, whether old members have left, and whether all members are present at every session. It is important to know if the group has a specific time limit for existence. If the group has a clearly stated goal or purpose, you should learn what that goal is.

Analyzing Group Processes

Analyzing group process is complex. To do a thorough study, you often must be an outside observer rather than a participant. However, you can study some of the group process while remaining a participant. You will need to look at each of the factors discussed previously and identify patterns of behavior. Which group members have assigned roles? Do these people complete their assigned roles well? What functional roles are members of the group assuming? Are these functional roles facilitating the work of the group or blocking the work of the group?

Power and influence can often be determined by examining communication patterns. A tool known as the sociogram is often used for this task. Draw a diagram of the group. Each time an individual speaks, draw an arrow out from that person on the diagram toward the person to whom the speaker is directing his or her remarks. After a while you will be able to see to whom most of the remarks are directed, which individuals do most of the talking, and who remains silent. The person to whom most of the remarks are directed is usually the person with the most power in the group. A single individual may direct most of his or her remarks to the person who has the most influence over him or herself (Fig. 14-5).

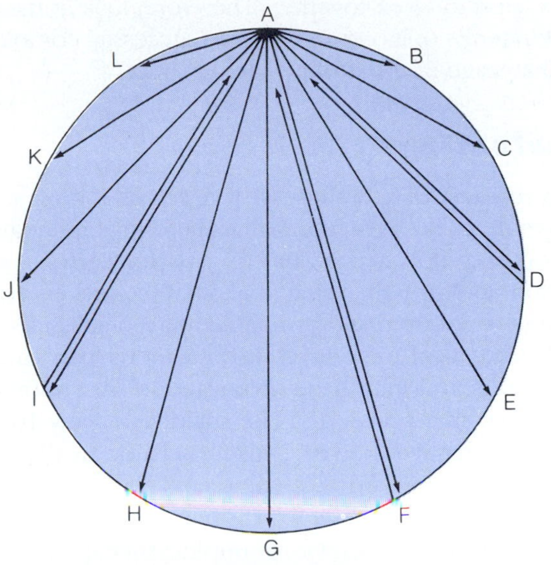

Figure 14-5. A sociogram of a 12-person group. This depiction of a short interaction demonstrates that person A is doing most of the talking and all other remarks are directed to person A. This pattern reveals that person A has power and influence in the group.

Some norms in a group are clearly stated, but many norms must be identified by observing how the individuals in the group behave. What behaviors are accepted or even rewarded? What behaviors are discouraged or ignored? The decision-making method may not be apparent if no decisions are made at a particular meeting. You might ask group members how decisions are made or pose a small problem and ask them for a decision to observe the process used.

Cohesion is not a concrete, observable behavior. Cohesion must often be inferred from the behavior and comments of the group. Generally, you can determine that cohesion is sufficient when group members faithfully attend meetings, when they are willing to take on tasks for the group, and when they express pleasure at being part of it. Cohesion may be lacking when members frequently miss meetings, are unwilling to accept tasks, or act uninterested and bored at meetings.

You will want to examine the leadership style and how that leadership is carried through. Does the stated leadership style match the leadership style actually being used? For example, an official statement may indicate that the group is democratic, while an authoritarian mode is actually operating. In another instance, you may see a group with an appointed authoritarian leader who does not function, so that the group actually operates with laissez-faire leadership. The lack of congruence between the stated leadership style and the actual leadership style is sometimes the reason why a group is ineffective.

Focusing on the Content

To evaluate the *content* of the group interactions, you will need to know the stage of the group. Time spent in orientation, although not apparently directed toward the goal, will in the end enhance the group's ability to function. Actions that do not appear to be goal-directed may be important in the accommodation process as members learn to work together. Therefore, look at the content in terms of its contribution to successful completion of that stage of the group's life.

Evaluating Effectiveness

The real test of the success of a group is how well it meets its goals. Remember that there may be goals for action accomplished and also goals for personal satisfaction and growth. Some goals may be met even if all are not. A group that was unable to accomplish its original stated goal may have allowed individuals to learn new skills and may have given people an opportunity for social interaction and the making of new friends, and thus may be viewed with satisfaction by the members. Another group that completed the tasks and accomplished the concrete goal may have left members feeling that the group was an unpleasant experience because unstated goals related to personal relationships were not met.

Another factor that must be looked at in evaluating effectiveness is the time expended by the group. Do the group members believe that the time was appropriate, or do they feel that the value of the time used was greater than the value of the goal accomplished? This is a subjective evaluation, but one that is important in determining future action. In a group consisting of employees of an agency, if the members are functioning on time for which they are paid, the cost of the time can be calculated for a budget. If too much time is spent, the employer may decide that use of a group for some tasks is not financially responsible. Some goals are time specific. A school group might be completing a project for an end-of-semester grade. No matter how good the project, it will be less valuable if not completed until after the end of the semester.

A group might evaluate itself on an ongoing basis to improve its functioning. In this case, group members might be asked to look at structure and process and to provide feedback to the group to permit constructive change. Groups that expect to continue, those that are aimed at meeting interpersonal needs, and those that are having difficulties in completing tasks might especially consider this approach. The evaluation must be carefully thought out to be seen by group members as a positive step in improving group functioning rather than a threat.

Nursing Care Study
Group Decision-Making For Care

Martha Wilson, an 80-year-old woman with a history of Alzheimer's disease was admitted on the evening shift after a fall that resulted in a fractured hip. Throughout the night she has been noisy, yelling out, and disturbing others on the unit. She was incontinent and the night nurse expressed concern that Mrs. Wilson's skin would not tolerate this added irritation.

Jennifer Lopez was the team leader for the team assigned to care for Mrs. Wilson during the day shift. Jennifer notified her team that Mrs. Wilson would be the major topic of their conference that morning. She asked that each person think about what their plan of care should include.

After initial assessments were completed, the team met in the conference room. Jennifer came down the hall with a tired-looking, middle-aged woman. She introduced the staff to Mrs. Wilson's daughter, Mrs. Simmons, and suggested that with her help they would be able to plan more effectively. Jennifer encouraged Mrs. Wilson's daughter to tell them how they managed at home. The rest of the team then made suggestions. Gradually they combined their suggestions and decided together on a plan of care. When they had completed the plan, Jennifer turned to Mrs. Simmons and said, "I really think you need to go home and get some rest. This has been a difficult night for you." Mrs. Simmons replied, "I didn't think I would be willing to leave her, but planning with you has really been helpful. Now I know that everyone understands her problems and I think I can go home."

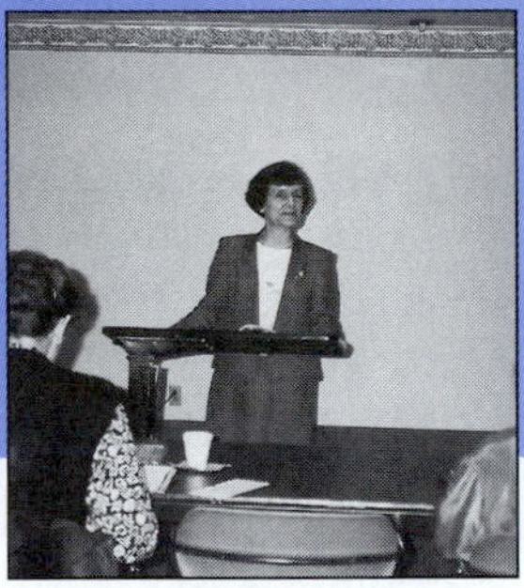

Key Points

- A primary group is the most important personal group of the individual. Secondary groups are those groups a person joins for a limited time; they can be informal, semiformal, or formal.
- Group structure involves the size of the group, its membership, its meeting times, and the stability of the relationships and roles within it.
- Group process or group dynamics refers to the way in which the group functions. Aspects of group process include assigned roles, functional roles, power, influence, norms, the decision-making method, and group cohesion.
- Leadership in a group may be autocratic or leader-centered, democratic, laissez-faire, or a combination of these. The appropriate leadership pattern depends largely on the nature of the group and its goals.
- Groups move through stages as they function. Orientation is the formation of the group and the establishment of goals. Accommodation is the beginning of working together. Negotiation is the decision-making stage of group life. Operation is the action phase in which the decisions are carried out. Dissolution or termination is the process of ending the group and its relationships.
- The functioning of a group may be facilitated by the members and its leader. Meeting the physical and psychosocial needs of the group will enhance function. Physical needs include time, space, and comfort. Psychosocial needs include common goals, action, a sense of accomplishment, and personal satisfaction in the group.
- An effective group member understands the group, is willing to compromise, is focused on the group goal, expresses concern for others, is direct and honest in communication, shares responsibility, and accepts tasks.
- The effective group leader must take a broad view of the group, plan for the physical needs of the group, and facilitate the movement of the group through its various stages. Competition, lack of motivation, blocking behaviors, and conflict all interfere with the group function.
- To work more effectively with a group, the nurse needs to study its structure, its function, the group process, and the content of the group's interaction. This helps the nurse to become a more effective participant in groups and a more effective leader.

Study Questions

1. Describe a situation in which you have worked with a group as a student.
2. List the size, membership, and meeting time of the above group and describe the stability of the relationships.
3. What is a functional role in a group?
4. Describe two functional roles that tend to enhance group function?
5. Describe two functional roles that tend to inhibit group function?
6. How does a laissez-faire group make decisions?
7. How could a group member help the group to cope with a person who continually puts down others?
8. What can a group member do to ensure achievement of the goal?
9. What are three of the special functions of the group leader?
10. How can conflict be constructive in a group?
11. How does competition interfere with group function?
12. List the aspects you should consider when analyzing a group.

Critical Thinking Activities

1. Analyze a group to which you belong. What is the leadership style of that group? List all the characteristics of the group that influenced your decision about leadership style.
2. In a group meeting, analyze behaviors and statements of group members in relationship to the roles each person fills. What roles discussed in the chapter were present in that group? Identify the roles that were not present.
3. Review your own participation in your clinical or discussion group. Evaluate your own behavior by comparing it with the characteristics of an effective group member given in the text. If you identify any areas in which you need growth, plan how you might change your own behavior to enhance the functioning of your group.

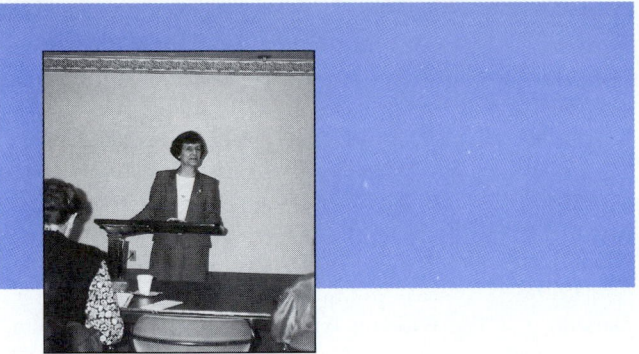

4. In your clinical or discussion group, appoint one person as process recorder and another as content recorder. After the session ends (or at the beginning of your next meeting), review the process and content of your group.

References and Readings

Bass, B. M. *Leadership, Psychology, and Organizational Behavior.* New York: Harper & Row, 1973.

Bass, B. M. and Stogdill, R. M. *Stogdill's Handbook of Leadership,* 3rd ed. New York: Macmillan, 1981.

Beeber, L. S., and Schmitt, M. H. "Cohesiveness in Groups: A Concept in Search of a Definition." *Advances in Nursing Science* 8, 2 (January 1986): 1–11.

Cartwright, D., and Zander, A. *Group Dynamics.* New York: Harper & Row, 1968.

Clark, C. C. *The Nurse as Group Leader.* 2nd edition. New York: Springer Publishing, 1987.

Ellis, J. R., and Hartley, C. L. *Managing and Coordinating Nursing Care.* Philadelphia: J. B. Lippincott, 1991.

Fontes, H. C. "Small Group Work: A Strategy to Promote Active Learning." *Journal of Nursing Education* 26, 5 (May 1987): 212–213.

Hare, P. *Handbook of Small Group Research.* New York: Free Press, 1962.

Hare, P., Borgette, E., and Balec, R. *Small Groups: Studies in Social Interaction.* New York: Alfred A. Knopf, 1962.

Hershey, P., and Duldt, B. W. *Situational Leadership In Nursing.* Norwalk, Conn.: Appleton-Lange, 1988.

Johnson, D., and Johnson, F. *Joining Together Group Theory and Group Skills.* Englewood Cliffs, N.J.: Prentice-Hall, 1975.

Kron, T. "How to Become a Better Leader." *Nursing '76* 6 (October 1976): 67–68.

Larson, M. L., and Williams, R. A. "How to Become a Better Group Leader: Learn to Recognize the Strange Things That Happen to Some People in Groups." *Nursing '78* 8 (August 1978): 65–72.

Loomis, M. E. *Group Process for Nurses.* St. Louis: C. V. Mosby, 1979.

Mariano, C. "The Case for Inter-Disciplinary Collaboration." *Nursing Outlook* 37, 6 (June 1989): 285–288.

Olmstead, M. *The Small Group.* New York: Random House, 1959.

Robbins, S. P. *Managing Organizational Conflict.* Englewood Cliffs, N.J.: Prentice-Hall, 1974.

Roseman, E. "Improving Your Interpersonal Skills: Understanding Your Role in Group Dynamics: Part 4." *Medical Laboratory Observer* 10 (July 1978): 47–52.

Sampson, E., and Marthas, M. *Group Process for the Health Professions.* 2nd edition. New York: John Wiley and Sons, 1981.

Small, L. L. "Finding Your Leadership Style in Groups." *American Journal of Nursing* 80, 7 (July 1980): 1301–1303.

Smith, W. S. *Group Problem-Solving Through Discussion.* Indianapolis: Bobbs-Merrill, 1965.

Trojan, A. "Benefits of Self-Help Groups: A Survey of 232 Members from 65 Disease-Related Groups." *Social Science and Medicine* 29, 2 (February 1989): 225–232.

Whitman, H. H., Gustafson, J. P., and Coleman, F. W. "Leaders and Members." *American Journal of Nursing* 79 (May 1979): 910–913.

Coordinating Care

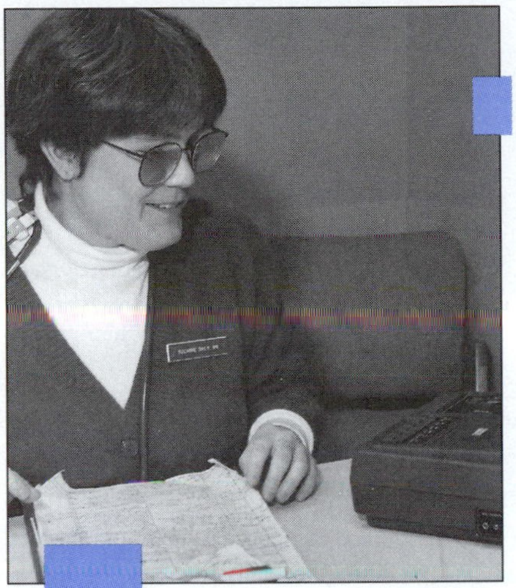

15

Objectives

After completing this chapter, you should be able to:

1. Identify essential elements for the student to communicate when reporting on and off duty.
2. Identify essential elements of an intershift report.
3. Explain the focus of team conferences.
4. State the purposes of the patient/client record.
5. Differentiate between traditional narrative charting, the problem-oriented record, and charting by exception.
6. Identify a variety of ways to support the effective functioning of a nursing team.
7. Explain how the nurse can coordinate care provided by various health care disciplines.
8. List ways a nurse can ensure continuity of care.
9. Outline ways in which the nurse can act as a patient advocate.

Study Terms

advocate
coordination of care
data base
discharge planner
flow sheets
incident report
initial plan
intershift report
narrative charting
problem list
problem-oriented record (POR)
progress notes
report
SOAPing
walking rounds

Outline

Verbal Communication in the Coordination of Care

Reporting On and Off Duty
Intershift Reports
Communication With the Physician

Written Communication in the Coordination of Care

Written Plans for Nursing Care
Documenting Care in the Chart or Record
Computerized Records
Quality Assurance or Incident Reports

Working with a Nursing Team

Team Conferences
Sharing Knowledge

Ellis, Nowlis: Nursing: A Human Needs Approach, 5th ed. © 1994 J.B. Lippincott Company

Delegating Care
Supporting Colleagues
Encouraging Growth

Coordinating Care of Other Disciplines

Scheduling Procedures
Interdisciplinary Teamwork

Ensuring Continuity of Care

Teaching for Home Care
Community Resources
Discharge Planning
Making a Referral

Acting as a Patient Advocate

Coordination of care means facilitating the functioning of the health care team to provide better care. It is primarily based on effective communication within the health care team. Some communication with other personnel will be oral and some written. Clarity and accuracy of both spoken and written communication are crucial concerns in health care because of the potential adverse consequences of poor or failed communication.

Beginning nurses often mistakenly think that coordination is a function only of nurses in supervisory or administrative positions. On the contrary, any nurse must be concerned from the outset with the total context of the health care situation and its impact on the patient. In all daily activities, you can help the system function more effectively for the patient's benefit.

Verbal Communication in the Coordination of Care

Your first experiences in coordinating care are likely to involve verbal **reports**, which you give to another nurse when you are reporting on and off duty and which are used for giving and receiving intershift reports. Everything you know and will learn about communication will be pertinent to this aspect of your practice. You will use skills of questioning, giving information, encouraging others to speak, and other pertinent skills.

Reporting On and Off Duty

When you arrive as a student on a unit to care for patients, you are in a unique position because you are not part of the current staff of that unit. You may be unfamiliar with the routines of the facility and the location of equipment, and the regular staff will not know you or your abilities. Although your instructor will communicate with the staff on your behalf, this cannot take the place of your own communication with staff members.

A staff nurse will have been assigned to each of your patients. This staff nurse has ultimate responsibility for care delivered. Find out who this staff person is and arrange a meeting. Communicate clearly what your abilities and responsibilities are. State straightforwardly the limits of your own abilities and what you expect to accomplish with the patient. If the patient has needs you are not yet prepared to fulfill (such as need for a procedure you have not yet learned), clarify this with the other caregiver. This staff member should be informed throughout the day if any changes occur. In addition, the staff nurse is a resource for questions you may have. If you will be on the unit for less than a full shift, it is important to find out who will be responsible for all aspects of care of your patients after you leave. You may need to communicate with more than one person if a registered nurse is responsible for overall care and another team member will be doing some aspects of the care.

When you leave the unit, whether for a break or at the end of your assigned stay, you must again contact the staff person to outline what has been accomplished and to communicate the patient's status. You may also be expected to report off to a team leader or charge nurse, in addition to the person assigned for care. Conscientiously maintaining clear communication with the staff will support positive relationships among all students and staff members.

Intershift Reports

Most health care facilities require an oral report between one shift and the next (such as the night shift and the day shift), called an **intershift report**. The purpose of the intershift report is to ensure continuity of care for the patient. To do this, the departing nurse provides essential assessment data and a brief overview of essential care needs for each patient.

When you are receiving a report, the extent of the notes you take will be determined by the nature of your responsibilities. If your responsibility is clearly limited to one or two patients, you will want to note carefully all information about those patients. If your responsibilities include answering call lights and serving meals to other patients, you will need to take notes on the diagnosis, activity level, and diet of each patient. Figure 15-1 illustrates a form on which you might record information received at an intershift report.

If you are responsible for giving a report, you must prepare carefully. Some facilities specify the information to be included; others rely on the individual nurse to decide what to include. The intershift report form might also be used to record information you wish to include when giving a report.

After reviewing or deciding what to include, make careful notes so that you have all the facts at hand. In giving reports nurses usually use a card index or notebook containing basic care information on all the patients. Proceed through the card index carefully, checking your notes periodically so that you do not forget any important information. Go slowly enough to allow those to whom you are reporting to take notes and ask questions. Although time should not be wasted, hurrying can cause incomplete communication.

Some facilities ask that nurses tape-record their intershift reports (Fig. 15-2). Doing this allows the nurse to prepare the report away from the distractions and interruptions of the change of shift period; it may also result in a decrease in socialization during the report time, so that time is used more efficiently. If you will be preparing a tape-recorded report, prepare ahead of time just as for an oral report. Most units identify essential information they wish to have included because there will be no opportunities for asking questions. Always double-check the tape recorder to be sure you have a tape, and if you are the first person to begin taping, that it has been rewound. Check the controls to be sure you know how to start and stop recording. Be sure to speak clearly into the microphone. Do not rush because this may make your speech less intelligible. If you must pause to collect your thoughts, check notes, or find needed data, stop the recorder temporarily (usually a pause button is available for this purpose) and restart the recorder when you are ready to resume speaking. This eliminates time-wasting waits for the listeners. When you are first learning to tape reports, it is wise to listen to your own recordings. This will help you to recognize areas in which you need to improve.

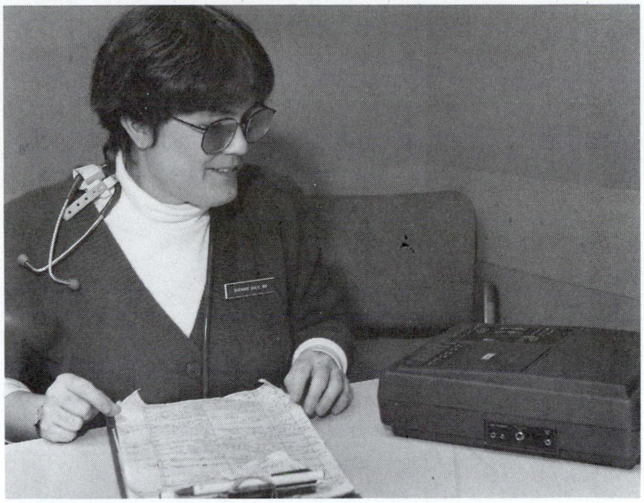

Figure 15-2. Tape-recording an intershift report allows the nurse to prepare the report away from the distractions and interruptions of the change-of-shift period.

Walking rounds are used for intershift report in some facilities. In **walking rounds**, the nurse who is leaving escorts the oncoming nurse to the patient's bedside. The report is given there with specific observations directly pointed out, and the patient is included in the conversation. Care must be taken to explain unfamiliar terminology and encourage the patient to ask questions. Under no circumstances should conversations occur over the patient as if the individual were not capable of hearing or participating. Such conduct may make the patient angry or anxious. If information that could be anxiety producing needs to be communicated between staff members, it should be discussed before entering

Room	Name	Diagnosis Surg & Date	Physician	Activity	Diet	Pertinent Assessment Data I & O	Drsg.	Tubes Drains	I.V.	Other
208	John James	Diabetic Ing. hernia Rep. 12/5	Evans	up ad lib	Reg	—	Clean + Dry	—	—	no pain
209A	Stella Washington	Chole 12/6	Jefferson	Chair t.i.d.	NPO	V, O.K. 250/1175	Clean + dry	N.G. to suction	D5W	
209B	Vacant									
210A	Judy Brown	abd. hyst. 12/5	Cole	up	soft	950-(low) 820	mod. sero. sang.		out ⓒ10	Gas

Figure 15-1. Intershift report form.

the room, while out of the patient's hearing. Walking rounds may be more time consuming than a conventional report, but the direct interaction with the patient promotes cooperative planning of care and includes the patient as a full participant in the health care process. Walking rounds also support a high level of continuity of care.

Communication With the Physician

Effective communication between the nurse and the physician is critical to high-quality care. Because the nurse must ensure that medical prescriptions are carried out, nurses must clarify any aspects of the medical plan they do not clearly understand. The nurse must clearly communicate observations and concerns that arise when the physician is not present. Routine information about such matters as stable vital signs, a wound that is progressing as expected, the patient's response to a medication, and so forth is communicated in the patient's chart. However, even for routine matters, personal communication is often more effective in ensuring that the physician has received information important to medical decision-making.

Many nursing students are reluctant to communicate with physicians because as students they lack self-confidence or are unsure of how the physician will respond to a student. If you consider the patient as your first priority and plan your communication carefully, you will generally find that the physician welcomes communication that will help to support high-quality care.

When you have information you believe should be communicated, you may feel more sure of yourself if you first check with your instructor or the staff nurse caring for the patient. Make sure that your data are correct and that you have all of the relevant information. Consider your purpose and whether you are asking the physician to take action. If so, you need to be clear as to what you are asking. Consider whether the information should be shared in front of the patient or out of the patient's hearing. Determine whether the information needs to be communicated immediately by telephone or whether it can wait until the next time the physician visits the patient. To gain self-confidence, you may find it helpful to rehearse your message with your instructor or the staff nurse.

Written Communication in the Coordination of Care

Many different types of written communication are used in health care. Although nurses understandably get frustrated when excessive time is consumed with paperwork, most agree that clear, accurate records are necessary to providing quality care. Time spent on these records is by no means wasted; it is part of patient care. As a practicing nurse, you will, of course, want to facilitate any effort to make record-keeping more efficient and less time consuming, so that it does not detract from direct care.

Written Plans for Nursing Care

The primary purpose of a written plan for nursing care is to communicate to the entire nursing care team what is to be done for the patient. Its secondary purpose is to serve as evidence that the patient is receiving ongoing and appropriate nursing care based on the nursing process. Written documentation is being required more and more by the federal government (through Medicare and Medicaid) and insurance carriers for purposes of evaluating health care. Nurses also use written records to evaluate and improve patient care; care reviews are routinely undertaken by nursing committees within the employing institution. Finally, accrediting bodies require documentation of the plan for nursing care for each patient.

The initial nursing care plan, usually written by the nurse responsible for admitting the patient, is based on the initial nursing history and examination. Figure 11-3 illustrates how a standard nursing care plan may be adapted for use with an individual patient.

The nursing care plan must be updated and reviewed on an ongoing basis. This responsibility may be assigned to the primary nurse, who is responsible and accountable for the patient's care, or it may be shared by all the nurses who care for the patient. In general, the nursing care plan is more likely to be kept up-to-date if one nurse is responsible.

Whether or not one person is responsible, others can contribute ideas and information to the nursing care plan. As a nursing student, you have a responsibility to determine the appropriate procedure for updating a care plan. Then, when you feel you have something to contribute, you can follow through by consulting with the appropriate nurse.

Because the nursing care plan is the nurse's responsibility, nurses must be able to appraise both content and form critically to ascertain whether the plan is fulfilling its purposes adequately. In evaluating any written nursing care plan, you may use the following questions as guidelines:

1. Can the patient's current problems be quickly discerned?
2. Are the desired patient outcomes, both immediate and long term, identified and clearly stated and measurable?

3. Are the prescribed nursing actions based on sound rationale?
4. Are the prescribed nursing actions stated clearly enough that anyone responsible for care can follow them accurately?

The written plan for nursing care may be in a card index (Kardex), on a separate sheet on the chart, or in any of a variety of other locations. The only requirement is that the plan be available to those who care for the patient. In some settings, nursing care plans are erased, changed, and eventually discarded when the patient is discharged. Although this approach makes it easier to change the care plan as the patient's needs change, it greatly hampers continuing review of the situation and subsequent evaluation. Sample nursing care plans were presented in the chapters on the nursing process and will be used as examples throughout the text.

Documenting Care in the Chart or Record

The patient's chart or record is a tool for communication among health care team members about the patient's illness, therapies, tests, and response to care. It is the legal record of care and as such may be used in a court proceeding. The chart is also used for monitoring quality of care and for conducting research.

All members of the health care team have responsibilities for the patient's official record, but nurses are usually charged with primary responsibility for seeing that the record is properly set up, that all pertinent forms and records are added when they become available, and that the chart accompanies a patient who moves within the health care system for treatments and tests. After the patient has been discharged, the medical records department assumes responsibility for the record, reviews it for completeness, obtains missing information, and stores the record for use in various evaluation, statistical, and research programs. The record is available for reference if the patient is readmitted.

In addition to assuming overall responsibility for the chart, the nurse must also record data related to the nursing process: assessment data, including subjective and objective information and problems; nursing actions; and evaluation of the effectiveness of those actions. Keep in mind that you need to record enough information to communicate adequately with other members of the health care team and to demonstrate the level of care provided. Many evaluation systems operate on the assumption that actions not recorded have not been performed. Adequate recording is also a legal safeguard for you personally. If questions arise about the appropriateness or adequacy of care, the chart is accepted as proof of the care given. See *Modules for Basic Nursing Skills*, Volume I, Module 6, Documentation, for detailed directions on charting techniques.

Traditional Narrative Charting

Traditional **narrative charting** provides separate forms for each discipline caring for the patient: doctor's progress notes, nurse's notes, a physical therapy record, and others involved in the patient's care. Each discipline records information gathered and actions taken on the appropriate form. Routine information is also recorded on a variety of graphs and checklists (Fig. 15-3).

The nurse's notes are usually organized chronologically. For each shift, the nurse notes both subjective and objective assessment data, problems identified, actions taken, and evaluation of those actions. The narrative may be modified to organize information around body systems, human needs, or in any other manner agreed on by the facility.

Most people find traditional narrative notes easier to write than those requiring a special format. This may increase their willingness to make appropriate entries in the chart. New types of information can be included in the narration without difficulty. For precisely the same

DATE ▶ ▼ TIME ▼	5/22/94 NURSING PROGRESS RECORD
09	CV BP remains stable, H.R. reg @ 64-68, slight ankle
	edema noted on both extremities over malleoli.
	Resp Lungs clear to auscultation, RR @ 16-20.
	NO S.O.B. states breathing much better than
	yesterday. Occ. prod cough with clear, white mucus.
	A. Richard RN

Figure 15-3. Traditional narrative charting.

reasons, however, a narrative record may be disorganized; it may be difficult to find needed information without reading through paragraphs of irrelevant narration. Module 6, Documentation, includes examples of adaptations of narrative charting that make it more organized.

Problem-Oriented Records

The **problem-oriented record (POR)**, or problem-oriented medical record (POMR) as it is sometimes called, is designed to encourage all members of the health care team to use a problem-solving approach to patient care and to organize the record so that information is readily available (Weed, 1970).

The basic components of the POR are 1) the data base, 2) the problem list, 3) the initial plan, 4) progress notes, and 5) flow sheets. The **data base** consists of all initial information on the patient, the physician's history and physical examination, the nursing admission interview and examination, and the admitting laboratory work. The patient's admitting problems are identified from the data base and are stated with as much specificity as possible. If later information provides more insight or allows for more accurate labeling of a problem, the statement of that problem will be revised. Each problem is then numbered and titled, and the resulting **problem list** serves as a combined table of contents and index to the record (Fig. 15-4). If further problems are identified, they are added to the list; when problems are resolved, their resolution is noted on the problem list.

The **initial plan** outlines what will be done for the patient initially, including any further diagnostic studies, specific treatment, plans for patient education, or plans for eventual discharge. The physician usually writes the initial problem list and plan.

Progress notes are written by all members of the health care team and are organized in a specific manner commonly referred to as **SOAPing**—an acronym for the order in which information is entered in the progress note (Fig. 15-5). First, the problem under discussion is identified by number and title. Then *S*ubjective information (symptoms) is recorded, followed by *O*bjective information. Next comes an *A*nalysis of the data (Weed calls this step assessment, a slightly different use of the term than is common in nursing). This might include the initial nursing diagnosis or statement of the problem. After the initial note, there is an evaluation of progress made toward resolving the problem or additional information regarding etiology of the problem. Finally, a *P*lan of action is specified. Progress notes need not always contain all these elements. For example, if the patient is unable to respond, no subjective data would be recorded. Similarly, if you have nothing new to add to the analysis of data, you would not include that section in your progress note. Module 6, Documentation, includes examples and directions for writing SOAP prog-

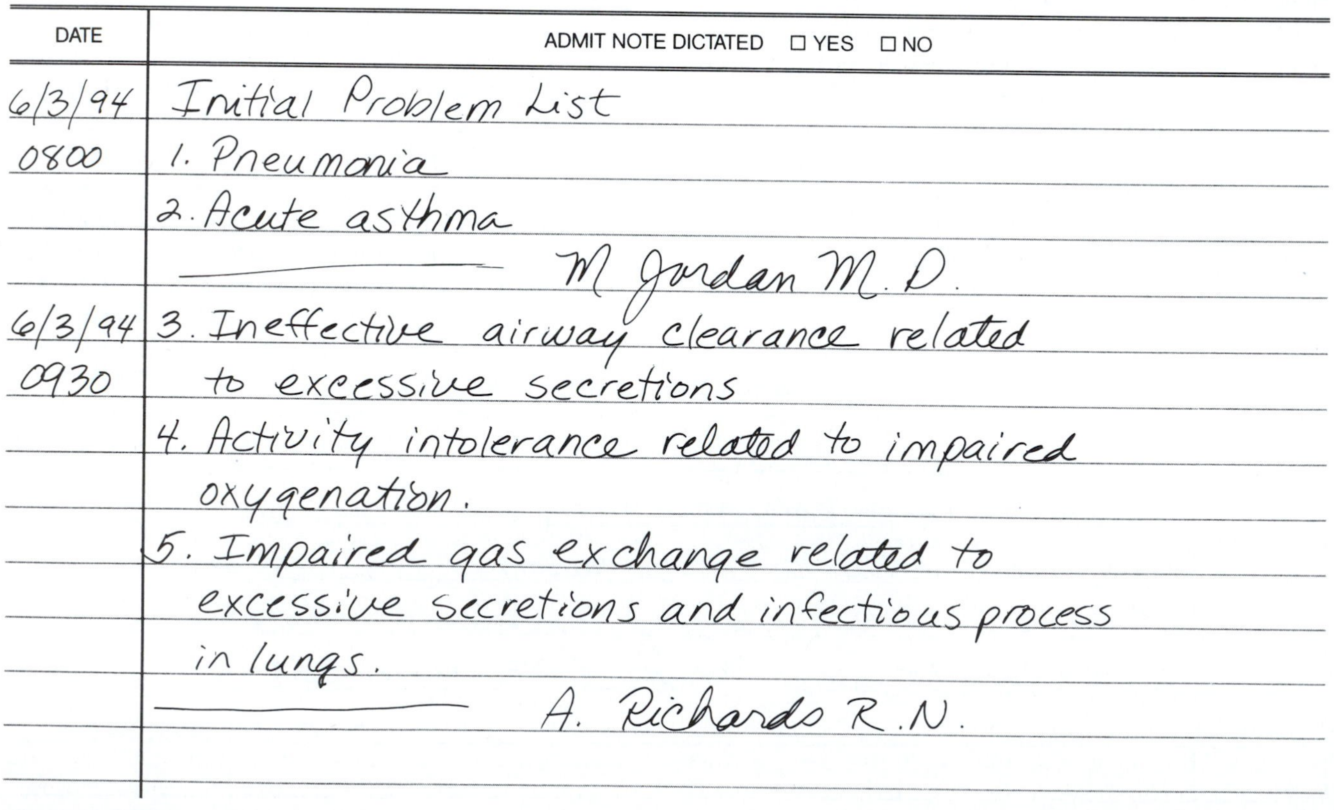
DATE	ADMIT NOTE DICTATED ☐ YES ☐ NO
6/3/94	Initial Problem List
0800	1. Pneumonia
	2. Acute asthma
	M Jordan M.D.
6/3/94	3. Ineffective airway clearance related
0930	to excessive secretions
	4. Activity intolerance related to impaired
	oxygenation.
	5. Impaired gas exchange related to
	excessive secretions and infectious process
	in lungs.
	A. Richards R.N.

Figure 15-4. Master problem list.

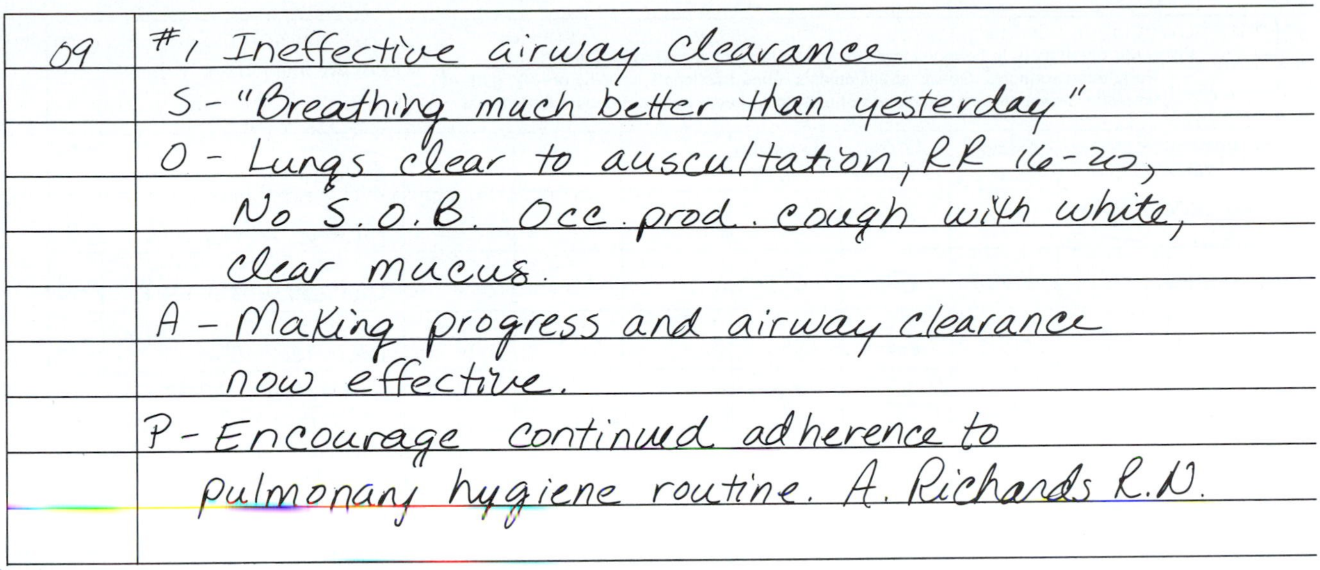
09 #1 Ineffective airway clearance
S - "Breathing much better than yesterday"
O - Lungs clear to auscultation, RR 16-20, No S.O.B. Occ. prod. cough with white, clear mucus.
A - Making progress and airway clearance now effective.
P - Encourage continued adherence to pulmonary hygiene routine. A. Richards R.N.

Figure 15-5. POMR progress note.

ress notes. Some hospitals have expanded the SOAP notation to include a section labeled "I" for *I*ntervention. In Weed's original work, the expected interventions would be recorded on flow sheets. Some hospitals have also added a section labeled "E" for *E*valuation. In Weed's format the data underlying the evaluation would be recorded under "S" and "O." The summary analyzing that data would be recorded under "A."

The last part of the POR consists of **flow sheets**—graphs and charts used to record simple data most easily absorbed in that form. Flow sheets reduce the volume of narration and the bulk of the chart while providing a record of important information (Fig. 15-6). They are commonly used for recurring information such as activity, vital signs, neurologic checks, and wound condition.

The advantages of the POR are that it encourages a problem-solving approach, all team members record on the same form and thus see one another's comments, redundancy is reduced, and the chart is less voluminous. Another advantage is the ease with which the course of a specific problem may be followed through the record.

A disadvantage is that POR charting is new to many health care providers and thus extensive in-service education may be needed to implement it. Another potential drawback is that people occasionally omit information that they believe should be recorded because they cannot find a place for it within the structure of the chart. The solution to this dilemma is to consult with others to decide where the information can be added, even if it means beginning a new flow sheet or checklist. Recording one-time actions may also be a problem on a POR because they do not fit easily into the progress note or merit a flow sheet. This problem may be solved by recording on the progress note that the action is planned and then adding a date, time, signature, and the word "done" when it is completed.

Perhaps the biggest problem arises when a particular item of data is pertinent to a number of problems, such as in the case of a critically ill patient. In this situation, data might be organized by body systems and all relevant problems charted together. The POR is most successful when such difficulties are approached creatively and not treated as stumbling blocks.

Charting by Exception

To make charting effective but less time consuming, some facilities have adopted a system called *charting by exception.* In this charting system, a standard data base is established along with a description of norms for each area of the standard data base. In all areas in which the patient exhibits the norms, the nurse simply checks a box or in some other way indicates that this area was assessed. Only in those areas in which the patient does not meet the norms, that is an *exception* exists, is a more extensive note made. In addition, if the same data persist, the nurse does not need to rewrite the description, but indicates by an arrow or asterisk or some other sign that the same condition continues. The nurse has much less writing to do because the majority of areas of assessment will be normal. Charting time is then used to describe those areas that are problematic and not used for repetitive recording of factors that have not changed.

Focus Charting

Another approach to decrease the time invested in record-keeping is *focus charting.* Focus charting is similar to problem-oriented charting in that the narrative record is limited and flow sheets are used for routine information. In this style of charting, the areas of concern for

PARAMETER FLOW SHEET

Fill in the parameters to be monitored. Refer to Standard & Individual Care Plans.
Parameter examples: Guaiac stools/emesis, urine fractionals, specific gravity, girth of limb/abd, bowel sounds, circulation of extremity, pedal pulses, frequent lab values.

Parameters		Routine Insulin	Blood Glucose	urine Acetone	Insulin Cover				Dietary Intake	Initial
Date	Time									
5/26/94	0630	Lente 22U	110	0	0				BKfst - Ate all	PB
	1130		140	0	0				Lunch - Ate all	AR
	1630		130	0	0				Dinner - Ate All	CG
	2030		180	0	Reg. 2u				Evening snack - Ate all	CG

Identify Initials with Signature:	4.	8.
1. PB P. Bonham RN	5.	9.
2. AR A. Reynolds RN	6.	10.
3. CG C. Gray RN	7.	11.

ADDRESSOGRAPH:
John O. Doe
000-00-0000

SWEDISH HOSPITAL MEDICAL CENTER
Seattle, Washington

NU-1549 Nursing Rev. 3/86 FC/SHMC SN-6115

PARAMETER FLOW SHEET

Figure 15-6. Flow sheet.

the patient are considered areas of focus. This is a somewhat broader concept than the problem-oriented method. Charting structure is not as formalized as in the problem-oriented format.

Abbreviations and Charting Style

The typically extensive use of abbreviations and incomplete statements in patients' charts and care plans often makes them hard to read. Module 6, Documentation, illustrates how to simplify statements when charting. Appendix B consists of a list of common abbreviations; you may also wish to ask whether your facility has a list of approved abbreviations. Appendix C provides a list of abbreviations of common medical diagnoses. You may need to look up an abbreviated diagnosis in this list before consulting your other reference books for information on nursing care. Appendix D lists prefixes and suffixes combined to form medical terms. Familiarity with these terms will make it much easier to understand patients' charts.

Computerized Records

Many health care facilities are computerizing their records for convenience and ease of retrieval. Usually the business and finance offices are the first areas to use computerized records. Ancillary services such as the pharmacy and the laboratory are often the next to begin using computers. Many nurses first become involved in using computerized records because of their contact with the laboratory. Laboratory data may be available on a computer terminal at the nursing station as soon as the test is completed, eliminating the lag time between the completion of the test and the delivery of the written report to the unit. A computer printer may be placed on the nursing unit, and routine medication records, census forms, and other such items may be printed as needed. The last area to put its records on the computer may be nursing.

Some hospitals are moving toward placing all nursing records in computers, in which case nurses must learn the new skills required to use the computer (Fig. 15-7). Many nurses fear this change unnecessarily because they believe that they will be expected to become computer experts. Just as those who write nursing notes do not need the skills of an author or a publisher, those who use computers do not need extensive skills related to computer programming and language. All they need is an open and inquiring mind, a willingness to use a keyboard instead of a pen, and careful attention to precise instructions.

Computers can be helpful in many areas, including the preparation of nursing care plans. A computer can store an extensive list of carefully written nursing diagnoses along with a list of the defining characteristics of each diagnosis and nursing actions that might be appropriate. A nurse might enter assessment data regarding the patient and then be presented with one or several nursing diagnoses containing defining characteristics that appeared in the data. After the nurse has chosen the appropriate diagnosis, the computer could be asked to generate a list of possible nursing activities. From this list the nurse could select those appropriate to the patient, modify them as needed, and then enter additional actions specific to this patient. The nurse could then have the computer print the total nursing care plan for the patient, including the current problem and all problems entered previously.

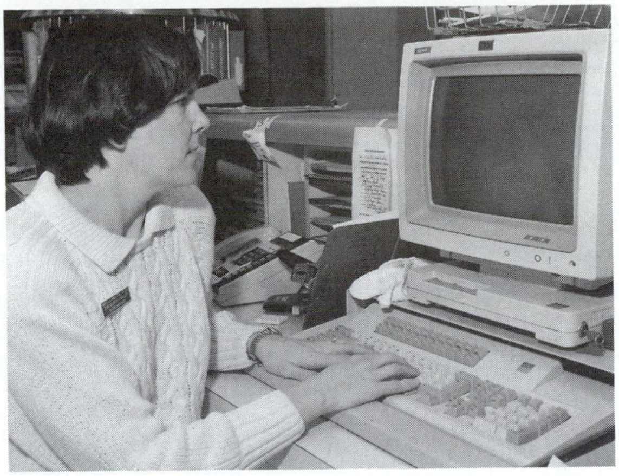

Figure 15-7. Nurses are learning to keep patient records on computers.

Patient charts can also be converted to computer. Instead of writing information, the nurse could sit at the computer and call up any patient's record. The correct information would then be entered via the keyboard. If entries were omitted, the computer could even prompt the nurse, such as reminding the nurse to fill in a section related to intake and output. Each nurse might have an individual code to verify access to records and to identify the "signature." Additional safeguards to protect confidentiality would also be needed.

Although use of computer records in nursing is costly to initiate, hospitals are moving in the direction of increased computerization and changes are occurring rapidly. Problems need to be solved and no system will ever be without flaws, but computers have the potential to assist nurses in providing high-quality care and to reduce the time spent in paperwork.

Quality Assurance or Incident Reports

Whenever an accident or error occurs in a health care facility, the nurse has two roles. The first role is providing immediate care and attention to any individual, whether patient, staff member, or visitor, who is injured. This care must always take precedence over routine concerns. The entire nursing process is required: assessment, planning for immediate intervention, determining whether a physician is necessary immediately, and carrying out the actions planned.

The second responsibility is related to preventing the same type of incident from being repeated and safeguarding the facility in case of legal action. This is usually accomplished by filing an **incident report** (sometimes called a quality assurance report), which is for the internal use of the facility in reviewing the incident, identifying ways it could have been prevented, and keeping a record of the facts for future use. Each facility has a specific form used to report untoward incidents. Incident reports should be clear, concise presentations of the facts of the situation. Opinions or conclusions are usually not wanted on an incident report; they may be asked for on a separate section, which is then detached from the factual document. Ideally, incident reports are used to collect information, to identify trends or special problem areas, and then to institute remedial action through education, new procedures, or structural changes (see Chapter 3).

Working with a Nursing Team

In the hospital, care is provided by nursing staff for 24 hours every day and 7 days every week. A high degree of coordination creates nursing care of consistently high quality. Even if team nursing is not the primary mode of care, the various nurses who care for a given patient constitute a team. Working effectively with this team is an important aspect of nursing. When you take part in team conferences and committees on nursing policies and procedures, reviewing the information on groups in Chapter 14 will help you participate most effectively.

Team Conferences

In facilities that use the team method of patient care, whereby a group of staff members work together to care for a group of patients, team conferences are held regularly. The purpose of such conferences may vary. Often the team conference is used to review the plans for the day and assign responsibilities to the team members. Some team conferences are devoted to discussing the care of a patient who presents particularly difficult nursing problems. Another purpose of the team conference is to explore a given aspect of care that may affect many patients, such as the admission nursing interview. Such a conference is more educational in intent.

A problem-oriented or educational team conference is an occasion for sharing. The better prepared each individual is to contribute, the more valuable the conference will be. To prepare, consider the topic or patient to be discussed. If a particular patient is involved, review the patient's chart. Then think about what you might contribute and about questions the team might discuss. If the conference has no predetermined subject, you might raise problems or topics you would like to have discussed. When you participate in team conferences, recall what you have learned about effective functioning in groups. Review Chapter 14 and consider how you can be supportive of the group's purpose.

Sharing Knowledge

On occasion an individual nurse is asked to lead a continuing education session for other nursing personnel. If, for example, a patient on your unit has a new type of colostomy irrigation and all staff members need to learn how it is to be done, one nurse may be asked to examine the literature on the subject, plan a presentation, and lead the class. As you become more experienced, this is a way you can contribute to the team. Using the teaching–learning principles outlined in Chapter 16, you will need to plan appropriate goals and objectives, select teaching methods suitable to the type of learning in question, and develop a means of evaluating learning. It is usually best to evaluate progress in such a way that only the person being evaluated knows his or her own evaluation results; this approach preserves the self-esteem of those having difficulties. You should also devise a method of evaluating your effectiveness as a teacher.

Delegating Care

Even if you are not a team leader, charge nurse, or head nurse, it sometimes becomes necessary to direct others in care. For example, you may have to direct a single nursing assistant with whom you are working or several students less experienced than yourself. A nursing process approach is suitable to such situations.

The first step in the nursing process approach to directing others is to assess carefully the abilities of those with whom you are working; spend a few minutes talking with the individuals about their past experience or consulting with other nurses. You will also need to know what the facility expects of an individual with a given job title. Is there a job description for nursing assistants? What kind of in-service preparation do nursing assistants in your facility receive?

The next step is to analyze the level of difficulty of each component of the task or assignment and decide what you will ask someone else to do and what you will need to do yourself. You should also plan a method of self-evaluation so that, after implementing your plan, you can evaluate the effectiveness of your decisions and actions.

Authoritarian relationships—in which the person in

charge simply tells other people what to do and checks to see that they have done it—tend to be effective in accomplishing many tasks in a short time. They are notably less effective, however, in terms of creating long-term job satisfaction. A more democratic and cooperative working relationship thus has important benefits for the patient as well as the health care worker. When people are satisfied with their jobs, they are more likely to manifest a positive attitude in their work and to apply their own problem-solving and creative abilities to improving patient care. Chapter 14 describes the functioning of a democratic group.

Supporting Colleagues

Occasionally some of your colleagues will experience problems related to working with patients. Many stressful events occur in health care facilities, and the demands on the emotional stability of caregivers can be extreme. Be sensitive to the feelings of those around you. People often need a genuinely concerned listener to help them sort out their feelings. Nurses can be helpful to one another by offering active listening when the occasion requires. For example, when a patient is difficult to care for or criticizes the nursing staff, some members of the nursing staff may become discouraged or self-doubting. By actively listening you can help them identify effective ways of responding, and by pointing out what they do well you can reinforce their feelings of self-esteem. In settings where nurses provide this kind of support to one another and to other caregivers, staff turnover is minimized and working relationships are more effective.

Encouraging Growth

Nursing is a highly demanding profession, and all nurses need to grow continually in knowledge and ability to care for patients. We can encourage one another in such growth by praising those who do well, acknowledging those who pursue continuing education, and refraining from personal criticism. When you notice that someone is not functioning appropriately, make an effort to point out better methods of practice without appearing unduly critical. When your work is criticized constructively, try to keep in mind that the criticism is not directed at you as a person; it is an effort to help you improve your practice.

Nurses are sometimes guilty of expecting excellence from one another but failing to acknowledge excellence when they see it. Learn to be free with praise. Receiving praise for your nursing care enhances your self-esteem, and the result is usually renewed effort to maintain high-quality care.

Coordinating Care of Other Disciplines

Because nurses are present at all times, they have accepted the responsibility for coordinating care given by members of other health care disciplines as well as for coordinating nursing care. Planning schedules, consulting, and communicating information are all part of this role. In the home care setting, nurses visit clients, assess for needs, and serve as coordinators of health care.

Scheduling Procedures

Scheduling of diagnostic examinations, physical therapy treatments, and a variety of other aspects of health care is usually the responsibility of the nurse. Each of these health care workers needs access to the patient at appropriate times; each has an important role to fulfill. However, they need to be scheduled in ways that still allow for rest and meeting basic needs of the patient. The nurse must consider meal schedules, whether the patient needs to eat before or after the examination, whether medication schedules need to be adapted, and

Nursing Issues and Trends: *Who Will Be The Case Manager?*

As more and more health care organizations and third-party payers move toward a managed care approach, the question arises as to who should be the case manager. The case manager has many responsibilities for monitoring progress and ensuring that appropriate care is provided in a timely fashion. In addition, the case manager may have the authority to approve or disapprove proposed plans for care. In some settings the physician assumes the role of case manager. Because of the physician's other responsibilities and the fact that the physician is most commonly an independent practitioner, many agencies are turning to professional nurses to perform the role of case manager. This role demands a highly skilled and well prepared nurse.

a host of other factors. To schedule effectively, the nurse must confer with others and negotiate in the best interests of the patient.

Interdisciplinary Teamwork

The understanding of people you have acquired to prepare you for patient care will also be of value as you work with health care team members from other disciplines. Insight into the feelings and motivations that influence people's behavior, familiarity with the functioning of groups, and highly developed communication skills are extremely useful.

Interdisciplinary team conferences are a characteristic of rehabilitation and long-term care settings. In these conferences, members of various disciplines (*eg*, dietary, physical therapy, medicine, and nursing) will share information and discuss approaches to care. Increasingly, the patient and sometimes even the family are included in these conferences. In the acute care facility, these relationships may be more informal, but they are just as important. Care is improved when information is shared and joint planning occurs.

Ensuring Continuity of Care

It is the nurse's responsibility to ensure that needed care continues when a patient is discharged from a health care facility. Patients discharged from acute care facilities while still in need of nursing care and rehabilitative support that cannot be provided by their family and friends will need referral to an appropriate health care agency. If the patient has improved, this may mean care in a less restrictive environment or even home care. If the patient has been in a long-term care facility, acute illness may require transfer to an acute care hospital.

Teaching for Home Care

Many patients who leave a health care facility are not completely recovered. They have completed the acute stage, in which professional care was necessary, but must continue to manage care at home in such a way as to promote complete recovery. Some patients even have extensive care procedures that must be continued at home. In Chapter 16, appropriate ways to help a patient learn those skills needed after discharge are discussed. This teaching should begin as early in hospitalization as possible. Here we would merely like to point out that teaching self-care skills is a nursing responsibility and requires careful planning. Figure 15-8 is an example of a form used to write down the discharge instructions for a patient. Written discharge instructions are extremely important. In the stressful and often hurried discharge situation, oral instructions may be forgotten or remembered incorrectly. Having a written record for referral at home is essential. Module 14, Admission, Transfer, and Discharge, contains more extensive information on discharging a patient.

Community Resources

Most communities have a wide variety of resources available to support individuals with health and adjustment problems. The nurse often takes a major role in helping the patient and family to identify those community resources that they feel would be beneficial. Community resources may include a supermarket chain that provides personal shopping and delivery of groceries for a fee, the transit company that provides special transportation for the disabled, or a congregate meal center for elderly persons. These types of resources are specific to a community. You will want to investigate what is available for your patients.

In addition to these local resources, national organizations with local chapters in many areas sponsor support groups and provide a wide variety of services. Appendix E presents names and addresses of many of these organizations. They will provide you with information about their services and direct you to your nearest local group.

Discharge Planning

Many hospitals give responsibility for discharge planning to a nurse known as the **discharge planner**. This nurse may follow patients' progress throughout hospi-

Nursing Research: *Implications for Practice*

Hall, M., Brandys, C., and Yetman, L. "Multidisciplinary approaches to management of acute head injury." *Journal of Neuroscience Nursing* 24 (4): 199–204, August 1992.

A multidisciplinary team was formed to follow head-injury patients from admission to the critical care unit through their rehabilitation. Treatment focused on physical, cognitive, and psychosocial areas. Cooperation of the various professionals facilitated earlier and more comprehensive treatment of the patients and their families.

DISCHARGE INSTRUCTIONS: CARDIAC MEDICAL

(Follow your doctor's orders if they differ from these instructions)

1. **DISCHARGE PLAN:** (Please Circle) ECF Home Health Agency Sustaining Care Other
   Follow-up plan not indicated because: (independent) family and/or friends will assist refused

2. **DIET:** Decrease cholesterol/fat. Decrease sodium/salt.
   Fiber and fruits in your diet will help prevent constipation.
   Recommended Reading:
   1. American Heart Association pamphlets
   2. Choices for a Healthy Heart
   3. Don't Eat Your Heart Out Cookbook

3. **ACTIVITY:**
   1. Follow your doctor's orders for increasing activity.
   2. Pace activity to avoid fatigue.
   3. Rest one hour after meals and between activities.
   4. Avoid heavy arm work, straining or extreme temperature changes.

4. **MEDICATIONS:** ____ OWN MEDICATIONS ____ PHARMACY ✓ PRESCRIPTION ✓ MED INFORMATION GIVEN
   1) Take the medications as listed on your medication schedule sheet.
   2) Do not take any other drugs before informing your doctor or pharmacist.

5. **TREATMENTS:** None

6. **EQUIPMENT AND SUPPLIES:** None

7. **SYMPTOMS TO REPORT TO YOUR DOCTOR:**
   1) Pressure, tightness or discomfort in chest, arm, throat (new or prolonged) unrelieved by rest and/or nitroglycerin under the tongue every 5 minutes × 3.
   2) Shortness of breath unrelieved by rest.
   3) Heart rate range: 60-90 beats per minute
   4) Dizziness, fainting, cold sweats, undue fatigue, palpitations, and weight gain over 2 pounds/week.
   5) Ankle swelling, new or increased.

8. **OTHER INSTRUCTIONS:**
   1) Take pulse if above symptoms occur.
   2) Take pulse daily.
   3) Weight before breakfast 2 times/week.
   4) Call 911 for unrelieved chest pain.
   5) Avoid constipation; consult your doctor for assistance.

9. **APPOINTMENTS:**
   WITH: Dr. Johnson WHEN: 1 week – Call his office for appointment
   WITH: WHEN:

I have received and understand the above instructions.

DATE: 6/14/94 PATIENT: John Sherman

WITNESS: M. Rogers RN PATIENT'S AGENT OR REPRESENTATIVE: ____________

ADDRESSOGRAPH
John Sherman
000-00-0000

SWEDISH HOSPITAL MEDICAL CENTER
SEATTLE, WASHINGTON

CCU-2 4/89 FC/SHMC

Figure 15-8. Patient discharge record.

talization or may depend on the referrals of staff nurses to identify patients in need of discharge planning services. The discharge planner meets with the patient and family to explore alternatives for continuing care. Such alternatives include home health aides, who assist with routine personal care and household tasks for a limited time; visiting nurses, who can provide skilled care; and residential skilled nursing facilities. Once a decision is made, the discharge planner makes the arrangements for posthospital care and transfer of care to the agency selected.

In a facility without a discharge planner, responsibility for planning discharge is typically diffused among the staff members responsible for the patient's care. The physician may meet with the patient and family to plan appropriate postdischarge care. A social worker may arrange the placement if a residential facility is needed; the nurse may arrange for visiting nurse services. The referral form is usually made out by the staff nurse. In some localities, the community health nurse visits the patient before discharge to facilitate continuity of care.

Making a Referral

There are various alternative approaches to officially making a referral. Although most require a physician's approval, it is often the nurse who indicates the most appropriate source of help and makes the referral. This requires that the nurse know the resources available in the local community.

When a patient is ready for discharge, it is the staff nurse's responsibility to complete a *referral form.* At this time it is both appropriate and legally permissible to share information about the patient with individuals outside the facility; the agency that will be responsible for the patient's care needs such information to provide care. By accepting a referral, the patient gives implied consent for appropriate information to be shared with the agency. Appropriate information is defined as that which is pertinent to care needs.

The patient's condition at the time of discharge is summarized, often in the form of a brief system review of all data pertaining to each body system. Current nursing care problems and planned interventions are then outlined. Information on special needs, such as a technique for transfer, a means of communication, or food habits, should be included. The form also provides for the physician to write discharge orders. In some settings, the nurse fills out the form, after clarifying with the physician which current medications and orders are to be continued. The physician then simply signs the form. Many hospitals fax these forms to the referral agency to ensure that information for care is promptly available.

Acting as a Patient Advocate

An **advocate** is a person who speaks on behalf of another. Because their illness makes them vulnerable, patients often need someone else to speak on their behalf in today's complex health care system. Although the family or significant others may assume this task, they often lack expertise in health care and so are limited in the advocacy they can provide. Because nurses may learn to know patients well and have an opportunity to identify their patients' concerns and difficulties, nurses are often in a position to be effective advocates. Most advocacy is related to upholding patient rights in the health care setting.

One area in which you might be an advocate is in regard to informed consent. You may learn that a patient does not understand a scheduled procedure or test. As an advocate you would contact the physician and ask that the patient be given further information. Another area of advocacy concerns treating the patient as an individual with dignity. You might become aware that care providers have stereotyped the patient and that this is interfering with providing optimum care. You might speak with those involved or ask that a care conference be held to bring your concern to the attention of all. Sometimes a patient needs an advocate to provide support with regard to a decision the patient made. An individual may have refused a blood transfusion because of cherished spiritual values. Although this was not a sound *medical* decision, an advocate may work with the staff, helping them to understand that this is an appropriate decision from the *patient's* viewpoint, so that the patient continues to receive caring support.

Remember that being a patient advocate requires skill in interpersonal relationships as well as a knowledge of patient rights. An effective advocate is able to initiate change without antagonizing others. If others perceive the advocate as being inappropriately aggressive or "the enemy," they will resist change even though they might objectively recognize that the advocate is correct. When acting as an advocate, try to approach others as responsible, caring people who also want what is best for the patient. This approach tends to bring out their best characteristics. Use appropriate channels of communication within the facility. Failure to do so may anger those in positions of authority and jeopardize your goal. The information in Chapter 13 will be valuable to you in being a patient advocate.

Nursing Care Study
Assisting with a Physical Therapy Treatment

Mrs. Jones, an elderly woman with severe arthritis in both hands, is a newly admitted patient. Ms. Schultz, the registered nurse, checks the physician's orders and notes that physical therapy treatment involving the application of hot wax to both hands is to take place daily to reduce pain.

Assessment. Ms. Schultz calls the Physical Therapy Department to arrange appointments for Mrs. Jones and at the same time inquires about the exact manner in which the procedure will be carried out. This is Ms. Schultz's first experience with such a treatment since her employment at General Hospital. She also checks the chart and identifies that this is the first hospital admission for Mrs. Jones.

Nursing Diagnosis. Ms. Schultz determines that Mrs. Jones is at High Risk for Anxiety related to new treatment plan and unfamiliar hospitalization and that Mrs. Jones has Knowledge Deficit related to new treatment plan. In this instance, the nurse decides that these diagnoses do not need to be entered onto the written plan but will probably be resolved by her own intervention.

Planning. The first part of Ms. Schultz's planning includes ensuring that the approach to the medical treatment plan is coordinated. Ms. Schultz enters the planned therapy and the scheduled time on the patient care Kardex so that other staff members will be aware of the scheduled treatment. She decides that a wheelchair is the most appropriate means of transporting Mrs. Jones to physical therapy, so she enters that decision on the Kardex. She adapts the nursing care plan so that morning care will be given to Mrs. Jones after treatment; this schedule allows time for the pain relief afforded by the treatment to become effective before Mrs. Jones tries to perform self-care.

Ms. Schultz plans to explain the procedure to Mrs. Jones so that Mrs. Jones will understand what is happening and why the nursing care plan is being adapted. She also plans to spend time with Mrs. Jones to ensure that any anxiety is relieved.

Implementation. Ms. Schultz then goes into Mrs. Jones's room to explain the treatment and discuss her concerns. The next morning Ms. Schultz prepares Mrs. Jones to go to physical therapy. The treatment itself is performed by the physical therapist, who also records complete information on Mrs. Jones's chart. When the patient returns to the unit, Ms. Schultz makes her comfortable.

Evaluation. After Mrs. Jones's return, her fatigue level is noted. Ms. Schultz inquires about the pain relief experienced and watches for any untoward results such as skin irritation. Mrs. Jones's understanding of her treatment and her level of anxiety are also evaluated.

Documentation. Ms. Schultz then records her observations on Mrs. Jones's record in the following manner (narrative charting): "Verbalizes understanding of goals and methods of hot wax therapy. On return from P.T., appeared pale and exhausted. Stated the hot wax decreased pain in hands. Skin appears pink and smooth. No irritation of skin noted. H. Schultz, R.N."

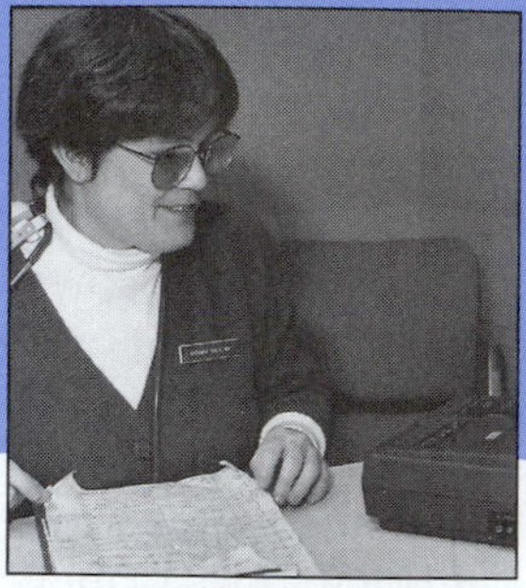

Key Points

- Coordination of care is a function of nurses at every level. Communication skills are a critical aspect of the nurse's role in providing and coordinating care. Verbal reports that nurses provide for each other at change of shift help to ensure continuity of care.
- Written records of care are legal documents and provide communication among all members of the health care team. The two most common types of chart organization are traditional narrative charting and the problem-oriented record system.
- Nursing care plans are used to provide continuity of nursing care. Ideally, the nursing care plan is clear and direct—the problems are identified, the patient goals or objectives of care are clearly stated and measurable, and the prescribed nursing actions are precisely detailed. In time, computerized records may relieve nurses of some of the paperwork that takes them away from direct care.
- Team conferences help the nursing team to coordinate their work roles and communicate in regard to patient care. A nursing process approach can be used when working with others. Consideration for the feelings of others and encouraging others in growth are important aspects of the nurse's interaction with team members.
- Nurses are usually responsible for coordinating care among the many different health care disciplines in the care setting, including scheduling for tests and therapy. Schedules must consider the needs of the patient as well as the demands on the professional.
- For patients who need continuing care following discharge from an acute care facility, nursing responsibilities include planning this care while the person is still in the hospital, contacting other health care professionals, teaching the patient and family self-care, and providing appropriate referrals.
- Nurses are often advocates for their patients. An advocate speaks on behalf of another person. Most advocacy is related to upholding patient rights.

Study Questions

1. List major points to be included when you report off.
2. What are the essential elements of an intershift report?
3. What is the focus of discussion at a nursing team conference?
4. Why is a written record for the patient/client essential?
5. In what ways is a problem-oriented patient record different from a narrative patient record? How do both of these differ from "charting by exception"?
6. What are four ways you can contribute to effective functioning of a nursing team?
7. What are three criteria for a good nursing care plan?
8. When should planning for discharge begin?

Critical Thinking Activities

1. Review the written records available for a patient in the facility where you have clinical experiences. Analyze the records to determine what type of charting is being used. Evaluate the entries for the last 24 hours in terms of clarity, brevity, and completeness.
2. Review the incident report or quality assurance report used in your facility. Analyze an incident and formulate a proposal for preventing its reoccurrence.
3. Attend a team conference. Apply your knowledge of group process in an analysis of the team's interaction. Identify barriers to effective function in this team.
4. Draw an organizational chart of the nursing staff in the facility to which you are assigned. Identify the individuals to whom you are responsible.
5. Go to an intershift report. Take notes. In a discussion in your clinical group, review and evaluate the information you received. Identify any information you needed but did not receive.
6. Accompany a patient to another department for a procedure (such as radiology or physical therapy). Identify any nursing actions that could be taken before and after to assist the staff in the other department and the patient. Share your information and ideas with your clinical group.
7. Attend an interdisciplinary team conference. Observe the roles of the various people present. Report on your analysis to your clinical group.

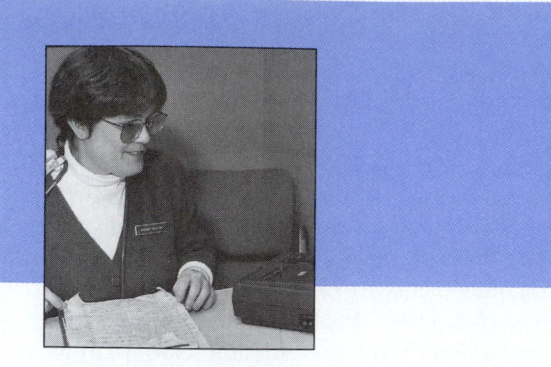

8. Identify a way in which you see a nurse acting as a patient advocate.

Relevant Sections in Modules for Basic Nursing Skills

Volume 1 Module

- An Approach to Nursing Skills 1
- Safety 3
- Documentation 6
- Admission, Transfer, and Discharge 14

References and Readings

Brennan, P. F., and Romano, C. A. "Computers and Nursing Diagnosis: Issues in Implementing Nursing Diagnoses." *Nursing Clinics of North America* 22, 4 (December 1987): 935–942.

Brill, C., and Hill, L. "Giving the Help That Goes On Giving." *Nursing '85* 15, 5 (May 1985): 44–47.

Donaghue, A. M. and Reilly, P. J. "Some Do's and Don't's for Giving Reports." *Nursing '81* 11 (November 1981): 117.

Group Health Cooperative of Puget Sound. *A Guidebook for Employees on the Consumer Bill of Rights.* Seattle: Group Health Cooperative, 1977.

Hansen, R., and Washburn, M. "What Do You Say When You Delegate Work to Others?" *American Journal of Nursing* 92, 7 (July 1992): 48.

———. "Tips for Delegating to the Right Person." *American Journal of Nursing* 92, 6 (June 1992): 64–65.

Kerr, A. H. "How the Write Stuff Can Go Wrong." *Nursing '87* 17, 1 (January 1987): 48–50.

Kerr, S. H. "A Comparison of Four Nursing Documentation Systems." *Journal of Nursing Staff Development* 8, 1 (Jan–Feb, 1992): 26–31.

Mehmert, P. A. "A Nursing Information System: The Outcome of Implementing Nursing Diagnoses." *Nursing Clinics of North America* 22, 4 (December 1987): 943–954.

Mowry, M. M., Korpman, R. A., and Armstrong, M. "Computer Consult: The Paper-Free Chart." *American Journal of Nursing* 86, 6 (June 1987): 848–849.

Newbern, V. B. "Computer Literacy in Nursing Education." *Nursing Clinics of North America* 20, 3 (September 1985): 549–556.

Northrup, C. "Filling in Charting Gaps in Court." *Nursing '87* 17, 1 (January 1987): 43.

Reed, C. "Patient Care Conferences: 3 Fast Steps to Better Patient Care Plans." *Nursing '87* 17, 3 (March 1987): 66.

Rehm, M. "How to Plan and Conduct a Patient Care Conference." *Nursing '87* 17, 10 (December 1987): 64–66.

Rich, P. L. "Make the Most of Your Charting Time." *Nursing '87* 17, 5 (May 1987): 68–73.

———. "With This Flow Sheet, Less Is More." *Nursing '85* 15, 7 (July 1985): 25–29.

Schaffer, C. L. "Documenting Special Legal Situations." *Nursing 92* 22, 5 (May, 1992): 32 C–D.

Tirk, J. "Determining Discharge Priorities." *Nursing '92* 22, 7 (July 1992): 55.

Valinga, T. M. "It's Time for Nurses to Begin Nursing Nurses." *Nursing and Health Care* 5 (June 1984): 331–335.

Weed, L. L. *Medical Records, Medical Education and Patient Care.* Cleveland: Case Western Reserve University Press, 1970.

Health Teaching

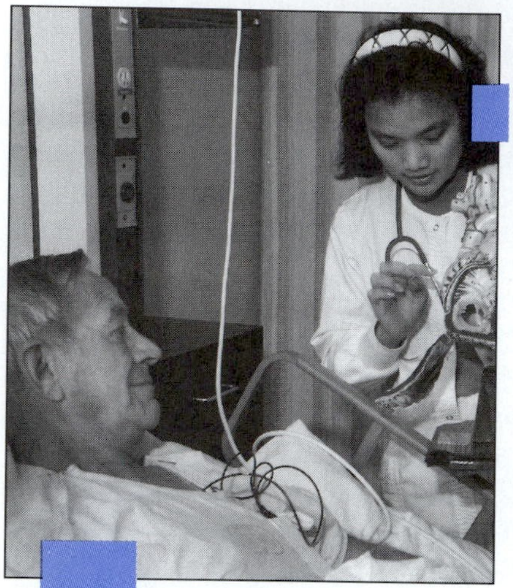

16

Objectives

After completing this chapter, you should be able to:

1. Define learning.
2. Explain why health teaching is an important responsibility of the nurse.
3. Compare and contrast three types of learning.
4. List internal and external influences on learning.
5. List basic principles of learning and relate them to planning for teaching.
6. Specify assessment data needed to identify a knowledge deficit.
7. Outline the essential components of a teaching plan.
8. Explain how evaluation relates to the type of learning desired.
9. Discuss how teaching groups differs from teaching individuals.

Study Terms

active participation
affective learning
application
audiovisual aids
behavior modification
cognitive learning
environment
external influences on learning
feedback
field-dependent
field-independent
internal influences on learning
knowledge deficit
learning
learning need
learning style
motivation
objective
physiologic status
practice
primary prevention
psychomotor learning
readiness to learn
reinforcement
secondary prevention
sequence
synthesis
teaching–learning process
understanding
vocabulary level

Outline

Ellis, Nowlis: Nursing: A Human Needs Approach, 5th ed. © 1994 J.B. Lippincott Company

Implementation
Evaluation
Behavior Modification and Nursing Practice
Teaching Groups
Advantages of Group Teaching
Disadvantages of Group Teaching
Planning Group Teaching
Evaluating Learning in a Group

Health teaching is helping people learn what they need to know to maintain or regain health. As life expectancy increases, more people must learn to live with complex regimens for managing chronic illnesses. At the same time, healthy people are increasingly eager for information about how best to maintain and enhance their own and their families' health. Thus, both the opportunities and the responsibilities of the nurse continue to grow. Nurses' knowledge of health and illness, as well as their constant interaction with patients, makes them particularly well suited to do health teaching. In turn, health teaching provides for a unique and fruitful application of the nursing process. In your role as a health teacher, you will 1) assess the patient and the situation, 2) determine the patient's learning needs and readiness to learn, 3) select goals and devise a teaching plan to meet them, 4) implement the plan, and 5) evaluate whether the desired learning outcomes have been achieved. In addition, you will want to evaluate your own performance as a teacher.

As you progress in nursing, your opportunities for involvement in health teaching will grow. It is a mistake to undertake large projects independently until you have had a chance to teach on a limited scale or with someone else. As patients in your care become increasingly self-directed as a result of skills and information you have taught them, you will begin to understand why some writers consider health teaching the most important function of the nursing practitioner.

Most health teaching is pursued with one learner at a time. However, nurses also teach groups of people, an undertaking that requires skill and experience in working with groups (see Chapter 14) as well as mastery of the material to be taught and familiarity with the **teaching–learning process**. Clearly, this chapter can be no more than a foundation for the teaching skills you will develop over time.

The Importance of Health Teaching

Individuals both want and need information and skills for health promotion and illness prevention, for overcoming illness, and for self-care in the presence of ongoing health problems. Early research in nursing focused a great deal on health teaching. Some of these studies revealed that patients themselves identify a need for learning (Linahan, 1966; Skipper and Tagliacozzo, 1964). Since these studies were completed, health care has grown more complex, and today's population probably feels a greater need for health education.

Clients need health education to provide for better outcomes. Hospital stays are shorter, complications are fewer, and symptoms are lessened in individuals who have had appropriate health teaching. This has been most extensively demonstrated through the years in regard to surgical patients but has also been shown to be important to individuals with chronic illnesses such as arthritis.

Clients also need knowledge to protect themselves against exploitation by those who pretend to be experts or to have specialized information and do not. From fad diets to fake cures for diseases, consumers are bombarded with pseudoscientific sales promotions. Correct information is the best defense against being misled by these persuasive sales efforts.

Patients/clients have a right to health education. Informed consent to care is a legal and an ethical requirement. Without education, consent may be uninformed or misinformed. Adequate teaching to ensure that patients/clients understand what they must observe and report to their health care provider as well as what they must do for self-care, has been considered by courts as fundamental to meeting standards of care. State nurse practice acts may specifically state that health teaching is a nursing responsibility.

Learning

Learning is the gaining of skill, knowledge, or attitudes. Individuals with health problems may have a particular need to make changes in their lifestyles, understand and administer therapies, or manage signs and symptoms of disease. As a nurse you will be identifying these **learning needs** and planning for ways to promote patient learning.

Types of Learning

Three types of learning are identified. **Psychomotor learning** is the acquisition of physical skills. **Cognitive learning** is gaining knowledge or intellectual under-

> **Nursing Issues and Trends:** *Time for Health Teaching?*
>
> As the pressure for cost control rises and hospital stays become ever shorter, nurses may find time for health teaching severely limited. Individuals who have learned to care for themselves competently will have fewer complications and will need fewer high-cost health care interventions. Because preventive care does not always present immediate and visible cost savings, its importance may be overlooked. Nurses need to continue to be advocates for the long-term value and cost effectiveness of appropriate health teaching.

standing. **Affective learning** is developing new attitudes or beliefs. All three types of learning occur continually throughout the life span as aspects of normal development, as well as in planned learning situations.

Psychomotor Learning

Learning physical skills requires the development of the motor pathways to enable coordinated motion as well as knowledge of the correct steps to take. Patients/clients often need to learn new physical skills, such as giving themselves injections or changing dressings. As a nursing student who is currently working on the development of new psychomotor skills, you are aware that opportunities for practice are essential to accomplish this type of learning. Evaluation of psychomotor learning is based on determining whether or not the person can perform the necessary skill (Fig. 16-1).

Cognitive Learning

The focus in cognitive learning is not simply memorization of facts, but rather **understanding**, which is demonstrated by the ability to reframe the information in one's own words, and **application**, which is the ability to use the information in new situations. Even more advanced are **synthesis,** the ability to put together information from different sources and use it in new ways and **evaluation,** the ability to weigh information against standards and determine its worth or significance. For many individuals with complex health problems, these higher levels of cognitive learning are essential to the future successful management of their problems. For example, in the course of your career, you will meet diabetics who know more about diabetes in general and their own specific diabetic situation than you know. You should try not to feel intimidated by clients with this level of cognitive learning but recognize them as individuals who can be effective partners in their own health care. You should also recognize that this level of knowledge and ability usually occurs as the result of attention to health teaching by many health care workers.

Affective Learning

Acquisition of new attitudes and values is usually the most gradual type of learning as well as the most difficult to measure. A patient learning to cope with a particular health problem may master new psychomotor skills and knowledge well before new attitudes are firmly established. Affective learning involves working through one's feelings about presently held attitudes and beliefs as well as the new values being considered. Learning has occurred when new beliefs are accepted. Participation in therapeutic interactions or group discussions is helpful to the process of affective learning (Fig. 16-2).

Factors Affecting Learning

To plan effectively for health teaching, you will need to understand the factors that affect learning. We have grouped these factors into internal ones and external (outside the person) ones.

Internal Influences on Learning

The first considerations in planning patient teaching are the **internal influences on learning**: 1) previous ed-

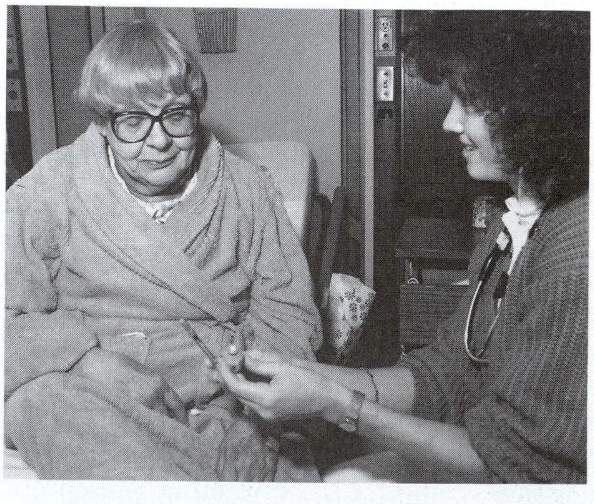

Figure 16-1. Psychomotor learning is acquiring new skills.

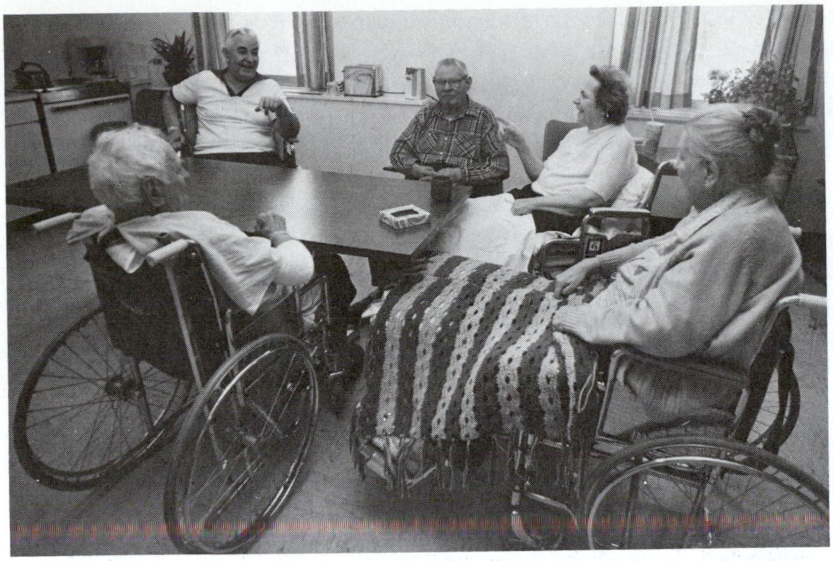

Figure 16-2. Affective learning is adopting new beliefs and attitudes.

ucation and experience, 2) physiologic status, 3) vocabulary level, 4) anxiety level, 5) motivation, 6) learning style, 7) readiness to learn, 8) support system, 9) culture and values, and 10) developmental level (Display 16-1).

Previous education and experience. *Previous education and experience* make a great deal of difference in the patient's approach to health learning. An individual who has enjoyed school and other types of learning may enjoy this new challenge. A person who associates education with shame and failure, however, will be hesitant to embark on new learning. A patient whose college work included extensive study of the biologic sciences will respond to learning how illness is affecting the body's functioning differently from a person who has avoided anything scientific and knows little about normal functioning of the human body. A parent of three small children has a different preparation for learning to care for a handicapped baby from that of a person who has never cared for an infant. Sometimes the desired learning will occur only if you provide basic background information; for example, you may need to teach normal nutrition to teach about a special diet.

Physiologic status. **Physiologic status,** that is, the status of the body in relation to physiologic needs that must be met, is affected by fatigue, hunger, lack of oxygen, altered blood components, drugs, and the like, which in turn significantly affects learning. This factor is a matter of particular concern to nurses because many patients have physiologic problems. Adaptations in teaching may have to be made to accommodate such problems. To not tire the patient, you may have to pursue teaching in small segments. You may need to reassure the patient that slow learning is a result of illness and fatigue, not an indication of lack of ability or effort. If the pace is so slow as to frustrate both the patient and the nurse, teaching may have to be postponed until the patient's condition improves. Remember Maslow's hierarchy of needs; immediate needs must be met before secondary needs can be addressed. A patient whose mind is absorbed with the effort of breathing is not likely to be interested in learning about a new diet. By planning for rest, providing medication for pain relief, and promoting comfort, you may be able to minimize the effects of physiologic factors.

Other physiologic factors such as vision and hearing also affect learning. If the patient's vision is poor, you may not be able to use some prepared written materials or audiovisual aids, and you will need to make special adaptations to demonstrate a skill. If hearing is decreased, you may need to rely on more visual aids and to validate carefully that what you say is understood.

Vocabulary. The learner's **vocabulary level**, that is, the level of difficulty of words used or understood, affects the person's ability to understand written material and oral explanations. Additionally the extent or breadth of vocabulary will be significant. The individual

Display 16–1
Internal Influences on Learning

Factors	
Previous education and experience	Readiness to learn
Physiologic status	
Vocabulary	
Anxiety	
Motivation	
Learning style	
Culture and values	
Support system	
Age and development	

may interpret some words differently from the way you do. As a beginning nursing student encountering a new vocabulary, you ought to have a heightened sensitivity to the patient's unfamiliarity with medical language. Sometimes the desired learning will occur only if you first explain the terms you are using. Those individuals, such as new immigrants, who speak English as a second language (often referred to as ESL) may speak English poorly or not at all. Even those with considerable English language proficiency may have difficulty with medical terminology. Often you may need to seek a knowledgeable translator to assist with teaching. When a translator is not available, you will need to proceed slowly and check frequently for understanding.

Anxiety. Mild anxiety may facilitate learning by focusing the learner's full attention on the task. Higher levels of anxiety interfere with learning by diffusing attention or focusing it on only a part of the situation. An individual who is extremely anxious may leap from one thought to another, unable to concentrate on a single idea. High anxiety also tends to orient the individual to the present rather than the future. A therapeutic interaction may help to lower the patient's anxiety. Sometimes anxiety-relieving medications are given to make learning more effective. If, on the other hand, the patient demonstrates total lack of anxiety and concern, pointing out potential problems that could be solved by the proposed learning may elicit enough anxiety to facilitate learning.

Motivation. **Motivation** is a tendency or desire to learn. Motivation is greatest when the individual feels a need and recognizes that the proposed learning would satisfy it. For example, a person living in a foreign country needs to learn its language to relate to others. Because the need to learn is great, effort and attention will be correspondingly great. But needs for new knowledge are often less readily obvious. A man who is to eat a special diet at home but expects his wife to plan and cook all his meals may not perceive a need to know about the diet. As a result, he would be likely to devote minimal effort and attention to learning about it. Trying to motivate an individual to learn is a challenging task. Merely pointing out a person's needs does not guarantee that the person will perceive them as needs. The most effective strategy is usually to help the person think through the situation and arrive at an independent decision that a need exists.

Learning style. **Learning styles** are the differing ways in which different individuals learn best. One aspect of learning style is the various responses to different modes of sensory input. Some individuals learn best from hearing, others from seeing or reading, and still others from hands-on contact. For many, multiple modes of input work best. Because it is not really possible for you to test each patient for his or her preferred mode, you will do the best job if you allow for a variety of types of sensory input.

Another aspect of learning style is whether one learns best by seeing the whole general outline of the situation and then learning segments, or by approaching material in careful order, learning about the segments first and then learning about the whole situation. The person who learns best by starting with the whole situation is termed a **field-dependent person**. The one who learns best by starting with the segments is called a **field-independent person**. Again, the tests to measure a person's orientation are complex and not suited to most nursing situations. However, you can ask your patients/clients how they prefer to approach material. Most people tend to teach in the way that they learn best. If you are a field-dependent person, you will most commonly provide an overview of the whole subject before moving to specific material. A field-independent patient may respond by saying, "Don't confuse me with all of that; let's take it one step at a time." On the other hand, a field-dependent patient would not respond well to the one-step-at-a-time approach. This person might respond, "Where are we going? How does this fit together? Give me the big picture." An understanding of this concept can help you recognize why a patient is having difficulty with your approach and guide you in modifying your teaching plan.

Culture and values. In Chapters 33 and 36, we will look more closely at how culture and values affect the individual. Just as they affect every other area of life, they affect the individual's approach to learning. If the goal of the learning is not compatible with personal values or would interfere with a cultural pattern of life, the individual will not focus on learning. You should consider cultural influences when you establish a teaching plan. Does this person's culture value self-reliance and independence? Is a change in diet acceptable from a cultural point of view? What is the response of this culture to scientific health care? Does this person believe that life is controllable, or is this person fatalistic about life? The person who is fatalistic will often see little value in trying to alter lifestyle to change the possible outcomes.

Support systems. Knowing about the patient's available *support systems* will help you to plan. Who is available to assist the person both during the learning period and later? Are there others who should be included in any teaching plan, both to assist the patient and to gain the knowledge necessary to manage aspects of care for the patient? The person who has a strong support system will be better able to focus on learning. Support persons can often provide encouragement and feedback to the learner and thus enhance the learning process.

Age and development level. Age and developmental level obviously affect the vocabulary a person uses and the experiences a person has had; they also affect the concepts the person can understand. For example, a young child thinks in concrete, specific terms and is not able to grasp future possibilities. A young child also has an inaccurate view of the body, how it works, and how the various parts relate to one another. There are differences between any two ages and developmental levels. The overview of Piaget's cognitive developmental levels presented in Chapter 17 will help you to identify appropriate teaching for various levels.

Readiness to learn. **Readiness to learn** is determined by the combined effect on the person of the internal influences on learning. The teacher, as facilitator of the learning process, is responsible for assessing the internal influences described in the previous paragraphs and determining the patient's degree of readiness to learn. If readiness is at a low level, it may be necessary to postpone teaching. In other instances, the teacher can alter or affect internal factors sufficiently to enable the person to learn.

External Influences on Patient Learning

The teacher can also facilitate learning by changing or adapting factors *external* to the learner, that is, the **external influences on learning**: 1) physical environment, 2) privacy, 3) timing, and 4) the teacher's vocabulary (Display 16-2).

Physical environment. The physical **environment** may need to be modified to ensure that temperature, light, noise, and the like are at levels compatible with optimum functioning. It may be necessary to find another setting for teaching or to consult with those responsible for the physical plant. Simply opening windows or doors to provide ventilation may help. If the learner will need to read or to examine a fine scale, such as on a syringe, the lighting should be appropriate.

Privacy. The nature of the task or the material to be taught will determine the degree of privacy required. It may be necessary to wait until the patient's roommate is absent or visitors have left to provide the necessary privacy. In other cases, however, it might be helpful for a family member to be present. Sometimes closing the curtains or shutting the door ensures adequate privacy. A task such as colostomy irrigation may be taught in a bathroom to protect the patient's privacy.

Timing. The timing of teaching is too often determined by the nurse's convenience rather than appropriateness to learning. For example, the arthritic patient who is stiff and sore on first arising may need to learn manual skills later in the day. The elderly diabetic woman who typically arises early, while other patients are still asleep, may learn best then, when she is rested and most alert. Scheduled diagnostic tests and other procedures should also be considered. Of course, if your teaching involves the test itself, the teaching should be scheduled to occur before the test. If the material to be taught concerns something else, the patient's preoccupation with the test may make the period preceding it inappropriate for teaching. Teaching scheduled too far in advance of the patient's need for the information may seem unimportant to the patient or provoke anxiety. If, on the other hand, the teaching is scheduled immediately before the knowledge is needed, there may not be sufficient time for learning.

Vocabulary level. The teacher should suit the vocabulary level used in explanations to the understanding of the learner. Consider the patient's education and socioeconomic background, as well as cultural factors, when determining what vocabulary to use. However, remember that many otherwise educated people are not familiar with such medical terms as void or stool specimen. Rather than asking whether the patient understands the words you are using, you might ask the patient to restate what you have said. This approach reveals whether you are conveying your message satisfactorily and provides you with a sample of the patient's vocabulary.

The following situation, in which a student nurse once found herself, exemplifies communication breakdown due to vocabulary differences. An elderly man hospitalized for diagnostic tests was friendly and anxious to please, but his English was difficult to understand. His physician ordered a stool specimen, which the nurses repeatedly explained to the patient. Over and over he smiled and nodded, but then later he walked to the bathroom, had a bowel movement, and flushed it down the toilet. The staff was becoming upset. The student nurse reviewed her information on the patient and found that he had worked at manual labor all his life and had little education. Concluding that he probably did not understand what was wanted, she tried a variety of terms—to no avail. Finally, in desperation, she said, "Shit in the pan," and pointed at the bedpan. The patient's face lit up. "Sure!" he said, and the problem

Display 16–2
External Influences on Learning

Physical environment
Privacy
Timing
The teacher's vocabulary

was solved. This was not the student's customary vocabulary—but it *was* the patient's.

Principles of Learning

The following have been shown to promote learning. Keep them in mind as you plan your teaching and select methods and materials (Display 16-3).

Reinforcement. **Reinforcement,** that is, rewarding the learner for making the desired response, is considered by many learning theorists to be the primary basis for learning. Anything the learner perceives as rewarding can be a reinforcement. Praise is the most common reinforcement because most people have learned to value it. For some individuals, a more tangible reward—such as reading a story to a child or allowing a teenager extra time to talk on the telephone—may be more appropriate. The most effective reinforcement follows immediately after the desired response, without delay. Punishment for inappropriate responses has less effect on behavior than does reward for appropriate responses. In fact, many theorists believe that ignoring inappropriate responses eliminates them more effectively than punishment.

Practice. The opportunity to **practice**, that is, frequent repetition of a new skill, increases the rate of learning. Practice spread out over time is generally more effective than a single long session because fatigue can undermine performance. Practice immediately following instruction is more helpful than delayed practice because less material is forgotten.

Feedback. **Feedback,** which is information provided to the learner that compares his or her performance during practice to the desired objective, promotes rapid learning. Without feedback, the learner may be inadvertently practicing and therefore learning incorrectly. Feedback also helps support motivation to learn by focusing attention on the learner.

Active participation. Personal involvement in a task, that is, **active participation,** facilitates learning. The learner can exercise several modes of input—touch, motor action, hearing, sight, and so on—by practicing each segment of the skill as it is explained. Writing down important points is another means of active participation; some learners benefit considerably from doing so.

Audiovisual aids. **Audiovisual aids** are alternative modes of communication that can enhance direct verbal interaction, particularly if the aids relate to the learner's previous knowledge or experience (Fig. 16-3). Many audiovisual aids for health teaching, including slide or tape presentations, films, and posters, are produced commercially and by voluntary associations. Anatomic models may help the person visualize the parts of the body being discussed. Some hospitals stock many such aids and a number of pamphlets and books appropriate for health teaching. It is a nursing responsibility to determine what audiovisual aids are needed and to communicate these needs to the administration of the health care facility. One may do so individually or through serving on special patient care committees.

Sequence of material. The **sequence**, or order, in which material is presented can have a direct effect on the rate and extent of learning. Proceeding from familiar to unfamiliar material helps the learner put new information in perspective. To proceed in this way, you must first find out what the learner already knows. Never make assumptions about a person's level of knowledge—whether the patient is a physician or a laborer,

Display 16–3
Basic Principles of Learning

1. Reinforcement enhances learning.
2. Frequent opportunities to practice new skills will increase the rate of learning.
3. Feedback facilitates learning.
4. Active participation promotes learning by providing for several modes of input: touch, motor action, hearing, and observation.
5. Audiovisual aids are an alternative mode of communicating that can supplement direct verbal interaction.
6. Appropriate sequencing facilitates learning. Information should proceed from
   a. simple to complex
   b. known to unknown
   c. well to ill
   d. normal to abnormal

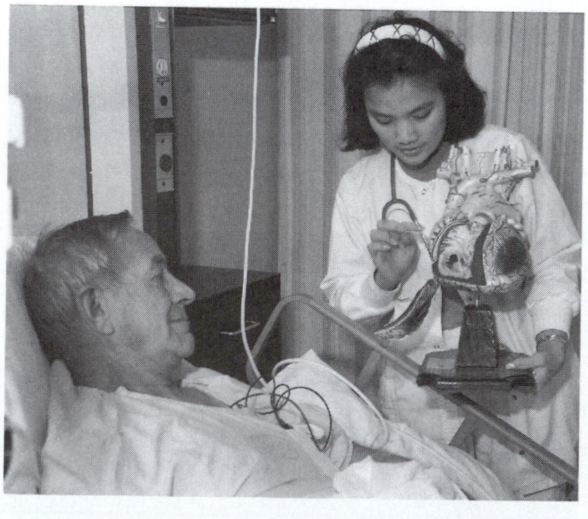

Figure 16-3. Audiovisual aids can facilitate learning.

an individualized assessment is needed. A dermatologist, for example, may be totally unfamiliar with routine preparations for kidney x-rays in a particular hospital, yet a laborer may have undergone such x-rays on a number of previous occasions and be aware of the routine. Be sure to validate your impressions of the patient's knowledge before you proceed.

In general, proceeding from *simple* ideas to *complex* ones, from what is *known* to what is *unknown*, from an understanding of the *normal* to an understanding of the *abnormal*, and from concepts involving *wellness* to concepts pertaining to *illness* helps the learner absorb new information in an orderly way.

Assessment

Assessing for Potential Health Knowledge Needs

When you are assessing an individual's health knowledge needs, you will look at those special needs created by growth and developmental level, the presence of illness, and the necessity for behavioral change. The three major categories to consider are health promotion and illness prevention needs, needs related to overcoming illness, and needs associated with self-care for persons with ongoing health problems.

Health Promotion and Illness Prevention

Health promotion includes all of those activities that create better health. They may include exercise, healthful diet, and stress reduction, as well as many other activities. For the pregnant patient, they might include the diet that will contribute to the optimum development of the fetus, and for the young family, they might include information on child development and parenting skills to enhance the well-being of all family members.

Society as a whole provides many resources for health promotion learning. Books, magazine articles, television, and all other media constantly present information on healthful living. Classes and instruction are also available from a wide variety of places. Nurses may participate in developing learning materials, provide classes and instruction, and serve as resource persons to assist patients/clients in evaluating resources.

Primary prevention of disease is preventing disease from occurring. Disease prevention instruction is usually directed at specific populations known to be at risk as well as at the general population. Information on immunizations to prevent communicable diseases is directed at parents of children and at travelers planning trips to areas where preventable communicable diseases occur. Information on tetanus immunization needs is usually given to those being treated for injuries. Those with a family history of heart disease may be encouraged to manage diet so as to decrease cholesterol levels. Smokers are encouraged to quit smoking to prevent both lung and heart damage.

Secondary prevention means detecting disease in its early stages so that it may be treated and cured, thereby preventing complications and even death. All women are taught the importance of regular examinations to detect cervical and breast cancer, and men are taught the importance of examinations for testicular and prostate cancer. Those with a family history of certain cancers may be taught to have more frequent and more extensive testing procedures because early detection may lead to cure.

Overcoming Illness

When illness is present, individuals need information to help them participate effectively in overcoming the illness. From taking medications to participating in complex treatment regimens, patients will regain health more rapidly when they participate. They need information about the disease condition itself, including the causes, if known, what signs and symptoms may be ex-

Nursing Research: *Implications for Practice*

Fowler, B. "A health education program for inner city high school youth: promoting positive health behaviors through intervention." *Association of Black Nursing Faculty Journal* 2 (3): 53–58, Summer, 1991.

The health behaviors of inner city youths, age 14–17, before and after a 7-week health education program were studied by this nurse researcher. A shift in reported health behaviors from high-risk to low-risk following completion of the health education program was identified. The researcher concluded that the nurse in this setting was in an excellent position to develop creative nursing interventions for promoting health behaviors in young people.

perienced, and what outcome is expected. They need information also about treatment they will receive, such as medications, tests, and surgical procedures.

Information about the care environment and the health care system may be essential. The person who understands the system and how it works will be less anxious and more able to use the system effectively. Such information includes knowledge about the resources in the system as a whole as well as about the specific patient unit in a hospital.

Families also may need information to participate effectively in the care of an ill family member. This is especially true when children are ill and much of the care may be performed by parents, with the assistance and support of the nurse. However, adults may also need help from family or friends. Remember to define family broadly and include those whom the client regards as family members and wishes to include.

The knowledge needed to participate effectively in overcoming illness may change as the course of the illness changes. In the acute phase of an illness, information needs may be confined to simple understanding of what health care personnel will be doing for the individual. Later, the focus will change as the patient becomes more capable of actually carrying out self-care or working cooperatively with the nurse.

As stated in Chapter 5, health is a complex phenomenon, and the individual who has an illness may at the same time experience health in many other areas. Efforts at maintaining and enhancing good health also continue while the individual is ill.

Self-care with Ongoing Health Problems

Those who have chronic health problems often need to learn special methods of accomplishing self-care activities, or their continuing self-care may require the use of special procedures and treatments. The person with diabetes is responsible for self-management of that disease and treatment on a continuing basis. To accomplish this successfully, the person will need extensive information and the ability to apply that information to an individual life situation. Problem-solving skills will also be necessary to enable the person to decide when self-care is adequate and when to seek the assistance of health professionals. In dealing with the hospitalized patient, the following questions may help you to identify health learning needs.

Must the patient perform a new task or use a new skill? For example, a person on crutches must walk in an unfamiliar way. Stairs, ramps, and doorways all require new movements and means of balance. Instruction in these skills is needed. Similarly, the mother of a first baby will be expected to bathe, change, and feed the infant when she goes home. Does she know how? Has she ever done these things before? Situations such as these abound in a hospital.

Will the patient's pattern of daily living have to change? A woman with a serious heart problem may need to rest during the day and avoid strenuous activities. What is she allowed to do? What specific exertions should be avoided? The diabetic patient needs to adopt a stable pattern of meals and activity. Does this mean that each day must be exactly like every other? How are necessary variations provided? Of course, teaching the patient to adopt a new lifestyle is not your only responsibility. You can also help the person deal with feelings aroused by such a change, as outlined in Chapter 34.

Does the patient need information on which to base judgments? The diabetic individual may be instructed to carry a carbohydrate supplement for use in an emergency. What constitutes an emergency? How much candy is enough? When must a physician be called? Many similar, if less dramatic, judgments need to be made. A mother must decide when a child is ill enough to require a visit to the physician. She must decide when to increase an infant's food intake. The health-related decisions we make throughout our lives need to be based on sound information.

Will the current problem be of continuing concern? Short-term problems call for different teaching than do long-term problems. Joint disability due to a sprain requires different adaptations and planning from joint disability due to rheumatoid arthritis, which is a lifetime health problem.

Is the immediate situation unfamiliar to the patient? A person who is about to undergo a diagnostic test needs to know what is to be done, how it will feel, what he or she is expected to do, how long it will take, and so forth. The person scheduled for surgery needs to know about preparation for surgery, recuperation, and expectations for his or her behavior.

Has the physician prescribed any specific drugs, diet, or activities? Although these are prescribed by the physician, the nurse commonly does the related teaching for the patient to understand how to follow the prescription.

Assessing Current Level of Knowledge or Ability

The second step in assessing learning needs is determining the patient's current knowledge, degree of skill, and attitudes. If you assume no prior knowledge of sound dietary habits or the components of a special diet the patient may have been adhering to for years, the individual may justifiably feel insulted or patronized. Sometimes nurses fail to recognize when the patient's learning need is not for information (such as learning about a special diet) but for a change in attitude (such as learning to value adherence to the diet).

To assess for current level of knowledge you will use interviewing strategies. It is usually best to ask patients/clients to tell you what they currently know and then to listen carefully. This allows you to determine the accuracy as well as the extent of the knowledge base.

Use nondirective techniques (Chapter 13) to encourage the client to explore the topic fully. If you ask questions that can be answered by yes or no, you may not receive a clear or accurate view of the client's knowledge base. If the learning need is related to a skill, you might ask the client to demonstrate his or her current technique. This will allow you to tailor your teaching to those specific areas in which a knowledge deficit is apparent.

The Patient's View of the Learning Needs

Once you have determined that a learning need exists, you must determine whether the patient also recognizes the need. If the patient does not perceive a learning need, your best efforts at teaching may be unsuccessful. You will find the techniques of therapeutic interaction helpful in this aspect of assessment. Using therapeutic interaction, you may be able to help the patient consider the situation and acknowledge learning needs. For example, a patient might recognize a need for affective learning by showing willingness to discuss feelings and concerns.

Identifying Internal Influences on Patient Learning

Once a knowledge deficit has been diagnosed, internal factors that affect learning—fatigue, vocabulary, anxiety, and the like, discussed above—must be assessed before you embark on your teaching plan. Otherwise your planning may be unrealistic or inappropriate for the patient in question.

Nursing Diagnosis

The North American Nursing Diagnosis Association has accepted one general category related to learning needs; it is entitled Alteration in Knowledge, and the nursing diagnosis specified within that category is Knowledge Deficit. When this diagnosis is written, it must be followed by more specific information, such as Knowledge Deficit related to low-sodium diet or Knowledge Deficit related to care of newborn infant.

Health teaching is needed when the nursing diagnosis of knowledge deficit has been made. A **knowledge deficit** is present when the person needs information, skills, or attitudes for health care that he or she does not currently have. Identifying the presence of a knowledge deficit requires two general areas of assessment. The first is identifying whether the person needs information, skills, or a change in attitudes for health care. The second area of assessment involves identifying whether the individual already possesses these attributes or has a deficit in one of these areas.

Nursing Diagnoses Related to Health Teaching Needs

Knowledge Deficit related to preoperative and postoperative care

Knowledge Deficit related to diagnostic tests for (specify health problem)

Knowledge Deficit related to need for special diet (specify diet needed)

Knowledge Deficit related to home management of (specify health problem)

Parental Knowledge Deficit related to care of child with (specify health problem)

Parental Knowledge Deficit related to normal growth and development pattern of child aged (specify age)

Planning

When a learning need has been mutually acknowledged, specific desired outcomes (often termed learning **objectives**) and a plan for achieving and evaluating them must be established in cooperation with the patient.

Establishing Desired Outcomes

In planning teaching, you will first need to determine the appropriate desired outcomes or objectives and then identify a way to evaluate their attainment. Desired outcomes and their evaluation should be based on the type of learning you have determined is necessary. For cognitive learning the desired outcome will be a statement that reflects that the client has gained knowledge and understanding. For example, if you have determined that the person needs to gain knowledge about a special diet, you will write the desired outcome as "lists foods to include and those that should be omitted from diet." Further understanding might be demonstrated by "plans a menu for one day that contains the basic food groups, includes those foods needed for the special diet, and does not include any of the prohibited foods." To evaluate the attainment of these outcomes you would provide materials and have the patient plan a day's menu.

If you have determined that the person needs to gain a skill (psychomotor learning), the desired outcome is that the person perform the skill. When skills are complex, they can be divided into several steps with each step stated as a separate outcome. This helps the person to see progress even when it is gradual. If the skill is that the person administer his or her own insulin injection, the desired outcome might be stated "administers own insulin correctly." Under that broad statement you might write: "1) Selects ordered type of insulin and prepares vial with alcohol. 2) Draws up ordered insulin dosage maintaining sterility. 3) Chooses correct site for injection, based on planned rotation. 4) Cleans injection site with alcohol. 5) Injects insulin at 90° angle. 6) Applies pressure to site after injection." To evaluate this type of outcome you would need to observe the patient performing the skill.

Writing desired outcomes for affective learning is more difficult. Attitudes and beliefs cannot be seen. Therefore, you will need to determine what statements or behaviors would indicate the change you hoped to facilitate. If you would like the patient to accept staying on a special diabetic diet as a value, you might write "states a belief that maintaining the prescribed diet will contribute to long-term health" or "states he has decided to maintain better dietary control of diabetes" as desired outcomes. Evaluation is more difficult for affective objectives. Conversation may be analyzed to identify values; behaviors may be observed over the long term to determine whether the patient has made a commitment to a new way of life.

Nurses commonly err by trying to impart to the patient all the information they themselves possess on a given subject. An effective way to correct this tendency is to be alert for nonverbal cues from the patient as to the information he or she will use and can absorb at the time. For example, a patient who is worried about giving himself an injection may be uninterested in considering any other aspect of his care until he has mastered that skill. Immediate needs must be addressed first.

In some cases it may be advisable to outline a series of objectives, recognizing that you are only beginning the teaching process. The patient may then continue learning at a later time, either independently or with another teacher. For example, the patient who has a complicated medication regimen to understand may spend an hour discussing her learning needs and formulating objectives with you. The next day she might initiate further discussion with the nurse who administers her morning medication. The nurse working in the evening might help her devise a means of keeping track of when medications are due. Thus, the entire team might become involved.

Such team involvement may be planned in advance and facilitated by a health teaching flow sheet on the patient's record. The objectives are listed on the flow sheet, and each nurse involved in teaching records what has been accomplished. The more specifically the goals and objectives are stated, the easier it will be for the patient to plan and pursue learning and to measure and evaluate progress. A goal as general as "to learn about the prescribed medications," although accurate, provides too little direction for someone who does not know what is important to know about medications. More specific objectives might be "1) to know the name and dosage schedule for each medication, 2) to know the purpose of each medication, and 3) to know what untoward signs and symptoms should be reported to the physician." This kind of objective enables the patient to ask appropriate questions and to personally evaluate learning. The patient can review the medications and determine whether or not more learning is needed. A patient who is discharged from the hospital before completing the objectives will also be able to continue learning with a nurse in the physician's office, a public health nurse, or another health care provider.

Planning the Teaching Process

After you have written desired outcomes, you will develop your teaching plan. A complete teaching plan includes specific content to be taught, specific methods that will be used, environmental adaptations that you will make, and a time sequence.

An outline of specific content should be complete enough so that you know exactly what will be included. Your methods might require that you seek out written materials or an anatomic model. Your plan should include opportunities for active participation, if possible, and feedback on the person's progress. You will also plan the type of reinforcement to be used for the individual. The environment might be modified by increasing lighting for better vision, providing privacy, or by arranging for a practice area. The time sequence will specify what will be done first, second, and so forth. You will also need to plan how much time you will need to carry out each section of your planned teaching. Review the Sample Nursing Care Plan for Individualized Health Teaching.

Informal Teaching

In many situations in nursing, teaching is conducted informally. No complex assessment process or carefully written plan is used, but the teaching is nevertheless important. Your assessment may be brief and acted on immediately. You may see that a patient needs to cough more effectively and immediately show the patient how this coughing should be done, then ask the patient to try coughing again using the new technique. Each time you explain what you are doing, you are teaching. Each time you give patients a rationale for what they need to do, you are teaching. Informal teaching is important in overall patient care. One error that often occurs in an informal teaching situation is the failure to make any assessment. It is a good habit to ask patients routinely what they understand before telling them what they may al-

Nursing Care Plan

Sample Nursing Care Plan for Individualized Health Teaching

Nursing Diagnosis

Knowledge Deficit related to self-care of new colostomy.

Supporting data:

New colostomy surgery.

Colostomy will be permanent.

To be managed with a continuous bag and no irrigation.

Desired Patient Outcomes

Independent in care of colostomy by discharge as indicated by the following behaviors:

1. Uses correct terms to describe ostomy and appliances.
2. Empties pouch correctly.
3. Cleans and deodorizes pouch.
4. Removes appliance correctly.
5. Applies new pouch correctly.

Nursing Action	Rationale
1. Explain each step and demonstrate as bag is emptied and cleaned and bag changed.	Providing information and demonstrating a skill enhances learning.
2. Provide booklet on colostomy care.	Multiple methods of input (oral and written) contribute to learning.
3. On Thurs. review booklet with patient and answer questions.	Opportunity for feedback in learning facilitates progress.
4. On Fri. have patient assist with all pouch emptying and cleaning.	Active involvement facilitates learning. Sequencing learning from simple to complex facilitates learning.
5. On Sat. have patient assist with removing old appliance and applying new one.	
6. After Sat. allow patient to assume responsibility for care. Be there and provide support by answering questions and giving verbal instructions.	Emotional support reduces anxiety and may facilitate learning.
7. Be sure to give patient lots of positive feedback for all efforts at self-care.	Reinforcement facilitates learning.

ready know. For example, you might say, "Can you explain why we're asking you to cough and deep breathe so often?" or "Do you understand why you are supposed to drink so much fluid?" When giving medications, you might say, "This is your digoxin; do you know what it is for?" This technique allows you to find out what the patient knows and gives the patient recognition for the learning that has already occurred.

Standardized Teaching Plans

Some situations for patient teaching recur so frequently in hospitals that standardized teaching plans have been developed. A standardized preoperative teaching plan (Fig. 16-4) is one of the most common. Many patients come to the hospital for surgery. Research (Reading, 1979) has clearly demonstrated that those with knowledge of the procedure and the postoperative care have a better recovery than those who do not have this knowledge. The standardized plan lessens work for nurses and makes recording much easier.

The greatest disadvantage of the standardized plan is that nurses are tempted to use it without first assessing the individual to determine what the patient's knowledge level already is and whether all of the information

TEACHING MAY INCLUDE: Pathophysiology, Treatments, Nutrition, Medications, Side Effects, Procedures, Symptoms to report, Home Management, Preventative Health, etc.

TEACHING CONTENT PRE-OPERATIVE TEACHING	PATIENT RESPONSE Indicates Understanding	 Needs Reinforcement	 Return Demonstration	 Able to Perform Independently
1. Understands surgical procedure and expected outcome. Bowel Resection	6/10 CW			
2. Immediate Post-op	6/10 CW			
a. Recovery room	✓			
b. Frequent monitoring of vital signs	✓			
c. Return to floor/ICU	✓			
3. Diet	6/10 CW			
a. Pre-op (i.e. clear liquids)	✓			
b. NPO after midnight	✓			
c. Progression after surgery	✓			
4. Medications	6/10 CW	6/10 CW		
a. Sedation at H.S.	✓			
b. Pre-op medication day of surgery	✓			
c. Post-op medications (analgesics, antibiotics, other)	✓			
5. Pre-op Preparation	6/10 CW			
a. Skin prep	✓			
b. Bowel prep	✓			
c. other	✓			
6. Equipment				
a. Intravenous	6/10 CW			
b. Foley catheter	6/10 CW			
c. Naso-gastric tube	6/10 CW			
d. Drains	6/10 CW			
e. Dressings	6/10 CW			
f. Cast/splints	N/A			
g. Other				
7. Activity Post-Op				
a. Positioning	6/11 WJ	6/10 CW	6/10 CW 6/11 WJ	6/11 WJ
b. Exercises	6/11 WJ	6/10 CW	6/10 CW 6/11 WJ	6/11 WJ
c. Restrictions				
8. Pulmonary Care	6/11 WJ	6/10 CW	6/10 CW 6/11 WJ	6/11 WJ

Identify Initials with Signature:	2. W. Jackson WJ	4.	6.
1. C. Wiley CW	3.	5.	7.

ADDRESSOGRAPH:
Wysocki, Gregory M.
612-72-9584

SWEDISH HOSPITAL MEDICAL CENTER
SEATTLE, WASHINGTON

NU-1551-C 12/81 FC/SHMC SN-6120

Figure 16–4. A standardized health teaching plan.

is needed, and then making adjustments in the plan to individualize it. Based on your assessment of the individual, you will need to modify these plans, taking into account the person's knowledge level, language level, physical condition, and previous education and skills.

Long-term Teaching Plans

Some teaching plans are long term—they must be carried out throughout the patient's hospital stay and continued even after the patient has returned to the community. In these situations you will want to write short-term goals as well as long-term goals. The short-term goals will help to prevent discouragement over the long process, but the long-term goals are essential to identify what the desired end point will be. You should take special care with a long-term teaching plan because of the number of different people who will need to be involved in carrying it out. You will also need to communicate this plan to care providers in the community through a written referral (see Chapter 15).

Long-term learning needs require a written plan. The more specific the plan, the more easily it will be implemented by the members of the team. The plan should specify the material to be taught, the objectives or goals to be reached, the methods to be used, the individuals who will do the teaching, and the duration of time in which it is to be accomplished. The more detailed your attention to external factors that are subject to modification, the greater will be the continuity of the teaching–learning process.

Writing the Teaching Plan

If the learning need is simple, it may be sufficient to write the teaching plan as part of the overall nursing care plan. Enter the nursing diagnosis related to the learning need and write out the goals with specific dates for attainment. Under the planned actions, write specific instructions for what is to be taught and the teaching methods to be used. If the plan is complex, you might find it convenient to use a teaching flow sheet in the chart, on which you enter the specific content for teaching and then initial the appropriate items when material is presented, demonstrations are returned, and goals are reached. Your teaching plan on the nursing care plan would emphasize the methods of teaching you chose, based on your assessment of the patient.

If there is a standardized teaching plan for the situation, such as for preoperative teaching, you could simply write, "See preoperative teaching plan in chart." If modifications of the standard plan are needed, be sure to enter those as prescribed in your facility.

For teaching that is only one part of the intervention

Nursing Care Plan
Sample Nursing Care Plan With Health Teaching Included

Nursing Diagnosis	Ineffective Breathing Pattern related to abdominal surgery. **Supporting data:** Respirations are 24 and shallow. Does not take periodic deep breaths. Surgical incision extends to area under the diaphragm.
Desired Patient Outcomes	Lungs remain clear to auscultation. Deep breathes ten times qh for 24 h postop and then q2h while awake.

Nursing Action	Rationale
1. Explain effect of deep breathing on lung function.	Understanding the purpose of learning may increase motivation.
2. Demonstrate splinting technique.	Demonstration provides visual input for learning.
3. Demonstrate deep breathing.	
4. Assist patient with deep breathing qh for 24 h postop and then q2h (even hours) while awake.	Deep breathing will expand alveoli, prevent atelectasis, and provide enhanced oxygenation for energy and healing.

for a particular diagnosis, it would be included with that diagnosis rather than separately. For example, if one of the patient's nursing diagnoses is Ineffective Breathing Pattern related to abdominal surgery, and you note that the patient does use appropriate techniques for deep breathing, one of your planned actions might be "Demonstrate splinting technique." Detailed instructions about techniques for teaching are not needed. This teaching would be one part of your intervention for the patient's breathing problem. See the sample Nursing Care Plan With Health Teaching Included.

Implementation

When you carry out your teaching plan, remain alert to the patient's needs and responses. It may be necessary to modify the pace or some other aspect of your teaching in light of the patient's progress. For example, if the patient is more fatigued than you expected, you will have to shorten your teaching time. Similarly, if you find that a skill is much more difficult for a patient than you had anticipated, you will have to plan additional time for practice.

The relationship you have previously established with the patient will be important to your effectiveness. You will find that a warm interpersonal relationship will enhance your teaching effectiveness.

Whenever possible, involve the members of a patient's family or other support system in the teaching plan. This involvement will help them to participate in care and reinforce learning for the patient. Often the support of others provides motivation to learn even when the illness itself seems overwhelming.

Evaluation

Evaluation involves comparing the learner's achievement to the outcomes or objectives initially specified. It may be necessary to devise tests or trials to evaluate learning adequately. In the case of psychomotor learning, such a test might consist of demonstrating the skill; cognitive learning might be tested by recitation; and affective learning might be tested by the successful assumption of certain responsibilities.

To be most helpful, evaluation of progress in learning should occur during the teaching process as well as at its completion. Ongoing evaluation allows you to modify your teaching plan if necessary and gives the learner helpful feedback regarding progress. If an opportunity for feedback is not provided at each step, the person may learn misinformation or practice incorrectly.

Success should be praised freely because praise tends to motivate further achievement. Praise should focus on specific accomplishments and learning, not personality traits. To a child learning to give an injection, you might say, "You did a good job of measuring the medicine. You showed real skill!" Do *not* say, "Good girl!" which appears to focus on personal traits rather than accomplishment. Make a conscious effort to enlarge your vocabulary of praise to include clear and specific indications of what was done well.

Be cautious with regard to failure. After pointing out errors, encourage renewed efforts in a nonthreatening way; failure can lead to depression and withdrawal. Criticism can easily be interpreted as personal rejection if it is not phrased with care. If learning fails to occur or if the rate of learning is too slow, reassess the internal and external factors affecting the teaching–learning situation and replan your teaching.

Learners should be encouraged to evaluate their own learning, a task that necessitates familiarity with the desired outcomes. Learners may need your assistance in comparing their performance with the desired outcomes.

Behavior Modification and Nursing Practice

Behavior modification is a method of teaching characterized by an explicitly stated behavioral objective, systematic reinforcement of the desired behavior, and ignoring (or other negative treatment) of undesired responses. The objective is to increase the incidence of desired behavior and decrease that of undesired behavior.

Behavior modification is extremely clear-cut methodologically. There are techniques to evoke the desired behavior at the outset, to identify an appropriate means of reinforcement, and to respond to undesired behavior. A number of good texts on behavior modification are available.

Behavior modification is widely used in health care and has proven particularly successful in helping the mentally retarded, the disabled, and people in chronic pain. Success appears to be greatest when behavior modification is part of a total team approach to care. For a fuller discussion of behavior modification in health care, see the text by Berni and Fordyce (1978).

Some nursing writers view behavior modification as mechanistic and thus fundamentally at odds with the humanistic mission of nursing. Questions have also been raised about the ethics of undertaking behavior modification without the knowledge and consent of the patient. Behavior modification without consent might be considered manipulative and an infringement on individual human rights. Because the success of such techniques is in no way compromised by informing the patient fully, most facilities that use behavior modification have policies of full disclosure, allowing the patient to decide whether or not to participate.

Teaching Groups

We have thus far focused exclusively on teaching individuals. Although most health teaching is one to one, nurses also teach groups of people, such as families and groups of patients with the same health problem.

Advantages of Group Teaching

Teaching groups offers some significant benefits in addition to simply saving time. Sharing of feelings and problems within the group helps meet the individual group members' psychosocial needs for support, self-esteem, and a sense of belonging. The wide-ranging discussion of issues possible in a group is particularly valuable in promoting affective learning (Fig. 16-5).

As members of the group raise questions, pertinent information is introduced and cognitive learning is fostered. Members who have coped successfully with a given problem in the past may have helpful and concrete suggestions to offer. For example, a group of people with diabetes may share hints about how to adhere to a special diet when eating at a restaurant, as well as their feelings about being set apart by their special diet.

In practicing new skills, some patients may be encouraged by the company of other beginners; for others, self-consciousness and fear of failure make practice in a group setting threatening.

Group teaching may also be an economic advantage to the health care institution. Groups of individuals preparing for surgery may be taught together. This allows one nurse to teach all at one time, rather than having several nurses repeat the same preoperative preparation to different patients. Other groups of patients may be taught together to maximize use of audiovisual materials.

Individuals who wish to learn about their own health problems may pay to attend classes. The cost of classes is less than the cost of individual instruction from a health care professional. Many classes, such as those about chronic lung disease or childbearing, are offered by hospitals to the community.

When group teaching is planned, objectives are written that can be communicated to potential participants or those who might refer clients to the classes. Clients and the referring person can then evaluate the applicability of these specific objectives to their own learning needs.

Disadvantages of Group Teaching

Teaching a group requires greater interpersonal skill on the part of the teacher than does individual teaching. Maintaining interaction with five, ten, or more people at once poses a complex and constantly varying challenge.

Group size is a major factor in the effectiveness of teaching. Ten to 15 people is probably the largest group that allows for a free interchange of feelings and an opportunity for all to participate. A larger group may need to be subdivided. A group of five or six people may be optimal for establishing the trust necessary to share feelings as well as thoughts.

When you teach a group of people, the possibility always exists that the material presented will be irrelevant to some members. By definition, group teaching cannot be as individualized or personal as one-to-one teaching can be. Remember, in addition, that some individuals are intimidated by groups and are reluctant to ask questions or appear less than competent in front of others. Evaluation may be more difficult in a group. It is also difficult to prevent feelings of failure on the part of individuals who perform less well. If one person is con-

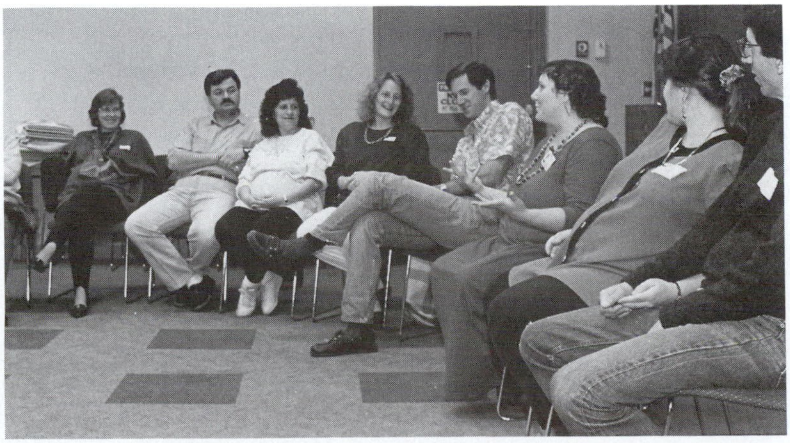

Figure 16-5. A nurse teaching a group of expectant parents.

sistently less able than others in the group, his or her self-esteem may be impaired.

Planning Group Teaching

The basic principles that guide individual health teaching apply equally to group teaching.

Group teaching always requires a formal written plan. The characteristics of the group should be spelled out, and goals and objectives specified with that particular group in mind. Sharing the written goals and objectives with prospective class members will enable them to decide for themselves whether the group will meet a personal learning need.

Your plan for teaching should allot sufficient time for every member of the group to participate at every stage in the teaching process. Ordinarily, therefore, group teaching requires a longer time span than individual teaching.

The setting for group meetings merits thought. Keep in mind the number of people in the group and the learning activities you have planned. Too large a space may inhibit discussion and participation, and too small a space will constrict activity and comfort. Sometimes the space available dictates the maximum size of the class.

Group meetings should be scheduled for a time of day when most of the individuals you hope to reach will be able to participate. If you are planning to teach a family, the evening is likely to be best. For a group of inpatients, an afternoon after all routine daily care is finished might be optimal.

The interpersonal relationships that develop within the group will be crucial to its success. You will need to assume leadership in fostering positive relationships and controlling members who would otherwise monopolize discussion or undermine others' self-esteem through criticism. Referring to the material on group interaction in Chapter 14 will help you plan effective group teaching.

Evaluating Learning in a Group

Evaluation of a group requires ample time—considerably more time than evaluation of individual learning. More formal techniques may also be necessary, such as a written quiz instead of an informal discussion. If psychomotor skills are to be evaluated, each person in the group will need an opportunity to demonstrate accomplishment.

Nursing Care Study
Teaching About a CAT Scan

Mr. Stokes has been admitted to the medical unit for diagnostic tests. His admitting problem is "Lower GI bleeding." His orders specify "Abdominal CAT scan in AM."

Mr. Kyle, a registered nurse, is assigned to care for Mr. Stokes. In the process of taking a nursing history, Mr. Kyle notes that this is Mr. Stokes's first hospitalization, that he is upset, and that he has a high school education and is currently employed as a salesman. The nurse asks what Mr. Stokes knows about the planned tests and decides on the basis of his answers that Mr. Stokes has a knowledge deficit related to the CAT scan. He thus formulates a tentative goal and plan and discusses it with the patient.

NURSE: "Mr. Stokes, it seems that you would like to know a little more about what is going to be happening."

MR. STOKES: "Sure would!"

NURSE: "Right now I must pass 4:00 medications. I'll come back at 5:00, and we'll discuss what will be done here before you go for the test, and exactly what will happen during the test. While I'm gone, you can think of any specific questions you'd like to ask. I'll leave a pencil and paper so you can jot things down if you'd like."

When Mr. Kyle returns, he gives Mr. Stokes a printed form outlining the CAT scan procedure and goes over it with him point by point. He answers all Mr. Stokes's questions about his test and makes simple anatomic drawings to clarify information.

Later that evening, Mr. Kyle approaches Mr. Stokes to review what they discussed earlier. Mr. Kyle clarifies a few points that were not clear to Mr. Stokes.

Mr. Kyle then records his assessment of the learning need, the teaching he performed, and the patient's learning.

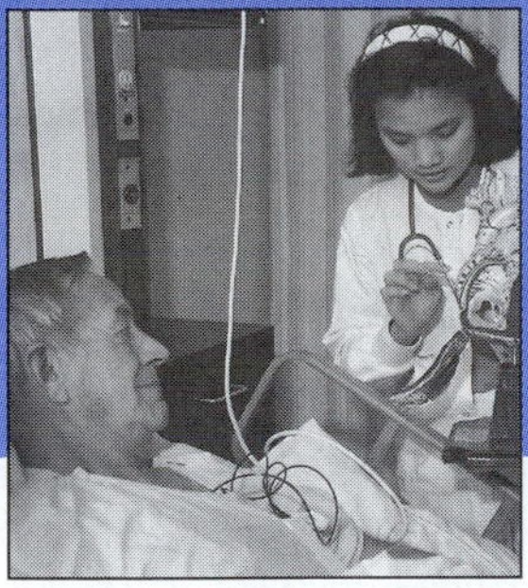

Key Points

- Nurses carry out health teaching both with individuals and with groups.
- Psychomotor learning involves learning physical skills; cognitive learning is gaining knowledge; affective learning is the acquisition of new attitudes and values.
- Internal influences on learning include previous education and experience, physiologic status, vocabulary level, anxiety level, motivation, learning style, support system, culture and values, developmental level, and readiness to learn.
- External influences on patient learning include the physical environment, privacy, timing, and the teacher's vocabulary.
- Teaching strategies can be based on the following principles of learning: 1) reinforcement, 2) frequent opportunities to practice new skills, 3) feedback during practice, 4) active participation, 5) audiovisual aids, and 6) sequencing from familiar to unfamiliar and from simple to complex.
- The nursing process is used in health teaching: assessment of knowledge deficits and learning needs; identification of a precise area of knowledge deficit; planning what is to be taught, using specific desired outcomes or behavioral objectives; and evaluation of learning.
- Establishing short-term objectives as interim steps in a long-term teaching plan helps to prevent discouragement.
- Teaching plans are subject to change, depending on the patient's progress.
- Family or other support persons should be involved in the teaching plan.
- Evaluation of learning is ongoing. Cognitive learning may be tested by recitation, psychomotor learning by the demonstration of a skill, and affective learning by changes in subsequent behaviors.
- Behavior modification is a specialized technique for establishing new behaviors. It is used particularly with the retarded, the disabled, and those with chronic pain.
- Behavior modification requires careful attention to consent from the patient.
- Group teaching requires a formal written plan that takes into account a wide variety of needs, and it requires a formal evaluation of learning.

Study Questions

1. Define affective learning, cognitive learning, and psychomotor learning.
2. In what ways does physiologic status affect learning?
3. How does anxiety affect learning?
4. How does the physical environment affect learning?
5. What is reinforcement, and how does it affect learning?
6. List three principles of learning, and give an example of how each can be used.
7. Explain how you might identify a patient's learning need?
8. Give one example of a nursing diagnosis related to a learning need with appropriate supporting data.
9. For the nursing diagnosis identified above, write desired outcomes or objectives individualized to a hypothetical patient.
9. Differentiate primary and secondary prevention.
10. How can you measure affective learning?
11. List two advantages and two disadvantages of group teaching.
12. How is behavior modification used in nursing?

Critical Thinking Activities

1. Review the card index (Kardex) in the clinical area to identify at least three patients who might be expected to have learning needs. Be prepared to describe and discuss these patients, their learning needs, and your rationale for choosing them.
2. If your clinical facility has a health teaching record or flow sheet, make a copy and demonstrate its use to record a teaching plan for a patient you have cared for.
3. Identify a community-based agency or program that has as its goal primary or secondary prevention. Examine promotional materials. Evaluate the listed objectives and identify individuals for whom this might be an appropriate referral.
4. Design a health teaching flow sheet for use in your clinical facility that cues the individual nurse to include all essential information.
5. For a patient in the clinical area:

a. Identify a knowledge deficit (choose a simple one, written up or reported verbally).
b. Identify the desired outcome or objective.
c. Plan the teaching.
d. Carry out the teaching.
e. Evaluate its effectiveness.

References and Readings

Armstrong, M. I. "Orchestrating the Process of Patient Education." *Nursing Clinics of North America* 24, 2 (1989): 597–604.

Berni, R., and Fordyce, W. *Behavior Modification and the Nursing Process.* 2nd edition. St. Louis: C. V. Mosby, 1978.

Collins, R. D. "Problem-Solving: A Tool for Patients, Too." *American Journal of Nursing* 68 (July 1968): 1483–1485.

Doak, C. C., Doak, L. G., and Root, J. H. *Teaching Patients With Low Literacy Skills.* Philadelphia: J. B. Lippincott, 1985.

Dobberstein, K. "Patient Education: Computer Assisted Patient Education." *American Journal of Nursing* 87, 5 (May 1987): 697.

Donohue-Porter, P. "Diabetes Now: Patient Education Makes All the Difference." *RN* 52, 11 (November 1989): 56–60.

Durback, E., Goodall, R., and Wilkinson, D. "Instructional Objectives in Patient Education." *Nursing Outlook* 35, 2 (March-April 1987): 82–83.

Dziurbejko, M. M. and Larkin, J. C. "Including the Family in Preoperative Teaching." *American Journal of Nursing* 78 (November 1978): 1892–1894.

Gibbs, R. D., and Gibbs, P. H. "Patient Misunderstanding of Medical Terms." *Pediatric Basics.* Fremont, Mich.: Gerber Medical Services, December 1987, p. 48.

Gonzalez, V. M., Goeppinger, J., and Lorig, K. "Four Psychosocial Theories and Their Application to Patient Education and Clinical Practice." *Arthritis Care and Research* 3, 3 (September 1990): 132–143.

Haferkorn, V. "Assessing Individual Learning Needs as a Basis for Patient Teaching." *Nursing Clinics of North America* 6, 1 (1971): 199–209.

Johnson, E. A., and Jackson, J. E. "Teaching the Home Care Client." *Nursing Clinics of North America* 24, 2 (1989): 589–595.

Kick, E. "Patient Teaching for Elders." *Nursing Clinics of North America* 24, 2 (1989): 681–687.

King, L., and Tarsitano, B. "The Effect of Structured and Unstructured Preoperative Teaching: A Replication." *Nursing Research* 31, 6 (November-December 1982): 324–329.

Kruger, S. "A Review of Patient Education in Nursing." *Journal of Nursing Staff Development* 6, 2 (March-April 1990): 71–74, 78.

Lindeman, C. A. "Nursing Interventions with the Presurgical Patient." *Nursing Research* 21, 2 (March–April, 1972): 196–209.

Lorig, K. *Arthritis Self-Help Course Leader's Manual.* Atlanta: Arthritis Foundation, 1981.

Loughrey, L. "Dealing with the Illiterate Patient . . . You Can't Read Him Like a Book." *Nursing* 13 (January 1983): 65.

Monroe, D. "Patient Teaching for Xray and Other Diagnostics." *RN* (A series of four clip-and-carry instruction guides listed below:)
#1 "Upper G.I. Series, Small Bowel Series, and Barium Enema." 52, 12 (December 1989): 36–40.
#2 "Cholecystography." 53, 4 (April 1990): 52–56.
#3 "Urography." 53, 9 (September 1990): 42–44.
#4 "Heart Catheterization." 54, 2 (February 1991): 44–46.

Nihil, J. "Community Education Programs Help Clients to Help Themselves." *Nursing and Health Care* 8, 2 (February 1987): 113–115.

Palmer, M. E., and Deck, E. S. "Teaching Your Patients to Assert Their Rights." *American Journal of Nursing* 87, 5 (May 1987): 651–654.

Pinner, J. "Patient Teaching for Xray and Other Diagnostics: Stress Tests." *RN* 54, 3 (March 1991): 32–36.

Plankey, E., and Knauf, J. "What Patients Need to Know About Magnetic Resonance Imaging." *American Journal of Nursing* 90, 1 (January 1990): 27–28.

Reading, E. A. "The Short-Term Effects of Psychological Preparation for Surgery." *Social Science and Medicine* 13A (March, 1979): 641–654.

Redman, B. *The Process of Patient Education.* 6th edition. St. Louis: C. V. Mosby, 1988.

Skipper, J. D., Tagliacozzo, D., and Mauksch, H. "What Communication Means to Patients." *American Journal of Nursing* 64, 1 (January, 1964): 101.

Smith, C. E. "Patient Teaching: It's the Law." *Nursing '87* 17, 7 (July 1987): 67–68.

Spees, C. M. "Knowledge of Medical Terminology Among Clients and Families." *Image* 23, 4 (Winter, 1991): 225–229.

Tripp-Reimer, T. "Cross-Cultural Perspectives on Patient Teaching." *Nursing Clinics of North America* 24, 2 (1989): 597–604.

Changing Needs Throughout the Life Span

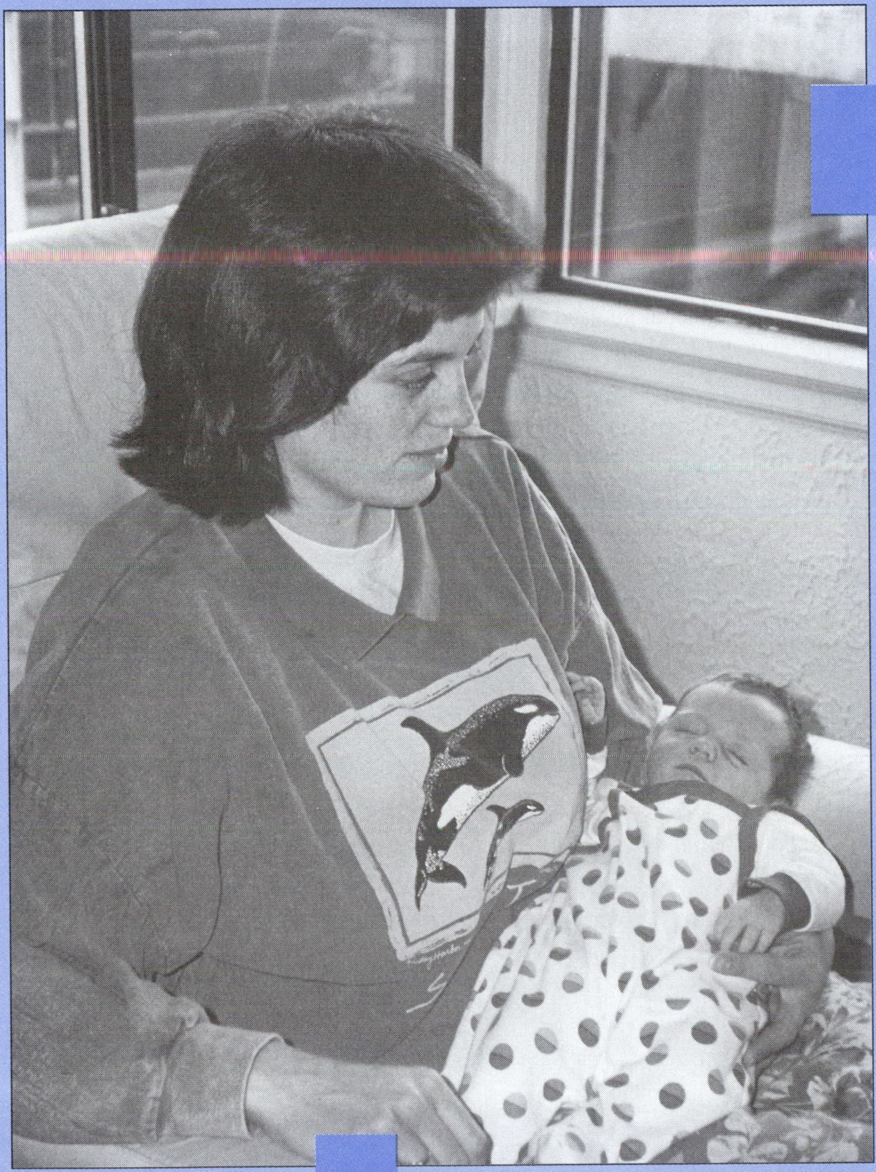

V

General Concepts of Growth and Development

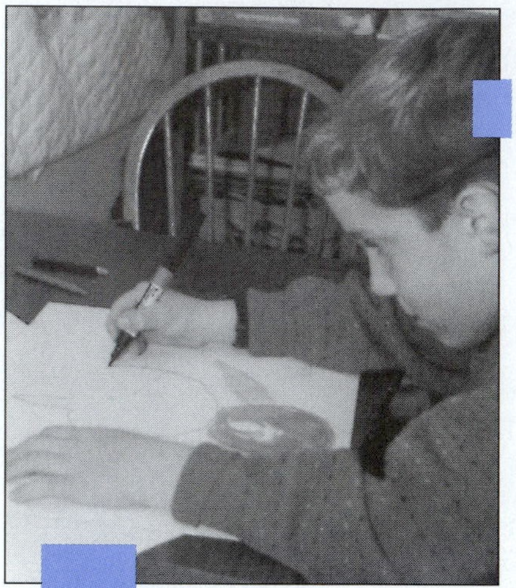

17

Objectives

After completing this chapter, you should be able to:

1. Define growth, development, and maturation.
2. Give examples of how heredity and environment can be important factors in influencing a person's growth and development.
3. Discuss, in general terms, seven concepts of growth and development.
4. List the reasons why a basic knowledge of the stages of the life span is useful to nurses.
5. Briefly discuss the theories of Erikson, Havighurst, Peck, Freud, Piaget, Kohlberg, Gilligan, and Westerhoff.

Study Terms

accommodation
assimilation
centering
chromosomes
concrete operational stage
congenital defects
development
ego
egocentrism
equilibration
formal operational stage
gene
genetic defect
growth
id
maturation
placenta
placental barrier
preoperational stage
psychosexual development
psychosocial tasks
sensorimotor stage
superego
unconscious

Outline

Definitions
Early Developmental Theory
Controversies in Developmental Theory
Heredity Versus Environment
Gender Differences in Development
Concepts of Growth and Development
Developmental Theories Useful in Nursing Practice
Physical Development
Psychosocial Development
Psychosexual Development
Cognitive Development
Moral Development
Faith Development
Life Span Considerations and the Nursing Process

Ellis, Nowlis: Nursing: A Human Needs Approach, 5th ed. © 1994 J.B. Lippincott Company

It is said that the events most unique and significant for human beings are birth and death. But between the moment of conception and the final breath of life comes a progression of changes that we call growth and development. As people change throughout the years of life, so do their needs. The society in which one lives has some influence on one's needs at various stages of life. However, some human needs change as a function of age regardless of the surrounding culture. For example, a basic need of all small children is to have food supplied to them by others. Young adults, regardless of culture, have a need to seek out some form of fulfilling education or work.

Needs can be more clearly met if you have basic descriptive knowledge of each stage of the life span and the factors that influence it. "It is also significant for nurses to know that there are characteristic health problems peculiar to each major phase of development" (Whaley and Wong, 1990, p. 76).

Within our society, the range of ages encompassing the span of life is fairly static. However, sociologic influences have altered previously predictable roles. Examples of these changes abound although the reasons for their occurrence are far too complex to discuss here in any length.

The family structure has changed so that many more children today are raised in one-parent homes, often with the presiding parent having to work outside the home. Even in two-parent homes, both parents may be required to work outside the home for economic reasons. For children, the process of bonding to parents, establishing individual identity, and accepting discipline may be difficult. As children move into the school-age years, the availability of alcohol and drugs, peer pressures, and lack of respect for authority figures, including teachers, are issues that have changed during the past two decades.

The drop-out rate of students from public schools has led to many young adults being unprepared to secure a job in the labor force and ineligible to enter institutions of higher education. For those who are able to pursue higher education, the high cost has forced many young adults to delay plans preparing for a profession or career.

The high rate of unemployment has cut deeply into the life plans of both young and middle-aged adults. Often middle-aged adults have had to look for work that did not provide wages previously earned so that lifestyles have to be altered at a time in life when economic and psychological stabilization is important.

A new occurrence has been the increasing number of middle-aged adults who have accepted the task of raising grandchildren when the adult child has failed to provide an appropriate home. These same individuals may also be caring for their own parents who have reached advanced age.

Finally, as people live longer, they may be less vigorous and develop debilitating diseases that make independent living impossible. Some families are unable to care for dependent elderly persons and nursing home placement is the only option.

Definitions

The meanings of *growth*, *development*, and *maturation* are different. **Growth** is an enlargement of or a change in the actual size of the tissues and organs of the human body. Growth can be measured in terms of weight, height, formation of teeth, density of bones, and evidence of sexual characteristics. There is also comparable growth of the internal organs.

Development is more complex than growth. Development refers to "a pattern of changes that are regarded as positive and functional for a living system . . . a change in the organization of the structure" (Reed, 1983, p. 19). Some of the theorists we discussed earlier in this text referred to the human as a system that interacts with the environment. It is, then, the human organism's refinement of responses to the physical, psychological, and social environment that constitutes the development of the individual. You may also hear the term **maturation**, meaning that the person matures, that is, growth changes as well as developmental changes occur. As the person ages throughout the life span, the ability to adapt increases. The importance of this change in complexity allows higher level functioning.

Early Developmental Theory

The early theorists had a narrow view of child development, in that they considered prenatal, hereditary characteristics as the dominant determinants of future personhood and performance. In light of their views, it is interesting that we are again looking at "coding," or predicting a person's future health and illness by identifying certain hereditary aspects.

Jean-Jacques Rousseau, the Swiss-born French philosopher, wrote of development as a prearranged design (1762). In the early 1930s, Arnold Gesell attributed to genetic influences not only physical growth patterns but the learned behavior of the infant and child. He considered the environment as a factor that could only support or modify what has been predetermined.

Daniel Levinson and his associates (1978) described growth and development as "life structure" or a "basic pattern or design of a person's life at a given time"

(p. 41). Although they describe a standard sequence of "periods," they maintain that there are times of relative stability and times of change in development. Many of these changes have to do with personal choices, such as marriage, family, or career selection, and with the death of significant persons. This theory of sequential but uneven development is also contained in the work of Kalkman and Davis (1974), who recognized that "in some areas of development, such as in the cognitive realm or in physical growth, there may be sudden, discontinuous changes, whereas simultaneously in other areas the changes toward maturity may be more gradual" (p. 45).

Many theories about growth and development are based on the assumption that the life span consists of increasing and decreasing faculties. These theories assume that in early years, young people accumulate increasing body stature, cognitive ability, and skill; then, as persons advance in age, they experience both a physical and a cognitive decline. The older person has the advantage of learning to organize and integrate life experiences over a longer period of time, so that transformation can occur. The concept of development, then, means qualitative or complexity rather than just an enlargement in size.

Controversies in Developmental Theory

Heredity Versus Environment

Strong argument continues among developmental theorists as to whether heredity or environment is the more important determinant of a person's developmental pattern. Most theorists feel that both are involved but some consider one more important; numerous studies have been done to substantiate one position or the other. As nurses, we must carefully consider both.

Heredity

A newborn's inherited characteristics derive from the genetic heritage of both parents. The infant is not a mere mixture of the parents' attributes but may inherit genetic characteristics that the parents themselves do not manifest.

The sex of the unborn child is determined through a pairing of **chromosomes**, the portion of a cell that determines inborn characteristics. In simple terms, the female carries two chromosomes, designated X and X. The male carries an unmatched pair, X and Y. If the X from the male unites with the female X, a girl is born; if the Y chromosome unites with the female's X, a boy is born. Thus, the first stage of life begins with determination of sex.

A pooling of **genes**, which are the units of a chromosome, also determines many of the physical characteristics of the individual. Among these are eye color, skin and hair pigmentation, limb length, and general appearance. How much intelligence and special abilities are inherited remains in dispute. Studies of identical twins suggest that heredity plays an important role in determining intelligence. Many researchers propose that mental traits, such as personality or disposition, are inherited as well as abilities in areas such as art, music, writing, and mathematics (Fig. 17-1). Those who oppose this view suggest that parental or environmental influences are responsible for such development. Nevertheless, human life, with all of its needs, begins long before the first vigorous cry at birth.

Genetic defects occur when an abnormality of the *genes* occurs. This abnormality causes inherited problems that can be structural, such as deformed fingers or toes, or more serious, such as some forms of retardation. Genetic tendencies toward certain diseases, such as diabetes, migraine headaches, rheumatoid arthritis, heart disease, and high blood pressure (hypertension), often are not apparent at birth but develop later in life.

An exciting aspect in the area of genetic study is the preliminary finding that codes or markers can be identified at birth and even before birth, which are predictors for future biologic abnormalities such as diabetes and hypertension. The availability of this information would allow earlier intervention to forestall or even eliminate some undesirable health states. As vigorous research continues, much more will be known about hereditary or genetic influences on growth and development.

Environment

Environmental factors can affect the health of the unborn child. Such factors as air pollution, water and soil

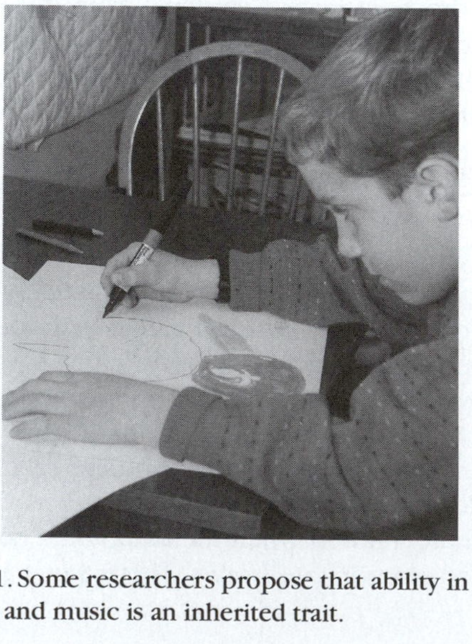

Figure 17-1. Some researchers propose that ability in such areas as art and music is an inherited trait.

contamination with chemicals, and even the toxic environmental elements in the parents' workplaces are being investigated.

It is also clear that parental behavior can alter infant well-being. Evidence has been found that children who live in an environment with a smoker have an increase in respiratory problems. Drug and alcohol abuse by either parent, particularly by the mother, can lead to low birth weight and heightened vulnerability to disease. Unsafe behaviors that lead to human immunodeficiency virus infection in the mother places the unborn child at risk of acquiring the infection. Environmental research continues, and we will probably have both unpleasant surprises about prenatal influences as well as discoveries of new ways to avoid or minimize birth defects.

Congenital defects are conditions present at birth that are not inherited. Certain viral infections contracted by the mother early in pregnancy, such as rubella (German measles), can lead to malformation or death of the fetus. However, immunization for measles has greatly decreased the occurrence of this problem. It has long been recognized that poor nutrition and poor health on the part of the mother affect the health of the infant. Infants who are deprived of protein are smaller, may have a reduced brain weight, and are less able to resist infection and disease. The **placenta**, a structure on the inner wall of the uterus that provides circulatory exchange between mother and fetus, has the capacity to withhold or allow passage of substances from mother to child through the separating membrane. This capacity is known as the **placental barrier**. We now have evidence that components of alcohol, certain drugs, and even the effects of smoking can cross this barrier to the fetal circulation, causing signs of substance withdrawal at birth for the exposed infant and even serious long-term consequences for the child. For these reasons, pregnant women are advised not to ingest alcohol or other drugs and to avoid smoking. Researchers have also been looking at possible fetal effects if the father is a smoker or user of alcohol or other drugs.

Environmental factors can also be psychological, social, or cultural in nature. The successful bonding of infant to parent can be the beginning of psychological and social comfort (Fig. 17-2). The presence or absence of warmth and love in the home adds to or detracts from the security of the child. It has been recognized that the home environment can have serious adverse effects (*eg*, those who are child abusers are often those who have been abused themselves). On a more positive note, in youth and adult life, social networking of friends adds to social comfort and identifying with one's unique culture and incorporating it into one's life enhances psychological well-being. The natural world, too, can influence development. Some studies suggest that a person's creativity can be promoted by the beauty of the natural environment.

Gender Differences in Development

Many of the theorists of growth and development studied only one sex and sometimes only persons of one gender and only a certain age. At times, these methods

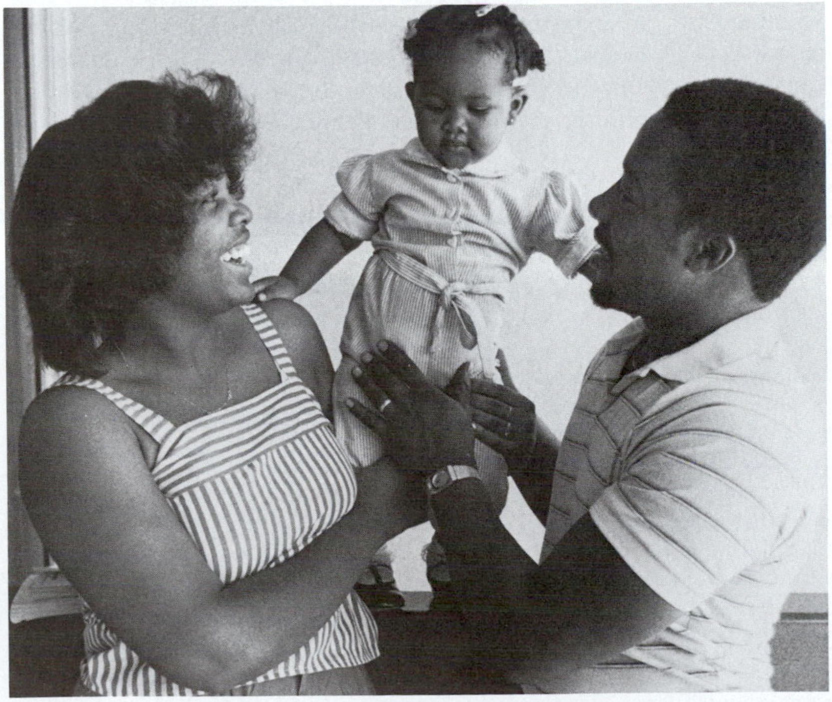

Figure 17-2. The presence of emotional closeness and love in the home adds to the child's feelings of security.

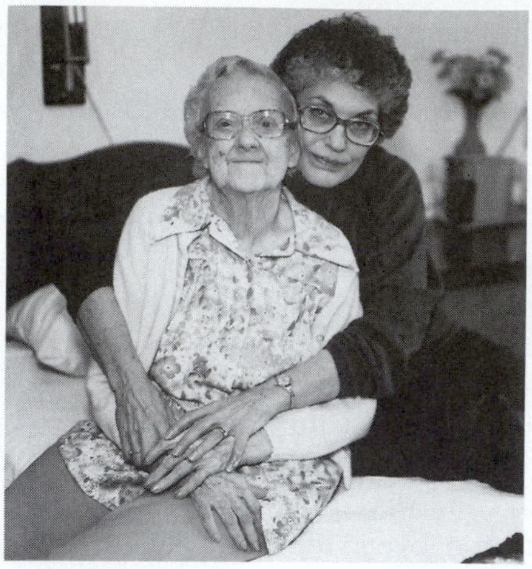

Figure 17-3. In contemporary society, women more often fulfill the care provider role than men.

built in biases and weakened the conclusions. In our contemporary world, many of the apparent differences in the development of males and females are environmental or societal. Women have been portrayed as more concerned with relationships than are men and, therefore, they more often fulfill the care provider role (Fig. 17-3). The International Association of Gerontology, in a message to the Assembly on Aging of the United Nations (1982), recognized that traditionally, the responsibility of caring for elders has fallen to women. A positive change has occurred with regard to women being accepted into more key positions in society where they can demonstrate autonomous thinking, effective decision-making skills, and an innate caring attitude.

Experiments have been conducted on children of both sexes of a standard age to determine whether or not certain behaviors are genetically determined. Several studies have shown that males generally may have a predisposition for numerical calculations. This in no way implies that all males are more proficient in mathematics than are females. Artistic and musical talent has also been explored from a genetic viewpoint, with some conclusions that suggest that not gender but rather individual predisposition influences such gifts.

Concepts of Growth and Development

A variety of theorists have offered definitions of and theories about growth and development. Some are divergent, but many of these concepts share similar premises. Most of the theorists hold one or more of the following to be true:

1. We are most alike at birth; after that, we begin to develop complexities that differentiate us from one another.
2. There is a predictable sequence to growth and development.
3. The rate of growth and development is unique to the individual.
4. Both growth and development are unidirectional, that is, they move from conception to death.
5. Both the environment and heredity can strongly influence growth and development.
6. Although growth may be controlled by age and certain conditions, there are unknown possibilities for the development of the individual.

The concepts just cited are important for your understanding of growth and development. It is true that in infancy we are most alike. There is a range of birth weight, height, and behavior that is almost universal. One need only travel to other parts of the world and observe infants in diverse areas to accept this fact. The

Nursing Issues and Trends: *More Caution Needed in Using Standard Charts on Growth and Development*

We need to recognize that the long-used standard charts relative to growth and development were written at a time when Caucasians were considered the major ethnic group in our society. The measurements were unintentionally culturally biased. Presently, ethnic diversity is more evident in western societies. This fact makes it imperative that we understand that these charts measure the growth and development of only one circumscribed group. Caution is suggested when we apply the charts to discern what is "normal" growth and development for a non-Caucasian person. For example, many children from Asian ethnic groups are shorter in height than are those from Caucasian groups. We need to have knowledge of ethnic differences so that any information used can be used more accurately.

infant turns the head to track the familiar sight or sound of a loving person or clutches the finger of the adult for security. Regardless of the language spoken by the adult world, the infant's response is the same. From this point on, certain hereditary characteristics may become apparent, as well as differences in the environment that elicit different responses.

There is a predictable sequence to growth and development. Infants stand at approximately the same age and take their first steps at about the same time. They move on to develop coordination and perform their own activities of daily living. Adolescence encompasses the period of time when puberty begins and individuals attain the ability to procreate. Families are formed within certain years of life and relationships continue to change throughout life. The desire for meaningful work is a universal quest for the young adult and continues into the advanced years as the life span increases.

Despite this universality, the rate of growth and development is unique to the individual. One has only to visit a classroom of third graders to see many differences in physical development. Education also recognizes that each person learns at his or her own speed and often performs tasks well depending on individual interest in performance. Some persons develop reading skills early in life, whereas others develop them later or not at all.

Because growth and development are unidirectional, we are at our simplest and most similar at birth. As the life span continues from that point, we develop both physical and psychological complexities. The refinement of these complexities allows us to cope with and adapt to the changes in our environment to maintain our stability.

Besides chromosomal makeup and gene patterns, which predetermine some aspects of life, environmental factors—physical, psychological, social, or cultural—have a role. It is the integration of these many factors that largely determines the development of the person.

Finally, one fascinating aspect of theories on growth and development is that there are few absolutes. This leaves open the possibility of developing the potentials within each person. It is this concept that allows individuals to successfully change roles within the life span; roles may be difficult but the potential exists for making a change that requires ability, strength, and adaptation. Often, the changes and demands of new roles go unrewarded except for inner satisfaction. In other instances, fulfilling one's potential is much more dramatic. For example, the intellectual lethargy of Albert Einstein as a child, which later developed into an intellectual capacity of gigantic proportions, is a situation few of us can realize. But on a lesser scale, life experience carries with it the excitement of exploring the potentials in each of us.

Developmental Theories Useful in Nursing Practice

It is helpful for nurses to be aware of the work of several developmental theorists. Their ideas are discussed here in terms of physical, psychosocial, psychosexual, cognitive, moral, and faith development.

Physical Development

Most of the studies on physical development deal with children. It is important to realize, however, that the majority of this work was based on middle-class white children, so it may not be applicable to minority children or those who are ethnically different. The Denver Developmental Screening Test is one guide that has proved reliable; this test measures children aged 1 month to 6 years in four areas: psychosocial, fine motor adaptive, language, and gross motor. Another helpful scale is that designed by the Child Evaluation Clinic of Cedar Rapids, Iowa. This test evaluates a child's motor and language skills and personal–social adaptation. This evaluation scale is presented and discussed in more detail in Chapter 18.

Psychosocial Development

Erikson

In *Childhood and Society* (1963), psychiatrist Erik H. Erikson describes the human life span as composed of eight stages, each accompanied by a characteristic "crisis," with a hoped-for or expected outcome or an unfavorable outcome that could result if certain conditions for growth are absent. Erikson considers psychosocial development a lifelong process. In contrast, Freud and Piaget whom we discuss later, treat sexual and cognitive development as virtually complete at puberty. Successful resolution of each crisis is necessary for optimal functioning at later stages. Whether a person experiences a positive or a negative resolution depends primarily, although not exclusively, on interaction with the world in general and with "significant persons." In a sense, then, the subject of Erikson's early writings is what we now call "conflict resolution" (Table 17-1).

Havighurst

Robert Havighurst's theory (1972) is that life consists of tasks to be learned rather than crises to be overcome to progress satisfactorily along the life span. Havighurst views life as one of continual learning through six stages of growth and development. The tasks described for early infancy and early childhood are physical, for example, learning to walk and talk as well as establishing bowel and bladder control. In the later stages of middle

Table 17–1. Stages of the Life Cycle (Erikson)

Stage	Age	Crisis	Significant Persons	Tasks	Typical Response to Illness
Infancy	0–1	Trust vs. mistrust	Mother or mother substitute	Expressing frustrations. Dependence on mother.	Physiologic irritation. Fear of environment.
Toddler	1–3	Autonomy vs. shame and doubt	Parents	Speech. Walking. Assertion of wishes. Beginning the postponement of pleasure.	Fear of threats to the body and painful procedures. Stress of separation from mother.
Early childhood	3–6	Initiative vs. guilt	Entire family	Enlargement of vocabulary. Interaction with total family group. Beginning of peer involvement.	Equation of illness with being bad. Guilt.
Middle childhood	6–12	Industry vs. inferiority	School and neighborhood	Increased physical activity. Competitiveness. Dealing with authority in the school environment.	Anger over restrictions due to illness. Guilt over causing family crisis.
Adolescence	12–18	Identity vs. role confusion	Peers, national leadership models	Independence from family. Strong influence of peer group. Becoming sexually active. Beginning to choose life goals.	Anger over dependency due to illness.
Young adulthood	18–40	Intimacy vs. isolation	Intimates, usually of opposite sex	Carrying out life plans. Choosing a mate. Selecting a life's work.	Fear of possible change in the intimacy relationship. Depression over the interruption of plans.
Middle years	40–65	Generativity vs. stagnation	Expanded family, institutions	Forming ideas and plans for the next generation. Carrying out life goals. Assessment.	Depression over the interruption of work and separation from family.
Later years	65–	Integrity vs. despair	Those who promote sense of usefulness	Life review. Finding satisfactions. Setting new goals for retirement. Sharing knowledge with others.	Feelings of no longer being useful. Fear of threat to life. Despair.

childhood, adolescence, early adulthood, middle age, and later maturity, the tasks are primarily **psychosocial tasks**, those having to do with emotions, attitudes, and relationships with others (Display 17-1 and Fig. 17-4).

Two criticisms are made of Havighurst's psychosocial task premise. First, the theory leaves little room for individual differences; for example, a task of young adulthood is "starting a family." Young persons are not "learning" this task as universally as they once did, so, according to Havighurst, personal conscious choices may be disregarded or even considered an impediment to successful fulfillment of certain "learned tasks" of the life span. Secondly, Havighurst's theory is limited to a Western cultural focus and does not adapt to the special mores of other cultures. What is important to learn in midlife in this country may not have relevance in another culture. Havighurst offers us a standard that must be examined critically in regard to the limitations just mentioned.

Peck

Robert Peck focused his developmental theory on adults. Although longevity has greatly increased since he proposed his stages of transition through the adult years in 1968, the general categories he proposed still have relevance. According to his work, aging offers opportunities for compensatory adjustments. Some of the stages of the later years involve mental agility in the face of declining physical health. He uses language that emphasizes transcendence and recapturing meaning in life (Display 17-2).

Psychosexual Development

Freud

Psychosexual development, that is, the psychological aspect of sexuality as it develops in the individual, was first systematically described by Sigmund Freud (1856–1939), who started his career as an outstanding neuro-

Display 17–1

Psychosocial Development Theory (Havighurst)

Infancy and Early Childhood

- Learning to walk
- Learning to take solid foods
- Learning to talk
- Learning to control the elimination of body wastes
- Learning sex differences and sexual modesty
- Forming concepts and learning to describe social and physical reality
- Getting ready to read

Middle Childhood

- Learning physical skills necessary for ordinary games
- Building wholesome attitudes toward oneself as a growing organism
- Learning to get along with peers
- Learning an appropriate masculine or feminine social role
- Developing fundmental skills in reading, writing, and calculating
- Developing concepts necessary for everyday living
- Developing conscience, morality, and a scale of values
- Achieving personal independence
- Developing attitudes toward social groups and institutions

Adolescence

- Achieving new and more mature relations with age-mates of both sexes
- Achieving a masculine or feminine social role
- Accepting one's physique and using the body effectively
- Achieving emotional independence from parents and other adults
- Preparing for marriage and family life
- Preparing for an economic career
- Acquiring a set of values and an ethical system as a guide to behavior—developing an ideology
- Desiring and achieving socially responsible behavior

Early Adulthood

- Selecting a mate
- Learning to live with a marriage partner
- Starting a family
- Rearing children
- Managing a home
- Getting started in an occupation
- Taking on civic responsibility
- Finding a congenial social group

Middle Age

- Assisting teenage children to become responsible and happy adults
- Achieving adult social and civic responsibility
- Reaching and maintaining satisfactory performance in one's occupational career
- Developing adult leisure-time activities
- Relating oneself to one's spouse as a person
- Accepting and adjusting to the physiologic changes of middle age
- Adjusting to aging parents

Later Maturity

- Adjusting to decreasing physical strength and health
- Adjusting to retirement and reduced income
- Adjusting to death of a spouse
- Establishing an explicit affiliation with one's age group
- Adopting and adapting social roles in a flexible way
- Establishing satisfactory physical living arrangements

Source: Havighurst, R. J. *Developmental Tasks and Education*. 3rd edition. New York: Longman, Inc., 1972. Reprinted by permission.

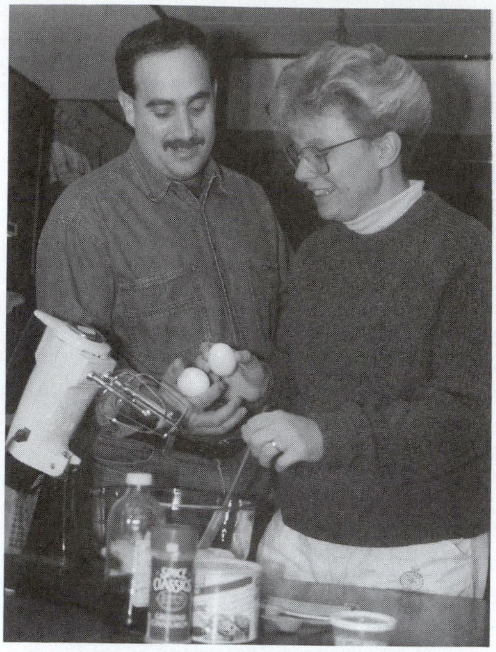

Figure 17–4. Learning to live with a partner is one of Havighurst's tasks of psychosocial development.

physiologist. Freud's work was modified by two younger colleagues, Carl Jung and Alfred Adler. Later, other psychosexual theorists offered other approaches.

Freud's early work was revolutionary for the Victorian times in which he lived. He postulated that much of our mental life occurs outside our awareness, in the part of the mind he called the **unconscious**. The human mind, according to Freud, has three main components: the **id**, motivated by primitive needs and impulses toward gratification and pleasure; the **ego**, the expressive self that consciously controls behavior and pursues goals and interprets reality; and the **superego**, or conscience. The ego is the force that mediates between the id and the superego.

Freud also strongly emphasized the importance of sexual development, postulating that many adult psychological problems are rooted in failure to resolve sexual conflicts at earlier stages of development (Table 17-2). Successful resolution allows the individual to achieve a mature sexual identity and a stable emotional life.

Freud's research has long been criticized for a number of reasons. First, it was designed on the basis of a population consisting strictly of women from the same cultural and social class. Second, these individuals all had sexual problems and, therefore, were not representative of the general population. Third, Freud's research ignored the stage of late puberty. However, Freud was the first to view sexuality as developmental, and using that important premise, others such as Piaget, Erikson,

Display 17–2
Tasks of Psychosocial Development (Peck)

Middle Age

1. Valuing wisdom over physical well-being. The ability to make effective choices based on intellectual perception and imagination.
2. Replacing sexuality with socialization in the male–female relationship.
3. Recognizing experience as an important guideline in one's life.
4. Redirecting emotional energy toward pursuing new relationships and activities as changes occur in life, such as changes in marital status, children becoming adults and leaving home, and friends becoming more distant.

Old Age

1. Finding self-esteem and pleasure in activities other than the work role. Ego differentiation versus work preoccupation.
2. Adjusting to a decline in physical health while maintaining a feeling of contentment and well-being.
3. Accepting the reality of one's eventual death with a sense of transcendence.

Table 17–2. Psychosexual Stages (Freud)

Age	Psychosexual Stage
Birth to 1 y	**Oral Stage** The mouth is the focus of stimulation and interaction; feeding and weaning are central.
1–3 y	**Anal Stage** The anus is the focus of stimulation and interaction; elimination and toilet training are central.
3–6 y	**Phallic** The genitals (penis, clitoris, and vagina) are the focus of stimulation; resolution of the oedipal conflict, sex role, and moral development are central.
6–12 y	**Latency** A period of suspended sexual activity follows oedipal conflict resolution; energies shift to physical and intellectual activities.
12–Adulthood	**Genital** The genitals are the focus of stimulation with the onset of puberty; mature sexual relationships develop.

Source: Seifert, K. L., and Hoffnung, R. J. *Child and Adolescent Development*. Copyright © 1987 by Houghton Mifflin Company. Adapted with permission.

and Kohlberg applied a developmental framework to the study of other aspects of the individual. In addition, Freud was the first to identify that we are influenced for psychological factors that lie outside of our consciousness.

Cognitive Development

Piaget

Jean Piaget, a Swiss educator and psychologist and a contemporary of Erikson, describes the life span in terms of cognitive or intellectual processes. Beginning in infancy, according to Piaget, human beings organize information into coherent systems of thought that determine how they interpret and adapt to their environment. The process by which information is absorbed Piaget calls **assimilation**. When new information conflicts with existing perceptions, one must make adjustments or **accommodations** in one's thinking to understand both familiar and new information. The process by which such accommodations are made, which Piaget calls **equilibration**, involves making apparently contradictory information consistent and returning to a state of mental comfort. Piaget considers intellectual growth of all ages to be dependent on these processes by which experience is transformed into concepts (Table 17-3).

Young children, age 2 and under, primarily use their senses to ascertain the properties of objects; by handling a ball, for example, the child experiences roundness. Piaget called this period the **sensorimotor stage**.

Between ages 2 and 7 years, the child is at the **preoperational stage**, which Piaget describes as characterized by egocentrism and centering. **Egocentrism** is perceiving oneself as the central focus of all experience. At this stage, physical objects and other people are seen as directly associated to oneself; for example, the child may expect others to be aware of his or her unexpressed thoughts. **Centering** is inability to see beyond the immediate aspects of a situation. For example, at this age a child cannot understand that a painful injection will reduce an infection. Rather, the immediate ex-

Table 17–3. Phases of Cognitive Development (Piaget)

Phases and Stages	Age	Significant Behavior
Sensorimotor	Birth to 2 y	
Stage 1 Use of reflexes	Birth to 2 mo	Most action is reflexive.
Stage 2 Primary circular reaction	1–4 mo	Perception of events is centered on the body. Objects are extension of self.
Stage 3 Secondary circular reaction	4–8 mo	Acknowledges the external environment. Actively makes changes in the environment.
Stage 4 Coordination of secondary schemata	8–12 mo	Can distinguish a goal from a means of attaining it.
Stage 5 Tertiary circular reaction	12–18 mo	Tries and discovers new goals and ways to attain goals. Rituals are important.
Stage 6 Inventions of new means	18–24 mo	Interprets the environment by mental image. Uses make-believe and pretend play.
Preconceptual	2–4y	Uses an egocentric approach to accommodate the demands of an environment. Everything is significant and relates to "me." Explores the environment. Language development is rapid. Associates words with objects.
Intuitive thought	4–7 y	Egocentric thinking diminishes. Thinks of one idea at a time. Includes others in the environment. Words express thoughts.
Concrete operations	7–11 y	Solves concrete problems. Begins to understand relationships such as size. Understands right and left. Cognizant of viewpoints.
Formal operations	11–15 y	Uses rational thinking. Reasoning is deductive and futuristic.

Source: Adapted from Piaget, J. *The Origin of Intelligence in Children*. New York: International Universities Press, Inc. Copyright © 1966. Used by permission.

perience is predominant. Egocentrism and centering are natural components of this stage. Reasoning, imagery, and representation become part of the cognitive process at this stage. The child can mentally picture a ball and compare the letter O to a ball. If an orange is mentioned, the child thinks of the shape.

The concrete operational stage usually begins around age 7 and continues until age 11 or so. The child can now carry knowledge of the specific ball we have been describing to a state of what Piaget calls *reversibility.* If an orange were cut into pieces, the older child could mentally envision it as it once was, or reverse the image. In this **concrete operational stage**, the child is able to perform acts or "operations" on specific objects in such a way as to begin to understand how the physical environment works.

Finally, at about the age of 11, the child progresses to the **formal operational stage** of cognitive development, in which abstract thought becomes possible; for example, the child can think about the roundness of the planets and can understand an analogy comparing the relative sizes of the earth and the sun to the sizes of a cherry and an orange. Piaget offers nurses a valuable view of the evolving intellectual capacity of the individual.

Moral Development

Several researchers have studied moral development during the early years of the life span. Two of the more prominent theorists are Lawrence Kohlberg and Carol Gilligan. Although Kohlberg acknowledges gender differences in moral development, Gilligan emphasizes the importance in recognizing that the decision-making process is different in boys and girls.

Kohlberg

On the basis of extensive longitudinal and cross-cultural studies, Lawrence Kohlberg, a developmental psychologist and educator, in 1963 identified three levels of moral development: *preconventional, conventional,* and *postconventional.* Each of these levels has within it two stages, so that, in all, six stages of moral development were described (Table 17-4). Although the greater part of his work was concerned with cognitive development, Piaget had earlier defined certain parameters of conscience development by using stories of moral questions with young children. Against this background, Kohlberg concluded that there were in fact three levels reaching from early childhood into adolescence. He did not believe in rigid age determinations in relation to the stages, but rather that each person moves through the stages sequentially and with some consistency.

In 1978, Kohlberg revised his original theory to include the possibility of a seventh stage. This subsequent research on the presence of later stages is optimistic because it implies that an individual has the potential to continue to grow morally into middle and later life.

Kohlberg's stages of moral development are defined as:

Level I—Preconventional

STAGE 1. The punishment–obedience orientation is a simple moral equation for the child. Punishment is to be expected if one is bad; the function of moral behavior is to escape punishment. Stage 1 is largely controlled by the parent as the authority figure. Reasons given for the punishment are largely inconsequential to the child, whose primary goal is to avoid punishment.

STAGE 2. Still a stage of the preschool years, stage 2 represents the beginning of egocentricity. The child sees that being good has benefits besides the avoidance of punishment: being good brings about certain rewards and is therefore self-serving. "Tradeoffs" constitute contract morality: one is good to get something desirable.

Level II—Conventional

STAGE 3. Moral behavior at this stage is important because of its effects on others. One has a desire to be good because being good is affirmed by authorities and peers. Since rules are still not clearly understood, rituals play a part. Bad luck/good luck rituals, such as not breaking a mirror, keep the world safer and maintain the individual's good behavior. Ritual behavior oftentimes assuages the child's beginning feelings of guilt (Dennis and Hassol, 1983, p. 139).

STAGE 4. Stage 4 is called the "law-and-order" stage. The child, now school age, understands more clearly the rules and laws of society and seeks to be a good citizen and person. Kohlberg states that some persons never progress beyond this stage, increasingly challenging society's rules to such an extent that they often become members of our prison population.

Level III—Postconventional

STAGE 5. This stage of young adulthood is more advanced and lacks the egocentricity of the earlier stages. Here the ethical principle of utilitarianism prevails (see Chapter 3 on ethics for a fuller discussion of this term). To be moral is to bring about the greatest good for the greatest number of people. Social ethics and a sense of altruism become significant in determining what is moral.

STAGE 6. The sixth stage and the highest, according to Kohlberg's early work, is much more encompassing. Universal law and principles are at play in molding a person's sense of justice. Essential to this stage is the protection of human rights within the framework of one's own conscience.

STAGE 7. Kohlberg and Shulik, exploring the possibility that a seventh stage exists, wrote that stage 6 appears not to provide total moral resolution for some

Table 17–4. Levels of Moral Development (Kohlberg)

Level and Stage	What is Right	Rationale for Right Behavior
Level I—Preconventional		
Stage 1. Punishment and obedience orientation	Do not do anything for which you might be punished.	Punishment is avoided.
Stage 2. Instrumental relativist orientation	Right doing is when you get something out of it. It is also when there is an equal exchange so that both gain.	It helps get you what you want in a world where everyone has needs and wants that need to be recognized. Desire for reward outweighs fear of punishment.
Level II—Conventional		
Stage 3. "Good boy, good girl" orientation	"Being good" is the goal for right behavior. Living up to what is expected of you is necessary. Bad luck/good luck rituals keep the world safer and maintain the individual's good behavior.	You are a good person in your own eyes and in the eyes of others.
Stage 4. The law-and-order orientation	Right behavior is obeying the law and the rules.	Laws and rules are necessary to the social system to avoid its breakdown.
Level III—Postconventional		
Stage 5. The social contract orientation	Right conduct is what results in the greatest amount of good for the greatest number of people in the society. Good is therefore this type of general consensus . . . a social contract.	To live in a society is to undertake the obligation for abiding by the laws that offer greatest welfare and protection of everyone's rights.
Stage 6. The universal ethical principle orientation	There are certain universal principles that transcend even what a given society may have designated as right. The individual is obligated to live by these principles, which include justice and equality of human rights.	To be a truly rational human being, it is necessary to believe in and abide by universal principles according to one's own conscience.
Stage 7. Mystical and religious reflection	As in stage 6, but deeper insight affects moral choices.	Greater reliance on intuitive rather than concrete reasoning. Potential for moral growth to continue throughout lifetime.

rather selective sensitive adults who move on to a stage 7, in which there is mystical and religious reflection on the reasons for one's morality. Stage 7 is similar to Maslow's stage of self-actualization (see Chapter 4) in that it provides a goal that many strive for but only some attain.

It is clear that Kohlberg has been significant in the understanding of moral development. Gilligan and others, however, have viewed his work as being flawed because it appears to pertain to the moral development of males in our society more than of females.

Gilligan

Carol Gilligan's text, *In A Different Voice* (1982), was based on a study of equally matched males and females throughout the life span from ages 6 to 60. She also conducted exhaustive interviews regarding moral issues and recorded verbatim responses from males and females. From this work and the work of other moral theorists, she concluded that males and females approach ethical dilemmas and solve moral problems in different ways. She attributes many of the differences to the manner in which society considers gender roles.

Gilligan writes of women's moral posture as being one of responsibility "not to hurt," whether it is the self or others. She believes that the conflict between the needs of self and others constitutes the central moral problem for women. Gilligan described moral development as being in three stages. After each stage comes a period of reconsideration or transition that leads to the next stage (Table 17-5).

STAGE 1. During this stage, the person views the survival of self as paramount in importance. Although this has been termed "selfishness" by some readers and even by Gilligan herself, the love and respect of self may understandably provide the firm base for morally supporting others.

STAGE 2. This stage is composed of the realization by the individual that there is a need for connectiveness or relationship with others and with this goes the re-

Table 17–5. Stages of Moral Development (Gilligan)

Stage	Age	Task
Stage I	Very young child	Egocentricism, survival of self guides morality. The love and respect of self provides the foundation for future moral support of others.
Stage II	Middle-age child through adolescence	The stage of "care ethics" during which there is a need for connectiveness, which results in a willingness to care about others.
Stage III	Young adult through advanced age	The time of moral responsibility with an emphasis on avoidance of hurting others

sponsibility to care. Gilligan uses the term "care ethics" when describing this stage. There is the recognition that even though one's own needs have to be met, there is also an obligation and a willingness to care for and about others. Through the transition period, the third stage is reached.

STAGE 3. The third stage incorporates a sense of responsibility for a position that is protective of one's own moral ethics and actively protects others from being hurt. Here, the avoidance of hurting others becomes all important and guides mature moral decision making.

Gilligan's theories regarding moral development aspire to heighten our awareness that gender is a factor in deciding moral dilemmas in life. She observes that the moral dilemmas females face are far different from those faced by males. "Only when life cycle theorists divide their attention and begin to live with women as they have lived with men will their vision encompass the experience of both sexes and their theories become more fertile" (p. 23).

Faith Development

When considering religious affiliation, the parameters are broad because the world's population embraces a wide variety of beliefs (see Chapter 36). Whether the development of this area is called the development of religion, values, or faith is perhaps not of concern. The important fact is that a need of all human beings is the integration of a value system that allows us to interact effectively with those around us.

Westerhoff

Westerhoff outlined another dimension of human life, which he called faith development. Some have considered this the development of values, although Westerhoff refers to four stages of the growth of faith. His theory might also be called the development of spirituality (Table 17-6).

STAGE 1. *Experiencing Faith*. Westerhoff calls this stage the experience of faith which takes place in the very young child who is becoming cognizant of the world and people around him. The stage continues through early adolescence and consists of experiencing faith of those significant family members, particularly the parents. Love and respect of one member for the other could be examples of this stage.

STAGE 2. *Affiliating with Faith*. During this period in late adolescence, the person begins the process of affiliation with a particular faith and as evidence, participates in the rituals and observances of that faith. For example, the young Jewish person may accompany the family to Friday night services and if male, wear the traditional skull cap, or yarmulke. This is the age when mysticism of a faith may be experienced and the person begins to incorporate a particular value system into life. There is a sense of identity with a group holding the same faith or religion.

Table 17–6. Stages of Faith Development (Westerhoff)

Stage	Age	Task
Stage I: Experiencing faith	Young child through early adolescence	Becoming cognizant of the world and the people around the individual. Sensing faith of family members.
Stage II: Affiliating with faith	Late adolescence	Begins affiliation with a particular faith, participates in rituals.
Stage III: Faith searching	Young adulthoodhood	An inspection and reconsideration of former religious choices.
Stage IV: Faith owned	Adult through advanced age	Acknowledgment of a personal belief system. Establishing unique values and spiritual concepts.

STAGE 3. *Faith Searching.* During young adulthood, there is an inspection of what one considers personal faith. The spiritual beliefs of the family, once highly protected, may come under scrutiny and be either discarded as no longer relevant or become more highly regarded. Through this questioning process, a strong belief system ensues which is highly personal.

STAGE 4. *Faith Owned.* Into adulthood and beyond, the individual acknowledges faith through openly practicing a set of unique values and spiritual concepts. These might be quite different from the family affiliation identified in stage 1. According to Westerhoff, it is no longer a matter of questioning, but of affirming one's faith by actions. Whether the development of this area is called the development of religion, values, or faith is perhaps not of concern. The important fact is that a need of all humans is the integration of a value system that allows us to interact effectively with those around us.

Life Span Considerations and the Nursing Process

It is important for nurses to be thoroughly familiar with the basics of developmental theory and thus the specific needs of the individual throughout the life span. The changing flow of life provides both challenge and opportunity to those of us who are in the care professions. The integration of an individual's physical, social, sexual, cognitive, and moral components results in a person different from any other individual. For care to be maximally effective, it should be tailored to the unique characteristics of its recipient.

Your assessments of all the characteristics of the patient are valid or meaningful only if you can make comparisons to what is usual. Notwithstanding the hazards of categorizing people, knowing the norms of social development will deepen your assessment abilities. For example, if the hospitalized 3-year-old child cries uncontrollably when the mother must leave the bedside to return home, you can give the child better support and assurance if you know that at this age the mother's presence is primary and even brief separation is devastating. With understanding of growth and development, you will gain insight into what is important to the patient. Knowing this will allow you to identify nursing diagnoses specific to the age-related needs of that person.

At each stage of the life span, a group of needs will either change completely or become more complex in the next stage. For example, the love needs of the infant may be the need to receive love rather than to offer it to others. But within only a few years, the youngster feels the pleasure of hugging or offering love. Later, the sexual love relationship of adults takes on a much more complex nature.

Understanding the interrelationship of needs with patterns of growth and development is also useful when planning interventions within the health care setting. One of the most interesting aspects of nursing is the variety of persons we care for, from newborns to the very aged. Therefore, familiarity with the life span allows nurses more clearly and realistically to identify concerns or problems in the care of patients.

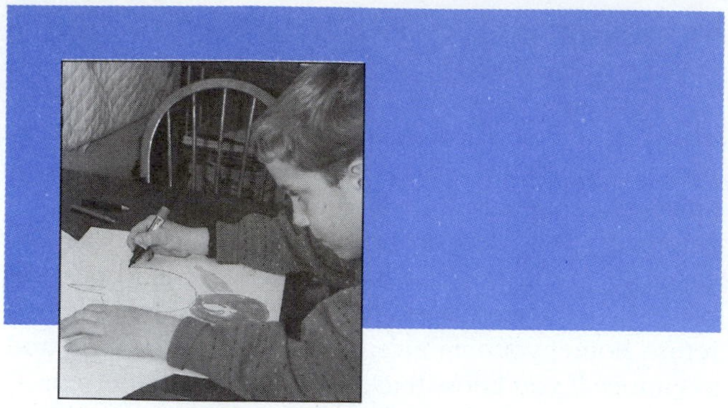

Key Points

- As human beings change throughout the life span, so do their needs. These changes relate to the organs of the body, the ability to think, emotions, moral and spiritual values. Nurses can more effectively meet the needs of patients when they have basic descriptive knowledge of each stage of the life span and the factors that influence it.
- There is ongoing discussion regarding the influence of heredity versus environment on the individual's development.
- Several theorists have developed frameworks for studying the life span. These theories can be categorized according to five aspects of development: psychosocial, psychosexual, cognitive, moral, and faith.
- Robert Havighurst's theory of development consists of six stages. The tasks to be learned during the first stages of life are primarily physical; the tasks of later years concern attitudes and relationships.
- Robert Peck focused on the middle and advanced adult years and looked on decline as an opportunity to call on and mobilize abilities and past coping experiences to transcend loss.
- Sigmund Freud's work continues to provide the classic definition of psychosexual development although some aspects of his theory are being challenged by today's research.
- Cognitive and intellectual development throughout the life span was outlined best by Jean Piaget. He described the development of the thought processes from birth through age 11, the age at which the ability to deal with abstractions and systematic problem-solving first appears.
- Lawrence Kohlberg described six stages of moral development, from the preconventional one of punishment–obedience to the sixth stage of recognition of the universal good. A possible seventh stage has been added, which allows one to reflect mystically on the moral meaning of life.
- Carol Gilligan expanded the concepts of moral development to include women and the differentiation of the resolution of moral problems for women compared with men. She outlined four stages of moral development for women.
- John Westerhoff described four stages of faith development, which begin in early childhood and result in a demonstration of a belief pattern in late adulthood. His theory can be thought of in terms of the development of spirituality in the individual, which is a universal need.
- The developmental theories can be used to describe the usual developmental pattern of the human life span. The integration of physical, psychosocial, psychosexual, cognitive, moral, and spiritual growth offers a holistic approach to studying the individual.

Study Questions

1. In your opinion, which of the definitions of growth and development is most accurate? Why?
2. What arguments are often given to substantiate whether heredity or environment is the most important factor influencing a person's growth and development?
3. Why do nurses need to have knowledge regarding human growth and development?
4. Briefly discuss and contrast the psychosocial theories of Erikson, Havighurst, and Peck.
5. How might Freud's theory of psychosexual development have relevance for today's nurse?
6. Discuss Kohlberg's seventh stage of moral development in terms of self-actualization.
7. Describe your experience with any gender differences in moral growth and development.
8. Using the four stages of Westerhoff, discuss how an individual in two of the world's main religions might demonstrate these stages.

Critical Thinking Activities

1. Analyze the moral developmental differences between males and females, according to Gilligan.
2. Find an article written by any of the eight theorists discussed in the chapter. Review the article in relationship to the general focus, who was studied, and the research conclusions. Do you believe the research is as relevant today as when it was written? Why or why not?

3. Identify the most important parts of the article and report to a small group of students.

References and Readings

American Journal of Nursing 75, 10 (October 1975). Seventy-fifth Anniversary Issue. (Entire issue devoted to the life span.)

Chally, P. S. "Theory Derivation in Moral Development." *Nursing and Health Care* 11, 6 (June 1990): 302–306.

Erikson, E. H. *Childhood and Society.* New York: W. W. Norton, 1963.

Freud, S. *The Ego and the Id* (1923). London: Hogarth Press, 1935.

Gesell, A. "The Ontogenesis of Infant Behavior." In *Manual of Child Psychology.* 2nd edition, edited by Leonard Carmichael. New York: John Wiley and Sons, 1954.

Gilligan, C. *In a Different Voice.* Cambridge: Harvard University Press, 1982.

Havighurst, R. J. *Developmental Tasks and Education.* 3rd edition. New York: Longman, 1972.

Kalkman, M. E., and Davis, A. J. *In Mental Health—Psychiatric Nursing.* New York: McGraw-Hill, 1974.

Kohlberg, L. "Moral Education in the Schools: A Developmental View." *School Review* 74 (1966): 1–30.

———. "Revisions in the Theory and Practice of Moral Development." In *Moral Development: New Directions for Child Development* (No. 2), pp. 10, 83–88, edited by W. Damon. San Francisco: Jossey-Bass, 1978.

Levinson, D. J., Darrow, C. N., Klein, E. B., and Levinson, M. H. *The Seasons of a Man's Life.* New York: Alfred A. Knopf, 1986.

Murray, R. B., and Zentner, J. P. *Nursing Assessment and Health Promotion Strategies Through the Life Span.* 4th edition. Englewood Cliffs, N.J.: Prentice-Hall, 1989.

Parker, R. S. "Measuring Nurses' Moral Judgments." *Image* 22, 4 (Winter 1990): 213–217.

Peck, R. "Psychological Developments in the Second Half of Life." In *Middle Age and Aging,* edited by B. L. Neugarten. Chicago: University of Chicago Press, 1968.

Piaget, J. *The Origins of Intelligence in Children.* New York: W. W. Norton, 1963.

Reed, P. "Implications of the Life-Span Developmental Framework for Well-Being in Adulthood and Aging." *Advances in Nursing Science* 6, 1 (October 1983): 18–25.

Rousseau, J-J. *Emile: Concerning Education* (1762). Translated by Rosalie Feltenstein. Great Neck, N.Y.: Barron's Educational Series.

Shulik, R. "The Aging Person as Philosopher: Moral Development and the Adult Years." Unpublished paper, Harvard University, 1981.

Westerhoff, J. *Will Our Children Have Faith?* New York: Seabury Press, 1976.

Whaley, L. F., and Wong, D. L. *Essentials of Pediatric Nursing.* 4th edition. St. Louis: C. V. Mosby, 1990.

Infancy Through Adolescence

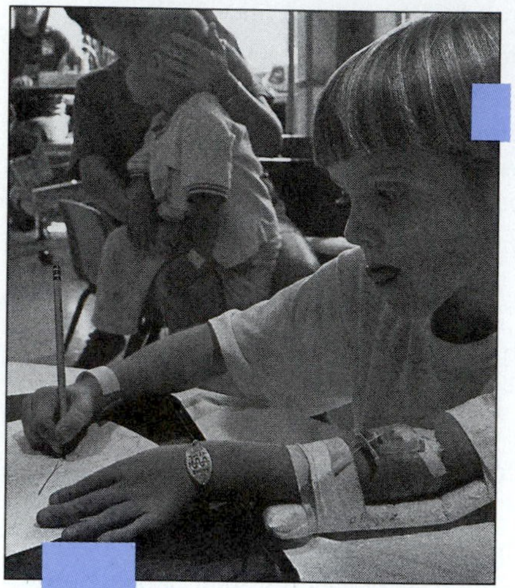

18

Objectives

After completing this chapter, you should be able to:

1. Discuss briefly the physical, psychosocial, psychosexual, cognitive, and moral development of the infant.
2. Discuss briefly the physical, psychosocial, psychosexual, cognitive, and moral development of the toddler, ages 1 to 3 years.
3. Discuss briefly the physical, psychosocial, psychosexual, cognitive, moral, and faith development of the child in early childhood, ages 3 to 6.
4. Discuss briefly the physical, psychosocial, psychosexual, cognitive, moral, and faith development of the child in middle childhood, ages 6 to 12.
5. Discuss briefly the physical, psychosocial, psychosexual, cognitive, moral, and faith development of the adolescent.
6. State why it is important for nurses to have basic knowledge regarding the development of the child in these age groups.
7. Outline the responses children in each of these age groups may have to hospitalization and illness.
8. Indicate ways in which the nurse can be effective in caring for patients in each age group.

Study Terms

adolescence
anal stage
asynchronous growth
autonomy versus shame and doubt stage
bilirubin
bonding
cephalocaudal development
deciduous teeth
identity versus role confusion stage
infancy
industry versus inferiority conflict
initiative versus guilt stage
latency period
menses
Moro reflex
neonate
oedipal stage
oral stage
phallic stage
plateaus
puberty
trust versus mistrust stage

Outline

Ellis, Nowlis: Nursing: A Human Needs Approach, 5th ed. © 1994 J.B. Lippincott Company

During your nursing career, you will be taking care of patients who are at different stages of the life span. Although individuals vary considerably, it is helpful to have knowledge concerning the expected responses to illness and hospitalization of persons of different ages when planning care.

The years from infancy to adolescence are crucial for exploring the immediate world, forming important lifelong relationships, and determining behavior. Some theorists have attributed much of adult behavior to the influences of the early years.

The nurse has an important role in caring for children in the hospital. Providing physical safety is essential. Adaptations are made in many procedures to consider the physical and psychological differences among pediatric patients.

Psychologically, the nurse builds on knowledge of each year of childhood to maximize the support needed to help a particular child to adapt to hospitalization without adverse effects. To better meet the needs of a variety of young patients, the nurse must have knowledge of the usual pattern of growth and development and the impact of hospitalization. As with all patients, nurses should focus on the individual's strengths rather than on weaknesses.

The person's stage within the life span is a crucial part of the data on which to build an appropriate nursing care plan. Assessment, nursing diagnoses, interventions, and evaluation may depend in large part on the age and expected responses of the client/patient. Pediatric nursing is beyond the scope of this text. However, within each age group of childhood, certain developmental factors are relevant for nursing care. This chapter explores those factors in terms of the developmental theories presented in Chapter 17.

Infancy: Birth to 1 Year

Physical Development

The departure of the *infant* from the warm, safe, fluid environment of its mother's womb initiates profound bodily changes or, in the words of Lawrence Frank, "violent alterations" that contribute to the establishment of physiologic homeostasis independent of the mother's body (1951).

During the first 28 days or month of life, the infant is designated a **neonate**. This is largely a clinical term and most nurses and families would refer to this age child as a newborn. For our purposes, we will define **infancy** as the stage from the time of birth through the first year of life. The infant grows proportionately more during the first month of life than at any other time but remains totally dependent on others in the environment to fulfill basic needs (Fig. 18-1).

The first assessment of normal physical development is done by determining the length, weight, and head circumference of the neonate. In Western countries, males tend to average approximately 20 to 21 inches in length (51–53.3 cm); females are approximately 19 to 20 inches long (48–51 cm). Birth weights average 7 to 8 pounds (15.4–17.6 kg), with males usually somewhat heavier than females. The circumference of the newborn's head is between 13 and 14 inches (33 and 35.5 cm). Nonwhite children may be somewhat

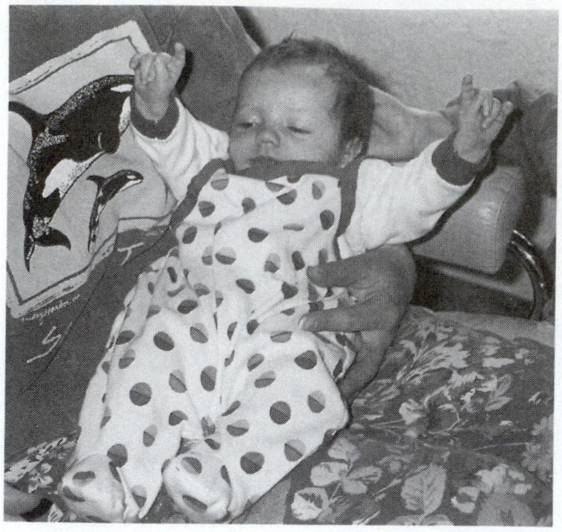

Figure 18-1. The infant is totally dependent on others to fulfill needs.

smaller at birth, perhaps because of ethnic factors such as the stature of the parents, nutritional, or environmental differences. Infants' vital signs, particularly breathing, are unstable. The infant's first cry expands the countless alveoli (tiny air sacs) of the lungs, initiating a lifelong dependence on the external environment for oxygen. Respirations fluctuate between 30 and 50/min, with short periods of apnea (no apparent breathing) between the actual breathing periods. Structural adaptations begin quickly in the heart at birth to complete the formation of the four chambers. The infant's heart rate is at its slowest during sleep, averaging about 90 beats/min, and highest with crying, about 150 beats/min. These strong rhythmic heart rate patterns, which began before birth, will gradually slow as they persist without interruption for 80 years or more. The infant is particularly vulnerable to the temperature of the environment and loses and gains body heat readily. Therefore, the infant's body temperature also fluctuates in response and is most stable in an environment of approximately 21° to 24°C or 70° to 75°F.

The need for nourishment is apparent shortly after birth. Stroking the infant's cheek elicits the rooting reflex, in which the head turns toward the stroked side in search of the breast. Infants begin early to put their fingers in their mouths and make sucking movements. Peristalsis, the wavelike movements of the intestines, ensues and the gastric secretions begin to flow in preparation for the first feeding.

Approximately 3 or 4 days after birth, the neonate's skin may take on a yellowish cast called jaundice, which is caused by serum bilirubin being deposited in the skin. **Bilirubin** originates from the breaking down of excess red blood cells accumulated from the mother during the embryonic period. Serum bilirubin is excreted by the liver, but the neonate is unable to excrete sufficient amounts. This normal newborn jaundice fades as the bilirubin is broken down and excreted. It is not normal for an infant to have this condition at the time of birth. Blood incompatibility between the infant and the mother could be the cause in this situation.

The posture of the infant is flexed most of the time during the first month as it was in utero. With stimulation, such as when being bathed, the newborn will stretch and extend the limbs. When a loud noise is heard, the infant's arms are suddenly abducted, or flung outward, and this is called the **Moro** (or startle) **reflex**, and disappears around the age of 4 months. A curling abdominal position, with the head turned to one side, is a comfortable sleeping position for the newborn.

The infant's awake-sleeping pattern is individual. Infants sleep from 15 to 20 hours out of 24, with the waking time devoted mostly to being fed and having soiled diapers changed. As the first month passes, sleep decreases and social activity increases.

Sight is blurred during the first weeks of life. At first, black and white objects are preferred to objects with bright colors. Shiny, flashing objects are appealing to the neonate, but the attention span is short, so that the gaze is quickly directed elsewhere. Accommodation develops so that the 3-month-old infant can distinguish faces at close range. At 4 to 5 months, distant vision is intact and medium to bright colors are preferred. Familiar faces can clearly be seen.

Hearing is intact in the infant, but differentiation occurs over months. Parents are encouraged to allow infants to see their faces at close range and provide both auditory and visual stimulation. Crying is normally a survival behavior, signaling discomfort, hunger, or fright (which can be brought on by loud noises or bright lights).

The infant's sensation of feeling is acute. Touching and closeness are important ways to bring about **bonding**, which is the forming of attachment to the significant person or persons caring for the infant, usually the parents. The technique of placing the newborn on the abdomen of the mother at the time of birth and allowing the father to be present in the birthing room are excellent ways to begin this important process. In many countries of the world, this has been an age-old practice; in others, the father is excluded but the mother–newborn contact is maintained.

From the first few months in life until the first year, physical growth is notable. The infant raises the head from the prone position at the end of 1 month, rolls from back to side at 4 months, and picks up objects at 6 months. Creeping begins at about 8 months. The infant is able to stand, supported by stable objects, at about 10 months. Many infants walk independently at 1 year.

At age 2 months, the child in the United States and Canada receives the first of many immunizations to prevent infectious diseases. It is important to adhere to a schedule that offers maximum protection (Table 18-1).

Table 18–1. Recommended Schedule for Immunization of Healthy Infants and Children*

Recommended Age†	Immunizations‡	Comments
2 mo	DTP, HbCV,§ OPV	DTP and OPV can be initiated as early as 4 wk after birth in areas of high endemicity or during epidemics
4 mo	DTP, HbCV,§ OPV	2-mo interval (minimum of 6 wk) desired for OPV to avoid interference from previous dose
6 mo	DTP, HbCV§	Third dose of OPV is not indicated in the U.S. but is desirable in other geographic areas where polio is endemic
15 mo	MMR,‖ HbCV¶	Tuberculin testing may be done at the same visit
15–18 mo	DTP,**'†† OPV#	(See footnotes)
4–6 y	DPT,§§ OPV, MMR¶¶	At or before school entry
11–12 y	MMR	At entry to middle school or junior high school
14–16 y	Td	Repeat every 10 y throughout life

* For all products used, consult manufacturer's package insert for instructions for storage, handling, dosage, and administration. Biologics prepared by different manufacturers may vary, and package inserts of the same manufacturer may change from time to time.
† These recommended ages should not be construed as absolute. For example, 2 mo can be 6–20 wk. However, MMR usually should not be given to children younger than 12 mo. (If measles vaccination is indicated, monovalent measles vaccine is recommended, and MMR should be given subsequently, at 15 mo.)
‡ DTP = diphtheria and tetanus toxoids with pertussis vaccine; HbCV = *Haemophilus b* conjugate vaccine; OPV = oral poliovirus vaccine containing attenuated poliovirus types 1, 2, and 3; MMR = live measles, mumps, and rubella viruses in a combined vaccine; Td = adult tetanus toxoid (full dose) and diphtheria toxoid (reduced dose) for adult use.
§ As of October 1990, only one HbCV (HbOC) is approved for use in children younger than 15 mo.
‖ May be given at 12 mo of age in areas with recurrent measles transmission.
¶ Any licensed *Haemophilus b* conjugate vaccine may be given.
** Should be given 6–12 mo after the third dose.
†† May be given simultaneously with MMR at 15 mo.
# May be given simultaneously with MMR and HbCV at 15 mo or at any time between 12 and 24 mo; priority should be given to administering MMR.
§§ Can be given up to the seventh birthday.
¶¶ Many states require MMR before school admission.
Source: Committee on Infectious Diseases. (1991). Report of the Committee for Infectious Diseases. Elk Grove Village, IL: American Academy of Pediatrics.

Other characteristics of increasing complexity emerge. At approximately 7 months, the 20 tiny teeth lying dormant within the gums begin to push their way, often painfully, through the surface of the gums. Chewing motions occur as preparation for the solid food soon to be introduced into the diet. The period from birth to 1 year is a time of active growing, with the birth weight doubling by 6 months and tripling by 1 year. The trunk and limbs elongate and the face becomes more lean with more distinctive and prominent features.

All growth and development is characterized by **plateaus** or periods during which change is slow or apparently nonexistent. The pace of growth and development is influenced by genetic background, general health, nutrition, glandular hormones, and psychological well-being.

An excellent developmental instrument (Displays 18-1 through 18-3) was designed by the Child Evaluation Clinic of Cedar Rapids, Iowa. This scale evaluates a child's motor skills and social adaptation month by month through the first year, every 3 months through the second year, and every 6 months until the fourth year, ending with usual behavior in the fifth year.

Psychosocial Development

Although physically separated from the mother and thus in a sense physically separate, the newborn is totally dependent on others for the gratification of all basic needs: sufficient air of a comfortable temperature, fluids and nutrients, a safe crib, and touch that conveys love.

The infant is *egocentric*, which means that the self is the most important. A soiled diaper or hunger contractions of the stomach wall signal distress and elicit a cry for help. The parent hurriedly responds, initiating an

(*Text continues on page 298*)

Display 18–1

Child Development from One Month to One Year of Age

1 month

Motor

1. Moro's reflex present.
2. Vigorous sucking reflex present.
3. Lying prone (face down); lifts head briefly so chin is off table.
4. Lying prone: makes crawling movements with legs.
5. Held in sitting position: back is rounded, head held up momentarily only.
6. Hands tightly fisted.
7. Reflex grasp of object with palm.

Language

8. Startled by sound; quieted by voice.
9. Small throaty noises or vocalizations.

Personal-social-adaptive

10. Ringing bell produces decrease of activity.
11. May follow dangling object with eyes to midline.
12. Lying on back: will briefly look at examiner or change activity.
13. Reacts with generalized body movements when tissue paper is placed on face.

2 months

Motor

1. Kicks vigorously.
2. Energetic arm movements.
3. Vigorous head turning.
4. Held in ventral suspension (prone): no head droop.
5. Lying prone: lifts head so face makes an approximate 45° angle with table.
6. Held in sitting position: head erect, but bobs.
7. Hand goes to mouth.
8. Hand often open (not clenched).

Language

9. Is cooing.
10. Vocalizes single vowel sounds, such as: ah-eh-uh.

Personal-social-adaptive

11. Head and eyes search for sound.
12. Listens to bell ringing.
13. Follows dangling object past midline.
14. Alert expression.
15. Follows moving person with eyes.
16. Smiles back when talked to.

3 months

Motor

1. Lying prone: lifts head to 90° angle.
2. Lifts head when lying on back (supine).
3. Moro's reflex begins to disappear.
4. Grasp reflex nearly gone.
5. Rolls side to back (3–4 mo).

Language

6. Chuckling, squealing, grunting, especially when talked to.
7. Listens to music.
8. Vocalizes with two different syllables, such as: a-a, la-la (not distinct), oo-oo.

Personal-social-adaptive

9. Reaches for but misses objects.
10. Holds toy with active grasp when put into hand.
11. Sucks and inspects fingers.
12. Pulls at clothes.
13. Follows object (toy) side to side (and 180°).
14. Looks predominantly at examiner.
15. Glances at toy when put into hand.
16. Recognizes mother and bottle.
17. Smiles spontaneously.

4 months

Motor

1. Sits well when supported.
2. No head lag when pulled to sitting position.
3. Turns head at sound of voice.
4. Lifts head (in supine position) in effort to sit.
5. Lifts head and chest when prone, using hands and forearms.
6. Held erect: pushes feet against table.

Language

7. Laughs aloud (4–5 mo).
8. Uses sound, such as: m-p-b-.
9. Repeats series of same sounds.

Display 18–1 (continued)
Child Development from One Month to One Year of Age

Personal-social-adaptive
10. Grasps rattle.
11. Plays with own fingers.
12. Reaches for object in front of self with both hands.
13. Transfers object from hand to hand.
14. Pulls dress over face.
15. Smiles spontaneously at people.
16. Regards raisin (or pellet).

5 months

Motor
1. Moro's reflex gone.
2. Rolls side to side.
3. Rolls back to front.
4. Full head control when pulled to or held in sitting position.
5. Briefly supports most of own weight on legs.
6. Scratches on table top.

Language
7. Squeals with high voice.
8. Recognizes familiar voices.
9. Coos and/or stops crying on hearing music.

Personal-social-adaptive
10. Grasps dangling object.
11. Reaches for toy with both hands.
12. Smiles at mirror image.
13. Turns head deliberately to bell.
14. Obviously enjoys being played with.

6 months

Motor
1. Supine: lifts head spontaneously.
2. Bounces on feet when held standing.
3. Sits briefly (tripod fashion).
4. Rolls front to back (6–7 mo).
5. Grasps foot and plays with toes.
6. Grasps cube with palm.

Language
7. Vocalizes at mirror image.
8. Makes four or more different sounds.
9. Localizes source of sound (bell, voice).
10. Vague, formless babble (especially with family members).

Personal-social-adaptive
11. Holds one cube in each hand.
12. Puts cube into mouth.
13. Re-secures dropped cube.
14. Transfers cube from hand to hand.
15. Conscious of strange sights and persons.
16. Consistent regard of object or person (6–7 mo).
17. Uses raking movement to secure raisin or pellet.
18. Resists having toy taken away.
19. Stretches out arms to be taken up (6–8 mo).

8 months

Motor
1. Sits alone (6–8 mo).
2. Early stepping movements.
3. Tries to crawl.
4. Stands few seconds, holding on to object.
5. Leans forward to get an object.

Language
6. Two-syllable babble, such as: a-la, ba-ba, oo-goo, a-ma, mama, dada (8–10 mo).
7. Listens to conversation (8–10 mo).
8. "Shouts" for attention (8–10 mo).

Personal-social-adaptive
9. Works to get toy out of reach.
10. Scoops pellet.
11. Rings bell purposely (8–10 mo).
12. Drinks from cup.
13. Plays peek-a-boo.
14. Looks for dropped object.
15. Bites and chews toys.
16. Pats mirror image.
17. Bangs spoon on table.
18. Manipulates paper or string.
19. Secures ring by pulling on the string.
20. Feeds self crackers.

10 months

Motor
1. Gets self into sitting position.
2. Sits steadily (long time).
3. Pulls self to standing position (on bed railing).
4. Crawls on hands and knees.
5. Walks when held or around furniture.
6. Turns around when left on floor.

(*continued*)

Display 18–1 *(continued)*
Child Development from One Month to One Year of Age

Language
7. Imitates speech sounds.
8. Shakes head for "no."
9. Waves "bye-bye."
10. Responds to name.
11. Vocalizes in varied jargon patterns (10–12 mo).

Personal-social-adaptive
12. Plays "pat-a-cake."
13. Picks up pellet with finger and thumb.
14. Bangs toys together.
15. Extends toy to a person.
16. Holds own bottle.
17. Removes cube from cup.
18. Drops one cube to get another.
19. Uses handle to lift cup.
20. Initially shy with strangers.

1 year

Motor
1. Walks with one hand held.
2. Stands alone (or with support).
3. Secures small object with good pincer grasp.
4. Pivots in sitting position.
5. Grasps two cubes in one hand.

Language
6. Uses "mama" or "dada" with specific meaning.
7. "Talks" to toys and people, using fairly long verbal patterns.
8. Has vocabulary of two words besides "mama" and "dada."
9. Babbles to self when alone.
10. Obeys simple requests, such as "Give me the cup."
11. Reacts to music.

Personal-social-adaptive
12. Cooperates with dressing.
13. Plays with cup, spoon, saucer.
14. Points with index finger.
15. Pokes finger (into stethoscope) to explore.
16. Releases toy into your hand.
17. Tries to take cube out of box.
18. Unwraps a cube.
19. Holds cup to drink.
20. Holds crayon.
21. Tries to imitate scribble.
22. Imitates beating two cubes together.
23. Gives affection.

Source: Block, W. M., and Fitzgerald, J. Child Evaluation Clinic of Cedar Rapids, Iowa, 1972.

emotional as well as a physical dependence that is the most meaningful relationship during the early years of life. Erikson calls this the **trust versus mistrust stage**. If the parent–infant relationship is characterized by consistency and genuine affection, the baby perceives the world as trustworthy, safe, and dependable. If, on the other hand, care of the child is inconsistent or neglectful, the infant displays fear, suspicion, and agitation.

Peck did not apply his developmental theories to infants. Havighurst begins his construct with the learning task of walking. It might be surmised that the learning tasks Havighurst would have assigned to the younger infant would be those of sucking, rolling over, and grasping.

Psychosexual Development

Although the infant is unaware of sexuality as adults experience it, stimulation of its body parts is pleasurable. Initially, the infant's mouth is its primary source of gratification, which Freud calls the **oral stage** of sexual development. The young infant may also accidentally explore the genitals and feel pleasure.

Although not pronounced, behavioral differences between the sexes have been noted early in life. Females appear to be more vocal as infants, and in later life they prove somewhat more adept at verbal skills and less prone to speech difficulties than males. Male infants are superior in motor skills, although fine muscle coordination develops earlier in girls. Thus, subtle sexual differences are evident even in the first few months of life.

Cognitive Development

Piaget describes the infant's cognition as consisting primarily of exploration of the body and immediate surroundings through the senses. The time when learning takes place through the senses and motor activity, he called the sensorimotor stage (see Chapter 17). Various external stimuli also are important in elementary cognition.

Display 18–2
Child Development from Fifteen Months to Thirty Months

15 months

Motor

1. Stands alone.
2. Creeps upstairs.
3. Kneels on floor or chair.
4. Gets off floor and walks alone with good balance.
5. Bends over to pick up toy without holding on to furniture.

Language

6. May speak four to six words (15–18 mo).
7. Uses jargon.
8. Indicates wants by vocalizing.
9. Knows own name.
10. Enjoys rhymes or jingles.

Personal-social-adaptive

11. Tilts cup to drink.
12. Uses spoon, but spills.
13. Builds tower of two cubes.
14. Drops cubes into cup.
15. Helps turn page in book, pats picture.
16. Shows or offers toys.
17. Helps pull off clothes.
18. Puts pellet into bottle without demonstration.
19. Opens lid of box.
20. Likes to push wheeled toys.

18 months

Motor

1. Runs (stiffly).
2. Walks upstairs—one hand held.
3. Walks backward.
4. Climbs into chair.
5. Hurls ball.

Language

6. May say 6–10 words (18–21 mo).
7. Points to at least one body part.
8. Can say "hello" and "thank you."
9. Carries out two directions (one at a time), for instance, "Get ball from table." "Give ball to Mother."
10. Identifies two objects by pointing (or picking up), such as cup, spoon, dog, car, chair.

Personal-social-adaptive

11. Turns pages.
12. Builds tower of three to four cubes.
13. Puts 10 cubes into cup.
14. Carries or hugs a doll.
15. Takes off shoes and socks.
16. Pulls string toy.
17. Scribbles spontaneously.
18. Dumps raisin from bottle after demonstration.
19. Uses spoon with little spilling.

21 months

Motor

1. Runs well.
2. Walks downstairs—one hand held.
3. Walks upstairs alone or holding onto rail.
4. Kicks large ball (when demonstrated).

Language

5. May speak 15–20 words (21–24 mo).
6. May combine two or three words.
7. Asks for food, drink.
8. Echoes two or more words.
9. Takes three directions (one at a time), for instance, "Take ball from table." "Give ball to Mommy." "Put ball on floor."
10. Points to three or more body parts.

Personal-social-adaptive

11. Builds tower to five to six cubes.
12. Folds paper once when shown.
13. Helps with simple household tasks (21–24 mo).
14. Removes some clothing purposefully (besides hat or socks).
15. Pulls person to show something.

24 months

Motor

1. Runs without falling.
2. Walks up and down stairs.
3. Kicks large ball (without demonstration).
4. Throws ball overhand.
5. Claps hands.
6. Opens door.
7. Turns pages in book, singly.

(*continued*)

Display 18–2 (continued)
Child Development from Fifteen Months to Thirty Months

Language

8. Says simple phrases.
9. Says at least one sentence or phrase of four or more syllables.
10. Can repeat four to five syllables.
11. May reproduce about five to six consonant sounds. (Typically m-p-b-h-w.)
12. Points to four parts of body on command.
13. Asks for things at table by name.
14. Refers to self by name.
15. May use personal pronouns, such as I-me-you (24–30 mo).

Personal-social-adaptive

16. Builds five- to seven-cube tower.
17. May cut with scissors.
18. Spontaneously dumps raisin from bottle (without demonstration).
19. Throws ball into box.
20. Imitates drawing vertical line from demonstration.
21. Parallel play predominant.

30 months

Motor

1. Jumps in place with both feet.
2. Tries standing on one foot (may not be successful).
3. Holds crayon by fingers.
4. Imitates walking on tiptoe.

Language

5. Refers to self by pronoun (rather than name).
6. Names common objects when asked (key, penny, shoe, box, book).
7. Repeats two digits (one of three trials).
8. Answers simple questions, such as "What is this?" "What does the kitty say?"

Personal-social-adaptive

9. Builds tower of eight cubes.
10. Pushes toy with good steering.
11. Helps put things away.
12. Can carry breakable objects.
13. Puts on clothing.
14. Washes and dries hands.
15. Eats with fork.
16. Imitates drawing a horizontal line from demonstration.
17. May imitate drawing a circle from demonstration.

Source: Block, W. M., and Fitzgerald, J. Child Evaluation Clinic of Cedar Rapids, Iowa, 1972.

The infant initially responds to the internal stimuli of pain and hunger without distinguishing between them. Gradually, the infant begins to identify feelings of discomfort that are relieved by food and to distinguish them from other feelings. The same process occurs with all internal stimuli, and the infant gradually learns to trust his or her body and to develop an understanding of its signals.

External stimuli also help infants identify their own bodies. Small babies may cause themselves pain by biting their own toes because they do not know their own boundaries. The touch of those who care for the infant also helps to differentiate self from others.

Moral Development

Adult morality is absent in infants. Because ethical orientation derives in part from the trust engendered by the gratification of one's needs, the infant is beginning to experience feelings that will eventually set the stage for the ethical give-and-take of interaction with others.

The first year is characterized by alternating frustration and pleasure and by the inability to postpone gratification. Infants receive pleasure, give nothing consciously in return, and are unaware of the unique pleasure their existence gives their parents and others.

Responses to Illness and Hospitalization

Infants respond instinctively to the environment. If bright lights, loud noises, and strange tactile stimuli are present, infants may become irritable, fearful, and anxious. Even without the ability to understand illness, infants feel systemically unwell and expresses this feeling in their behavior. Sleep and eating behaviors may be affected by it.

Infants need closeness with others in the environ-

Display 18–3
Child Development from Three Years to Five Years

3 years

Motor

1. Stands on one foot for at least one second.
2. Jumps from bottom stair.
3. Alternates feet going upstairs.
4. Pours from a pitcher.
5. Can undo two buttons.
6. Pedals a tricycle.

Language

7. Repeats six syllables, for instance: "I have a little dog."
8. Names three or more objects in a picture.
9. Gives sex. ("Are you a boy or a girl?")
10. Gives full name.
11. Repeats three digits (one of three trials).
12. Knows a few rhymes.
13. Gives appropriate answers to "What swims-flies-shoots-boils-bites-melts?"
14. Uses plurals.
15. Knows at least one color.
16. Can reply to questions in at least three-word sentences.
17. May have vocabulary of 750 to 1,000 (3–3½ years).

Personal-social-adaptive

18. Understands taking turns.
19. Copies a circle (from model, without demonstration).
20. Builds three-block pyramid.
21. Dresses with supervision.
22. Puts 10 pellets into bottle in 30 s.
23. Separates easily from mother.
24. Feeds self well.
25. Plays interactive games, such as tag.

4 years

Motor

1. Stands on one foot for at least 5 s (two of three trials).
2. Hops at least twice on one foot.
3. Can walk heel-to-toe for four or more steps (with heel one inch or less in front of toe).
4. Can button coat or dress; may lace shoes.

Language

5. Repeats 10-word sentences without errors.
6. Counts three objects, pointing correctly.
7. Repeats three to four digits (4–5 y).
8. Comprehends: "What do you do if you are hungry-sleepy-cold?"
9. Spontaneous sentences, four to five words long.
10. Likes to ask questions.
11. Understands preposition, such as on-under-behind, etc. ("Put the block on the table.")
12. Can point to three out of four colors (red, blue, green, yellow).
13. Speech is now an effective communicative tool.

Personal-social-adaptive

14. Copies cross (+) without demonstration.
15. Imitates oblique cross (×).
16. Draws a man with four parts.
17. Cooperates with other children in play.
18. Dresses and undresses self (mostly without supervision).
19. Brushes teeth, washes face.
20. Compares lines: "Which is longer?"
21. Folds paper two to three times.
22. Can select heavier from lighter object.
23. Cares for self at toilet.

5 years

Motor

1. Balances on one foot for 8 to 10 s.
2. Skips, using feet alternatively.
3. May be able to tie a knot.
4. Catches bounced ball with hands (not arms) in two of three trials.

Language

5. Knows age ("How old are you?")
6. Performs three tasks (with one command), for instance, "Put pen on table—close door—bring me the ball."
7. Knows four colors.
8. Defines use for fork, horse, key, pencil, etc.
9. Identifies by name nickel, dime, penny.
10. Asks meaning of words.
11. Asks many "why" questions.
12. Relatively few speech errors remain—90% of consonant sounds are made correctly.
13. Counts number of fingers correctly.
14. Counts by rote to 10.
15. Comments on pictures (descriptions and interpretations).

(continued)

Display 18–3 *(continued)*
Child Development from Three Years to Five Years

Personal-social-adaptive

16. Copies a square.
17. Copies oblique cross (×) without demonstration.
18. May print a few letters (5–5½ years).
19. Draws man with at least six identifiable parts.
20. Builds a six-block pyramid from demonstration.
21. Transports things in a wagon.
22. Plays with coloring set, construction toys, puzzles.
23. Participates well in group play.

Source: Block, W. M., and Fitzgerald, J. Child Evaluation Clinic of Cedar Rapids, Iowa, 1972.

ment. They also need to feel safe. When illness or injury limits the contact of the infant with parents, nurses can fulfill these needs. Knowledge of the life span aids us in identifying appropriate nursing actions.

Nursing Considerations When Caring for the Infant

The nurse should provide a physically safe environment for the infant. This should include a crib from which the infant cannot fall, moderate temperatures, and air that is free of toxicity. Repeated studies have shown that both touch and voice stimulation promote not only Piaget's cognitive ability but social development of the infant as well.

Nursing staff members frequently talk and sing to infants in their care. Touch should be generously provided. These are ways in which the nurse can provide sensory stimulation to the hospitalized ill infant. The parents should be given ample time to hold, cuddle, and talk to the baby. These actions are so important that they should become part of the plan of care.

When working with parents of the newborn, the nurse can emphasize the importance of breast-feeding. Breast milk is the best natural nutrient for infants. It contains all the essential elements needed for normal growth except vitamins C and D and iron. These components can be supplemented by oral preparations. Another important advantage of human milk is that it contains immunoglobulins and antibodies that are transmitted to the infant, offering limited protection against some pathogens.

However, the virus for acquired immunodeficiency syndrome can be transmitted to the infant by breast milk so mothers who are positive for human immunodeficiency virus should not breast-feed. Parents should be encouraged to have their children immunized against common communicable diseases beginning in infancy (see Table 18-1). The introduction of solid food is now recommended at a later time than formerly because infants are able to store iron for as long as 6 months and readily develop allergies to many solid foods. For these reasons, it is recommended that solid food be introduced when the infant is 5 to 6 months old.

The Toddler: 1 to 3 Years

Physical Development

Between the ages of 1 and 3 years, the child achieves a degree of freedom from total dependence on the parents. Physical freedom results largely from mastery of the art of walking (Fig. 18-2). Everyone knows the wonderful game in which the toddler runs from the pursuing parent with laughter and squeals of delight. If not pursued, the youngster stops, forlorn, only to find reassurance in the welcoming arms of the waiting parent.

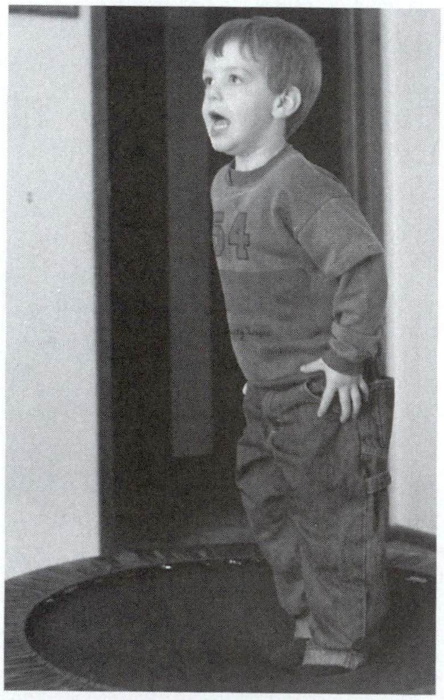

Figure 18–2. The toddler is physically active.

Physically, the toddler grows at a rate that is slower than infancy but still very rapid (see Display 18-2). Physical growth and development are uneven. Until about the age of 2, neuromuscular motor development proceeds from control of the head gradually downward to the feet. For example, a child can throw a ball from the sitting position before he or she can walk. This sequence is called **cephalocaudal development**. The physical growth of body parts is also disproportionate and is termed **asynchronous growth**. By the time a child reaches the age of 2, the weight of the brain and the circumference of the head approximate those of the adult. The skeletal system and muscles grow rapidly from infancy to adulthood, experiencing particularly vigorous growth during adolescence.

The average weight of toddlers is about 20 pounds. The average height is 34 inches, or about one-half the expected adult height. The physiologic responses have matured so that, in proportion to body stature, the child's lung capacity and circulation are normal. The ability to maintain body temperature has stabilized, with the normal body temperature at 37.1°C or 98.8°F, slightly above that for the normal adult. The passages of the throat, nose, and ear shorten, so the toddler is susceptible to organisms that cause ear and respiratory infections.

The toddler is physically active and characterized by gross body movements. Fine muscular agility has not yet developed well. The body loses some of its "baby fat" and becomes more elongated. Skin texture becomes more course. Visual acuity approximates that of the adult. Sphincter control is gradually achieved. The child can now eat with minimal assistance.

Psychosocial Development

At this age the youngster strives toward psychological independence. A part of this process is the toddler's confrontation with the parents and society. Needs are no longer promptly satisfied. A gain for the toddler, however, is the ability to decide whether to cooperate with parents in meeting the demands of a situation. "The battle of the potty chair" can become a confrontation of wills; the parent imposes conformity and the child discovers a new power to manipulate or control. If the rewards exceed the punishments, the child gains pleasure from the parents' approval (love) of the new behavior and from a growing sense of control over the environment. The child begins to understand what is expected and is increasingly aware of being a distinct individual with the ability to affect the surroundings. The toddler sees for the first time that pleasure postponed can be pleasure gained.

Erikson calls this the **autonomy versus shame and doubt stage**. If capabilities are acknowledged, according to Erikson, the child will develop a lasting sense of confidence and autonomy. If thwarted, the child may develop an unhealthy doubt of his or her own capabilities and, in turn, of other people and the environment.

Peck's theory did not address the learning tasks of the toddler. Havighurst's theory of developmental tasks looked at the toddler in terms of learning to walk, taking solid foods, talking, and learning to control the elimination of body wastes (see Display 17-1).

Psychosexual Development

Control over elimination gives the child a sense of power, which can be used manipulatively at times in relation to the parents. Wanting to please may be translated into using the toilet or potty chair; anger at the parents may be displayed by refusing to do so. Freud calls this period the **anal stage** of sexual development, when the anal and urethral areas provide sensual satisfaction.

The toddler does not yet have a firm grasp of differences between boys and girls. Young children derive pleasure from touching themselves and from the cuddling and fondling by their parents. In fact, many psychiatrists believe that early childhood is the most crucial period in sexual development because the child receives open love from the mother or father and learns—or fails to learn—to love and give to another. Some unfortunate children are punished for touching their genitals and made to believe that all sexual matters are taboo. Other children become confused about the contradictory reactions of adults, who may convey conflicting messages by promoting sexual attractiveness in the child (coyness, flirtation, cuteness) but reacting to overt sexuality with silence and secretiveness.

Cognitive Development

The thought processes of the toddler center on the immediate physical world or what is happening at the moment. The amazing energy and mobility of the toddler allow exploration of the physical environment. Touching, kicking, and throwing objects define the properties of an object through the delight of play.

Certainly the most important cognitive development of this age is the beginning of language. In language, the toddler and parent have a new, exciting form of communication. Being able to use a word (symbolism) for an object gives the child of about 2 years of age a new dimension of control over the environment because needs can be more effectively communicated. Various theories have been offered regarding the acquisition of language. The parent patterns language in toddlers by showing pleasure when the child mimics a word. Because of the obvious approval shown by the parent, the child feels rewarded and repeats the word. It has been documented that many children who have considerable language ability have parents who spend a large amount of time with them in verbal communication. However, deaf children who can hear neither their own voices nor those of parents do develop a verbal pattern of sounds. This demonstrates that speech does not entirely depend on teaching by adults. We might conclude that some form of verbal communication is a human cognitive need.

Vocabulary begins around the first year with single repetitious words and progresses to sentences of a few words—for example, "big ball," "give drink," "go now," or "see snow come down." Children master more than 1,000 words by the end of the third year.

Moral Development

The toddler has not yet reached Kohlberg's (1966) preconventional level of morality although behavior is influenced by parental approval and disapproval. Positive reinforcement from significant persons promotes beginning moral or ethical awareness by strengthening the concept of self. Gilligan would refer to this beginning moral stage as one of attaining self-respect and love.

Responses to Illness and Hospitalization

The toddler experiences separation anxiety when separated from the primary caregiver for a prolonged time. This is characterized by three behavioral reactions: protest, despair, and detachment (Whaley and Wong, 1989, p. 583). The toddler may feel acute psychological pain because of separation from parents. Cries of protest, kicking, striking out, and attempting to escape to find the parent may all be reactions at this stage. Following protest and the inability to locate the parents, the child may fall into despair, which is manifested by quiet, uninterested, passive behavior. Finally, the third stage, a period of detachment, occurs, characterized by some renewed interest in the events of the surroundings. This should not be interpreted as adjustment to separation. Detachment that persists for a long period of time can interfere with emotional development. Studies have shown that toddlers suffering from this reaction may have difficulty with forming relationships later in life.

The toddler has gained a new independence, and the restrictions imposed by hospitalization are frightening. Pain is often interpreted by the toddler as punishment, which incurs a sense of guilt.

Nursing Considerations When Caring for the Toddler

The nurse can be instrumental in meeting the special needs of the ill toddler by communicating that feeling sick is unrelated to having done something bad. It is also important for nurses who care for toddlers to recognize that this is the age in which separation anxiety becomes intense. Hospitals are becoming increasingly aware of the importance of this stressor on the child and as they do so, they allow parents to be with the child as long as they wish. However, the 18-month-old child will cry loudly when the parent or care provider leaves. The leaving is interpreted as abandonment. For the older toddler who has established an even tighter bond with the parent, it is devastating to have the parent leave, regardless of explanations. It is also hard for parents to subject their toddler to such distress although their absence is often a necessity. Nurses can be helpful in encouraging parents to be loving but firm when taking their leave. Although the toddler may loudly protest amid tearful outbursts, touching and consoling the youngster is an appropriate action for the nurse.

Medical procedures, particularly painful ones, pose a threat to the body in the mind of the young child. It is also difficult for the parents and the medical staff when painful procedures must be performed. The child aged 1 to 3 may not understand the rationale and explanations. However, 3-year-old children can understand simple explanations given in language within their grasp. Explanations should be honest; lying to a child—or any other patient—is inappropriate and counterproductive because it destroys trust. Procedures should be carried out promptly so that the anxiety they cause is minimized. Swaddling or restraining the youngster may be necessary to avoid injury. If a procedure is painful or upsetting to watch, the parent may not wish to attend and should not be encouraged to do so. After any procedure, the parent or nurse should offer comfort to the child.

Early Childhood: 3 to 6 Years

Physical Development

Early childhood is characterized by intense physical and mental activity (see Display 18-3). Physical growth is slower than during the first 3 years. The child is continuing to shed "baby fat" and acquiring the lean, tall body build of the school-age child. Both height and weight steadily progress during these years (Table 18-2). Boys and girls tend to grow similarly in height and weight until about the sixth year, when boys become somewhat heavier and taller than girls. African American, Hispanic, and other nonwhite children may be somewhat smaller in stature because of the factors already discussed.

Vital signs move more toward adult values. Sleep needs are more than those of the adult. Activity increases in amount and type. Combined with this increase in activity is an insatiable curiosity that helps the

Table 18–2. Average Height and Weight Parameters, Ages 1 to 6 Years

Age	Average Height	Average Weight
1 year	29 inches (74 cm)	21 lb (9.5 kg)
2 y	34 inches (86.6 cm)	27 lb (12 kg)
3 y	37 inches (94 cm)	33 lb (15 kg)
4 y	41 inches (104 cm)	38 lb (17 kg)
5 y	50 inches (127 cm)	45 lb (20.45 kg)
6 y	46 inches (117 cm)	48 lb (21.75 kg) (boys) 46 lb (20.94 kg) (girls)

child explore the world but requires vigilance because it also places the child at risk of accidents and poisonings.

The 3-year-old child has some limitations in coordination. Physical activities include the ability to ride a tricycle, climb steps tenuously with alternate feet, and manage simple closures on clothing. There may be occasional accidents in toileting. The child sometimes has to be reminded to eat because of easy distractions. The 4-year-old runs and skips easily, enjoys new activities, and can put on simple clothing with minimal assistance. Elimination is controlled. The youngster enjoys finger food but may reject certain items that are on the family menu. By age 5, the youngster can maintain balance, jump, and rollerskate. The 5-year-old can dress independently, including the tying of shoelaces. The child goes to the bathroom for toileting independently and closes the door for privacy. "Junk food," or the food from commercial fast food outlets, becomes attractive. Television and peer pressure may strongly influence food preferences. Play becomes an important part of socialization (Fig. 18-3). Lever (1978) found gender differences in children's play and games. Boys played outdoors more and played games that were much more competitive than girls. Hand coordination is developing, so crafts are often a part of leisure activities. Toward the end of the sixth year, the first of the **deciduous** (temporary) **teeth** may loosen and fall out. This process usually interferes minimally with the ability to eat.

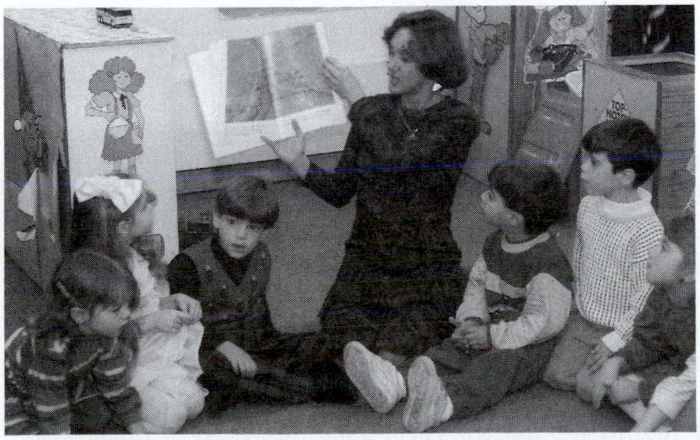

Figure 18-3. The teacher serves as a role model for three- to-six-year-old children.

Psychosocial Development

Erikson calls the period of early childhood the **initiative versus guilt stage**. The initiative of which Erikson speaks gives the youngster a feeling of accomplishment and thus diminishes rebelliousness. Children of this age tend toward orderliness and a willingness to perform household tasks, put away personal possessions, and bathe and dress themselves. Successful performance offsets feelings of guilt at not meeting parental expectations. The 3-year-old begins to demonstrate initiative through saying "no" to parental decisions.

Parental attitudes are crucial at this period. If the parents treat the child's activities and questions as significant, the child is encouraged to grow in response to such positive reinforcement. If the child's questions and explorations are treated flippantly or ridiculed, a sense of guilt may delay or undermine further emotional growth.

Peck did not extend his theory of development into the childhood years. Havighurst's theory of developmental tasks included psychological tasks such as learning sex differences and sexual modesty, forming concepts, and learning about social and physical reality. Young children identify with boy groups and girl groups early in development. A cognitive task, according to Havighurst, would be that of getting ready to read. He also included acquiring the physical skills needed for ordinary games (see Display 17-1).

Psychosexual Development

Freud subdivides the preschool years into two stages of sexual development. At age 3 or 4, the child enters the **phallic stage**, a period during which both girls and boys experience sensual pleasure in their genitals and may masturbate.

Freud's **oedipal stage**, which occurs at about age 4 or 5, is characterized by a heightened attachment to the parent of the opposite sex and identification with the parent of the same sex. For example, children of this age may see themselves as "little adults," the boy pretending to be like his father and the girl imitating her mother. According to Freud, sexual attraction to the parent of the opposite sex is a conflict resolved only by further emotional development.

Parents tend to encourage children to adopt sexual identities. For example, a boy may be given a football to play with, whereas a girl is given a doll. Boys are often dressed in masculine clothing and girls in dresses long before apparel has much meaning to youngsters. In recent years, parents have been widely encouraged to minimize the sexual patterning of children's behavior to allow for the development of individual interests and abilities.

The 3- to 6-year-old has a natural curiosity about the body and soon discovers that boys and girls are different. The proximity of the genitals to the organs of elimination, as well as the attitudes of adults, may cause the child to think of the sexual organs as unclean. Learning that nudity is not generally accepted in our culture may further mystify the child about sex.

Cognitive Development

Piaget portrays the 3- to 6-year-old as preoperational, continuing to be centered on the self. Because opinions are regarded as absolutes, the child is reluctant to alter decisions in the face of opposing views. Children at this age display the new ability to consider two ideas at the same time—for example, "If you eat your lunch now, we will be able to spend some time in the park." The child is developing the ability to deal with written symbols, such as the alphabet and numbers, and is learning to read a few words and to count using basic numbers. Questions are asked about the physical world: "Where does the sun go at night?" or "What makes a rainbow?"

The process of thinking also expands to include *fantasy.* The imagination can encompass wonderful things, sometimes replacing that which is unpleasant in life. To imagine that one has a special friend no one else can see is comforting to a lonely child. For the child who has a full life with family and friends, fantasy adventures offer unusual excitement. Recent texts on the value of fantasy suggest that children who are allowed to indulge in fantasy display more creativity in later life and that fantasy should also be encouraged in adults as long as they function adequately in the real world.

Moral Development

The preschooler reasons on the preconventional level; fear of punishment molds behavior. Pleasing parents is important, not for its own sake but to bring about desirable consequences. By the time the child reaches the upper levels of this age group (age 5 or 6) and enters school, the second stage of Kohlberg's preconventional level has been reached. The punishment–consequences idea of morality is refined to consider that being good allows you to feel good about yourself (relieving guilt) and to be in the favor of those for whom you care. According to Gilligan, this age child is experiencing the second stage, that of "care ethics" during which there is a desire for relationship and a need not to hurt others.

Westerhoff describes this age as capable of stage I beginning faith development. The young child is now aware of the surrounding world and sensing the faith of significant others.

Responses to Illness and Hospitalization

The preschooler continues to feel a deep sense of loss when separated from home and family. However, the child of this age has mobilized a variety of beginning coping skills to deal with the separation more constructively. Protests still occur but usually not as noisy outbursts. The child still feels a sense of guilt connected with illness. The preschooler is sensitive to the threat of bodily harm. Pain is often managed with a facade of being a good boy or girl. The preschool child often reacts to pain, stress, or fear with aggression or dependency. The aggression may be verbal and focused toward the nurse as the care provider. The dependency can take the form of regression to a level that is more comfortable for the child and requires less control.

Nursing Considerations When Caring for the Preschooler

Many hospitals have "play-persons" (sometimes referred to as *play therapists*) who either are paid by the hospital or are volunteers. Special play areas are designed for the young child. Encourage young patients who are well enough to make use of these areas. If a play area is not available, the parents can bring in treasured toys or diversions from home. Play persons should not be confused with "play nurses," who are specially trained pediatric psychiatric nurses. Through the use of play, they help identify the fears and concerns of the child.

If the child exhibits aggressive behavior, accept it as a normal response but set appropriate limits. The preschooler loves to play games, and some of this negative expression may be vented with game playing. Roommates are great diversion and company for the lonely, unhappy institutionalized child.

Preschoolers are concerned about their bodies and have great capacity for fantasy. Because of these facts, health care professionals should use language carefully so that misinterpretations are not made. For example, a nurse came to the bedside of a preschool patient with an order to discontinue the intravenous infusion. Glancing down at the tape, she remarked, "Well, we'll just have to take this off now." The wide eyes and look of terror told her immediately that the youngster had misinterpreted her casual remark and feared for his limb.

Like the toddler, the preschooler may have periods of aggression and regression, but preschoolers are more controlled in expressing these feelings. Some youngsters are stoic about pain but may try to bargain or delay injections and other painful procedures. It is best to move ahead with procedures in a timely but caring fashion.

Middle Childhood: 6 to 12 Years

Physical Development

Entrance into school is an important mark in the life span. Schools in this country and Canada have programs for monitoring physical development and often identify health problems, which are reported to the parents. Immunization programs continue under the auspices of schools. In some states, children may not be admitted to the classroom unless they have been immunized against certain diseases.

The physical growth rate of the child from 6 to 12 is steady except for a spurt just before puberty. Girls are frequently taller and more developed than boys by age 12. The brain reaches adult size by age 12, and the vital signs are close to the adult range. Except for the second molars and wisdom teeth, the permanent teeth have all erupted. The face begins to show adult characteristics. Coordination improves, and some children seek out competitive sports.

Nutritionists consider good dietary practices in these years essential to establishing good eating habits. Lowering the content of saturated fats in the diet may help decrease the chances of contracting cardiovascular disease later in life. Good nutrition can also aid the management of obesity in children, which can contribute to high blood pressure (hypertension). Six percent of children under the age of 12 are hypertensive. The National Heart, Lung, and Blood Institute has designed a grid to aid in identifying hypertensive children within this age group. The sudden rapid increase in physical growth must also be balanced with sufficient sleep and rest.

Psychosocial Development

For both girls and boys, friends and other peers assume great importance in this stage of development. Team sports channel the aggression common at this age into competitive agility. Fighting and wrestling dissipate energy. Girls' groups are usually less aggressively oriented. Girls do, however, form highly competitive basketball, soccer, baseball, and other sports teams.

Erikson defines the middle childhood years as devoted to resolving the **industry versus inferiority conflict**, that is, if the child's industry is praised and the child is allowed to undertake and complete tasks, the resolution of this stage will be healthy. A child whose efforts are ridiculed and criticized becomes discouraged and feels unworthy and inferior.

Peck does not focus on developmental tasks for this age group. Havighurst lists several tasks, most having to do with developing one's identity and social role. He emphasizes the following:

1. Building wholesome attitudes toward oneself as a growing organism.
2. Learning to get along with peers.
3. Learning an appropriate masculine or feminine social role.
4. Developing fundamental skills in reading, writing, and calculating.
5. Developing concepts necessary for everyday living.
6. Developing conscience, morality, and a scale of values.
7. Achieving personal independence.
8. Developing attitudes toward social groups and institutions.

Psychosexual Development

Freud calls this stage the **latency period**, that is, a period of quiescence of sexual feelings toward the opposite sex. The oedipal conflict has been resolved, and the child aligns with peers and authority figures of the same sex. Usually, boys form all-boy groups and girls socialize only with girls. Despite such voluntary separation, boys often perform feats of daring and bravery to gain the admiration not only of their male peers but also of girls. Girls are aware of the boys' antics and many express role identification by experimenting with lipstick or asking to learn to sew or cook. It is unclear whether recent trends toward less strictly defined sex roles among adults and the advent of large numbers of women in professions once exclusively for men, and to a lesser extent the reverse, are influencing children of this age to identify less with the parent of the same sex.

Cognitive Development

Many educators regard the years from 6 to 12 as the most important period for cognitive development. These are the "doing" years. Teachers share responsibility for the child's development because the youngster in this age group substitutes the teacher's authority for much of the parents'. The encouragement of a sensitive teacher can have a lasting impact.

Piaget characterizes the cognitive stage of the school-age child as "concrete operational," that is, the child deals best with concrete phenomena and situations but can consider others' ideas and can communicate in a controlled, articulate way. These children understand clear-cut relationships, such as those involving size and locations of objects. Questioning and curiosity about life begin, promoting future learning for the youngster. In school skills preadolescent girls frequently do better than boys of the same age in such areas as reading, spelling, and writing, but boys catch up in early adolescence.

Moral Development

The school years are an important period in ethical development (Fig. 18-4). In general, self-serving motives and avoidance of punishment have been superseded as sources of moral decisions. In the elementary years, conventional level reasoning begins. Kohlberg (1966) calls this stage the "good-boy morality of maintaining good relations, approval of others." Authority (teachers, parents, the law) is beginning to influence behavior. Gilligan believed that stage II, "care ethics," continues through middle childhood when the child is not only seeking approval but genuinely desires not to harm others.

According the Westerhoff, a child of this age continues to experience the faith of the family and may participate in the rituals of a formal religion.

Responses to Illness and Hospitalization

This active stage may be translated by illness or hospitalization into one of depression and passive submission for the school-age child. These quiet, withdrawn periods may be interspersed with periods of hostility or bargaining. Lack of stimulation brings on boredom. The child attempts to act brave, particularly when the parents are present. Privacy is a concern, as well as painful procedures, which the child interprets as endangering the body.

Nursing Considerations When Caring for the School-age Child

The ill school-age youngster keenly resents the restrictive atmosphere of the hospital and the limitations it places on exploratory activities, a major need of this age group. Letting the child visit outdoor areas or the snack bar or cafeteria with the family or a staff companion is an excellent way to relieve this feeling (Fig. 18-5). Peers and friends from school should be encouraged to visit. The parents can also bring in favorite books, records, or other pastimes.

Mainly because of the child's boredom, the less understanding nurse may find the school-age child a demanding and boisterous patient. It is important to plan time to allow the child to talk about the frustrations present. Such attention and sympathy can help the child and encourage participation in the plan of care.

When painful procedures are necessary, tell the child that being brave is not necessary. When describing procedures, honesty is essential to develop and maintain trust with the young patient. Touch is usually appreciated at these difficult times.

It is crucial to protect privacy and ask permission to enter rooms with closed doors and bathrooms. Explain what you are going to do in clear terms to lessen the youngster's fear of being threatened.

If school studies are interrupted, refer the parents to the school so that a tutor or school aide can be secured.

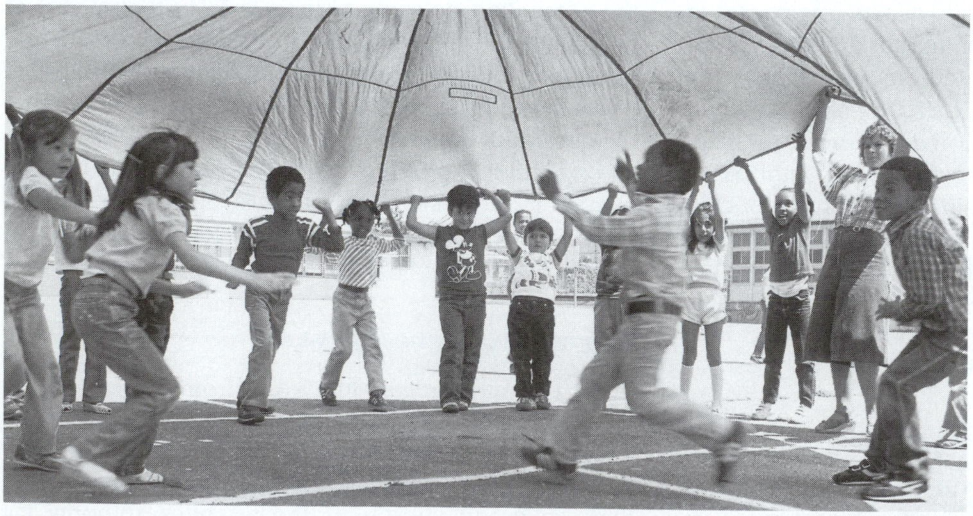

Figure 18-4. School-age children are developing values and attitudes.

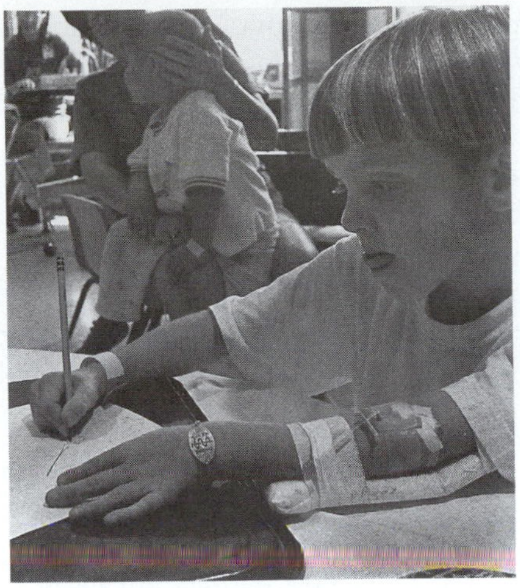

Figure 18-5. Nurses can use a hospital play area to provide a warm and comforting environment.

Continuing school lessons, if the child is able to do so, signals hope for recovery and is sometimes a surprising relief from the tedious routine of the hospital.

Adolescence: 12 to 18 Years

The term adolescence is an arbitrary one. Some resources give the years of this stage of life from 11 to 20. For our purposes, we will consider **adolescence** as generally between the time of **puberty** (the development of secondary sexual characteristics) and the end of physical growth, at approximately 18 years of age. Perhaps more than any other period of the life span, adolescence is a time of transition. During this movement from childhood to adulthood, youngsters mature and prepare for their meaningful place in life.

Adolescence can be exciting but unsettling (Fig. 18-6). Today's adolescents are taller, healthier, and more independent than their ancestors, but their freedom of access to automobiles, sexual experiences, and substance abuse can demand a high level of maturity for rational decision-making. Rising divorce rates place additional stress on all youngsters in single-parent homes, including adolescents. The rise in teenage suicide is of grave concern to community mental health professionals.

Physical Development

Many physical changes, both overt and internal, are occurring in the adolescent. Physical growth, initially rapid, ceases in late adolescence, when dreams of what might be must be reconciled with reality. Rapid growth can cause awkwardness and a sense of unfamiliarity with one's body; furniture can be a stumbling block to large feet and uncoordinated legs. Physical activity and exercise can help teenagers overcome these difficulties.

Because of their rapid growth, adolescents have increased nutritional needs. The typical teenage appetite for "junk food" can make obesity as well as skin disturbances a problem. Many teenagers are adopting healthier diets because of public education regarding decreasing fat consumption and increasing intake of fruits and vegetables.

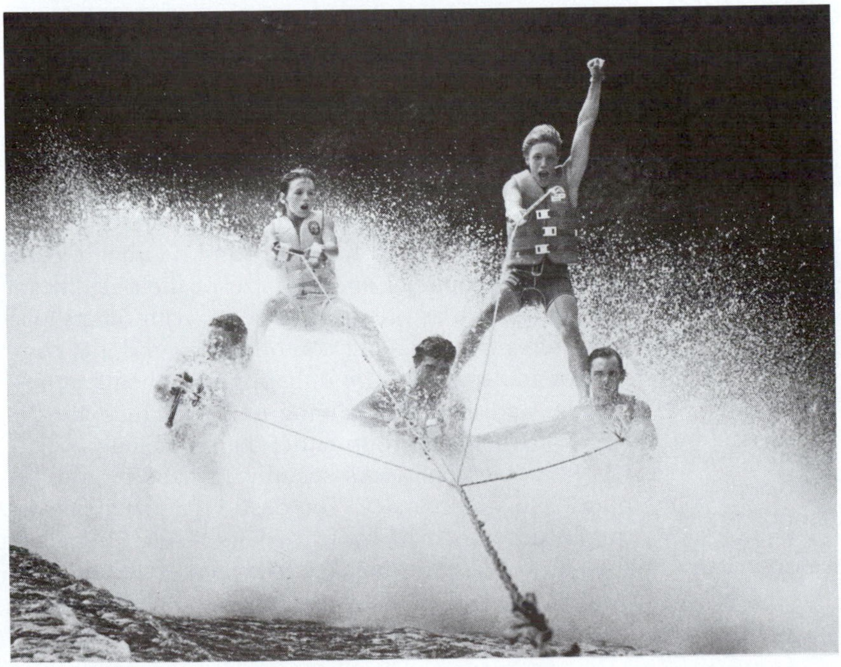

Figure 18-6. Adolescents are often risk takers.

Puberty—the maturing of the sexual organs—takes place during adolescence. **Menses** (menstruation) begins in girls, often erratically at first, but the cycle usually becomes fairly regular at an average of 28 days. Boys typically experience nocturnal emissions, or "wet dreams," during which semen is expelled. Both the onset of menses and nocturnal emissions can cause anxiety, which an understanding parent or other adult can allay.

Psychosocial Development

Erikson characterizes the adolescent crisis in psychosocial development as the **identity versus role confusion stage**. A sense of individual identity evolves during these years, setting the stage for adulthood, largely through the process of reconciling one's changing self-image ("Who am I?" "What kind of person am I?") with the image presented to family and friends ("How do other people see me?"). The strengthening of identity is accompanied by a need to separate oneself psychologically from one's family. Family outings become less popular and peer activities increasingly important. A period of emotional distance between adolescents and their parents can occur related to lifestyle and values. Although teenagers often appear sullen and rebellious in the eyes of their parents, solid parental support remains essential. Setting limits for the youngster becomes more difficult but must not be abandoned.

Interest in finding a life partner and vocation may begin. Using the reactions of parents and peers as guideposts, the teenager can gradually achieve the security of a valid role identity, that is, a satisfactory self-image congruent with the views of others. If this delicate balance cannot be attained, Erikson tells us, role confusion results. Youngsters who fail to establish identity in adolescence typically lack direction and have difficulty making decisions about such important matters as education, work, sexual orientation, and moral and spiritual values. Adolescents need acceptable role models on whom to pattern themselves. Parents who exercise too much or too little control cannot function as satisfactory role models; as a result, the confused young person may grasp at any available identity, such as drug use, sexual precocity, or defiance of authority. Such desperate efforts to "be somebody" can lead to serious problems.

Havighurst (1972) lists several developmental tasks for the adolescent. Many of these are further development of the tasks described for middle childhood.

1. Achieving new and more mature relations with peers of both sexes.
2. Achieving a masculine or feminine social role.
3. Accepting one's physique and using the body effectively.
4. Achieving emotional independence from parents and other adults.
5. Preparing for a relationship with a lifetime partner and family life.
6. Preparing for an economic career.
7. Acquiring a set of values and an ethical system as a guide to behavior—developing an ideology.
8. Desiring and achieving socially responsible behavior.

Cognitive Development

Adolescents have reached Piaget's phase of formal operations. They have attained maximum ability to process information and learn. An essential part of this learning is to question and formulate independent ideas. The adolescent can participate in thought which is hypothetical, scientific, and deals with the past, present, and future. There is a high propensity for creativity and participation in complex games. Imagination and fantasy are common components of the thinking patterns of adolescents. Exposure to the multimedia of society leads to the formation of opinions on issues, opinions that may be counter to those of the parents. "Parents sometimes underestimate the cognitive abilities of the adolescent. Parents can learn from adolescents, just as adolescents learn from parents" (Murray and Zentner, 1989, p. 345). Nurses should encourage parents to spend time with adolescents in order to share mutual views. The expanding proficiency in thinking and formulating ideas is the natural forerunner to the future and determining life goals.

Psychosexual Development

Freud treats adolescence as synonymous with puberty, which he defines as the conciliation of physical and emotional needs into a sexual identity. Adolescents tend to be preoccupied with normality and constantly compare the development and the size of their significant body parts, such as breasts and penis, with others'. Facial features take on adult conformation, and it is common for adolescents to be unhappy with their features. Attitudes and values pertaining to appearance are derived from the peer group rather than the family.

The adolescent seeks security in handling the responsibilities of intimacy. The desire for sexual activity may be accompanied by fear of its results. In recent years, however, many teenagers have failed to fulfill this task. The availability of contraception has altered sexual behavior. Many young people have viewed contraceptive pills, the use of condoms to avoid sexually transmitted diseases, and abortion as methods for releasing sexuality from unwelcome consequences. However, the alarming rise in teenage pregnancy continues to be a concern. Additionally, many adolescents find themselves unprepared for the emotional consequences of sexual intimacy. The issues of whether sex education and condoms should be available in schools and whether parents should be notified when those under age seek contraceptive counseling remain sensitive and controversial.

Moral Development

When a person enters adolescence, most morals have been established on the basis of those of the parents and other adult authority figures. During the adolescent years, these positions may be critically reexamined. If the parents have not maintained a strong moral base, adolescents may be adversely affected, even though they are, at the same time, seeking independence from parental influences. The values of these adults may be rejected or may become more firmly a part of the adolescent's moral philosophy. Many adolescents become idealistic and support political or social causes. These adolescents are developing a level of morality that Kohlberg (1966) describes as the postconventional level. At a time when adolescents are becoming emancipated at an earlier age, the development of a sound and caring moral base is even more important. Gilligan's view of the adolescent's moral behavior is that the stage of "care ethics" continues. Chapter 17 presents a more detailed discussion of the various theorists.

Faith Development

Westerhoff's stage I of experiencing faith continues. There is a tempered acceptance with the beginning of evaluation of a particular faith and its value. Some adolescents express their independence by renouncing the religion in which they were raised or adopting a religious affiliation different from that of their parents.

Responses to Illness and Hospitalization

The adolescent is closely allied with the peer group and feels isolated when in the hospital. Although there is a degree of separation anxiety for parents and home, "missing out on the action" of the peer group is distressing to these youngsters. Adolescence is a time of independence and control of one's own behavior. The constraints of illness and the institution are threatening to the self-concept of the teenager, who fears giving up control. In our society, responses to pain may be different in boys and girls. Boys may feel obligated to be brave and not show fear and distress at the prospect of pain or painful procedures. Crying is more accepted by society as female behavior and allows adolescent girls to release their fears of painful procedures and pain by weeping. However, the nurse must allow male and female adolescents alike to express pain in whatever way best meets their needs, without social judgment.

The hospital is an intrusion on privacy, which only adds to the discomfort of illness. Both adolescent boys and girls are conscious of their bodies and may have some hesitancy in revealing themselves to care providers or to other patients.

Nursing Considerations When Caring for the Adolescent

For the adolescent, illness interrupts an exciting time of life. For the young person hospitalized for a long period, academic studies and social function participation are disrupted. As a nurse, you can encourage peers not only to visit but to enjoy and feel comfortable about visiting. Although your role is not that of a friend to the patient, you can be supportive of the young person and his or her friends. Schools often provide tutors for those who are confined so that studies are not neglected. You may suggest this or other appropriate resources to the family.

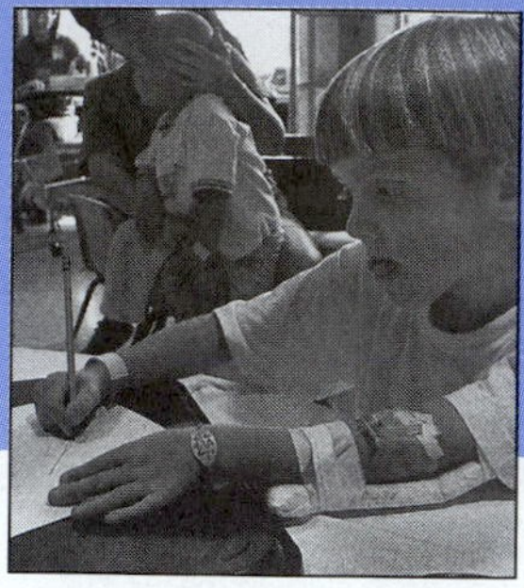

Key Points

- During the neonatal period, that is the first month of life, the human undergoes rapid physical growth and stabilization of vital functions and sleeps for most of each 24-hour period.
- During the remainder of the infant's first year, growth is rapid and social interaction begins.
- Touching is vital to the bonding of the infant to the parents.
- By the end of the first year of life, the infant's birth weight has tripled, walking has begun, and visual acuity is closer to that of an adult.
- The toddler stage is one during which there is great physical activity, the development of language skills, and toilet training. The child has little concept of either sexuality or morality.
- Early childhood is a time when vital functions approximate the adult's, and the family diet becomes more acceptable to the child. Parental attitudes are crucial at this time to encourage growth, and setting limits is essential to provide safety, guidance, and discipline.
- Middle childhood is a time of greater cognitive growth, the beginning of limited independence, and a beginning interest in participating in rituals. Gender differences are recognized but there is not overt interest.
- During middle childhood, the child continues to be egocentric, and morality is focused on pleasing, that is, being the good boy or good girl. Faith development involves observation of the way in which parents express their faith.
- Adolescence is turbulent but gratifying in the attainment of new skills, recognition of gender roles, and preparation for a life career. It is a time of questioning and evaluating moral and faith issues.
- Rebellion during adolescence may indicate a search for identity and can eventually result in purposeful goals.
- Knowledge of the usual development that occurs from infancy through adolescence can give the nurse valuable clues for planning appropriate and effective care. The most important role of the nurse may be to provide support and encouragement of the natural coping skills of the child, regardless of age.

Study Questions

1. Name the factors that determine the sex of the unborn child and the process that determines many physical characteristics.
2. Identify the primary needs of the infant.
3. What are three motor skills of the 2-year-old?
4. Name three of the motor skills of the 5-year-old.
5. What cognitive skills described by Piaget as "concrete operational" are present during the school-age years?
6. What moral influences does the adolescent derive from parents and other adult authority figures? How might an adolescent react to these influences?
7. What four stages are important in faith development?
8. Select two stages of child development and discuss the care the nurse provides for children in these age groups.
9. We recognize that the child is a part of the family and community. Discuss why remembering this is important for nurses who care for hospitalized children.
10. List some of the concerns you had as an adolescent.

Critical Thinking Activities

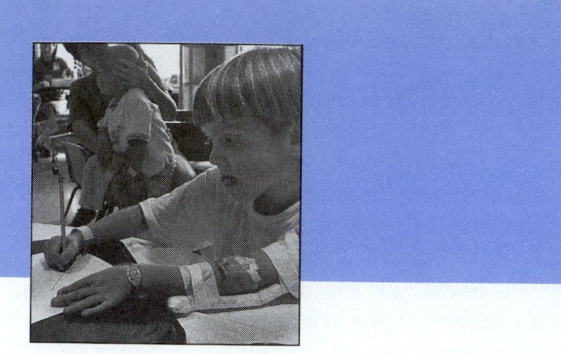

1. Compare the motor characteristics of a 6-month-old infant to those of a 5-year-old child.
2. Contrast the language acquisition of a 1-year-old with that of a 4-year-old.
3. From a list of the members of your family or a neighbor's family, select one child you know well. Using the work of the eight theorists, assess that person in relation to physical, psychosocial, psychosexual, cognitive, moral, and faith development.
4. Identify the nursing diagnoses that would be most commonly seen in each age group.
5. With prior arrangement, visit a preschool or elementary classroom and report in writing your observations of the children as they relate to developmental theory.
6. Invite a pediatric nurse to a small group of your fellow students. Prepare a thoughtful list of ques-

tions regarding the care of the hospitalized child and lead the discussion.

References and Readings

American Journal of Nursing 75, 10 (October 1975). Seventy-fifth Anniversary Issue. (Entire issue devoted to the life span.)

Craft, M. J., and Denehy, J. A. *Nursing Interventions for Infants and Children.* Philadelphia: W. B. Saunders, 1990.

Eisenberg, A., Murkoff, H., and Hathaway, S. *What to Expect the First Year.* New York: Workman Publishers, 1989.

Erikson, E. H. *Childhood and Society.* New York: W. W. Norton, 1963.

Frank, L. K. *Nature and Human Nature.* New Brunswick, N.J.: University Press, 1951.

Freud, S. *The Ego and the Id* (1923). London: Hogarth Press, 1935.

Gilligan, C. *In a Different Voice.* Cambridge: Harvard University Press, 1982.

Greenberger, E., and Steinberg, L. *When Teenagers Work: The Psychological and Social Costs of Adolescent Employment.* New York: Basic Books, 1988.

Havighurst, R. J. *Developmental Tasks and Education.* 3rd edition. New York: Longman, 1972.

Jurgrau, A. "Why Aren't We Protecting Our Children?" *RN* 53, 11 (November 1990): 30–34.

Kohlberg, L. "Moral Education in the Schools: A Developmental View." *School Review* 74 (1966): 1–30.

Kosfer, M. K. "Self-Care: Health Behavior for the School Age Child." *Topics in Clinical Nursing* 5 (April 1983): 199–212.

Lever, J. "Sex Differences in the Complexity of Children's Play and Games." *American Sociological Review* 43 (1978): 471–483.

Mahon, N. E. "Developmental Changes and Loneliness During Adolescence." *Topics in Clinical Nursing* 5 (April 1983): 66–76.

Murray, R., and Zentner, J. *Nursing Assessment and Health Promotion Strategies Through the Life Span.* 4th edition. Englewood Cliffs, N.J.: Prentice-Hall, 1989.

Peck, R. "Psychological Developments in the Second Half of Life." In *Middle Age and Aging,* edited by B. L. Neugarten. Chicago: University of Chicago Press, 1968.

Piaget, J. *The Origins of Intelligence in Children.* New York: W. W. Norton, 1963.

Westerhoff, J. *Will Our Children Have Faith?* New York: Seabury Press, 1983.

Whaley, L. F., and Wong, D. L. *Essentials of Pediatric Nursing.* 4th edition. St. Louis: C. V. Mosby, 1993.

Adulthood

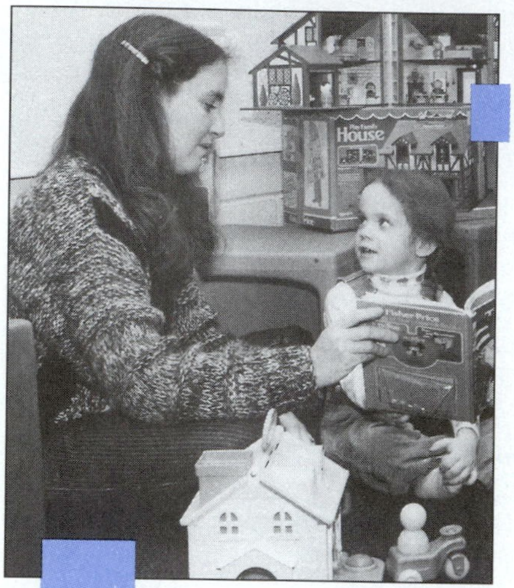

19

Objectives

After completing this chapter, you should be able to:

1. Briefly discuss the physical, psychosocial, psychosexual, cognitive, moral, and faith development of the young adult.
2. Briefly discuss the physical, psychosocial, psychosexual, cognitive, moral, and faith development of the middle adult.
3. Briefly discuss the physical, psychosocial, psychosexual, cognitive, moral, and faith development of the older adult.
4. Outline the responses each of these age groups may have to illness and hospitalization.
5. Discuss the special aspects that should be considered when planning care for each age group.

Study Terms

Alzheimer's disease
body image
climacteric
generativity versus stagnation
integrity versus despair
intimacy versus isolation
kyphosis
menopause
presbyopia
postconventional level
sandwich generation
sebaceous glands
sensory overload
young adulthood

Outline

The Young Adult: 18 to 44 Years

Physical Development
Psychosocial Development
Psychosexual Development
Cognitive Development
Moral Development
Faith Development
Responses to Illness and Hospitalization
Nursing Considerations When Caring for the Young Adult

The Middle Adult: 45 to 64 Years

Physical Development
Psychosocial Development
Psychosexual Development
Cognitive Development
Moral Development
Responses to Illness and Hospitalization
Nursing Considerations When Caring for the Middle Adult

Ellis, Nowlis: Nursing: A Human Needs Approach, 5th ed. © 1994 J.B. Lippincott Company

Adulthood is a time in the life span during which the person has the opportunity for new experiences, responsibilities, and challenges. Reed (1983) states that adults have established a clear sense of identity and therefore are more equipped to engage in meaningful interactions with others (p. 20). Much of this interaction may involve the physical and psychological care of others: children, aging parents, or relatives. Although most adults are part of a family, the individual adult assumes an independent role in society and is looked on as a responsible member who interacts with and fulfills the responsibilities required by society.

In the United States, life roles have changed dramatically over the last 10 years, and the nurse needs to be aware of these role changes in relation to the conceptual theories presented in earlier research on the life span. At the same time, much of what has been written still provides a useful framework for discussion of the developmental tasks of the adult. As in caring for the child, the nurse must have a working knowledge of the usual pattern of development in the adult as well as its impact on the ill or disabled adult to provide the most suitable and effective nursing care.

The Young Adult: 18 to 44 Years

The ages considered as young adult vary according to the country and culture. In some cultures, the "child bride/groom" traditions are still in effect, so that a 14-year-old is considered a woman, marries, and begins a family with her partner, who may be much older. In other cultures, a woman or man may continue to reside in the family home much later than is the practice in our Western countries. Statistically, the United States and Canada consider persons aged 25 to 44 as young adults. **Young adulthood** for our purposes stretches from the time of emancipation from parents, at about 18 years of age, until the beginning of midlife, at 44 years.

Physical Development

Young adults are physically at the peak of development, with a healthy concept of the appearance of the body (**body image**). A great deal of this self-concept was derived during adolescence, when they became aware of how peers and others viewed them. Stereotyping can occur. Height, in our society, especially in men, is sometimes equated with competence or power. Persons who are not tall may compensate for this view by developing intellectual capabilities far above the level of their taller counterparts.

Generally, when the feedback from others is positive, the young adult will have a well-defined and accurate perception of the physical self. This perception also enhances feelings of psychological well-being. Systems are functioning effectively, and the outward appearance is pleasing and affirming. Physical appearance continues to be directly linked to the perceptions of others in the environment. The confidence generated by a healthy concept of the physical self can be an important factor in gaining what are perceived as one's life goals.

Because Western society is youth oriented, young adults are portrayed as at the height of physical attractiveness. This attitude is paramount in consumerism, where the majority of commercial advertisements portray young models and focus on the young adult purchaser. Only recently has the older model been visible in promoting consumer products.

Physical growth is completed during these years, nutritionally lowering the need of earlier years for energy-giving calories. Because stature is now fairly defined, obesity can occur if caloric intake is not moderated. Wide attention has been given to eating the healthy diet, and many adults are changing their dietary patterns for health reasons. This change is beneficial in reducing dietary fat and cholesterol, which decreases the risk of heart disease and stroke. A healthy diet also helps maintain acceptable body weight.

Both sexes may begin to have graying of the hair at this age. Some men over age 30 may experience premature hair loss. Body changes perceived as signaling the beginning of middle age may cause some anxiety.

Psychosocial Development

The social options for young adults have changed remarkably over the past 15 years. According to government statistics, both one-adult households and households of unmarried couples with or without children greatly increased from 1970 to 1989 (Fig. 19-1). One rea-

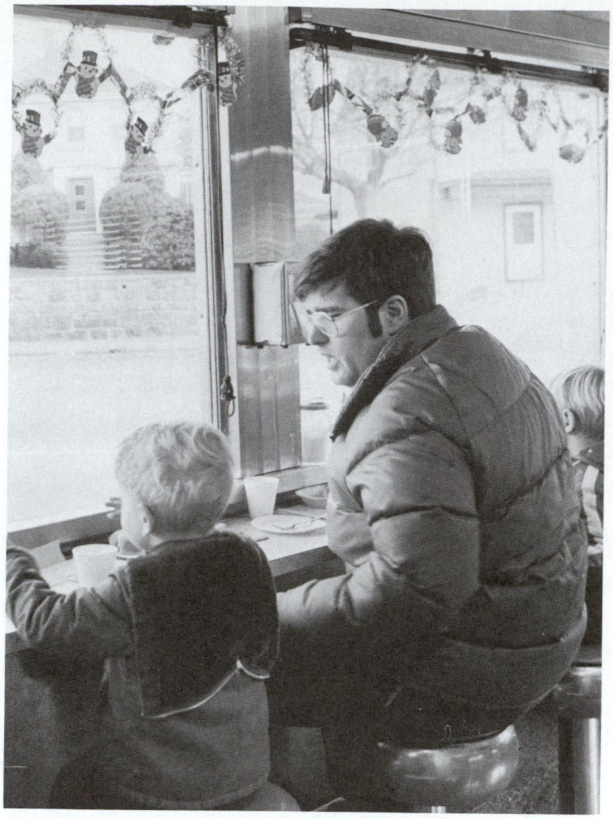

Figure 19-1. The number of single-parent households has increased dramatically.

son is that shared housing is on the increase, partly in response to rising housing costs. The most impoverished group in our society is that of young adults.

The majority of single households are headed by women and have greatly increased in number over the past 18 years. In 1970, female family householders with no spouse present totaled 25.4% and increased to 56.5% in 1989. Children lived in the majority of these single-parent households (Table 19-1).

Couples are having fewer children and having them later than a decade ago. Many couples are consciously choosing not to have children. A major factor contributing to these decisions is the prevalence of two-career households. Role and career reversal is also occurring, with increasing numbers of women entering formerly male occupations and men entering traditionally female ones. No longer is it uncommon to encounter a male telephone operator or nurse or a female mail carrier or physician. Although the range of alternatives is widening, high college tuition costs and unemployment rates restrict young adults in pursuit of their life goals.

During young adulthood, most individuals are pursuing and establishing meaningful long-term relationships. Because today many young adults, for a variety of reasons, do not have families of their own, they may have problems in meeting the need for intimacy. Erikson (1963) describes the conflict of young adulthood as **intimacy versus isolation**.

Although the intimacy desired by the young adult is usually a love relationship with a sexual component, this is not exclusively the case. The basic need is for closeness and relatedness to another person. Homosexual and bisexual people are finding growing acceptance in the mainstream of society and are increasingly being perceived in terms of their individual merits rather than mere sexual orientation.

The attainment of intimacy further enhances the identity first established in the teenage years. The young adult is a competitive, productive, creative person who sees the results—and, one hopes, the rewards—of decision-making. Erikson states that isolation can occur if "intimacy, competitive and combative relations are experienced with and against the selfsame people."

Havighurst's developmental theory (1964) lists the tasks for the young adult as both those concerning family and home and those relative to work and the larger community. More specifically, those having to do with family and home are selecting and learning to live with a life partner, starting a family, rearing children, and managing a home (Fig. 19-2). Beginning an occupation, accepting civic responsibilities, and finding a congenial social group are all young adult tasks that involve work life and the community.

The tasks as outlined by Murray and Zentner (1989) are much more adaptable to the various lifestyles and goals of young adults in society today. Among the additional tasks they define are "accepting self, establishing independence from the parental home, establishing an intimate bond with another through marriage or with a close friend and deciding whether or not to have a family and parenting" (p. 426).

Psychosexual Development

Young adulthood may be characterized by sexual fulfillment in long-term relationships of satisfying intimacy. However, it has been suggested that many young adults have unrealistic expectations of romantic love and intimacy and find long-term sexual involvement dull and disappointing. Nevertheless, the young adult typically embraces the sexual role and looks for security in a love relationship.

Men are at the peak of their sexual performance during the early young adult years, approximately 18 to 20 years of age. Women achieve their maximum sexual performance much later, at approximately 40 years. This gender difference may be a factor in determining the satisfaction or dissatisfaction of sexual adjustment.

A current legal and ethical issue is that of sexual harassment, which is the unwelcome overt or subtle

Table 19–1. Female Family Householders With No Spouse Present—Characteristics, by Race: 1970–1989

Characteritic	Unit	White					African American				
		1970	*1980*	*1985*	*1988*	*1989*	*1970*	*1980*	*1985*	*1988*	*1989*
Female family householder . . .	1,000	4,185	6,052	6,941	7,235	7,342	1,349	2,495	2,964	3,074	3,223
Percent of all families	Percent . .	9.1	11.6	12.8	12.9	13.0	28.3	40.3	43.7	42.8	43.5
Median age	Years . .	50.4	43.7	42.7	42.2	42.5	41.3	37.4	38.0	38.1	37.2
Marital status:											
Single (never married)	Percent . .	9.2	10.6	11.9	15.1	15.7	16.2	27.3	33.4	35.9	38.5
Married, spouse absent	Percent . .	18.5	16.9	16.0	15.7	14.7	39.7	28.6	21.1	23.2	22.2
Separated	Percent . .	11.4	13.9	13.8	12.6	12.2	33.8	26.8	19.3	20.3	19.3
Other	Percent . .	7.2	3.0	2.1	3.0	2.5	5.9	1.8	1.7	2.9	2.9
Widowed	Percent . .	47.0	32.7	28.3	27.0	26.7	29.9	22.2	21.2	18.8	17.3
Divorced	Percent . .	25.3	39.8	43.8	42.2	43.0	14.2	21.9	24.5	22.1	22.0
Presence of children under 18:											
No own children	Percent . .	52.0	41.2	43.5	43.8	43.6	33.5	28.1	34.5	34.3	32.7
With own children	Percent . .	48.0	58.8	56.5	56.2	56.4	66.6	71.9	65.5	65.7	67.3
1 child	Percent . .	18.8	28.1	28.9	28.5	28.9	19.1	26.3	27.5	28.1	29.8
2 children	Percent . .	15.0	19.9	18.6	18.9	18.7	14.4	23.2	21.6	20.2	19.7
3 children	Percent . .	7.8	7.4	6.4	6.4	6.4	12.5	11.1	10.1	10.5	10.8
4 or more children	Percent . .	6.4	3.4	2.6	2.4	2.4	20.6	11.3	6.3	6.9	7.0
Children per family	Number . .	1.00	1.03	0.96	0.94	0.95	1.83	1.51	1.29	1.23	1.24

As of March. 1970 covers persons 14 y old and over; beginning 1980, covers persons 15 y old and over. Based on Current Population Survey. Source: U.S. Bureau of the Census, *Current Population Reports*, series P-20, No. 447 and earlier reports.

sexual overture to another. Sexual harassment can be the presence of offensive language in the workplace or actual touching or fondling. Much of this behavior may be learned from societal expectations of gender relationships.

Health professionals, including nurses, must maintain a nonjudgmental approach to sexual activity while at the same time teaching about healthy and safe sexual practices. If an individual nurse is uncomfortable discussing sexual matters, knowledge of resources could be useful in providing information of a sexual nature.

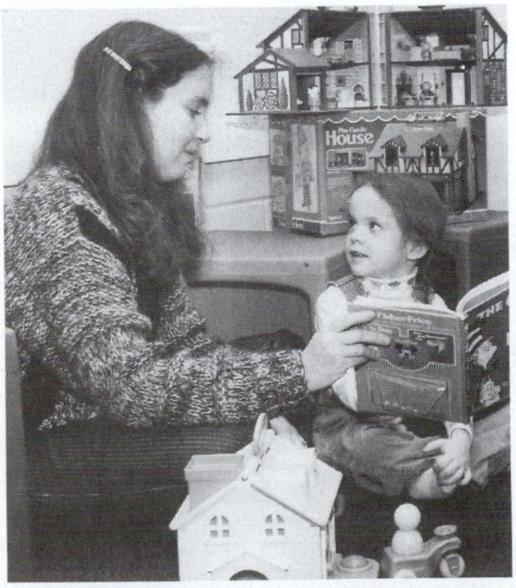

Figure 19-2. Young adults enjoy being with their children.

Cognitive Development

The young adult is typically preoccupied with developing and applying the practical and professional skills necessary to build a satisfying adult life. Completion of schooling and the advent of working allow financial independence from the parental family. Independence in turn brings responsibilities that require substantial skill at planning, coping, foreseeing problems, and interpreting reality.

Although the slogans and abstractions that often dominate adolescent thought processes may not be forsaken, they are likely to be reinterpreted in terms of the practicalities of life. Ordinary thinking may gradually become more systematic, decisive, and task oriented. At the same time, thinking, fantasizing, and emoting may become more smoothly integrated than during adolescence.

By this stage in the life span, men's and women's overall cognitive abilities are equal, if not precisely identical. Opportunities for women to use their full capacities in the world of work are growing strikingly, and women are conclusively demonstrating their equal ability to perform. Recent research has indicated that certain neurophysiologic differences between men and women may make some types of learning easier for one sex than the other.

Generally, young adults are energetic, forward looking, and ambitious. However, emotional conflicts about identity, dependence/independence, and other issues of adulthood can interfere with the thrust of cognitive development, and many young adults experience an extended period of indecision, rebellion, or relative passivity before resolving such conflicts and wholeheartedly pursuing adult lives.

Moral Development

The age of young adulthood brings about a search for an ethical philosophy that may be religious in nature. For some, moral certainty and self-righteousness, accompanied by scorn of divergent beliefs and behavior, give way over time to tolerance and respect for others' convictions. Young adults typically invest a great deal of thought in coming to terms with personal and social ethical issues.

The young adult often attains Kohlberg's higher levels of moral development, in which there is belief in a universal good. This moral position may be translated into membership in not only a religion but in a political action group. On a personal level, emotions of this age group run high relative to the issue of abortion. Reactions against world hunger or aggression may be expressed. Preservation of the natural environment of the world and the animals who live within it is another issue often championed by young adults. Young adults apply their moral convictions to a wider range of issues than they did during their adolescent years.

Gilligan defines the moral development of the young adult as being the realization of the obligation for responsibility toward others. The emphasis is on avoiding harm to others.

Faith Development

Westerhoff describes the time of young adulthood as particularly important in faith development. It is a time when the acceptance of a genuine spiritual position is arrived at through a careful consideration of religious choices.

Responses to Illness and Hospitalization

Injury or illness interrupts the essential flow of life for the young adult. Persons of this age are at risk for injuries and for illnesses caused by infection, heart problems, diabetes, and many other chronic diseases.

Young adults may feel most acutely the consequent interruption in productivity. Work-time loss may also bring about fears of loss of employment at a time when unemployment is high. Anxiety can then occur, revolving around the possible necessity for a change in lifestyle and for regaining health to find new employment. If they have a family and children, feelings of guilt may arise for the restrictions the illness imposes on them.

The person may also fear change in the quality or character of the intimate relationship. The relinquishing of social and sexual responsibilities may only intensify already present feelings of guilt. Because injury, illness, or hospitalization hampers fulfillment of what young adults find important in life, many feel angry and powerless over their situation.

Another important consideration is the altering of body image. Physical appearance is a high priority to the person in this age group. To neither feel nor look well lowers the esteem of a person of any age, but more so for those in early adulthood. Change in body weight or skin color or having mutilating procedures performed causes great fear and sadness in young adults.

Nursing Considerations When Caring for the Young Adult

Most nurses in the acute care setting are themselves young adults and can readily understand the problems and concerns of patients within that age group. It is important, then, for the nurse to acknowledge that care is not just for the young adult patient as an individual but also for that person in the context of family and community. The nurse should consider the coping skills and strengths the patient possesses. With this information, help can be given by encouraging the person to explore options and choices in response to illness. Being an attentive listener is an effective way to accomplish this. The nurse can also listen to the concerns of family members and provide support at a time when it is most needed.

In terms of health teaching, the nurse can also be helpful by sharing knowledge of community resources. Knowing about the various programs and agencies designed to support ill persons and their families and how to contact such groups is an invaluable service. The need may concern finances, maintenance of the household, or the psychological well-being of individual members of the family or other relatives.

Another subject for health teaching concerns the alarming statistics indicating that many young adults drink alcohol heavily and use illicit drugs. Major physical and psychological problems, including increased rates of suicide and accidents, occur with the consumption of large amounts of alcohol as well as with the use of illicit drugs. Of primary concern is the fact that this is

Nursing Issues and Trends: *Nurses as Role Models for Health*

For 17 years, the Nurses Health Study followed more than 100,000 nurses. The nurses in the group who were smokers demonstrated an increased risk for stroke. Even though the number of people in the study who smoked decreased over the 17-year period, it remained surprisingly high. Smokers suffered stroke two and one-half times more often than did nonsmokers. It is clear that smoking causes significant health risk but it is also clear that cessation brings with it a sudden decrease in risk. As nurses, we should encourage our patients to stop smoking and serve as role models by being nonsmokers.

the age of childbearing, and current research links low birth weight and a variety of more serious birth defects to parental intake of toxic substances.

The nurse can also be instrumental in educating adults about "safe" sex and not sharing needles as preventive measures against sexually transmitted diseases and acquired immunodeficiency syndrome. A major educational program has been developed to educate young adults and others regarding prevention or transmission of these serious diseases.

The Middle Adult: 45 to 64 Years

With the extension in life expectancy, middle age is now considered to encompass many more years than previously. Those of advanced years may live into their eighties or beyond. Approximately one-fourth of the population of the United States and Canada is middle aged. The years of middle age are years of comparative health and productivity. Middle-aged persons "earn most of the money, pay the higher percentage of taxes, and have a higher voter participation than people of other ages." Therefore, they are instrumental in making many of the decisions that guide national policy. "The power in government, politics, education, religion, science, business, industry and communication is often wielded not by the young or the old, but by the middle-aged" (Murray and Zentner, 1989, p. 458).

The term "middle age" is more than a cliché because individuals aged 45 to 64 are indeed in the middle between two other groups in the life span. Many have children who may themselves be reaching adulthood. On the other side of the spectrum, middle-aged persons are often the primary relationship persons or even care providers for elderly parents. Sometimes, middle-aged persons who are the adult children of older parents have health problems of their own that detract from the energy needed to care for the older parents. In earlier generations, a middle-aged couple could plan on caring for one of their four parents in old age because of the shorter life span. People live much longer today so that this same couple may be caring for three or four parents. When these adults also have teenagers or young adults living in the household, they are sometimes referred to as the **sandwich generation**. Misunderstandings may arise between the more youthful members of the family and the older members. Midlife persons who are in touch with both their children and older parents can find efforts at intergenerational reconciliation difficult. On the other hand, great satisfaction can occur with good intergenerational relationships.

Decisions regarding alternative lifestyles and personal philosophy may ideologically distance some middle-aged persons from their children. Others find these years a time of great joy and discover that communication is not only that of familial affection but one of mutual respect and friendship. "What we will continue to have in common with our children through the years, however, will be much more important than anything that may seem to divide us" (Vickery, 1978, p. 78).

The gender differences among middle-aged persons are diminishing, although "gender is a primary aspect of anyone's social existence" (Allen and Whatley, 1986, p. 7). Many more women are in the work force, and household tasks are shared more equally between partners.

A great deal has been written about the "midlife crisis." Facing midlife and the changes it brings can be stressful for both men and women. Men and women may face unemployment due to layoffs within the work force. It is particularly difficult for these long-employed people to find employment replacement opportunities because of general high unemployment. Self-help sharing groups and commercial business companies have developed strategies to help with this problem. As health care professionals, it is important to know that a strong link has been made between unemployment and health status (Abraham and Krowchuk, 1986, p. 38). Although declining health may not be an issue, midlife is a time when health problems such as arthritis and cardiovascular, vision, and hearing problems may arise. Both men and women reexamine their respective roles and sometimes feel that the goals they set for themselves during the preceding years have not been accomplished.

The care and death of older parents also produce stress. Regardless of whether the relationship of the adult child with the older parent was positive or negative, the death of parents forces a confrontation relative to the reality of one's own mortality.

Widowhood is also an issue because it is more likely to occur in middle age, with more women being widowed than men. Studies show that mortality rates for widowed and married women are about the same but are significantly higher for widowed men who choose to not remarry (Murray and Zentner, 1989, p. 462).

Divorce is now more common and socially acceptable in midlife than it once was. Although midlife can be a time for finding new challenges in life, it can also be a financially trying period, particularly for women. The standard of living for divorced women decreases 73%, whereas that of divorced men decreases only 41% (Leslie and Swider, 1986, p. 117).

Near the end of the years of middle life, retirement from employment becomes a possibility. The unemployment problem in our country has led to the encouragement of early retirement for persons in their middle years. Retiring from the work force early can be an exciting time if one has developed skills for finding meaningful ways to spend leisure time. Some people who retire early have long-existing talents that can be converted into money-making ventures, whereas others find pleasure having time to enjoy relationships and recreational experiences. Economic difficulties make early retirement impractical for a large segment of the population, and thus younger people are prevented from securing positions in the work force. For the person in midlife, whose longevity is predicted to be increasing, a new task may be to prepare carefully so that the later years are more individually satisfying.

Retirement can become a major stressor, particularly for men who centered their lives and esteem around their work. There appears to be a direct relationship between being out of work and cardiovascular disease (Abraham and Krowchuk, 1986, p. 38). Psychological problems or stress resulting from unemployment can also lead to increased use of alcohol and drugs and weight gain. The suicide rate among middle-aged and older men is five times that of women of the same age, a fact that may be related to the so-called work ethic.

Physical Development

During midlife both women and men experience a **climacteric** (referred to as **menopause** in women) during which a complex interaction of endocrine, somatic, and psychic changes occurs. Both men and women may display labile emotions, as well as physical hormonal changes. "Although the possibility of a hormonal basis for behavioral changes occurring at any time of menopause cannot be ignored, studies conducted to date have not supported the widely held view of woman as victim of her hormones," states Nolan (1986, p. 153). Women usually experience menopause sometime between 40 and 50 years of age. A decrease in the estrogen level may bring on some discomfort such as "hot flashes," mild depression, and dryness of the vaginal vault. If symptoms persist, some physicians prescribe vaginal estrogen creams or oral estrogen. Recent data suggest the decreasing incidence of osteoporosis in postmenopausal women who have been placed on oral estrogen replacement therapy (Blanchard, 1990). However, the link between hormonal replacement and the occurrence of uterine and breast cancer remains under investigation.

The testicles of the man become less firm. In about 25% of men, the prostate enlarges and encroaches on the urethra so that problems in urination may occur. Many men must have surgical intervention to correct this condition. Although women are no longer fertile after menopause, men can continue to father children. Both may find some delay in reaching orgasm.

Heart disease is the second leading cause of death for those in the middle-aged group. This has been attributed to lifelong poor eating habits and a sedentary lifestyle. As people select healthier diets earlier in their lives and increase physical exercise, it is hoped this risk will decrease.

Hearing and visual acuity may decline. **Presbyopia**, difficulty in accommodating the eye to nearby objects, becomes increasingly evident as a result of an age-related flattening of the anterior surface of the eyes. Corrective lenses may have to be worn for the first time. The blood pressure rises, so that a chronic state of hypertension may occur. Arthritic changes may begin in the joints as well.

Because of the extreme emphasis on youth in Western culture, many individuals have difficulty facing these age-related changes, and some make massive efforts to continue looking young. Such individuals may dress in a youthful manner, use cosmetics to cover signs of aging, and undergo cosmetic surgery. These activities are not harmful in themselves but may indicate that a person has difficulty accepting body changes. A few individuals react in the opposite way, simply giving up at the first signs of aging. They may refer to themselves as old, wear clothing characteristic of elderly people, and withdraw from physical activity. This response only accelerates the aging process.

The current emphasis on physical fitness has had a great positive impact on individuals in their middle years. Neighbors are walking or running together on a regular basis, and health clubs have drawn large numbers of members from this age group. How much this will improve the general health of the midlife person is still controversial.

Psychosocial Development

Erikson identifies the middle years as characterized by a crisis of **generativity versus stagnation**. This conflict may begin as early as age 30 for some people. They review past accomplishments and assess what remains to be done, a process that can arouse satisfaction or disappointment. They may make the desirable psychological adjustment of considering capacities and accomplishments in light of their value to the younger generation. The development of such a sense of generativity does not require that they have children of their own; it is more a matter of psychologically "parenting" all youth (Fig. 19-3). Productivity and political and social responsibility in the middle years provide ways of striving to help young people grow.

If, in the middle of life, adults can assess themselves realistically and at the same time concern themselves with the needs of the younger members of society, they can achieve a state of generativity that makes for contentment. If this encompassing view of life is lacking, self-pity, self-interest, and sadness may result.

Havighurst's theory lists several tasks for the person in middle years. Some have to do with the physical self or family: accepting and adjusting to the psychological changes of middle age, relating to one's spouse or life partner as a person, assisting teenage children to become responsible adults, and adjusting to aging parents. Other tasks are reaching and maintaining satisfactory performance in one's occupational career, developing adult leisure activities, and achieving adult social and civic responsibility.

Psychosexual Development

Sexual activity can be highly gratifying during the middle years. A woman whose children are reaching adulthood may find new joy in her sexuality. However, if she feels unfulfilled and remote from or unappreciated by her partner, sexual pleasure is unlikely to fill emotional voids.

The middle-aged man may experience brief episodes of impotence, often psychological in origin. The realization that he may not accomplish all he intended can cause him to feel sexually inadequate. If his sexual partner is understanding and supportive, such problems

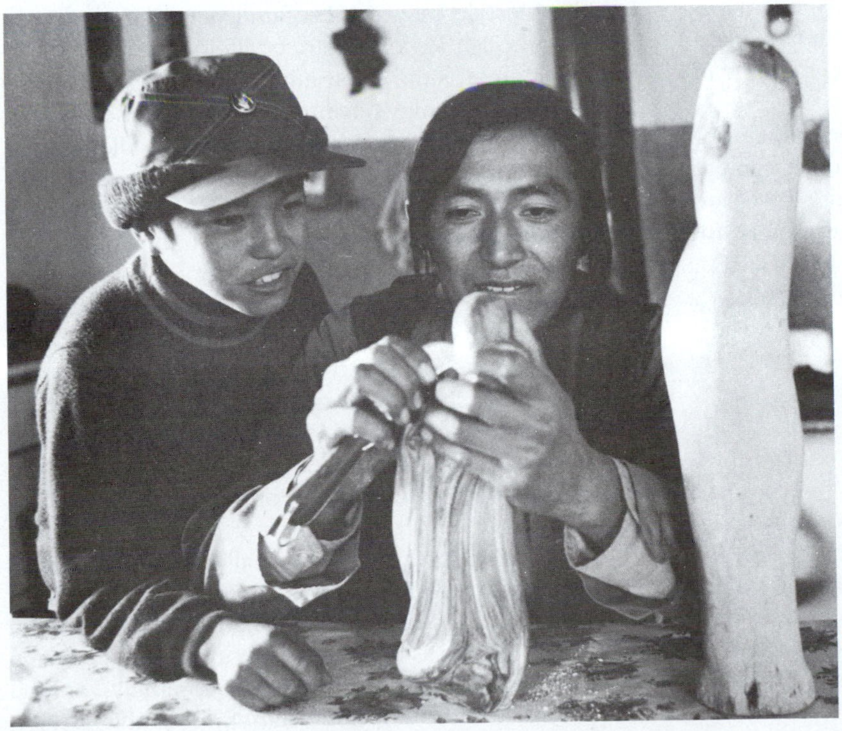

Figure 19-3. The middle years: a "parenting" of all youth.

can be fleeting. If they persist, however, professional counseling may be needed. Despite the potential problems of middle age, sex may be more satisfying than at any other time in life. When the responsibility for childrearing is past, partners have more time to appreciate one another.

Cognitive Development

Cognitive capacity is unimpaired in middle age and motivation to learn is typically high. Career advancement may require the individual to develop new skills—often administrative, computer, or teaching skills. With the advances in technology, workers may be required to apply in a new way skills already mastered. In conjunction with such goal-oriented learning, the wish to enjoy life to the fullest prompts many middle-aged people to make time for more recreational activities: reading, music, art, enjoyable projects, and new interests. Both types of learning experiences can be pursued in continuing education, which many middle-aged people find an extraordinarily rewarding resource.

Moral Development

Ethical judgments in middle age are typically based on the adult's past experience and established belief system, which may be either conventional or postconventional. At the **postconventional level**, the person becomes thoughtful about ethical issues. An individual's moral development can progress or regress in response to an emotional crisis. For example, serious illness may elicit a retreat to superstition or an unprecedented maturity and appreciation of life, not to mention possible intermediate reactions.

Kohlberg and Shulik (1981) picture the midlife person as not only postconventional in moral development, but uncomfortable with many who are at the lower levels (some may be adults). At these higher levels, the ability to feel empathy is strong. Morality may be on a formal or informal religious basis. Seeing oneself as a part of the larger community produces a need to help those who are disadvantaged.

Responses to Illness and Hospitalization

The middle adult has more stresses but also better coping skills than a younger person. Work may be intense and demanding and problems of teenage or young adult children an ongoing concern. The person may view injury or illness as a precursor of old age and, if these fears are not dealt with effectively, may be frightened. Sometimes the ideas and plans so essential to this age must be put aside in deference to illness. Cardiac problems, hypertension, and skeletal problems such as degenerative joint disease are common during the middle years. These problems may restrict some of the desired activities of the person and compromise, to some extent, quality of life. The disruption of family and community activities becomes a major concern for this age group.

Concern over adult children or aging parents may intensify feelings of powerlessness and motivate the person to call on long-held coping skills. If depression occurs and interferes with treatment or rehabilitation efforts, the course of the illness may persist much longer than it would have with an optimistic outlook.

Nursing Considerations When Caring for the Middle Adult

Because many nurses practicing in acute care settings are young adults, they may view the middle-aged adult patient as a surrogate parent, which produces some apprehension. It is important to listen closely to the concerns of both the midlife patient and the family. Middle age is a time of independent decision-making and being comfortable with having control over one's life. The nurse should allow the person to participate in the plan of care to meet the goal of regaining health or adjusting to illness.

Middle age is also a precarious time for the occurrence of accidents or illness. Many of the more current recommendations for accident prevention and living a healthy lifestyle may not be familiar to the person in midlife who is the beneficiary of lifelong habits. Something as simple as the conscientious wearing of seatbelts in an automobile may have to be newly learned behavior. Decreasing saturated fats and salt in the diet may be difficult for the person who has always cooked from family recipes that disregarded this advice. Your sharing information with the patient and the family would be of great benefit.

You can most effectively care for people in midlife by supporting individual coping skills and affirming their abilities to adapt to the changes of aging without viewing these changes as decline. Letting them know that they are doing a good job in response to life's demands is extremely important. This often relates to the relationship with adult children or the care of parents of advanced age.

In addition to caring emotionally for the patient in middle age, you will be providing care relative to the person's medical condition. The plan of care should be as comprehensive as it would be for a patient of any age with any adaptations the patient, the family, or you think appropriate. An understanding of this person within the life span framework will guide your plan of care in an individualized manner.

The Older Adult: 65 Years and Older

The older adult in this country has unique and special problems. The expected life span has increased so that the 65-year-old person is considered by some to be in midlife rather than old age. These younger older adults statistically have years ahead in which to enjoy recreational pursuits and travel for which previously they had little time. The early and even late years of old age can be fulfilling and enjoyable.

The statistically fastest growing group of persons is comprised of those 85 years and older, often called the "old–old." These expanded years, although joyful ones for many persons, may also bring increased risk of acute and chronic illness. How the government and the health care system meet these challenges is a complex issue and one we will discuss further in the next chapter.

Modern developmental theorists have changed the view of aging from one of unavoidable decline to one of developing competence in dealing with problems through the application of a lifetime of experiences. Frenkel-Brunswik (1963) states that the "psychological functions, such as knowledge, experience, training, which, because they help toward a rise in capability, counteract the biological decline" (p. 166). The adult's sense of well-being is based significantly on the "increasing ability to purposefully transform the current context with all of its problems and contradictions into energy for development" (Reed, 1983, p. 19).

Physical Development

The physical conditions of older adults vary markedly. Factors affecting this complexity may be heredity, emotional outlook, lifelong nutritional practices, levels of physical activity, and previous or current illness or disease. All body systems undergo some change during the aging process. The skin may thin and become more dry and scaly because of less activity of the **sebaceous glands**. Wrinkling of the skin occurs. The hair also becomes dry and less lustrous. Many men experience alopecia (baldness), and women may also experience thinning of the hair. Body hair may become more sparse with aging. Gum disease, not decay, is the leading cause of tooth loss. The nails may thicken and become discolored.

Muscle mass decreases and muscle strength diminishes. Body fat is redistributed from the extremities to the trunk. Some decalcification of bone occurs, causing a decrease in body height and placing the person at increased risk for fractures. Some older adults experience an abnormal increase in the convexity (outward curvature) of the upper spine, resulting in a noticeable **kyphosis** ("humpback"). Some plaque buildup occurs within the blood vessels, with a resulting loss of elasticity, so that both the diastolic and systolic blood pressures rise. The rib cage becomes more rigid, decreasing lung expansion. In response, the respiratory rate rises. Saliva and gastric secretions decrease. Food intolerances are frequent, particularly for spicy foods. The motility of the bowel slows, resulting in constipation. Renal flow is somewhat compromised, causing a decrease in urinary output. The muscles of the bladder wall and orifices are less reactive, so nocturia and urinary control problems may arise. This situation, combined with a less active immune system, may be a precursor for repeated bladder infections. Hearing problems in older adults are more prevalent than are problems of sight. Hearing high-pitched sounds may be difficult due to changes in the cochlea, decreased number of fibers in the auditory nerve, and deterioration within the auditory center in the cerebral cortex. Taste and smell also decrease in acuity, but touch is generally unaffected (Kopac, 1983).

The testicles diminish in size, secretion of testosterone decreases, and erection and ejaculation time may be delayed. The decline of estrogen levels in women continues. Dryness of the vaginal walls may result in dyspareunia (painful intercourse). If the individuals are sexually active, intercourse may be less frequent although libido and performance are maintained. Older women are less sexually active than are older men, primarily because of the absence of a partner, because women statistically far outnumber men in our society.

The brain undergoes changes that are still being explored. There is some decline in the responses of the autonomic nervous system. It is thought that temperature regulation changes in such a way that the older adult feels cold more readily. Another factor may be that with redistribution of body fat, the extremities feel cold. Whether or not pain sensitivity decreases is controversial. Cognition and alertness are sometimes altered in older persons who undergo a shrinkage in brain mass, but the reasons for this are not clearly understood. **Alzheimer's disease**, a condition in which there is progressive loss of functioning brain tissue and the development of abnormal neurofibrillary tangles and plaques, may begin as early as age 50, but its symptoms and effects are most prominent later in life. It is the leading cause of dementia in elderly persons (Given et al., 1988).

As the advanced years approach, the person responds to stress less efficiently. The immune system is not as effective so that fighting various infections becomes a concern. It must be emphasized that because one older individual varies greatly from another, the above outline of the various systemic changes should be used only as a guide when assessing the older person.

Psychosocial Development

The conflict of aging, according to Erikson (1963), is **integrity versus despair**. Changes that occur with age must be incorporated into the body image and a realistic adaptation must be made if the elderly person is to participate optimally in life. But lack of trust in one's body, fear of chronic illness, and anxiety about dependence make this a difficult task. Older individuals suffering from ill health, alienation or separation from loved ones, and financial difficulties can understandably succumb to despair. Depression is not uncommon in individuals over the age of 60. As with adolescents, the reactions of others greatly influence how elderly people feel about themselves. The older person who is looked on as useless feels of no use.

By reviewing achievements and disappointments, the older person searches out the meaning of his or her individual life. Many older people make a point of undertaking new ventures and projects, broadening their perspectives and circle of friends.

Havighurst's developmental tasks for the older adult (1972) are ones of adjustment and adaptation of social and civic life. The tasks include adjusting to decreasing physical strength and health, adjusting to retirement and reduced income, and facing the possible death of a spouse or lifelong partner (Fig. 19-4). He also sees importance in establishing a satisfactory living arrangement, developing an explicit affiliation with one's age group, and becoming more flexible in adopting social roles.

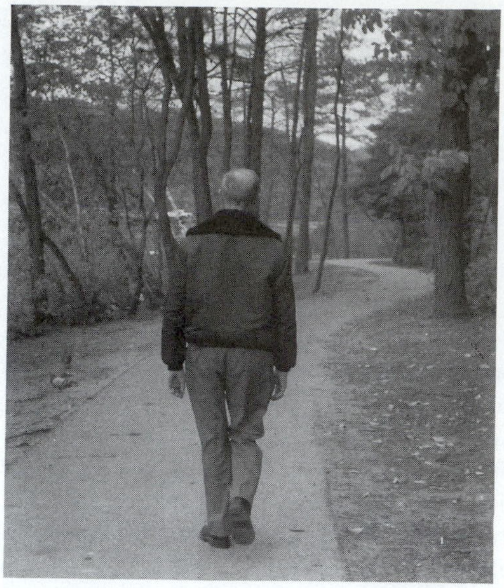

Figure 19-4. Many older adults are interested in maintaining maximum health.

Psychosexual Development

The reproductive systems of older adults have changed. The woman can no longer bear children, but procreation may continue for the man. New research has shown that when men of advanced years father children, defective sperm may be a factor in an increased risk for birth defects.

An important change for elders in recent years has been a much more liberal societal attitude toward their sexual behavior. In conjunction with this change in attitude, older persons need no longer feel it is wrong to have sexual feelings or be sexually active. Although sexual activity may become somewhat less frequent, it can remain pleasurable and meaningful. With adult children establishing their own homes and older adults entering the stage of retirement, older adults have time to focus on the sexual aspects of life. Whether or not older adults are sexually active, it is important for nurses to recognize that people remain sexual beings until the end of life.

Cognitive Development

Prior opinion to the contrary, elderly people's minds remain agile, undergoing only slight decline very late in life, unless affected by such physiologic changes as decreased circulation to the brain because of arteriosclerosis. Any slowing of thought that does occur is often compensated for by problem-solving ability based on life experience. Some evidence indicates that older people who have used their minds most actively throughout their lives experience the least diminution of mental ability. It is clinically demonstrable that intellectual stimulation promotes and maintains alertness.

Moral Development

A lifetime of moral assessment and experience and observation leads many older adults to ethical clarity and strong convictions. Many achieve Kohlberg's highest level (1981), postconventional ethical thought, and view morality as a matter of individual rights and principles of conscience. Some older people, on the other hand, tend to be judgmental about other people's behavior.

During the later years, the individual has enormous opportunity to fully develop morally. According to

Kohlberg and Shulik (1981), older adults can possess a realistic feeling of having survived the years (age sense) and a sense of renewal that transcends the body and leads to a reaffirmation of their philosophy of living. Not everyone, however, reaches this special state.

Gilligan (1982) believes that the stage III moral affirmation that developed in young adulthood continues with a well established philosophy. To not harm others takes precedence over persuasions that are more self-serving. To not harm others may be translated into helping others. The older person may contribute considerable time, money, or both to charitable organizations.

Faith Development

According to Westerhoff (1983), the older adult continues in stage IV faith development. This person has continued to practice and "own" a particular faith, which represents the values important to the individual. Facing the later years may require that the person's faith become even more established and steadfast than in earlier years.

Responses to Illness and Hospitalization

In the mind of the older adult, illness may be an indicator of permanent disability or a decline toward death. Even if this is an inaccurate assessment of the situation, this view can cause the individual anxiety and fear. The dependency associated with illness can intensify these feelings. At a time in life when being useful and independent are important issues, the restrictions on activities of daily living and social responsibilities can be disturbing.

The restrictions imposed by the health care setting can also cause feelings of isolation and loneliness. The patient may look forward to visits by the family but, at the same time, may feel guilty about both encroaching on others' time and about the worry the illness has caused individual family members.

The older adult may be unfamiliar with policies of the facility and associate "rules" with being "treated like a child," and, therefore, losing dignity. Responses vary, but they may be negative, such as irritability or unreasonable demands for attention. Some older persons become withdrawn and uncomplaining. Either response can be a manifestation of fear.

The intensity of care needed may cause **sensory overload**, the presence of more sensory stimuli during a given period than can be tolerated. Because most older adults live fairly quiet, regulated lives, the many visitors, staff personnel, procedures, and equipment within the facility can become an unmanageable amount of input. The response to this can be confusion and disorientation. The nurse has an important role to play in decreasing these negative responses by older patients to illness.

Nursing Considerations When Caring for the Older Adult

First and foremost, nurses who care for older persons must have a positive attitude toward aging. This may not be easy in our society, and it may take a conscious effort to dispel long-held myths. A strong knowledge base about the development of the older adult is also useful.

An important way to minimize feelings of loneliness and uselessness is to include the older patient in the plan of care, beginning with explanations given in a manner that respects the patient as a thoughtful, mature, and capable individual. The patient should be included in decision-making whenever possible.

Policies of the hospital should be explained so they become reasonable and acceptable to the person's lifestyle and philosophy of health care. If the patient is irritable or withdrawn, planning to spend extra time with that person, expressing your observations of the person's behavior and providing sympathetic listening, can be helpful.

To minimize sensory overload, you can write a care plan that gives the person sufficient time to rest between procedures and tests. Providing nursing care in time blocks and allowing ill persons to become participants in care helps make input more meaningful, in turn offsetting excessive extraneous stimulation from the health care environment.

Many older adults are spiritual persons. It may be appropriate for members of the clergy to visit the patient and the family to provide comfort and affirmation of their spiritual values. The nurse may ask whether a clergy person would be a comfort during a time of illness. The clergy should not be contacted unless the patient and family are receptive to the referral (see Chapter 36).

Supporting the family of the ill individual in other ways is an important nursing task. The family may not only be worried about the outcome of the illness but also concerned about discharge plans that may involve them. Referring the patient and family to the discharge planner to explore options can aid them in making some crucial decisions.

New trends in housing can maximize the lifestyle of the older adult. Retirement communities, condominiums that offer easier living with fewer physical demands, and shared living arrangements can be alternatives to long-term care facilities, if appropriate.

The growth of organizations and programs for elderly persons is enhancing the quality of many people's lives. Community resources can be valuable in aiding the patient and the family temporarily or permanently in a time of crisis. Many of the institutions of higher learning offer classes specifically designed for older people and using resident faculty. Subjects are presented that many have never had time to explore and can now find interesting and informative. Inexpensive travel programs, many with knowledgeable persons, are also available to those retired and free to travel. Accommodations are made for those with disabilities. Nurses should be aware of programs available in their communities.

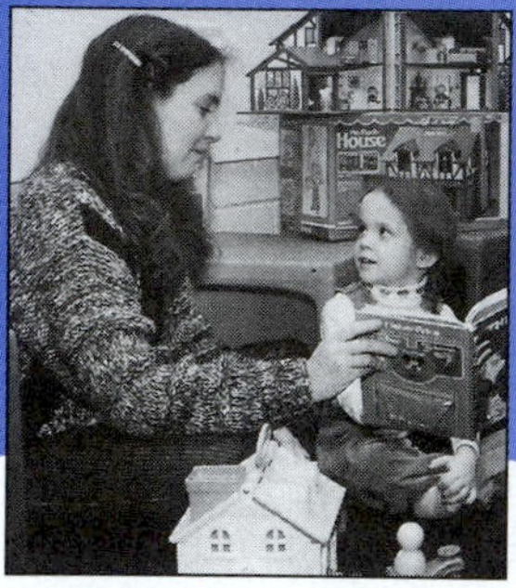

Key Points

- In caring for young adults, the role of the nurse is often one of sharing concerns that are familiar and that have been experienced within his or her own life. Nurses often find caring for young adults rewarding because most staff persons are of this age group and share common hopes and concerns.
- Because the young adult is in the years of peak performance both physically and psychologically, nurses often have an optimism and hope for recovery that may or may not be warranted.
- The middle-aged patient is involved in a productive time of life with commitments to social responsibilities. The disruption imposed by illness or injury may be disturbing and may have great impact on the financial and psychological well-being of the family.
- Nurses who care for older persons need to have a positive attitude toward aging. A strong knowledge base concerning the developmental tasks of this age group as well as age-related changes and their effect on daily living is vital in providing nursing care for the older adult.
- An understanding of the concerns of persons in young adulthood, the middle years, and in advanced age, enables the nurse to provide effective and individualized nursing care.

Study Questions

1. What are some of the lifestyle changes that have taken place in our society for adults within the last 10 years?
2. What are some of the current concerns of young adults in society?
3. List some of the concerns you have as a young or middle adult.
4. What tasks should be done during the stage of young adulthood to resolve the crisis of intimacy versus isolation?
5. What tasks should be done during the stage of middle adulthood to resolve the crisis of generativity versus stagnation?
6. What tasks should be done during the stage of older adulthood to resolve the crisis of integrity versus despair?
7. Why is it important for nurses to have knowledge of the stages of adulthood? Give two examples.

Critical Thinking Activities

1. Contrast the physical development of the young, middle, and older adult.
2. If you were writing a nursing care plan, what data relative to growth and development of the young adult would it be important for you to collect?
3. If you were writing a nursing care plan, what data relative to growth and development of the middle adult would it be important for you to collect?
4. If you were writing a nursing care plan, what data relative to growth and development of the older adult would it be important for you to collect?
5. Visit one of the following:
   a. food bank
   b. community program for the prevention of sexually transmitted diseases
   c. political action or religious group
   d. senior citizens center

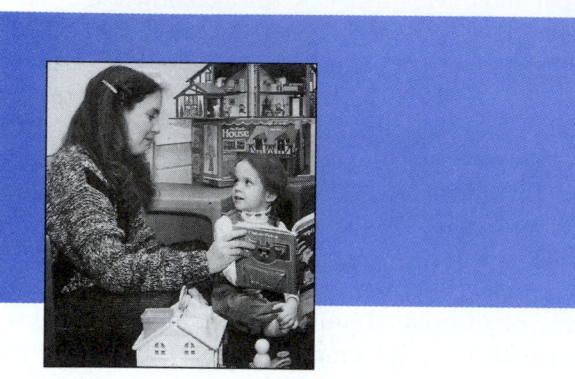

In writing, analyze what age group participated, and why you believe this resource is needed or valuable for that age group.

References and Readings

Abraham, L. L., and Krowchuk, H. V. "Unemployment and Health." *Nursing Clinics of North America* 21, 1 (March 1986): 37–47.

Allen, D. N., and Whatley, M. "Nursing and Men's Health." *Nursing Clinics of North America* 21, 1 (March 1986): 3–13.

Blanchard, D. "What Women Can Do to Protect Against Osteoporosis." *RN* 53, 10 (October 1990): 60–64.

Brodoff, A. S. "Assessing Marital Stress by Life Stages." *Patient Care* 15 (March 1983): 140, 145, 148–149.

Carroll, J. S. "Middle Age Does Not Mean Menopause." *Topics in Clinical Nursing* 4 (January 1983): 38–44.

Doress, P. B., and Siegal, D. L. *Ourselves, Growing Older.* New York: Simon and Schuster, 1987.

Ebersole, P., and Hess, P. *Toward Healthy Aging: Human Needs and Nursing Response.* 3rd edition. St. Louis: C. V. Mosby, 1990.

Erikson, E. H. *Childhood and Society.* New York: W. W. Norton, 1963.

Frenkel-Brunswik, E. "Adjustments and Reorientation in the Course of the Life Span." In *Psychological Studies in Human Development* (rev. ed.), edited by R. G. Kuhlen and G. D. Thompson. New York: Appleton-Century-Crofts, 1963, pp. 161–171.

Gilligan, C. *In a Different Voice.* Cambridge: Harvard University Press, 1982.

Given, C. W., Collins, C. E., and Given, B. A. "Source of Stress of Among Families Caring for Relatives with Alzheimer's Disease." *Nursing Clinics of North America.* 23, 1 (March 1988): 69–82.

Guyton, A. C. *Human Physiology and Mechanisms of Disease.* 5th edition. Philadelphia: W. B. Saunders, 1992.

Havighurst, R. J. *Developmental Tasks and Educations.* 2nd edition. New York: David McKay Company, 1964.

Kohlberg, L., and Shulik, R. "The Aging Person as Philosopher: Moral Development in the Adult Years." Unpublished paper, Harvard University, 1981.

Kopac, C. A. "Sensory Loss in the Aged: The Role of the Nurse and the Family." *Nursing Clinics of North America* 18, 2 (June 1983): 373–384.

Leslie, L. A., and Swider, S. M. "Changing Factors and Changing Needs." *Nursing Clinics of North America* 21, 1 (March 1986): 111–123.

Levinson, D. J., Darrow, C. N., Klein, E. B., Levinson, M. H., and McKee, B. *The Seasons of a Man's Life.* New York: Alfred A. Knopf, 1986.

Murray, R., and Zentner, J. *Nursing Assessment and Health Promotion Strategies Through the Life Span.* 4th edition. Englewood Cliffs, N.J.: Prentice-Hall, 1989.

Nolan, J. W. "Developmental Concerns and the Health of Midlife Woman." *Nursing Clinics of North America* 21, 1 (March 1986): 151–159.

Reed, P. "Implications of the Life-Span Developmental Framework for Well-Being in Adulthood and Aging." *Advances in Nursing Science* 6, 1 (October 1983): 18–25.

U.S. Department of Commerce, Bureau of the Census. *Statistical Abstract of the United States.* 111th edition, 1991.

Vickery, F. *Old and Growing.* Springfield, Ill.: Charles C. Thomas, 1978.

Westerhoff, J. *Will Our Children Have Faith?* New York: Seabury Press, 1983.

Special Needs of the Older Adult

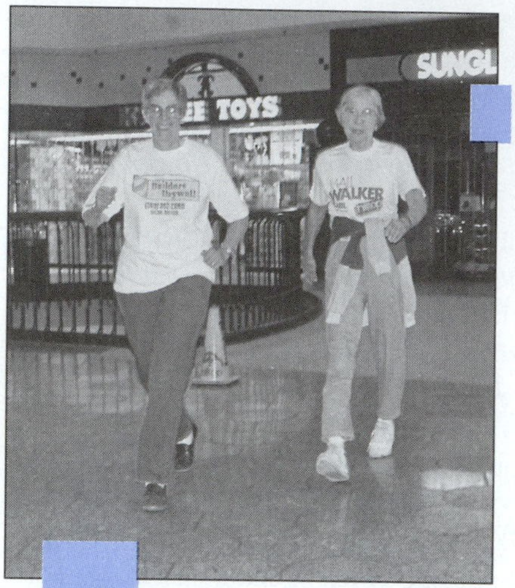

20

Objectives

After completing this chapter, you should be able to:

1. Explain two theories of aging.
2. Discuss the elderly population in terms of health status, family, finances, and housing.
3. Describe the physical changes that occur in the various body systems with aging.
4. Describe the psychosocial changes that accompany aging.
5. List the types and characteristics of long-term care settings available to older people.
6. Discuss concerns related to institutionalization, communication, confusion, and safety for the patient in the long-term care setting.
7. Explore the attitudes of nurses toward the older adult.
8. Describe services that can be provided by organizations for the elderly.
9. Write a nursing care plan related to the older person in a health care setting.

Study Terms

ageism
alopecia
arteriosclerosis
assisted living centers
atherosclerosis
cataract
continuing care community (CCC)
elder abuse
geriatrics
gerontology
glaucoma
long-term care (LTC) facility
nursing home
osteoarthritis
osteoporosis
retirement residence
senile dementia
shared housing

Outline

Ellis, Nowlis: Nursing: A Human Needs Approach, 5th ed. © 1994 J.B. Lippincott Company

Growing old in Western society is far from the valued experience it appears to be in some Asian countries, where age elicits respect and the young solicit the wisdom of the old. The irony of aging is "that everyone wants to live as long as possible, but no one wants to grow old" (Lancaster, 1981 p. 31). Many myths surround aging: older people cannot learn new tasks, most older persons "end up in nursing homes," and older people are depressed and irritable (Table 20-1).

Pamela Reed states (1983, p. 19) that aging has been far too long associated with decline rather than with development. Rather than "running out of steam," older adults have increased capacity for new understandings. They have a higher level of integration so life experiences can be used to cope with and solve problems.

For nurses in general practice, care of the older adult is extremely important because the majority of patients entering the acute care setting are over 60 years of age. This fact has obvious implications for nursing education. Schools of nursing have recognized the importance of providing nursing students with clinical experience in caring for geriatric (aging) patients. Two specialties concerned with the older adult are **geriatrics**, health care of the aged patient, and **gerontology**, the study of the aging process, including the illnesses and diseases of old age.

As people age, they must accommodate themselves to certain normal changes. For purposes of assessment, nurses must have some knowledge of the physical and psychosocial changes that accompany the aging process, yet set aside any preconceived ideas of the characteristics of aging people.

The skills of caring for the aging patient are essentially the same skills the nurse offers every patient, adapted to the physical changes and limitations that may accompany aging. In addition, special attention must be given to the psychological needs of the older person. Although the student nurse may not wish to pursue a career in geriatric nursing, knowledge of older patients and their needs is essential because interacting with older persons is inherent to nursing.

The Demographics of Aging

Information and predictions about changes in population reveal the fact that older adults as a group are increasing in number more than any other age group. The "baby boom" of the 1940s has literally evolved into an "aging boom." The latest U.S. Census revealed some interesting facts. It is predicted that by the middle of the next century, the proportion of young persons under age 19 will approximately equal that of persons over age 65, or about 22%. Those of advanced age, above 85, make up the fastest growing age group (Table 20-2). The increase in longevity is attributed to social changes and modern technology. Social changes have brought about better health care in general, more service organizations, and improved nutrition. Modern technology has provided medical interventions for extending the lives of the aged as was never before believed possible. Although females have a longer life expectancy at birth than do males, the life expectancy of both is constantly rising.

Elderly women now outnumber elderly men by three to two. This figure becomes even more disproportionate over the age of 85, when there are only 40 men to 100 women. Perhaps because older women have been, by number, more visible, "older women have been the victims of negative social stereotyping" (McElmurry and LiBrizzi, 1986, p. 170). In artistic presentations, the old woman is often portrayed as aggressive and unpleasant, whereas older men are often viewed as attractive. Despite this stereotyping, most older women manage their lives competently and are independent and capable of self-care (McElmurry and LiBrizzi, p. 169). The emphasis on womens' health care has been

Table 20–1. Fight Ageism With Facts

Myths	The Truth of the Matter
1. Old age begins at 65.	1. The concept of being old is an "unrealizable reality" that is gradually accepted through its application by outsiders.
2. The old nonproductive, unemployable, "finished."	2. Older workers are valued for their 20% better absentee records and fewer on-the-job accidents. The need for older workers is steadily increasing.
3. The ability to learn declines with old age.	3. New skills take longer to learn but are retained longer. The brain can grow with experience chemically and structurally. "Use or lose" is a significant concept.
4. The old are more forgetful.	4. True, the brain cannot scan and retrieve as fast, but defects in memory may result from physical causes that can be corrected by supplying needed substances to the brain.
5. Old age inevitably results in senility.	5. "Senility" is a catch-all term for everything from mild confusion to mental deterioration. As many as 100 physiologic and psychological causes of confusion in elderly persons can be diagnosed and treated.
6. Old age means becoming ill and going to a nursing home.	6. Despite chronic health problems, as many as 70% of elderly persons stay in their own homes. Only 5% are in nursing homes, a figure remaining substantially the same.
7. Elderly persons are more rigid in thought and action—more "set in their ways."	7. It takes courage and adaptation for elderly persons to have survived through wars, depression, and unprecedented social technologic changes.
8. The old are not interested in sex (and it's disgusting when they are).	8. Not only do letters to "Dear Abby" attest to the interest and performance of sexually active elders, but articles by health professionals encourage sexual activity as normal and healthy at any age.
9. Older people today enjoy a greater acceptance in society.	9. Not true. They are often rendered invisible by a society obsessed with "gerontophobia." At best, when noticed, older people are patronized, and at worst, may be subject to abuse.
10. Most of today's elders have incomes adequate for their needs.	10. If they must enter a nursing home, two-thirds of elderly persons become eligible within 13 weeks for Medicaid. Two-thirds of elderly persons in poverty are women, depending on Social Security for 90% of their income.
11. Old people are pretty much alike.	11. Unlike newborn babies and adolescents who strive to be exactly like their peers, elders are individuals above all, the sum of personal triumphs and mistakes, rewards and triumphs. Celebrate their differences.
12. The old have "one foot in the grave."	12. EVERYbody has one foot in the grave. We all grow old; we all die. A gentle physical decline begins with the 30th birthday, not the 65th. No one ever died of old age.

Source: Prepared by Margaret Svec, Professor Emeritus, Shoreline Community College, Seattle, Washington.

one response to the existence of large numbers of women, particularly older women, in our population.

Because of the prospective Medicare payment regulations discussed in Chapter 2, elderly patients may be discharged earlier from hospitals and continue their convalescence at home or in a chronic care setting. Nursing responsibilities related to older patients will not decrease, however, for it has been proven that people who have good nursing care within the hospital suffer fewer complications after discharge.

The number of older persons within our society will continue to increase, a trend that will continue throughout the professional life of those practicing nursing today. Because so many patients/clients are of advanced age, nurses must have sound knowledge of both the development of and care of older adults.

Attitudes Toward the Older Adult

Even though each of us in nursing comes from a family and a community with attitudes toward social issues, as individuals we are responsible for our own attitudes. Certainly one's attitude toward aging persons is crucial in a profession that provides health care. **Ageism** is a societal attitude of prejudice against the elderly that is

Table 20–2. Population 65 Years Old and Over, by Age Group and Sex, 1960–1989, and Projections, 2000

Age Group and Sex	Number (1,000)					Percent Distribution				
	1960	*1970*	*1980*	*1989*	*2000, proj.*	*1960*	*1970*	*1980*	*1989*	*2000, proj.*
Persons 65 y and over . . .	16,675	20,107	25,704	30,984	34,882	100.0	100.0	100.0	100.0	100.0
65–69 y	6,280	7,026	8,812	10,170	9,491	37.7	34.9	34.3	32.8	27.2
70–74 y	4,773	5,467	6,841	8,012	8,752	28.6	27.2	26.6	25.9	25.1
75–79 y	3,080	3,871	4,828	6,033	7,282	18.5	19.3	18.8	19.5	20.9
80–84 y	1,601	2,312	2,954	3,728	4,735	9.6	11.5	11.5	12.0	13.6
85 y and over	940	1,430	2,269	3,042	4,622	5.6	7.1	8.8	9.8	13.2
Males, 65 y and over	7,542	8,413	10,366	12,636	14,273	100.0	100.0	100.0	100.0	100.0
65–69 y	2,936	3,139	3,919	4,631	4,382	38.9	37.3	37.8	36.7	30.7
70–74 y	2,197	2,322	2,873	3,464	3,860	29.1	27.6	27.7	27.4	27.0
75–79 y	1,370	1,573	1,862	2,385	2,971	18.2	18.7	18.0	18.9	20.8
80–84 y	673	883	1,026	1,306	1,739	8.9	10.5	9.9	10.3	12.2
85 y and over	366	496	688	850	1,322	4.9	5.9	6.6	6.7	9.3
Females, 65 y and over. . . .	9,133	11,693	15,338	18,348	20,608	100.0	100.0	100.0	100.0	100.0
65–69 y	3,344	3,887	4,894	5,538	5,109	36.6	33.2	31.9	30.2	24.8
70–74 y	2,577	3,145	3,968	4,549	4,892	28.2	26.9	25.9	24.8	23.7
75–79 y	1,711	2,298	2,966	3,648	4,311	18.7	19.7	19.3	19.9	20.9
80–84 y	928	1,429	1,928	2,422	2,996	10.2	12.2	12.6	13.2	14.5
85 y and over.	574	934	1,582	2,192	3,300	6.3	8.0	10.3	11.9	16.0

As of July 1. Includes Armed Forces overseas. These projections were prepared prior to the release of 1990 census results and are therefore not based on 1990 census data.
Source: U.S. Bureau of the Census, *Current Population Reports,* series P-25, Nos. 519, 917, 1018, and 1057.

exhibited in biased language, consumerism, and policies. To say simply that we must change our personal attitudes toward older people is naive because such attitudes are deeply engrained in family attitudes and in relationships of childhood. Some nurses have never known an older person intimately and have little knowledge on which to build or change attitudes. Regardless of our background and contact with older persons, we should attempt to expel old myths.

Just as you have learned that basic care focuses on fulfilling physical and psychosocial needs, you will also learn methods to adapt your nursing actions to meet the specific needs of the person of advanced age. As a student, you will probably have experience in the long-term care setting. Before you begin such an experience, examine your own attitudes toward the elderly. How quickly and how well you relate to the older patient depends largely on past experiences with elderly people. A nurse whose elderly aunt or grandparent has been cantankerous or disruptive to the family might find it harder to be empathic and close to an elderly patient than would a nurse who has had a cherished relationship with an older relative.

Nurses must guard against stereotyping the aged. Often a patient's age elicits an unfortunate response before the person even arrives, a response expressed in such remarks as "Oh, but she's 91. What are we supposed to do?" It sometimes appears that the limitations age imposes on good recovery promote lack of interest on the part of the nurse.

Because our behavior is directly influenced by attitudes, nurses must develop positive attitudes for providing care for the elderly (La Monica, 1979). As nurses, we can offer respect so that the aging can maintain dignity. Your older patient has been a child, a teenager, a student. Your older patient has loved, had friends, taught others, and acquired wisdom and skills. Your older patient has feelings much like your own. By caring, you can provide your patient with what you would want and need in the same circumstances—meaningful human contact.

Positive Aspects of Aging

Because of the growing numbers of aging persons in society and because each of us will join this age group in time, we must maximize the quality of life for older adults. Most of us will be in a relationship with older persons and will need to become familiar with their strengths as well as their vulnerabilities.

In the last chapter, we discussed some "trade offs" that bring about a satisfying final stage of the life span. Raising children in the physical sense is no longer a task for the older person. However, many older adults are becoming surrogate parents in single-adult households with children, allowing the parent to work outside the home. Having adult children can enrich the later years of life. "Our lives (older persons) will remain inextricably and profoundly bound to theirs (adult childrens'). Our concern for their welfare and pride in their accomplishments and careers will continue to be one of our major life interests, their continuing love and affection one of our deepest needs" (Vickery, 1978, p. 77). Giving direction to social and political groups through a lifetime of experience and wisdom can be rewarding for many older people. The natural environment in which we live often takes on a new meaning for older persons who structure their time to enjoy what has hastily been passed by in earlier years.

However, we must not lose sight of the fact that the vast majority of older persons are living in the community, successfully coping with life changes. A number of satisfactions are connected with growing older. Erikson's conflict of later life, that of integrity versus despair, means that in reality most older persons gain, with passing years, a renewed sense of integrity. This feeling often comes from the satisfaction of having attained goals set earlier in life and enjoying the results that have come from them. Many women who devoted their earlier years primarily to the traditional role of being mothers feel increasing pride in the accomplishments of their children and continue to serve as role models and advisers as they grow older. The older man can share in this joy as well as take pride in his own accomplishments in the work force. Even before the recent trend toward role reversal, some older persons forged ahead in nontraditional roles, and they now gain satisfaction from having been pioneers in establishing new social values.

Many of the developmental tasks outlined by Havighurst and mentioned in previous chapters are achieved through the remarkable resiliency of advanced age. These tasks include adjusting to deteriorated health status, retirement, and the death of others and establishing affiliation with one's own age group, meeting social obligations, and living comfortably within the physical environment.

New motivation and opportunities for learning are continually arising. The names of many community-based programs reflect their purpose of continuing education and lifelong learning. Physical fitness programs focused on the aging population, many of which are offered by nonprofit organizations, encourage social as well as physical well-being.

Although some families suffer intergenerational disruption, which we briefly discussed in Chapter 19 and will talk about later in the chapter, more often the presence of older persons enriches the family and mutual love grows as the life of the older person shortens.

The older adults we discuss in this chapter are primarily those whose needs are not being adequately met because of illness, increasing disability, or changes in their life situation. Most of the chapter is devoted to discussing the problems of these older adults and how, as nurses, we might assist those persons and their families in more fully meeting their needs.

Theories of Aging

Although many theories of aging have been offered, no one knows precisely why some people age more rapidly than others. Selye (1956) and others have postulated that each person has an individual "aging clock" whose rate depends on inherited adaptive energies. Selye further suggests that one's degree of ability to cope with stress is a central factor in aging. In other words, aging is seen by Selye as a function of life stress and the degree to which one can successfully resolve or adapt to stressors.

Another theory of aging postulates that the autoimmune system of the body, which protects us from disease and combats injury by producing antibodies and hormones that have a homeostatic action, becomes less responsive with age, allowing structural deterioration and diseases to increase in occurrence.

According to the complicated cross-linkage theory, aging is accompanied by an increase in accidental crossings-over, or linkages, between the intracellular and extracellular molecules, resulting in a stiffening of all of the connective tissues of the body. This phenomenon is accompanied by a realignment of DNA particles, an essential component of all living cells. Perhaps easier to grasp is the "wear-and-tear" theory, according to which all plant and animal life is subject to wearing out after a certain period of time.

No single theory of aging has been proven; aging may possibly be attributable to a combination of factors. It is certain, however, that aging, like all other human experiences, is individual. Consider for a moment the 83-year-old retired attorney, hospitalized for minor surgery, who sits up at night studying computer skills, because, as she says, "It's so exciting. There's so much to know." At the other end of the spectrum is the 68-year-old woman lying impassive in a nursing home bed, staring blankly at a rain-spattered window. Why do people age so differently? Variations appear to depend on such factors as the patient's heredity, previous mental attitudes, health, and nutritional status, as well as the support of the family.

The Health Status of the Older Adult

Individuals within each stage of the life span differ greatly from each other in health status. However, this range may be widest among the elderly. One government study reported that almost one-third of the older persons saw themselves as reasonably healthy.

Self-help groups are useful in promoting physical health and emotional well-being. Similarly, senior citizen centers and an emphasis on self-care have also increased the quality of life. Self-care refers to the criteria outlined in Belloc and Breslow's (1972) study of 7,000 elderly Californians. The criteria were health practices such as maintaining proper nutrition and a recommended weight level, engaging in adequate activity and rest, having no or only occasional alcohol, and not smoking. These principles have been incorporated into the practices of hundreds of sharing or self-care groups for the elderly throughout the country.

However, as many people become older, their health does decline to some degree. With extended age come more chronic illnesses as systems undergo change. Chronic diseases like arthritis and heart conditions, which 50 years ago accounted for 30% of all illnesses, today represent more than 80%. Ouslander and Beck (1982, p. 56), admitting that it is difficult to measure health in the aged, indicate that persons over age 65 account for 30% of the $160 billion spent annually on health care and purchase one-fourth of all prescription drugs. However, despite advancing years and decreased physical health, only 8% of those 65 to 74 years of age have difficulty performing their own activities of daily living (ADLs). This number increases only to 18% over the age of 75.

The Family of the Older Adult

Although the family always plays an important role in caring for a patient, the family becomes particularly important when the patient is an older adult. Older persons with self-care deficits may require help with ADLs, and this task often falls to the adult children. The increased longevity of the elderly now places more family members in the role of care providers, and most of them lovingly fulfill the older adult's needs.

In a message to the Assembly on Aging of the United Nations in 1982, the International Association of Gerontology recognized that traditionally the responsibility of caring for the elderly has fallen to women. The association pointed out the problems arising from this practice in today's world, with its changing role for women and increased reliance on women as part of the work force.

The extension of the life span has also affected the adult children of the elderly in that they too are older than those of previous generations. Many of the persons who are caring for older family members are themselves reaching late middle age and experiencing declining health as well as declining resources. Cicirelli (1982) found that divorce was higher among couples who were caring for elderly persons, the assumption being that parental conflict was a contributing factor in the divorce.

Some disturbing research has been conducted on a subject that directly affects nursing—abuse of the elderly. Although documentation of the extent of this problem is incomplete, the magnitude of the abuse is probably substantial. As with wife and child abuse, the topic is extremely sensitive, with difficulties regarding accurate reporting.

There are two kinds of **elder abuse**. The first is physical and can involve withholding medical care, confinement, abandonment, or even beating. The second is psychological abuse, which can be equally destructive, and may take the form of verbal abuse or threats: anything imposed by the care provider that produces fear in the older adult (Falcioni, 1982, p. 208).

Recently, abuse of clients has been reported in chronic care settings. Resident abuse may take the form of either of the two types just described. Oversedation, unnecessary restraint, physical and psychological isolation, and, in some unfortunate situations, actual physical injury may occur. In some states, an appointed ombudsman hears and investigates the complaints of patients and residents as well as family members. In many states, if evidence of the abuse of residents in chronic care settings is substantiated, the licensing of these facilities can be rescinded and the residents moved to a safer environment. Because the ill or infirm elderly are often defenseless, it is the responsibility of each person, particularly nurses, to report any evidence of abuse in a timely manner so that all older adults can be protected. It is unclear how often elder abuse happens, but even one instance is unacceptable to the mission of providing sensitive nursing care to the older person.

More often, fortunately, intergenerational relationships are warm and positive. Olsen and Kahn (1980, p. 154) state that the family is the greatest resource an older person has. The elderly and their families can share happy memories and find new growth experiences together.

Financial Status of the Older Adult

Finances affect health status in that they influence both nutrition and housing. Nurses should look beyond the bedside to understand more clearly the needs of their older patients.

What are the causes of financial distress on the part of the elderly? First, although most have accumulated retirement income through the federal Social Security program, these funds alone have proven inadequate to meet the high cost of living today, and employment savings plans were relatively uncommon during their working years. Second, money put aside years ago has been severely devalued by inflation. Furthermore, people are living longer, and any savings they have accumulated must last longer.

Having to live on a fixed income has penalized many older citizens. Increased Social Security and Medicare payments have not kept pace with spiraling price increases resulting from inflation as well as increases in medication and health care costs not covered by Medicare. Although health care in Canada is much more comprehensive for the elderly than it is in the United States, inflation has caused a rise in the cost of consumer products and general services in both countries.

In 1988, 12% of people over the age of 65 in the United States lived at or below the poverty level. Although this is an alarming figure, it has not risen higher partly because since 1975 the government has annually enacted cost of living adjustments (COLAs) in Social Security payments.

Lack of money also affects the diets of older people, for whom adequate nutrition should be a priority. Because food costs have risen steeply in the last few years, elderly people spend approximately one-third of their incomes on food. The older population has been found to have a high incidence of chronic malnutrition due largely to food costs, the difficulties of shopping, longstanding poor eating habits, and poor meal planning. Breitung (1980, p. 19) found deficits in both the nutrition and the subsistence level of the older population she studied. More than one-half of those investigated lived on $5,000 a year or less. Many were unaware that they were eligible for food stamps and did not know where to go for such assistance. Pride also played a large part in the decision not to seek help.

Housing for the Older Adult

Housing for the elderly is a problem of considerable magnitude. Many who have lived in the inner city for years no longer find their neighborhoods desirable or even safe. Many cities are developing the inner cities, building apartments and condominiums designed for young professional people and the financially advantaged elderly. Only a few cities in the United States and Canada are planning low income housing in the inner city. For those who live in suburban areas, deteriorating neighborhoods, theft, and street violence have placed undue stress on older citizens and forced them to secure their homes or live with relatives. Finding adequate housing on a fixed income is difficult. Large homes with high maintenance costs must often be traded for smaller, less expensive apartments. Some elderly people purchase mobile homes and form their own retirement communities; others must accommodate themselves to small furnished or unfurnished rooms with minimal cooking facilities. The U.S. Department of Housing and

Nursing Issues and Trends: *Health Insurance for Older Adults*

The Medicare program, passed by Congress in 1965, has consistently run at a fiscal "deficit." The system attempted to correct this with the introduction of "DRGs" in 1983 which was a prospective payment system for health care agencies which cared for older patients. (See other chapters of this text for a more detailed explanation of these plans.) The implementation of DRGs has not been totally successful. An issue currently confronting all providers of health care is the question of how to best integrate the Medicare system with proposals for universal health care for all. As the population ages and more older people seek services, we must encourage health care for all but at the same time, we must not lower the standards of care or coverage deserved by older members of society.

Urban Development (HUD) has subsidized a limited number of low and moderately priced public housing units, but the waiting lists for such accommodations are long.

Eighty-four percent of older adults state that they would prefer to live in their own homes. One survey (Nowlis, 1983) found that of 100 older adults, 38% live alone, 28% live with adult children, 14% live with a spouse, and 20% live with persons other than family. The longevity of older adults plus declining health and finances may greatly increase the number of persons living with adult children or relatives in the years to come (Table 20-3).

Shared Housing

In several parts of the country with large elderly populations, it is becoming increasingly common for older people to establish a living arrangement called **shared housing**, often in the home of one member of the group. This is often called *home sharing for the elderly.* Sharing expenses and responsibilities in this way allows some people to remain independent longer than they otherwise could.

Table 20–3. Housing Arrangements for Older Adults

Shared Housing	House owner shares dwelling with other older adults who contribute to expenses and assume responsibilities of independent living.
Retirement Residencies	Usually apartments or condominiums that provide privacy for residents. Some household help may be available. Persons are capable of managing independently.
Assisted Living Centers	Provides minimal levels of personal care, meals, and housekeeping. Designed for persons who need minimal help with meeting personal daily needs but who cannot manage alone.
Continuing Care Communities (CCC)	Offers a variety of living options from private apartments to extended care. May require residents to financially invest in agency.
Nursing Homes (LTC)	Long-term care facilities (LTC) provide supervisory care to elders who can no longer meet their personal needs. Persons may be those who are independent but need supervision, as well as the chronically ill.

Retirement Residences

Retirement residences are homes or apartments specifically designed for the older population. Retirement apartments provide for privacy within a community. For such an arrangement to be suitable, the older person must be able to perform all ordinary ADLs, including meal preparation. In some facilities, limited household help is available. Many also sponsor social activities.

Retirement homes have become popular. Each resident has a private room and bath and sometimes a small kitchenette. Served meals are available for people who cannot prepare their own. Some homes provide all meals; others offer only one or two meals a day. Some require payment for all meals, whether or not they are eaten in the dining room. Some retirement homes provide household services although residents take care of their own personal needs. Emergency medical services may be available.

Assisted Living Centers

Assisted living centers provide minimal levels of personal care as well as meals and housekeeping. They offer primarily supervisory care, such as helping residents maintain hygiene and supervising medications. They are appropriate for people who do not need a great deal of help fulfilling their needs but cannot manage totally alone. The need for assisted living centers is growing.

Continuing Care Communities

The **continuing care community (CCC)** is a multipurpose agency that offers a variety of living options. These planned communities often require the person to invest money in the plan but offer services that range from retirement apartments and homes to nursing home levels of health care. A more complete discussion of nursing home living is presented later in the chapter.

Nursing Homes

Nursing homes are sometimes referred to as **long-term care (LTC) facilities** and provide a variety of levels of care ranging from supervisory care for the more independent resident to total care for the resident with debilitating or serious long-term illness. A complex payment system often defines "skilled nursing care" as a criteria for payment. Skilled nursing care means that the patient requires a level of care given by a registered nurse. The majority of residents in nursing homes are elderly but many younger persons with chronic illness or catastrophic injury may reside long term or perma-

Nursing Care Plan

Sample Nursing Care Plan Related to Relocation of the Older Adult

Nursing Diagnosis

Relocation Stress Syndrome related to movement from home to long-term care.

Supportive data:

Admitted to long-term care facility 2 days ago.

Widowed 4 months ago.

Lived in own home for 41 years; alone since husband's death.

Prefers to stay in own room, eats only one-half of meals, and awakens frequently at night.

Son travels and is unable to have mother live with him.

Desired Patient Outcomes

The patient will:

Express sorrow at having to leave own home.

Be able to share memories of past home.

Interact with people in new environment by end of month.

Participate in activities, resume usual eating and sleeping pattern.

Communicate feelings of acceptance of new environment and reduced frustration.

Nursing Action	Rationale
1. Provide time to visit and listen to resident's concerns.	Active listening conveys a caring attitude on the part of the nurse and promotes trust.
2. Talk with resident and son, focusing on memories of living in own home.	Verbalizing both satisfactions and regrets provides a basis for resolution of feelings related to loss of independence.
3. Provide information regarding activities in the facility.	Acting as a resource provides choices for patient to consider.
4. Introduce resident to other residents who have successfully made the transition to living in the facility.	Seeing and meeting others who have made a transition successfully facilitates adaptation to one's own transition.
5. Accompany resident to the dining room and plan seating with suitable companions.	All individuals function as members of social groups. Assisting the person to find suitable companions may foster lasting friendships.
6. Have staff visit at bedtime to identify ways for resident to sleep more effectively.	Adapting the sleep environment and resolving anxiety enhances the ability to sleep effectively.
7. Make frequent contact with resident.	Frequent contact maintains open communication.

nently in a nursing home. The concerns and stages of adjustment for clients are discussed later in this chapter (see sample Nursing Care Plan Related to the Relocation of the Older Adult).

Physiologic Changes of Aging

In Chapter 19, we briefly discussed the physical development of the older adult. Here, we focus more precisely on physical changes as they affect the function of persons in the later years of life (Display 20-1). Caution must be used not to generalize these changes, which occur to some degree in all body systems, to all older individuals. Some changes happen almost imperceptibly; others, particularly when they affect function and require adaptations, are more apparent.

The body of a young person makes the adaptations necessary to maintain homeostasis rather quickly. Because of cellular and tissue changes, the elderly adapt more slowly to physiologic changes and thus have more difficulty maintaining a state of balance.

When assessing the older patient/client, you must understand that what you may consider significant alterations in laboratory values may actually be normal changes caused by the aging process. Garner (1989, p. 144) makes an interesting point by stating that normal laboratory values are based on the physiology of 10- to 40-year-olds so that interpreting laboratory values in elders is extremely complex.

Display 20–1
Physical Changes of Aging

Circulation

Thickening of walls of blood vessels
Narrowing of lumen of vessels
Loss of vessel elasticity
Lower cardiac output

Oxygenation

Rigidity of chest wall reducing recoil
Fewer alveoli

Mobility and Activity

Decreased muscle mass with more fat cells
Decalcification of bones
Degenerative joint changes

Nutrition

Periodontal disease, loss of teeth
Decrease in secretion of digestive juices
Food intolerances

Skin Integrity

Loss of subcutaneous fat layers
Decreased number of oil, moisture, and sweat glands
Intolerance of heat and cold
Hair whitens, becomes sparse
Nails contain more keratin, become thick

Urinary Elimination

Decreased renal blood flow
Less bladder capacity, sphincter control

Regulation

Pancreas not as active, so decreased production of insulin increases blood glucose
Women lose ability to procreate
Men retain ability to procreate but sperm count diminishes

Sensation and Perception

Learning occurs as well but more slowly
Some degree of recent memory loss
Decreased proprioception

Vision

Pupils decrease in size, admit less light
Decreased accommodation, lens darkens

Hearing

Thickening of tympanic membrane
Sclerosis of inner ear

Smell

Degeneration of olfactory bulb decreases ability to smell

Touch

Decrease in skin receptors

Taste

Fewer taste buds on tongue and mouth

Another area in which you must carefully adapt and validate your care is the administration of medications. "Aging changes interfere with the ability to absorb or excrete drugs. As a result, there is a toxic buildup which increases the effects and side effects of drugs to levels that impair the elderly patient's performance" (Spellbring, Gannon, Kleckner, and Conway, 1988, p. 32.) Older adults are particularly vulnerable to drug reactions because of changes related to the aging process. First, lowered cardiac output can decrease absorption of parenterally administered drugs. Second, there may be toxic effects because the blood contains fewer proteins for the binding of certain drugs, which leads to a greater concentration of unbound drug. Last, the liver cannot detoxify drugs as efficiently as before, so the older person can accumulate dangerous levels in the blood. A pharmacologic text will give you more details on safe drug administration for the older patient/client.

With each system described below, we discuss the most common health problems. Andresen (1989, p. 28) warns us that we should never dismiss a complaint on the basis that "it is just because of age." Elderly persons show the greatest diversity of all age groups. It is for this reason that we should resist the temptation to relate problems all too quickly to age. "Aged patients (60–90 years old) have a wide and unpredictable spectrum of responses to illness: whenever possible, compare the patient to himself, not to a younger counterpart" (Bender, 1992).

In response to the nursing diagnoses, interventions or actions can be taken that attempt to relieve the problems identified.

Circulation

One of every two adults over the age of 65 has heart disease. Forty percent of all drugs prescribed for the elderly are for cardiac problems. Cardiovascular conditions are the leading cause of death among the elderly; 70% of all people who die of heart attacks are over the age of 65 (Gawlinski and Jensen, 1991).

Changes in the cardiovascular system are complex. The most generalized complication that arises in the elderly is **arteriosclerosis**, a thickening of the middle wall of blood vessels that narrows the opening through which the blood flows. A more severe form of vascular compromise occurs with **atherosclerosis**, an additional thickening of the inner wall of arteries caused by the presence of deposits. This condition, which makes the vessels even more rigid and narrows the *lumen* (the interior of the vessels), affects every system of the body by diminishing the blood supply to all organs.

The heart muscle itself is less efficient because of decreased blood supply, and a weaker beat, often described as "thready," results. In conjunction with degenerative changes in the vessels supplying the heart muscle, the valves of the heart calcify so that they do not close as tightly as they once did. What are the consequences of all this for the patient? The blood pressure rises as a result of the increased force with which an unchanged volume of blood is pushed through a smaller lumen in the vessels. Because circulation is slow, the patient feels cold. Standing for a long period of time causes blood to pool in the lower extremities and may cause dizziness. Lying on the extremities causes tingling and can disturb rest.

The muscles stiffen, the muscles of respiration are no longer as vigorous, and overexertion can quickly exhaust the individual. The kidneys also receive less blood supply and are less productive than before. The patient may be prescribed special drugs to facilitate functioning of the cardiovascular system, perhaps for the rest of the person's life.

When assessing the older adult, you might find alterations in heart rate and rhythm and blood pressure. You could also detect edema, coldness of the extremities, fatigue, difficulty breathing, safety risks, and many other symptoms related to poor tissue perfusion.

Using the nursing process, you may be writing diagnoses concerning problems arising from the person's decreased cardiac output or problems with daily living that stem from poor tissue perfusion. Throughout the text, you will find specific examples of nursing diagnoses related to each human need.

Interventions may be indirect but effective. Although the structural changes in the heart cannot be modified, you can plan nursing actions to help alleviate the problem. Allowing the person time to rest between periods of activity and to make changes in position slowly will help prevent this problem. Assisting the person when standing and monitoring the person's ability to ambulate alone are essential.

The older adult should be monitored closely for drug side effects. These persons may exhibit drug reactions rarely seen in younger persons, and any change in vital signs or body systems should be promptly reported to the physician. Drugs should not be discontinued unless you are imminently concerned about the person's well-being because the sudden withdrawal of many drugs can cause serious consequences for the patient.

Oxygenation

The respiratory system is affected by changes in the musculoskeletal system. Bone and muscle changes decrease actual chest size. There are also fewer alveoli, and those present become larger and less elastic. Chest wall rigidity causes decreased *recoil* (springing back of the lung during expiration), which is one of the factors leading to decreased *vital capacity* and *tidal volume.*

Nursing Diagnoses Related to the Older Adult

Circulation

Decreased Cardiac Output related to bradycardia

Activity Intolerance related to decreased muscle strength

Self-care Deficit, partial or complete

Altered Health Maintenance related to deficits in cerebral circulation

High Risk for Peripheral Neurovascular Dysfunction

High Risk for Injury: Falls related to dizziness

Oxygenation

Impaired Gas Exhchange related to narrowed bronchial airways

Ineffective Breathing Pattern: Hyperventilation related to anxiety

Ineffective Airway Clearance related to decreased ability to cough

High Risk for Injury: Falls related to fatigue

Mobility and Activity

Impaired Physical Mobility related to decreased ability to move joints and muscles

Impaired Physical Mobility related to joint pain caused by osteoarthritis

Chronic pain related to osteoarthritis

Nutrition and Bowel Elimination

Altered Nutrition: Less than Body Requirements related to anorexia caused by depression

Altered Nutrition: More than Body Requirements related to sedentary lifestyle

Altered Oral Mucous Membrane related to inadequate oral hygiene

Self-care Deficit, feeding

High Risk for Injury: Aspiration related to impaired swallowing reflex

Constipation related to medications, sedentary life-style, and decreased intestinal motility

Diarrhea related to relocation stress and anxiety

Bowel Incontinence related to decreased sphincter control

Skin Integrity

Impaired Skin Integrity related to cracking caused by dryness

Altered Comfort: Pruritus related to dry skin

Body Image Disturbance related to baldness

High Risk for Infection related to scratching

Urinary Elimination

Altered Urinary Elimination

Urge Incontinence

Stress Incontinence

Functional Incontinence related to decreased bladder capacity/incomplete emptying/residual urine

Urinary Retention

Pain on urination

High Risk for Infection related to presence of indwelling catheter

Regulation and Sexuality

Altered Sexuality Patterns related to
presence of chronic illness
loss of sexual partner

Sexual Dysfunction related to
inadequate erectile ability
lack of libido caused by depression

Sensation and Perception

Sensory/Perceptual Alteration: Sensory overload related to high acuity of care needed

Sensory/Perceptual Alteration: Sensory deprivation related to social isolation

Impaired Verbal Communication related to
effects of aphasia
effects of hearing impairment

Sleep Pattern Disturbance related to frequent wakenings

High Risk for Altered Nutrition: Less then Body Requirements related to
decreased taste
decreased smell

High Risk for Injury related to visual impairment; proprioceptual impairment; tactile impairment

Mental Status

Self-esteem Disturbance related to declining health

Dysfunctional Grieving related to loss of long-term family home

Relocation Stress Syndrome related to recent move from home to long-term care setting

Altered Thought Processes related to effects of dementia

High Risk for Injury related to altered thought processes

The *dead air space* and *residual volume* then increase. These terms are discussed more fully in Chapter 28. To compensate for these changes, the older person breathes slightly faster than the younger person. Breaths may be more shallow. Careful assessment should include the rate and depth of respiration, the patient's skin color, and the presence of any pain with breathing. More important than a decrease in actual chest size is a decrease in the ability to cough. The collection of secretions that are not *expectorated* (spat out) is often a source of infection. Encouraging patients, especially those who are bedridden, to cough and deep breathe can help ward off respiratory complications.

A number of signs and symptoms form a basis for the nursing diagnoses for persons with respiratory problems. Some are the same for both the cardiovascular system and the respiratory system because these two systems are so closely interrelated. Daily deep-breathing exercises are helpful in maintaining lung expansion. Sometimes, just teaching the patient to breathe more

Nursing Care Plan

Sample Nursing Care Plan Related to Physiologic Changes of Aging

Nursing Diagnosis

Activity Intolerance related to long-term sedentary lifestyle and presence of arthritis.

Supportive data:

79 year-old man.

Able to dress self and perform own care.

Osteoarthritis in neck, knees, and hips.

States, "I get tired if I do too much so I just mostly rest."

Sits in chair most of day.

Walks to bathroom and dining room.

Desired Patient Outcomes

Participates in chair exercises.

Progresses to walking activities within facility.

Joins group for "mall" walking by end of month.

Nursing Action	**Rationale**
1. Discuss goal and plan with resident.	Allowing resident to participate in goal setting and planning leads to greater motivation and willingness.
2. Teach chair exercises per unit protocol.	For those with restricted activity, chair exercises provide maintenance of joint mobility and muscle strength.
3. Remind client to do chair exercises 3X day at 9 AM, 1 PM and 7 PM, beginning 1/7.	Reminders cue resident to importance of frequency of exercises which lead to a more positive outcome.
4. Beginning 1/14, have resident join exercise class that meets daily.	Group exercise may increase motivation through social intervention.
5. On 1/21, begin regular walks in hall 2X day.	Regular walks will provide more active exercise.
6. Inform resident of "mall" walking group and encourage him to try it.	"Mall" walking will continue active exercise as well as provide social interchange outside of the facility.
7. Beginning 1/28, arrange for resident to accompany small walking group 3X week.	Small walking group advances level of activity and provides opportunity for resident to be with others who offer companionship and motivation.

slowly and deeply is useful. Breathing can also be improved by relieving fear and pain. Explore the orders for pain management and carry out any appropriate actions. Providing a calm attitude and touching and staying with the patient can slow breathing and help relieve respiratory distress. Changing the position of those who are bedridden is essential in preventing respiratory complications. By far the best intervention for respiratory impairment is activity, which increases blood supply and deepens breathing. Such activity must, of course, be within the tolerance level of the individual.

Mobility and Activity

Muscle mass decreases with aging as muscle cells are replaced with fat cells. This change often gives the musculature a "flabby" appearance. It has been shown, however, that the active, healthy older person need not lose more than 30% of muscle strength through aging. Lack of exercise and improper diet often cause older people to lose a much greater proportion of their muscle strength and tone than necessary (see sample Nursing Care Plan Related to Physiologic Changes of Aging).

Weakened muscles increase the danger of breaking bones because they cannot provide adequate support. Bones themselves also undergo degenerative changes with aging. The most common condition is **osteoporosis**, a metabolic failure to replace bone tissue, which leads to thin, porous bones that fracture easily. Although this condition occurs primarily in older women, because of the reduction of estrogens, it also afflicts men. Symptoms include low back pain, weakness, stooped posture, and a tendency to fracture bones. It has been speculated that in many cases of hip fracture, the hip fractures spontaneously and causes the fall, rather than the fall causing the fracture.

Hormonal supplement therapy for women after menopause appears encouraging for the prevention of osteoporosis. However, this therapy may have adverse side effects and, therefore, needs to be discussed thoroughly with the health care provider. Recent research has shown that sufficient calcium taken early in life provides the best protection against osteoporosis. Experts are now recommending that adult women take 1,000 to 1,200 mg of calcium per day before menopause and 1,500 mg/day after menopause (Urrows, Freston, and Pryor, 1991).

Most geriatric patients have some degree of **osteoarthritis**, which is assumed to be caused by the wearing of joint cartilage until the underlying bone is exposed. This condition causes pain and immobility and sometimes swelling of the joint. Almost every person over the age of 40 has some osteoarthritis in the cervical spine or neck, which may be asymptomatic until later in life, when joints of the extremities also become involved.

Important information to gather includes the degree of understanding regarding diet, usual amount of exercise tolerated, desired activities, and the presence of any pain in the muscles or joints. This assessment is essential because as persons age, they tend to experience arthritic pain and less joint mobility. Because of pain, they become more sedentary, and in turn, exercise the muscle groups less. Most nursing diagnoses revolve around pain or impairment of function.

Because bones under stress decalcify less than bones at rest, an exercise program diminishes bone destruction. Frequent active assistive range-of-motion exercises may be substituted when absolutely necessary. A diet sufficient in protein and calcium also helps maintain musculature. In general, the diet should contain adequate calcium, protein, and vitamin D.

The nurse must take extra precautions to protect a patient with osteoporosis against accidents that could lead to fractures. If osteoporosis is severe, even grasping the long bones to turn the bedridden patient can result in a fracture.

Treatment of arthritis consists of moderate exercise to maintain mobility, medications for inflammation and pain, and special heat therapy. When caring for the person with arthritis, use gentle touch. The patient may be able to tell you how he or she moves most easily. Nursing actions such as health teaching regarding exercise and diet and involving the patient in the plan of care are useful in maintaining musculoskeletal function.

Nutrition and Bowel Elimination

More teeth are lost in the advanced years due to *gingivitis* (gum disease) than to decay. The loss of teeth causes difficulty in mastication (chewing), and dentures may fit poorly. Decreased production of saliva in the mouth and of hydrochloric acid in the stomach may cause food intolerances. Motility of the esophagus, stomach, and intestines also slows. Older persons may develop gallstones because of reduction in the ability of the gallbladder to secrete bile.

Although the gastrointestinal tract undergoes fewer major changes than do many of the other systems, gastrointestinal problems probably cause the elderly more distress than even problems of joints. Constipation in the elderly is often caused by early and continued use of laxatives, decreased activity, and lack of fiber in the diet. It occurs much more frequently than diarrhea. With old age and its accompanying muscular changes, the bowel becomes less responsive and laxatives less efficient.

Nursing diagnoses related to the gastrointestinal

tract are specific to the individual. Some older adults are lonely and eat to relieve those feelings. Overeating or hormonal changes may bring on obesity. In other individuals, loneliness can bring on *anorexia* (loss of appetite). These persons eat less than what is required. These data may lead to a nursing diagnosis concerning nutrition when there is less than or more than body requirements. Constipation is also a common nursing diagnosis for the older patient.

Several nursing actions can be taken to address the poor intake of food. Diets planned with color and interesting consistency in mind enhance appetite and are no more expensive to prepare than bland, colorless diets. Using assessment data regarding favorite food items in diet selection can also affect the patient's food consumption. The family may suggest or bring to the patient foods the patient will particularly enjoy. Because eating alone undermines appetite, sharing a meal with a visitor or family member may improve food intake.

A bowel program that includes high fluid intake levels, sufficient fiber in the diet, and optimal exercise will offset much of the constipation suffered by older people. It is sometimes difficult to eliminate the use of laxatives, however, once they have been used for many years and become a habit.

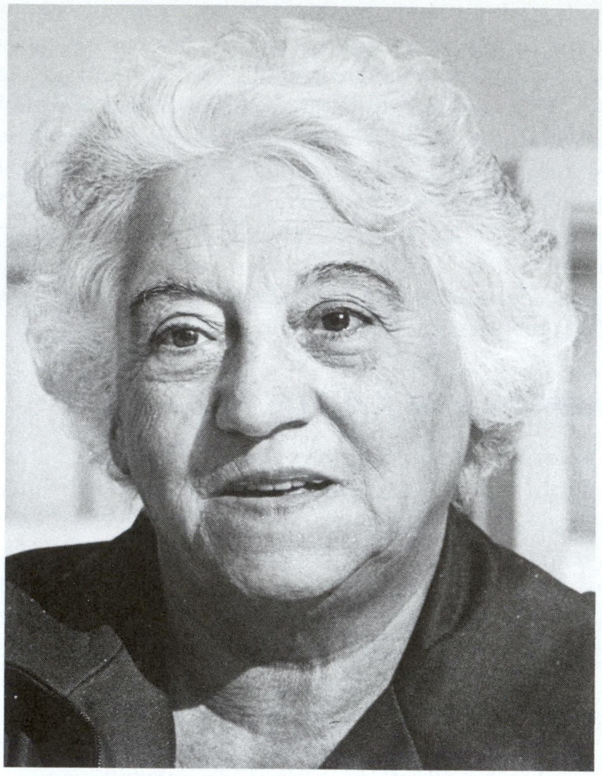

Figure 20-1. Changes in hair and skin accompanying aging.

Skin Integrity

The integument (skin) changes considerably with aging. The subcutaneous fat layers that provide insulation decrease, bringing on wrinkles and placing older people at risk for intolerance to cold. Although some wrinkling is inevitable, smoking, poor diet, and exposure to sun and weather hasten the process. The decrease in natural oils in the skin causes dryness, decreasing turgor (fullness) and increasing the risk of irritation and infection. Reduction in the number of sweat glands decreases the body's ability to regulate heat. The skin of persons of color stays more supple and better lubricated and retains better turgor with aging than does the lighter skin of whites (Fig. 20-1).

Many older persons develop areas of pigmentation of the skin, which are often referred to as age spots. If these areas become darker in color or change in texture, a physician should be consulted because these signs may indicate a cancerous growth. Hair grays or whitens with age through loss of pigment. Hair may also change in texture, becoming curlier or straighter. **Alopecia**, loss of hair, is another common result of aging. Not only scalp hair but also hair in the axilla and genital area and general body hair become sparse. Baldness, though more common in older men, also occurs in women. In women, baldness of the scalp is often patchy. It has been suggested that excessive shampooing, tight hats, and the practice of setting the hair tightly all promote balding, but evidence is not conclusive. Much male baldness is genetic and cannot be prevented. Baldness is important only in its effect on the patient's body image.

The nails become thicker and brittle from increased keratin. Ridges may appear, and the color may darken to yellow or tan. Splitting caused by lack of calcium and poor circulation to the fingers is common.

A variety of nursing diagnoses have to do with the integument. Body image may be affected if the woman has bald areas on the scalp. A more common nursing diagnosis for older adults is that of dry skin. Itching may be intense and scratching can lead to skin infection.

Because skin becomes thin and dry as it ages, it is helpful to add oils directly to the bath water and to apply palliative oils or lotions sparingly to the skin immediately after the bath. Patients need not be bathed daily because bathing is drying to the skin. Many older patients are used to bathing only once a week and become upset at what they consider undue emphasis on cleanliness. Use care when placing an identification armband on the wrist of an elderly patient. An overly snug band can cause an abrasion as can a tight watchband. Rubbing on sheets, lying on wrinkled bedding, and striking a side rail can also cause skin damage to the elderly. The slightest redness may be the forerunner of a difficult-to-heal decubitus ulcer (pressure sore).

For patients with skin problems you may wish to wrap side rails, if they are being used, or loosely apply soft dressings around vulnerable areas of the patient's arms or legs. Frequent inspection of the skin is essential to prevent problems.

Hair should be shampooed only when necessary rather than daily to prevent chilling the patient and drying the scalp. Simple hair arrangements are appropriate for women so that hair follicles are not pulled, leading to loss of hair.

The nails should be inspected for rough areas and cracks that can abrade the skin. If nails are too thick to clip, filing will decrease the length and provide a smooth contour that will prevent catching on clothing and linens.

Urinary Elimination

Between age 20 and age 90, a person experiences a 50% decline in kidney function. The vessels and renal arteries narrow, and the filtering process is less efficient. However, the volume of urine produced in a day remains relatively stable throughout life. Studies show that bladder capacity lessens with age, necessitating more frequent emptying. Getting up at night to urinate is common but interrupts the patient's rest. The sphincter, because it is muscular, loses some of its elasticity, and urine leakage can occur in both men and women. This is understandably disturbing to the patient, and a solution is not easily found. Muscular deterioration can also prevent the bladder from emptying completely, encouraging the growth of bacteria. Infections and the formation of stones (calculi) can occur.

Nursing diagnoses center around problems of urinary elimination, which may be disturbing to the daily routine of the older person. Older patients/clients may have a variety of urinary symptoms. Burning or pain is sometimes present on urination, which may indicate the presence of a bladder infection. Nocturia (having to urinate during the night) may disturb sleep. Urgency and frequency may create difficult social problems. For some, incontinence or retention may be present. The best long-range and most helpful intervention for the person with urinary incontinence is a bladder retraining program. This takes patience and dedication on the part of the individual and the nurse.

Because older individuals are at risk of urinary infections, one of the best interventions is to encourage fluid intake. An increase in fluid intake can readily be accomplished through careful planning, which should, if possible, include the patient. You can make a list of beverages preferred by the person and use them to supplement the intake of water. It is best to encourage high fluid intake throughout the day, when the older person has toileting facilities close at hand, rather than during evening hours. The intake of fluids during the evening may cause the patient to awaken frequently during the night for elimination purposes and disturb sleep.

Sexuality and Reproduction

The woman's ability to produce children ends at menopause. The man's ability to produce sperm persists throughout life although the number of sperm diminishes. Thus, the man can procreate well into his eighth decade. There is little reason, physically, on the part of either sex, for libido (sexual desire) to decrease in later life. Frequency of intercourse may decline and it may take longer to reach orgasm, but libido remains.

Estrogen deficiency in the woman may cause thinning of the vaginal walls and decreased lubrication. Vaginal creams are available to alleviate this problem. Some physicians believe that the administration of supplemental estrogens is helpful.

When identifying nursing diagnoses, many of the defining characteristics you need to consider are subjective, especially regarding sexual function. The man may express feelings of being devalued because he cannot attain the sexual performance he once enjoyed. Women may feel frustration on losing a partner or may experience painful intercourse due to drying and atrophying of the vaginal vault.

Some individuals are not aware that the aging process may bring about changes in sexual performance. Sharing information and health teaching may be all that is required to resolve simple problems. If sexual problems are more complex, not all nurses are comfortable with discussing them nor have the special training to help patients. However, part of the nursing role is to be an attentive listener and share community resources that have the expertise to work with individuals or couples regarding their sexual problems.

Perception and Cognition

Although brain mass (weight) diminishes in later life and cerebrovascular changes may result in decreased blood flow to the brain, a direct link between these conditions and reasoning and thinking has not been established. Brain function depends on many factors. The physiologic changes described above, as well as motivation and stimulation, may affect the ability to think and learn. Older people tend to learn more slowly than the young but can learn as well. The synapses (connections) of the spinal column with the peripheral nerves may lengthen, slowing reaction time. For this reason, precautions should be taken in the operation of motor vehicles and machinery.

Senile dementia is a broad term used to describe the impairment of cognition in an older person. Research has shown that in some people this process can be reversed because the impairment can be caused by conditions that respond to treatment. Fluid and electrolyte imbalances, hormonal irregularities, and subclinical infections can lead to what appears to be senile dementia.

As mentioned earlier, a recent and immense worldwide concern is that so many older people are developing Alzheimer's disease, first described in 1907. It is unclear whether the apparent increase in this disease is due to actual acceleration in incidence or better diagnostic techniques. The cause appears to be the formation of plaquelike areas in portions of the brain rather than deterioration of the cortex itself.

Other diseases also cause irreversible dementia, which can be associated with a variety of problems such as impaired language and motor function, memory loss, inability to perform adequate personal hygiene, and intellectual impairment, particularly regarding decision-making. These diseases have adversely affected the quality of life for many older people. The increasing burden and pain experienced by older people and their families has prompted the formation of a national organization, the Alzheimer's Disease and Related Disorders Association. See Appendix E for information regarding this voluntary organization.

Because of the vast complexity of the nervous system, a variety of nursing diagnoses are possible. Many of them focus on safety when gait, balance, or the senses are impaired. The patient can also show deficits in memory or judgment. The nursing diagnoses should be written as appropriate for the individual. Nursing actions should be congruent with the neurologic deficit specific to the patient/client.

Regulation and Sensation

Some older adults may experience increased levels of glucose in the blood because the pancreas is less active than in earlier years and releases insufficient amounts of insulin. Proprioception, balance, and gait are often affected with aging. Many problems are due to changes within the muscles, joints, and inner ear.

The five senses—seeing, hearing, smelling, tasting, and touching—diminish to some extent with age. It is thought that these alterations occur because of degeneration of nerves, vascular irregularities, or local tissue changes. In some patients such diminishment is almost undiscernible; in others it is profound. Although it may be obvious that a patient is partially blind or hard of hearing, you may overlook decreased sensitivity of taste, smell, and touch. When the patient has suffered a significant loss in one or more senses, a degree of sensory deprivation can result, which can in turn cause psychological depression (see Chapter 31). Patients are sometimes defensive about a loss of hearing or sight, and some frankly deny it.

The pupils of elderly people's eyes become smaller, admitting less light to the retina. The vitreous humor becomes more liquid. The lens may darken somewhat and not be as clear as previously. The lens on one or both eyes of many older persons becomes opaque or cloudy. This condition is known as a **cataract** and is corrected by surgery.

The elderly also have a high incidence of **glaucoma**, which is characterized by increased intraocular pressure. If untreated, blindness can result. Diagnosis is vital because the condition can be satisfactorily controlled by medical treatment, which usually includes eye drops.

Loss of hearing is far more common among the elderly than is loss of sight. It has been estimated that one of four people over age 60 has a sufficient degree of hearing loss to be characterized "medically deaf." Among the several causes of deafness are disturbances of the auditory nerve or cerebral cortex and changes in the structure of the ear itself. One of these changes is a thickening and sclerosis of the tympanic membrane, which decreases sound conduction. Older persons have less ability than younger people to hear high-frequency sounds.

The ability to smell diminishes with age, largely because of degeneration in the olfactory bulb, the sensing organ. Because smell is a major factor in appetite, anorexia is in part attributable to olfactory impairment. Some older people, mainly women, use fragrances excessively because of a loss of olfactory acuity. Inability to smell smoke in time to flee from a fire could affect an older person's safety.

Age-related changes in tactile ability are caused largely by decreases in receptors on the outer skin and increased conduction time to the brain. Although a tactile deficit rarely interferes with daily living, it poses safety dangers because pain and temperature are not easily perceived. The taste buds on the tongue and roof of the mouth decrease in number with age. Some also seem to become more sensitive than others. This may explain changes in food preferences as aging occurs; one person will crave sweets, yet another who has always been fond of sweet foods will no longer find them appealing. Because of decreased sensitivity to tastes, many find food generally less appetizing, a situation that can lead to inadequate food intake.

Nursing diagnoses are usually written to address the person's specific sensory deficits. Some of these focus on comfort and others relate to safety risks. Nurses cannot change the underlying pathology, but they can take actions to protect the person who has sensory impairment.

Many of the nursing actions surrounding sensory

deficits concern patient safety. These must be individualized to fit the particular patient and deficit.

Care of the patient with visual and auditory deficits is discussed in Chapter 31. Ways to offset taste impairment were discussed in connection with the gastrointestinal system. For people with tactile deficits, some measures can be taken to reduce frustration and reduce safety hazards. The primary problem posed by impairment of touch is the possibility of injury from sharp or hot objects. Such accidents might be prevented by setting hot water heaters to a lower temperature and by wearing shoes at all times to protect the feet. A deficit in touch could also cause a person to overlook an injury and go without care. Older people should be encouraged to examine the extremities daily for signs of injury.

Psychosocial Changes of Aging

The attitudes of society impose many problems on the elderly. Social restrictions may bring on more significant psychological problems than does the aging process itself (Display 20-2). However, our society is becoming increasing responsible and initiating programs to help meet the needs of the aging.

Adjusting to Declining Physical and Psychological Health

Although adjustments have to be made to the gradual or uneven decline in the physical and psychosocial aspects of the life of the older person, these adaptations need not necessarily decrease the quality of life. For example, sometimes these adjustments involve no more than wearing lenses to see the newsprint or the phone book. For others with more serious eye problems, the adjustment may require listening to books and magazines on records or tapes procured through the free services of libraries. The joy of reading can continue with modifications.

Certainly adjusting to declining health is often painful and discouraging, but the person can make it less so by exploring ways to compensate for what is lost. Finding new ways to be creative and meeting new people can help enormously. Finding other persons with the same problems or groups that understand the problems can make the adjustment more comfortable.

Taking steps to live a healthful life and remembering that a belief system is important to life can diminish feelings of loss when health is jeopardized. Many useful coping mechanisms are discussed more fully in Chapter 34.

Display 20–2
Psychosocial Adjustments to Aging

- Adjusting to declining physical and psychological health
- Adjusting to retirement
- Adjusting to reduced income
- Finding appropriate living arrangements
- Resolving the deaths of others
- Being a member of the community
- Maintaining independence and productivity

Adjusting to Retirement

Traditionally, retirement age was fixed at 65, regardless of whether or not the individual was able and wanted to continue working. Fortunately, this practice is changing; some places of employment allow the age of retirement to be extended to 70 if doing so is mutually desirable. On the other hand, the possibility of early retirement has attracted those who look forward to retirement with long-standing interests in hobbies and other leisure activities (Fig. 20-2). People who have devoted themselves wholeheartedly to their jobs may find that retirement brings on feelings of worthlessness and depression. The adjustment can be equally traumatic for the retiree's partner. Both may find it unnatural for the worker to be around the house all day with little to do, and conflicts can result. Preparation for retirement helps to alleviate these problems.

Retirement often disrupts established social patterns and may require the making of new friends. Ideally, these new contacts include people of all ages. Many

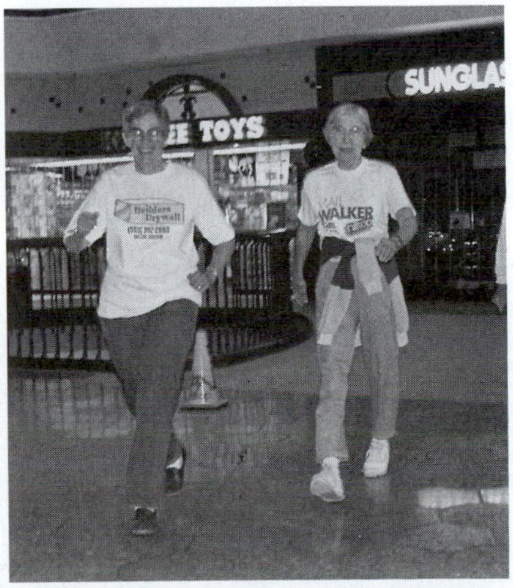

Figure 20-2. Many active older adults continue to enjoy group activity.

older people make younger friends by attending classes on college campuses or in the community (Fig. 20-3).

Adjusting to Reduced Income

We have discussed the dilemma of today's older population with respect to shrinking financial resources. Social legislation enacted for the benefit of others on more liberal incomes compounds the problem. An example is the constant raising of taxes on such commodities as gasoline and telephones. For the older person, still being able to operate a vehicle may not only promote independence but may also be a necessity for interaction with a family who lives many miles away. Possession of a telephone may be essential for health and safety reasons. To continue to drive and also keep a phone, the older adult may have to eliminate other valuable parts of life.

Health care workers should assume a more active role in advocacy for the elderly. Although Medicare has been helpful in assisting the older population with health costs, it does not pay for drugs and imposes limits on payment for other care, which is often a considerable expenditure for the elderly. Caring for older people may include finding assistance for financial planning and being knowledgeable about social legislation and possible reforms that would be beneficial to the older population.

Finding Appropriate Living Arrangements

We have mentioned several options for the elderly regarding housing. The following are general but important guidelines that can aid the older person to find housing that is appropriate.

Housing for the elderly should be located in an area with easy access to transportation, shopping, and social contacts. Pets should be permitted because they can be a great comfort to those who live alone. Homes must be in good repair to prevent injury. Ramps can be easily constructed for wheelchairs. A number of elderly people may need occasional help from "chore" agencies to maintain the cleanliness of their homes.

With the rising costs of maintaining a home, many older people are having to sell homes in which they have lived most of their lives, giving up beloved gardens and pets. A significant number of older persons are forced to live with adult children. Intergenerational living can be a positive experience for everyone, or it can result in conflict. Counseling services are sometimes needed.

Resolving the Deaths of Others

Limited diversions and isolation often make adjustment to the loss of a lifelong spouse or friend particularly hard for the elderly. The family of a bereaved person can facilitate the process of emotional reinvestment by offering love and care and by encouraging as much independence as is appropriate. Sometimes rapidly relocating the survivor before the active grieving period is completed and making all decisions for the person only intensify the feelings of depression and despair.

Resolution is most difficult for the elderly. A large proportion of elderly persons have spent 40 or 50 years in a traditional marriage in which the woman did not work outside the home and the man did not perform routine household tasks. The death of one partner thus requires an enormous adjustment to the loss. Also, the restitution process may be hampered by real or perceived limitations on the elderly person's options: re-

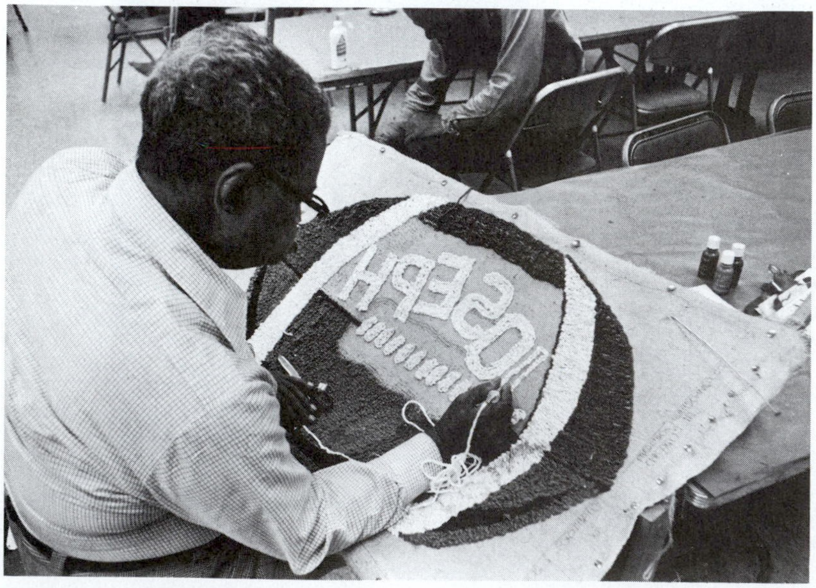

Figure 20-3. Learning new skills adds meaning to life.

marriage or returning to school, for example, may not be desired or feasible. The literature on widowhood reports that the death rate of surviving spouses within 6 to 12 months of the death is higher than that of the same age group in the general population. Nurses who recognize the particular dilemma of the elderly survivor can help provide the special support and counseling that may be needed (see Chapter 41).

Being a Member of the Community

Establishing relationships with others in the community is necessary throughout life but becomes even more important in the later years when persons tend to feel isolated. Participating in social and civic activities places individuals in contact with those who have similar interests and goals (Fig. 20-4). With an increase in leisure time, the older person may be in a better position to join various groups for either recreation or community projects. You may notice that older citizens often work at voting stations. The chairpersons of numerous community committees and groups are older people who generously give their time and energy.

Other Tasks of Longevity

Older adults have a need to be independent as well as productive. Creativity is also part of living fully. One need not participate in a specific art form but may enjoy the beauty of music, writing, or art. Creativity can also be expressed through gardening or cooking.

The older person needs time for reflection on the value of life. Through reflection can come an awareness of security and a positive outlook on the remaining years.

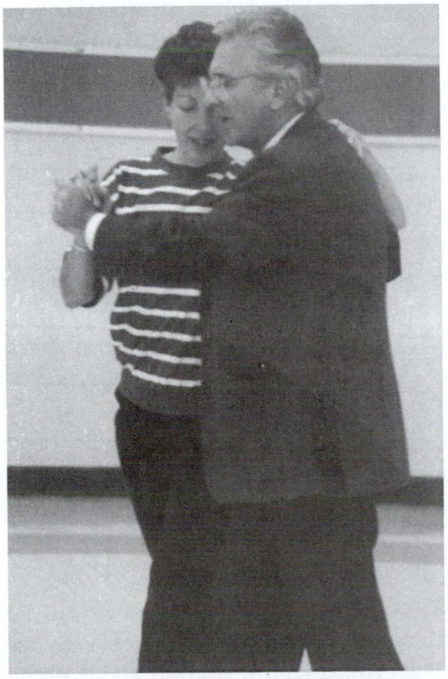

Figure 20-4. Older adults find enjoyment and companionship in social events.

As a nurse, you may not be able directly or independently to carry out nursing actions that will change the causes of psychosocial problems, but you may be helpful by focusing your actions on the assessments you observe. You may simply add your diagnosis to the plan of care or seek resources for the patient or the family.

Concerns Regarding Long-term Care

Nursing homes exist to meet the needs of elderly people and others who need supervisory or skilled nursing care for physical or psychological reasons. The quality of care in nursing homes varies from excellent to poor. Complex economic issues, particularly those involving public funding, have fed national controversy over the nursing home industry and the ways in which government and the private sector can best serve the aging. The answers are neither simple nor easy.

Although long-term placement has many benefits for persons in need of this type of care, it gives rise to many problems as well. The nurse in a long-term care facility needs to know how to minimize the impact of institutionalization, communicate effectively with the elderly, cope with confusion, and ensure safety.

This chapter has explored many of the reasons, both physical and psychosocial, why an older patient may be placed in a long-term care setting other than the home. The decision to move oneself or place a loved one in a restricted setting is a difficult one because it realistically may mean not only separation from family but also personal loss of control over life. Regardless of the setting—and some are only minimally restrictive—the decision is not to be taken lightly.

Minimizing the Impact of Institutionalization

Relocation to a chronic care institution on a long-term basis can be unsettling for the older adult. Recent studies have found increased mortality rates among recent arrivals to long-term care facilities, especially when the move was not voluntary.

Brooke (1989) has defined four stages of adjusting to a nursing home (Fig. 20-5). The first is *disorganization* during which the elder feels displaced and abandoned. During the second stage, *reorganization*, there is a conscious effort to problem solve, to resolve and justify being in the long-term care setting. The third stage, *relationship building*, is important because it incorporates those in the immediate environment into the

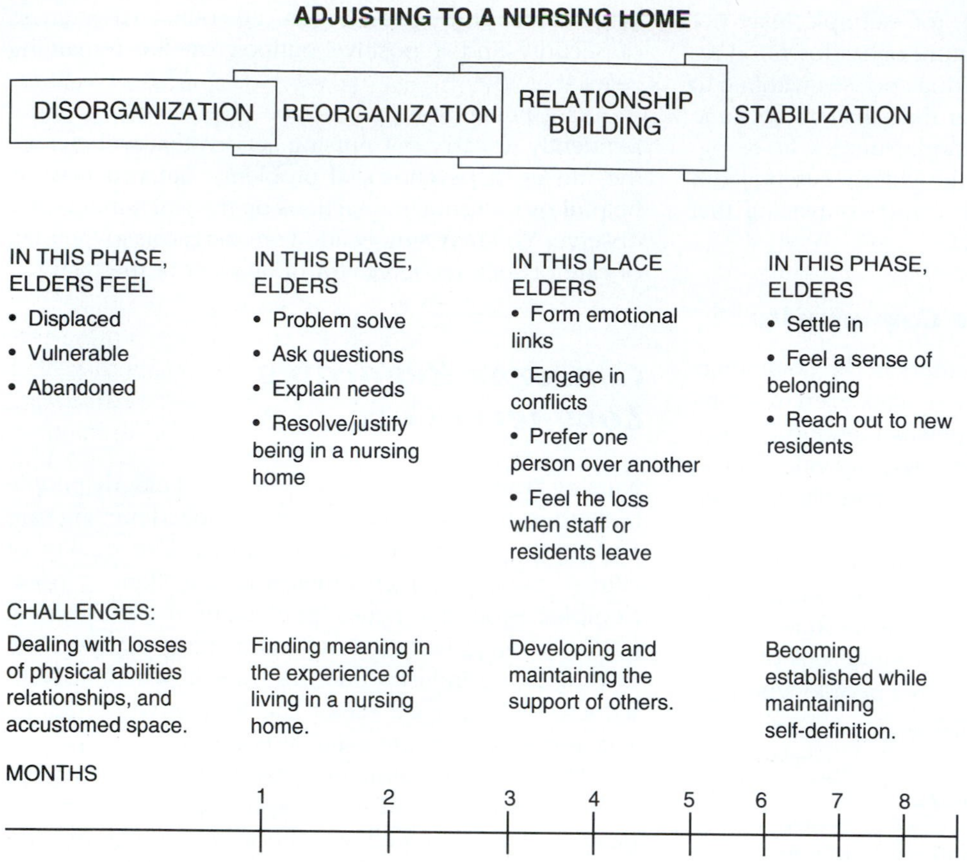

ADJUSTING TO A NURSING HOME
DISORGANIZATION
REORGANIZATION
RELATIONSHIP BUILDING
STABILIZATION
IN THIS PHASE, ELDERS FEEL
• Displaced
• Vulnerable
• Abandoned
IN THIS PHASE, ELDERS
• Problem solve
• Ask questions
• Explain needs
• Resolve/justify being in a nursing home
IN THIS PLACE ELDERS
• Form emotional links
• Engage in conflicts
• Prefer one person over another
• Feel the loss when staff or residents leave
IN THIS PHASE, ELDERS
• Settle in
• Feel a sense of belonging
• Reach out to new residents
CHALLENGES:
Dealing with losses of physical abilities relationships, and accustomed space.
Finding meaning in the experience of living in a nursing home.
Developing and maintaining the support of others.
Becoming established while maintaining self-definition.
MONTHS
1
2
3
4
5
6
7
8

Figure 20-5. Adjusting to a nursing home. (Brooke, V. "Your Helping Hand." *Geriatric Nursing* 10, 3 (May/June 1989).

life of the resident. People who become important in this stage may be staff members or other residents. Finally, the fourth stage, *stabilization*, brings about a sense of belonging with psychological enfolding of other new residents. A feeling of "settling in" makes the move successful. The nursing staff can help substantially in this process of adjustment by treating the person with respect, recognizing individuality, capitalizing on strengths, and allowing for personal decision-making.

Compliance, another consequence of institutionalization, is often welcomed by a hard-working staff but may increase the patient's despair. Total compliance, even with nonpriority routines like hygiene, may not be healthy because it promotes dependence.

It is important to stress that many long-term care facilities offer personalized and sensitive care. Most provide a wide range of crafts, classes, and social activities and encourage residents to maintain interest in the wider community. Many now allow pets. Inclusion of the family in the care program has high priority in many long-term care facilities.

Communicating Effectively

The suggestions for effective communication below are appropriate when interacting with any patient/resident. However, certain adaptations more specifically serve the elderly. When communicating with the older person, it is beneficial to speak of the past, the present, and the future. The past is familiar, the present keeps one's thinking current, and the future—even the near future—suggests hope. Some nurses complain that care of the elderly is time-consuming because older patients seem to talk endlessly or not at all. Remember that either response may signal that the patient is lonely and really cherishes the nurse's presence for even a short time. If the nurse visits the patient frequently when care is not needed, communication will be improved.

Overly familiar communication can undermine a potential good relationship with an elderly patient. Most older patients were raised with much more social formality than is usual now. First names were not used casually. Thus, it is best to address the older patient by the appropriate title and last name until the patient requests that you do otherwise. Although hospitals are becoming increasingly informal and many nurses and patients are on a first-name basis, it is prudent to show respect in this way. Another unfortunate common practice is "talking down" to the elderly as if they were children. Terms such as "honey" and "dear" may be interpreted as degrading by the patient. The inclusive "let's do that" is also inappropriate because it intrudes on the dignity of the patient and suggests dependence. For more on communication, see Chapter 13.

Coping with Confusion

For a variety of reasons, including the anxiety of relocation, confusion is common in the geriatric patient. Often the patient recognizes this confusion and is frightened by it. Such a situation is not easily remedied, but you can help. An older patient who is able to be of service in some manner will benefit from feeling needed. One older woman became much less confused and depressed when she was asked to help fold linen. Another patient wrote a letter for a fellow patient who could not write. A creative approach in developing the nursing care plan can do a great deal to alleviate confusion.

Intervention is essential for the confused older patient because confusion often increases if nothing is done about it. If the patient is confused about time and place, informing the patient of the location and time, including the day and month, is helpful. You might ask the family to bring a large-faced clock and a large-print calendar as aids to orientation. Sometimes confusion is evident only at night. A nightlight can give the patient a feeling of security and enhance safety. Any necessary changes in routine should be undertaken slowly because confused patients adapt poorly to sudden change. Another helpful technique is to make a daily schedule, written in large print, which allows the patient to keep track of the day's plan and to know what to expect at a given hour. Unrealistic plans and behavior should not be supported by the nurse. For example, if a patient tells you that he is going on a picnic and the snowy weather obviously makes such a plan impossible, it is not a kindness to agree but you might reply, "Picnics are enjoyable. Tell me about picnics you remember." This response focuses on positive communication, encourages skills such as long-term memory, and validates the person as valued.

It is poor practice to tell an elderly patient you will do something or be back at a specified time and not do so. Such a practice not only confuses the patient but also rapidly destroys trust. Specifying a time is good but only if it is followed. Five minutes may seem like 20 minutes to the inactive patient. It is wise when you inform the patient that you will return in 5 minutes to suggest watching the clock. This practice calls on the patient's sense of time and enhances confidence that you will return as promised. These suggestions may seem insignificant, but they are valuable to the aged.

Ensuring Safety

Accidental injury or trauma sustained by the older patient is a particularly serious problem. The older patient heals slowly and may develop pneumonia because of immobilization during recovery. Safety demands that you constantly observe the patient and the environment for potential hazards.

In a state of confusion, overzealous independence, or night disorientation, the patient may try to get out of bed unaided. In some institutions side rails are mandatory at night for older residents unless a waiver has been signed by the patient or the family. If the nurse describes this practice to the patient as a form of protection and not a punitive action, the patient will more easily accept it. Some patients are also restrained. Recent research has shown that both side rails and restraints should be applied more selectively and with caution. Evans and Strumpf (1990) report that injuries often occur with side rails or restraints in place. Residents fall attempting to crawl over an upright side rail. Fighting or resisting restraints can lead to fractures of extremities or falls. When either device is used, the call bell must always be placed so that the restrained patient can summon the nurse. Federal legislation now mandates that patients be cared for in the least restrictive environment. This means that both chemical (drugs) and physical restraints should only be used as a last resort. Many nursing homes are developing restraint-free policies and report no higher incidence of falls and injuries.

Other measures can prevent falls. Properly fitted,

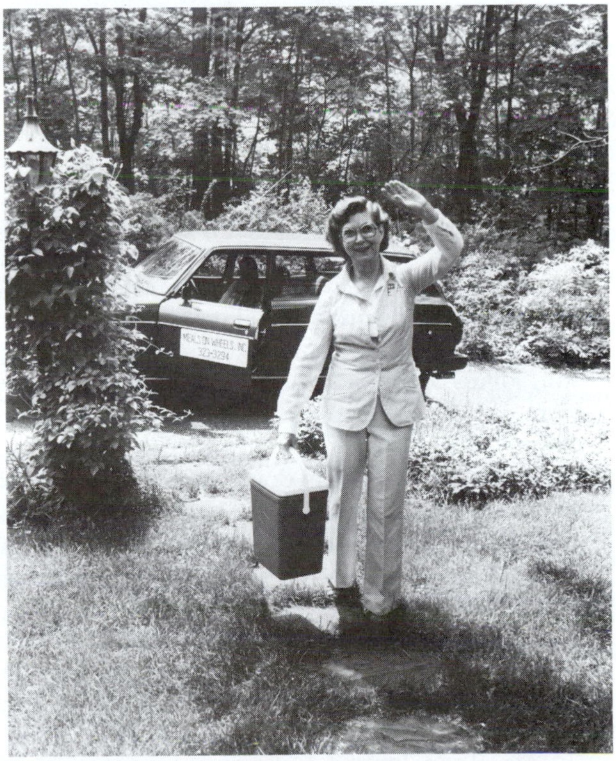

Figure 20-6. Many services for elderly persons are provided by community organizations.

hard-soled leather shoes are safest for older people. Bedroom slippers are often slippery, tend to fit poorly, and give inadequate support; tennis shoes "catch" because of the rubber sole covering and do not provide enough support. Spills can be dangerous for both patients and nurses and should be wiped up immediately. Loose floor tiles, throw rugs, and small items such as bobby pins on the floor may all imperil the patient. Furniture should not obstruct passageways. Showers and tubs can also be dangerous; a bath towel placed on the bottom of the tub provides for better footing. Handrails on bathroom walls also offer support to the unsteady person. Good lighting is essential for safety in all areas.

Other hazards include electrical appliances with worn cords or connections, which may cause a shock or start a fire. Smoking is distinctly dangerous, and most facilities have rules controlling it. Smoking in bed, dangerous for anyone, is particularly so for the older person whose reflexes may be impaired. Ensuring the patient's safety is imperative, and perpetual vigilance by care providers is indispensable.

Organizations for the Elderly

The realization that older citizens can, with proper organization, influence economic change and promote consumer rights has brought into being a number of organizations geared to the interests of the elderly (Fig. 20-6). By the late 1970s, about six million older Americans were active in such organizations, 24 times as many as during the previous decade (Aiken, 1978).

In addition to groups devoted to political change, many informal groups stress social interaction. Dues are usually modest in amount. Retired and elderly people who live in rural areas should be encouraged to start such groups in their area and many have done so. Younger people can be helpful by supporting the efforts of these organizations and by making such contributions as volunteering to transport aging citizens to voting polls. Appendix E lists a few of the larger organizations and agencies, both federal and private, devoted to the interests of the elderly. Each state also has its own organizations with which you should become familiar.

Nursing Care Study
The Value of Occupational Therapy for Older Adults

Nursing student Susan Tapp suddenly realized how sad she felt. In the past 3 weeks, while practicing in a long-term care setting, she had grown very fond of Mrs. Aldrich, a 91-year-old patient. She had not know either of her grandmothers, who had both died when she was an infant. She realized now how nice it would have been to have had a grandmother like Mrs. Aldrich.

Mrs. Aldrich was a quiet, gentle lady who missed her only grandson and his family, who lived in California, and particularly her only great-grandson, Mike. The holidays had just ended and they were not planning to visit until summer. Mrs. Aldrich talked a great deal about the arthritis in her hands that kept her from doing any fine handiwork. The diminished strength of her legs kept her wheelchair bound most of the day, which seemed to increase her depression. "I feel so worthless, no good to anybody," she had remarked one day. Ms. Tapp had read the Bible with Mrs. Aldrich at her request and taken her to the activities room, but Mrs. Aldrich had shown little interest in participating, saying, "There is nothing for me to do there."

Ms. Tapp looked back over her assessment. Mrs. Aldrich certainly had strengths. She liked to work with her hands and was alert and communicative. She had a family who cared about her although they were far away. Mrs. Aldrich needed a short-term goal, perhaps something to do, and also a way of communicating with her family, particularly Mike. Ms. Tapp decided to work further on her plan that evening. Perhaps she'd think of something.

As she hurried down the hallway to her car, Ms. Tapp glanced into the ceramics room. A friend of Mrs. Aldrich and several other women and a man were making clay mugs. A plan began to form in Ms. Tapp's mind: a mug for Mike!

The following day, she could hardly wait to start on her plan. She told Mrs. Aldrich about the ceramics room, which they then visited together. She showed Mrs. Aldrich how easy and how much fun it was to mold the clay and set up a schedule so that she could accompany Mrs. Aldrich to the ceramics class twice a week.

Several weeks were spent sharing the creation of a loving gift for Mike. The gray clay was rounded and formed, mainly by Mrs. Aldrich. Then came the drying period and the selection of a deep blue glaze. When the mug emerged from the kiln, all

(*continued*)

Nursing Care Study (continued)
The Value of Occupational Therapy for Older Adults

agreed that it was beautiful. Ms. Tapp and Mrs. Aldrich celebrated with coffee. Mrs. Aldrich reacted with enthusiasm when Ms. Tapp suggested making the mug unmistakably Mike's by painting his name on it. With Ms. Tapp's encouragement, Mrs. Aldrich lettered MIKE around the side in white paint.

Ms. Tapp and Mrs. Aldrich gave the mug a special place in her room to await Mike's next visit. Ms. Tapp promised to return for the presentation to meet Mike and the family.

Seven weeks later, Ms. Tapp thought back over her experience. Mrs. Aldrich had changed in several ways. She had become more talkative about matters other than her problems. She seemed more optimistic and, best of all, she had decided to continue going to the ceramics classes. "I hope she doesn't stop when I leave," thought Ms. Tapp.

That afternoon after her clinical experience ended, Ms. Tapp ran into her friend Ginny Colbert. "Ginny, aren't you going to be at Meadowdale next quarter?" Ginny Colbert nodded her head affirmatively. "Well, I'd really like to have coffee with you soon and tell you about a patient of mine you could help."

"Sure, Susan, let's do that."

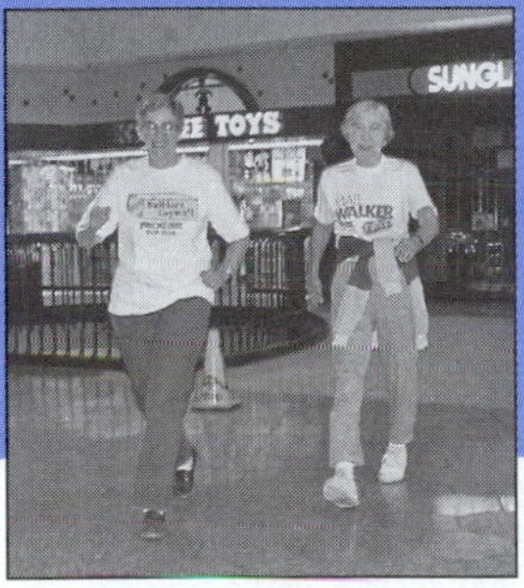

Key Points

- The growing number of elderly people makes it more essential than ever for nurses to gain skill in the care of the older adult.
- Most older adults are living in the community rather than the nursing home environment and cope well with the age-related changes in their lives.
- Among the many positive aspects of growing older is the satisfaction derived from the achievement of goals and accomplishments, continuing relationships with younger members of the family and community, and the opportunity to explore new learning experiences.
- Because of the increase in life expectancy, the incidence of chronic illnesses of years past in the elderly has been exceeded by chronic illnesses such as cardiac, respiratory, and musculoskeletal conditions.
- The adult children of the elderly, who are sometimes needed by the elderly parent to provide care, are themselves reaching late middle age and experiencing a decline in health as well as financial resources.
- Because of inflation's erosion of funds that have been saved for the retirement years, the older adult is finding it increasingly difficult to live on a fixed income. Poor housing and deficiencies in nutrition are results of this situation.
- All body systems are affected by the aging process, and most persons do remarkably well in integrating these changes into their daily lives.
- When illness occurs, changes brought on by the aging process can make recovery more difficult.
- One of the most disturbing problems is the increased incidence of Alzheimer's disease, a condition that is difficult for families to handle and often requiring institutionalization.
- The psychosocial challenges of aging include coping with aging, adjusting to declining physical and psychological health, adjusting to retirement, adjusting to reduced income, finding appropriate living arrangements, resolving the deaths of others, being an active member of the community, participating in creative activities, and reflecting on the value of life.
- Planning care for the older adult often involves consideration of high-risk states because the elderly person is more prone to physical injury and susceptible to infection and illness.
- Nursing actions for the elderly should be creative and individualized to meet their needs without stereotyping.
- For older persons who cannot be cared for in the home, options for living range from supervised apartments to chronic care facilities.

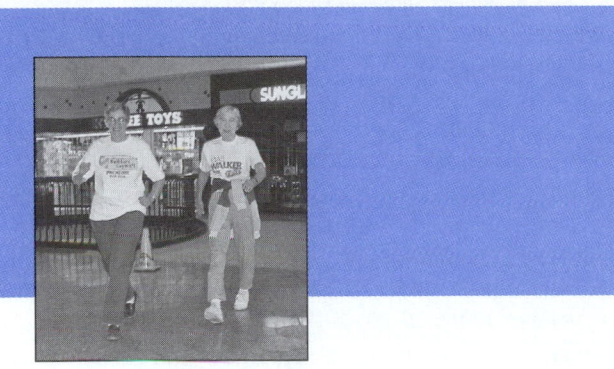

Study Questions

1. What is Selye's theory of aging?
2. How has the extended longevity of older persons affected their health status?
3. How have the changes within the family affected the older adults in today's society?
4. What has affected the financial and housing situation of older persons in the last few years?
5. Briefly describe the changes in systems that normally accompany the aging process.
6. What are some of the tasks involved in successfully coping with aging?
7. List and briefly describe the various living and care options available to older adults.
8. Discuss the main problems that arise with those who are institutionalized.
9. What are some actions nurses can take regarding their own attitudes to best relate to the elderly person in the health care facility?
10. Describe several community services that are available to older persons.

Critical Thinking Activities

1. Interview an older person who is in good health and one who is hospitalized concerning their satisfactions and concerns in life. Compare the viewpoints of the two persons according to the tasks listed for that age group.
2. Find an article in a recent periodical regarding a current issue for older people. Identify the most important parts of the article and the impact of the issue on the quality of life for older adults. Discuss this in a small group.
3. Visit a community resource designed to help the elderly.
4. While caring for an elderly patient in the clinical area, write a nursing care plan specific to aging.
5. In a small group, compare your attitudes toward aging persons before you were a student nurse and your present attitudes. Have your attitudes changed in any way?

References and Readings

Abrutyn, E., Berk, S. L., and Raff, M. J. "High Risk Infections in the Elderly." *Patient Care* 22, 6 (March 1988): 9–12.

Aiken, L. *Later Life.* 3rd edition. Philadelphia: W. B. Saunders, 1989.

Andresen, G. P. "A Fresh Look at Assessing the Elderly." *RN* 52, 6 (June 1989): 28–34.

Belloc, N. B., and Breslow, L. "Relationship of Physical Health Status and Health Practices." *Preventive Medicine* (August 1972): 409–421.

Bender, P. "Deceptive Distress in the Elderly." *American Journal of Nursing* 92, 10 (October 1992): 29–33.

Breitung, J. "A Nutritional Survey of the Well Older Adult." *Perspectives on Aging* (November-December 1980): 409–421.

Brooke, V. "Your Helping Hand." *Geriatric Nursing* 10, 3 (May-June 1989): 126–132.

Carpenito, L. J. *Nursing Diagnosis: Application to Nursing Practice.* 4th edition. Philadelphia: J. B. Lippincott, 1992.

Cicirelli, V. G. Study funded by the AARP Andrus Foundation, Purdue University, 1982.

Clevenger, F. F. "Interviewing the Elderly Client." *Advances in Clinical Care* 5, 6 (November-December 1990): 26–27.

Duffy, M. E. "Determinants of Health-Promoting Lifestyles in Older Persons." *Image* 15, 1 (Spring, 1993): 23–28.

Evans, L. K., and Strumpf, N. E. "Myths About Elderly Restraint." *Image* 22, 2 (Spring 1990): 124–127.

Falcioni, D. "Assessing the Abused Elderly." *Journal of Gerontological Nursing* 8, 4 (April 1982): 208–212.

Fielo, S. B., and M. A. Rizzolo. "Handle With Caring: Meeting Elderly Clients' Special Learning Needs." *Nursing and Health Care* 9, 4 (April 1988): 192–195.

Garner, B. C. "Guide to Changing Lab Values in Elders." *Geriatric Nursing* 10, 3 (May-June 1989): 144–145.

Gawlinski, A., and Jensen, G. A. "Complications of Cardiovascular Aging." *American Journal of Nursing* 91, 11 (November 1991): 26–30.

Gortner, S. R., Dirks, J., and Wolfe, M. M. "The Road to Recovery for Elders After CABG." *American Journal of Nursing* 92, 8 (August 1992): 44–49.

Holzapfel, S. K. "The Importance of Personal Possessions in the Lives of the Institutionalized Elderly." *Journal of Gerontological Nursing* 18 (March 1982): 156–158.

Joel, L. A., and Patterson, J. E. "Nursing Homes Can't Afford Cheap Nursing Care." *RN* 53, 4 (April 1990): 57–60.

La Monica, E. L. "The Nurse and the Aging Client: Positive Attitude Formation." *Nurse Educator* 4 (December 1979): 23–26.

Lancaster, J. "Maximizing Psychological Adaptation in an Aging Population." *Topics in Clinical Nursing* 3 (April 1981): 31–43.

Mahoney, C. "Return to Independence: Lessons from a Hospital Long-Term Care Unit." *American Journal of Nursing* 91, 3 (March 1991): 44–48.

Matzo, M. "Confusion in Older Adults: Assessment and Differential Diagnosis." *Nurse Practitioner* 15, 9 (September 1990): 32–36, 39–46.

McElmurry, B. J., and LiBrizzi, S. J. "The Health of Older Women." *Nursing Clinics of North America* 21, 1 (March 1986): 161–171.

Nowlis, E. A. "A Study to Determine How Care Providers for the Elderly Perceive and Use Informational Resources."

Unpublished doctoral dissertation, Seattle University, 1983.

Olsen, J. K., and Kahn, B. W. "Helping Families Cope." *Journal of Gerontological Nursing* 6 (March 1980): 152–154.

Ouslander, J. G., and Beck, J. C. "Defining the Health Problems of the Elderly." *Annual Review of Public Health* 3 (March 1982): 55–83.

Pritchard, V. "Geriatric Infections: The Gastrointestinal Tract." *RN* 51, 4 (April 1988): 58–60.

Rantz, M., and Egan, K. "Reducing Death from Translocation Syndrome." *American Journal of Nursing* 87, 10 (October 1987): 1351–1352.

Reed, P. G. "Implications of the Life-Span Developmental Framework for Well-Being in Adulthood and Aging." *Advances in Nursing Science* 6, 1 (October 1983): 18–25.

Resnick, B. M. "Geriatric Motivation: Helping the Elderly to Comply." *Journal of Gerontological Nursing* 17, 5 (May 1991): 17–20.

Rice, L. " Do We Discriminate Against the Elderly?" *Nursing '88* 18 (March 1988): 44–45.

Routzahn, J. M. "Conflicts in Managing Elderly Clients and Elderly Parents: The Dual Role of Health Professionals." *Physical and Occupational Therapy in Geriatrics* 9, 3/4 (March-April 1991): 107–112.

Santo-Novak, D., and Edwards, R. M. "Rx: Take Caution with Drugs for Elders." *Geriatric Nursing* 10, 2 (March-April 1989): 72–75.

Selye, H. *The Stress of Life.* New York: McGraw-Hill, 1956.

Spellbring, A. M., Gannon, M. E., Kleckner, T., and Conway, K. "Improving Safety for Hospitalized Elderly." *Journal of Gerontological Nursing* 14, 2 (February 1988): 31–37.

Steinke, E. E. "Older Adults' Knowledge and Attitudes About Sexuality and Aging." *Image* 20, 2 (Summer 1988): 93–95.

Strome, T., and Howell, T. "How Antipsychotics Affect the Elderly." *American Journal of Nursing* 91, 5 (May 1991): 46–49.

Urrows, S. T., Freston, M. S., and Pryor, D. L. "Profiles in Osteoporosis." *American Journal of Nursing* 91, 12 (December, 1991): 32–37.

U.S. Department of Commerce, Bureau of the Census, 111th edition. 1991.

Waltman, R. E. "Dealing with Older Patients and Their Families." *Nursing '91* 21, 10 (October 1991): 66–68.

Vickery, F. *Old and Growing.* Springfield, Ill.: Charles C. Thomas, 1978.

Physiologic Needs

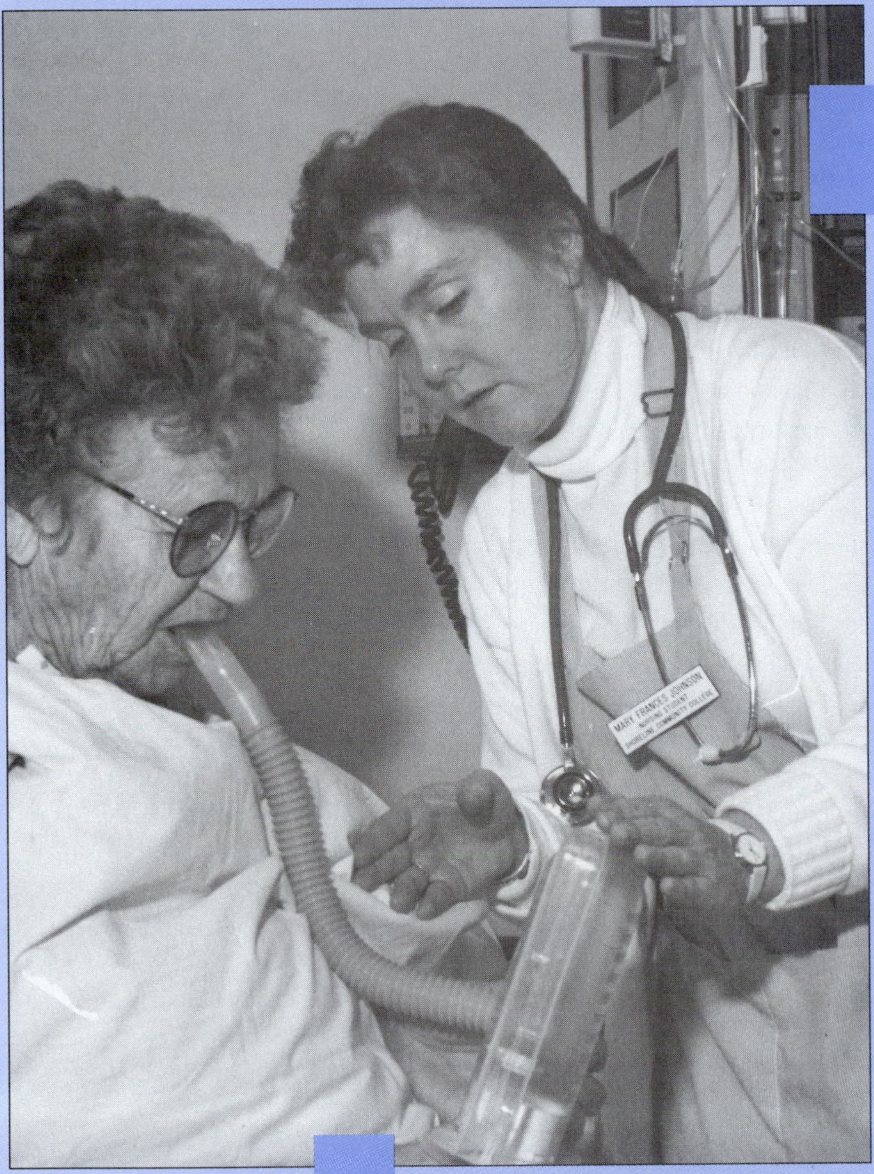

VI

Safety in the Environment

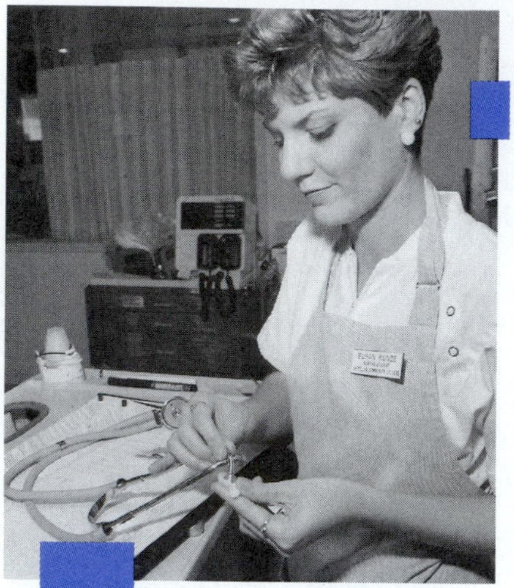

21

Objectives

After completing this chapter, you should be able to:

1. Identify the characteristics of a safe physical and psychological environment for the patient and the nurse.
2. Name five pathogens capable of causing infection.
3. Diagram and explain the movement of pathogens through the infection chain.
4. Identify and differentiate the roles and purposes of four organizations for the prevention and control of infection.
5. Discuss the responsibilities of the infection control nurse.
6. Explain what is meant by nosocomial infections.
7. List the three categories of drugs commonly used to treat infection.
8. Briefly explain the body's defenses against infection.
9. Explain the importance of immunization as a method to control infection.
10. Describe patients who may be at high risk of infection or injury.
11. Discuss the control of infection through the use of medical and surgical asepsis.
12. Outline the current Centers for Disease Control and Prevention (CDC) and Occupational and Safety Health Administration (OSHA) regulations as they affect employers and employees of health care facilities.
13. Describe strict, respiratory, and protective isolation and when their use is appropriate for prevention of infection.
14. Discuss the psychological impact of isolation on the patient and identify nursing interventions to support psychological homeostasis.
15. Use the nursing process to prevent the transmission of infection.

Study Terms

acid mantle
antigens
blood-borne pathogens
colonization
helminthic infections
iatrogenic infections
nosocomial infections
purulent drainage
seropositive
spore
vector
yeasts

Ellis, Nowlis: Nursing: A Human Needs Approach, 5th ed. © 1994 J.B. Lippincott Company

Outline

One of the human needs cited by Maslow is safety (see Chapter 5). He places this at the most basic level. All human beings need to be and feel safe, both physically and psychologically. Most of us feel safe in our own homes and protect ourselves within the changing environment by functioning as healthy individuals who make decisions in a reasonable manner. Many of the theorists discussed in Chapter 7 defined health and illness in a way that included the environment. The interaction with and accommodation to the environment was one measurement of health versus illness. For our purposes, safety means feeling secure from physical, mental, or emotional harm, danger, injury, or risk.

When the individual becomes a patient in an acute care setting or a resident in a long-term care setting, the new environment is strange and unsettling. Often, illness or impairment makes the person depend on others for maintaining safety. An unsafe environment can undermine those important feelings of security. Not only must the environment be made safe and free of infection for those in our care, but as nurses, we also need to have a safe workplace in which to practice. This chapter discusses how we can provide safety for others and how we can protect ourselves from the hazards that constantly confront us in the profession we have chosen.

Providing Safety for the Patient

The hospital unit, the room, and often the bed alone become the patient's environment. The variety of people making up the health care team also become part of the environment. Certain physical and psychological factors are important to consider.

Physical Safety

A safe hospital unit should be neat and well organized so that ambulatory patients and staff can move about freely without cumbersome equipment obstructing the way. Good lighting and ventilation are essential. Dropped objects and spills should be picked up or wiped up immediately before they can cause a fall. The first person to observe an unsafe situation should be the person responsible for taking care of the problem. Putting it off or delegating action could lead to the situation not being taken care of and someone being injured.

Within the patient's room, the temperature should be comfortable for the person, neither too warm nor too cold. Certain patients such as those who are postoperative, seriously ill, or very old or very young may need a warm environment to maintain body temperature. Because most patients are less active than nurses, remember that you may feel uncomfortably warm while giving care, even though the patient is comfortable. There should be sufficient air flow because adequate ventilation allows odors to dissipate, making the room smell fresh and clean. Lighting within the room should be bright enough to allow the person to see clearly and the nurse to identify the patient, assess accurately and thoroughly, and safely perform procedures and administer medications.

Not only should the nursing unit be kept neat and uncluttered to prevent injury, the patient's room should also be kept orderly. Interior doors should be closed, floor surfaces and electrical outlets kept clean and in good repair, and uneaten food removed promptly. If oxygen or other special treatments are ordered that require special equipment, you should consult the hospital policy for safe operation guidelines.

The low position should be used for occupied beds because it is easier to get in and out of bed so that a fall is less likely to happen. Raised side rails and physical restraints should only be used when necessary and with caution. Many falls occur with attempts to climb over side rails, and injuries can occur due to resisting restraints even when they are properly placed. See Chapter 20 for information on the use of these devices. A list of modules related to safety appears at the end of this chapter.

Psychological Safety

Nowhere is there more chance that one might feel psychologically unsafe than when assuming the patient role (see Chapter 15). The fact that the environment is strange and that the people within it are unfamiliar causes each patient some degree of uncertainty. Not having personal possessions about and wearing hospital gowns required by the facility can cause the patient to have feelings of anxiety that are associated with psychological safety.

Nursing Research: *Implications for Practice*

Wheson, M. B., and Shedd, P. "Prediction and Prevention of Patient Falls." *Image*, 21,2 (Summer 1989): 108–114.

The investigators reviewed 12 risk profiles, developed specifically to identify patients at risk of falls so that preventive measures could be taken. These profiles varied and "most did not specifically test its usefulness or state clearly its overall contribution to reducing falls" (p. 110). Interventions were frequently based on policy to avoid liability rather than on scientific research. One instance was the use of side rails, which is known to increase rather than decrease falls.

The authors found that integrating safety into the plan of care for those at risk was most helpful. Nurses should emphasize specific preventive interventions for avoiding patient injury when writing the care plan. The researchers conclude that it is not nurses' lack of knowledge that contributes to falls. They recommend raising staff awareness as the single most important measure to prevent patient injury.

The fear that basic needs will not be met can be a realistic concern. Tests and procedures may engender fear, particularly when the patient wonders whether or not they will produce pain or that a test result will reveal that something serious is wrong with the body. A common fear for those experiencing surgery may be that of sufficient pain control. Possible loss of privacy can cause the patient to feel psychologically unsafe as well.

The patient may fear that physicians, nurses, and others on the health care team are unsure or incompetent. Patients need to feel safe with the care provided within the environment. Most patients have no medical background, yet their degree of trust that care will be delivered safely is surprising. Many do not question the medications given to them nor the procedures being performed. Other patients hesitate to confront the nurse or even to ask questions about the safety of their care. By being offered information and reasonable explanations, all patients feel more psychologically safe. They need to know also that their communication with the nurse and others on the health care team will be dealt with in a confidential manner and that any negative feelings they express will be accepted without rebuke or personal rejection. Also important to psychological safety is that the patient receives respect and has a feeling of control by being included in decision-making. Studies have shown that the most effective means for providing psychological safety for the patient is for nurses to reflect knowledge, competence, and sensitivity (Fig. 21-1).

Maintaining Safety for the Nurse

Nurses need both physical and psychological safety in the workplace. The behavior of the nurse can greatly determine the degree of safety at work.

One way nurses' behavior can guard against injury is by the conscientious use of body mechanics when lifting or moving patients. Many nurses develop chronic back problems because they use proper body mechanics inconsistently.

Another recent concern related to the safety of nurses has been the issue of inhaled microdroplets of medications that have been aerosolized or nebulized for the patient. One example is an antiparasitic medication used to treat the type of pneumonia suffered by patients with acquired immunodeficiency syndrome (AIDS) and frequently delivered by aerosol mist. Persons sensitive to this medication can develop head pain, sore throat, and other symptoms merely by being near the patient undergoing the treatment. Because we do not know whether other inhalants might also cause undesirable effects in individuals who are sensitive to them, many

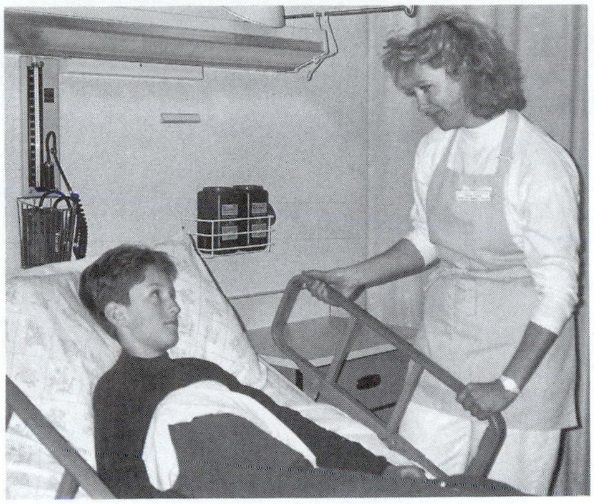

Figure 21-1. The nurse provides a safe environment for the patient.

respiratory therapists recommend that health care workers leave the room while these treatments are being performed. Whether or not nurses can suffer ill effects from dispersing microdroplets of medications into the air while holding the syringe up to dispel the air is unknown at this time. It is possible that the administration of other categories of drugs may prove hazardous. Therefore, you should avoid inhaling any medication.

Chemotherapeutic agents may pose a hazard to those handling them. Research is ongoing regarding safety of the fetus when a pregnant nurse administers these drugs. Everyone who administers chemotherapeutic drugs should follow prescribed procedures to prevent skin contact. Remaining free of infection is currently an important area of safety for nurses and will be discussed in more detail later.

Nurses also need to feel psychologically safe in the workplace. The support of peers and supervisors can foster psychological equilibrium (Fig. 21-2). In turn, each nurse can become an important part of the support of others in the work environment. Nurses need to work in situations for which they possess appropriate skills and feel competent and comfortable when delivering care to the patient. Legal and psychological hazards arise if nurses practice beyond the scope of their preparation. Some stress and burnout can be avoided when the nurse feels adequate and prepared. With career ladders (discussed in Chapter 1) and recognition, nurses feel more professionally safe.

Nursing education programs consider safety of the student and the patient to be a serious matter. Actions that place the patient or another person in jeopardy bring about a verbal or written warning. Safety errors are not acceptable, and repeated errors may lead to dismissal. The faculties of nursing programs view this action not as punishment but as responsibility for the protection of patients and care providers.

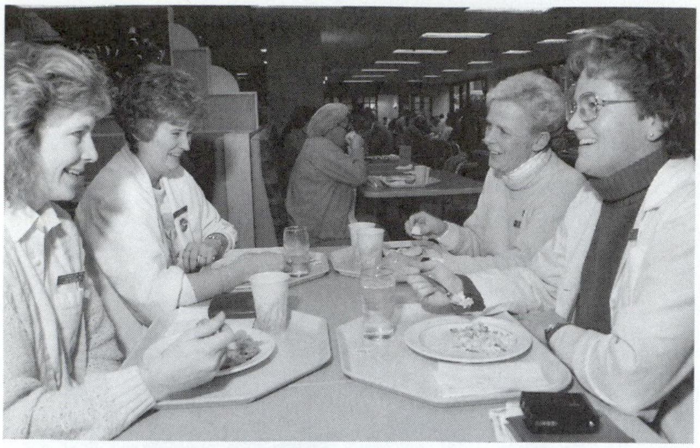

Figure 21-2. Companionship provides psychological safety for the nurse.

Maintaining Institutional Safety

A wide variety of federal, state, and local regulations protect patients/residents, staff members, and visitors within institutions. Such regulations grouped together are sometimes referred to as codes. Fire and disaster codes are mandated so that if an emergency arises, a plan of action can be implemented quickly. Tests, or simulations, take place regularly so that all those involved have an opportunity to perform their roles as if the emergency were an actual event.

In addition to codes and disaster plans, institutions include various departments that protect personnel and patients. Engineers control environmental heating and cooling by overseeing the power sources. Other workers in the maintenance department inspect and make recommendations regarding electrical devices and small appliances. Nutritionists, as managers of food services, guard safe food storage and preparation. Most large institutions have a security staff. These security personnel have a call system that brings about a quick response in cases that cause a threatening situation within the facility.

Safety and the Role of the Nurse

In many ways, the nurse is the manager of the patient's care within the institution. With this comes the responsibility of providing a safe and infection-free environment. Patients in the hospital may have all levels of impairment. Some people experience only mild anxiety produced by a minor health problem, which requires a short stay in the hospital. Others may have more serious impairments requiring you to continually make assessments for unsafe conditions that may endanger persons who cannot protect themselves. Some hazards are more apparent than are others; a spill on the floor or a half-open door visibly alert you to take action to prevent someone being injured. The risk and transmission of infection may be less obvious. To adequately protect the patient and yourself, you must stay current and vigilant in respect to infection control management (see sample Nursing Care Plan Related to Safety).

Infection and the Environment

An important component of the safety needs of human beings is protection from infection in the environment. Throughout the human life span, health is threatened by infection. Many people are admitted to the hospital because they have contracted an infection. More often than health care workers would like, patients who are in the health care facility for surgery or treatment of a medical condition develop secondary infections.

These infections are called **nosocomial**, or hospital-acquired, **infections**. It is estimated that nosocomial infections occur in approximately 5% of all hospitalized patients. These infections cause patients considerable unnecessary pain and, in some cases, even cause their deaths (Mooney and Armington, 1987). Another alarming problem is that over half the categories used for the recent prospective Medicare reimbursement plan (diagnosis-related groups) do not provide reimbursement to the hospitals for these infections, so large amounts of revenue are lost at a time when health care costs are increasing.

The best health care includes careful measures for protection from infection. These measures comprise mobilizing the protective mechanisms of the individual and, at the same time, minimizing the environmental causes of infection. Nurses have a responsibility to see that patients remain infection free while they are in their care.

The rest of this chapter focuses on the causes of infection, the body's internal and external protective mechanisms, and the factors in the environment that can cause or help prevent infection. A lengthy discussion will be presented concerning the newly mandated OSHA regulations. These regulations directly affect every health care facility and the infection control practices of every student and registered nurse.

A Brief History of Infection

Means to prevent and control infection were virtually unknown until the 1800s, when the methods for transmission of disease organisms began to be understood.

Nursing Care Plan

Sample Nursing Care Plan Related to Safety

Nursing Diagnosis	High Risk for Injury: Falls related to confusion, postanesthesia, and pain meds **Supportive data:** Woman, age 67 Surgery this morning with 4-h inhaled anesthesia. Medicated with morphine sulfate 2× since surgery. States, "Am I at home or in the hospital?"
Desired Patient Outcomes	**Short term:** The patient will not attempt to get out of bed without assistance. **Long term:** The patient will have no falls while in the hospital or after discharge.

Nursing Action	Rationale
1. Check patient frequently and orient to the environment.	Frequent checks will allow the nurse to prevent unsafe behavior that may result in a fall. Reorienting helps the client to maintain safe behavior.
2. Maintain side rails in upright position.	Raised siderails prevent the patient from rolling out of bed.
3. Have call light within patient's reach at all times.	Availability of call light promotes a feeling of security and allows the person to call for assistance and not attempt unsafe activity independently.
4. Remind patient to call if she is not comfortable or needs anything.	The nurse's willingness to respond will encourage the use of the call light.
5. Caution patient to remain in bed.	Remaining in bed provides a safe environment for the confused postoperative patient. Reminders help the patient to avoid unsafe behavior.
6. If confusion continues, apply Posey restraint and notify physician.	Temporarily applying restraints prevents patient injury. The physician provides a written order.

However, in earlier times it had been observed that previously healthy people who touched or came in contact with the ill often became ill themselves, and isolation of the sick thus was common.

As long as human beings have existed, their wounds have been accompanied by infection. Although attempts were made to contain it, infection was long thought to be a natural component of healing. The ancient Romans dressed wounds with pastes of molds and yeasts, called poultices, spread on cloth. These mixtures slowed the infection process although it was not understood why. Not until the twentieth century was it discovered—by Sir Alexander Fleming, a Scottish bacteriologist—that penicillin, a compound derived from a mold, is effective in the treatment of many infections. Penicillin and its derivatives are the most widely used antibiotics in the world today.

In the 1840s, Ignaz Semmelweis, a Hungarian obstetrician, demonstrated that germs could be transmitted from the hands of one person to another person. Physicians routinely had examined pregnant women immediately after examining cadavers, without washing their hands, and Semmelweis observed that these women became infected and often died of what was known as "childbed fever." In 1862, Louis Pasteur, a French chemist, first proved the germ theory of disease.

Before the advent of aseptic surgical practice, a surgeon might wear the same soiled frock coat for several surgical procedures. Clean gowns came into use in 1880. Ten years later Dr. William Halsted introduced the use of sterile gloves. The understanding of infection and its control through asepsis thus expanded gradually, eventually giving rise to scientific principles with important implications for the health care team.

Causes of Infection

Extremely small animals and plants called *microorganisms* exist throughout the human body. Many of these tiny organisms are beneficial, but some are not. Those that are beneficial, called *normal flora,* prevent the growth of disease-producing microorganisms within a particular area of the body, such as the nose, throat, intestinal tract, and vagina. Disease-producing microorganisms are called *pathogens.*

Both types of microorganisms, the beneficial normal flora and the pathogens, coexist to a degree in most individuals. In healthy people with intact immune systems, the small number of pathogens within the body do not cause disease.

When pathogens multiply within the body to the point of causing signs and symptoms, the individual is said to have an infection. There are many classifications of the known pathogens. The new infections that appear occasionally are thought to be caused by as yet unidentified pathogens. The six types of known pathogens (infectious agents) are bacteria, viruses, fungi, protozoa, parasitic worms, and rickettsiae. Some of these pathogens cause disease more often in some parts of the world than in others. In the Western world, bacteria and viruses are more common causes of infection among the general population than are parasitic worms. Yet in areas of the world lacking adequate sanitation, worms and protozoa still cause many infections.

Several factors determine how harmful infectious agents are within the body. First, the number of pathogens is significant. The body may be able to tolerate a few such organisms for extended periods of time, but it is incapable of resisting large numbers of the same pathogen, which are likely to be present if the pathogen multiplies rapidly. Second, the pathogen's ability to find susceptible body tissue is a factor in infection. For example, one bacterium, staphylococcus, can be relatively harmless on the skin but causes serious infection in lung tissue. Finally, some strains of the same pathogen are more virulent than others. A pathogen's virulence is its potency or the strength of its ability to cause disease. In any given person, the strain must be virulent enough to cause an infection.

Bacteria

The most numerous of all the pathogens, *bacteria* are one-celled microorganisms. Bacteria that can live only in the presence of free oxygen are called *aerobic. Anaerobic* bacteria do not multiply in the presence of oxygen. Harmless bacteria far outnumber those that are harmful. Among the human diseases caused by bacteria are food poisoning, tuberculosis, some types of pneumonia, urinary tract infections, and some sexually transmitted diseases (STDs). Some bacteria, when dormant (quiet), form **spores** with thick, resistant walls, which make them extremely difficult to kill. Tetanus is caused by spore-forming bacteria.

Viruses

The smallest of all microorganisms, many *viruses* are observable only with powerful electron microscopes. Some diseases are assumed to be caused by viruses that cannot be visualized at present. Viruses cause many infections, such as one type of pneumonia, measles, mumps, influenzas, and the common cold. Viruses can lie dormant within the body until certain conditions, such as a person's decreased resistance, encourage them to grow and become active. The *herpes* "family" of viruses provides one example of this phenomenon. The familiar "cold sore" recurs from the herpes virus, which continues to live in the tissues. More serious are congenital herpes infections.

Of current worldwide concern is the apparent appearance of a newly identified virus, the human immunodeficiency virus (HIV) that is dormant in a person for a protracted period of time before causing the disease we know as AIDS. A major effort is underway to find a vaccine against this virus or develop improved medications that can control the progress of this disease.

Fungi

Moldlike pathogens, fungi, can also cause infections that are difficult to subdue. Fungi grow best in moist climates, and infections caused by fungi are prevalent in wet tropical areas. Athlete's foot and ringworm are both *fungus* infections.

Yeasts are unicellular, rounded fungi. Yeasts called candida cause infections such as "thrush" in the mouths of infants and immunocompromised individuals. Yeast infections also occur on the skin, in the intestines, and in the genital area.

Protozoa

There are over 15,000 species of *protozoa,* large single-celled microorganisms that live in fresh or ocean water (particularly stagnant water) and in soil. Malaria is one of the common diseases caused by protozoa. The protozoa that cause malaria are carried from one individual to another by the mosquito.

Parasitic Worms

Parasitic worms are not technically microorganisms but small, disease-causing invertebrate animals that cannot exist unless they feed off a host or microorganism. Infections caused by parasitic worms are called **helminthic infections**. Pinworm and hookworm are parasitic worms.

Rickettsiae

Rickettsiae are small bacteria transmitted by bloodsucking parasites such as ticks, lice, and fleas. Rocky Mountain spotted fever and typhus are rickettsial diseases. Insect and rodent control are the most effective means of preventing diseases caused by rickettsiae.

The Infection Chain

To understand how pathogens cause infection, look closely at Figure 21-3, which illustrates the chain reaction that spreads infection. The infection chain is the way pathogens pass between human beings.

First of all, an *infectious agent* (pathogen) must be present. The pathogen grows in a place, called a *reservoir*, where the conditions for its reproduction are optimal. The pathogen leaves the reservoir through what is called a *portal of exit*. The pathogen then moves by some *means of transmission* to a person (*host*) who is susceptible to it. The pathogen enters the host through a *portal of entry*, usually a body opening, and may or may not multiply further. If not extinguished within the host, it may exit through the same or a different portal.

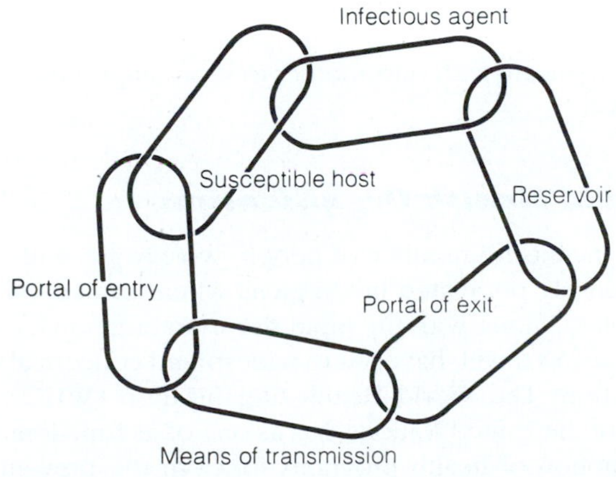

Figure 21-3. The infection chain.

For example, an organism taken in through the respiratory tract may exit through the same portal by means of a cough or sneeze. Or the portals of entry and exit may differ: an organism that enters by mouth may exit through the bowel.

Each link is essential to the chain. If the chain is interrupted at any point, by chance or because of deliberate intervention, the pathogen is inactivated. Let us examine each link in more detail.

Infectious Agents

We have already described the six most common classifications of pathogens that comprise the infectious agent in the chain. These infectious agents are present in the environment and on and within the bodies of people and animals. How to prevent and control infection depends largely on the type of infectious agent.

The Reservoir

The reservoir is the place where infectious agents or pathogens multiply. Common reservoirs are water, food, body tissues, excreta, body fluids, and contaminated objects such as basins, equipment, and dressings.

Microorganisms need one or more of a variety of conditions to multiply: the presence or absence of oxygen, light or darkness, compatible temperature, moisture, a specific pH, and some form of nourishment. A pH (acid–base balance) above 5, slightly alkaline, promotes the growth of many pathogens.

Portal of Exit

When body tissue harbors the organism, a pathway for pathogens to leave the body, a portal of exit, can be identified. Pathogens may exit through the orifices of the respiratory tract in the form of secretions, the gastrointestinal tract in the form of vomitus or feces, or the genitourinary tract in the form of urine. Wound drainage, blood, and other body fluids can also provide a portal of exit. If the reservoir is outside the body, the portal of exit is the point at which the organism leaves the food, water, or other substance.

Means of Transmission

The means of transmission, or means by which pathogens move from one person to another, is the link in the infection chain at which intervention is often most effective. We will discuss this concept later in relation to the practice of universal precautions.

Some pathogens can be transmitted by only one

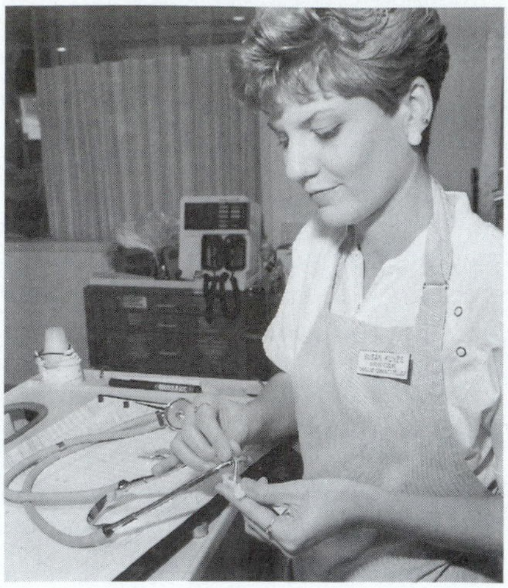

Figure 21-4. Unwashed hands and equipment can transmit pathogens between patients.

means. Others use more than one means of transmission. In general, there are four routes of transmission.

Contact, the first route, may be *direct* or *indirect*. Direct contact is a means of transmission with particular pertinence for nurses who provide hygienic care or perform procedures. Touching another person during these procedures is a way to transmit pathogens by direct contact. Transmission of pathogens by *droplet*—the projection of moisture by coughing or sneezing—is also considered direct contact. Indirect contact is transmission of a pathogen on linen or equipment that has been contaminated. Using inadequately cleaned equipment from one patient to another is a breach of proper technique (Fig. 21-4).

Pathogens are also transmitted by *vehicles*—substances in or on which they are conveyed. Food and water serve as vehicles for some organisms. Food poisoning is an infection caused by the staphylococcus bacterium and transmitted by the vehicle of spoiled food. Blood, semen, and vaginal secretions can also serve as vehicles for the spread of certain pathogens. An example is the virus that causes hepatitis B, or serum hepatitis, which can be transmitted in blood transfusions. The HIV virus can be transmitted through semen, vaginal secretions, blood, and breast milk.

Pathogens can also be *airborne*, carried on dust particles surrounded by moisture and suspended in the air. Pathogens projected by a sneeze can become attached to dust particles and remain airborne.

Finally, pathogens can be transmitted by vectors. **Vectors** are nonhuman species that can carry an organism that produces disease in human beings. Some vectors are insects (such as the malarial mosquito) and animals such as birds, rats, or mosquitoes. Rat control measures have greatly reduced the incidence of vector-transmitted infections.

Portal of Entry

The pathogen enters the body of a *susceptible host* through a portal of entry. Any of the *orifices*, or opening, of the body, such as those of the respiratory, gastrointestinal, and genitourinary tracts, can serve as portals of entry. A person's circulatory system can serve as a portal of entry also because infected blood from one person can enter the circulatory system of another person through transfusion. Skin that is no longer intact is another important portal of entry. Even small skin abrasions may serve as portals of entry as can larger wounds and decubitus ulcers (pressure sores).

The Susceptible Host

The person in whom the organism is present is called the host. In some persons, the pathogens never reach a high enough level to cause an active infection in that person but are harbored and can be passed to someone else. Such a person is called a *carrier*. One type of carrier is the person who colonizes bacteria. This means that a person has a mass of organisms growing on tissue (**colonization**) but remains disease free. However, this person can transmit the organism to a susceptible host. More specifically, for a person to become ill, not only must the strain be virulent to that person, but also the host must be susceptible to the organism. Some people are more susceptible to infection than others for reasons that will be mentioned later.

Organizations for the Prevention and Control of Infection

Because infective agents know no national boundaries, efforts to control the spread of infection have involved organizations on the international, national, and regional levels. To facilitate the establishment of effective programs, these organizations have worked diligently to communicate with one another to share important information.

World Health Organization

The increasing number of people worldwide who live in densely populated urban areas where sanitation is a problem, along with the rapid rise in international commerce and travel, have led to widespread concern about infection. The World Health Organization (WHO), an arm of the United Nations, has as one of its functions the promotion of health programs for both the prevention and treatment of infection. Through international cooperation for developing immunization programs, significant progress has been made in infection control. The complete eradication of the deadly disease smallpox during the past decade was a major victory for those concerned with the spread of disease throughout the world. However, several diseases, such as meningitis, trachoma, and influenza continue to affect people in countries throughout the world.

International attention is currently focused on the continuing spread of HIV infection. First identified in 1979, it has reached endemic proportions without abatement. Each year, an international conference is held with presentations by the world's leading researchers in an attempt to better understand this disease so that ways can be found to contain or eliminate it.

Centers for Disease Control and Prevention

The national Centers for Disease Control and Prevention (CDC), located in Atlanta, Georgia, and supported by federal funds, has a variety of functions. This organization provides information and education on infection issues to individuals and health care agencies throughout the United States. It also acts as a liaison with WHO, relaying incidence-of-disease information that has been gathered by a computerized surveillance system. Using scientifically based research, CDC issues guidelines on health practices for health care facilities and recommendations for the general population. The CDC is viewed as one of the most important resources for obtaining information relating to health issues, but it has no regulatory power.

Occupational and Safety Health Administration

One of the most authoritative agencies developed under federal mandate is the Occupational and Safety Health Administration (OSHA). Canada has similar agencies under provincial statutory law. Established under the 1970 Occupational and Safety Health Act, its mission is to issue policies that protect people in the workplace from injury and disease. This agency has full regulatory power with the authority to fine those facilities who endanger others because of noncompliance. The current OSHA regulations will be outlined in the final portion of this chapter.

State and County Departments of Public Health

On the state and county levels, public health departments have epidemiologists (physicians and others with special education) who gather statistical information and carry out research on the transmission of disease. These persons share their findings with other national and international groups from which come recommendations for infection prevention and control. Public health departments maintain immunization programs, particularly for school-age children. These programs vary from state to state and province to province.

The Health Care Facility Infection Control Committee

The Joint Commission on Accreditation of Healthcare Organizations (JCAHO) requires that every accredited health care facility have a multidisciplinary committee with responsibility for the control of infection within the hospital. These committees have the responsibility for surveillance and policy implementation. These multidisciplinary committees should be composed of persons having expertise in the area of epidemiology (the study of infectious diseases). Epidemiology is a recognized nursing specialty area. The most effective infection control committees are multidisciplinary ones with nursing well represented. These committees need the autonomy to establish policy and adequate funding to carry out effective surveillance programs. Infection rate data are reported to the CDC for statistical purposes. Many hold staff development presentations to educate workers regarding safe practices.

The infection control nurse needs knowledge of microbiology and statistics. An important responsibility of the infection control nurse is to recognize and document all cases of infection within the facility. A report is then made to the Infection Control Committee on a regular basis. Ching and Seto (1990, p. 1130) emphasize the fact that providing education is an essential role in being an effective infection control nurse. This entails educating the staff and patients regarding safe practices to prevent infection. The infection control nurse may also help write policies regarding infection control practices and will assume expanded responsibilities implementing new federal guidelines. The infection control nurse may also have responsibilities in the area of personnel health, particularly if there is a concern about infection transmission.

To stay current in the prevention and management of infection takes considerable interest and energy for all nurses. Infection control committees and the nurses who work in this specialty contribute significantly to making the hospital a safer place for both patients and staff.

The Body's Defenses Against Infection

The body has a variety of defenses against invasion by pathogens that can cause infection. The structure and physiology of the body is designed to ward off threats by microorganisms. In addition, one can live a lifestyle that encourages health and makes infection less likely.

Structural and Physiologic Defenses

The structure of the human body provides protection against the invasion of pathogens. The skin, with its several layers, provides a mechanical *barrier* if it is intact. Perspiration moves organisms along the skin surface, and the slightly acid pH, sometimes referred to as the **acid mantle**, retards the growth of microorganisms. More will be said about the skin in Chapter 22.

The mucosal tissue lining the nose, mouth, pharynx, trachea, and bronchi also serves as a barrier. The top surface of this tissue consists of tall, hairlike mucous-secreting cells that constantly wave in an upward direction, clearing unwanted particles and organisms from the lower respiratory tract. The microbes in the normal flora of this area also play a role in annihilating harmful microorganisms.

Within the stomach, the hydrochloric acid content of gastric secretions creates a hostile environment for growing organisms. The emptying of the stomach contents at regular intervals and the peristaltic movement of the intestinal tract remove pathogens from the body. Secretion of mucus by the tract also walls off organisms until they can be expelled. Although it has no normal flora to ward off attack, the urinary tract has a formidable defense in the copious flow of urine. In addition, the bladder wall has resistance. Like the skin, urine normally has a slightly acidic pH, which helps defend the tract against the growth of any organisms that may be inadvertently introduced. Finally, if pathogens get past the various body defenses and enter the bloodstream (**blood-borne pathogens**), the macrophages of the reticuloendothelial system are designed to neutralize or destroy them.

Lifestyle Defenses

Studies show that one's lifestyle can indeed protect against infection. Healthy patterns of living can make one an unlikely candidate for harboring pathogens, that is, they can make one a nonsusceptible host (Fig. 21-5).

Adequate nutrition that is high in protein maintains tissue integrity, which helps prevent infection. Sufficient fluid intake provides the tissues and the circulatory and urinary systems with adequate fluid volume, which helps dilute and move invading organisms. Exercise tones muscles and stimulates the systems of respiration and elimination, allowing the body to maintain optimum functioning of these systems, which play a role in resistance to infection. Sufficient rest and sleep enable a person to fight off infection by preparing the body to cope with stress. Controlling the amount of stress in one's life or successfully coping with stress can help to make the body a nonsusceptible host. Good personal hygiene such as adequate bathing, handwashing, and nail, hair, and oral care contribute significantly to lowering the risk of infection.

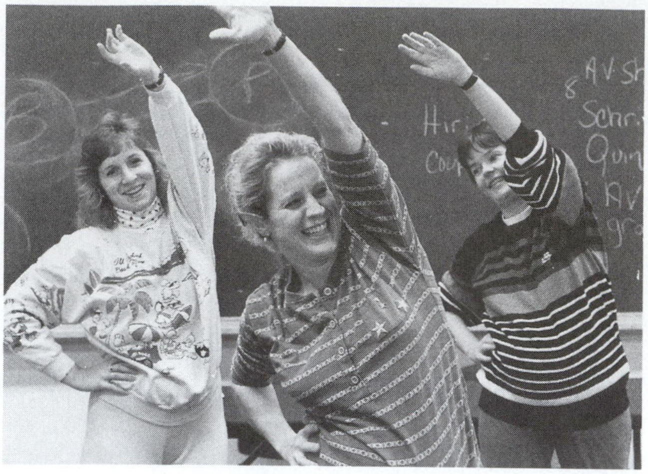

Figure 21-5. A healthy lifestyle can help protect against infection.

The most effective protection against HIV infection and other blood-borne diseases such as hepatitis is to live a lifestyle without drug abuse or sexual partners who have been exposed. It is now clear that sharing unclean needles and syringes can lead to the transmission of HIV infection or hepatitis. Unsafe sexual practices may also cause HIV infection or the occurrence of STDs (see Chapter 37).

These lifestyle defenses against infection apply to nurses as well as to patients. Nursing is demanding, both physically and emotionally. Nurses need to remind themselves constantly that they, too, can guard against infection by programming into their personal lives the various lifestyle defenses.

Immunization

It is far better to prevent infection than to attempt to contain it or eradicate it within the body. Immunization only became possible when scientists gained knowledge concerning the body's natural defenses against infection, such as the skin and the body's internal immune system. In 1796, Edward Jenner, an English physician, injected a small boy with a vaccine made from cowpox serum, and it proved effective against smallpox. This giant step gave the health care profession its first opportunity to prevent, rather than simply treat, infections.

As we now know, the *immune process* is an important mechanism of the body to resistant infection and maintain homeostasis. The response of this complicated body system is currently being carefully studied. Many diseases involve alterations or impairments of the immune system, which place the person at high risk for infection. Our rapidly expanding knowledge of this system may greatly aid in the control or prevention of many of these dreaded diseases. The immune system and its response were discussed in detail in Chapter 6.

Inoculation refers to the purposeful introduction of substances or microorganisms into the body to stimulate the production of antibodies for immunity. Inoculation can be done by injections or orally, as with polio vaccine. *Vaccines* are made up of dead or attenuated (weakened) microorganisms that have the ability to stimulate the body's production of antibodies and thus protect the person against disease. Vaccines are the most commonly used anti-infective agents. *Toxoids* are derived from the toxins produced by microorganisms. Because the toxins are too dangerous to be given without alteration, heat or chemicals are applied to toxins to make them safe for human injection as toxoids.

Two points are worth mentioning. First, naturally acquired immunity (the body's primary response to invasion) is longer lasting and more effective than artificially acquired immunity (that gained through the introduction of vaccines and toxoids). Therefore, the use of "serial" inoculations (reinoculating at specific times to prolong immunity) is often recommended.

Advances in immune research and the development and refinement of new vaccines and toxoids have prevented many communicable diseases (see Chapter 18 for immunization schedule).

Immunization programs throughout the world have completely altered patterns of morbidity (illness). As new infections emerge, the emphasis shifts to subduing these new threatening agents. There has been a dramatic decrease in communicable diseases in the United States since the advent of widespread vaccination (Fig. 21-6).

A few religious groups resist immunization practices, not only for school-age children but in general, believing that immunization interferes with the will of God. Their views make it difficult to enforce immunization legislation thoroughly. At times parents have raised some resistance to mandatory inoculation on the grounds that it violates parental authority or conflicts with religious beliefs. The courts, however, have consistently ruled that these programs are sound ones for the protection of children and the community.

The thinking of health authorities in government is that immunization programs are effective only if all comply. Nurses have a clear responsibility to use their knowledge about immune processes and the processes of transmission of infection to encourage people actively to take advantage of immunization programs within their community.

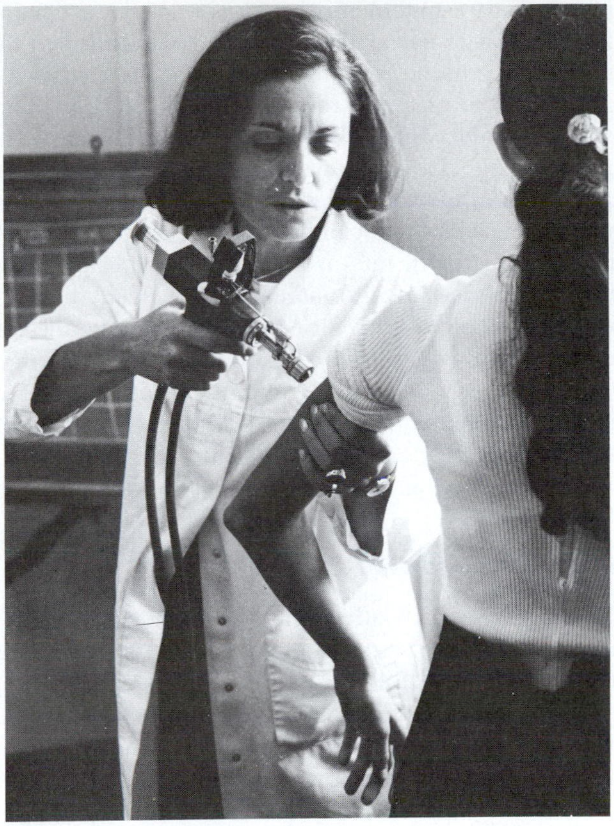

Figure 21-6. Immunization is an important part of the prevention of infection.

Persons at Risk of Infection

Despite immunization and attention to lifestyles, some people are at more risk of infection than others, for one or a variety of factors. Although we will mention these factors separately, the more factors present within a single individual, the more that person is at risk. This fact is particularly important for nurses to consider when assessing, diagnosing, and planning care.

Infants, Young Children, and the Elderly

Although the infant receives from the mother partial immunity from certain infections across the placental barrier, the infant's immune system remains immature until many months have passed. The infant is gradually exposed to organisms within the environment that can be dealt with without causing infection, and this gradual exposure leads to antibody formation. The passages of the respiratory system are short in the infant, facilitating the entrance of pathogens and this, combined with the immature immune system, causes infants to have a larger number of upper respiratory tract infections than people of other ages. The young child, particularly the one entering school, shows a resurgence of infections, primarily because of the sudden exposure to a large number of school-age children as well as to the exceedingly rapid growth rate at this age, which can deplete energy and resistance to infection. The elderly have an increased chance of infection because their immune systems are not as vigorous as they were in the younger years. There is a delay in the immune response to infection and an inadequate response to the stress of an infection. These factors alter the normal inflammatory response to infection. (Murray and Zentner, 1989).

The Chronically Ill

Chronic illness can affect many of the activities of a healthy lifestyle. The person may not be able to eat regularly or exercise fully. Coughing and deep breathing may be less active, leading to increased numbers of respiratory infections. With alterations in function, the person's general health may be less good than is desired.

Because people are living much longer than in the past, more older adults are developing chronic illnesses. However, a person with a chronic illness, regardless of age, is at risk for infection because one or more body systems are involved and their function is compromised. Therefore, decreased resistance often leads to invasion by pathogens.

Chronic illness may also involve the need for the presence of an indwelling catheter, which can lead to infections. The importance of proper practice is illustrated by the disturbing number of infections involving urinary catheters. The CDC cites the presence of a catheter as the primary reason for infections involving the urinary tract. This fact is especially important for nurses because catheterization and care of the catheterized patient are nursing responsibilities. For specific procedures, refer to Module 39, Catheterization. Even without catheterization, the person with a spinal cord injury, for example, may acquire repeated bladder infections because the bladder cannot empty sufficiently and therefore provides a reservoir for organisms (see Chapter 42).

Patients in the Care Setting

Nosocomial infections occur far too frequently. Because they can easily transmit these infections, nurses must be instrumental in decreasing the rate of hospital-acquired infections. Despite their appearance, hospitals are not clean places. Many people from many different environments are confined to a fairly restricted facility in which they can hardly avoid contact with one another. Thus, patients become exposed to a wide variety of unfamiliar organisms. Also, patients' other health problems weaken their resistance to infection. Many patients have open wounds, which offer entry for pathogens.

Patients Having Tests and Procedures

Whenever a test or procedure carried out in the plan of care is *invasive*—that is, enters the interior of the body in some manner—infection becomes a risk. Infections that occur because of this invasion are called **iatrogenic infections**—that is, caused by the plan of care.

Patients on Drugs That Suppress the Immune System

Certain medications encourage infection by suppressing the body's immune system. The large class of drugs known as steroids and some chemotherapeutic agents used to treat cancer are examples. The use of such drugs, in conjunction with the patient's already decreased ability to fight infection, makes infection an ever-present danger. Patients taking such medications are known as *immunosuppressed* patients. Another term frequently used is *compromised host.* We will talk later about measures to protect these persons, who have such a high risk for infection.

Surgical Patients

Surgical procedures require incisions that interrupt the integrity of the integument (skin) and mucous membranes, major barriers against infection. When organs and body tissues are exposed, even in operating rooms where the environment is controlled as strictly as possible, pathogens can enter.

Many surgeons order prophylactic antibiotics before surgery to prevent postoperative infection. Despite such action, wound infections do occur. Diabetic patients and those in poor nutritional status or those with chronic illness are most susceptible.

Postoperatively, the risk of infection is also heightened whenever dressings are changed or any special equipment is used. The psychological stress that surgical patients experience may also lessen resistance.

Preventing Infection

The outstanding factor in the spread of infections in hospitals, states the CDC, is patient care practices. Studies have shown how organisms are transferred from one patient to another by members of the health care team and by equipment used in giving care.

Following Prescribed Guidelines

Because they provide the majority of direct care to patients, nurses can be extremely effective in preventing the incidence of nosocomial infections by consistently washing their hands and following the guidelines issued by the federal government. These guidelines focus on practicing universal "blood and body fluid precautions," discussed later in this chapter. Because both the new OSHA regulations and the CDC recommendations focus on providing barriers to infection by nurses' actions, such as wearing gloves and taking other precautions more frequently when giving care, it is estimated that the rate of nosocomial infection will decrease.

Another way to prevent and control nosocomial infection is by constant surveillance of the hospital environment. Both the CDC and OSHA offer extensive written guidelines on cleaning and disinfecting equipment. These agencies also have material on surveying personnel to identify individuals who harbor infections, so that they cannot pass pathogens on to patients who have lowered resistance to infection.

Aseptic Conscience

It is essential for you as a nurse to develop an *aseptic conscience*, or a strict, rigid, and constant monitoring of your own adherence to technique. Aseptic conscience can apply to both medical and surgical techniques. If, for example, you have begun to prepare a patient's tray for feeding and suddenly remember that you have not washed your hands since leaving the patient in the next bed, your aseptic conscience directs you to leave the tray and go directly to the nearest sink to wash, offering your patient at least partial protection from pathogens. If, while performing a catheterization, you inadvertently touch the surrounding unsterile drape with the tip of the catheter, your aseptic conscience tells you to secure another catheter and discard the first.

Remedying deviations from technique—and every nurse does at times fail to conform to technique—often takes time and is inconvenient. Although the patient will not always develop an infection as a result, the outcome cannot be predicted; the patient may be subjected to pain and further suffering caused by infection resulting from just such a lapse. A nurse who knows that medical or surgical technique has been broken and does not rectify the deviation is a poor representative of the profession. If you observe a lapse in aseptic technique by someone else, you are equally obligated to see that the lapse is rectified to protect the patient. Simply commenting that contamination has taken place and offering to secure new equipment will usually be sufficient. Sometimes the other person does not know such a lapse has occurred and will appreciate your intervention. Even if the nurse only suspects that aseptic technique has been breached, steps must be taken to correct the possible lapse. With regard to asepsis, nothing is assumed.

Medical and Surgical Asepsis

Asepsis is the absence of all disease-producing microorganisms. Asepsis is the key to protecting hospitalized patients from infection and preventing the spread of infection from a patient who is already infected.

Nurses and other health care team members differentiate between two kinds of asepsis. *Medical asepsis* is designed to reduce the number of pathogens in an area and decrease the likelihood of their transfer. It is often referred to as *clean technique*. Microorganisms may continue to be present, but a threshold of safety has been established. During a given day, a nurse's hands may touch numerous patients and a variety of equipment, perform various procedures, and attend to elimination needs. Each contact or task represents a potential transfer of microorganisms. Because you must move quickly from patient to patient, it is easy to forget to wash your hands properly between patients. Although it is hard, it is necessary for beginning student nurses to remember to wash their hands. Handwashing must always be the last task performed before going to the patient and the last performed when leaving. The hands must be washed with flowing warm water over a sink. A good soap or detergent is applied, accompanied by brisk friction. If the hands are dirty, they are rinsed from the wrist downward, the elbows held high to allow microorganisms to be rinsed off the fingers into the sink. This procedure is called *medical asepsis handwashing*. Hands should also be washed after removing sterile gloves because the hands may have microorganisms even though covered with gloves.

If, on the other hand, the hands are uncontaminated and are being washed before putting on sterile gloves or working within a sterile field, *surgical asepsis handwashing* is performed. The hands are thoroughly washed, sometimes with a brush, and rinsed with the elbows low over the sink so that the fingers are rinsed first and the water flows off the elbows into the sink. This procedure makes the fingers the cleanest part of the hands. The aim of *surgical asepsis* is not simply to reduce the number of pathogens but to make the object or person free of all microorganisms. Also known as *sterile technique*, surgical asepsis is reserved primarily for such procedures as changing sterile dressings, performing catheterizations, and maintaining intravenous infusions (see Module 2, Basic Infection Control).

Official Guidelines Affecting Health Care

Hospitals and other health care facilities used to survey and monitor their own rates of infection and wrote independent guidelines to decrease the occurrence of cases. This is no longer the case. Infection control was sometimes lax, causing additional discomfort to the patient and added costs to health care. Currently, throughout the United States and Canada, the governments have assumed the role and responsibility for establishing infection control guidelines and regulations for all aspects of health care.

CDC Guidelines

Basic guidelines for infection control are formulated by the CDC of the U.S. Department of Health. Recognizing that HIV and hepatitis B virus are transmitted through infected blood and body fluids, this agency made recommendations that the procedures in *Universal Precautions for Blood and Body Fluids* be observed by all health care workers in *all* patient situations (Display 21-1). The rationale was the realization that infected persons could not be identified, so that universal protection was necessary. Substances included when using universal precautions are blood, semen, vaginal secretions, cerebrospinal fluid, synovial fluid, pleural fluid, peritoneal fluid, pericardial fluid, amniotic fluid, and other body substances when they contain visible blood.

In addition to these universal precautions, most health care facilities also require the wearing of protective gloves when the health care provider comes in contact with other body substances such as sputum, urine, feces, nasal secretions, and vomitus. This is called body substance precautions. Gloves are worn not only for aesthetic reasons but because these substances contain organisms that can cause nosocomial infections. If visible blood is observed in any of these substances, universal precautions must be observed.

Display 21–1

Substances Included in Universal Precautions for Blood and Body Fluids

Blood	Pleural fluid
Semen	Peritoneal fluid
Vaginal secretions	Pericardial fluid
Cerebrospinal fluid	Amniotic fluid
Synovial fluid	

OSHA Regulations

In 1988, OSHA began formulating new infection control standards for health care facilities that mandated the CDC guidelines. The regulations focused on the use of universal precautions by all health care workers. With a firm "target date" of Spring 1992 for implementation, the written regulations were sent to all health care facilities in the United States. Noncompliance would result in substantial fines being levied against the facility. Universal precautions operates on the assumption that all patients and all medical staff are potentially infected. Although this sounds harsh, in reality it protects possible transmission of harmful organisms from one person to another, regardless of role. The rationale underlying universal precautions follows the principle of setting up barriers to interrupt the chain of infection primarily at the transmission link so that pathogens cannot be transferred. (Review the section earlier in this chapter on the infection chain.) The following guidelines are statements of the OSHA regulations that will directly affect your nursing practice:

1. *Exposure control plan*: Requires employers to identify in writing, tasks and procedures where occupational exposure to blood occurs.
2. *Methods of compliance*: Mandates handwashing and universal precautions that treat body fluids and materials as infected. Sets forth procedures to minimize needle sticks, minimize splashing of blood, and ensure appropriate packaging of specimens and regulated wastes. Employers must provide (at no cost) and require employees to use appropriate personal protective equipment (gloves, masks, mouthpieces, and resuscitation bags; Fig. 21-7).
3. *Hepatitis B vaccination*: Requires hepatitis B vacci-

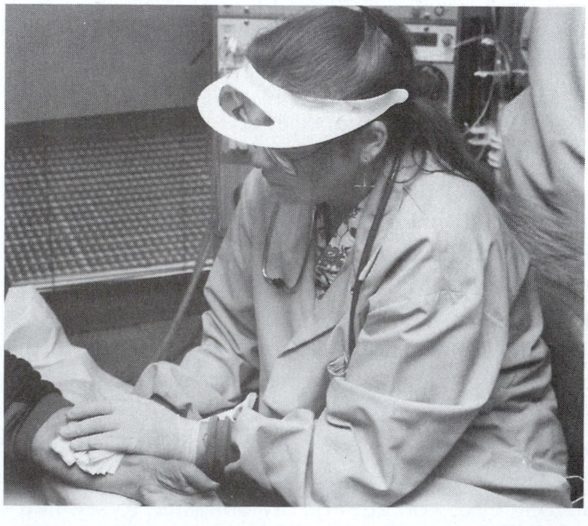

Figure 21-7. Nurse in gloves and face shield is protected from blood splashes.

nation, without prescreening or cost, to be made available to all employees who have occupational exposure to blood within 10 working days of assignment. This should follow the latest recommendation of the U.S. Public Health Service. Employees must sign a declination form if they choose not to be vaccinated. (The American Association of Colleges of Nursing recommends that nursing students be required to have hepatitis B vaccine before beginning clinical practice.)

4. *Postexposure evaluation and follow-up*: Specifies procedures be made available to all employees who have had an exposure incident, including any necessary laboratory tests at no cost. All reporting and testing is to remain confidential.
5. *Hazard communication*: Requires warning labels, including the orange or orange-red biohazard symbol, affixed to containers of regulated waste, refrigerators, freezers, and other containers used to store or transport blood or other potentially infectious materials. Red bags may be used as a substitute for labeling. When a facility uses universal precautions with all specimens, labeling is not required. When all laundry is handled with universal precautions, laundry need not be labelled (Fig. 21-8).
6. *Information and training*: Mandates training within 90 days of effective date, initially on assignment and annually. Employees who have received appropriate training within the past year need to receive training in items not previously covered. The trainer must be knowledgeable and there must be opportunity for questions and answers.
7. *Recordkeeping*: Requires that confidential medical records be kept on each employee with occupational exposure for the duration of employment plus 30 years. Training records must be maintained for 3 years. All records must be made available to the subject employee and will not be released to the employer. They will be made available to anyone with the written consent of the employee or to OSHA. Any disposal of records must be in compliance with OSHA's standards.
8. *Other considerations*: The choice of gloves to be worn is under study. Latex or vinyl gloves are available. The Food and Drug Administration is authorized to test all gloves for production quality. It should be understood that neither glove protects you from needle sticks, making the recommendation to never recap needles even more important. Although both types of gloves cost about the same, you should choose the type that is most appropriate for the task you are performing. Latex is more flexible and more durable than vinyl. For tasks where you need ultimate protection, latex gloves are probably the better choice. However, vinyl gloves are adequate for routine, short-term tasks (Korniewicz, Kirwin, and Larson, 1991, p. 39).

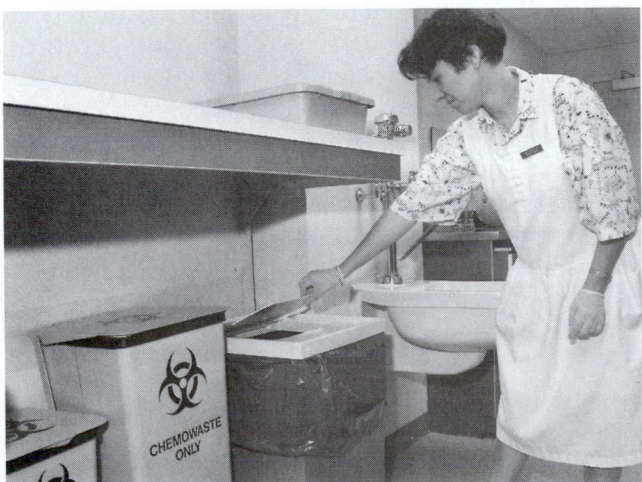

Figure 21-8. Hazardous materials must be disposed of properly.

Another consideration is patient education. The extensive wearing of gloves during the administration of care is new to many patients, making them feel uncomfortable or unclean. Once patients understand that the precautions are not only to protect the caregiver but the patient as well, resistance usually turns to ready acceptance.

Importance of the OSHA Regulations

Although the language of the regulations implies importance for the "employer" and "employee," it is essential that you understand that they apply to you as a student and as a member of the health care team. The intent of the OSHA regulations is to prevent and contain the spread of blood-borne infections, and it is crucial that everyone involved in direct patient care comply. It only takes one person who does not follow the guidelines to disrupt the effectiveness of this infection control plan. Some state nursing boards have policies that outline the responsibility of nurses to report other health care workers, including other nurses, if the regulations are not followed. You will have to consult the policies of your state or province nursing board regarding this matter. The intent is to educate rather than take punitive action.

Representatives from OSHA will conduct unannounced inspections of health care facilities to ensure compliance. Fines will be levied if infractions are found. It should be clear that the purpose for your personal compliance is not to avoid having your institution fined but to practice safety. Remember that the guidelines actually afford mutual protection—protecting staff from potentially infected patients and protecting patients from potentially infected staff.

Let there be no question as to the seriousness of these new federal regulations. You should begin your nursing experience incorporating these preventive measures into your daily care of all patients.

Other Infection Control Methods

Other than universal precautions, which are intended to become a part of the plan of care for *all* patients, on occasion it is appropriate to use other methods of infection control. You should become familiar with these other systems and know when they are appropriate for your patients.

Strict Isolation

Strict isolation is indicated when the organism can be transmitted by both contact and air. Strict isolation means that other patients cannot share the room, and all who enter must protect their clothing as well as the respiratory tract. This protection is achieved by wearing gowns and masks. Because indirect contact is also a consideration, equipment must be guarded against contamination.

Certain strains of meningitis and pneumonia require strict isolation until drugs are effectively instituted. A recent concern is the emergence of methicillin-resistant *Staphylococcus aureus* (MRSA). This is a strain of staphylococcus that has become resistant to the drug, methicillin. Methicillin was, for a period of time, the drug of choice to treat "staph" infections until this strain of organism became resistant. The drug, gentamicin, was then used effectively for a period of time until the organism developed resistance to this drug as well. Other drugs are now used for this infection. The infection is passed primarily from patient to patient by the hands of health care workers (Czurylo, Pfeiffer, and Steffen, 1991, p. 68.) Most at risk are patients with wounds, with suppressed immune systems, and with any drainage tubes in place. For specific techniques for carrying out isolation practices, refer to Module 34, Isolation Technique.

Respiratory Isolation

Respiratory isolation is carried out when the organism is transmitted through the air by droplet formation. It is particularly important in this type of isolation to provide health teaching regarding patient handwashing and the use and disposal of tissues the patient uses when coughing because the organism may also be transmitted by direct contact.

Protective Isolation

Protective isolation in the past was referred to as *reverse isolation*. This type of isolation is designed to protect those whose immune systems are compromised. The word "protection" means that the environment around these individuals poses a considerable threat of infection. Protecting the patient from infection involves that only clean persons and items enter the patient's room. Universal precautions are observed regarding contaminated items from leaving the patient's room. Protective isolation is not used in many hospitals because its effectiveness and necessity are questioned.

Specialized medical centers that perform bone marrow transplants and similar procedures have special laminar air-flow rooms to protect patients who are at extremely high risk of infection. Specially filtered air enters the closed room through one vent, flows through the room, and exits at another vent. The air is constantly circulating and as free of contaminants as possible. Pharmacists often mix and process intravenous medications under laminar air-flow hoods to minimize contamination. In all types of isolation, stringent and conscientious handwashing remains the single most effective measure.

Providing Psychological Comfort for the Isolated Patient

Because communication through masks is difficult and because garbing for isolation is inconvenient, the isolated patient rarely receives as much attention and interchange as a nonisolated patient. Holding the hand of a severely ill or depressed patient through a glove is not a wholly satisfying experience for either nurse or patient. As a result of lack of attention, such patients can become irritable, restless, and depressed.

The nurse can help minimize the emotional and sensory deprivation the isolated patient experiences by spending extra time with the patient, in addition to the time devoted to physical care. Some ideas for creative intervention are offered in Module 34, Isolation Technique.

The patient's self-concept frequently suffers as a result of being considered infectious. Psychological support for the patient throughout this difficult experience is an essential part of total care. Care providers sometimes carelessly use words that may be overheard by the patient, such as "dirty" or "contaminated" when referring to areas of isolation. A patient who overhears such a remark may construe it to mean that he or she is dirty and a danger to others. Comments of this kind should be avoided.

Drugs Used to Treat Infection

There are several hundred *antimicrobial* drugs, many of them simply variations of one another. The antimicrobial drugs that were developed and first used in the 1950s are referred to as first-generation drugs. Organisms became resistant to some of these drugs, making them ineffective. Other drugs were developed, some variations of the first. This group became the second-generation drugs. Concurrently, a third or new generation of antimicrobials is in use along with the development of even of a fourth-generation group. As some of these drugs are withdrawn and later reinstated for treatment of infection, they often regain their effectiveness so that you will see a variety of drug combinations being used for patients.

In general, the antimicrobials are subdivided into three large categories. These three categories should not be confused with their generation or the time they were developed. The *sulfonamides*, low-cost synthetics usually given orally, have an antibacterial effect. The second group consists of the *antibiotics*, both natural and synthetic. Natural antibiotics are derived from yeasts and molds that have a destructive effect on the more virulent pathogens. The *antifungals*, the third group, are agents used specifically against fungal infections.

When you administer these preparations, it is your responsibility to know not only their actions but also their contraindications and side effects (see Chapters 1 and Chapter 39). Because these drugs have varied and potentially dangerous side effects, close observation is always necessary. Besides watching for the allergic reactions that may occur in response to antimicrobials, you will be monitoring the effect of a particular drug on the patient and his or her progress. You might note, for example, a diminishing fever, lessening of the general malaise that frequently accompanies an infection, the improved appearance of an infected wound, or the patient's reported feeling of increased well-being.

Assessment

The patient's need, first and foremost, is to be protected from infection. Thus, identifying those at high risk for infection should be of prime concern in addition to recognizing the signs and symptoms of infection in patients under your care.

Interview

In identifying both those at risk for infection and those who have an infection, the information obtained from a careful history is as important as the information gained from the physical assessment and laboratory tests. Although signs and symptoms of infection are well documented, they can be manifested differently in various persons and age groups.

Obtaining as much information as possible about a patient's complaint of pain is important because this symptom can provide the major clue to infection even before physical assessment or laboratory tests indicate its presence. Critical information about high-risk states can also be obtained during the interview.

Physical Assessment

The first step in assessment is to identify patients who may be at high risk for infection. Although any patient within the care setting is at some risk for infection, some are in more danger than others. We have already discussed many of the patients in the high-risk category: the very young (because their immune systems are immature) and the elderly (because their immune systems are less vigorous). Other persons at risk are those who have chronic illness or suppressed immunity, patients having invasive tests or procedures performed, surgical patients, and those with equipment such as intravenous infusions, catheters, or drains. The incontinent patient can also be in jeopardy because of difficulty in maintaining standards of personal hygiene. Any patient with a decreased white blood cell count, whether it is an effect of medication or a complication of the illness, is at risk for infection.

The second step in assessment is to identify the presence of an infection. In caring for some patients, it is important for the nurse to be constantly vigilant for early signs of infection to ensure that medical and nursing interventions begin promptly. If the infection is localized to a specific part of the body, you may find that the area reveals **inflammation** as well as an infection. The infected area may be warm to the touch, reddened, swollen, painful, and, if it is an extremity, difficult to move. There may also be drainage or an exudate. Some bacteria cause a serous exudate, whereas more serious infections often produce **purulent drainage** (drainage with pus). See Chapter 6 for a further discussion of inflammation. Although a generalized infection may not be as apparent as one that is localized, it can be very serious and even life threatening. If large numbers of bacteria enter the blood, a dangerous condition called *septicemia* can result. Signs and symptoms of a generalized infection include *malaise*, weakness, fever, head pain, anorexia, and swelling of the lymph nodes.

Diagnostic Testing

Identifying the microorganism involved in an infection is vital to successful treatment. Culture and sensitivity testing of the affected tissue is ordered by the physician so that the correct antibiotic can be administered to the patient. As a nurse, it is important for you to know what bacteria have been identified so that you have a better understanding of the drugs being used for treatment.

Blood tests are also a part of the patient's work-up, an elevated white blood cell count being one of the body's first defenses against both localized and generalized infection. Increased or decreased levels of other blood components can also be used by the physician in the diagnosis of infection.

Nursing Diagnosis

The North American Nursing Diagnosis Association (NANDA) has accepted the diagnosis High Risk for Infection. An etiology should be added. The diagnosis High Risk for Infection may be related to a variety of health problems or situations that could lead to the development of an infection.

A related factor may be a concurrent disease or a condition that places the person at risk, such as malnutrition, diabetes, or AIDS. Another risk factor could be related to invasive procedures or devices such as total parenteral nutrition or dialysis. The elderly with chronic disease and children who are not protected by immunization make up maturational factors that may lead to infection.

Nursing Diagnoses Related to Infection

High Risk for Infection related to
- altered immune response
- altered production of leukocytes
- advanced age

High Risk for Infection: Wound related to surgical incision

High Risk for Infection: Urinary tract related to presence of indwelling catheter

Pain: Burning on urination related to urinary tract infection

Activity Intolerance related to infected leg ulcer

Self-care Deficit: Bathing/Hygiene related to extreme malaise caused by infection

High Risk for Infection Transmission

Another nursing diagnosis regarding infection, High Risk for Infection Transmission, is not, as yet, NANDA approved. This diagnosis also needs a statement of etiology. This diagnosis is appropriate when there is potential for activating the infection chain so that pathogens could be transferred. This diagnosis would be appropriate for a patient with a blood-borne infection or one with copious wound drainage. Other objective data that could lead to this diagnosis might be the presence of infected respiratory secretions or a systemic viral infection.

Knowledge Deficit

The patient with an infection or who is at high risk of an infection needs health teaching that will provide adequate knowledge concerning infection. Through simple handwashing and hygiene, the patient can learn to be more protective regarding infection. If the person has an infection, knowledge can be gained regarding implementation that can help resolve the infection.

Other Nursing Diagnoses Related to Infection

For patients with an infection, nursing diagnoses should be written to identify patient problems caused by the symptoms of the infection process. It is useful to be as specific as possible. Patient problems related to the presence of infection include discomfort in the form of muscle cramps, pain, or cough. Fever is often used as a diagnosis because a common cause is infection. An activity or self-care deficit caused by the presence of infection may appropriately be stated as a nursing diagnosis.

By using these diagnoses, the nurse can plan the first step in either preventing an infection in a susceptible individual or in preventing the spread of infection to another.

Planning and Implementation

Planning and intervention should relate directly to the nursing diagnosis. When the nursing diagnosis is High Risk for Infection, the desired outcome is a patient who remains infection free. If there is danger of transmission of disease, the outcome is the containment of infection to the involved patient. When there is an actual infection, the infection management measures should lead to a complete resolution of infection. Desired outcomes should also consider the patient's need for relief from discomfort and from the debilitating effects of fluid loss and immobility.

The interventions needed for these outcomes to occur are a combination of both general comfort measures and specific infection control techniques. These techniques have as their purpose the interruption of the infection chain, and many of them, such as handwashing, are nursing actions that become an integral part of the care given to every patient (Table 21-l). Care of the patient with infection is also an area of nursing in which collaborative management often comes into play.

Protecting the Patient From Infection

Planning and intervention should relate directly to the nursing diagnosis. When there is a nursing diagnosis for high risk, intervention should be aimed at protecting the patient and preventing infection (see sample Nursing Care Plan Related to Infection). If transmission is a danger, intervention is focused toward establishing barriers and if an actual infection is present, infection management measures are taken. Interventions address the prevention of transmission of infection as well as the management of symptoms. Interventions can be designed to protect the patient from infection or to protect others.

The symptoms of infection often cause the patient discomfort for which interventions are needed. Actions involve carrying out nursing judgments and participating in the medical plan of care. If the patient had a low white blood count or a compromised immune system for some reason, the nursing intervention used in the past was to place the patient in protective isolation. However, this practice was not effective in most cases. These patients may currently be identified as "compromised hosts," and simpler precautions are taken, such as strict handwashing and keeping the patient away from persons known to have an infection. Severely immunocompromised patients (such as bone marrow transplant recipients) are placed in specially controlled protective environments. If your assessment indicates the possibility that an infection is present, you may need to place a patient in some type of isolation until the patient's status can be determined with more certainty.

Interventions are also designed to prevent nosocomial infections. Many intervention plans stress the need for using sterile technique when doing surgical dressings or inserting catheters. Actions such as encouraging activity and the intake of fluids by the patient at risk of pneumonia are also appropriate interventions.

Table 21–1. Interruption of the Infection Chain

Link in the Infection Chain	Nursing Action
Infectious agent	Knowledge of the characteristics of pathogens Sterilization techniques
Reservoir	Surveillance of reservoirs in the hospital Handwashing and, when appropriate, surgical asepsis Personal cleanliness
Transmission	Knowledge of pathogens' routes of transmission Routine medical asepsis Isolation, when appropriate
Susceptible host	Knowledge of factors affecting susceptibility Identification of high-risk patients Knowledge of pharmacology relative to antibiotics Clean environment Support of body's own defenses
Portal of entry	Precautions to ensure food and equipment are free of contamination Measures to keep integument intact Sterile technique when skin is not intact and for invasive procedures
Portal of exit	Proper handling of secretions and excreta Special precautions with needles and syringes, when appropriate Proper disposal of linens and equipment

Providing Care for the Patient With an Infection

The ill person needs adequate rest, and an ill person with an infection needs additional rest and sleep. Providing for such rest sometimes requires ingenious planning of nursing care. Because infection makes increased demands on the body, the diet must not be deficient. Intake of protein and carbohydrates is especially important: protein helps in healing damaged tissue, and carbohydrates help to meet the increased metabolic requirements caused by infection. High fluid intake prevents dehydration resulting from fever and aids in the excretion of toxins (poisonous protein substances produced by pathogens) from the body (see Chapter 25).

Meticulous hygiene should be observed when caring for a patient suffering from an infection. Such patients are often *diaphoretic* (perspiring) because of fever, which necessitates frequent bathing. General malaise may prevent the patient from performing adequate self-hygiene. Infection can also cause foul odors, unpleasant to the patient and the staff alike, which can be alleviated by frequent and adequate hygiene. For exam-

Nursing Care Plan

Sample Nursing Care Plan Related to Infection

Nursing Diagnosis	High Risk for Infection: Urinary tract related to presence of indwelling catheter **Supportive data:** Indwelling catheter inserted.
Desired Patient Outcomes	**The patient will remain free of urinary tract infection during time of indwelling urinary catheter, as evidenced by:** No fever. Continuous urinary output. Clear-appearing urine. No urinary tract discomfort.

Nursing Action	Rationale
1. Encourage 3,000 ml of fluid per day. a. 1,200 ml during day shift b. 800 ml during evening shift c. 400 ml during night shift	High fluid intake facilitates kidney function, decreasing risk for infection. Providing fluids during the day will allow elimination to occur during the waking hours while limiting fluid intake in the evening will decrease the need to void during sleep.
2. Hygiene of perineal area once per shift.	Removing pathogens from the perineal area prevents contamination of the urinary tract.
3. Keep catheter collection bag below level of bladder.	Keeping the collection device positioned below the level of the bladder prevents the backflow of urine from the tubing.
4. Monitor patient for signs of urinary tract infection: fever, cloudy urine, burning around catheter, or abdominal/flank pain.	Regularly monitoring the patient for signs of infection allows early intervention if signs are present.

ple, the plan of care of a patient with a *suppurating* (pus-discharging) wound should also specify frequent dressing changes and cleansing of the wound area. The patient suffering a severe throat infection needs extra oral care.

Providing Comfort Measures and Fluids

Nursing interventions for patient discomfort caused by infection may be simple comfort measures, such as keeping the room at a cool but comfortable temperature for the patient with a cough. In this case, you might also intervene by administering medications ordered by the physician to subdue the cough. Sometimes the same intervention can be used with both the patient at risk and the patient who is infected. For example, the interventions mentioned above for the patient at risk of pneumonia—encouraging activity and intake of fluids—also assist the patient with a respiratory infection: the increased fluids help liquefy secretions, and activity at an appropriate level increases the ability to move and expectorate the secretions from the tract.

Administering Antimicrobials

The nurse will collaborate with the medical plan of care by administering any ordered antimicrobials. These drugs are instituted to subdue the organisms causing the infection. Before a particular drug is chosen, the patient may have a culture and sensitivity laboratory test to determine which of a variety of drugs will be most effective in eradicating a certain organism. It is important to administer the medications at the prescribed time and for the prescribed course of doses so that the blood level of the drug remains constant. Any untoward reactions to a drug should be reported immediately.

Providing Emotional Support

Finally, the patient with an infection needs emotional support from the nurse and family. Infection is a psychological as well as physical assault on the body. The patient often interprets an infection to mean that things are not going well or as planned. Infection is frequently called a *complication*, which understandably makes the patient anxious. An explanation of the vigorous efforts being made to treat and control the infection usually reassures the patient.

Health Teaching

In any situation related to infection, whether it is risk for infection or the presence of infection, teaching good handwashing and hygiene is an important task for the nurse. There are many areas for health teaching the patient and the family or those significant to the patient. Effectively taking medications for the infection or the proper disposal of secretions may be a part of health teaching. Techniques to be used when performing procedures, such as how to maintain clean or sterile technique, are also areas commonly taught.

Evaluation

Evaluation must always be patient centered and focus on desired outcomes. Evaluation should be a continuing process, directed toward the changing status of the patient: the patient continues to be free of infection, the patient's infection is resolving, or the patient has not infected anyone else.

Nursing Care Study
A Patient in Isolation

A call from the admitting department said that John Marcus, an alert 70-year-old retired gardener was to be admitted to the medical unit for management of his diabetes. It was also on the record that he had a methicillin-resistant staphylococcus infection (MRSA) of a leg ulcer, which required strict isolation. Joan Sealy, staff nurse, consulted the infection control manual for that infection. It stated that a private room was needed and that gowns and gloves were to be worn. Masks were not necessary unless the patient or nurse had an active respiratory infection. Isolation was to remain in effect for 7 to 10 days while the antimicrobial therapy was being given. An instruction card was obtained, appropriately filled out, and attached to the door.

Joan's assessment revealed that John was quite ill, with a fluctuating high blood glucose level, fever, and a beginning leg ulcer. Joan administered the ordered drug along with an antipyretic to reduce the fever. She sat and talked with John; they chatted briefly about music and sports. Then Joan, wearing isolation garb, explained what MRSA was and why isolation was necessary. Joan assured John that his family and friends would be able to visit later when John felt better and could enjoy seeing them more. Joan explained that all visitors should follow the instructions on the door card advising them to report to the nurse's station first, so that the isolation procedure could be explained and they could garb properly for protection. She also told John that isolation makes some patients feel neglected and they get bored, so maybe John might like to watch the television mounted high on the wall, read newspapers or magazines, and have friends call.

Joan wrote the care plan, incorporating the data from her interview with John and the isolation precautions. She shared this at team report and added a comment that reasonable visits should be made to John's room to check with him and see if anything was needed.

Four days later, John began to improve, his diabetes was stabilizing, and his leg ulcer was healing. The fifth day, isolation was discontinued and the care plan altered. John, with great relief, said he felt much better now that they were no longer asking everyone to wear masks and gowns. He commented, "This was all so new to me and I must admit that when we first met, I was really scared. Thank you for explaining things so well."

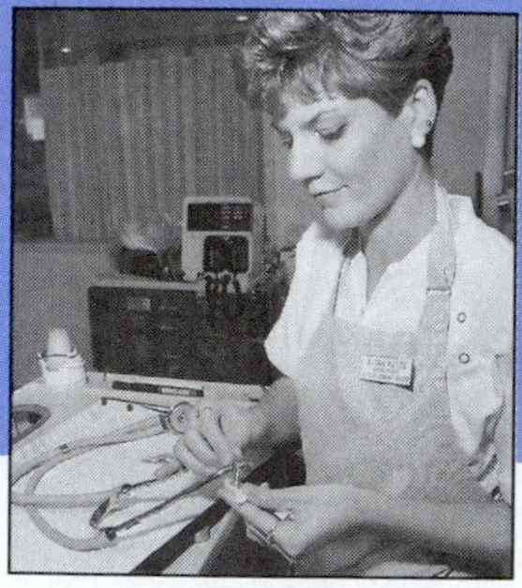

Key Points

- Nurses have the fundamental responsibility of ensuring basic physical and psychological safety for each person under care.
- Both nurses and patients can be exposed to a variety of potentially unsafe situations in the care setting. Therefore, nurses must protect both patients and themselves from harm.
- Because nurses give the majority of direct care to patients, they need to have extensive knowledge about and skill in prevention and control of infection.
- There are six major categories of microorganisms: bacteria, viruses, fungi, protozoa, parasitic worms, and rickettsia. Pathogens are microorganisms capable of causing infections.
- Pathogens infect people by a process referred to as the infection chain. Interruption of the infection chain is the basic goal of nurses' efforts to protect patients from infection.
- The WHO, CDC, and OSHA are organizations involved in the prevention and control of infection.
- OSHA has set standards for the prevention of the spread of blood- and fluid-borne disease that must be implemented by all health care facilities.
- The infection control committee within each facility internally monitors and makes recommendations for protection of patients and staff.
- The body's structure and physiology are important in protecting it from infection, for example, the skin, the mucosal tissues, and gastric secretions.
- The immune system and a healthy lifestyle also protect the body from invading microorganisms.
- Those at particular risk of infection include the very young, the very old, those with a chronic illness, and those whose immune systems have been suppressed by disease or the administration of certain drugs.
- All hospitalized patients are at risk of nosocomial infection.
- Meticulous attention to handwashing is the most important defense against the spread of infection.
- Infection is usually treated by the administration of drugs, including sulfonamides, antibiotics, and antifungals.
- Nurses have an important role, both as practitioners and health teachers, in providing a safe and infection-free environment that satisfies the patient's basic need for safety.

Study Questions

1. Describe the characteristics of a safe patient's room.
2. What patients in the hospital setting would you identify as most at risk for physical injury?
3. What factors within the health care facility might lead to the patient's feeling psychologically unsafe?
4. Name some of the safety hazards in the workplace for nurses.
5. What are the smallest of all microorganisms, and what are three infections they cause?
6. When using "universal precautions," you are focusing on what part of the infection chain?
7. Name and describe persons who are most at risk of infection.
8. Name three areas of the body that are natural barriers to pathogens, and explain why this is so.
9. Briefly discuss the immune process and how it protects people from invasion by microorganisms.
10. What lifestyle factors are helpful in warding off infections?
11. Discuss three important functions of the infection control nurse.
12. What measures will you take to follow the OSHA infection control guidelines?

Critical Thinking Activities

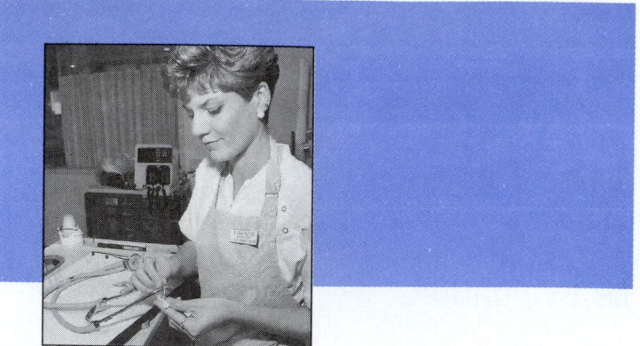

1. Focusing on visits to the laundry, kitchen, and medical laboratory of your facility, analyze the actions taken in each setting to treat contaminated articles, preventing infection. Include the type of organism, its route of transmission, and the method used for cleaning.
2. Give a brief presentation on the topic of "aseptic conscience." Relate it to professional values and its importance to the nursing role.
3. Write a nursing care plan for a patient with bacterial pneumonia. What nursing diagnoses are possible and what nursing actions can be taken?
4. With a small group of students, take the position FOR universal immunization in the health care sys-

tem. Incorporate the benefits to society as well as the economic impact nationally.

5. Find an article in a recent periodical regarding the increase of one type of infection. Identify the most important parts of the article, such as what causes the infection, how it is spread and community efforts to control or eradicate the infection. How serious to health is the outbreak, what pathogens are involved and are suggestions for control adequate?

Relevant Sections in Modules for Basic Nursing Skills

Volume I Module
- Basic Infection Control 2
- Safety 3
- Assisting with Elimination and Perineal Care 10
- Hygiene 11
- Using Physical Restraints 21

Volume II Module
- Isolation Technique 34
- Sterile Technique 35
- Surgical Asepsis: Scrubbing, Gowning, and Gloving 36
- Wound Care 37

References and Readings

Besler, C. "The Greening of Hospitals. . . Joining the Fight to Save the Environment." *RN* 2, 1 (February 1990): 12–16.

Blakeslee, J. A. "Untie the Elderly." *American Journal of Nursing* 88, 6 (June 1988): 833–834.

Brennan, L. "The Battle Against AIDS." *Nursing '88* 18, 4 (April 1988): 60–64.

Carpenito, L. J. *Nursing Diagnosis: Application to Clinical Practice.* 4th edition. Philadelphia: J. B. Lippincott, 1992.

Ching, T. Y., and Seto, W. H. "The Efficacy of the Infection Control Liaison Nurse in the Hospital." *Journal of Advanced Nursing* 15, 10 (October 1990): 1128–1131.

Cornell, C. C. "Tuberculosis in Hospital Employees." *American Journal of Nursing* 88, 4 (April 1988): 484–485.

Craft, K. "Do You Really Know How to Handle Sharps." *RN* 53, 8 (August 1990): 33–35.

Cuzzell, J. Z., and Stotts, N. A. "Wound Care: Trial and Error Yields to Knowledge." *American Journal of Nursing* 90, 10 (October 1990): 53–60.

Czurylo, K., Pfeiffer, A., and Steffen, M. "Dealing with a Hidden Hazard: MRSA." *Nursing '91* 21, 12 (December 1991): 68–69.

Doan-Johnson, S. "Taking a Closer Look at Needle-Sticks." *Nursing '92* 22, 8 (August 1992): 24–27.

Eagan, J. "Measles: An Infection Control Nightmare." *RN* 54, 6 (June 1991): 26–29.

Elliot, P. "Handwashing: A Process of Judgment and Effective Decision-Making." *Professional Nurse* 7, 5 (February 1992): 292–296.

Evra, G. "Danger . . . Hospital at Work: Nurses in the OR." *Revolution.* 2, 2 (Summer 1992): 64–66.

Fletcher, K. R. "Restraints Should be a Last Resort." *RN* 53, 1 (January 1990): 52–56.

Gropper, E. I. "Florence Nightingale: Nursing's First Environmental Theorist." *Nursing Forum* 25, 3 (March 1990): 30–33.

Hilton, A. "The Hospital Racket: How Noisy Is Your Unit?" *American Journal of Nursing* 87, 1 (January 1987): 59–61.

Jackson, M. M., and Lynch, P. "Infection Control: In Search of a Rational Approach." *American Journal of Nursing* 90, 10 (October 1990): 65–73.

Jacobson, E. "New Hospital Hazards: How to Protect Yourself." Part 1. *American Journal of Nursing* 90, 2 (February 1990): 36–41.

———. "Hospital Hazards: How to Protect Yourself." Part 2 *American Journal of Nursing* 90, 4 (April 1990): 48–53.

Jurgrau, A. "Why Aren't We Protecting our Children?" *RN* 53, 11 (November 1990): 30–34.

Korniewicz, D., Kirwin, M., and Larson, E. "Do Your Gloves Fit the Task?" *American Journal of Nursing* 91, 6 (June 1991): 38–40.

Larson, E. "Handwashing: It's Essential—Even When You Use Gloves." *American Journal of Nursing* 89, 7 (July 1989): 834–839.

Lemmink, J. A. "Infection Control: When A Surgical Wound Becomes Infected." *RN* 50, 9 (September 1987): 24–27.

Marchiondo, K. "Flu Vaccine: Give it, Get it." *RN* 54, 10 (October 1991): 59–62.

Millam, D. "Avoiding Needle-Stick Injuries." *Nursing '90* 20, 1 (January 1990): 61–63.

Mooney, B. R., and Armington, L. C. "Infection Control: How to Prevent Nosocomial Infections." *RN* 50, 9 (September 1987): 20–23.

Morton, D. "Five Years of Fewer Falls." *American Journal of Nursing* 89, 2 (February 1989): 204–205.

Murray, R., and Zentner, J. *Nursing Assessment and Health Promotion Strategies Through the Life Span.* 4th edition. Norwalk, Conn.: Appleton and Lange, 1989.

Rogers, B., and Travers, P. "Overview of Work-Related Hazards in Nursing: Health and Safety Needs." *Journal of Critical Care* 20, 9 (September 1991): 486–499.

Ruscitti, C. "Caring for a Combative Patient." *Nursing '92* 22, 9 (September 1992): 50–51.

Shovein, J. "MRSA: An infection Control Crisis Comes Home." *RN* 52, 7 (July 1989): 42–48.

Stilling, L. "The Pros and Cons of Physical Restraints and Behavior Controls." *Psychosocial Nursing* 30, 3 (March 1992): 18–20.

Walz, J. A. "A Simulated Disaster Drill." *American Journal of Nursing* 88, 3 (March 1988): 301–303.

Skin Integrity and Hygiene

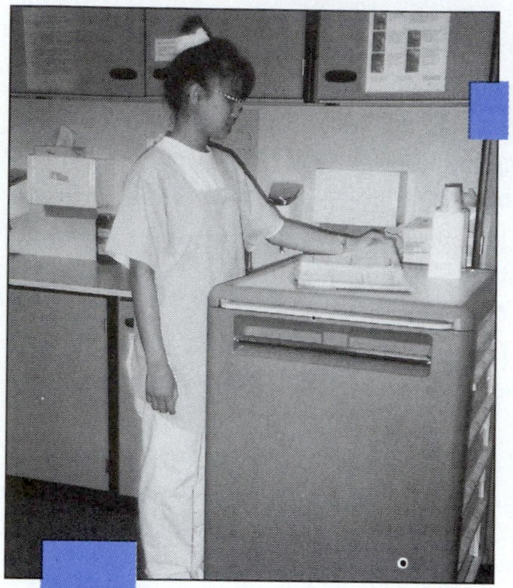

22

Objectives

After completing this chapter, you should be able to:

1. Name the three goals of hygiene.
2. Outline components of hygienic care for the patient.
3. Describe structures of the integumentary system.
4. Discuss skin assessment, comparing normal and abnormal characteristics.
5. List nursing diagnoses and nursing actions related to maintaining skin integrity.
6. Identify characteristics of patients at risk of pressure ulcers.
7. Explain nursing actions that can prevent the development of pressure ulcers.
8. Explain independent and collaborative nursing actions used to treat pressure ulcers.
9. Describe the appearance of a nurse who practices good hygiene and looks professional.

Study Terms

artificial tears
blanching
caries
clubbed fingers
debridement
deciduous teeth
desquamation
ecchymosis
eschar
hexachlorophene
hygiene
jaundice
keratin
maceration
pressure ulcer
smegma
turgor

Outline

The Integumentary System

Skin
- Composition of the Skin
- Function of the Skin
- Appearance of Normal Skin

Accessory Parts of the Integument
- Hair
- Nails

Teeth

Common Problems Affecting Skin Integrity

Chronic and Acute Skin Disorders
Surgical or Traumatic Wounds
Pressure Ulcers

Assessment Related to the Integumentary System

- Interview
- Physical Assessment
- Patients at Risk of Pressure Ulcers

Ellis, Nowlis: Nursing: A Human Needs Approach, 5th ed. © 1994 J.B. Lippincott Company

Maintaining adequate hygiene and skin integrity are basic to the practice of nursing. The nurse must be a role model in maintaining impeccable hygiene when caring for others. It is also important for the nurse and the patient to have the skin protected against breaks or blemishes that may allow the entrance of microorganisms. This chapter provides guidelines for maintaining and administering hygiene to the patient. The integumentary system is discussed relative to assessment and care of the skin of those who have limited mobility or are ill.

The Integumentary System

The integumentary system is composed of the outer coverings of the body. It protects the vital organs that lie within the body. For purposes of giving hygienic care, nurses focus on the skin, mucous membranes, hair, nails, and teeth.

Skin

The skin is actually an organ of the body. It is a bodily structure that fulfills a certain purpose—encasing the other organs. Additional functions of the skin are discussed later. Another name for the skin is the *integument.* The skin accounts for 16% of total body weight (Delancy and North, 1983) and is the largest organ of the body. The skin is also one of the fastest growing tissues in the human body and is constantly replacing itself (Dossey, 1983; Fig. 22-1).

Composition of the Skin

The skin has two distinct layers, the epidermis, or outer layer, and the dermis, which lies beneath. The *epidermis,* which is made up of epithelial tissue containing no blood vessels, consists of four layers over most of the body and a fifth layer that covers the palms of the hands and the soles of the feet. The two layers of the epidermis that we will discuss are the stratum corneum and the stratum germinativum. In the outer layer, or *stratum corneum,* dead cells change into a protein substance called **keratin**. This substance flakes off in a process called **desquamation**. In the deepest layer, or *stratum germinativum,* new cells are produced at the same rate as those above are desquamated. These new cells continually move upward through the outer layers until they, too, are keratinized and flake off. The lower level, or *dermis,* contains blood and lymphatic vessels, nerve

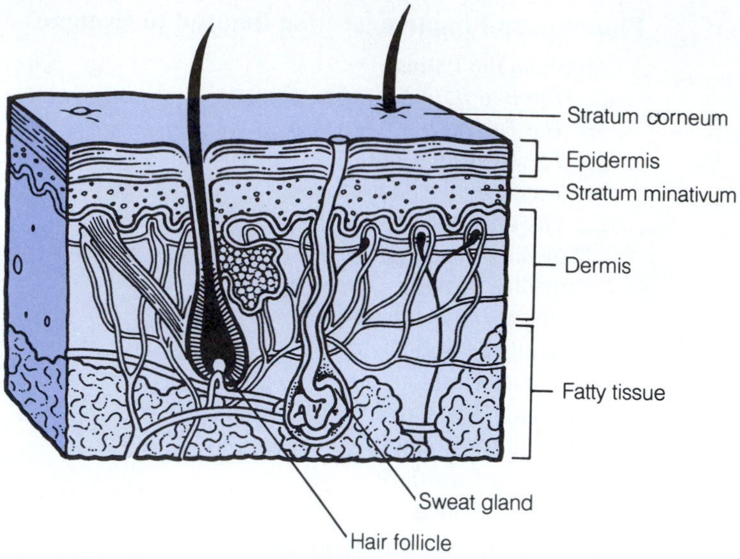

Figure 22-1. Cross-section of the skin.

endings, glands, and hair follicles. This lower layer is important in skin healing because it is where new tissue growth occurs.

Function of the Skin

The intact skin protects the body from invasive organisms (see Chapter 21). The constant flaking off of the top layer makes it difficult for organisms to reside on the surface, and the slightly acid pH of the skin creates an inhospitable climate for microbial growth. The fifth, thicker layer of skin on the palms of the hands and the soles of the feet provides extra protection from sharp, potentially piercing objects.

The skin contains water and fat, which help regulate body temperature. In fact "goose bumps," which occur when a person is exposed to cold, are produced by the body in an attempt to conserve body heat; the sudden constriction of the tiny *arrector pili muscles* that surround hair follicles causes a tightening of the skin. This tightening prevents the evaporation of moisture, which cools the body. When a person is too warm or has a fever, sweat ducts in the skin emit moisture so that the patient perspires; the moisture evaporates and cools the body. Secreting large amounts of perspiration is called *diaphoresis*.

Skin coloring affords some degree of protection against the direct rays of the sun, which can be found in some of the most southern parts of the world, and against wind and harsh climates, such as those found in the arctic regions. The color of an individual's skin is determined by heredity; the skin's coloring agent is a pigment called *melanin*, which is deposited in the epidermis.

The nerves of the skin are important as receptors, transmitting such sensations as temperature, pain, tickle, and itch. These sensations are conveyed to the brain and then to other body systems for the body to take compensatory actions to protect the person.

Dossey refers to the skin as "the main organ of communication" for some individuals. Furthermore, he surmises that touching "generates a cascade of biochemical events whose reverberations in the body are more pervasive and complex than might be imagined" (Dossey, 1983, p. 2). We recognize the value of *therapeutic touch* as a mechanism for mobilizing effective body responses to stressors. Research has demonstrated physiologic changes from therapeutic touch. The handshake of friendship, the stroking of an infant, and the touch between a nurse or family member and the patient are alike in that the feeling of another human's skin conveys what sometimes cannot be said.

Appearance of Normal Skin

Normal skin should be smooth and supple with good **turgor**, meaning that the texture is elastic and movable. Good turgor requires sufficient moisture. Skin is normally soft in texture and warm to the touch. The skin of white persons is usually a faint pink, and the mucous membranes are a deeper pink. People who are not white have a variety of skin colors, from yellow to shades of brown ranging from light tan to deep brown. The skin should not be *mottled*; that is, the skin should not have splotches of red or blue coloring, which are evidence of impaired circulation. Finally, the skin should be intact, without blemishes or lesions, because any break or impaired area can lead to invasion by

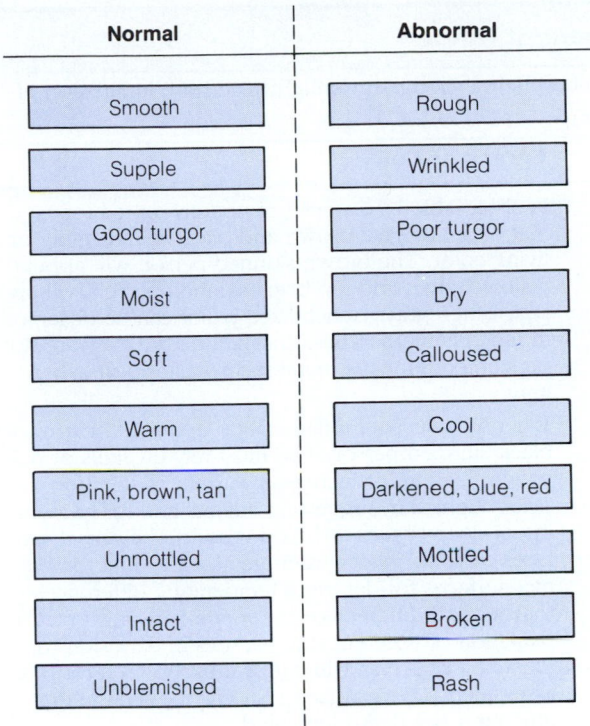

Normal	Abnormal
Smooth	Rough
Supple	Wrinkled
Good turgor	Poor turgor
Moist	Dry
Soft	Calloused
Warm	Cool
Pink, brown, tan	Darkened, blue, red
Unmottled	Mottled
Intact	Broken
Unblemished	Rash

Figure 22-2. Characteristics of normal and abnormal skin.

pathogens, endangering other systems. Residing on the surface of normal skin are 3 million bacteria per square centimeter (Gould, 1991). Figure 22-2 lists the characteristics of normal and abnormal skin and Table 22-1 presents a guide for assessing comparative skin color changes.

The *mucous membranes* are contiguous with the skin; they line the passageways of the body that open to the exterior, such as the mouth and digestive tract, and the respiratory and genitourinary tracts. (Serous membranes line those passageways that do not open to the exterior of the body.) Mucous membranes not only protect the body against the invasion of pathogens, but also secrete *mucus*, a lubricating agent that mixes with and moistens food and absorbs water, salts, and other substances and in the lungs, and traps foreign material.

Accessory Parts of the Integument

The hair and nails are accessory organs to the skin. Nurses care for these areas as well as the skin, and some basic knowledge about them is useful.

Hair

Except for the palms of the hands and the soles of the feet, the entire body is covered by hair. Like the skin, the hair is in layers, the lower layer producing new cells that push upward and undergo the keratinizing process. The visible part of a hair is called the *shaft*, and the part rooted in the dermis, or deeper layer of the skin, is termed the *follicle*. As long as the follicle with its attached blood capillaries remains healthy, the hair, even if cut or shaved to skin level, will regrow. The hair is kept soft by the *sebaceous gland's* secretion of oil. The lashes around the eyes and the fine hairs of the nose and ears protect those organs from dust and insects.

Nails

The nails are composed of keratinized *epithelial cells*, which, because of their hardness, protect the digits (fingers and toes). Historically, early human beings used the nails to protect themselves, scratch for grains, or prepare food.

The normal nail is hard in texture and should be smooth without ridges. The nail bed shows beneath the nail but is not part of the nail itself. The nail bed in white people is pink; in persons of color, the nail bed is a pinkish tan. The angle of the nail to the finger is also important in assessment; it is normally approximately 160° (Fig. 22-3). A person whose nails curve upward (*spoon shape*) could have an iron deficiency anemia. When the fingers "club," the nails flatten and the angle of the nail to the finger increases so that it resembles a club (**clubbed fingers**). Persons with clubbed fingers have had a long-standing problem with oxygenation such as that occurring with emphysema. Precisely why this change occurs in the fingers is not clearly understood. The color of the nail beds can be a tool for assessing circulation. Paleness is one sign of poor tissue perfusion.

The fingernails and toenails of many older adults are thickened and ridged because of age-related changes. The skin around the nails should be intact, protecting them from local infection. Infection can spread underneath the nail to the nail bed, where it is more difficult to treat.

Teeth

Although the teeth are not an accessory organ of the skin, their care is also an important aspect of hygiene. The first of the deciduous teeth usually erupts by the time a child reaches the age of 6 months. By the age of 24 months, a child generally has all 20 of the deciduous teeth. These teeth allow the individual to chew (masticate) until the permanent teeth forming beneath the gums push their way upward, causing the shallow-rooted deciduous teeth to be shed. Between the ages of 6 and 14, a child acquires 32 permanent teeth to replace

Table 22–1. Comparative Skin Color Change Assessment Guide

The best time to do skin assessment is when bathing the patient. The best light is nonglare sunlight. The soft illumination of most overhead lights is inadequate for observing subtle skin changes.

	White Person	**Person of Color**
Pallor	Occurs when the cutaneous vessels are severely constricted. The skin takes on the color of the subcutaneous connective tissue, which is composed mainly of collagen fibers and has a whitish hue.	Is observable by absence of underlying red tones that normally give brown and black skin its glow or living color. The brown-skinned person will appear yellow-brown and the black-skinned person will appear ashen gray. Generalized pallor can be observed in mucous membranes, lips, nail beds if they are not pigmented. Mucous membranes will appear ashen gray.
Erythema	Means redness caused by vasodilation of the cutaneous blood vessels that brings more blood to the surface layer of the skin as the body attempts to lose internal heat.	When you suspect inflammation in a dark brown- or black-skinned person, you must rely on skills of palpation: feeling for increased warmth of skin, for "slick" tight skin suggesting edema, and for hardening of deep tissues or blood vessels. The dorsal surfaces of your fingers are more sensitive that the palmar surfaces for detecting temperature differences (use several different areas for comparison). Practice palpation of different skin textures in dark skin to identify a skin rash (fingertips must be used for this assessment). Generalized rash may be seen in oral mucosa if not dark-pigmented.
Cyanosis	Hypoxia or lack of oxygen in the late stages causes a bluish tinge of the skin. The color is the result of excessive amounts of deoxygenated hemoglobin in the cutaneous blood vessels. It is best observed in the earlobes, lips, around the mouth, cheeks, nail beds (pinch the fingertips; if capillary filling is normal, the nail beds will remain pink). Other observations should be made: assess person's behavior (appropriate vs. inappropriate), level of consciousness, rate, rhythm, and regularity of respirations, presence of secretions causing obstruction.	This is the most difficult clinical sign to observe in dark-skinned persons. Become familiar with the precyanotic color of the patient. Closely inspect lips, tongue, conjunctivae, palms, soles of feet at regular intervals. When cyanosis is questionable, apply light pressure to create pallor. In cyanosis, tissue color returns slowly by spreading from the periphery to the center. Normally, the color returns in less than one second, appearing to return below the pallid spot and the periphery. The lips and tongue become ashen gray color in a black person who is cyanotic.
Ecchymosis	Medical term for "bruise." When a blood vessel is broken, the blood, which quickly becomes deoxygenated, seeps out into the subcutaneous tissues, turning purple-blue color or blue color. As this is reabsorbed, the color changes to yellow and yellow-green. "Purpura" refers to large areas of ecchymosis.	It is difficult to assess in dark skin. You must depend on the history of trauma or accompanying discomfort that suggests the presence of ecchymosis unless it is complicated by the presence of a hematoma (swelling), which can be felt on skin surface. It can also be observed in the oral mucosa on conjunctiva if trauma occurs in these areas.
Petechiae	These are round, pinpoint spots of purplish red color which result from intradermal or submucosal bleeding.	The oral mucosa or conjunctivae should be assessed in dark skin, since petechiae cannot be seen on a dark-pigmented person's skin.
Jaundice	The excessive accumulation of bilirubin in the tissues produces a yellow color. Jaundice occurs when bile pigments discolor plasma, skin, and mucous membranes. It is usually noticed in the sclera of the eye and skin. It may be difficult to assess in edematous persons; the inner aspect of the forearm is another good place to check. Light stools and dark urine often occur with jaundice.	To assess dark-pigmented skin for jaundice, you must check the sclera of the eye for yellow discoloration, mucous membranes of the buccal mucosa (hard palate), the palms of the hands and soles of the feet for yellow discoloration. *Two limitations:* carotene deposits in the sclera of the eye, and dark-pigmented mucous membranes.

Reprinted with permission from the November issue of *Nursing '72*. Copyright © 1972 Springhouse Corporation.

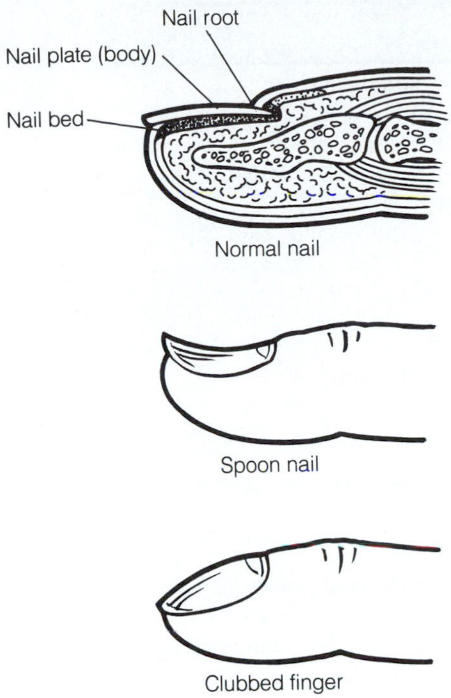

Figure 22-3. Identifying abnormal nails.

the deciduous teeth. Finally, the last stage of tooth development is the eruption of the third molars, or wisdom teeth, which occurs when an individual is about 17 years old. The wisdom teeth are often absent or may be small or misaligned, a problem that may later necessitate their removal.

The most common dental problems are the development of **caries** (decay), gum disease (periodontal disease), and malocclusion. Each can lead to loss of teeth. Caries can be prevented or controlled through less frequent ingestion of simple sugars and regular dental supervision. The addition of fluoride, either applied topically or added to drinking water, has benefit in the prevention of caries. Fluoride does not make the enamel harder but makes it less soluble so that it cannot be penetrated by bacteria, which can cause caries (Guyton, 1991, p. 602). Periodontal disease can begin in early adulthood. Conscientious brushing and flossing of teeth plus a nutritious diet can help control this condition. Malocclusion means abnormal alignment of the upper teeth to the lower. This can result in poor chewing action leading to problems with digestion. Eventually, the maloccluded teeth can become eroded and diseased. Orthodontic correction, although expensive, is often undertaken in childhood. If the teeth are healthy and in good repair, correction of malocclusion can also be done in adulthood.

Many older adults are edentulous (without teeth) primarily because of periodontal disease. Fifty percent of older adults (over age 65) have lost their teeth and 90% of those who have teeth have periodontal disease. Gum disease, decaying teeth, and having to wear dentures may contribute to nutritional deficiencies in elderly persons. Such deficiencies can be largely prevented through lifelong good nutrition, oral and dental hygiene, and dental therapy (Murray and Zentner, 1989, p. 509).

Common Problems Affecting Skin Integrity

Whenever the integrity of the skin is interrupted, microorganisms from the environment can enter and invade the tissues. Many people have chronic or acute skin disorders. Even if the person is generally healthy, an infection can occur. Certainly, persons who have surgical wounds or are debilitated so that they have pressure ulcers have impairment of skin integrity and are at high risk for infection.

Chronic and Acute Skin Disorders

Many people have chronic skin disorders that have periods of remission and exacerbation (Table 22-2). Some disorders are age related such as the *acne* of adolescence. *Psoriasis* is a disorder of persons in the middle or older adult years that causes red, leathery patches to appear on various areas of the skin of the body. The widespread use of over-the-counter medications and prescribed drugs has resulted in increased allergic reactions, often manifested in acute skin lesions.

New methods have been developed for treatment of many chronic disorders, making consultation with a physician appropriate. If the condition is an allergic reaction to a medication, merely discontinuing its use or substituting another pharmacologic agent often corrects the condition.

Surgical or Traumatic Wounds

Performing an incision during a surgical procedure interrupts the normal protection of the body provided by the skin. Because of the danger of infection, antimicrobial drugs are often given to the patient before surgery. These drugs are continued for several days after the surgical procedure to avoid wound infection.

People who sustain traumatic wounds such as accidental lacerations or penetrating injury have an increased risk for infection because the wound may be unclean from dirt or other objects that have penetrated the broken surface. The wound is cleaned as thoroughly

Table 22–2. Common Skin Lesions

Abrasion	A scraped area on the skin often caused by friction
Birthmark	An irregular permanent purplish discoloration of the skin referred to as a "port-wine birthmark" or a bright red permanent discoloration called a "strawberry birthmark." These blemishes are present at birth and benign.
Blister	A thin, circular, fluid-filled swelling on the skin
Bulla	A large fluid-filled vesicle
Cyst	Small mass containing fluid
Ecchymosis	A bruise
Erythema	Redness of the skin with warmth and swelling
Excoriation	An abrasion with destruction of the top layer of the skin
Fissure	A crack or break in the skin's surface
Keloid	A raised overgrowth of scar tissue, found more often in blacks
Macule	A flat, colored, circular lesion less than 1 cm in diameter, much like a freckle
Maculopapular	A fine raised rash such as is seen in rubeola (measles)
Nodule	A small hard mass that may or may not be movable
Papule	A small, raised, inflamed lesion less than 1 cm in diameter, much like a pimple
Petechiae	Tiny red spots on the skin or mucous membrane caused by minute hemorrhages
Pustule	A papule filled with pus
Scar	A thick fibrous area formed as a result of injury or a surgical incision
Ulcer	A circular, inflammatory, often necrotic indented lesion of the skin affecting deeper tissues
Vesicle	A blister that is serum filled
Wheal	Any confined acute swelling of the skin

as possible and antimicrobial drugs are given. Even with these measures, it is often difficult to avoid infection.

Pressure Ulcers

One of the most troublesome and difficult to cure skin lesions is the **pressure ulcer**. Pressure ulcers are also called *decubitus ulcers*, pressure sores, or bedsores. Decubitus means lying down, and, indeed, persons who are immobile or lying down are at high risk of such lesions. Fortunately, prevention of pressure sores is possible with nursing actions that focus on relieving pressure on tissues and health teaching.

When pressure above the normal arterial capillary pressure of 32 mm Hg is exerted on subcutaneous tissue, the small vessels collapse and the tissue becomes ischemic (lacking in blood). If pressure is quickly alleviated, blood supply is restored and the cells recover. However, if the blood supply is interrupted for a period of time (as short a duration with some patients as 2 hours), cells are unable to recover and necrosis, or cell death, occurs. Pressure ulcers occur more often over the bony prominences of the body such as the coccyx, trochanter, scapulae, ankles, and elbows, where soft tissues are more prone to compression. An ulcer may also occur over the ischial spine from prolonged sitting or over an ankle bone from lying on the side for long periods of time. However, pressure ulcers can appear on any body surface.

A pressure ulcer usually begins as an area of reddened skin. If the redness disappears when massaged, a process called **blanching**, permanent tissue damage has not yet occurred. If the redness does not disappear, some tissue damage has occurred and an incipient pressure ulcer is present. This is sometimes referred to as a *stage I* pressure ulcer. Although further breakdown may be prevented by aggressive nursing care, damage to deeper tissues may have already occurred. If this is the case, surface tissue may continue to break down despite nursing action. The epidermis and dermis become involved, and the skin is no longer intact. This is called *stage II*. If further breakdown occurs, the ulcer has progressed to *stage III* in which the muscle layers beneath the skin become necrotic, and healing becomes more difficult. Finally, during *stage IV*, a pressure ulcer can progress to the bone as the skin and muscle slough away. Display 22-1 summarizes the stages of pressure ulcer development.

Display 22–1
Stages of Pressure Ulcer Development

Stage I (Incipient)
Circumscribed area of reddened skin that does not blanch when massaged

Stage II
Break in skin; epidermis and dermis involved

Stage III
Lower muscle layers involved; necrotic tissue is apparent

Stage IV
Bone tissue is involved with sloughing of muscle and skin

Assessment Related to the Integumentary System

Because many patients in the hospital are immobile, maintaining skin integrity becomes an important part of nursing care. The nursing process offers a framework for assessing, planning, and assisting patients with potential or real skin problems.

Interview

First, the patient may be able to give you assessment clues in an interview. A history of skin problems can be elicited this way. The following are some of the questions you should ask during the interview:

1. Has the patient or the family had a history of skin problems?
2. Obtain general information relative to nutrition, bathing habits, smoking, or exposure to environmental irritants or smoke.
3. How would the person describe the current problem?
4. How long has the condition been present and does the patient know what caused it?
5. What symptoms or signs affect daily living?
6. What factors make the condition better or worse?

Physical Assessment

The person's age will be important because so many skin disorders are age related. For example, the infant often has chafing or blistering caused by contact with urine or feces, often referred to as diaper rash. The hormonal adjustments of the adolescent can lead to skin manifestations. Young people and young adults can sustain injury that impairs skin integrity. Persons of advanced years experience increasing dryness of the skin, which can lead to itching. If scratching occurs in response to this, the skin can be disrupted.

Next, you can make general observations of the skin. One organized and systematic method is to make a head-to-toe assessment. The mucous membranes should be inspected and the teeth observed for caries. Refer to Tables 22-1 and 22-2 for guidance regarding assessment of comparative skin color and skin lesions. There may be other discolorations of the skin such as **ecchymosis** (a bruise) or generalized **jaundice** (a yellowing of the skin). The temperature of the skin should be warm, a sign of adequate circulation to the area. Turgor should be tested to see if the skin and underlying tissues are well hydrated. For this test, gently pinch a small area of skin between your thumb and index finger. Lift and let go. The skin should flatten immediately. If it continues to remain at all raised, fluid distribution is disturbed or inadequate.

Check for skin lesions even though none have been mentioned during the interview. The recommended practice is to go from head to toe, inspecting from the scalp and hair to the feet. Skin folds under pendulous breasts, the axilla, and the perineal area should be inspected. Is there a single lesion or multiple ones? Are lesions confined to one part of the body? What shape are they? How fine are they? What color are the lesions? Are they raised or flat? Is there pain or itching? If you cannot decide which term identifies what you find, simply describe what you see as carefully as possible. If there is a reddened area, massage it to check for blanching. If the area does not blanch, potential for the development of a decubitus ulcer is present.

Finally, touch the skin's surfaces to ascertain whether sensation is intact. The patient should be able to feel light touch. The skin could be hypersensitive so that even light touch is uncomfortable. Clearly identify which areas are involved if a deficit is noted.

Patients at Risk of Pressure Ulcers

Assessment for the risk of developing pressure ulcers is essential for all patients but particularly for those confined to a bed or chair for any length of time. It is important to realize that the beginning of a pressure ulcer can be evident within 24 hours if pressure is placed on tissue. Regardless of age, any person can develop pressure ulcers under certain conditions, but the older adult is particularly at risk because of the skin changes of aging. These persons have decreased skin turgor and less of the underlying fat tissue that protects bony prominences from pressure. The dermis becomes less elastic and, therefore, gives less when pressure is applied (Fitzsimons, 1983 p. 34). Because of perceptual changes in the skin, older persons may not sense discomfort as readily as younger people and may not change position to relieve pressure. Other people who also have decreased awareness of peripheral sensation include patients with diabetes, persons who have had strokes, and those with spinal cord injuries.

Persons who are malnourished and lack such nutrients as protein, vitamins, minerals, and calories are also prone to ulcer formation. "Alterations in nutritional status occur in almost 50 percent of the older population. Deficiencies in vitamins A and C and in iron are common in older persons" (Fitzsimons, 1983, p. 36). Pressure ulcers sometimes develop in the aged and others who have slowed metabolism and circulation because their cell nutrition may be inadequate to allow cells to recover from even minor damage.

Other factors can increase the risk of ulcers in elders and others. Although fat tissue pads the skin from sharp, bony prominences, those who are obese with excess fatty tissue can have undue pressure from the added weight over prominences. Pressure ulcers can also occur in the overweight person when body surfaces rub together or are in contact and hold moisture. Dehydrated persons may have dry, cracked skin that can precede ulcer formation.

Any incontinent patient whose skin is exposed to the chemical irritation of urine or stool is at risk. Drainage from wounds can also expose the skin to irritation, which can lead to pressure ulcers. Casts and appliances that rub on the skin and impinge on joints also encourage pressure ulcer formation.

Bergstrom and colleagues (1987) state that the critical factors in pressure ulcer development are "intensity and duration of pressure and the tolerance of the skin and its supporting structure for pressure." With others, they developed a useful scale for predicting pressure sore risk. Known as the Braden Scale for Predicting Pressure Sore Risk, the scale considers the patient's mobility, activity status, and sensory perception (Fig. 22-4). Other conditions included in the scale are such extrinsic factors as degree of moisture and amount of friction and shear and intrinsic factors such as nutritional status, age, and other variables specific to the individual being assessed.

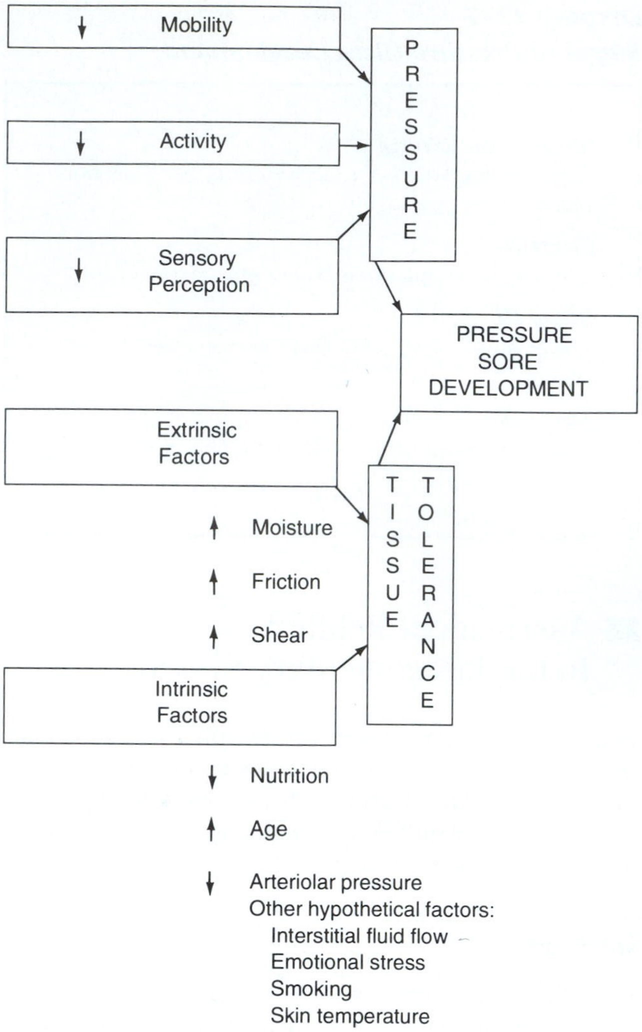

Figure 22-4. The Braden model for predicting pressure sore development. Reprinted from *Rehabilitation Nursing*, volume 12, Issue 1, with permission of the Association of Rehabilitation Nurses, 5700 Old Orchard Road, First Floor, Skokie, IL 60077-1057. Copyright 1987 Association of Rehabilitation Nurses.

Nursing Diagnoses Related to the Integumentary System

A priority for planning individualized skin care for a patient is accurate nursing diagnosis. Diagnosis should include risk states so that implementation can also focus on prevention of skin breakdown. The North American Nursing Diagnosis Association (NANDA) has defined three general categories for problems of skin integrity: High Risk for Impaired Skin Integrity and Impaired Skin Integrity. In 1992, NANDA added the nursing diagnosis, High Risk for Peripheral Neurovascular Dysfunction. For each of these categories, the etiology must be identified.

High Risk for Impaired Skin Integrity

A diagnosis of High Risk for Impaired Skin Integrity becomes more meaningful when the cause of the risk is defined. This diagnosis is also appropriate when assessment reveals an abnormal color to the skin or the presence of lesions that constitute a potential impairment.

Nursing Diagnoses Related to the Integumentary System

High Risk for Impaired Skin Integrity
- related to urinary incontinence
- related to mobility impairment
- related to inability to turn self
- related to inadequate nutritional status

Impaired Skin Integrity
- related to pressure ulcer over coccyx
- related to immobility
- related to fine skin rash possibly secondary to medications
- related to pruritus secondary to rash
- weeping skin lesion underneath left breast fold related to close skin surface

Body Image Disturbance
- related to generalized jaundice

The etiologies for this diagnosis could state that, for example, the risk is related to urinary incontinence, mobility impairment, inability to turn self, or inadequate nutritional status. This diagnosis could also be used if the person is at risk for scratching the skin or if the person of advanced years has fragile skin and is wearing a tight wristwatch or a patient identification band that may erode the skin.

This diagnosis is appropriate when the patient is at risk of disruption in circulation, sensation, or motion. An example of risk factors would be fractures that necessitate the use of a cast or brace. These devices exert mechanical pressure that can compromise circulation.

Impaired Skin Integrity

A diagnosis of Impaired Skin Integrity is appropriate when lesions are actually present or an incision has been made through the skin. Assessment will reveal the presence of lesions or an incision. The etiology may be the presence of pressure ulcers or restrictions on mobility. Persons with impaired skin integrity may also have the related diagnosis, High Risk for Infection because the skin barrier to microorganisms has been disrupted.

Body Image Disturbance

Great emphasis is placed on the value of healthy, unblemished skin in our society. For the teenager whose face is visibly flawed by the lesions of acne, for example, or the person whose skin is yellowed because of jaundice, body image disturbance is a serious consideration. The diagnosis may be stated as a risk for or actual situation depending on the assessment.

Planning and Implementation Related to the Integumentary System

The most critical desired outcomes in the care of the patient's skin are for the patient to remain free of skin infection (as from wounds or surgery) and to remain at low risk for the development of pressure sores. Depending on the individual circumstances of the patient, other outcomes could include eliminating itching or dermatitis and decreasing dry skin.

Regardless of the skin problem, an important part of planning care is adequate, individualized hygiene. Hygiene tasks consume a large segment of the staff nurse's time and remain an important aspect of the care of patients.

If skin lesions are present, the plan may involve maintaining a comfortably cool environment to decrease itching, reviewing the medication regimen to identify potential causes that can be reported to the physician, and administering drugs that may be ordered to reverse or alleviate the condition (see the sample Nursing Care Plan Related to Skin Integrity).

Providing Wound Care

If a wound is present, wound and skin care would be part of your plan. If a surgical wound has been made, the policy of the surgeon or that of the institution should be followed. Various dressing materials are available. Sterility must be maintained until the wound surface is sealed closed against the entry of microorganisms. Wounds heal more rapidly with less scarring in a moist environment than in one that is dry (Krasner, 1992).

Prevention and Treatment of Pressure Ulcers

The United States Congress has formed the Agency for Health Care Policy and Research (AHCPR), which sets guidelines for the prevention and treatment of health care conditions. Prevention and treatment of pressure ulcers in adults is one of the first conditions for which guidelines were established. Care providers can take a variety of actions to prevent and treat pressure ulcers. The appropriate nursing actions for potential pressure problems may include placing a special mattress on the bed, initiating a turning and skin inspection schedule, and reviewing the patient's nutritional and fluid status. If the person is incontinent, establishing and following

Nursing Care Plan

Sample Nursing Care Plan Related to Skin Integrity

Nursing Diagnosis

Impaired Skin Integrity: Pressure ulcer related to inability to turn self.

Supportive data:

Unable to turn self.

3 cm reddened open area over coccyx.

Skin dry.

Low fluid intake.

Desired Patient Outcomes

Short term:

For ulcer border to not extend nor increase in size, evidenced by granulation taking place.

Long term:

For ulcer to heal so that skin is once again intact.

Nursing Action	Rationale
1. Clean around ulcer area once each shift.	Cleansing decreases and therefore helps prevent infection.
2. Irrigate ulcer with hydrogen peroxide qd per order for 20 min.	Irrigation removes dead tissue which can foster infection and antiseptic solution impedes colonization of microorganisms.
3. Turn q2h using turn sheet.	Changing position relieves pressure on the area. The use of a turn sheet helps move patient and prevents shearing of the skin.
4. Encourage fluid intake to 3,000 mL.	Increasing fluid intake helps treat infection by keeping tissue well hydrated, preventing further breakdown, and facilitating removal of toxins produced by microorganisms.
5. Encourage intake of protein items in diet for healing.	Protein is necessary for tissue-building.
6. Give special hygiene after defecation.	Special hygiene will prevent contamination of the area by pathogens contained in the feces.

guidelines for frequent and conscientious perineal care is an important part of the plan and implementation of care.

Prevention of Pressure Ulcers

The keymark in prevention is identifying persons at risk and being aware of early signs of breakdown. This can be done by ongoing inspection by the nurse within the facility or the family at home. Immediate action should be taken if there is any indication of pending skin breakdown.

Conscientious and regular cleansing of the skin prevents breakdown. Perspiration, urine, and feces, if left on the surface of the skin, encourage skin integrity interruption due to chemical action. Good general hygiene is essential for any patient but particularly for those at risk of developing pressure ulcers.

Any factor that leads to drying of the skin should be avoided. Also, the skin should not be exposed to prolonged moisture. Excessive bathing should be avoided to prevent drying and providing lubricating lotion after bathing is helpful in keeping the skin supple and in good condition.

Any patient on bed rest must turn or be turned at

least every 2 hours. Turn sheets and a lifting motion should be used to prevent the patient's skin from being sheared against a bottom sheet. The skin surfaces should also be regularly massaged to stimulate circulation although current research advises that one not massage directly over bony prominences, which can actually reduce blood flow.

Distributing the patient's body weight by having a firm mattress underneath is helpful. Bottom linen should be tight and unwrinkled. Some fairly simple and inexpensive devices are available to prevent undue pressure on tissues. Among these are foam rubber mattress pads, silicone gel, and synthetic sheepskin (lamb's wool) pads.

A soft foam-rubber pad with a convoluted surface characterized by many small (approximately 1-inch high) fingerlike projections (often called an egg-crate mattress) may be placed over the regular mattress. The pad's irregular surface allows air to circulate near the skin, helping alleviate skin **maceration** (softening and wearing away) due to perspiration. The pad's softness allows pressure to be distributed over a wider area, thus relieving some of the pressure on bony prominences. Such pads are produced in small sizes to fit under the buttocks or in wheelchairs and in large sizes to cover the entire bed.

Silicone gel pads are used most frequently under the buttocks. These devices, similar in density to body fat, provide padding and distribute pressure across the entire body surface, preventing its concentration on any one point. Lessened pressure prevents blocked circulation and tissue damage. The pad must usually be rotated regularly to prevent permanent ridges from occurring on the surface. Such pads are encased in easily cleaned plastic and may be covered with protective padding.

Sheepskins, both natural and synthetic, have been used under bony prominences to provide a soft surface that does not abrade (rub open) the skin. The fleecy surface also allows for air circulation and distribution of weight. Commercial sheepskins are completely washable and are only effective when in direct contact with the patient's skin.

Chair-bound persons should have sufficient padding under areas where pressure is applied to bony prominences. If possible, these persons should be removed from the chair every 2 hours for change of position. For areas of the body that are most prone to pressure ulcer problems, see Figure 22-5.

If the patient is on continual bed rest, the head of the bed should be no higher than medically indicated. The higher the head of the bed, the more pressure on the buttocks and hips.

Adequate nutrition and fluids are essential. Well nourished skin is less likely to break down.

Treatment of Pressure Ulcers

Consult others on the health care team when you note evidence of a pressure ulcer. The physician and nurse often share the care plan and are receptive to each other's ideas about assisting the patient in the healing process. Physical therapists may offer help with special frames and devices. An enterostomy nurse or therapist who teaches and cares for patients with urinary and fecal diversions (see Module 38, Ostomy Care) may add guidance regarding special care of the skin. The nutritionist can give valuable advice concerning an appropriate diet to promote healing. If the ulcer is extensive, more involved special mattresses, frames, or beds may be necessary for treatment. For specific types of equipment and guidelines for using them, refer to Module 25, Special Mattresses, Frames, and Beds.

If an advanced ulcer is present, necrotic material should be debrided because it provides a reservoir for increased colonization of pathogens. All measures used

Nursing Research: *Implications for Practice*

Frantz, R. A., and G. C. Xakellis. "Characterists of Skin Blood Flow Over the Trochanter Under Constant, Prolonged Pressure." *American Journal of Physical Medicine and Rehabilitation* 68, 6 (December 1989): 272–276.

Using a laser Doppler flowmeter, 19 healthy adults placed on supportive air mattresses were measured for their ability to maintain adequate blood flow when constant pressure was exerted on the trochanter. Subjects were in the supine and left lateral positions with subsequent return to the supine position.

Results showed that response is individualized; not all individuals maintained the same ability of maintaining adequate circulation on exertion of pressure on the area. Secondly and importantly for nurses, 30 minutes or more was required to adequately return to preload blood flow in these healthy persons. This study emphasizes the need for nurses to accurately assess and provide a plan of care that protects the ill person from having undue pressure exerted on bony prominences.

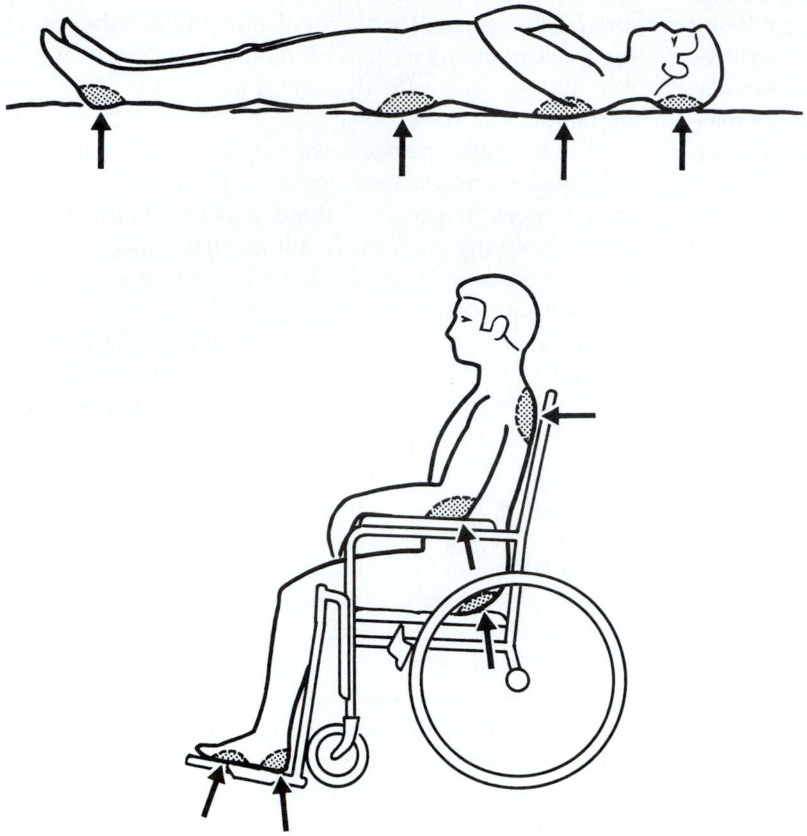

Figure 22-5. Common areas prone to development of pressure ulcers.

for **debridement** (removal) are ordered by the physician. If the ulcer is deep and purulent, surgical debridement is sometimes necessary. For serious but less extensive ulcers, the use of a whirlpool bath (which must be ordered by the physician) has proved helpful. The whirlpool has the disadvantages of adding to medical costs and necessitating the cumbersome cleaning that must be done before and after a patient receives a treatment. Topical medications consisting of *enzyme* agents are sometimes used for debridement. In general, these compounds break down collagen material, which is connective tissue protein. These substances need moisture to be activated. Some irrigants and solutions, however, inactivate the agents. Be sure to read the manufacturer's instructions carefully when using any enzymatic substance. Some require saline irrigations before instillation. The surrounding skin must also be protected against the enzyme action by a coating of petroleum jelly. After the debridement has been completed, saline irrigations are used to remove the enzyme and desquamated tissue. Absorbent granules such as Debrisan (molecular dextran) and vegetable gum wafers such as Stomadhesive and gum karaya can be used to form an **eschar**, or thick scab, in noninfected ulcers. These agents are not used with infected ulcers because the agents can localize and encapsulate the infection, making it difficult to cure.

A great deal of research has been done to determine whether ulcers resolve better when kept wet or when kept dry although it has been established that other types of wounds heal better when kept moist. Many techniques have been used to keep pressure ulcers dry, such as applying heat lamps or exposing the ulcers to air. Dressings moistened with various solutions have been packed into the wound to facilitate moist healing. The current thinking is that pressure ulcers heal best if covered with a sealed dressing to preserve a moist surface. One study used both dry and moist techniques. The application of a moisture vapor-permeable transparent dressing sealed in place over the ulcer proved to be the most "safe and effective" treatment. (Kurzuk-Howard, Simpson, and Palmieri, 1985). The rationale for using a sealed dressing is that it acts as a pseudoskin, protecting the ulcer from pathogens and promoting more rapid epithelialization. The dressing is placed and allowed to remain undisturbed for several days before changing. The surface beneath remains moist but "breathes" through the special dressing material.

The Kurzuk-Howard study found that although the healing time was about the same with either treatment, wet or dry, the staff time was much less when a sealed dressing was used, and if the ulcer formation was in the beginning stage, the moist treatment was more likely to prevent the ulcer from progressing.

When an ulcer is infected, it is better to use a light gauze dressing to protect it. A culture is taken to determine what organism is present so that antibiotic therapy can be started. Sometimes the patient is placed on wound and skin precautions to prevent spread of the infection as well as to protect other patients and staff members.

Finally, the risk, prevention, or presence of a pressure ulcer should be documented in the plan of care so that health care members can offer continuity of care that incorporates appropriate and ongoing action.

Pressure ulcers can become life threatening, usually because the patient becomes toxic from the presence of bacteria in the blood (bacteremia). If this happens, aggressive action is taken to subdue the infection and heal the ulcers.

Health Teaching

Effective health teaching can not only prevent the development of pressure ulcers but can also effect earlier treatment and more rapid resolution of the problem. This is particularly true for those persons who have been identified "at risk." For example, if a person is elderly and has skin that is fragile so that breakdown is more likely than in those who are younger, the nurse in the hospital or the care provider at home can take actions which will protect the skin so that pressure ulcers will not occur.

Daily inspection of the skin may reveal early signs of breakdown due to pressure. If the person is unable to perform self-inspection, a family member or health care provider can fulfill this important function.

Evaluation Related to the Integumentary System

The evaluation of risk-state diagnoses will demonstrate a positive outcome when the patient's skin shows no evidence of interruption of skin integrity and healing or decrease of any lesions that cause skin integrity impairment.

If a rash or skin lesion such as a decubitus ulcer is present, evaluation will focus on whether the rash decreases in intensity or disappears. The desired outcome related to a pressure ulcer may be for the ulcer to decrease in size or diameter. The depth of the ulcer will also be part of evaluation. Demonstration that a pressure ulcer is contained or its borders have not been extended would at times be considered a successful outcome. Further nursing intervention may be needed to bring about a totally positive outcome such as complete healing.

Hygiene

Among the most basic and important tasks of nursing is assisting the patient to carry out hygiene-related activities. This consists of helping patients maintain skin integrity and caring for the hair, nails, and teeth. The nurse may be performing these activities for the patient who is unable to do this independently. At times, the nurse may teach techniques for hygiene. This part of nursing never loses its importance. Basic hygiene contributes to body image and comfort and protects from infection.

Hygiene may be defined as those practices that bring about personal cleanliness, comfort, and feelings of well-being. The way a nurse manages the patient's/client's and his or her own hygiene communicates a great deal. Because hygiene practices vary greatly from one setting to another, you should take hygiene seriously when making decisions about your own appearance.

By practicing good hygiene yourself, you emphasize its importance. In the hospital setting, your being clean, tasteful, and neat conveys to the patient that you know the importance of good personal hygiene. Although general appearance such as nurses' apparel may be somewhat different in urban and rural outpatient settings, standards of hygiene remain high for all those who care for ill persons.

If you administer skillful and knowledgeable hygiene, the patient will have more confidence in your ability to perform other tasks. Helping patients maintain hygiene tells them that you care about their comfort.

Culture and Hygiene

One has only to walk through European palaces and castles to understand what kept their early occupants from bathing frequently—cold and dampness. Burning herbs and fragrances was a common practice, both to ward off disease and to disguise unpleasant odors resulting from poor hygiene. As late as the beginning of this century, bathing was infrequent; in fact, many people believed that frequent bathing was injurious to health.

During the last 30 years, people have become much more conscious of hygiene. The development and sale of hygiene products is an enormous national business. Central heating and ample supplies of hot water have made daily bathing more feasible than in the past, and the traditional "Saturday night bath" is no longer a way of life. Showers supplement or replace bathtubs in many homes. Deodorants, shampoos, oils, powders, lotions, and a wide variety of soaps, some antibacterial in nature, enhance individual hygienic practices. Among the many patients who do not regard a daily bath as healthful or necessary may be the economically disadvantaged person whose dwelling does not provide proper bathing facilities or privacy and the elderly person with dry, fragile skin.

Dry skin is a chronic problem for many people, young and old, partly because of the warmth and dryness typical of American homes. This may be exacerbated by frequent bathing with hot water and strong soaps. It is a problem particularly with older white adults. The skin of those with darker color contains more oil so the problem of dryness is not as apparent. The person with dry skin can disrupt skin integrity by scratching, which can lead to infection. Unless oils are used, daily bathing can aggravate dry skin. Many older adults avoid frequent bathing for this reason. They also avoid bathing because of the chances of chilling and because they perspire less than do younger persons. Finally, people who were not taught as children to bathe daily do not make it a practice as adults.

The Goals of Hygiene

The administration of hygiene has three main goals, the first of which is to maintain healthy skin. Massaging and cleansing increases circulation, which helps cellular nutrition and therefore, keeps the skin intact as a defense against infection. Second, hygiene removes transient microorganisms from the body, decreasing the chances of infection. Third, hygiene contributes to the patient's comfort. Feeling refreshed and clean contributes to subjective well-being and self-esteem. Encouraging women who normally use makeup to continue to do so in the hospital and encouraging men to shave or trim their hair or beards regularly will also enhance self-worth.

Besides bathing, complete hygiene also includes the use of deodorants, bath powders, and soaps; perineal care; the backrub; shaving; oral, eye, nail, and hair care; and care of the patient's bed.

Although we will discuss the various aspects of hygiene in this chapter, for procedures to assist with hygiene, see Modules 2, Basic Infection Control; 3, Safety; 7, Bedmaking; 10, Elimination and Perineal Care; and 11, Hygiene.

Hospital Routines for Hygiene

In most hospitals it has long been the policy to bathe each patient completely every day. In nursing homes, where staff–patient ratios are lower, patients are necessarily bathed less frequently. Some hospitals are beginning to modify the rigid policy of daily bathing.

Complete morning care usually consists of a bath or shower with perineal care; a backrub; and care of the mouth, hair, and nails. Bed linens are inspected and, if needed, changed. Only linens in direct contact with the patient's body or soiled are changed. The budgets of health care facilities have to be tightly controlled and using linen when it is not needed adds a financial burden. The unit is made neat, and unused items are discarded or sent for cleaning or laundering. Items are never returned from the patient to the general unit supplies to prevent transfer of microorganisms. Personal items are straightened or moved only with the patient's permission.

Partial care involves washing of particularly soiled areas of the body, usually the face, neck, hands, *axillae* (armpits), and perineum. Oral care and hair care are also provided, and a backrub may be included. The unit is made neat as with complete care, and soiled linens are changed. It is a thoughtful practice to change the pillowcase to give the patient a sense of freshness.

Both complete care and partial care are sometimes referred to as "AM care." The practice of bathing patients in the morning disregards the wishes of the individual who prefers to bathe in the evening or just before bedtime, and some facilities offer bathing at times other than the morning. This practice helps relieve the strain on staff time during the busy morning hours and accommodates the patient who sleeps better after an evening bath.

Early AM care often provided by the night staff before the nurses' report in the morning, is preparation for the morning meal. Toilet facilities are offered, and the patient's face and hands are washed. The stand is straightened and cleared to make room for the food tray. Oral hygiene, the cleaning of teeth or dentures, may be done. It is also appropriate to clean eyeglasses before giving them to the patients.

Evening or bedtime care, called HS care, is given in the evening just before sleep. If you think of the things you like done before sleep, you will recognize the importance to the patient of evening care. A clean gown or pajamas is often appropriate. The face, hands, and back are washed, and a relaxing backrub is given. Glasses and dentures are carefully put away for the night if the patient cannot do this independently, and soiled dressings or linens are replaced. Oral care is given.

Hygiene is also appropriate at other times. Handwashing before eating should be encouraged. After using a bedpan, urinal, or toilet, the patient should be given the opportunity to wash his or her hands to remove microorganisms. If the nurse has assisted, the nurse's hands should also be washed even though gloves were worn.

Care of the Patient's Bed

The patient's bed is his or her environment. Because patients spend long periods of time in bed, nurses must pay careful attention to making the bed a place of comfort and safety.

Proper placement of linens, such as incontinent pads and turn sheets, allows the bed's cleanliness to be easily maintained and saves the nurse and the patient the inconvenience of having to change the entire bed. Draw sheets, small sheets placed under the main portions of the trunk, often with a waterproof sheet beneath, are no longer used routinely. For the patient who cannot turn without help, a *turn sheet* can be made from a bath blanket folded in quarters or a draw sheet folded in half and placed under the heavier portion of the patient's body. It is much easier to turn a patient by grasping the sides of this piece of linen than by grasping the patient's extremities. This method is also more comfortable and safer for the patient.

When making a bed, whether or not the patient is in the bed at the time, you should keep four goals in mind. First, the surface under the patient should be smooth and free of wrinkles. The patient with sensitive skin can develop pressure sores (decubitus ulcers) from the slightest wrinkle. Even wrinkles in the underbedding—the mattress pad, bottom sheet, or draw sheet—must be smoothed. Second, all surfaces that touch the patient must be meticulously clean. To protect the patient from microorganisms, the linens nearest to the body must be changed as necessary. Third, enough bedding should be used to keep the patient warm. The physical work you do may make you feel warm, but you should not assume that the patient resting quietly in bed is equally warm. Although a single blanket is usually enough, because hospitals are kept warm, asking patients how many blankets they want provides a good check. Finally, the bed must give the patient adequate room for movement. Preparing an overly neat bed that constricts movement is not a service to the patient. Loosening the bedding over the feet is especially important so when the patient is lying on the back, the feet need not be in constant extension, but remain in a relaxed position, the toes pointing upward.

Comfort and safety are more important considerations, but a neat appearance should also be a goal. It is possible to make a neat bed without ignoring the more important factors.

Assessment Related to Hygiene

Nursing process is particularly helpful when one is planning hygiene for the patient. Patient deficits and strengths are identified so that care can be individualized to more closely meet the patient's needs. Assessment usually includes pertinent data regarding deficits in body systems. For example, a deficit in muscle strength may prevent the patient from assisting with hygiene.

For some patients, particularly those admitted to the surgical unit where the presence of organisms can be especially harmful and cause infection, facility policy may dictate that the patient have an admission bath. To assess the patient for this initial procedure, you will need to know several things. What is the patient's diagnosis? If the patient is in pain, has difficulty breathing, or appears fatigued, you should not cause further fatigue by performing extensive hygiene. If the patient has come directly from home and is clean, comfortable, and rested, you may choose to delay or omit the bath. If, on the other hand, the patient was admitted with dust or dirt on the skin, for example, after a pedestrian accident, immediate special hygiene may be indicated.

How does the patient view needs for hygiene, and how can these needs be incorporated into the hospital routine most easily and comfortably for the patient? Does the patient prefer a shower or does fatigue make a bed bath more appropriate? Would the patient like a shampoo? If possible, let the patient help you plan care for hygiene. Patients have far too few decisions to make in the hospital and should be given some control over their care whenever possible.

With regard to an established inpatient, evaluate the hygiene the patient has been receiving. Read the record to determine whether there have been problems and identify them clearly. How might you modify care? For example, if a patient with an indwelling catheter has been given tub baths but since yesterday has developed a fever from a bladder infection, a bed bath with cool but comfortable water is appropriate. Another patient who has been showering may have reported fatigue after the shower yesterday and slept through most of the lunch hour so you may decide to give a partial bath to allow the patient to rest.

Nursing Diagnoses Related to Hygiene

Nursing diagnoses related to hygiene may pertain to risk states related to care, deficits in self-care, or to special needs for hygiene as defined by NANDA.

High Risk for Injury

Hygiene practices can place some patients at risk of injury. Because of deficits in muscle strength or coordination, patients can fall in showers or when getting into or out of bathtubs. Long periods of bed rest can result in postural hypotension, a temporary pooling of blood in the lower part of the body on rising, a condition that can

Nursing Diagnoses Related to Hygiene

High Risk for Injury: falling in shower related to intermittent dizziness

Self-care Deficit: Total, related to unconscious state

Self-care Deficit: Hygiene, inability to perform own perineal care related to visual impairment

Self-care Deficit: Dressing/grooming related to incoordination of upper extremities

Situational Low self-esteem related to inability to perform own activities of daily living

lead to unsteadiness or falls when patients attempt to get up too quickly to shower or bathe.

Self-care Deficit

Many of the NANDA diagnoses related to hygiene focus on deficits in self-care. Such diagnoses are appropriate for the patient in a lower level of awareness who cannot perform any aspects of hygiene and for patients who cannot perform some part of their own hygiene for physical or emotional reasons. A patient who has had a stroke may be unable to floss the teeth. Some patients who are immobilized may not be able to manage their own perineal care or to wash their feet adequately. It is useful to define clearly the specific aspects of care that cannot be performed.

Special Needs for Hygiene

A nursing diagnosis may also identify a special need for hygiene related to the condition of a particular patient. Diaphoretic or obese patients may need extra care to protect skin integrity. Incontinent patients may need extra hygienic measures beyond what is usually provided.

Planning and Implementation Related to Hygiene

After needs have been carefully assessed and nursing diagnoses established, your planning will address the hygienic needs of a particular patient. The person should be allowed to participate actively in hygienic procedures whenever possible. The desired outcomes for the patient are cleanliness and comfort, provided in a safe and efficient manner, and an overall enhanced body image and sense of well-being.

Because of the personal nature of this kind of care, you will need to be aware of the possibility that some patients will consider the hygiene care you provide to be an invasion of privacy or, at the very least, embarrassing. The patient may also experience negative feelings of dependency.

You will probably be assessing and providing hygiene for more than one patient. You will need to be well organized and to plan carefully so that all patients receive the hygiene needed. If, for example, you are to administer morning care, you should have determined, through assessment, which patients need a complete bath and which might appropriately be given a partial bath (assuming, of course, that your facility allows you to make such decisions and does not require daily morning baths for all patients). If you are to administer morning care to as many as five or six patients, giving each a complete bed bath would be difficult. Often patients can perform part of their own care. Allowing patients to participate in their own care helps promote and maintain a sense of independence and can be beneficial psychologically. Some patients who are free of drainage and body odor do not need a complete bath daily. Others may need to bathe more than once a day. In addition to the patient's needs, the nurse's time must also be considered. You must weigh the two factors together to use your time as advantageously as possible for the patients under your care.

In practice, you may choose to strip the bed of top linen, replacing it with the blanket, and bring the bath water and other items needed for one patient to perform self-care while you administer a bed bath to another. Communicating this procedure clearly to the patients involved allows such scheduling to run smoothly.

Bathing the Patient

Bathing affords generalized physiologic benefits to the patient. The activity and movement bathing elicits stimulate the respiratory system and improve circulation. The movement of muscles and joints maintains and promotes mobility. Because the muscles are relaxed by exposure to warm water, it is appropriate for the patient to perform range-of-motion exercises in the bathtub (see Chapter 23).

Bathing provides an excellent opportunity to assess the patient further. Physical assessment can focus on the patient's general appearance or on such specifics as relative strength and the presence or absence of stiff joints. Muscles may be observed for muscle strength and skin for turgor, color, dryness, and the presence of lesions. The condition of the hair, nails, teeth, and gums may also become apparent in the course of care. The time spent with the patient can also be an occasion for psychological assessment and interaction, allowing you to explore tactfully the patient's feelings and concerns.

States of confusion, depression, contentment, and elation can all become apparent to the nurse who is sensitive to others' feelings. The time spent with the patient can also be valuable for mutual communication. It should be an unhurried and pleasant time (Fig. 22-6).

Depending on your assessment of the hygiene needs of the individual patient, one of several types of baths can be selected: the bed bath, the tub bath, the hydraulic tub for those more incapacitated, the standing shower, or the chair shower. Assessment will be discussed later in this chapter.

Whatever type of bath is decided on, with or without the patient's participation, safety is a prime consideration. Water temperature poses a possible hazard and must be carefully checked. Tubs are filled and showers run before the patient enters, and water for the bed bath is checked before it is applied to the patient. A bath thermometer is sometimes difficult to find, but if you are unsure of the temperature, an ordinary thermometer can be used. With practice, most nurses become adept at recognizing safe temperatures by testing the water on their wrists; until you become skilled at doing so, always test the water with a thermometer. It is advisable to ask patients whether or not they use soap on their faces. Soap can be irritating, and it can be dangerous to the eyes if not used with care. Many soaps are drying, so oil might be added to the bath water for patients with obviously dry skin. The patient who showers could apply a small amount of oil after the shower. Most facilities have installed hand rails in the tub or shower area, and the patient should be encouraged to use them (see sample Nursing Care Plan Related to Hygiene).

The Bed Bath

A nurse or other staff person performs a bed bath by using basins of warm water to bathe the patient in bed. Special draping prevents the patient from being chilled or unduly exposed. Washing is accomplished in long, smooth strokes, moving from the cleaner parts of the body to the more soiled parts to decrease the spread of microorganisms.

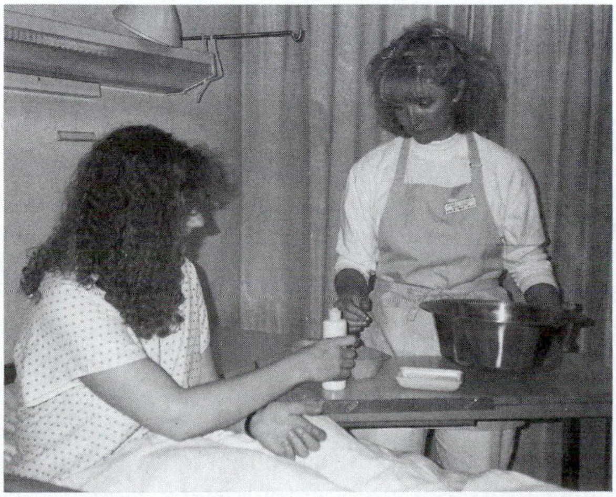

Figure 22-6. Providing skin care for a hospitalized patient.

The Tub Bath

A tub bath is virtually the same as a bath the patient would take at home. The water temperature should be carefully monitored; very cool water may chill the patient because most body surfaces are in contact with the water, and extremely warm or hot water can be dangerous to the circulatory system, particularly in the elderly patient. A bath towel on the bottom of the tub prevents slipping. Transferring a patient to the tub from a wheelchair is facilitated by positioning the wheelchair at the back of the tub or facing its side. The patient's legs can easily be lifted over the lip of the tub and a two-person assist used to lift the person into the water. Module 22, Transfer, describes and illustrates techniques for transferring a patient.

The Hydraulic Tub

The hydraulic tub, frequently used in chronic care settings, consists of a plastic chair in which the patient sits. Straps are fastened to secure the patient, and the entire chair then locks to a hydraulic lift, which raises, turns, and lowers the chair into a high tub that can accommodate the sitting patient. A special oil soap is added to the water, and the patient can be bathed or whirlpool outlets can be activated to stimulate and further clean the body surfaces.

The Standing Shower

Showers are the most thorough method of cleansing because the water is rinsed from the body, carrying off microorganisms. Before arranging a shower, be sure the patient feels strong enough to undertake it. You may wish to place a chair nearby in case the patient feels sudden fatigue. Use a bath mat to prevent slipping and place the call signal in an accessible spot, explaining its presence and use to the patient. A bath mat may also be placed outside the shower so that the patient does not slip.

The Chair Shower

A chair shower is administered in a cabinet that allows the patient to remain seated in a shower chair. A waist-high partition may enclose the shower area, permitting the nurse to assist while remaining dry. Whether the nurse can give an effective shower from such a position, however, is questionable. A newly available device consists of a horizontal shower cabinet that allows a bedridden patient to be showered on a special stretcher.

Nursing Care Plan

Sample Nursing Care Plan Related to Hygiene

Nursing Diagnosis	Self-care Deficit: Bathing/Hygiene related to weakness. **Supporting data:** 32-year-old man. Diagnosis of AIDS. Attempted to bathe self yesterday but became fatigued and short of breath. States he is just too weak to bathe self.
Desired Patient Outcomes	**Short term:** Patient states he feels clean and comfortable and not unduly fatigued. **Long term:** Patient resumes self-hygiene when no longer so fatigued.

Nursing Action	Rationale
1. Give bedbath in morning before visitors arrive.	Assisting with hygiene in the morning conserves patient's energy for visitors, enhances appearance, and makes patient feel refreshed.
2. Allow patient to wash face or give any part of care he wishes, but monitor for fatigue.	Participation in self-care increases self-esteem and minimizes feelings of dependency. Monitoring the patient for signs of fatigue provides opportunity for early intervention if fatigue does occur.
3. Record patient's ability to participate and fatigue level.	Documentation provides a record for the health care team so that useful interventions can continue as part of the patient's plan of care.

Providing Deodorants, Bath Powders, and Soaps

Individuals respond differently to products like deodorants and bath powders. If a person regularly uses a certain product, there is probably no danger of toxicity. But if such a product is new to the patient, use it sparingly until its safety has been established for that person.

The active ingredient in many antibacterial soaps and hygiene products is **hexachlorophene**. In the early 1970s, a study revealed that use of this chemical in high concentration caused brain lesions in newborn monkeys. Although such serious effects have not been demonstrated in human beings, the U.S. Food and Drug Administration issued a warning that hexachlorophene in concentrations of more than 3% should not be used on newborns. The policy of limiting hexachlorophene to 3% has since been extended to most over-the-counter hygiene products today, making them safe to use.

Growing preoccupation with meticulous hygiene has created a market for what advertisements call feminine hygiene products. These products are, in fact, perineal deodorant products whose value is questionable. They can be irritating to some women and have caused severe reactions in a few.

Providing Perineal Care

Clean gloves are always worn to protect the nurse when giving perineal care or any other care that potentially exposes the nurse to body fluids. The perineal area requires meticulous care. It is characterized by a heavy concentration of bacteria because the excretion of feces and urine and the deep creases of the groin provide a moist and warm environment in which bacteria can grow. A thick, cheesy secretion called **smegma**, largely composed of dead epithelial cells in the area of the perineum, can act as a reservoir for bacteria. Good perineal care is a matter of careful cleansing. Cleansing is always performed from front to back, or from the urinary orifice to the intestinal orifice, to prevent contamination of the urinary tract with intestinal organisms. The importance of frequent perineal care for the patient who has an indwelling catheter in place cannot be overemphasized. The region around the catheter should be cleaned well with soap and water before the remainder of the area is cleaned.

Patients who are able should be given the opportunity to perform their own perineal care. While providing the patient with clean water, soap, a cloth, and a towel, you might ask, "Would you like to finish your own bath now?" " . . . wash between your legs?" " . . . wash your genitals?" or " . . . wash the crotch area?" Use words the patient is likely to understand and allow sufficient time and privacy. If the patient is unable to perform this task unaided, your undertaking it in a professional, efficient manner will help relieve anxiety and embarrassment. This aspect of care may discomfit the inexperienced student, but practice makes it a more routine matter; patients will become more relaxed as you do. Module 10, Assisting with Elimination and Perineal Care, provides more detailed directions on giving perineal care.

A *douche* is an irrigation of the vagina. The fluid used may be a commercial product, a mild vinegar solution, or tap water. Because douches can destroy the normal *flora*, or usual residing organisms in the vagina, leading to infection, douching is regarded as unnecessary for the normal healthy woman.

Giving the Backrub

The backrub is a cherished nursing art and one that has been abandoned occasionally because of time pressures (Fig. 22-7). This is unfortunate if a backrub is performed properly. If not done well, a patient may be disconcerted when a nurse pours a bit of lotion in the hand, briskly rubs up and down the patient's back, and considers the patient to have had a backrub. A backrub or massage is given for two purposes: stimulation and relaxation. A backrub after a morning bath may be given to stimulate the skin and muscles; before sleep, a soothing backrub encourages rest. If the patient falls asleep during a relaxing backrub, the nurse should feel a sense of success. Both the extent of the backrub and the type of stroke used, including the amount of pressure, will determine the effect on the patient.

The backrub is a part of the administration of the bath and should be considered as such. When a backrub is offered, the patient may decline on the basis that "it's too much trouble" for the nurse. The nurse should explain that it is no trouble because the patient's skin, which is in contact with the bed, needs such care. Most patients enjoy backrubs, and many ask for the procedure. Because a backrub brings pleasure to the patient, the nurse may also enjoy it. A backrub is often an opportune occasion to talk quietly with the patient and convey a caring attitude.

Shaving the Patient

You may prefer to shave the male patient before beginning a bed bath. Alternatively, placing warm, moist hand towels over the patient's face while you are administering a bed bath feels comforting to the patient and softens the hair follicles for easier shaving. Bed patients should always be shaved before the bottom linen is changed because small hairs that fall into the bed can cause discomfort.

Daily shaving is necessary for many men to appear and feel well groomed (Fig. 22-8). Some men with beards shave the edges to give their beard the shape

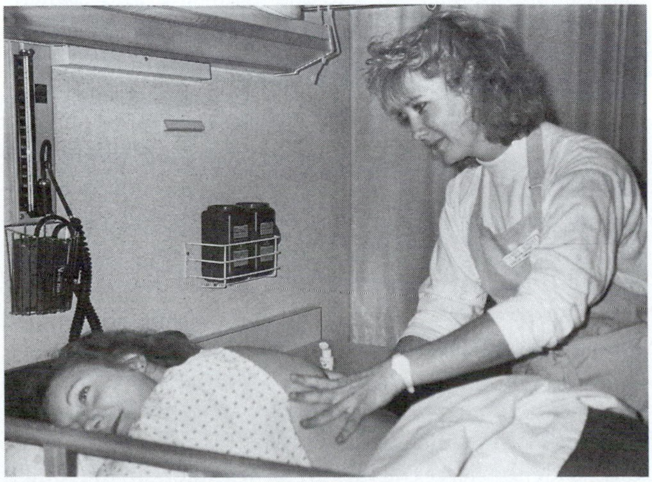

Figure 22-7. A backrub can be a satisfying experience for both the patient and the nurse.

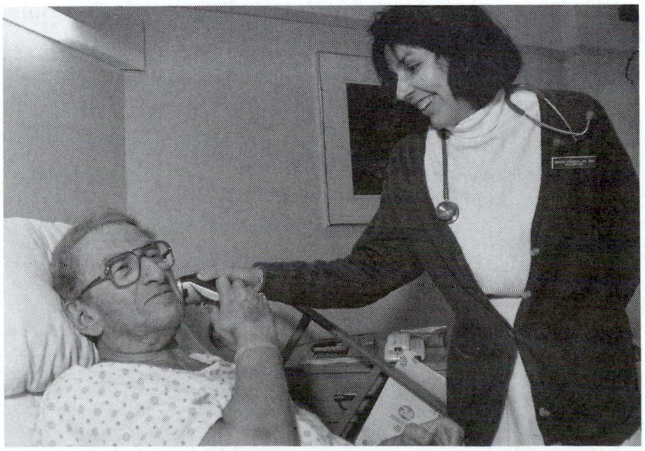

Figure 22-8. Shaving the patient enhances personal comfort.

they desire. Furthermore, some patients develop skin irritations if they do not shave; the hairs hold perspiration on the skin, causing a fine rash. Men often bring their own shaving equipment to the hospital, but some hospital units have electric razors available for patient's use. The blades of such communal razors must be soaked in disinfectant solution between patients. Alternatively, disposable safety razors designed for one-time use are inexpensive and appropriate for the hospital setting. If you stretch the skin slightly taut, shaving a patient is not a difficult task. The shaving soap the patient customarily uses is the best choice. An electric razor is preferable for use with any patient who has bleeding tendencies or is taking anticoagulant medication because the danger of nicks is reduced.

Providing Oral Care

Oral care consists of assessment, treatment, and care of the teeth, mouth, and gums. Illness and contingent problems involving diet and fluids cause the patient's mouth to need more frequent attention. To care for patients unable to perform their own oral care, a number of techniques are needed. Clean gloves are always worn (see Module 11, Hygiene).

If the patient can hold water in the mouth and spit it back out without choking, the nurse may perform regular oral care with a toothbrush and dental floss. The patient may also wish to use a commercial mouthwash. Some nurses provide solutions for administering oral care. Nurses have different preferences as to solutions they use for oral care. A diluted solution of hydrogen peroxide, with a small amount of mouthwash added for esthetic purposes, has good cleaning properties.

A proprietary product, a mouth-moistening salivary supplement called Moi-Stir, is now being used in many facilities. This substance has the same pH level and electrolytes as the body's saliva. A study comparing the use of a lemon and glycerin product and Moi-Stir overwhelmingly confirmed Moi-Stir as the preferred substance. A group of patients used each product and rated the effectiveness after 7 days of intense application. With the use of lemon and glycerin in combination, 9% improved, 75% reported no change, and 16% worsened. When Moi-Stir was used, 62% improved, 37% reported no change, and 1% worsened (Poland, 1987).

If the patient's lips are dry, a light coating of a *water-soluble* jelly, A&D Ointment (containing the vitamins A and D, which promote healing of irritations), or petroleum jelly may be applied. These should always be applied sparingly because inhalation of insoluble products can obstruct lung tissue and cause serious pneumonia. Patients who are receiving oxygen or have gastric intubation (a tube inserted through the nose) need more frequent oral care. Oxygen is drying, and patients who are short of breath tend to breathe through their mouths, thereby drying the tissues of the mouth. When this occurs, there is an increased accumulation of sordes, which can cause the mucous membrane to form cracks.

Providing Eye Care

Most patients' eyes do not need special care because the tears produced by the lacrimal glands constantly wash over the surfaces of the eyes, freeing them of dust or other contaminants. At times, however, eye care is needed. If a discharge is present, the eye can be irrigated with sterile water or normal saline solution. This procedure is described in Module 48, Irrigations. Crust on the lashes or lids composed of dried discharge material can be removed with moistened gauze.

The eyes of an unconscious patient should be frequently inspected and irrigated, if necessary. The physician may order that a solution of **artificial tears**, a neutral, sterile lubricating agent, be instilled if natural tearing is deficient. If one or both eyes of an unconscious patient remain open and unblinking, an eye pad and protective shield can be applied to prevent drying of the surfaces and injury. However, it is important to inspect the eyes frequently for signs of irritation or infection.

Occasionally a patient will have a prosthetic (artificial) eye. If the patient is unable to care for the prosthesis, the nurse must do so. Open the eye, place a clean finger under the lower edge to break the suction, and then remove the glass or plastic eyeball. The eye can then be washed in normal saline solution and replaced by opening the lid and placing the prosthesis firmly under the upper lid. The prosthesis will fall into place and reseal.

Many patients wear contact lenses. Lenses may be hard, semisoft, or soft, and the cleansing and storage procedures vary accordingly. If you are unsure of the type, consult with the patient or family. An optometrist would also be able to tell you how to care for a particular type of lens. A sterile, cotton-tipped applicator moistened with normal saline can be used to remove hard or semisoft contacts. With the tip, gently push downward on the lower edge of the lens. This will raise the top edge of the lens so you can remove it. Small, suction devices are also available for this purpose. The larger soft lenses are removed by bending them between the fingers and lifting outward. Lenses should be stored according to directions. To replace a lens, first wet the surface with a commercial wetting solution. Then hold the eyelid open with the fingers of one hand and, with the lens on the tip of a finger of the other hand, place it directly onto the middle of the *cornea* (the convex surface of the eye).

Providing Nail Care

Complete hygiene includes attention to the nails. Pointed nail cleaners are often kept on hospital units for the purpose of cleaning under patients' nails, where secretions, loose skin, and pathogens can collect. Many institutions allow only a registered nurse or a *podiatrist* (specialist in care of the feet) to trim the nails of diabetic patients because the tiniest nick may result in serious infection for the patient. Filing the nails of diabetic patients is considered safer than cutting. Filing is also preferable in the case of the older patient with extremely hard and thick toenails, which can be almost impossible to cut with scissors or clippers. Soaking the nails before cutting is usually beneficial. It is important to examine the patient closely for rough nails, which can cause abrasions of the skin if the patient should scratch.

Providing Hair Care

Hair can become a significant problem in the hospital, for both the patient and the staff. Long hair quickly becomes matted from rubbing against bedding. Applying a small amount of alcohol or vinegar to the hair and then brushing will usually remove such tangles, but alcohol dries the hair and should be used only occasionally. To avoid problems, arrange the patient's hair in an attractive and convenient manner of the patient's choosing soon after admission. Braiding the hair or tying it back or to one side are popular ways of arranging long hair. You can usually assess the frequency of the patient's need for shampooing. Most hair need not be washed every day. Dry shampoos are available for use with bed patients, but they are less than satisfactory because they may cause itching of the scalp and discomfort. Some patients can be placed on a stretcher and taken to a basin where, with padding under the head, the scalp and hair are washed. Commercial hair shampoo sets can usually be obtained from the central service department of most hospitals. There may, however, be a charge because it is requisitioned for a particular patient. It should be stored at the bedside so that it can be used again with that patient. Many patients report that being unable to shampoo the hair is a major irritant in being hospitalized. Assessing the need for a shampoo and performing it efficiently is an essential part of providing hygiene.

A white nurse may feel uncertain about caring for the hair of an African American patient because of unfamiliarity with its texture and style. If the patient's hair is elaborately styled, as in "cornrows" (intricate, tiny head braids), be sure to ask for permission before dismantling the style. The patient and family may object because such styles are time consuming and expensive to arrange. If you shampoo curly black hair, style it before it is completely dry because it becomes more difficult to manage when dry. Comb small sections of the hair away from the scalp, taking care not to put undue tension on the hair roots. The smooth hair of Native Americans and Asians is easier to arrange. Consult the patient or family, if possible, when caring for the hair of a person from an ethnic group other than your own (Fig. 22-9).

Health Teaching

Health teaching about hygiene begins within the family. It is essential for good health but also is both culturally and socially linked. For those who are ill, teaching hygiene becomes even more important so that they do not spread infection to others and do not receive pathogens from the environment, the staff, or other patients. First, rationale must be provided regarding the necessity for good hygiene. For example, teaching good handwashing techniques maintains the body's first line of defense against pathogens. Secondly, the person should be taught the types of hygiene practice that are appropriate and reasonable for that individual. In many situations, the nurse or others may need to provide assistance. The older patient may have difficulty using a tub shower because it requires raising the legs over the side of the tub. This type of hygiene may be possible with the help of another person. A shower also may be unsafe unless a chair can be provided for sitting. Third, hygiene practices are equally important in the home so that when discharge is planned, the nurse can incorporate health teaching for the patient and the family, emphasizing the importance of hygiene.

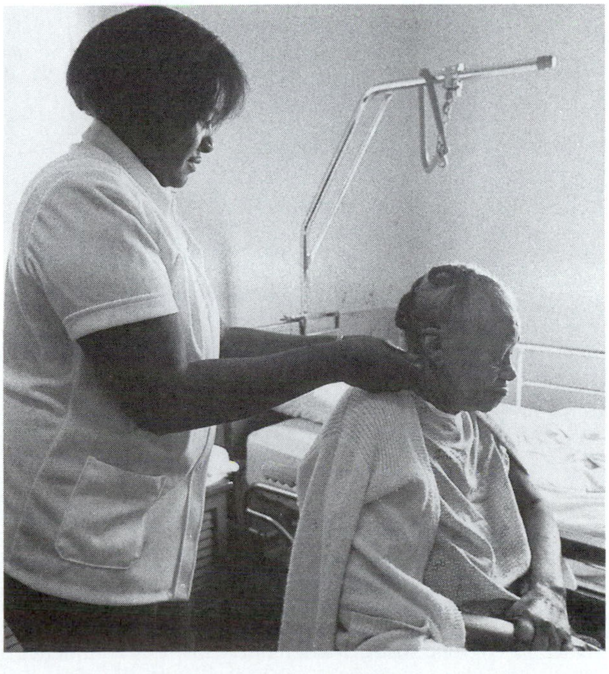

Figure 22-9. Caring for the hair of an African American patient.

Evaluation Related to Hygiene

Evaluation should be based on the desired outcomes or goals for hygiene. It should include input from the patient regarding further needs and the degree of satisfaction with care. If safety was maintained throughout and the patient is clean and comfortable, the outcome is positive. If your evaluation determines that a change in the plan of care for hygiene is needed, you should communicate this need to the health care team.

The Nurse's Personal Hygiene and Appearance

Nurses are in a profession that requires close contact with patients, their families, and coworkers. Nurses must be role models for maintaining personal hygiene (Fig. 22-10).

In addition to meeting the patient's need for hygiene, nurses are teachers of hygiene and should exemplify healthful living. One of their responsibilities is to practice personal hygiene conscientiously so that the closeness required in giving care is always pleasant and never offensive. A nurse who is neat and clean also protects patients and others from the unnecessary spread of pathogens. Personal cleanliness is essential for nurses, regardless of their work setting. Many nurses bathe immediately after arriving home from work to remove any pathogens that might have been transmitted to them. This is a prudent practice.

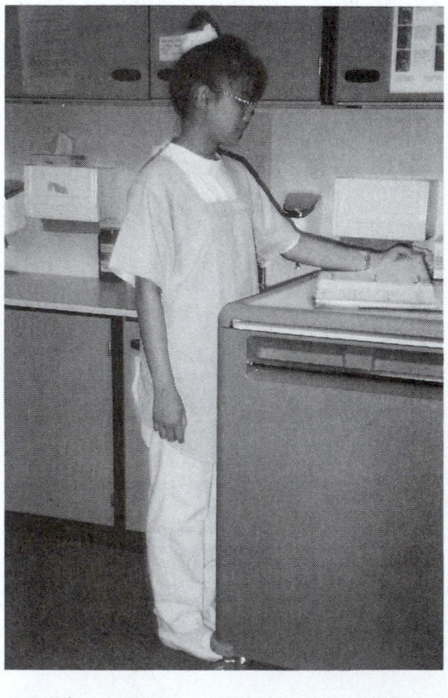

Figure 22-10. The well-groomed nurse inspires confidence.

Uniforms

Uniforms reflect a degree of proficiency in providing care as well as professional identification of the nurse to the patient. Regardless of current moves toward establishing a variety of dress codes, when patients were surveyed regarding uniforms for women nurses, they preferred nurses in white dress uniforms with caps. This attire was less favored by nurses themselves (Mangum, Garrison, Thackeray, Lind, and Wyatt, 1991).

Your uniform should be clean when you enter the clinical area so you will not bring microorganisms to the susceptible patient. Some hospitals provide locker facilities where nurses may change clothes. Pediatric units and other specialty settings may have uniform codes different from standard nursing units but nevertheless, adhere to principles of hygiene.

Many of the functions nurses perform are physical in nature, and stimulate more perspiration than do sedentary tasks. Synthetic uniforms, which do not "breathe" as cotton fabrics do, allow perspiration to remain on the skin and *deteriorate*, sometimes causing unpleasant odors. It is advisable to wear a uniform only once before laundering it and to remove it immediately on arriving home. Like bathing, this practice prevents pathogens from being spread to the home environment. Concern for the welfare of others also suggests that a uniform worn in the hospital should not be worn in other settings, such as stores and offices.

Oral Care

The nurse should practice good oral care. Brushing the teeth and flossing regularly makes the mouth clean and odor free. Caries can be prevented. If they do occur, they should be repaired promptly; carious teeth create a persistent mouth odor not relieved by brushing or mouthwash. Although smoking behavior has generally decreased in the population, nurses who smoke should brush their teeth even more often than nonsmokers. The use of chewing gum to mask mouth odor is discouraged because it is distracting to patients and other workers; good oral hygiene is far preferable.

Hair

For both men and women in nursing, hair should be worn short or secured close to the head to prevent it from falling forward and obscuring your vision. In addition to being convenient and neat, such styling makes it unnecessary to use your hands to rearrange your hair. Touching the hair is unhygienic because it transmits microorganisms from hands to hair and vice versa and can scatter organisms about the immediate surroundings.

Long, loose hair can also hang over patient's food trays and over open wounds when dressings are being changed, creating a general hazard of transmittal of microorganisms. Beards and mustaches should be short and well groomed. Regular shampooing gives all hair a shiny, healthy look.

Fingernails

Trimmed and filed fingernails are easy to keep clean and unlikely to scratch a patient. Because nail polish can chip and fall into a patient's bed, or worse, into a sterile field, its use is generally discouraged. If worn, nail polish must be in good repair and of an undistracting pale shade.

Jewelry

The nurse should wear little personal jewelry in the hospital setting. Acceptable items are a wedding band, watch, and studs with posts in pierced ears. Excessive jewelry not only is unprofessional, but it can be damaged or lost in the practice of nursing. Jewelry also presents the more serious danger of scratching a patient's skin or catching rings or bracelets in a patient's hair. If hoop earrings accidentally catch in hanging equipment or are grasped by an agitated patient, the nurse's ear lobes could be lacerated. Jewelry should usually be reserved for a social setting.

Identification Pins

Proper identification of health care personnel is crucial because there are so many different providers. A name pin that designates the wearer's role is an official part of the nurse's uniform and should always be worn. Patients greatly appreciate knowing the name and function of care providers; the name pin is a reinforcement to a verbal introduction.

Caps

The wearing of nursing caps by female nurses has become controversial. Although some facilities require the wearing of caps by all female nursing personnel as a matter of policy, caps are worn infrequently or not at all in other facilities. Female nurses may question the need for caps because they are often inconvenient to wear while administering care and because there are now many men in nursing for whom caps have never been designed or required.

Dress Code for Nonhospital Settings

The uniform traditionally worn by hospital-based nurses is not appropriate in many schools, community health clinics, and other agencies that employ nurses. Nurses in such facilities often wear street clothes, sometimes covered by a lab coat for asepsis and appearance. If you wear street clothes, they should be appropriately tailored and your name pin clearly displayed. Regardless of the setting, personal hygiene and appearance are important for nurses in their professional roles.

Nursing Care Study
A Patient at Risk for Impairment of Skin Integrity

Jana Morita reviewed her care plan for Teresa Schaefer over coffee in the empty conference room of the orthopedic unit on which Jana worked. Teresa had been on her way to work yesterday morning when her car collided with a panel truck. She sustained some minor facial abrasions and a compound fracture of the left leg. After surgery, she had arrived on the unit in leg traction. Jana had provided her with an orthopedic bed on which had been placed an egg-carton mattress. Teresa had some discomfort during the night but appeared to be resting quietly this morning. After reviewing the plan, Jana decided she would make further assessment. Pain and High Risk for Skin Integrity Impairment were the two high-priority nursing diagnoses on the plan. Pain would probably be adequately controlled and should, Jana knew, decrease after the first day or so. But the skin integrity problem could be troublesome unless the plan was complete, shared with the entire health care team, and adhered to until Teresa was mobile again.

After greeting Teresa and explaining that she would like to gather more information, Jana asked if any skin surfaces were painful or even uncomfortable. Teresa said she was surprised after so short a time how pink and mildly uncomfortable her elbows were from rubbing on the sheet. Jana noted

(continued)

Nursing Care Study (continued)
A Patient at Risk for Impairment of Skin Integrity

this on the care plan and told Teresa that she should always mention any degree of discomfort so that they could forestall more serious skin problems. Jana then asked Teresa to pull her body up, using the trapeze device hanging from the frame of the bed, so that she could inspect her back. Except for some creases caused by a wrinkle in the sheet, which Jana pulled tight and straightened, the skin of the back appeared to be normal. The cast, however, was another matter. It was not yet dry and seemed to impinge somewhat on the adjacent skin, particularly circling the thigh. Jana noted this along with her other observations. Last, Jana looked at the rest of Teresa's skin and found it clear and intact. Jana noticed that light crusts had formed over the facial abrasions.

After washing her own hands, Jana shared the care plan with Teresa, emphasizing the importance of skin care. Jana left the room to gather the equipment she would need to implement her plan. It certainly would have to include good hygiene as well, she decided. Jana reentered Teresa's room and applied lamb's wool elbow pads. Next she tucked strips of padding around the top and bottom of the cast. Gently Jana cleaned the edges of the abraded areas on Teresa's face with hydrogen peroxide. Finally, she asked Teresa to rise up as far as possible while she washed her back and massaged the area. Teresa remembered the fragrant skin lotion she had received for her birthday and asked if she might have someone bring it to her so that she could enjoy it while in the hospital. Jana thought this was a good idea. After instructing Teresa about toe exercises to increase circulation in the injured leg and enhance skin integrity, Jana went to finish her care plan and get ready to share it at team report.

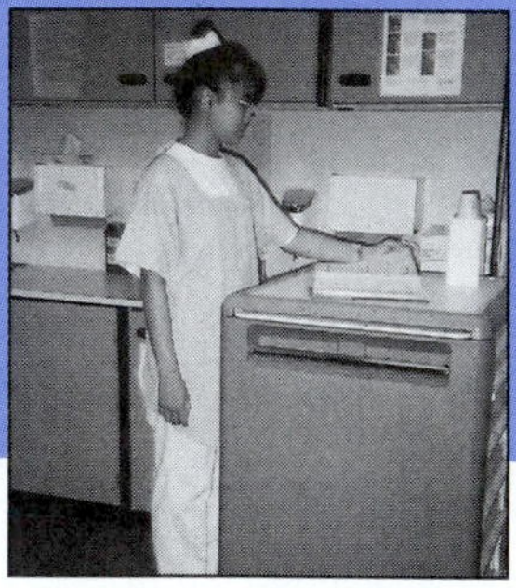

Key Points

- Because the skin serves so many functions, maintenance of skin integrity is a basic need of all human beings.
- The functions of the skin include protecting the vital organs that lie beneath it, protecting the body from invasive organisms, maintaining body temperature, and providing sensory communication with the environment.
- The integumentary system is composed of the skin and the mucous membranes, hair, nails, and teeth. By far the largest organ of the body, the skin constitutes 16% of total body weight.
- Normal skin is smooth and supple with good turgor, is warm to the touch, and is of a color appropriate to the person's ethnic heritage.
- It is important to prevent or reduce the incidence of skin lesions that may impair skin integrity.
- Mucous membranes, which are contiguous with the skin and line the passageways of the body that open to the exterior, should also be cared for in the maintenance of skin integrity.
- Care of the integumentary system includes keeping the hair clean and healthy in appearance, the nails neatly trimmed and smooth without being brittle, and teeth clean and free of gum disease and caries.
- Hygiene is defined as those practices associated with the integumentary system that bring about personal cleanliness, comfort, and a sense of well-being.
- What is considered appropriate hygiene differs from one culture to another, and nurses must keep this in mind when caring for persons from different cultures than their own.
- The goals of hygiene are to maintain healthy, intact skin; to remove transient microorganisms; and to provide feelings of comfort.
- Hygiene care can be given as complete or partial and can be administered early in the morning, during the day, or at bedtime, depending on the needs of the patient and the routine of the health care facility.
- Bathing provides an excellent opportunity for assessment and interaction with the patient. Choices

for bathing include a bed bath, tub bath, hydraulic tub bath, and standing or sitting shower.

- Along with the bath, the nurse may also administer special perineal care, a backrub, or a shave in addition to oral, eye, nail, or hair care.
- The patient's bed is also the nurse's responsibility and should be kept clean, wrinkle free, and neat.
- Application of the nursing process is useful in providing hygiene. Many patients have a self-care deficit so the nurse must perform what the patient is unable to accomplish.
- The risk to skin integrity posed by pressure ulcers is a special concern for the nurse. The guidelines released by the Agency for Health Care Policy and Research have set standards of care for the prevention of pressure ulcers.
- The Braden Scale is another tool that is useful in assessment of those at risk of developing pressure ulcers.
- Nurses are in close contact with patients, and they have a responsibility to maintain good personal hygiene so that they are never hygienically offensive. The nurse's appearance should also be appropriate to the work setting.
- Maintaining skin integrity is one of the most important goals of patient care. For a positive outcome, the nurse must have knowledge of body structure, the risks imposed by illness, and practices that can aid in prevention of skin breakdown and the restoration of skin integrity.

Study Questions

1. Name the five parts of the integumentary system.
2. Why is skin integrity so important?
3. What are the three basic functions of the skin?
4. Describe the characteristics of normal skin.
5. List the questions you would ask during the assessment interview for skin integrity.
6. What is a pressure ulcer?
7. List five factors that place a person at risk of pressure ulcer.
8. Discuss some of the actions you might take to prevent or treat a pressure ulcer.
9. If you were assigned a patient for complete morning hygiene, what tasks would you perform?
10. In deciding what kind of bath to give a patient, what factors would you consider?
11. What benefit for the patient does a backrub provide?
12. What are the two main considerations when making a bed for a patient?
13. Describe the characteristics necessary for a nurse's appearance to be classified as professional.
14. Why should nurses not wear excessive jewelry?

Critical Thinking Activities

1. Make a general assessment of your own skin. Then do a similar skin assessment of an older member of your family or an older patient; compare the two assessments.
2. Identify a small skin lesion you have (this might be a freckle, wart, or pimple). Pair up with a classmate and, without showing it, describe the lesion. Ask how accurate your description was when the classmate observes the lesion. Reverse roles with your classmate.
3. When writing a nursing care plan for a patient for whom you have cared, what assessment data would be important in order for you to identify risk factors for developing a pressure ulcer?
4. Find two advertisements in the media displaying hygienic products. Interpret what message is intended and the possible response of the reader. Discuss your findings in a small group of students.
5. Analyze your own habits of hygiene and professional appearance. What changes would you like to make?

Relevant Sections in Modules for Basic Nursing Skills

References and Readings

American Journal of Nursing. "How to Predict and Prevent Pressure Ulcers." Clinical Guidelines. 92, 7 (July 1992): 52–60.

American Nurse. "Guideline Released on Pressure Ulcers." 24, 6 (July-August 1992): 17.

Anastasi, J. K., and Rivera, J. "Identifying the Skin Manifestations of H.I.V." *Nursing '92* 22, 11 (November 1992): 58–61.

Barnes, H. R. "Alternating Transparent and Hydrocolloid Dressings—A Difficult Case." *Nursing 93* 23, 3 (March, 1993): 59–61.

Barnum, B. "Wear Your Designer Clothes on Duty." *Nursing and Health Care* 11, 9 (November 1990): 484–485.

Bergstrom, N., Braden, B. J., Luguzza, A., and Holman, V. "The Braden Scale for Predicting Pressure Sore Risk." *Nursing Research* 36, 4 (July-August 1987): 205–210.

Braden, B. "A Conceptual Schema for the Study of the Etiology of Pressure Sores." *Rehabilitation Nursing* 12, 1 (January-February 1987): 8–16.

Carpenito, L. J. *Nursing Diagnosis: Application to Clinical Practice.* 4th edition. Philadelphia: J. B. Lippincott, 1992.

Chagares, R., and Jackson, B. S. "Sitting Easy: How Six Pressure-Relieving Devices Stack Up." *American Journal of Nursing* 87, 2 (February 1987): 191–193.

Colburn, L. "Preventing Pressure Ulcers: How to Recognize and Care for Patients at Risk." *Nursing '90* 20, 12 (December 1990): 60–63.

Conforti, C. "Pressure Sores: Dressed for Successful Healing." *Nursing '89* 19, 3 (March 1989): 58–61.

Cuzzell, J. "Clues: Itching and Burning in Skin Folds." *American Journal of Nursing* 90, 1 (January 1990): 23–24.

———. "Clues: Bruised, Torn Skin." *American Journal of Nursing* 90, 3 (March 1990): 16–18.

Delancy, V. L. and North C. "Skin Assessment." *Topics in Clinical Nursing* 5, 2 (July, 1983): 5–10.

Dossey, L. "The Skin: What Is It?" *Topics in Clinical Nursing* 5, 2 (July 1983): 1–4.

Fitzsimons, V. M. "The Aging Integument: A Sensitive and Complex System." *Topics in Clinical Nursing* 5, 2 (July 1983): 32–38.

Gates, R. L. and Holloway, G. A. "A Comparison of Wound Environments." *Ostomy/Wound Management* 38, 8 (October, 1992): 34–36.

Gilchrest, B. A. "Skin Aging and Photoaging." *Dermatology Nursing* 2, 2 (April 1990): 79–82.

Gould, D. "Skin Bacteria: What is Normal?" *Nursing Standard* 5, 52 (May 1991): 26–28.

Guyton, A. C. *Human Physiology and Mechanisms of Disease.* 5th edition. Philadelphia: W. B. Saunders, 1992.

Hill, M. J. "The Skin: Anatomy and Physiology." *Dermatology Nursing* 2, 1 (February 1990): 13–17.

Iverson-Carpenter, M. S. "Impaired Skin Integrity." *Journal of Gerontological Nursing* 14, 3 (March 1988): 25–29.

Johnson, B. "The Meaning of Touch in Nursing." *Nursing Outlook* 13 (1965): 59.

Krasner, D. "The 12 Commandments of Wound Care." *Nursing '92* 22, 12 (December 1992): 34–41.

Kurzuk-Howard, G., Simpson, L., and Palmieri, A. "Decubitus Ulcer Care: A Comparative Study." *Western Journal of Nursing Research* 7, 1 (February 1985): 58–79.

Mangum, S., Garrison, C., Thackeray, R., Lind, C., and Wyatt, M. "Perceptions of Nurses' Uniforms." *Image* 23, 2 (Summer 1991): 127–130.

McConnell, E. "Assessing the Skin." *Nursing '92* 22, 4 (April 1992): 86.

Michelsen, D. "How to Give a Good Back Rub." *American Journal of Nursing* 76, 11 (November 1976): 1762–1764.

Murray, R., and Zentner, J. *Nursing Assessment and Health Promotion Strategies Through the Life Span.* 4th edition. Englewood Cliffs, N.J.: Prentice-Hall, 1989.

Poland, J. M., "Comparing Moi-Stir to Lemon-Glycerine Swabs." *American Journal of Nursing* 87, 4 (April 1987): 422, 424.

Rubin, M. "The Physiology of Bed Rest." *American Journal of Nursing* 88, 1 (January 1988): 50–56.

Schmidtling, R. E., Gordon, S., and Davenport, B. "Treating Pressure Sores With a Myocutaneous Flap." *Nursing '92* 22, 7 (July 1992): 56–59.

Sebern, M. "Home-Team Strategies for Treating Pressure Sores." *Nursing '87* 17, 4 (April 1987): 50–53.

Stotts, N. "Seeing Red . . . and Yellow . . . and Black: The Three Color Concept of Wound Care." *Nursing '90* 20, 2 (February 1990): 59–61.

Mobility and Activity

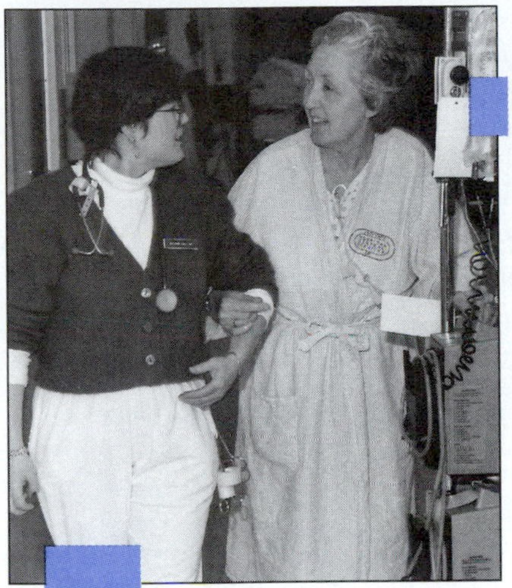

23

Objectives

After completing this chapter, you should be able to:

1. Describe the components of the musculoskeletal system.
2. Define and describe the basic patterns of activity.
3. Describe the benefits and hazards of exercise.
4. Identify groups of persons at risk for alteration in mobility.
5. Outline the data gathered as part of activity assessment.
6. List common nursing diagnoses related to mobility.
7. List actions that can be used for nursing intervention in problems of immobility.
8. Discuss the role of rehabilitation for maintaining the disabled to a maximum state of function.
9. Identify ways to evaluate response to activity.

Study Terms

active assistive exercise
active exercise
base of support
body mechanics
center of gravity
contracture
goniometer
internal girdle
isometric exercise
isotonic exercise
passive exercise
postural (orthostatic) hypotension
range-of-motion (ROM) exercise
resistive exercise

Outline

Ellis, Nowlis: Nursing: A Human Needs Approach, 5th ed. © 1994 J.B. Lippincott Company

Mobility and activity are not the same. Mobility is the ability to move. With human beings, it means to move all body parts and to move the body from one place to another. Activity can be the way in which mobility is expressed. Walking is an activity. When walking, the person is mobile, moving from one place to another, and receiving the physiological and psychological benefits of an activity. A wheelchair-bound person may not be viewed as "mobile," yet can be an active person, performing exercises that are an activity adapted to the level of functioning.

Activity of whatever kind is a basic human need (Fig. 23-1). Research indicates that, beginning at birth, human beings need activity for optimum development. If a child does not have physical activity, muscles, joints, and bones will not develop to maximum size and strength. The circulatory system will fail to develop the extensive network of small vessels that provides for additional circulation to meet stressful situations; the respiratory system will not develop additional lung capacity. Insufficient physical activity causes muscles to atrophy, joints to become stiff, and internal organs to function less effectively than they should. If this happens, the diminished strength of atrophied muscles undermines the systems they support. For example, weakened back muscles make the spine more liable to injury; weak abdominal muscles cause both the bladder and bowel to function less effectively.

Rest can be thought of as the opposite of activity. It is not the same thing as sleep. All body parts need regular rest, just as they need activity. Overused muscles are unable to rid themselves of all waste products and thus become painful and nonfunctioning. For example, using one's eyes to do detailed work for long hours may make them ache and temporarily impair one's vision. Thus, a balance between activity and rest is necessary for optimal health. Rest will be discussed in Chapter 24.

On either a temporary or permanent basis, activity may be profoundly affected by any illness. Often the patient experiences some degree of immobility, and the nurse must assume a major role in maintaining the patient's ability and functioning. As you assess the patient's activity status, identify particular problems and needs, and undertake nursing actions that will be most supportive, keeping in mind that your goal is assisting the patient to attain an optimal activity level.

The Musculoskeletal System

An understanding of the musculoskeletal system provides a foundation for understanding the needs for activity and rest. The bones and muscles work together to enable the body and its parts to move effectively. Without this capability, the body would be unable to meet its basic needs.

The musculoskeletal system is one of distinct components each of which interacts with other structures of the system. Movement requires coordinated activity of

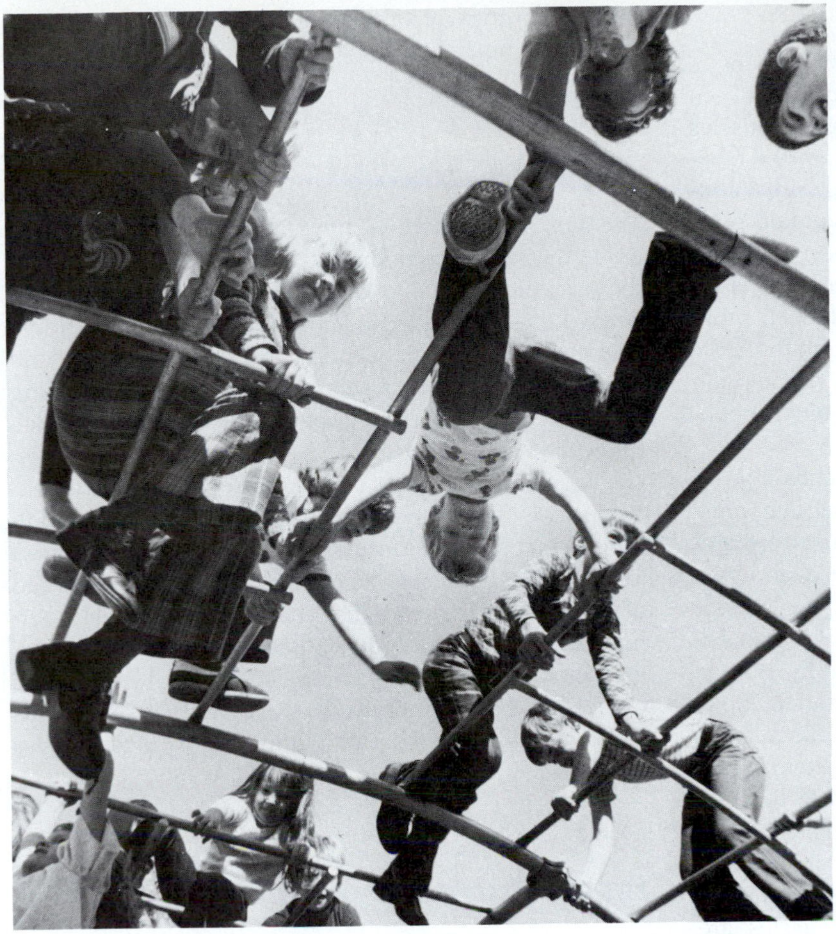

Figure 23-1. Children enjoy meeting their needs for activity.

each of these segments along with enervation by the nervous system.

Bones

The *bones* are the rigid, calcium-based tissue that form the support system for body tissue. In addition, bones protect the soft, vulnerable structures of the body by enclosing them. The skull protects the brain; the ribs protect the lungs; and the pelvis protects the bladder, the intestines, and the reproductive organs. The bones of the extremities are effective levers operated by the muscles to produce movement. Within the bones of the sternum, ribs, vertebral bodies, cranial bones, iliac bones, and growth points of the femur and the humerus is red bone marrow, which is a specialized tissue that produces all three types of blood cells.

The bone itself contains living cells as well as the nonliving rigid intracellular material. The intracellular material is made up of calcium salts and protein tissue. The living cells within the bone function continually, receiving nutrients, breaking down, and building up bony tissue. Therefore, circulation to bones is essential. Another important fact for health care providers is that the rate of bone deposition is directly related to bone stress (Guyton, 1992, p. 594). For example, if a patient has a fractured leg in a cast and that extremity is immobile, the bone layers will thin until such time as the leg has recovered sufficiently and can safely support increased weight (stress).

Cartilage

Cartilage is similar to bone, but it does not contain calcified tissue in the intracellular structure. Instead, a network of connective tissue fibers forms a tissue that is like firm plastic. Cartilage does not have a blood supply. Needed nutrients reach the few living cells of the cartilage by diffusing through the tissue. Cartilage covers the surface of the bones at the joints and provides a smooth surface that facilitates movement. Cartilage is also found between the vertebrae and between the bones of the pelvis, where the bones do not move across one another but need a connecting point with some flexion. Cartilage also provides structure for soft organs such as the nose and the ear.

Muscles

Muscles are responsible for effecting the movement of body parts. Movement is produced when muscles contract, exerting force on the bones. In addition, muscles produce most of the body's heat and maintain the position and alignment of body parts. Continued partial contraction of some muscles is necessary to maintain position and alignment. This partial contraction is called *muscle tone*. The constant activity of the muscles is responsible for producing heat as a by-product. If more heat is needed than is being produced through the basic activities of the muscles, the control centers of the brain induce shivering, which is a high-intensity muscle contraction that will increase heat production.

Muscles are composed of bundles of cells able to contract and expand. In their most expanded state, muscles are relaxed. However, conditioned muscles maintain a state of minimal contraction, or *tonus*, even when relaxed. This minimal contraction renders the muscle strong and prepared to act when necessary. It also enhances circulation in the muscle. The healthy muscle maintains enough tonus to be firm to the touch. *Atony* is complete lack of muscle tone, which sometimes accompanies paralysis of central nervous system (CNS) origin. The atonic muscle is flaccid. A muscle that has some tonus but is not fully firm is termed *hypotonic*; hypotonic muscles result from inactivity and insufficient exercise or from illness and fatigue. A hypotonic muscle is weak and easily injured. *Hypertonic* muscles are firmly contracted even when they are ostensibly at rest. They promote fatigue and muscular aches and pains and contribute to joint deformities. Hypertonic muscles may result from tension, disease, or injury.

Joints

There are several different ways in which bones are attached to one another, forming joints. Joints and their proper movement are essential to maintaining mobility and activity. Each of these types of joints moves in a specialized way.

Some joints lack a joint cavity, and the cartilage grows between the bones. These joints, which are called *fixed joints*, do not allow free movement, although they allow some flexibility. The connections between the ribs and sternum are a good example of fixed joints. They allow the ribs to flex outward for breathing but limit the amount of movement, creating a fairly fixed, strong structure.

Joints with free movement have a small space between the bony surfaces, which is filled with fluid secreted by a membrane lining the joint. The bones are attached by means of soft-tissue ligaments that hold the bones in proper relationship to one another. The knees, shoulders, hips, fingers, and toes are all examples of freely movable joints.

Connective Tissue

The muscles are covered by a thin sheath of connective tissue that comes together at the end of the muscle. If the structure at the end is narrow and cordlike, the connective tissue is called a *tendon*. The tendon is firmly attached to the bone. Tendons are strong tissues, and great force is required to tear them. The fibers wrapping a muscle may also come together in a broad flat structure called an *aponeurosis*. The aponeurosis holds muscles together in groups and stabilizes them. *Ligaments* are broad, flat connective tissues; they provide additional attachment of muscles to bones, and they support joints. These tissues all have some ability to stretch and then return to their original shape. This flexibility permits easy movement. If these tissues lose their flexibility, joint mobility is severely compromised. However, these tissues have definite limits on their flexibility; the limits increase stability in the joint but may allow the tissues to be damaged by excessive stretching.

Basic Patterns of Activity

Certain basic patterns of activity are essential to meeting the needs of the body for activity. Posture, body alignment, and various types of exercise are all parts of these basic patterns.

Neuromuscular Control

The muscles are controlled by voluntary and involuntary CNS processes. Involuntary movement, such as muscle tone or shivering, originates in the medulla. Reflex movement, such as withdrawal from a match flame, originates in the sensory nerve at the surface. Then, the impulse connects with the motor neuron in the spinal cord and immediately moves back out to the muscle without going through the cortex of the brain. Voluntary movement arises in the cerebral cortex where movements are coordinated in the cerebellum, and the impulse travels down the spinal cord.

Motor nerves conduct impulses from the CNS to the muscles. Although these motor nerves arise within several areas of the CNS, all the nerves for an individual muscle meet in the anterior horn area of the spinal cord and then follow a final common pathway to the muscle fiber.

Types of Movement

Joints permit basically seven types of movement. Some joints are capable of several types of movement; others are constructed so that only one type of movement is possible (Table 23-1).

Flexion is the simplest type of joint movement and consists of "bending" at the joint, thereby decreasing the angle between the surfaces of the bones. Flexion occurs at all freely movable joints. Bending the knee backward, making a fist of the fingers, and bending the head forward are examples of flexion.

Extension is a return to the original alignment from a flexed position. Extension is basically straightening of the body part. Continuing to move beyond the position of normal alignment is called *hyperextension.* Although some hyperextension is normal, excessive hyperextension may damage supporting tissues around the joint.

The terminology used to describe the joint movement of the ankle can sound confusing. Bending the ankle so that the foot moves forward and up toward the leg is an example of *dorsal flexion.* Extending the ankle so that the toes are pointing downward is called *plantar flexion.* Plantar flexion is actually a type of extension, but the former terminology has been in use a long time and continues to be considered standard.

Abduction moves the body part away from the midline of the body. A leg moved straight out to the side is in abduction. Moving the arm out to the side is abduction. *Adduction* is moving the body part toward the midline of the body—the opposite of abduction. Moving the arm back to the side after abduction is adduction. Continuing the movement from the normal position of the arm on across the body is a continuation of adduction. The two terms may be easier to remember if you note that adduction begins with "add," and you are "adding" the extremity to the body as a whole. When the terms for these two types of movement are spoken, it is often easy to misunderstand what is said. Therefore, you may hear the terms partially spelled out, as in "a-d-duction" or "a-b-duction."

Rotation is moving the extremity in a pivoting fashion on its own axis. Although this movement is sometimes likened to that of a top, it is really a much more limited movement because one can rotate only part of the way in one direction and part of the way in the opposite direction. Turning your head from side to side is considered rotation.

Circumduction is the movement of an extremity in a cone-shaped pattern. The proximal (close to the body) end of the bone is fixed in position. The distal (far from the body) end of the bone describes a circle. The joints capable of this movement are ball and socket in configuration, such as the hip and the shoulder.

Certain special movements are only possible in one type of joint because of the special construction of that joint. The jaw may be moved forward in *protraction* and moved back in *retraction.* The forearm may be turned so that the palm is down, called *pronation,* and then turned so that the palm is up, called *supination.* The ankle may be turned so that the sole of the foot is toward the midline, which is *inversion,* and so that the sole of the foot is toward the outside, which is *eversion.*

For a discussion of joint movement in relation to

Table 23–1. Types of Joint Movement

Type	Description
Flexion	Decreasing the angle between the surfaces of the bone, bending
Dorsal flexion	Bending the foot forward and up at the ankle
Extension	Returning to the original alignment
Hyperextension	Moving beyond normal alignment
Plantar flexion	Extending the ankle with the toes pointing downward
Abduction	Moving the body part away from the midline of the body
Adduction	Moving the body part toward the midline of the body
Rotation	Moving the extremity in a pivoting fashion on its own axis
Circumduction	Moving an extremity in a cone-shaped pattern with the proximal end fixed and the distal end scribing a circle
Special movement	Movement possible in only one type of joint
Protraction	Moving the jaw forward
Retraction	Moving the jaw backward
Pronation	Turning the palm downward
Supination	Turning the palm upward
Inversion	Turning the sole of the foot inward
Eversion	Turning the sole of the foot outward

range-of-motion (ROM) exercises, see Module 24, Range-of-Motion Exercises.

Gait and Ambulation

Gait is the manner in which a person walks. A normal gait involves placing the weight fully on each leg in turn. Normal gait consists of weight being on both feet for a brief period of time, shifting to one foot as the other is swung forward, shared by both feet briefly, and then shifting again to the second foot as the first foot is swung forward. All steps are the same length and take the same amount of time. The two sides show a symmetry of movement and all the related movements of the body are smoothly coordinated. The person appears to be well balanced, with the center of gravity moving smoothly forward over the supporting legs (Table 23-2).

Ambulation is walking. Although a simple exercise, walking accomplishes effectively all the purposes of exercise. It not only keeps joints flexible and strengthens muscles, but also stimulates the entire circulatory, respiratory, and gastrointestinal systems. Walking uses almost all the body's muscles. As an exercise, walking can be varied in speed and distance to accommodate the abilities of a wide variety of people, even those with severe disability. Hospitalized patients often require support or the use of such devices as walkers and crutches to ambulate. Considerable care must be taken to protect the safety of an ill person while ambulating. Module 23, Ambulation, describes how to help a patient ambulate and use assistive devices.

Posture and Body Alignment

Posture and body alignment are essential elements involving the basic patterns of activity. *Posture* is the position of the body parts relative to one another. To maintain posture, muscles must be constantly at work, balancing and adjusting. Ideal posture puts the least strain on body parts and is most functional. It is usually described with reference to the standing position. Posture in the standing position is also called *stance.*

Correct Posture and Body Alignment

In an ideal posture, the feet (in low-heeled or flat shoes) are placed slightly apart to provide a wide **base of support** for the body's weight. The abdominal muscles are contracting, supporting the abdominal organs. The buttocks are tucked in and down, somewhat flattening the curve of the lower back. Because the muscles support the abdomen and buttocks as a girdle does, this state is sometimes compared to wearing an **internal girdle**.

The alignment of body parts in relation to the spine is a critical aspect of good posture. This is sometimes referred to as anatomic position. The standing anatomic position is one in which the person stands erect with the

Table 23–2. Terminology Used to Describe Gait

Term	Description
Ataxic	There is a lack of balance: the person keeps the feet spread in a wide stance and appears to be in danger of falling.
Double-step	There is a clearly distinguishable difference between the length of steps taken with each foot. A pattern of step–half-step–step appears. The timing is such that on first glance the walker appears to be putting the same foot forward twice in a row.
Dragging	The foot is dragged along the surface rather than swung forward.
Propulsive	The upper body moves forward faster than the lower body, and the person begins to move rapidly to try to keep from falling forward. This is also called a festinating gait.
Spastic	The legs are held close together because of spasm of the flexor muscles. The person moves in a stiff manner because it is hard to overcome the rigidity of the flexor muscles. The person often rises up on the toes.
Staggering	The person veers from side to side.
Steppage	The foot is lifted high so that the toes clear the surface because the person is unable effectively to flex the foot dorsally.
Stumbling	The person does not lift the feet high enough with each step and stumbles on the surface.
Tabetic	This gait is basically ataxic with the feet characteristically slapping the ground as they are put down.
Waddling	There is exaggerated hip movement in which the hip is lifted and swung forward, giving a ducklike motion.

arms hanging at the sides with the feet slightly apart. The body is relaxed but in perfect balance. Twisting the pelvis, shoulders, or head to the side also twists the spine. Instead, in good posture, the head is held erect over the shoulders and faces straight ahead. The shoulders are held straight (often best achieved by pulling them back and then dropping them). In this position, the body's **center of gravity**, the point at which gravitational pull functions as if the body's entire weight were concentrated at that single point, is directly above the base of support. The center of gravity in the human body is approximately at the level of the pelvis.

Closely related to posture is *body alignment.* This term is more commonly used to describe the position of the body when the person is lying in bed. Proper body alignment prevents both discomfort and injury to the back and other body parts.

Factors That Affect Posture and Body Alignment

Age is a factor that affects posture and body alignment. Very young children normally have somewhat protruding abdomens and their lumbar spines show a backward curvature (swayback). To accommodate for this curvature, they learn to walk with the feet apart. Even though most teenagers have good posture and body alignment, their parents often admonish them "to stand up straight!" Some very tall young people who are self-conscious about their height tend to slump to look shorter. However, slumping can lead to permanent anterior curvature of the thoracic spine. Young adults are physically active and usually maintain good posture. Pregnant women tend to walk with the back tipped backward to compensate for the weight of the enlarged abdomen.

Persons of advanced years often develop contractures of the flexor muscles of the upper back, so that the upper spine is "humped," a condition referred to as *kyphosis.* The knees of the older person may be slightly bent because of *osteoarthritis* and to accommodate for sensory perceptual changes that can make them unsteady. Older persons may alter their posture and body alignment because they fear falls and injury. Because of these changes, older adults may have stooped posture and a shuffling gait.

The most common bone disease in adults is *osteoporosis,* in which the production of bone cell replacement is diminished. Osteoporosis can be caused by lack of stress on bones because of inactivity, protein depletion, lack of estrogens after menopause, or decreased production of growth hormone due to aging (Guyton, p 599, 1992). Nurses should have some knowledge of this condition because it accounts for about 90% of all fractures of the femur. In men, osteoporosis arises later in life and is not as severe as it is in women.

Some nutritional diseases can change posture and alignment. For example, *rickets* is a calcium and phosphate deficiency and occurs primarily in children. This disease weakens bones so that the long bones of the body become brittle. The long leg bones bend slightly, causing "bowing" of the legs and a distorted posture.

Emotions can also affect posture and body alignment. Depressed persons sometimes display a stooped appearance, with the eyes looking downward. Others, who are in a state of elation, may walk forcefully with the arms swinging at the sides and the head thrust slightly forward. A more detailed discussion on how the emotions alter appearance is given in Chapter 34.

Using Proper Body Mechanics

Body mechanics is the application of mechanical principles and knowledge of human anatomy to the action of body parts during activity. Study of body mechanics usually involves learning appropriate ways to move the body to accomplish tasks without stress or injury. Correct body mechanics helps protect joints and muscles from being forced beyond their capacities while allowing them to be used for maximum effectiveness. Body mechanics is important for everyone but particularly for the nurse whose profession entails a great deal of moving and lifting. A major reason some nurses leave practice is because of lower back problems. The nurse not only must use proper body mechanics but be able to teach patients to move the body correctly. Patients often need to be taught how to move safely and effectively. The nurse can promote proper body mechanics by such measures as placing the bedside stand in a position that does not require the patient to twist and demonstrating correct techniques for moving in and out of bed. Display 23-1 outlines basic principles of body mechanics, which are discussed more thoroughly in Module 4, Basic Body Mechanics. Following is a review of the major principles of body mechanics.

1. *Maintaining center of gravity over base of support*: Weight is balanced best when the center of gravity is directly above the base provided by the feet. When walking, bending from the knees, rather than the waist, or placing one foot in the direction of the bending enlarges the base of support, providing stability.
2. *Avoiding twisting*: Twisting, or torsion, of the spine lessens its ability to function effectively and can lead to injury. Rather than twisting, the entire body should be turned in one plane.
3. *Using leg muscles*: The large, thick muscles of the legs are better able to tolerate heavy loads than the broad, flat muscles of the back. Therefore, lifting is

Display 23–1
Basic Principles of Body Mechanics

1. Weight is balanced best when the center of gravity is directly above the base of support.
2. Enlarging the base of support increases the body's stability.
3. A body or object is more stable if its center of gravity is close to its base of support.
4. Enlarging the base of support in the direction of the force to be applied increases the amount of force that can be applied.
5. Tightening the abdominal muscles upward and the gluteal muscles downward before undertaking any activity decreases the likelihood of strain or injury.
6. Facing toward the task to be performed and turning the entire body in one plane, rather than twisting, lessens the back's susceptibility to injury.
7. Lifting is better undertaken by bending the legs and using the larger leg muscles than by using the back muscles.
8. Moving an object on a level surface requires less effort than moving it against the force of gravity.
9. Less energy is required to move an object when friction between the object and the surface on which it rests is minimized.
10. It takes less energy to hold an object close to the body than at a distance from the body.
11. The weight of the body can be used to facilitate lifting and moving.
12. Smooth, rhythmic movements at a moderate speed require the least energy.
13. When a soft object is pushed, it absorbs part of the force being exerted; pulling a soft object subtracts less of the force from the movement.

best undertaken by bending the legs and using the leg muscles.

4. *Pulling or sliding instead of lifting*: Before moving an object or a patient, consider whether the weight might be pulled or slid, rather than lifted, to the new position. Both alternatives require less strength. Friction of the surface under the object or person can be minimized by providing a smooth surface (such as tight bed sheets). A turning sheet placed under a patient is an effective aid.
5. *Contracting abdominal muscles*: Undue strain on the abdominal muscles can tear the muscle along a weakened point, causing a hernia. This outcome can be avoided by contracting the abdominal muscles—referred to earlier as wearing an internal girdle—before undertaking any effort.
6. *Using a counterweight*: Your weight and that of the object or person to be moved may be used to assist movement. Hold your body in a stable position and then rock back, using your entire weight, rather than simply your muscular strength, as a counterbalance to assist the patient to a standing position. To turn a patient from back to side, bend the knees up. The weight of the legs turning to the side will help pull the entire body over.

Exercise

Exercise is active movement of the body beyond that required to maintain muscle tone and posture. Exercise maintains joint mobility and function, as well as muscle strength and flexibility. Furthermore, physical exercise enhances the functioning of the gastrointestinal system by increasing appetite and promoting elimination. The metabolic rate increases during activity, exercising the temperature-regulating mechanisms and a wide variety of other physiologic processes.

According to Pender (1992), "frequent strenuous exercise associated with a continuous and significant elevation of pulse for 20 to 30 minutes helps protect individuals against the threat of heart attacks, improves physical well-being, and increases feelings of vitality" (see Chapter 29).

Exercise seems to enhance the ability to think clearly by stimulating circulation and promoting optimum ventilation. Activity also serves as an outlet for tension and anxiety. A game of tennis or a long walk may reduce tension and anxiety to manageable levels and permit one's energy to be focused on problem solving. Even asleep, people are physically active, moving their extremities, turning from side to side, and changing position repeatedly.

Active Exercise

The following types of exercise are normal components of daily living and may be adapted to the special needs of those with decreased energy and ability. **Active exercise** involves voluntary movement of a body part by means of muscular contraction and relaxation.

Normally, *position changes* are actually a type of active exercise. If the person's position is changed with the assistance of another person, it could be referred to as passive exercise. Position changes, such as from one sitting or lying position to another, are fundamental components of an exercise baseline. When people are well, they do not even think about their constant shifts and changes of position. Position changes alleviate pressure on supporting body parts, such as the buttocks, feet, and sacrum, and enhance circulation. Position changes also facilitate deep respirations, movement of lung secretions, drainage from the kidneys, and gastrointestinal functioning. Changing a person's position can alter circulatory patterns. Raising a person to a sitting position, for example, increases the heart rate and facilitates general circulation. Respiration is also enhanced. Sometimes a person can be helped to perform *activities of daily living* (ADLs) in a passive manner. Allowing the patient to wash the chest, for example, provides passive exercise and may lead to greater independence in ADLs.

Many ADLs consist of active exercise. These activities include feeding oneself, caring for one's own hygiene and elimination needs, dressing oneself, and performing other tasks necessary to meet one's basic needs. Performing ADLs will usually provide a minimum baseline of activity important in avoiding illness. Performing ADLs also supports self-esteem and a self-image as an independent individual. For these reasons, ADLs tend to be the first active exercises a recuperating patient is encouraged to perform, the exercises most likely to be allowed during the course of illness, and the first exercises taught in the course of rehabilitation.

Another type of active exercise is **isometric exercise**—also called static exercise—which involves contracting a muscle, keeping it tight, and then relaxing it without moving the joint. Isometric exercises strengthen muscles and effectively stimulate circulation, especially venous return. These exercises are particularly useful when joint mobility is not possible or desired, as in the case of a person with a joint disability. Isometric exercises may also be used to strengthen muscles in preparation for more strenuous active exercise. Patients who are confined to bed for long periods of time can be instructed to perform leg, thigh, and gluteal isometric exercises to promote venous return and prevent thrombosis.

A term used for active exercise is **isotonic exercise**. However, the term is most often used to refer to planned active movement. The ordinary daily activities of people with sedentary occupations may not be adequate to meet all the body's needs for exercise. For maximum health of the cardiovascular and respiratory systems, a person should engage in exercise that causes the pulse to rise and respirations to increase in sessions at least three times a week on a regular basis. Calisthenics, jogging, and tennis are examples of isotonic exercise. Exercising for cardiovascular health will be discussed more fully in Chapter 29.

Resistive exercise is a special type of isotonic exercise performed against resistance, such as a weight. Weight lifting is resistive exercise. Resistive exercise builds muscle volume and strength faster than more active isotonic exercise. Resistive exercise produces strong muscles in women, but, because of differing hormonal responses, the muscles produced in women are of a different shape and contour from those produced in men. Resistive exercise is a preferred mode of treatment in physical therapy when muscle strength is poor.

Range-of-motion-exercise (ROM) is the movement of the joint through its full extent. It may be done as *active ROM* by the patient. When carried out by the nurse or physical therapist, it is *passive ROM* (see the next section). Each joint in the body is capable of certain types of movement, and some joints can perform more than one type of movement. The full extent to which a joint can move in any direction is called its range of motion. Types of joint movement are defined in Table 23-1. Planned ROM is typically recommended when a person is in danger of losing the full extent of joint motion as a result of disease process or weakness.

The range of a joint may be determined by measuring the degree of the angle formed by the joint at each end of its movement. A structural change in a joint (shortened muscles and tendons and inflexible skin) that prevents full range of motion is termed a **contracture**. For example, a person with a permanently flexed elbow is said to have a contracture of the elbow. If bone deformity has also occurred and the two bones are fused together, the joint is termed *ankylosed*.

The ROM exercises are designed to maintain maximum joint mobility. The joints are moved to their full range or as far as possible without causing pain. A severely disabled person might need to do such exercises several times a day to maintain functional ability.

Any exercise in which the energy and movement are provided by a person other than the person exercising is called **passive exercise**. Passive exercise is usually performed to increase ROM and joint flexibility. Passive exercise serves fewer of the purposes of exercise than does active exercise, but it is a valuable alternative in some situations.

When an individual can perform some joint motion independently but needs help completing the motion, such help is termed **active assistive exercise**. Active and active assistive ROM provide for more complete exercise than does passive ROM, which provides only for joint mobility.

The Benefits of Exercise

There has been increasing interest during the last 5 years of the importance of regular exercise for every individual. Books and exercise programs are available in abundance. The goal is that each person develop a personal program of exercise appropriate to his or her age, lifestyle, and endurance.

Even though the profession of nursing involves strenuous physical movement, many health care facilities have programs devoted to group aerobics and other types of exercise programs. Many nurses have found that running relieves tension. Other nurses have found that participating in an exercise program helps them feel less stressed; they have increased energy and an increased feeling of well-being. If you do not exercise regularly, you may wish to ask about available programs in your facility. Any degree of exercise has hazards, which are mainly related to the intensity and duration of exercise and the person's health status. The possible hazards of vigorous exercise, such as running, may not be a problem for patients who are able to exercise vigorously on a regular basis and are in good health. Concern has been expressed regarding the harmful effects of extreme exertion, particularly if the person does not undertake the activity on a regular basis. Stroke and heart attack have been documented as serious hazards in these situations. Of a less serious but nevertheless disabling nature, of the estimated millions of Americans who jog or run, up to 70% will sustain a running-related injury (Brody, 1987). Many specialists who treat musculoskeletal disorders warn against running because of its repeated impact on the cartilage surrounding bone. It is thought that because cartilage does not replace itself, the continuous "impact injury" produced on ankles and knees by this kind of exercise can result in disability later in life. Exercise that produces the greatest benefit with the least risk is that which is at the moderate level and performed consistently.

Common Problems Related to Mobility and Activity

Loss of Muscle Strength

Muscle strength is an important aspect of motor function. Normally, a person is able to move the trunk, head, and all extremities strongly within their full range. Lack of muscle strength, which can involve any of the skeletal muscles of the body, may occur because nerve stimulus (innervation) to a particular muscle or group of muscles has been partially interrupted. This condition, known as *paresis*, is often accompanied by lack of coordination. With decreased use, the muscle itself may *atrophy*, becoming smaller in size.

Loss of Neuromuscular Control

Paralysis is inability to move a body part voluntarily. The most common causes of paralysis are cerebral vascular accident (stroke) and trauma to the spinal cord. Paralysis may or may not involve a disturbance in sensation. A paralyzed arm, for example, may have no sensation, normal levels of sensation, or hyperesthesia (increased sensation). Some patients experience pain in a paralyzed extremity.

Hemiplegia is paralysis of one side of the body. *Paraplegia* is paralysis of the lower part of the body. *Quadriplegia* is paralysis of all four extremities. Paralysis is usually readily apparent. The affected side of the face may droop. The extremities may be flaccid and unable to move. Keep in mind that paralysis may not be complete. For example, the fingers may be capable of slight movement even though the arm is paralyzed or the arm may be moved by lifting the shoulder. The patient may be able to lift a paralyzed arm with the unaffected hand or to grasp a partially paralyzed leg and pull it forward. *Coordination*—the ability to move and control the extremities and body parts in a balanced and effective manner—is disturbed in a variety of neurologic conditions. Abnormal gaits and poor ambulation may result from disorders of the musculoskeletal system or from disorders of the neuromuscular control system. A clear description of an abnormal gait may be helpful when one is making plans to provide support during ambulation. Gait may also be important to the physician's diagnosis of the medical condition. Table 23-2 provides a list of terms commonly used to describe gait. If you cannot remember the correct terminology, simply describe the gait in detail.

The fact that there is only one final common pathway for motor nerves has practical implications. If any damage occurs to the anterior horn area or to a motor nerve between this area and the muscle fiber, there will be no impulses at all to the muscle; both voluntary and involuntary movement will be destroyed. Damage in the CNS may damage some aspects of movement without damaging them all. For example, damage in the cerebellum might make movement uncoordinated, but voluntary control would still exist. Damage in the cerebrum could destroy voluntary movement completely, but involuntary movement would still be present and muscles would have tone and shivering capability. It is important for you to know that whether or not the patient's muscles are spastic or whether they are flaccid depends on the location of injury or disease. Generally, when upper motor neurons are damaged, rigid or spastic paralysis occurs. When lower motor neurons (those from the anterior horn cells on) are damaged, a flaccid paralysis occurs.

Dysphagia is inability to *swallow*, usually caused by partial paralysis of the esophagus. The patient with dysphagia may choke on fluids or food, aspirating the particles into the bronchi or lungs. The gag reflex, which protects us from aspiration by closing the epiglottis, may also be deficient. Patients with a deficient gag reflex may have difficulty not only in swallowing but also in expectorating food or foreign bodies. The resulting irritation and partial obstruction can lead to an infection called aspiration pneumonia, a serious condition that can be fatal.

Persons at Risk for Alterations in Mobility

Many patients are at risk of alteration in mobility. Illness, surgery, trauma, or advanced age can affect muscle strength, which leads to fatigue and a decreased feeling of general well-being.

The Patient with a Medical Condition

Regardless of the severity of an illness, there is some limitation to activity and mobility. When you are experiencing a cold, you may not feel like running for exercise as you do regularly. You may wish to delay this until you feel better. Similarly, when patients are ill, they may feel fatigue, generalized weakness, or depression, disrupting normal activities. Some patients have medical conditions that limit their tolerance for activity. Chronic arthritic and respiratory conditions as well as neuromuscular disease are three that can limit mobility. Even though the person with arthritis feels some degree of pain on movement and is tempted to be sedentary, the patient should be encouraged to participate in as much exercise as possible. Much of the patient's pain can be controlled with medications. People with neuromuscular disease commonly have problems with gait, balance, and weakness. Again, encouragement should be given to maximize mobility although, at the same time, maintaining safety. Persons with severe respiratory problems, such as emphysema, may not be able to tolerate strenuous exercise so you must plan with the patient for the optimum acceptable level.

It is uncommon for patients to be ordered on bed rest for any length of time because health care providers recognize the importance of physiologic and psychological exercise and mobility. Patients with heart problems may be placed on a mobility program with gradually increasing activities. Once recovery is certain, more vigorous exercise is prescribed under supervision. Specific programs are available for the person in cardiac recovery.

The Surgical Patient

Part of the experience of having surgery is the recognition that for most procedures, there may be at least temporary decrease in activity. This may be due to the inability to move about as readily as one could do preoperatively. Incisional pain, generalized fatigue, and the presence of dressings or appliances may hamper movement. It is not uncommon for the physician to order that a patient get out of bed and move to a chair for a short period of time 12 to 24 hours after a surgical procedure. The beneficial effects of early movement or ambulation after surgery have been well documented. Patients appear to have far fewer respiratory, circulatory, and elimination problems than previously when postoperative patients were placed on extended bed rest (see the sample Nursing Care Plan for Activity Following Surgery).

The Trauma Patient

Being injured is an extremely stressful event. One of the most frequently encountered problems is the disruption of exercise and activity. Certainly, we must recognize that the degree of impairment is different depending on the extent of the injury. For example, persons with back injury may face a lengthy period before they can move comfortably without pain through a long period of therapy focused toward recovery. Those who have sustained bone fractures may find that regaining mobility takes both patience and assistance from others because bones heal slowly and sufficient healing must occur before weight can be applied safely to bones.

The Older Adult

We have discussed some of the physiologic factors that realistically may limit the activity of the older adult to some degree. However, with an ongoing exercise program, elders are able to maintain much of the function and mobility they enjoyed earlier.

When your patient is of advanced years, your plan of care should consider the area of activity so that you can assist the patient to stay as mobile as possible within the constraints of the medical condition. "Wellness maintenance is a positive approach to life and well-being for older adults" (Forbes, 1992). This may take some thought on your part to plan an individualized activity program in which the patient will willingly participate. Although the younger patient may be fairly inactive and enjoy reading and television for several hospitalized days, only to resume normal activity after discharge, this is often not the case with elderly persons. They may see their activity limitations as an indication that they are "on a slide" and will never regain their former ability to move about. You should keep an optimistic view along with providing skills to achieve a positive outcome for the patient. For more discussion about the older person, see Chapter 20.

The Disabled Person

Persons who have a *disability* have been referred to as "handicapped" or "disabled." Some prefer one term over the other. It has been suggested that society should refer to persons with a disability as "the physically

Nursing Care Plan

Sample Nursing Care Plan for Activity Following Surgery

Nursing Diagnosis

Activity Intolerance related to recent surgery

Supportive data:

52-year-old female post-hysterectomy

States "feels all washed out."

Becomes pale and dizzy and pulse reaches 120 when up as long as she wishes.

Desired Patient Outcomes

Does not become overfatigued, as evidenced by:

1. Pulse no more than 80 when up.
2. Color remains pink.
3. No dizziness.

Gains activity tolerance needed for self-care by discharge:

1. Does own bath.
2. Ambulates around the hall twice in the AM, once in the afternoon, and once in the PM with no statements of excess fatigue and vital signs remaining within 10% of preactivity vitals.

Nursing Action	Rationale
1. Check pulse, blood pressure, and respiration before and after ambulation.	Checking vital signs before the activity ensures that the patient is physically able to ambulate safely. Using these as a baseline, the vital signs taken after ambulation provide a record of the degree of activity tolerance.
2. Ambulate 3 times a day. Increase distance each day until going around hall twice. Patient will keep track of distance.	Daily increase in activity will gradually strengthen muscles and raise endurance level. Allowing patient to keep track of progress will encourage participation.
3. Have patient do own bath each AM. Stay with patient and have her stop when she feels tired. Gradually increase independence.	Being involved in one's own care increases self-esteem.

Nursing Research: Implications for Practice

Blaylock, B. "Mobility and Ambulation: Not Easy Tasks for All Older Adults." *Advancing Clinical Care* 6, 6 (November–December 1991): 20–21.

Blaylock identified reasons for the rapid loss of muscle strength in acutely ill elderly patients in the acute care setting. The study further suggests that because these individuals are seriously ill, interventions to maintain muscle strength may be overlooked. Nursing actions focused toward maintaining muscle strength during the time of the illness are essential. The outcome is that on recovery the older person can return to independent functioning and regain the ability to perform activities of daily living.

challenged" rather than by either of the two former terms. The thinking behind this idea is good because these persons are often physically challenged in carrying out the ADL that most of us take for granted (Fig. 23-2). However, the term is not widely used, so we will refer to the disabled person, regardless of the kind or complexity of the disability. This subject will be discussed in more depth in Chapter 42.

Many people have one of a number of disabling conditions. These include congenital *disabilities* related to neuromuscular functioning, such as cerebral palsy, paraplegia or quadriplegia due to spinal cord injury, and hearing or vision impairment.

People with such problems do not usually consider themselves ill; they see themselves as having special conditions that necessitate adaptations in daily life. Until recently, society did not support the efforts of many disabled people to function independently. However, recent federal and state legislation has mandated equal opportunity for employment, which has opened doors to fuller participation in the workplace for the disabled person. Some employers are adapting the work environment by means of devices that print messages for the deaf and telephones with desk speakers for the visually impaired, enabling these disabled persons to become economically independent. In the United States, the Americans with Disabilities Act passed by the 1992 Congress states that all public buildings must now be designed or renovated to afford physical access to the disabled. Schools now must allow disabled children to attend regular classes whenever possible (a practice called mainstreaming).

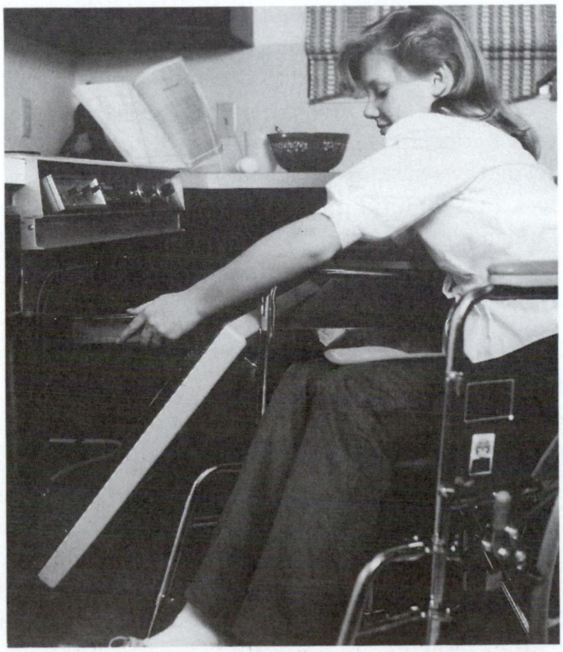

Figure 23-2. The disabled person can function independently.

When a person with a disability is admitted to a hospital for an illness or surgery, the staff commonly impose more dependence than is necessary. In fact, the disabled person may have a greater need than any other patient to maintain autonomy because that autonomy is often the result of considerable past effort by the disabled. Assessment of the disabled person's needs should involve determining what he or she can do independently and what adaptations can be made in the environment to facilitate independence. The disabled person who enters the hospital as a patient may have a better view of what is needed than does the nurse who provides care. Listening to the patient, rather than making abrupt assumptions, is useful to the nurse and the care of the patient. For example, crutches should not be stored in a closet but placed where they can be reached when needed. The quadriplegic who manages personal skin and bowel care at home should be allowed to continue to do so. If the person reports that bowels are kept functional by the use of stool softeners every day and a glycerin suppository every other day, your plan of care should provide for continuation of that routine. With regard to each ADL, you should consult with the individual and plan together for the adaptations that will be necessary in the hospital.

Assessment

Interview

Assessment of activity status requires careful interviewing of the patient and, if appropriate, family members. You need to know what has been the usual pattern of activity. Some individuals are much more active than are others. Knowing the patient's age may also add to your interview data because aging often changes levels of activity. All aspects of the musculoskeletal system and its functioning need to be considered. In addition, the nurse must assess the person's need of assistive devices, comfort level, options available for activity, motivation, and level of knowledge.

During the interview, you should inquire about the past medical problems of the patient and family. Does osteoarthritis occur in the family? You should elicit the patient's perceptions of the impact of activity limitations on daily living. What factors increase the degree of immobility and what factors are helpful? The interview also requires special assessment of those identified as being at risk for alteration in mobility.

Another important part of assessment is determining the patient's *activity level.* How much activity is the person actually undertaking? What is the usual patten of activity? Do the usual pattern and the current pattern differ? Is this variance causing the patient concern? Are there limitations on activity imposed on the individual, such as by a physician's order for restricted movement? Is illness in another body system, such as the circulatory or respiratory system, affecting the ability to engage in activity?

The person's *knowledge of the need for activity* and of the conditions that may change that need is a factor to be considered when you are conducting the interview for activity and rest patterns. You should also determine the person's knowledge of how to carry out desired activities safely.

For the patient and the nurse, the *comfort level* must be assessed. Health care problems can create discomfort in the musculoskeletal system in many different ways. This discomfort may be present constantly or only when the person moves. Clearly noting the location and the individual's description of the discomfort will aid in communication with the patient and the health care team.

Physical Assessment

First, assess the *appearance of the musculoskeletal system.* Assess posture and alignment. These are important both for the patient confined to bed and for the ambulatory person. Look for symmetry between the sides of the body so that you can identify a stronger side. Look for the shape and conformation of joints and bones, and note any abnormalities.

Assessment of Motor Function

Next, assess the *ability to move.* What parts of the body can the patient move independently? You can sometimes identify deficits by watching the person conduct ADLs. At other times, you will need to give the patient specific instructions about movement and then watch to see whether the directed activity can be done. It is helpful to ask the patients concerning their ability to move and what problems they have so that you can assist them during their hospitalization.

Characteristics of movement are also important. The ROM of a joint may be estimated by moving it gently through its full range. Range of motion is reported in terms of degrees that the joint will move. When precise information is needed, a **goniometer** may be used. This simple device, most commonly seen in physical therapy departments, is placed beside the joint, and the degree of angle is read from the scale on the instrument.

Gait is described after watching a person walk across the room. Gross incoordination is often easily assessed by observing how the patient walks. Is it steady and confident? Does the patient lurch? Does the person reach out for the wall or furniture for support? Difficulty with coordinating the gait is called *ataxia.* If the gait is unusual, you may need to observe the person several times to describe the gait clearly. Remember, you do not need to use special terminology for the gait to describe it clearly.

Tremors—involuntary shaking of a body part, an extremity, or the head—sometimes contribute to the coordination problem. Tremors are most common in the hands but may also be seen in the knees and feet. Other factors affecting motor function include balance and dizziness.

Coordination in movements other than walking is also an important consideration. You might watch the person handling a call light, a water pitcher, or a pencil to assess coordination. A more subtle sign of incoordination you might assess is difficulty locating the mouth with the toothbrush.

The body mechanics a person uses when moving can also be assessed. How does the person move in bed? Does the person twist or bend in ways that might cause injury to body parts?

Some muscle weakness can be assessed by observation. Does the patient drag one leg? Is there drooping of the eyelids (ptosis) or drooling at the mouth? Weakness can also be identified by means of simple testing. Ask the patient to grip both your hands and squeeze. Is the grip approximately equal on both sides or is one side much weaker than the other? You can assess the muscle strength of the shoulders and legs by asking the patient to push against your hand while you provide resistance. Muscle weakness is not true paralysis.

Lack of coordination may be limited to a single extremity, such as an arm that moves randomly or fingers that are unable to grasp objects. It may also be generalized, as in the case of a person severely handicapped from cerebral palsy.

Assessment of Physiologic Response to Activity

The individual's physiologic response to activity is an important indicator used to determine whether activity is appropriate for the person's physical condition. The major concern is the response of the cardiovascular and respiratory systems to activity. You will often need to check pulse, blood pressure, and respiratory rate before and after the activity. You should also look for changes in skin color, breathing pattern, coordination, or psychological distress.

Assessment of Swallowing Ability

Careful assessment is necessary when a patient or the family reports any degree of difficulty in swallowing. A sip of sterile water is an appropriate first step because it will be less injurious than any other fluid if aspirated. Some patients can swallow solid substances more easily than clear fluids, whereas others find thin liquids most acceptable. When testing during assessment, place the patient in high Fowler's position so that gravity flow can facilitate swallowing.

To assess for a normal, active gag reflex, you can touch the back of the throat with a cotton-tipped swab to elicit a gag. If the gag reflex is absent or significantly decreased, this stimulus will not elicit a response.

Nursing Diagnosis

Changes in the ability to maintain activity and mobility patterns are a major focus for nursing diagnosis. Careful consideration of the related factors is important because of the many causes of immobility and inactivity. Nursing diagnosis statements that are specific provide the basis for successful planning and implementation.

Activity Intolerance

Activity Intolerance is a nursing diagnosis for the person with restrictions of activity; it is approved by the North American Nursing Diagnosis Association (NANDA). The patient with the diagnosis of Activity Intolerance is unable to endure or tolerate an increase in activity. This diagnosis is often related to changes in body systems as outlined above. Activity intolerance might be related to pain experienced, to fatigue and weakness, or to any of a variety of physical factors. It might also be related to psychological factors such as depression, lack of motivation, or lifestyle. Activity intolerance might be identified by overt signs of fatigue and distress after activity, by statements made by the individual, or by physiologic responses to the activity.

Pulse rate is one indicator of response to activity. Either a too rapid pulse or a failure of the pulse to return to a resting rate would indicate this diagnosis. A pulse that is normally between 60 and 90 is not expected to be greater than 100 with ordinary activity. It should return to within six beats of the resting rate within 3 minutes. Activity Intolerance is also indicated if the pulse decreases in rate or strength or becomes irregular or weak during activity. Blood pressure is another indicator of activity tolerance. It should not rise to greater than 140 mm Hg systolic if the resting level is within normal limits. Respirations may increase, but should not be greater than 22/min. Respirations should not decrease in rate or be accompanied by shortness of breath.

Nursing Diagnoses Related to Mobility

- Activity Intolerance
- Impaired Physical Mobility
- High Risk for Disuse Syndrome
- High Risk for Injury
- Self-care Deficits
  - Self-care Deficit: Total
  - Self-care Deficit: Feeding
  - Self-care Deficit: Dressing self
  - Self-care Deficit: Toileting self
- Situational Low Self-Esteem
- Impaired Home Maintenance Management

Impaired Physical Mobility

Although not yet approved by NANDA, Impaired Physical Mobility is a major diagnostic category that reflects the potential for many problems in various body systems. Because the immobility itself is the major concern, you will often find that using this term as your nursing diagnosis makes planning easier. However, some nurses prefer to list the many high-risk problems related to immobility as individual nursing diagnoses. They believe that doing so encourages more specificity in planning. When specific complications of immobility do arise, the complications will need to be identified separately on the nursing care plan and additional actions related to resolving those problems planned.

You should identify immobility as a problem when the patient is unable to move because of a physiologic condition or when there is an order for rest that requires the person to refrain from the usual ADLs. Because the need for activity and the need for rest are both basic needs, restricting mobility has profound and far-reaching effects. Immobilization causes changes and deterioration in even a healthy person; the axiom "that which is not used is lost" is apt. However, nursing measures can help prevent deterioration.

A diagnosis of Impaired Physical Mobility can be made when the person has some limitation on physical movement and may be related to anatomic and functional changes in the upper extremities or the lower extremities. The etiology statement should reflect the anatomic or functional change present. For example, a diagnosis of Impaired Physical Mobility might be related to left-sided paralysis, to fracture of the right ankle, or to any of a number of other specific conditions. Common problems resulting from immobility will be discussed in terms of the affected body systems.

It is important to remember that no system is affected independently and that preventive measures addressed to one body system may also help prevent problems in others. You may wish to refer to the chapters focusing on particular physiologic needs to review normal functioning. The following are changes within systems that may lead to your writing specific nursing diagnoses. This is one of the most frequently used nursing diagnoses for patients with neuromuscular problems because so many of these conditions cause limitation in mobility. The defining characteristics should clearly identify the degree and type of limitation. This diagnosis may also be related to insufficient knowledge of ways to increase mobility or use assistive devices (Carpenito, 1992). In this instance, you could also write this as a Knowledge Deficit nursing diagnosis.

High Risk for Disuse Syndrome

This NANDA-approved nursing diagnosis is often stated as High Risk for Disuse Syndrome (Display 23-2). Its use is appropriate when the person has alteration of other body systems related to imposed or unavoidable immobility or inactivity (Carpenito, 1992, p 324).

Musculoskeletal System. Lack of exercise causes the muscles to become weaker, smaller, and even shorter, that is, they can *atrophy*. If immobility persists for a long enough period (variable from person to person), atrophy can limit the joint's ROM and eventually cause contracture of the joint. Because flexor muscles are stronger than extensors, the atrophied joint has a tendency to remain flexed. The flexor muscles then become shortened and the extensors lengthened.

When the stresses and strains imposed on the bones by normal movement and weight bearing are absent, the body begins to reabsorb calcium, and the bone becomes weak and porous. This condition may cause pain on stress and can result in easily fractured bones.

Integumentary System. Problems of the musculoskeletal system lead to nursing diagnoses of the integumentary system because the skin and subcutaneous tissue are not able to tolerate continued pressure in one area. When small blood vessels become occluded (blocked off) by such pressure, cells begin to suffer from *ischemia* (lack of blood supply to a tissue). If the blood supply is interrupted too long, cells are unable to recover and *necrosis* (cell death) begins. This situation is the origin of most *pressure ulcers* (see Chapter 22). Pressure ulcers may occur on any body surface as a result of maintaining any position for too long.

Urinary System. Position and activity directly affect the urinary system. Some people's ability to void is impaired by lying down. This is especially true of men, who are accustomed to urinating in a standing position. If a person cannot maintain a normal position to urinate, the bladder may not empty completely and urinary retention may occur. The overdistended bladder may also overflow, causing incontinence. Both of these situations may predispose to infection (see Chapter 27).

Normal kidney drainage is maintained by gravitational flow. If a person must remain supine, urine may pool in the renal (kidney) pelvis, also creating a climate for infection. Furthermore, the stagnant urine may be a source of kidney stones, which are minerals precipitated from the urine. This problem is aggravated by the necessity to excrete the excess calcium that is being reabsorbed from inactive bone. This calcium tends to precipitate out as kidney stones.

Display 23–2

Specific Risk States Related to Immobility

Musculoskeletal System

High Risk for Impaired Physical Mobility
- related to disuse of muscles
- related to fracture secondary to osteoporosis
- related to joint contractures secondary to not moving joints

Integumentary System

High Risk for Impaired Skin Integrity related to constant pressure on bony prominences

Urinary System

High Risk for Infection: Urinary, related to presence of indwelling catheter

High Risk for Altered Urinary Elimination related to renal calculi secondary to excess calcium

Gastrointestinal System

High Risk for Constipation related to lack of activity

Respiratory System

Impaired Gas Exchange related to shallow breathing

Ineffective Breathing Pattern related to difficulties with chest expansion while lying flat

Circulatory System

High Risk for Altered Peripheral Tissue Perfusion: Thrombophlebitis, related to venous stasis

High Risk for Injury: Falls, related to orthostatic hypotension

Psychological

High Risk for Altered Thought Processes related to sensory deprivation

Impaired Social Interaction related to family's inability to visit

Self-esteem Disturbance related to loss of independence

Powerlessness related to prolonged dependence

Ineffective Coping related to prolonged or enforced dependency

Gastrointestinal System. The progress of food through the gastrointestinal system is facilitated by gravity and the normal movement of abdominal muscles. When these forces are not functioning, the entire digestive process may be slowed. This situation can result in increased gas formation and the retention of stool for such a long time that excess fluid is reabsorbed, making the stool dry and hard. If a patient is required to use a bedpan, the normal position for defecation cannot be achieved. Lack of privacy also inhibits bowel function. Together, these factors may lead to constipation and even *impaction* of hardened feces in the rectum (see Chapter 26).

Respiratory System. Because the respiratory system is so important to muscle activity, this is another system appropriate for writing nursing diagnoses. Secretions in the lungs are usually moved from the alveoli by changes in gravity due to position change and the pressure of moving air. Once the secretions are in the bronchioles, cilia move them upward and out of the respiratory passages. When movement and position changes are minimal, secretions tend to pool in the dependent sections of the lungs, where they consolidate and can cause hypostatic pneumonia. This condition decreases the surface available for oxygen exchange and can be life threatening.

Circulatory System. Although the heart of the circulatory system pumps blood through the arterial system to the tissue, no pump exists to return blood to the heart. This return blood flow depends greatly on movement and pressure from muscles surrounding the veins, aided by a system of valves that maintains one-way flow. When muscle movement is decreased, blood moves sluggishly in the large veins, predisposing an individual to *thrombus* (clot) formation and *phlebitis* (inflammation of the vein). Clots dislodged by massaging the muscles, primarily of the legs, can become *emboli* (moving particles in the bloodstream), which can move through the circulatory system to the heart or lung where they lodge in the small vessels and block circulation or gas exchange. A *pulmonary embolism* is a serious threat to lung function and possibly to life. To prevent embolism, the leg muscles of immobilized patients are not massaged.

Ordinarily, the body compensates for changes in position and the resulting changes in the effect of gravity on circulation by constricting and dilating vessels as necessary to maintain constant blood flow. After a period of bed rest, during which these mechanisms are not used, they do not function as effectively. Thus, if the circulation is unable to make the rapid adjustment needed when rising to a sitting or standing position, blood pools in the lower extremities, causing *hypotension* (low blood pressure), diminished blood flow to the brain, dizziness, or fainting. Low blood pressure caused by position change is called **postural (orthostatic) hypotension**.

Other Effects. An immobilized person may experience a variety of psychological effects. First, the need for belonging may be disrupted. When individuals are unable to join in the mainstream of life, they may feel isolated. Loneliness or a sense of depression is not uncommon.

Self-esteem may suffer, possibly severely. Society usually values people for their accomplishments and an immobilized person is often unable to fulfill others' expectations such as work, family responsibilities, or socializing with friends. Suspension of these activities may diminish self-esteem and contribute to depression. Perception may also be affected. Decreased sensory input may make it difficult to remain oriented to time so that a few minutes may seem like half an hour to an immobilized person. If stimuli are greatly reduced, sensory deprivation can occur (see Chapter 31).

Dependence on others can create additional problems. Resultant anger may be directed at caregivers, who serve as constant reminders of dependence. Some people, on the other hand, submit to dependence so completely that they do not undertake independent activities of which they are capable. Such patients may exhibit an apparent lack of motivation either to work toward improvement or to learn.

When caregivers recognize these responses and continue to be accepting and supportive, a climate of trust is established in which constructive communication can help alleviate the immobilized patient's distress.

High Risk for Injury

Falls are one of the most common types of injuries. Many of the deficits we have discussed can contribute to an increased risk for falling. Lack of coordination makes the person more likely to fall where there are uneven walking surfaces or when a quick adjustment must be made. Comprehensive programs to prevent falls among patients or residents of care facilities are in place in many agencies. Falls increase the length of hospital stay and may contribute to further deficits and impairments. Impaired swallowing or dysphagia could also lead to injury because it can cause *aspiration.* If the patient cannot swallow well enough to eat a nutritious diet, another nursing diagnosis could be stated as Alteration in Nutrition: Less Than Body Requirements. Although this is not a nursing diagnosis related to injury of the patient, it is a diagnosis that may result from impaired swallowing.

Self-care Deficits

Self-care Deficits compose a major group of nursing diagnoses. Carpenito (1992, p 684) outlines four areas of self-care deficit (Display 23-3). The first is self-feeding in

Nursing Care Plan

Sample Nursing Care Plan Related to Immobility

Nursing Diagnosis

Impaired social interaction related to bedrest and isolation from family

Supportive data:

71-year-old female with right hip fracture.

Ordered on bedrest.

Physically active and lived in retirement apartment before hospitalization.

Family lives in eastern part of the state and has returned home after visiting patient.

Helped with an "envelope stuffing" project for a political group at the time of injury.

States, "I sure miss all my friends and the activities at the apartments."

Desired Patient Outcomes

Short term:

Patient welcomes visits from old friends and states she enjoys diversionary activities until more mobile.

Long term:

Patient returns to apartment, continues contact with friends, resumes activities.

Nursing Action	Rationale
1. Encourage friends to visit patient often.	Encouraging friends to visit provides an environment conducive to social interaction.
2. Ask patient if there are games or group projects she might enjoy.	By eliciting the patient's suggestions as to what games and projects she might enjoy, you can better individualize meeting her social needs.
3. Welcome friends of the patient and encourage them to join patient in a game or to bring along a project she might do with them.	A welcoming attitude on the part of the nurse encourages people to want to visit with patients. Suggestions for activities may help friends to feel more comfortable and thus increase frequency and length of visits.

which some degree of assistance is necessary to eat. The second is a deficit in self-bathing. This may include the inability to bathe or obtain equipment needed for bathing. Self-dressing deficits are the third category within this nursing diagnosis. The patient needs assistance with some aspect of dressing. Lastly, there may be a deficit in self-toileting. This may involve transfer, help with clothing, or carrying out the process of elimination. The patient's self-care deficits may include all four, the inability to feed, bathe, dress, or toilet self. This is then referred to an a total self-care deficit.

Whether or not the self-care deficit is total or partial, you will need to look specifically at what the person is able and willing to do in regard to self-care. Such factors as visual deficits, motor impairment, fatigue, and mental alertness might contribute to a self-care deficit diagnosis.

Impaired Home Maintenance Management

Impaired Home Maintenance Management is another NANDA nursing diagnosis. A nursing diagnosis of Impaired Home Maintenance Management may be a current concern for a person who is being cared for as an outpatient. For the person who is an inpatient, the diagnosis is related to needs that will arise after discharge.

Display 23–3
Levels of Self-care Deficit

Level 0:	Is independent in movement.
Level I:	Requires use of equipment or device.
Level II:	Requires help from another person(s): assistance, supervision, or teaching.
Level III:	Requires help from another person and equipment or device.
Level IV:	Is dependent and does not participate in movement.

From Gordon, M. *Manual of Nursing Diagnosis,* 1991–1992. St. Louis: Mosby-Year Book, 1991.

To make this diagnosis, you will have assessed the life style and demands on the individual, the help available, and the setting in which the person will live. You need to consider whether the person must prepare meals, clean the house, do the routine shopping, and care for all the other details of a household. You may need to consult with other agencies and resources as you plan with the patient to solve this problem.

Situational Low Self-esteem

Some patients are embarrassed about their neurologic deficits, referring to themselves as "walking like a drunk" or apologizing for their messiness at the table. This may lead to either situational or chronic low self-esteem. The person may see himself or herself as less valuable than others. When the deficits are a result of illness or accidents, the individual may compare the current reality with what was and this may also contribute to low self-esteem.

Impaired Social Interaction

The individual who has a chronic condition limiting mobility may find many of life's tasks very difficult. Dependence on others for support often is essential. This need for dependence at the same time that the individual seeks and values independence may undermine the quality of the interpersonal relationship, leading to negative, insufficient, or unsatisfactory responses from others. The individual experiencing impaired social interaction will report an inability to establish and/or maintain stable, supportive relationships. In addition, this person may exhibit excessively dependent behavior, lack of self-esteem, social isolation, and hopelessness.

Planning and Implementation

Recognizing desired activity outcomes for an individual patient will help you in planning and implementing your care. The outcome may be one of maintaining the present activity level. Desired outcome for other patients may be progressing the activity level. With both, an outcome would be that the patient will demonstrate tolerance for the activity. Tolerance is demonstrated by stable vital signs and no evidence of undue fatigue. Outcome criteria for the extremely incapacitated patient may be to achieve adaptation, and at the same time, actively participate in any restorative implementation available. The desired outcome with many patients is to experience increased strength and endurance to a higher level of mobility. Other etiologies focus on *ADL limitations.*

When planning nursing intervention, you will ordinarily aim your efforts at helping the patient to attain or maintain an activity level as near to normal for that person as possible. To achieve this goal, you will need to plan both the type and the frequency of a patient's activity.

In many situations, increased activity will be contraindicated by the patient's medical condition or impossible because of the individual's permanent disability. In these instances, you will be establishing ways of meeting needs for mobility in the current situation.

The physician usually writes an order for activity level based on the problems created by the disease state. The order may be general, such as "up ad lib," which means the person may perform general self-care and walk about the room or the unit as desired. This order leaves room for wide variation. When such an order has been written, do not make the mistake of thinking that planning is not a serious consideration. Based on your initial assessment, you will need to help the patient establish an activity level that provides for optimum health status.

The order for restricting activity may be more specific, such as the ones for cardiac patients. Even with a clearly defined order, the nurse must decide when activity is appropriate and how it should be integrated into the plan of care. The nurse must also discontinue an activity if there is an adverse response.

Determination of Appropriate Activity

The best means of combating the effects of immobility is activity—whatever activity the patient can pursue. When activity is not possible, alternative measures can be taken to combat the effects of immobility. The primary purpose of nursing care when the person has a mobility problem is to maintain maximum muscle strength and joint mobility. This objective might be pursued by means of either active or assistive ROM exercises, independent movement, or ambulation. Braces, canes, walkers, and crutches can facilitate movement and prevent unnecessary atrophy of muscles (Fig. 23-3). Continue to offer the patient encouragement and realistic hope—not for complete return of function, perhaps—but for maintenance of whatever function is present. In some instances a physician will write orders specifying a particular activity that is appropriate for the medical condition. More frequently, the physician's orders indicate the maximum amount of activity that can be undertaken, but do not specify each activity.

Range-of-Motion Exercises

A person unable to move one or more joints will require ROM exercises to maintain joint mobility of all joints unless a specific medical contraindication is present. As a nurse, you will determine when ROM exercises are needed if not contraindicated by the patient's condition. As a beginning student, specific diseases and pathologic problems may be unfamiliar so that in making this decision, you will need to consult with your instructor or another registered nurse.

Activities of Daily Living

You should encourage the patient's participation in performing ADLs whenever possible. The goal here is not to save the nurse time; in fact, it may be far more time consuming to help patients feed themselves or perform some aspect of personal hygiene than to do it for them. More important is that being independent in self-care promotes physical well-being as well as self-esteem.

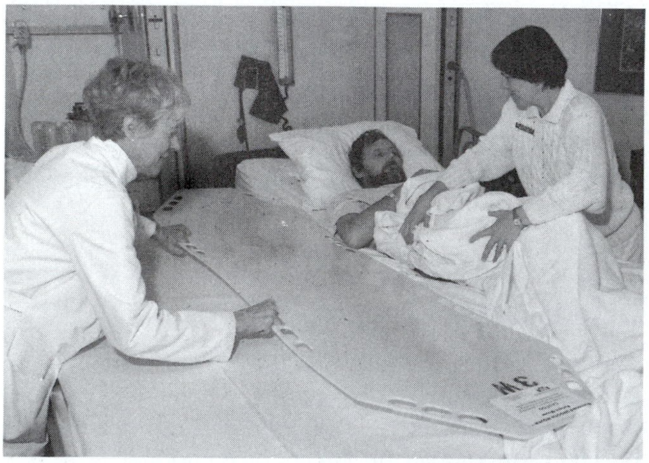

Figure 23-3. The nurse uses assistive devices to help the patient move and exercise.

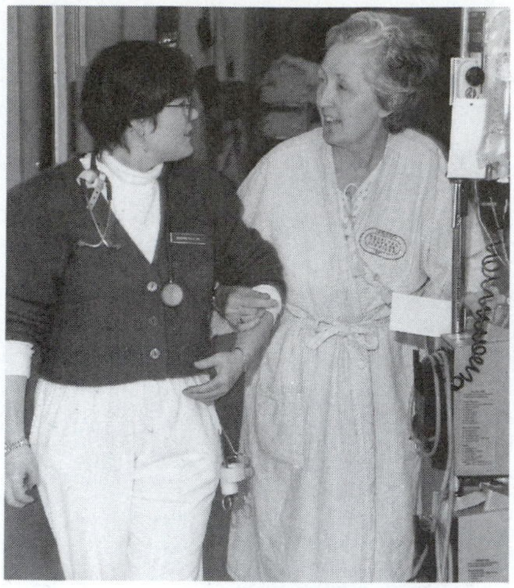

Figure 23-4. Ambulation effectively combats the effects of immobility.

Sitting in a chair is valuable even if the patient must be lifted into the chair. Sitting in a chair for meals often enhances appetite as well as providing for activity. At times you will need to choose from among several activities the one or two most valuable for the patient, because performing all of them would be too fatiguing. For example, you might choose to bathe a patient so as to let the patient conserve energy for sitting in a chair if you consider the change in posture and position more important for the patient than self-care.

When the goal is to increase activity progressively, a gradual approach is used. The first step may be *dangling*, that is, sitting with the legs hanging down over the edge of the bed. Standing at the bedside, which requires balance and strength, may be the next step. Then ambulation can begin, increasing only a few steps each time until the patient has achieved an optimal level of activity (Fig 23-4). Sometimes patients need to remain at a given level of activity for an extended time before proceeding further, or they may have to regress temporarily because of other problems associated with their illnesses. Helping these patients remain motivated to increase activity and not become discouraged by the slow pace of progress is a challenging task. A patient who is responding well to treatment, such as a person recovering from a common intestinal upset, may be able to make advances in activity at 4-hour intervals during the day.

Determination of Frequency of Activity

Activity is most effective when it is attempted with adequate rest periods. If a patient is to sit in a chair three times a day, a sound distribution of the activity might be once each morning, afternoon, and evening.

Ideally, passive ROM exercises should be performed four times a day or more. Realistically, it may be possible to schedule full ROM only twice a day.

Position changes are traditionally scheduled every 2 hours. This activity is essential to prevent the development of pressure ulcers. It is important to individualize planned position changes, which are as critical for the person who is wheelchair bound as it is for the person in bed.

Provision of Proper Body Alignment for the Patient

Maintaining correct posture while sitting and lying down—usually spoken of as good body *alignment*—is particularly important for the hospitalized patient. Rest and sleep are enhanced for the patient by good body alignment.

Sitting posture is important. The back muscles need to be well supported and the body should be flexed at the hips, not slumped along the spine. The person's feet should have a firm support, either the floor or a footstool, to prevent excess pressure behind the knees and to allow the knees to remain in a functional position. Arms need armrests so that their weight does not pull on the shoulders. The head must be either positioned vertically over the neck or supported because the neck muscles are not strong enough to support the head adequately against the pull of gravity.

The nurse is responsible for maintaining correct body alignment for the patient confined to bed. Several points need consideration to approximate optimal erect body posture for the patient who is lying down. Whether one or more pillows are used, they should be placed well under the shoulders as well as under the head. This is done to prevent flexion and strain on the neck. The shoulders and hips must be squarely aligned. Arms and legs are placed in relaxed but straight alignment. If arms are bent at the elbow or legs bent at the knees, small pillows can be placed to support the extremities and protect bony surfaces. Pillows should be placed under any extremity that is elevated.

If the patient must be immobile, change of position and activity are the most effective preventive measures for disuse syndrome. One aid to positioning the immobile patient is the action of *bridging.* Bridging is the use of pillows and cushions to support the body in such a way as to distribute weight and pressure over areas not normally exposed to pressure and to reduce pressure on areas usually subject to maximal pressure. The customary pressure points literally form a bridge between two pillows. For example, when the person is in the supine position, pillows and cushions are placed underneath the legs, back, and head, but a space is left under the sacrum. The weight is thus distributed on the pillows and the sacrum is entirely free of pressure. When pressure is alleviated, blood supply is restored and the cells recover.

Maintaining these same principles while the patient is in the side-lying position affords good body alignment. Caution should be taken, however, to make sure the patient is not putting pressure on the underlying arm. The arm can be brought forward and supported on a pillow. Legs are usually slightly bent with a pillow positioned lengthwise to avoid pressure being exerted on tissues.

Using the prone position (patient lying on the abdomen) is a useful alternative for changing the patient's position. A pillow for the head is not used and the head is turned to one side. The spine should always be in straight alignment. The arms rest at the side of the body. One arm or both can be bent and placed near the patient's head. To avoid extension of the feet, elevate the feet on a small roll placed under the ankles or extend the feet over the lower end of the mattress. The spine must be positioned in its normal curvature, avoiding twisting or torsion. Module 8, Moving the Patient in Bed and Positioning, demonstrates how to help a patient achieve good alignment.

Provision of Personal Care

Providing personal care to compensate for self-care deficits is many people's view of what nursing is all about. Identifying those aspects of personal care that the patient cannot or should not undertake and providing for those needs is an essential part of assisting with mobility. You will want to consider the patient's emotional and physical status to determine how best to meet needs without undermining the patient's self-esteem. Most patients find it easier to accept help with personal care if the help is freely offered and does not have to be requested each time it is needed. You should provide personal care in a manner and at a pace that is comfortable for the patient. Include the patient in decision-making whenever possible to support self-esteem.

Use of Assistive Devices to Increase Mobility

To help a patient ambulate, you may need to use such assistive devices as a walker, a cane, or crutches. Although assistive devices are usually ordered by the physician, this is not always the case. You may be the person who identifies the fact that a walker would benefit a patient by making ambulation more stable and increasing independence. Devices to assist with feeding, with grooming, and with other ADLs are available. The occupational therapist is a good resource for advice regarding potentially valuable assistive devices for personal care. Assistive devices may be needed on a short-term basis as the patient progresses, or they may be needed on an ongoing basis to facilitate maximum independence after discharge. Usually the physical therapist initiates instruction of the patient at the time when the device is issued. The nurse is then responsible for continuing assistance to the patient and monitoring progress. Module 23, Ambulation, explains the use of walkers, canes, and crutches.

Maintenance of Safety

If motor function or coordination is impaired, falls can occur. Falls can also happen to the patient with a visual impairment who cannot see furniture or equipment and is unfamiliar with the general environment. Although rare, the patient with a hearing or olfactory impairment may not hear an emergency announcement or smell smoke in the case of a fire.

Although you can do little about the underlying causes of these safety problems, you can help the patient accommodate. Caution patients with problems of coordination to ring for assistance when they want to get out of bed or to ambulate. Encourage patients to move slowly, and plan ahead on how you might help. Assistive devices, although designed primarily for patients with weakness in the legs, can also provide security to uncoordinated or visually impaired patients. A cane or a walker steadies the gait.

The patient whose hand coordination is impaired can use large-handled utensils and large mugs. Always make sure hot liquids are kept at a safe distance so they cannot be spilled by involuntary movements. Smoking behavior, if allowed, should be closely monitored for safety.

Great care should be taken to protect a paralyzed part from injury. Never grasp and lift a patient under the axilla of a paralyzed arm because the shoulder could become dislocated (subluxated). If the patient is in a wheelchair, be sure that no part of the body is in a position to be caught. A foot can be twisted under the chair as it moves forward; fingers can become entangled in the wheel as the chair is moved. Patients can be positioned in bed on the paralyzed side if proper alignment is maintained with no twisting of or pressure on the extremities. Injections should be administered in the unaffected side where there is often better perfusion of tissues for absorption. Heat and sharp objects should be kept away from paralyzed body areas. Edema may occur if paralyzed extremities are allowed to hang in a lowered position for long periods. Slings can be used to keep the arms nearer the level of the heart, and footrests and footstools help keep feet in a less dependent position. Again, braces and walking devices may make ambulation easier and joint mobility can be maintained with regular ROM exercises. Paralysis distorts body image and is usually difficult for the patient psychologically. Emphasizing the patient's strengths rather than weaknesses is a valuable aspect of nursing care.

Assistance With Swallowing Problems

Impairment of swallowing requires special skills on the part of the nurse. Using assessment, you can identify the types of food the patient can best manage. Some patients can swallow soft solid food, such as gelatin, more readily than liquids, whereas others can swallow small quantities of liquids but may gag on solid food. Careful selection of food and positioning the patient in the sitting position both help swallowing. Encourage small bites and portions; observe the patient carefully. If the gag reflex is greatly diminished or absent, do not attempt to feed the patient. Report this to the physician, who will decide on alternative methods to provide nutrition to the patient. Fear of choking is disturbing, and dysphagic patients need psychological support (see Module 9, Feeding Adult Patients).

Health Teaching

Health teaching is an essential part of fulfilling all human needs but particularly so when illness determines an individual's mobility and activity. As a vital part of health teaching, the patient needs to identify realistic goals and methods that will achieve those goals. Goal setting may be minimal at first with progression as more activity is tolerated. The patient should be taught to remain optimistic in the light of gradual progress.

The care provider or family must also be involved. The family can offer daily support and monitor progress. Others may be involved with assisting the affected person and will also need to be taught procedures to maximize their assistance. Assistive devices such as canes and walkers can also enhance mobility. To obtain these, the nurse can share resources within the community that help not only in gaining access to assistive devices but may also have programs for those with mobility problems.

An important part of health teaching is to emphasize physical safety. Adequate instruction for the patient and the family on procedures such as transfer, walking, and using devices can reduce the risk of injury for those who have impaired mobility.

Rehabilitation

Rehabilitation is the process by which an individual affected by a disabling condition returns to as nearly normal functioning as possible. In its most comprehensive sense, rehabilitation begins the moment the disabling illness or injury begins. Care that is planned from the outset with the person's eventual return to an acceptable level of function encompasses rehabilitation. When you preserve joint function through ROM exercises, encourage each small increment in self-feeding, or help a person keep track of intake and output, you are participating in rehabilitation. You can help the person facing many changes by offering encouragement, understanding, and a sense of humor as the person copes with deficits and learns new ways of functioning.

Comprehensive rehabilitation may require extensive team effort. In cases of major disabling illness, rehabilitation may be planned by a team composed of physicians, nurses, social workers, occupational therapists, physical therapists, and dietitians. The patient may be transferred to a special unit or even a special hospital whose staff has particular expertise in rehabilitation and whose facilities are especially designed for this purpose. In such a setting, the disabled person is helped to pursue independence and autonomy in all aspects of life. For example, the paraplegic, paralyzed from the waist down, may learn new ways of managing elimination and skin care as well as techniques for moving about. Vocational counseling and job placement may be an important part of the rehabilitation process as the patient progresses. Education for an occupation that can be pursued from a wheelchair may be undertaken. Personal counseling to help the patient resolve feelings about the tremendous changes in life is an essential part of a major rehabilitation program. Both the United States and Canada offer rehabilitation programs under their respective departments of health.

Evaluation

The outcomes you identified earlier are directly related to activity evaluation. Evaluation can be measured by whether or not the outcomes were reached.

Observation is essential at each step so that the effectiveness of the plan for the patient's activity and the outcome of tolerance by the patient can be evaluated and revised as needed. Whatever the order, the nurse is responsible for thorough observation of the patient's response to any activity undertaken. Measuring vital signs before and after activity may yield important information on the patient's response or tolerance. If pulse, respiration, or blood pressure rise more than 10% and do not return to the preactivity level within 3 minutes, the activity may have been too strenuous. Excessive dizziness may indicate that the activity was performed too rapidly. If severe fatigue occurs, you may be increasing the amount of activity too rapidly. Evaluation of the patient's response will enable you to replan your nursing actions.

Nursing Care Study
An Immobilized Patient

Joan Taylor, a student nurse, was assigned to care for Sarah Mitchell, a 92-year-old woman completely immobilized as a result of a cerebral vascular accident (stroke). In the course of her assessment, Joan noted that, although one leg and arm did flex slightly, Mrs. Mitchell did not change her position in bed at all. Her joints were somewhat stiff, but she did not appear to have any deficit in range of motion. The physician's order for Mrs. Mitchell was "activity as tolerated."

After consulting with her instructor, Joan decided to do complete passive range-of-motion exercises during bathing. Doing so would also present an opportunity to assess joint range accurately. After Mrs. Mitchell had rested, Joan would obtain assistance and move the patient into a chair. The student arranged for adequate pillows to support the patient's position and decided that a two-person lift would be needed for the transfer.

Joan carried out her plan for Mrs. Mitchell. As Joan observed the patient in the chair, she noted that Mrs. Mitchell's respirations were deeper than they had been in bed and that for the first time all morning she opened her eyes and was looking around as if interested in her surroundings. Joan concluded that this level of activity was beneficial to her and decided to consult with the team leader about entering it on the nursing care plan.

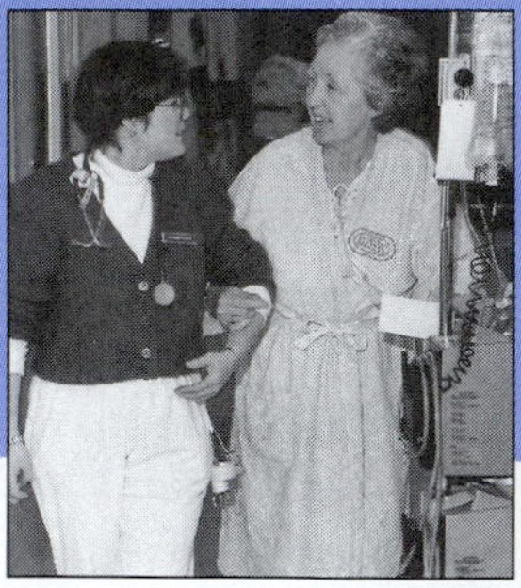

Key Points

- The musculoskeletal system is made up of bones, cartilage, muscles, and connective tissue. There are several different types of joints and differing types of joint movement.
- The actions of the musculoskeletal system are controlled by the CNS. The cerebrum controls voluntary movement; the cerebellum coordinates movement; and the medulla controls involuntary movement.
- All motor impulses go to the anterior horn cells of the spinal cord before moving down the last single motor nerve pathway to the muscle fiber. Damage to the anterior horn cells or the motor nerve to the muscle results in flaccid paralysis. Damage above the anterior horn cells may result in a loss of one aspect of movement without total loss of movement.
- Basic patterns of activity include posture, body mechanics, and exercise. Exercise may be active or passive. Active exercise may include isotonic exercise and isometric exercise.
- Persons with disabling conditions often do not consider themselves to be ill. Instead, many persons will make adaptations to live as nearly normal a lifestyle as possible. When a disabled person is hospitalized, every effort should be made to preserve maximum independence.
- To assess activity status, the nurse needs to consider the appearance of the musculoskeletal system, the ability to move, and the characteristics of movement. This includes the ROM of joints, gait, coordination, and body mechanics. An interview with the person to determine the presence of any discomfort, the usual activity pattern, and the person's knowledge regarding activity needs is also important.
- The physiologic response to activity is assessed by checking the individual's pulse, blood pressure, and respiratory rate before, during, and after the activity.
- Nursing diagnoses related to activity status include Activity Intolerance, Impaired Physical Mobility, High Risk for Disuse Syndrome, High Risk for Injury, Self-Care Deficits, Impaired Home Maintenance Management, and Situational Low Self-esteem. Immobility is characterized by changes in many different systems of the body.
- In planning and implementing actions to meet the patient's needs for mobility, you must plan the type of activity, its frequency, and its duration.
- When adding activities to a person's life is impossible, other actions may need to be taken to combat the effects of immobility on the body's system.
- Identifying whether any assistive devices are needed for ambulation or for personal care is also important. To evaluate activity, the nurse again checks pulse, blood pressure, and respirations, observes the person for fatigue, and questions the individual regarding discomfort or distress experienced. It may be the nurse's decision to discontinue the ordered activity if it is not tolerated until the physician can be consulted.
- Rehabilitation is a process for returning a person to as nearly normal functioning as is possible. At its best, rehabilitation begins at the outset of a disabling illness and continues in an individualized manner to maximize the person's quality of life.

Study Questions

1. What is anatomic position?
2. What is the difference between abduction and adduction?
3. List four groups of persons are at risk for alteration in mobility and activity?
4. How are the results of isometric exercises different from the results of isotonic exercises?
5. Name three special mobility needs of the disabled person.
6. How can you assess for mobility status?
7. List measures in addition to activity that can be used to combat immobility.
8. How does mobility aid urinary function?
9. What changes in blood pressure with exercise would indicate activity intolerance?
10. Describe the psychological effects of immobility.
11. Why is a wide base of support important when one is lifting and moving a heavy object?

Critical Thinking Activities

1. Stand in front of a mirror (full-length, if possible) and analyze your posture from the front and from

the side. Which features of your posture are correct? Incorrect? How can you improve your posture?

2. Visit the physical therapy department of your facility. Identify the exercises and movements which are performed by the clients. Analyze which joints and muscles are being exercised and the desired outcome for the therapy.
3. Assess the physical and psychological well-being of a patient with a chronic illness which limits mobility for whom you have cared.
4. Write a brief report regarding the impact of the Americans With Disabilities Act of 1992. What does the Act cover? In what ways can it help the person with impaired mobility who lives in the community?

Relevant Sections in Modules for Basic Nursing Skills

Volume 1 Module

- Basic Body Mechanics 4
- Moving the Patient in Bed and Positioning 8
- Feeding Adult Patients 9
- Using Physical Restraints 21
- Transfer 22
- Ambulation: Simple Assisted and Using Cane, Crutches, or Walker 23
- Range-of-Motion Exercises 24
- Caring for Patients with Casts and Braces 30
- Applying and Maintaining Traction 31

References and Readings

Armstrong, J. J. "A Brief Overview of Diabetes Mellitus and Exercise." *Diabetes Educator* 17, 3 (May-June 1991): 175–178.

Benison, B., and Hogstel, M. O. "Aging and Movement Therapy: Essential Interventions for the Immobile Elderly." *Journal of Gerontological Nursing* 12, 12 (December 1986): 8–16.

Blanchard, D. S. "What Women Can Do to Protect Against Osteoporosis." *RN* 53, 10 (October 1990): 60–65.

Bonheur, B., and Young, S. W. "Exercise as a Health-promoting Lifestyle Choice." *Applied Nursing Research* 4, 1 (February 1991): 2–6.

Braun, L. T. "Exercise Physiology and Cardiovascular Fitness." *Nursing Clinics of North America* 26, 1 (March 1991): 135–147.

Brody, D. M. "Running Injuries: Prevention and Management." *Clinical Symposia* 39, 3 (March 1987): 2–36.

Caranasos, G. J., and Israel, R. "Gait Disorders in the Elderly." *Hospital Practice* 26 (June 15, 1991): 67–94.

Carpenito, L. J. *Nursing Diagnosis: Application to Clinical Practice*, 4th edition. Philadelphia: J. B. Lippincott, 1992.

Collier, S. "Mrs. Hixon Was More Than 'The C.V.A. in 251'." *Nursing '92* 22, 5 (May 1992): 62–64.

Forbes, E. J. "Exercise: Wellness Maintenance for the Elderly Client." *Holistic Nursing Practice* 6, 2 (February 1992): 14–22.

Grainger, R. D. "Managing Fatigue." *American Journal of Nursing* 90, 3 (March 1990): 13.

Guyton, A. C. *Human Physiology and Mechanisms of Disease.* 5th edition. Philadelphia: W. B. Saunders, 1992.

Haty, L. K., and Freel, M. I., and Milde, F. K. "Fatique." *Nursing Clinics of North America.* 25, 4 (December 1990): 967–976.

Jones, C. A. "These Patients Really Need Our Help." *RN* 55, 10 (October 1992): 46–53.

Lane, P. L., and LeBlanc, R. "Crutch Walking." *Orthopedic Nursing* 9, 5 (September-October 1990): 31–38.

Mol, V. J., and Baker, C. A. "Activity Intolerance in the Geriatric Stroke Patient." *Rehabilitation Nursing* 16, 6 (November-December 1991): 337–344.

Mold, J. W., Nevins, M. A., Sherman, F. T., and Waltman, A. C. "What Weakness Means in the Elderly." *Patient Care* 24, 6 (March 30, 1990): 68–72, 77–78.

Murray, R. B., and Zentner, J. P. *Nursing Assessment and Health Promotion Strategies through the Life Span.* 4th edition. Englewood Cliffs, N.J.: Prentice-Hall, 1989.

Olson, E. V. "The Hazards of Immobility." *American Journal of Nursing* 90, 3 (March 1990): 43–48.

Ormiston, C. "Let's Get Physical . . . Exercise Helpful to People with Depression." *Nursing Times* 87, 19 (May 1991): 8–14.

Owen, B. D., and Garg, A. "Back Stress Isn't Part of the Job." *American Journal of Nursing* 93, 2 (February 1993): 48–51.

Passarella, P., and Gee, Z. "Starting Right After Stroke." *American Journal of Nursing* 87, 6 (June 1987): 802–808.

Pender, N. J. *Health Promotion in Nursing Practice.* 2nd edition. Norwalk, Conn.: Appleton-Century-Crofts, 1987.

Rapp, S., and Carlson, C. "Attitudes Toward Exercise in Institutions for Elderly Residents." *Journal of Visual Impairment and Blindness* 81, 7 (September 1987): 328–329.

Scheve, A. S. "Exercise in Continence." *Geriatric Nursing* 12, 3 (May-June 1991): 124.

Selcher, D. "Helping Your Patient Dress for Success." *RN* 54, 8 (August 1991): 43–45.

Smith, J. F., and Graham, M. D. "Exercise Helps These Postop Patients." *RN* 55, 2 (February 1992): 38–40.

Watson, P. G. "Family Issues in Rehabilitation." *Holistic Nursing Practice* 6, 2 (February 1992): 51–59.

Winningham, M. L. "Walking Program for People with Cancer." *Cancer Nursing* 14, 5 (October 1991): 270–276.

ZuWallack, R. L., Patel, K., Reardon, J. Z., Clark, B. A., Normandin, E. A. "Predictors of Improvement in the 12-minute Walking Distance Following a Six Week Pulmonary Rehabilitation Program." *Chest* 99, 4 (April 1991): 805–808.

Rest And Sleep

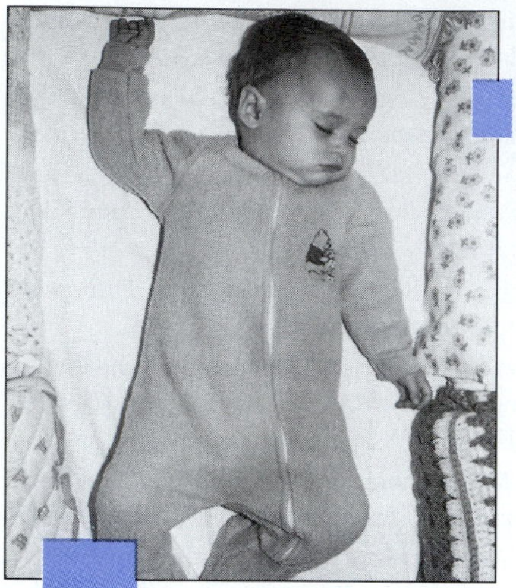

24

Objectives

After completing this chapter, you should be able to:

1. Differentiate rest from sleep and discuss the function each fulfills for the patient.
2. Incorporate rest effectively into the care plan.
3. Define biorhythms and describe changes in various body functions as the cycle progresses.
4. Describe briefly the five stages of sleep in sequence.
5. Relate age to the stages of sleep.
6. Discuss common causes and the effects of sleep deprivation in patients.
7. Describe briefly the following sleep disturbances: insomnia, somnambulism, enuresis, narcolepsy, sudden infant death syndrome, and sleep apnea.
8. Describe the effects of hypnotics, amphetamines, and alcohol on sleep.
9. Outline appropriate nursing measures for a patient experiencing sleep disturbance.
10. Recognize the possible sleep hazards created by shift work as a nurse.
11. Relate your knowledge of sleep to your life as a nurse.

Study Terms

biorhythms
circadian rhythm
enuresis
infradian rhythm
insomnia
narcolepsy
paradoxic sleep
rapid eye movement (REM) sleep
sleep apnea
somnambulism
sudden infant death syndrome (SIDS)
ultradian rhythm
uvulopalatopharyngoplasty (UPPP)

Outline

Ellis, Nowlis: Nursing: A Human Needs Approach, 5th ed. © 1994 J.B. Lippincott Company

Rest and sleep are basic human needs. However, rest and sleep are neither identical nor interchangeable, an important fact to remember when you care for patients. Some patients may have adequate rest but perhaps insufficient sleep. For example, the person with arthritis may rest at sufficient intervals throughout the day. Yet at night, possibly because of pain or discomfort caused by moving, the person's sleep needs are not met. On the other hand, many patients may have their sleep needs met but not their need for rest during the day. For example, a patient may sleep well and adequately during the night, but because of the interruptions necessary for care or tests, not have the need for rest met during the day.

Rest

Rest is a period of conscious inactivity. Either the entire body or a single body part may be rested. A sprained ankle, for example, is supported by elastic bandages and walking is curtailed to allow the ankle to rest.

Rest affords the body the opportunity to use all its resources to repair damaged cells, remove waste products, and restore tissue to maximum functional ability. Ideally, rest should be alternated with activity to allow the various body parts to recover completely from one activity before another is begun. This alternation is preferable to scheduling a lengthy, strenuous period of activity followed by a long rest.

If a physician orders rest as part of the plan of care, it is important to distinguish between rest of a specific body part and rest of the entire body. The patient on bed rest for a broken leg is still able to move the arms and the other leg and should be encouraged to do so. However, the patient on bed rest after an sudden heart attack is discouraged from moving about because any body activity requires increased cardiac output. Clarifying the exact meaning of an order for rest is the responsibility of the nurse. The meaning of any order for activity or rest must be carefully explained to the patient and arrangements should be made for the assistance necessary to comply with the order.

Therapeutic Rest

Therapeutic rest requires the person to be in a state of psychological comfort as well as physically inactive. Some rest is not restful for both the mind and the body. For example, a person fleeing from a threatening situation may have to rest to renew the capacity for escape. The fear and anxiety experienced make the resting period only a time to recuperate physical strength. A patient anxious about a pending surgery may appear to be resting but is not psychologically restful. This type of rest is not therapeutic. Care providers should be aware of several prerequisites to beneficial rest.

Therapeutic rest occurs only when persons feel that they are in a safe environment, free from threat. Not only must they feel physically safe, but they must also experience physical and psychological comfort, including freedom from pain. Usually, the patient has had a period of wakefulness or physical activity before resting, so that the individual feels a need for rest.

Rest in the Hospital Setting

Although the adult in Western society rarely plans rest periods during the day, they are often needed for the ill person to function well. Because some medical conditions increase the energy needs of the individual, additional rest is often required.

In the hospital setting, nurses often plan for patient activity and assume that the patient will be able to rest at other times. The reality of the modern hospital is far different. A patient may receive respiratory therapy and physical therapy treatments. Nursing procedures may be scheduled. Several physicians may each visit at different times. Meals are scheduled for serving convenience. Some observations must be made at specified intervals. Finding a place for rest in this schedule may demand extraordinary attention to detail, organization, and communication with many other members of the health care team. In making your plans, you will want to consider whether the patient can tolerate many activities grouped together without excessive fatigue.

Visitors may need to be considered in this plan. Some family members will be content to sit quietly and allow the patient to rest. Their presence may decrease anxiety and encourage resting. Other visitors may talk and continually bombard the patient with stimuli or make resting difficult by other behaviors. The nurse is responsible for identifying the effect of visitors on the patient and preparing a plan to meet the patient's needs in the most effective way. You may want to consult with the patient about curtailing phone calls, limiting visitors to 5 minutes, having only family members visit, or having all visitors check at the nurses' station to make sure a rest period is not being interrupted.

Assessment Related to Rest

Interview

The first step in the interview is to determine how much resting time the person engaged in when healthy. For example, if an elderly person generally rested for a short time after breakfast and again just before dinner, these rests should become part of the plan of care. If the individual never rested during the day, this pattern is also significant.

Second, the nurse should talk with and involve the patient in determining the amount of rest indicated for the patient's particular illness or incapacity. The person with serious respiratory limitations may need much more resting time than one with a dislocated shoulder. The patient's psychological state is also important. Anxiety and emotional turmoil make physical rest difficult.

Physical Assessment

The physical appearance of the person will add important data to your assessment. Patients may report that they get enough rest, yet they appear tired and anxious. The person may be thin and the skin pale. Persons without adequate rest often have difficulty following simple directions so that when you ask the patient to cooperate with measuring vital signs or testing reflexes, the person may appear distracted, disinterested, or angry. Insufficient rest can result in alterations of the person's breathing, heart rate, skin, appetite, and elimination.

Nursing Diagnoses Related to Rest

Because of the increased demands illness and injury make on the body and the need for care, rest problems are common among patients. You can arrive at nursing diagnoses that will help you plan actions to provide more rest for those with a rest deficit.

It would be appropriate for a nursing diagnosis directly related to rest be approved by the North American Nursing Diagnosis Association (NANDA). There is a proposed general category called Alteration in Rest. Another proposal is the use of "deficit" as a category for persons who are prevented from resting by illness, treatments, or other life events. Until there is an approved nursing diagnosis, you could identify nursing diagnoses that relate to patient problems derived from rest deficits.

Fatigue related to lack of rest

This nursing diagnosis identifies the individual who has inadequate activity because of rest problems. The fatigue is manifested when the patient attempts what has been a tolerated level of activity. It may also represent the patient who is on bed rest and not active, yet feels fatigued. Fatigue is often a subjective feeling of overwhelming exhaustion that prevents the person from per-

Nursing Diagnoses Related to Rest

Fatigue related to lack of rest secondary to intensity of care

Fatigue related to lack of rest secondary to anxiety

Activity Intolerance related to lack of rest

Ineffective Individual Coping related to lack of rest

forming physical and mental activities (Carpenito, 1992, p. 362).

Activity Intolerance related to lack of rest

Under this nursing diagnosis, fatigue is demonstrated by an intolerance for activity. Using this nursing diagnosis requires both subjective data or how rested the patient feels as well as objective data. The objective data would include determining what activity level is appropriate and comparing it to the subjective feelings of the patient.

Ineffective Individual Coping related to lack of rest

Because rest greatly affects the psychological well-being of the patient, coping with an illness may be made much more difficult if rest is inadequate. When nursing actions are taken to provide rest, the person's coping mechanisms may be revitalized so that necessary adjustments and adaptations to the illness can be made. Chapter 34 offers more information on coping strategies.

Planning and Implementation Related to Rest

The patient should be given the option of planning. The patient, then, could help you to ascertain periods of time when care is being given and the amount of free time during the day when rest periods can be initiated. Identifying specific nursing actions that relate directly to the nursing diagnosis provides a cohesive plan of care for the patient.

At this time you determine the desired outcomes for the patient. These may include the following: the patient is more alert and energetic during periods of activity; the patient is able to focus both physical and mental energy on getting well when rest periods are provided. If the patient has generalized weakness, from either advanced age or the disease process, planning resting times with the patient so that energy can be reserved for needed activity is important. Activity and rest may have to be balanced (see Chapter 23). If, however, you are implementing rest for a patient with fever and infection, you may have to provide for more rest than is usually needed. For the patient with an acute illness, you may need to plan not only more rest but rest that is prolonged in duration (see the sample Nursing Care Plan Related to Rest).

If other factors are interfering with rest, your actions may be focused on removing the causative factor. Decreasing anxiety through attentive listening and other measures will help prepare the patient for a state of relaxation and rest (see Chapter 34). If the patient is experiencing itching skin, providing a cool quiet environment and soothing lotion may improve the patient's ability to rest. If rest is being hindered by the intensity of care being given by the health care team, revising the plan of care so that care is given in "blocks" will allow sufficient time for rest.

Recognize that rest means different things to different people; a change in activity constitutes rest to some people. Such a change can be accomplished within the hospital setting. A patient may simply wish to listen to music with the eyes closed after participating in diet instruction. The change is, in itself, restful. Durham and Frost-Hartzer (1991) suggest a variety of methods for helping patients of different ages relax and feel rested. They emphasize that the use of music, story telling, and guided imagery take minimal work but do require creativity on the part of the nurse.

In general, implementation involves providing the amount of rest time needed by the individual in an environment conducive to rest. Implementation also entails inducing psychological readiness for rest on the part of the patient and removing factors that interfere with rest. The sleep section of this chapter lists nursing interventions that are applicable to rest as well.

Evaluation Related to Rest

Evaluation is done by reviewing the established desired outcomes. Patients may say that they feel better because of extra rest, which is subjective data, or you may notice that the patient has increased activity levels without untoward consequences, which is an objective evaluation. Both may relate directly to the desired outcomes.

Sleep

Rest and sleep are not the same. Therapeutic conscious resting, which involves muscular relaxation and mental calm, can prepare the individual to enter the unconscious sleep state. Sleep is a universal need. However, "as unique individuals we all have differing behavioral patterns relating to sleep, we all need and receive differing quantities and qualities of sleep, and we are all capable, more or less, of adapting to new sleeping environments and conditions" (Webster and Thompson, 1986, p. 447). This last is an important statement because the hospital environment can interfere with or alter normal sleep.

Sleep is a basic need and sleep management an in-

Nursing Care Plan
Sample Nursing Care Plan Related to Rest

Nursing Diagnosis

Fatigue related to lack of rest.

Supportive data:

Man, age 97.

History of increasing weakness at recent chronic care facility.

Activity tolerance level markedly less today than yesterday. Only able to ambulate to door of room with assistance.

States, "I feel tired and weak."

Desired Patient Outcomes

Rests at intervals throughout the day.

Participates in all activities.

Nursing Action	Rationale
1. Plan activity periods three times per day: 1) after hygiene, 2) late afternoon, and 3) just before sleep.	Spacing activities allows for regular times for rest.
2. Plan rest periods just before and after activity periods.	Rest periods will allow the patient to participate more fully in activity.
3. Observe patient closely during activities.	Observing for fatigue allows the nurse to prevent falls and other hazards.
4. Do not exceed tolerance levels.	If tolerance levels are exceeded, the patient may fall and be injured.
5. During periods of rest, provide a quiet, clean, safe environment.	This type of environment is conducive to rest because it is one which decreases stress and anxiety.
6. Encourage patient feedback regarding activity/rest balance.	Feedback will help the patient feel more included in the plan of care and provide valuable information so that the plan is more individualized in meeting the patient's needs.

tegral part of nursing care. Over the years, more attention has been given to the subject of sleep in the curricula of nursing programs. The medical literature has given considerable attention to sleep since the mid 1940s, and some of the conclusions are highly relevant to nursing. For example, it is not uncommon for a night nurse to chart that a patient slept well, only to discover that the following day the patient complained of fatigue and being irritable. Recent studies suggest that such a patient may be sleep deprived, appearances to the contrary. We shall return to this subject later in the chapter.

Sleep is also a central issue in the lives of nurses. Many nurses in hospital settings work variable shifts, necessitating continual adjustment of their sleeping hours. Continuing evidence suggests that nurses should look more closely at their sleep patterns. Research has provided answers to some of the questions about sleep most pertinent to nurses. How much sleep is adequate for a particular individual? Is all sleep alike? How can you help provide for adequate sleep for yourself and for the patients in your care?

Biorhythms

All human beings have **biorhythms**, that is, the cyclic occurrence of physiologic events. Some of the biorhythms within the body involve the activity–inactivity or wake–sleep rhythm, temperature regulation, cardiac output, and blood pressure levels (Fig. 24-1). What affects or controls the biorhythms of people is not clearly understood although environmental factors such as the rhythm of light and dark may have a role. Without scientific proof, some people attribute rhythmic activity to factors such as gravitational pull or an electromagnetic atmospheric capsule surrounding the body. Others believe that biorhythms partly control behavior although this belief is also without scientific foundation at this time. It is a fact, however, that biorhythms exist and that the body, through the process of homeostasis (see Chapter 4), allows the person to adapt with ease to most fluctuations of bodily functions. Additional research is being done regarding biorhythms, which will have practical application to nursing.

The most important biorhythm affecting sleep is the **circadian rhythm**, the cyclic repetition of a physiologic event approximately every 24 hours. Like plant and animal life, human existence is cyclic, which means that people experience sequentially patterned periods of activity and inactivity. Each day of life is composed of a period of awareness (wakefulness) and a period of relative unawareness (sleep), which comprises circadian rhythm. The term circadian, derived from Latin, means approximately a day. Most people identify themselves as "day people" or "night people," that is, more alert and productive in the morning or in the evening. Despite such differences, however, the 24-hour circadian cycle is uniform in human beings. People experimentally isolated without time-measuring devices of any type, for example, quickly establish schedules that approximate the 24-hour day.

It is useful to consider sleep as one end of a continuum the other extreme of which is wakefulness. In Figure 24-1, wakefulness is characterized by maximal functioning of the body systems. Muscular activity stimulates the respiratory system, food intake arouses the production of gastric and intestinal secretions, and the processes of elimination function actively. Furthermore, mental awareness is heightened, and the reflexes are active and prepared for a threat response (Chuman, 1983).

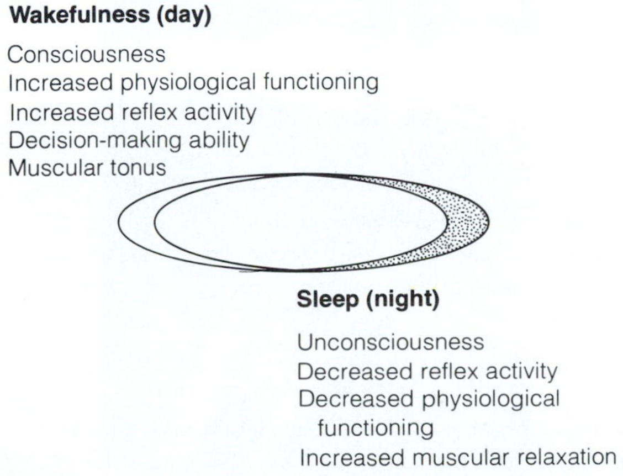

Figure 24-1. Physiological and psychological aspects of circadian rhythm.

Sleep is a less active state than wakefulness although it is not, as was once believed, a state of inactivity. Blood pressure, temperature, pulse, and respirations decrease; digestive juices subside to some degree; and the kidneys become less productive. The basal metabolism rate (BMR) decreases as muscle relaxation increases. Most of the reflexes weaken or disappear entirely, with the important exception of the cough reflex. The *cough reflex* prevents foreign bodies from lodging in the sleeping person's respiratory tract. During sleep, the mind focuses on its internal environment. The activities of the mind during sleep will be discussed in detail shortly.

Ultradian rhythms occur for shorter periods of time than a day, usually during the waking hours. The release of insulin and certain hormones produces an ultradian rhythm. Ultradian rhythms seem to differ from one individual to another.

Infradian rhythm is a term applied to a monthly cycle. Although only women during the childbearing years manifest an infradian cycle with menstruation, research indicates that men also have a monthly cycle of hormonal fluctuation. Some men experience mood swings and general discomfort once thought only to involve women.

Definitions and Causes of Sleep

Although we now know a great deal about the patterns of sleep, a precise definition of and the precise cause of sleep continue to elude us. A workable definition is that sleep is "unconsciousness from which the person can be aroused by sensory or other stimuli" (Guyton, 1992, p. 453). Several researchers have attempted to define sleep, but each included in the definition some aspect under study that failed to lead to an inclusive statement. Some of these persons referred to the *cyclic* nature of sleep; others stated that sleep was an alteration in the cortical patterns of the brain.

Just what causes sleep is unknown. What sustains consciousness, however, is known: excitation of the neurons within the *reticular activating system.* The reticular activating system is the "relay" system in the brain stem that receives impulses from the spinal cord and relays them through the thalamus to the cortex of the brain (see Chapter 31). The constant flow of impulses to the brain results in consciousness. The drugs that depress this system, such as the barbiturates, cause drowsiness and can induce sleep. The inquiry into more specific causes of sleep goes on. Various theorists have suggested that the origins of sleep are primarily chemical, neurohormonal, vascular, pituitary, feedback related, or instinctual.

The *chemical theory* focuses on two hypotheses. The first holds that sleep is brought on by an increase of carbon dioxide in the blood, which affects brain functioning. However, decreased physical activity could in turn account for the increase in carbon dioxide. Although drowsiness commonly develops in inadequately oxygenated surroundings, the carbon dioxide theory has proved inadequate for explaining the more complex findings about sleep.

The second theory involves normal alterations in neurohormones, which then produce sleep. Neurophysiologists, working on this *neurohormonal theory*, have demonstrated different levels of both serotonin and norepinephrine during periods of wakefulness and sleep. These hormones are neurotransmitters that relay information within the brain. With experimental animals, sleep occurs when these substances are injected directly into the cerebral vascular system.

The *vascular theory* assumes that the fall in blood pressure that occurs during sleep decreases the flow of blood within the brain, sustaining the state of unconsciousness. Current studies clearly show, however, that the opposite is the case; cerebrovascular blood flow increases during sleep.

It has long been thought that the *pituitary*, a small gland at the base of the brain, is a regulator of sleep, if not its primary activator. Nevertheless, people whose pituitary glands are removed surgically do not experience great changes in their sleep habits.

One of the most promising theories to date, a complicated one, is the *feedback theory*, which proposes that after a period of neuronal activity during which electrical impulses are relayed throughout the system, fatigue occurs at the synapses, or connections between nerve cells, bringing on sleep.

Finally, some dismiss the entire controversy by stating simply that sleep is *instinctual*.

Functions of Sleep

Whether or not we know the exact cause of sleep, we do know that sleep provides important functions that are closely allied to several of the theoretical causes of sleep. One of these is the *humoral* function of sleep. This theory proposes that the sleep period rids the body of toxins that have built up during the waking hours (Caravan, 1986, p. 321). Sleep has also been regarded as a restorative period for tissue regeneration and healing. Adrenaline, which is released during waking hours, appears to interfere with cell division and healing (Webster and Thompson, 1986, p. 449). Another possible function of sleep is that this state enhances learning and memory. However, this theory has been currently unsubstantiated except in situations of sleep deprivation when learning and memory levels clearly decline.

The Stages of Sleep

To the person who awakens in the morning feeling fairly well rested, sleep may seem no more or less than a period of unawareness and quiescence, highlighted by an occasional dream and the sensation of turning. However, sleep researchers have demonstrated that sleep is a far more active and complicated state than had been supposed.

Dement (1974), Kleitman (1963), and Oswald (1971), three prominent researchers working separately, have found that the character of sleep changes during a given sleeping episode, progressing through sequential *sleep stages*. Their findings are based on the use of the *electroencephalograph* (EEG), a device that measures and records the electrical energy produced by the cortex, the thin outer layer of the brain (Fig. 24-2). The recording is called an *electroencephalogram*, or tracing.

A typical episode of sleep consists of four to six complete cycles, each of which is composed of five stages. Each of the five stages has its own special characteristics (Fig. 24-3). Tracings of the *sleep cycle* are illustrated in Figure 24-4.

Stage I

Stage I most closely resembles wakefulness; it produces a recording of brain activity similar to that of a person who is awake, except for a few slow waves on the tracing. Muscles retain their tone although a slow rolling of the eyes takes place. If aroused during this stage, a person will often deny having slept, saying that he or she

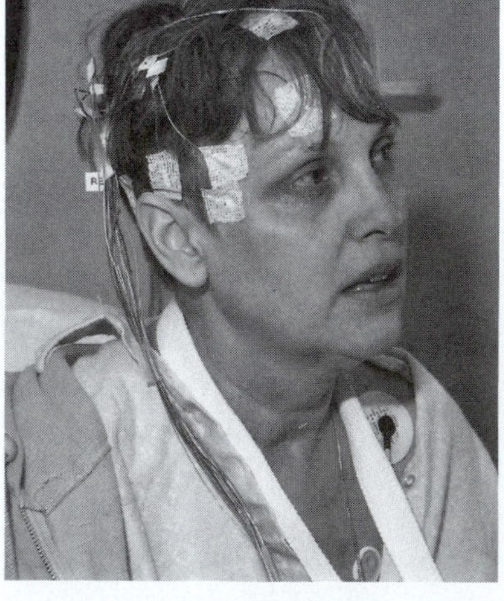

Figure 24–2. The electroencephalograph measures sleep patterns.

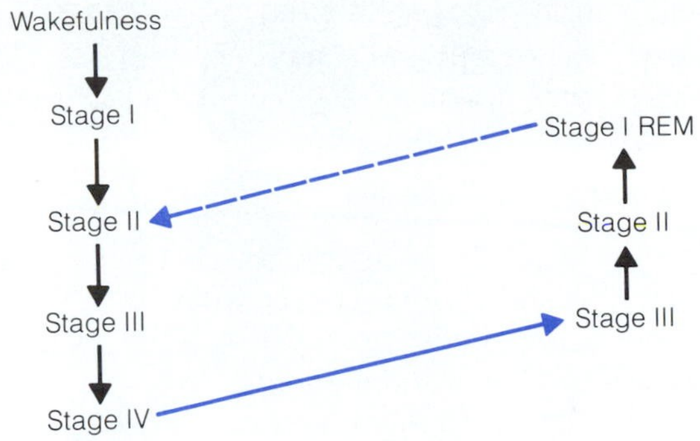

Figure 24-3. The sleep cycle.

was "just drifting off," although sleep had actually begun.

Stage II

Stage II marks the beginning of muscle relaxation. The EEG waves become more regular and rounded. Persons appear asleep but can still be aroused by the call of their name. Considerable turning and shifting in bed accompanies progression toward the next stage.

Stage III

Stage III consists of deeper sleep, manifested in further slowing and rounding of the EEG tracing and loss of muscle tone. Some reflexes diminish at this point, and snoring may occur. The person no longer responds to name call and can be aroused only by touch.

Stage IV

Stage IV, the period of deepest sleep, is characterized by total relaxation and the onset of dreaming. The EEG tracing appears as large, slow waves. The muscles are in their most relaxed state since the onset of sleep. The dreams that occur during this stage have a conventional, everyday quality and are typically extensions or revisions of the preceding day's events or familiar experiences. This is in distinct contrast to the dreams that occur during the next stage of sleep, rapid eye movement (REM) sleep.

Twenty to 30 minutes elapse between initially falling asleep and stage IV. At this point, the process is reversed. The sleeper begins an ascent from stage IV through stage III to stage II and then enters the most profound stage of sleep, REM sleep.

REM Sleep

Sometimes referred to as stage I REM, **REM sleep**, or rapid eye movement sleep, is a distinct phenomenon and quite different from stage I described above. The characteristics of REM sleep are dramatic. Both eyes move rapidly back and forth horizontally. Body twitching is common and one observer has reported occasional twitching of the ears. With the exception of the eyes, the muscles are almost totally relaxed. Reflexes are even more diminished than in stage IV. However, both blood pressure and respirations increase. Although the muscles are completely relaxed, cortical activity (activity in the outer, or thinking, portion of the brain) is high. The EEG tracing is varied and active, not unlike that of waking. The dreams that take place frequently during REM sleep are much more vividly detailed than those of stage IV and may be colorful, violent, or erotic. The contradiction between the relaxation of the muscles and the extreme activity of the brain leads some to refer to REM sleep as **paradoxic sleep**. This term is used interchangeably with REM and stage I REM. You may read about non-REM sleep, defined as sleep during all the stages except the stage of REM.

With the end of REM sleep, one sleep cycle has

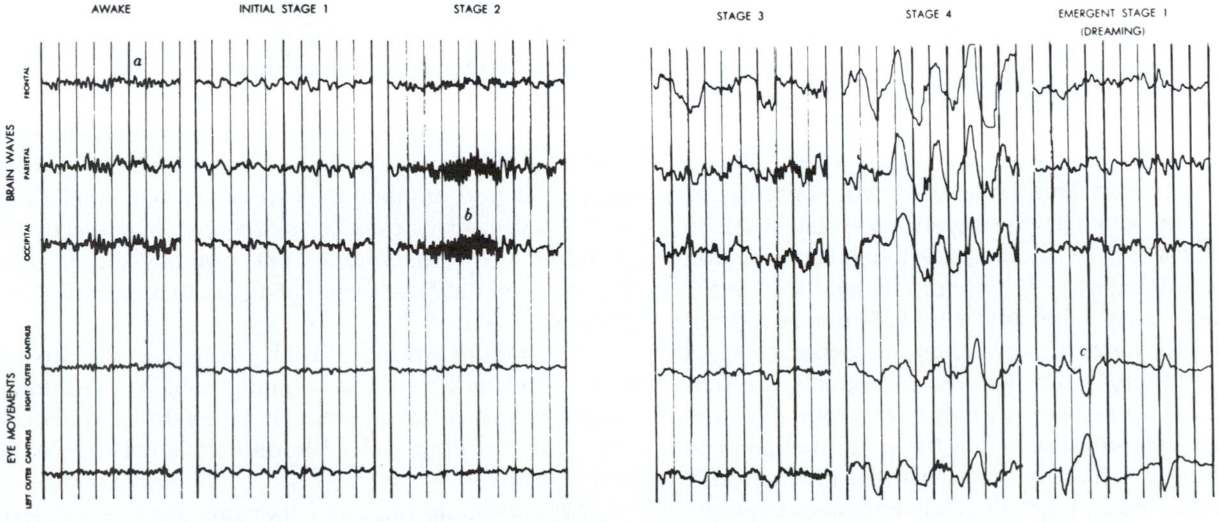

Figure 24-4. Electroencephalograph tracings of sleep stages.

been completed. The entire cycle usually takes about 90 minutes. The next cycle begins with entry into stage II sleep. As the night progresses, stages III and IV decrease in length and REM increases. Although scientists dispute the precise purpose of REM sleep, they seem to agree that it is essential.

Sleep research has demonstrated some interesting differences in sleep cycles. People suffering from schizophrenia experience much less REM sleep than do nonschizophrenics. A study of the causes of sudden infant death syndrome (SIDS) has led to one theory that respiratory failure in infants is caused by neurologic dysfunction during stage IV or REM sleep.

Sleep deprivation studies demonstrate that the duration of REM sleep is even more important than the total hours of sleep. Whether REM sleep is a psychic outlet for stress and tension accrued during the waking hours or is a data-processing mechanism that establishes new neural pathways is a fascinating question. However, these conjectures are less important to you as a nurse than is understanding that both stage IV and REM sleep are essential to human functioning in a manner that is not fully understood.

Research findings also suggest that people have "waking cycles" that correspond to sleep cycles. The human brain appears to become more active for a short period approximately every 90 minutes (Chase, 1979). Some individuals show minor variations in the sleep cycle.

Factors Affecting Sleep

Age

Sleep patterns change throughout the life span as maturation takes place and age-related characteristics occur. It is essential for nurses to understand that the age of a person often dictates the amount of sleep needed for optimal functioning.

Infants and young children. Almost as if resting in preparation for life's journey, the infant spends many more hours of the day sleeping than does the adult (Fig. 24-5). In fact, the newborn may sleep from 16 to 20 hours out of 24. Of this time, approximately 50% is spent in REM sleep. During the REM stages, grimacing, twitching, and sucking movements are frequent. Much waking time is spent meeting physiologic and comfort needs, such as being fed, held, or changed so that the body is kept warm. The child who is 3 months old has about 8 to 10 uninterrupted hours of sleep each night and three to four shorter periods of sleep and rest during the day. This pattern appears to be maturational in that it develops whether or not the parents attempt to alter sleeping and feeding times (Wardle, 1986). From 3 months until 1 year of age, the child lengthens the night sleep time by 1 to 2 hours and shortens the daytime sleeping hours.

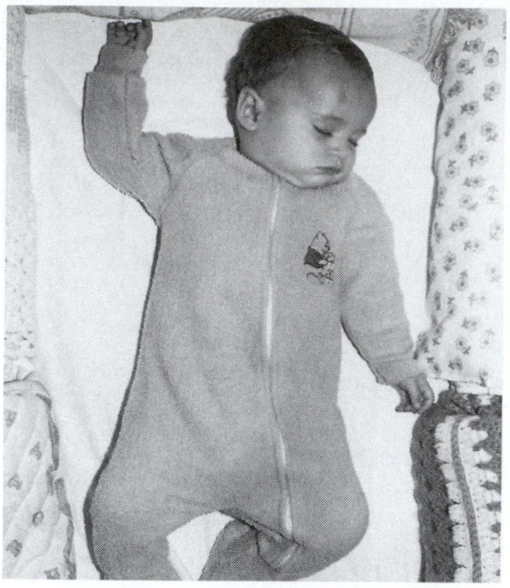

Figure 24-5. Infants' sleep patterns differ from those of adults.

As the child grows older, sleep demands decrease, as does the proportion of REM sleep. Many children are comforted and fall asleep more easily if they have a favorite stuffed animal or blanket in bed with them. Preschoolers usually need naps to meet their high energy demands. Dreaming begins between the ages of 1 to 2 years, when the child may suddenly awake, aroused and screaming (Wardle, 1986).

School-age children. By the time the child reaches school age, sleep consumes about 10 to 11 hours per night, with the REM sleep stage taking up about one-fifth of that time. Some children this age have difficulty falling asleep because of the stimulation of the day's activities. Parents can offset this problem by providing a relaxing period with music or stories just before bedtime.

Thirty percent of normal children report nightmares (frightening dreams), which occur at least once a month (Wardle, 1986). When a child reaches the age of 4 or 5 years, dreams can be recounted and they appear to be similar in content to those of adults.

Adolescents. The need for sleep time continues gradually to decrease, the adolescent needing about 8 to 9 hours of sleep per night, again with one-fifth of it REM sleep. Because of the adolescent lifestyle, including school and social activities, sleep time may electively become more erratic. Adolescents typically supplement regular sleep time by sleeping late in the morning when possible.

The middle adult. An adult needs 7 to 8 hours of sleep, containing four to six complete sleep cycles. REM sleep remains at approximately one-fifth of the total time. There is no appreciable difference between men and women.

The older adult. Older persons experience less stage III, stage IV, and REM sleep than do people of other ages. As little as 15% to 18% of total sleep may be

REM sleep, a decrease from younger years. Elderly persons have increased difficulty in sleeping. "The concern of the elderly is obvious in their demand for sleep medications, and the difficulty health professionals have in dealing with this occurrence can be measured by the number of prescriptions that are written to alleviate the problem" (Ross, Hare, and McPherson, 1986). Older adults have a variety of specific sleep problems, which we discuss in the next section.

The above figures are only averages; individual patterns for sleep vary considerably. It has now been well documented that some persons function well sleeping only 4 to 5 hours per night, whereas others have a definite need for 10 hours on a continuing basis. In planning care, nurses must consider these differences.

Drugs

The work of Evans and Ogunremi (1970) and others reveals that *hypnotics*, drugs used to induce sleep, shorten the REM sleep stage although the total duration of sleep may be lengthened. Many sleep medications, including the group called barbiturates, decrease REM sleep. None of the hypnotics induces natural sleep.

Amphetamines also inhibit REM sleep. This class of drugs, known colloquially as "speed" or "uppers," figures prominently in drug abuse and can cause aberrant behavior such as combativeness or agitation. The amphetamines are no longer a component of any over-the-counter medications and are restricted by law except when prescribed by a physician. Some drugs used in breathing disorders, such as aminophylline, also disturb sleep.

To a lesser degree, the use of alcohol shortens REM sleep. People who consume large quantities of alcohol over an extended period of time experience some of the same symptoms of REM deprivation as people on other drugs such as hypnotics and amphetamines.

Discontinuing any of these drugs causes abnormally extended periods of REM sleep, which is probably a catch-up mechanism. This phenomenon is called *REM rebound*. It is important for the nurse to know that the patient withdrawing from any of the REM inhibiting drugs frequently experiences vivid, frightening nightmares. If the person is made so uncomfortable by these episodes as to feel a need to return to the drug, a cycle of drug dependence can begin. Fortunately, the withdrawal period is relatively short. Talking with the patient about the feelings that accompany withdrawal and their cause may be valuable. Offering emotional support may prevent the patient from using drugs unnecessarily.

An important point made by research is that the hypnotics taken by elderly persons may be effective in decreasing frequent arousal during the sleeping hours but may be harmful to respiratory function. It is thought that the normal arousal periods during sleep clear the airway through coughing or swallowing. When they are taken away through the use of medications, the susceptible elderly may experience respiratory distress (Ross, Hare, and McPherson, 1986).

Disorders Associated With Sleep

Sleep disturbances may be long-term difficulties, developed long before an individual enters the hospital as a patient. Some people, however, who have never had difficulty sleeping may experience such difficulty in the care setting. It is often the nurse who first discovers that the patient has problems sleeping.

Sleep Deprivation

"Sleep deprivation, caused by overstuffed schedules and clinical sleep disorders, has become one of the nation's most pervasive health problems. It is one of the least recognized sources of disability, costing U.S. com-

Nursing Issues and Trends: *Over-the-Counter Sleeping Medications*

The perceived need for a "good night's sleep" is realistic for many Americans who attempt to balance many roles; that of parent, student, worker, and community member. Because of this, the media has devoted a great deal of attention toward promotion of OTC (over-the-counter) sleeping medications. These compounds are not hypnotics but do foster dependence and contain potentially harmful agents for some susceptible people. The variety of products now on the market has increased markedly over the past 10 years. Many contain "P.M." as part of their name to signify that they should be taken appropriately at bedtime to encourage sleep. Living a healthy daytime regimen which includes regular exercise, a nutritious diet, and especially managing stress well can lead to a feeling of natural relaxation and restful sleep without medication. The reliance and possible dependence on OTC sleeping medications are concerns for health care providers.

panies an estimated $70 billion annually in lost productivity, medical bills and industrial accidents" (Society of Neuroscience, 1991, p. 1).

The subject of sleep deprivation is particularly important for nurses in that many patients, because of either illness or the health care setting, are at risk for this problem. Sleep deprivation can occur when the duration of sleep is inadequate or when sleep time is repeatedly interrupted over an extended period, especially during stage IV or the REM stage. Patients may be sleep deprived because of pain, anxiety, drugs, or the necessity of having constant nursing care (Fig. 24-6).

Sleep deprivation studies have been conducted with volunteers sleeping in the laboratory. When the EEG indicates that the person is dreaming, usually during stage IV or REM, the subject is awakened and then allowed to return to sleep. This arousal at the onset of dreaming is repeated over and over until certain signs and behaviors indicate that the subject is experiencing sleep deprivation. Some studies do not allow the subject to sleep at all for long periods of time. The subjects in these experimental situations clearly demonstrated signs of sleep deprivation.

Signs of sleep deprivation include a decrease in attention span, irritability, slowed reactions, and heightened sensitivity to pain or a lowered pain threshold. Sleep deprivation also results in an inability to perform tasks that require fine motor skills so that a diabetic patient learning to give self-injections would, for example, have difficulty.

Many physiologic signs also accompany sleep deprivation. The body temperature of a sleep-deprived person fluctuates, the production of red blood cells decreases, and the body's chemistries are altered. For example, the potassium concentration in the urine is elevated by sleep loss. As deprivation becomes more pronounced, the behavioral and physiologic signs intensify. A patient may even become confused or disoriented. Some portion of the disorientation experienced by some patients may be a manifestation of sleep deprivation.

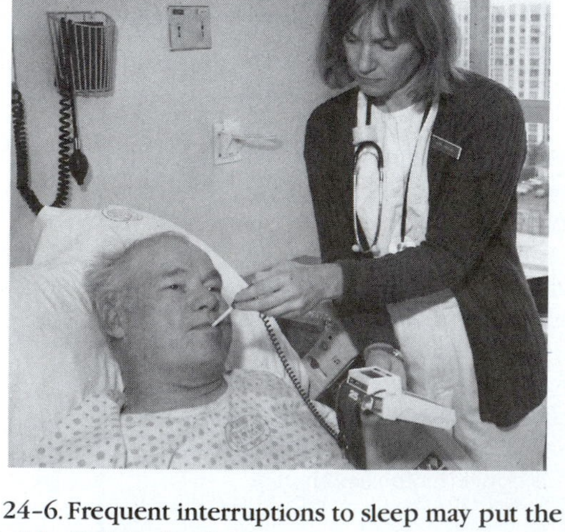

Figure 24-6. Frequent interruptions to sleep may put the patient at risk of sleep deprivation.

Insomnia

Insomnia (inability to sleep) is a relatively common problem and is defined as the inability to initiate and maintain sleep. Insomnia is the most frequently reported sleep disorder, affecting twice as many women as men. It is also more prevalent in elderly people and those of lower social classes (Jahanshahi, 1986). Persons suffering this disorder may have one or all of three states: difficulty in falling asleep, difficulty maintaining sleep throughout the night, or early awakenings.

Some insomnia is caused by such contributing factors as pain, emotional upset, and poor sleeping conditions. Eliminating the cause of such sleeplessness usually brings about relief. However, as much as 10% to 15% of the population suffers from chronic insomnia, a more troublesome phenomenon the cause of which is not so evident. It has been suggested that rigid parental expectations of sleep behavior may begin a person's sleep disturbance (Douglas, 1987). Other researchers have observed that persons complaining of insomnia are more tense and anxious than noninsomniacs. A chemical imbalance in the brain has also been suggested. Women experiencing menopause have a higher incidence of insomnia. Because this is such a common problem, research is continuing to try to find help for these persons.

A new and reportedly effective therapy for insomnia is *stimulus control therapy* (*SCT*). This is particularly helpful for people who use the bedroom for other activities such as eating and reading. It attempts to reinstate the bedroom as a place solely for sleep behavior so that it acts as a "sleep stimulus" (Jahanshahi, 1986). This therapy consists of instructing the person to 1) go to bed only when feeling sleepy, 2) not use the bedroom for activities other than sleeping, 3) get up after 10 minutes if unable to sleep and return to bed only when sleepy, 4) get up each morning at the same time, and 5) not nap during the day.

Regardless of one's regimen, insomnia is a complicated problem that requires changes in behavior. Insomnia is often a long-standing pattern on the part of the individual. The fear of being unable to sleep only intensifies the problem. Medical intervention, such as the use of drugs, may be necessary until new patterns are established. If used, sleep-inducing drugs should be carefully selected for suitability to the patient's particular problem. A short-acting drug may be sufficient for a patient who cannot fall asleep, whereas a longer-acting drug may be required for a patient unable to stay asleep.

Somnambulism

Somnambulism (sleepwalking) occurs mainly with children. Although myth suggests that sleepwalking places the young child or adolescent in danger, this is usually not true. Children sleepwalk most often because they are sleeping uncomfortably, perhaps because of the need to urinate or because the weather is unseasonably hot. When sleepwalking, children most often walk about in familiar daytime patterns and familiar spaces such as going to the kitchen or walking toward the living room or yard. The best way to manage sleepwalking persons is to remind them to return to bed and then, without abruptly awakening them, guide them in the appropriate direction. Sleepwalking is uncommon after puberty.

Enuresis

Enuresis (bedwetting) most often occurs in preadolescent children, boys more often than girls. Nocturnal urinary continence should be accomplished by age 4 (Whaley and Wong, 1989). Many physicians do not view enuresis as a disorder unless the child who has remained dry each night suddenly develops enuresis. When this happens, the cause of the enuresis could be a physiologic or a psychological problem. However, wetting the bed may upset the parents and the child and may curtail social overnight activities. For this reason, it may cause a problem despite the evidence that in most situations, it may be a *maturational* delay rather than a specific physical or psychological disturbance.

When enuresis occurs in adults, usually medical reasons are the cause. Many factors can cause enuresis in children. There may be a physical problem such as an incompetent or small bladder. Various researchers have proposed different possible psychological reasons for bedwetting. Some researchers suggest a threatening environment or hostility toward parents as a primary cause, whereas others stress anxiety-provoking toilet training as a factor.

Many interventions have been suggested, such as limiting fluids in the evening, interrupting sleep to take the child to the bathroom, and using devices that wake the child when enuresis occurs. In some instances, antidepressant and anticholinergic drugs have been used to slow the urinary reflex action.

Narcolepsy

Narcolepsy is a lifelong syndrome of sleep disturbance that does not threaten life and can be managed but not cured. It is uncommon but not rare, affecting approximately 1 in every 2,500 persons with its onset from childhood to midlife. Recent research has revealed a possible complicated mechanism in which the immune system of these individuals is overcome by stress, causing narcolepsy. Other studies focus on a weak family linkage, with more males affected than females.

Narcoleptics cannot resist falling asleep many times during the day. These sleeping periods are usually of short duration and are often associated with brief muscular paralysis. Despite short, frequent periods of sleep, the person feels weak and fatigued.

Several nursing actions are effective. Encouraging several short naps during the day appears to decrease the number of irresistible very short sleep periods. Stimulating drugs, such as amphetamines, prescribed by the physician provide some relief of symptoms. Research is continuing, focused on the use of newer drugs and methods for control.

The person who has narcolepsy needs sensitive care and understanding because the condition is unfamiliar to most people. The person with narcolepsy may be admitted to the health care facility for another reason so you must plan care in such a way that this condition is also given attention in the plan of care. Information regarding local support groups is available from the American Narcolepsy Association.

Sudden Infant Death Syndrome (SIDS)

Sudden infant death syndrome (SIDS), also known as crib death, has been associated, although tentatively, with sleep pathology. SIDS occurs in children of all races, slightly more often in African Americans and Native Americans and slightly less often in Asian children. More boys than girls are affected. Within the United States, SIDS is now the leading cause of death of children, age 1 week to 1 year (Whaley and Wong, 1989).

The syndrome refers to young, apparently healthy children dying suddenly while sleeping. The child at risk for SIDS appears to suffer prolonged periods of apnea during sleep. Many factors have been proposed as risk factors for SIDS. Some of these are prenatal causes such as poor health care, mothers under the age of 20, maternal smoking, and the use of illicit drugs. After birth, risk factors are prematurity, the presence of heart and lung problems, low birth weight, and having siblings who died of SIDS. The most recent research identifies the possibility of delay in the maturation of the brain stem as being a causative factor for SIDS (Kryger, Roth, and Dement, 1989).

Some children in the high-risk group are attached to a home respiratory monitoring unit, which signals the parents or care provider when breathing problems arise. There is, at present, much doubt that SIDS can be prevented. These monitors are not used with infants of low risk because they can create parental anxiety and can cause problems with parent–child bonding. Certainly, the parents and family of SIDS victims require sensitive, understanding care. The death of children is discussed in Chapter 41.

Obstructive Sleep Apnea Syndrome

Sleep apnea is a condition of sleep pathology in adults. Unlike SIDS, adult sleep apnea is considered an obstructive disorder. If not treated, it can cause death. Sleep apnea is sometimes confused with narcolepsy because of the presence of daytime sleepiness, which may be caused by multiple periods of sleep apnea during the night. The condition occurs more often in men than in women and may have a mild family linkage.

Symptoms of the syndrome include obesity, daytime somnolence, loud snoring unrelieved by change in position, and periods of apnea during sleep time. Drinking alcohol, taking antidepressant drugs, and changing sleep patterns can intensify the condition. The person may be unaware of the problem so the diagnosis is often made on the reporting of a bed partner or family member.

The precise mechanism of the obstruction is unknown, but it is thought that the occlusion is inspiratory and occurs at the level of the soft palate. Decreased respiratory muscular activity is present during REM sleep, whereas snoring is more prevalent during non-REM sleep periods (Jaquis, 1987). These two stages appear to be the most hazardous within the sleep cycle.

Several years ago, the treatment for those with life-threatening apnea was the performance of a preventive, elective *tracheostomy*, with the insertion of a permanent tube into the trachea, so that an airway was always patent. This procedure, which led to a high rate of infection and complications, is now considered unnecessary and is not commonly performed. Much simpler procedures are done to alter the anatomy of the upper airway. These include tonsillectomy, adenoidectomy, and **uvulopalatopharyngoplasty (UPPP)**, a reconstruction of the soft palate. Long-term respiratory distress can lead to psychological alterations; treatment may be a combined effort of surgery, medications, and psychotherapy (Jaquis, 1987). The person is also advised to lose excess weight and refrain from alcohol intake.

Assessment Related to Sleep

There are three basic ways to determine the quantity and quality of sleep: subjective (the patient's perception); objective (observing the person's sleep behavior); and measurement, using the EEG. In the hospital setting, subjective data, the person's perceptions of the quantity and quality of sleep, are important. Therefore, the first step in assessing the patient's sleep status is to determine how much sleep the individual usually needs for optimum functioning and how the illness or being hospitalized has affected sleep requirements. For example, if the patient, during the nursing interview, reports a usual sleep time of 6 hours each night and now has a serious infection, this patient's nightly sleep time may have to be extended at least 2 to 3 hours for the patient to gain sufficient sleep and feel rested. More nursing history forms are now asking about the patient's sleep patterns. If your facility does not ask for this information, you should add it to the record. Include such information as the number of hours of sleep the patient normally needs, usual bedtime, and factors conducive or disturbing to the patient's sleep. For example, a ticking clock soothes some people and irritates others.

Second, you will want to review the care plan to see if care is interfering with sleep and, if so, how a revision might be implemented. To be most effective, this assessment step should be carried out over an entire 24-hour period. Many other factors should be assessed regarding sleep disturbances. One factor is the adjustment patients must make to the unfamiliar environment of the hospital; most people sleep best in their own homes. The anxiety and physical discomfort of illness or injury are disturbing factors. Breathing problems such as *chronic obstructive pulmonary disease* (*COPD*) cause serious disturbances in sleep patterns as can the pain of arthritis in the patient.

Physical Assessment

Your observation of daytime behavior may be indicative of sleep disturbance. Irritability, intermittent dozing, lassitude, and fatigue during the day may be a sign of sleep deprivation. Frequent complaints of pain inconsistent in degree with the underlying condition may also be a sign of sleep problems. The irritable patient in pain may be simply a tired patient who needs understanding and better planning to allow for sufficient sleep. Nurses must be careful, however, to look for other signs of sleep deprivation as well, so that they do not misjudge the pain level of the patient.

Assessment of sleep disturbance is important if you plan any health teaching. Not only may the person be resistant to the plan if he or she lacks the energy required, but lack of concentration and memory impairment may present problems. It may be best to postpone plans for health teaching if the assessment suggests sleep problems.

In patients who become severely sleep deprived, such as those in intensive care units, hallucinations have been reported. Studies also show that prolonged sleep deprivation lowers the seizure threshold as well as the pain threshold. People with seizure disorders, such as epilepsy, may not have their seizures well controlled. Nurses should teach patients with seizure disorders to avoid sleep loss or jobs that require frequent changes in schedule. When people with epilepsy do have a seizure, they appear to experience much less REM sleep for several days after the seizure. Neurologic researchers have suggested that perhaps the seizure serves in some fashion as a compensatory mechanism for REM sleep in that individual.

If a patient of any age has a tight binder, cast, or dressing that causes discomfort, the possibility of sleep deprivation should be a nursing concern. Careful assessment can lead to practical solutions for decreasing discomfort.

Various conditions within the health care setting may interfere with normal sleep habits, and understanding the particular factors involved may help delineate the problem more clearly. One factor is that the hospital routine does not recognize that some persons are "day persons," whereas others are "night people." For example, if a person is a night person, being aroused for vital signs at 6 AM is an intrusion on this person's sleep although the morning person may not find this awakening at all upsetting. Patients who have difficulty fitting into a prescribed hospital schedule may find their sleep patterns disturbed.

The physical environment may cause interference with normal sleep. Noise, odors, and interruptions needed for the provision of care are just a few of these factors. The lighting, temperature of the room, and close proximity of others are also impediments to normal sleep. One researcher found that "staff talking" was particularly disturbing to those trying to sleep (Webster, 1986). The hospital bed is intimidating and unfamiliar to most patients. Unlike the bed at home, hospital beds are narrow and may have bed linens and blankets that feel different from those at home. Maintaining a comfortable position in such restricted bed space is also a common problem.

The patient's illness is a contributing factor to inadequate sleep so that pain and discomfort as well as the anxiety and stress brought on by illness or surgery become common causes of sleep disturbances.

Any one of these factors or a combination of them can place the patient at risk of sleep disturbance. The statements of etiology that identify risk states are useful in that they suggest nursing actions that may prevent sleep disturbance. Becoming more aware of factors that disrupt sleep and including risk states for sleep disturbance in your plan of care often deter the development of actual sleep problems.

Nursing Diagnosis Related to Sleep

Sleep Pattern Disturbance

The NANDA approved a general category of Sleep Pattern Disturbance for sleep disturbances defined as causing discomfort or interference with life's activities. This category is broad and needs to be more clearly defined to plan care.

The nursing diagnosis of Sleep Pattern Disturbance is used when the patient's usual pattern is disturbed, whether or not care providers think there is really adequate sleep. One night of inadequate sleep for a patient does not necessarily mean there is a long-term problem, but further assessment should be carried out.

Sleep disturbance is diagnosed when the individual lacks energy and alertness the next day because of lack of sleep. Sleep disturbance may include difficulty in getting to sleep, frequent awakenings, or early awakening.

Interference with sleep may be caused by a variety of factors. When you write the nursing diagnosis, you must specify the etiology so that nursing actions can be individualized for the particular patient. For example, if the disturbance is related to pruritus or itching, those nursing actions to relieve the discomfort would promote the person's sleep.

Nursing Research: *Implications for Practice*

Topf, M. "Effects of Personal Control of Hospital Noise on Sleep." *Research in Nursing and Health* 15, 1 (February 1992): 19–28.

More than 100 female volunteers where placed in a simulated high noise level hospital environment. Randomly selected subjects were given instruction in a noise control device; others were subjected to the simulated noise without control. Women who had no control over the noise level found alterations in overnight sleep that resulted in more difficulty falling asleep, staying asleep, and progressing from one sleep stage to another. There was also less total REM sleep.

This study affirms the importance of noise control within the clinical setting so that patients can receive adequate sleep. It also supports the importance of control of the environment for both patients and nursing staff.

Nursing Diagnoses Related to Sleep

Sleep Pattern Disturbance
- related to pruritus
- related to anxiety
- related to incisional pain
- related to intensity of care

Activity Intolerance related to lack of sleep
Fatigue related to lack of sleep
Ineffective Individual Coping related to lack of sleep

Other Nursing Diagnoses

As for the nursing diagnoses discussed for a deficit in rest, other nursing diagnoses resulting from a sleep deficit include Fatigue, Activity Intolerance, and Ineffective Individual Coping.

Planning and Implementation Related to Sleep

One of the desired outcomes for nursing interventions associated with sleep deficits would be recognition by the patient that a sleeping difficulty is present. Another desired outcome is the identification of the factors that interfere with sleep, with the result that there is a decrease in fatigue and increased activity tolerance and coping ability. Finally, the patient's understanding of those factors that promote sleep in his or her individual circumstances is a key desired outcome.

The planning of actions related to sleep problems is aimed at reducing or eliminating factors that are interfering with normal sleep patterns, creating an environment and comfort state conducive to sleep, and reinforcing sleep-conducive behavior by setting aside time for patient teaching (see the sample Nursing Care Plan Related to Sleep). The nursing interventions discussed in the following paragraphs can be effective in preventing sleep disturbance.

Modifying Care Schedule

One of the most creative and satisfying actions nurses can take to provide patients with sufficient sleep is to plan for nursing care to be delivered in specified time blocks. During these time blocks, nurse–patient communication, vital signs monitoring, procedures, and treatments can be performed. At other times, patients who need high-intensity care can sleep uninterrupted. Studies have repeatedly shown that at least some of the confusion and disorientation displayed by patients in intensive care units is caused by sleep deprivation resulting from constant interruption of stages III and IV and REM sleep. For all patients, a closer look at the intrusion of care on the essential sleep cycle is in order.

Providing a Conducive Environment

Although the bed, furniture, and room itself are far different from what the patient is used to, an effort can be made to personalize the surroundings of patients, particularly those in the hospital or extended care facility for long periods of time. Some patients use quilts or blankets from home, personal nightwear, and pictures, clocks, and books that have meaning; all contribute to a restful mind, which can bring on sleep.

Eliminating or minimizing disturbing factors in the hospital environment is also helpful. Unpleasant odors, excessively warm or cool temperatures, and unnecessary lights and noises, including conversation in proximity of the patient, may all prove distracting and interfere with sleep.

Providing Comfort Measures

The value of providing comfort measures cannot be overestimated. The nurse who spends time providing care before the patient's bedtime may considerably minimize the need for sleep medications. An unhurried backrub, the straightening or replacement of wrinkled or soiled linens, and a warm noncaffeinated beverage all enhance the ability to sleep. Offering the bedpan or urinal at bedtime prevents sleep from being interrupted.

If the person has been troubled by a cough, instruct the patient to breathe deeply and cough in the high Fowler's or sitting position (see Module 41, Respiratory Care Procedures) just before sleep. If the patient coughs and expectorates any secretions, sleep is less likely to be disturbed.

The recumbent position can increase bronchial and nasal secretions, aggravating a cough. Anticipating this outcome for the respiratory patient and securing an order for an appropriate cough medication before the patient's bedtime may prevent hours of sleeplessness.

Providing Emotional Support

As well as providing physical comfort, the nurse strives to provide for maximum peace of mind, remembering that stress and anxiety frequently cause restlessness or insomnia. Anxiety could be related to tests just performed or about to be performed, apprehension over the patient's condition, or the strangeness of the hospital environment. The nurse who listens and discusses such

Nursing Care Plan
Sample Nursing Care Plan Related to Sleep

Nursing Diagnosis

Sleep Pattern Disturbance related to nocturia.

Supportive data:

61-year-old man.
First hospitalization.
Immobilized due to hip replacement.
Reported at interview that he was a "light sleeper."
Voided 3× on night shift last 3 nights.
Stated he had difficulty falling asleep after being awakened.

Desired Patient Outcomes

For the patient to:

Interrupt sleep only once during night for voiding.
Sleep soundly for at least 5 h per night

Nursing Action	Rationale
1. Encourage patient to limit fluids after 9:00 in the evening.	Limiting fluids in the evening will decrease the quantity of urine produced during the sleeping hours.
2. Have patient void before retiring.	Emptying the bladder before sleep lengthens the time before a full bladder awakens the person.
3. Place urinal close to bedside, within reach of patient.	Sleep is minimally disturbed if a person does not have to walk to a bathroom when awakened by a full bladder.
4. Monitor sleep pattern and share with health care team.	Documentation of the sleep pattern and nursing actions aids the health care team to better meet the patient's need for uninterrupted sleep.

concerns with the patient is promoting sleep by providing maximum peace of mind.

Timing Administration of Prescribed Drugs

If your assessment indicates that drugs are a possible cause of sleep disturbance, you might consult the physician regarding the possibility of adjustment in medication. If the medication is essential, you can be ready to support the patient if unpleasant dreams or other side effects occur. You can also be helpful by using good judgment in making nursing decisions regarding PRN drugs ordered for a patient. For example, if sleep is disturbed by pain, administering the prescribed pain medication is much more sensible and useful to the patient than giving a sleeping medication. The relief of pain often allows sleep to ensue naturally. It is undesirable to give medication known to interfere with REM sleep if other alternatives are available.

Providing the Opportunity for Increased Activity

Persons who are alert and active throughout the day tend to sleep more easily at night. Boredom and the absence of the usual demands of work or home cause patients, particularly the bedridden, to sleep intermittently throughout the day. Because of interruptions, this sleep is often not of the duration or quality needed but may still interfere with night sleep. In time, sleep deprivation can occur. You might talk with the patient or contact the family or occupational therapy department concerning appropriate interesting and stimulating activities.

Preventing Restlessness

Sleep is not quiet. The well person is active throughout the sleeping period and has frequent movement. Some patients who are unable to turn experience muscular fatigue that interrupts sleep. The restless patient who is unable to turn independently should be repositioned every 2 hours to promote sound sleep and maintain skin integrity. More frequent turning may alter the sleep cycle and should be avoided.

Adjusting Binders, Dressings, Casts, and Equipment

Any patient with a binder, dressing, or cast, or with equipment that is noisy or has an alarm system, is at risk of having sleep disrupted. Simple nursing actions can often correct the problem. Rewrapping a binder, reinforcing or replacing soiled or uncomfortable dressings, and padding or repositioning a cast can lead to uninterrupted sleep. If equipment such as an intravenous infusion is in use, checking the flow rate and adding on solutions just before sleep may prevent alarm sounds from waking the patient.

Referring Patients to a Sleep Disorder Center

Finally, if the person has experienced extended or lifelong problems with sleep, you could act as a resource for possible referral to a sleep disorder center in your community. More than 150 centers in the United States study sleep disturbances and help persons with sleep disorders. The nearest large medical facility or university would be able to identify the center available to persons in your area. If your area does not have a sleep disorder center, there are professionals educated in providing therapy for long-term sleep problems.

Nurses should be aware that in addition to the numerous sleep disorder centers, several national organizations are concerned with special sleep disturbances. The American Narcolepsy Association in California and Project Sleep: National Program on Insomnia and Sleep Disorders, an arm of the U.S. Department of Health and Human Services, are but two.

Evaluation Related to Sleep

Evaluation for resolution of sleep disturbance or deprivation is both subjective and objective, relating back to desired patient outcomes. Subjectively, many patients openly verbalize a feeling of being more rested and more energetic. The patient who appeared depressed and unmotivated before implementation may now express renewed interest and motivation in the plan of care. You may observe less irritability or signs of confusion. If serious deprivation was present, you may observe greater mental agility and no signs of hallucinations.

Nurses and Sleep

Nurses are themselves susceptible to sleep disturbances and sleep deprivation because of irregular hours and shift changes (Fig. 24-7). Some nurses adjust more easily than others. A nurse who has worked the night shift for a number of years may adjust more easily into a pattern of night work punctuated by a 2-days-off rotation than a nurse who works 4 nights consecutively and then shifts back to the day shift after 2 days off. Studies show that it takes as long as 10 days for some individuals who have worked night shifts to revert to normal daytime body temperatures and urine potassium levels (Felton, 1976). It is also known that nurses who transfer from the night shift to day work experience less REM sleep for a short period of time (Lanuza, 1976).

Both quality and quantity of the sleep of night workers is "considerably inferior to the sleep of day workers" (Rose, 1984, p. 443). One reason the night worker is less proficient is that the person is working at a time when the body temperature is lowest, which is contrary to the usual circadian rhythm. Czeisler and colleagues (1982), using circadian rhythm principles, make several suggestions for improving sleep quality for night

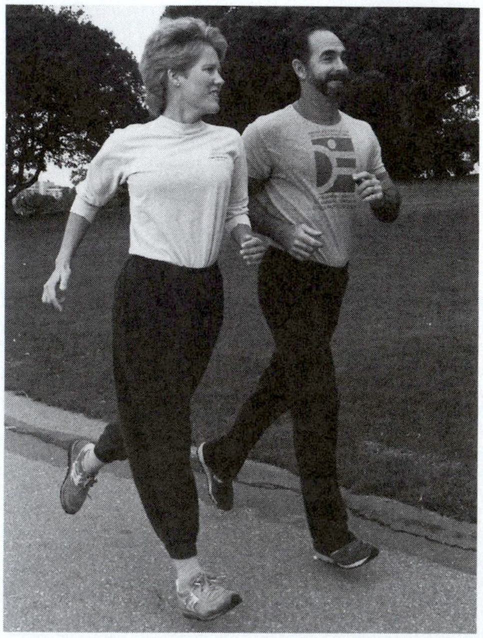

Figure 24-7. Nurses need exercise in order to relax and promote sleep.

workers. First, avoid shift work where possible (not feasible in nursing), and where shift work is necessary, provide long intervals between shift rotations to allow for maximum adjustment. Second, recognizing that some persons naturally adjust to shift changes more easily than others, nursing managers should select these persons for shift work if they are willing.

Even for those who appear to adapt easily to shift work, studies have indicated that these persons have a considerable sleep reduction. Part of this problem may be that "shift-workers often have the tendency to mix night work with normal social hours when not working, thus preventing the establishment of a consistent sleep pattern" (Caravan, 1986, p. 323). Impairment on tasks of night shift workers has been demonstrated in the laboratory.

Rose (1984) showed that where rotations are necessary, the body's inner clock works best if the shift is forward. For example, nurses who work nights should shift to days, with day personnel moving to afternoons and afternoon people moving to nights.

Nurses can lessen the effects of sleep deprivation on shift nursing. If possible, begin gradually adjusting your sleeping hours several days in advance of a shift change. Go to sleep an hour or two earlier or later, depending on what your new shift will be. Be sure to keep up your nutritional level and exercise.

A benefit for nurses' sleep patterns has been the increasing policy of 10- and 12-hour shifts. This allows three to four long working periods, followed by 3 to 4 days off. This work pattern with "overlapping" shifts provides better continuity of care for the patient and allows nurses more regular sleep periods. Although there is some concern at present regarding the fatigue factor of longer hours of work, the longer time off to regain sufficient sleep is considered an advantage. Studies are now being done to validate the benefits for patients and nurses.

As nurses, we must be cognizant of our usual sleep patterns and needs and how we individually react to sleep disturbances. Mild depression, for example, is common. Irritability may strain interpersonal relations. Medication errors and deviations from aseptic technique, endangering the patient, can occur if the nurse is overly tired. You should be particularly vigilant about any effects of fluctuating working hours that may jeopardize you or the patient. Avoiding sleep loss as much as possible promotes safe practice.

Nursing Care Study
Patient with Sleep Deprivation

Mrs. Julie Stafford is a 57-year-old patient with bronchitis and emphysema. Long a heavy smoker, Mrs. Stafford has experienced increasing respiratory difficulty over the past few years. In recent weeks, the infection has made breathing so difficult that Mrs. Stafford has become dependent on frequent use of a hand-held inhaler.

On admission Mrs. Stafford reported feeling anxious as well as "generally tired" and appeared pale. Her respirations were shallow and rapid. Mr. Stafford said his wife had been sleeping poorly for 2 to 3 weeks.

The physician's orders include bed rest, an antibiotic, a mild tranquilizer, pain medication, and respiratory therapy treatments every 2 hours. The staff nurse assigned to Mrs. Stafford begins her assessment by reading the data in the record, which note the history of sleeping poorly, tiredness, and anxiety, and the physician's orders. A visit to Mrs. Stafford confirms the persistence of the same concerns. The nurse notes the patient's exhausted appearance. A menu order lies on the bedside table unmarked. When asked if she would like to complete the form or needs help to do so, Mrs. Stafford replies, in a mildly irritated manner, "I really don't care what I eat. I just want to be left alone." When asked if her husband has left the hospital, she replies, "I really can't remember." She requests pain medication every 3 hours. Mrs. Stafford's sleep is being interrupted about once an hour and she appears to be experiencing sleep deprivation.

The staff nurse determines that nursing intervention is needed. Because the normal sleep cycle lasts about 90 minutes, she thinks the patient needs a more extended period of uninterrupted sleep. The nurse arranges to talk with the physician, to whom she describes the patient's sleep history and behavior. The physician and nurse examine the current pulmonary reports and, noting improvement, decide that the 2:00 PM respiratory treatment can be omitted. The physician writes the order to omit the treatment; the plan is explained to the patient. Mrs. Stafford seems to welcome the news. At 12:00 she receives her noon meal, medications, respiratory treatment, and a relaxing backrub. With the patient's permission, the hospital telephone operator is instructed not to put through calls to the pa-

(*continued*)

Nursing Care Study (continued) **Patient with Sleep Deprivation**

tient for 4 hours. The room is darkened. A sign noting the period during which the patient is not to be disturbed is posted on the door of the room. At 3:00, the plan is explained to the PM staff nurse.

Evaluation by the staff nurse at the 4:00 PM report is positive. Mrs. Stafford awakens from 4 hours of deep sleep stating that she feels "so much better." She appears to breathe more easily and requests a clean gown in preparation for evening visiting hours.

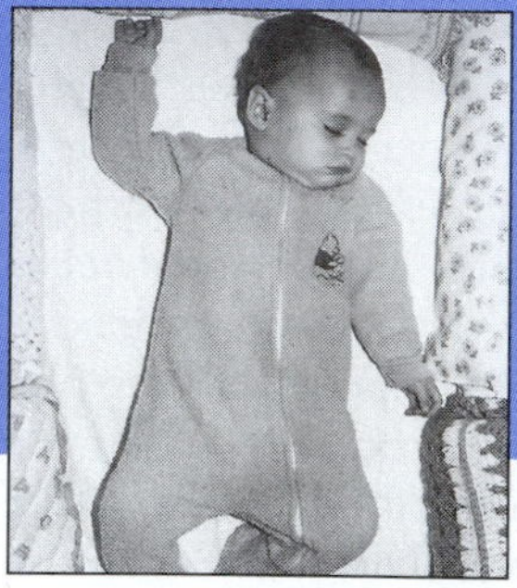

Key Points

- Rest and sleep are basic human needs. The stress caused by illness places undue demands on energy levels and the physiologic and psychological response systems of individuals.
- Sufficient rest and sleep are even more important for the ill than for people who are healthy.
- Rest provides a period for the body to restore tissues and psychological comfort. Because the many activities and interruptions within the health care setting make resting difficult for patients, the nurse should incorporate into the plan of care times when the patient can rest in an environment conducive to rest. This may include restriction of visiting time.
- When assessing the amount of rest an individual patient may need, one should consider the amount of rest the patient needs when well, the type of illness or incapacity being experienced, and the patient's psychological state.
- The nurse's knowledge of the circadian rhythm and the stages of sleep is essential in the management of sleep pattern disturbance.
- Prolonged sleep deprivation, particularly of REM stage sleep, has adverse physical and psychological effects.
- Age affects not only the amount of sleep needed but the length of the various stages of the sleep cycle. Infants need the most sleep and have the highest amount of REM stage sleep, whereas older persons need the least amount of sleep and have the least amount of REM stage sleep.
- Sleep disturbances range from sleep deprivation to obstructive sleep apnea. Nurses need to be knowledgeable about these disturbances as well as the effects of psychosocial factors and drugs on sleep.
- The nursing process is used to identify what is normal sleep for an individual, factors involved in illness or the plan of care that can interfere with sleep and appropriate nursing interventions.
- Nursing interventions for sleep pattern disturbance include minimizing unfamiliar surroundings, providing physical and psychological comfort, monitoring the effects of drugs on sleep patterns, and encouraging daytime activity. In addition, nurses can refer patients to sleep disorder centers for those with long-standing sleep problems.
- Because medication errors and incomplete care can often be attributed to nurses who are overtired from sleeplessness, nurses need adequate rest and sleep to provide safe and efficient care.

Study Questions

1. What function does rest fulfill for the patient?
2. Explain the importance of the circadian rhythm as it relates to planning care for the patient.
3. List the stages of the sleep cycle and the characteristics of each.
4. What specific actions might you take to help the patient obtain adequate amounts of REM sleep?
5. Briefly, how do the numbers of hours spent in sleep and in the REM stage change throughout the life span?
6. Name and define six sleep disturbances.
7. What data would indicate that a patient is sleep deprived?
8. Discuss how the day within the health care facility can restrict time for rest and sleep and how you might plan for these within the plan of care.
9. What factors might cause some degree of sleep deprivation in a surgical patient?

10. What effect do barbiturates have on sleep?
11. Discuss at least four nursing actions you might take to improve the overall sleep pattern of a person in the health care facility.
12. What are the main problems in relation to sleep for nurses assigned to shift work?
13. What are some of the potential problems for a patient if the nurse is sleep deprived?

Critical Thinking Activities

1. Keep a record of your hours of sleep per night for one typical week. Analyze your sleep pattern and determine if it is adequate. If not, decide ways you might adjust your schedule to provide optimum rest and sleep.
2. Analyze an article written within the last 5 years on the topic of sleep. Discuss the most important parts of the article with a small group of students.
3. Write a nursing care plan for either a patient for whom you have cared or a hypothetical patient who is sleep deprived. Determine what factors contributed to this condition and actions you might take to resolve the deprivation.

Relevant Sections in Modules for Basic Nursing Skills

References and Readings

Alward, R. R. "Are You a Lark or an Owl on the Night Shift?" *American Journal of Nursing* 88, 10 (October 1988): 1337–1339.

Banning, J. A. "Chronic Fatigue and Shift Work." *Canadian Nurse* 87, 8 (September 1991): 3.

Caravan, T. "The Functions of Sleep." *Nursing* (London) 3, 9 (September 1986): 321–324.

Carpenito, L. J. *Nursing Diagnosis: Application to Clinical Practice.* 4th ed. Philadelphia: J. B. Lippincott, 1992.

Chase, M. H. "Every Ninety Minutes, a Brainstorm." *Psychology Today* 13 (November 1979): 172.

Chuman, M. A. "The Neurological Basis of Sleep." *Heart and Lung* 12, 2 (March 1983): 177–182.

Cross, S. J. "Assessment of Sleep in Hospital Patients: A Review of Methods." *Journal of Advanced Nursing* 13, 4 (July 1988): 501–510.

Czeisler, C. A., Martin, C. M., and Coleman, R. M. "Rotating Shift Work Schedules That Disrupt Sleep Are Improved by Applying Circadian Principles." *Science* 217 (July 30, 1982): 460–463.

Dement, W. C. *Some Must Watch While Some Must Sleep: Explaining the World of Sleep.* New York: W. W. Norton, 1978.

Douglas, J. "Coping with Sleep Problems." *Health Visitor* 60 (February 1987): 52–53.

Durham, E., and Frost-Hartzer, P. "Relaxation Therapy Works." *RN* 54, 8 (August 1991): 40–42.

Evans, J. I., and Ogunremi, O. "Sleep and Hypnotics: Further Experiments." *British Medical Journal* (August 1970): 310–312.

Felton, G. "Body Rhythm Effects on Rotating Work Shifts." *Nursing Digest* 4 (April 1976): 29–32.

Guyton, A. C. *Human Physiology and Mechanisms of Disease.* 5th edition. Philadelphia: W. B. Saunders, 1992.

Hodgson, L. A. "Why Do We Need Sleep? Relating Theory to Nursing Practice." *Journal of Advanced Nursing.* 16, 12 (December, 1991): 1503–1510.

Hospital Employee Health. "Shift Work Indicated as Possible Health Hazard." 10, 6 (June 1991): 69–72.

Jahanshahi, M. "Insomnia." *Nursing* 9 (London) 3: 9 (September 1986): 328–332.

Jaquis, J. "Obstructive Sleep Apnea Syndrome." *Nurse Practitioner* 12, 6 (June 1987): 50–56.

Kales, A., and Kales, J. "Hypnotics and Altered Sleep-Dream Patterns." *Archives of General Psychiatry* 73 (September 1970): 211–218.

Kleitman, N. *Sleep and Wakefulness* (rev. ed.). Chicago: University of Chicago Press, 1963.

Kryger, M. H., Roth, R., and Dement, W. B. *Principles and Practice of Sleep Medicine.* Philadelphia: W. B. Saunders, 1989.

Lanuza, D. M. "Circadian Rhythms of Mental Efficiency and Performance." *Nursing Clinics of North America* 11 (December 1976): 583–593.

Murray, R. B., and Zentner, J. P. *Nursing Assessment and Health Promotion Strategies Through the Life Span.* 4th edition. Norwalk, Conn.: Appleton and Lange, 1989.

Morrison, J. L. "Working Nights? It Doesn't Have to be a Nightmare." *RN* 50, 9 (September 1987): 33–35.

Oesting, H. H., and Manza, R. J. "Sleep Apnea." *Geriatric Nursing* 9, 4 (April 1988): 232–233.

Oswald, I. "The Biological Clock and Shift-Work." *Nursing Times* 67 (September 1971): 1207–1208.

Roscoe, J., and Haig, N. "Planning Shift Patterns: Shift Work." *Nursing Times* 86, 38 (September 19-25, 1990): 31–33.

Rose, M. "Shift Work: How Does it Affect You?" *American Journal of Nursing* 84, 4 (April 1984): 442–447.

Ross, M. M., Hare, K., and McPherson, M. "When Sleep Won't Come: Helping Our Elderly Clients." *The Canadian Nurse* 82, 9 (October 1986): 14–18.

Sadler, C. "Shift Work: Beat the Clock." *Nursing Times* 86, 38 (September 19-25, 1990): 28–31.

Skipper, J. K., Jung, F. D., and Coffey, L. C. "Nurses and Shift Work: Effects of Physical Health and Mental Depression." *Journal of Advanced Nursing* 15, 7 (July 1990): 835–842.

Society for Neuroscience. "Brain Concepts: Sleep and Dreaming." 11 Dupont Circle, Washington, D.C., 1991.

Wardle, J. "The Chronology of Sleep." *Nursing* 9 (London) 3: 9 (September 1986): 325–326.

Webster, R. A., and Thompson, D. R. "Sleep in Hospital." *Journal of Advanced Nursing* 11 (November 1986): 447–457.

Whaley, L. F., and Wong, D. L. *Essentials of Pediatric Nursing.* 4th edition. St. Louis: C. V. Mosby, 1993.

Nutrition

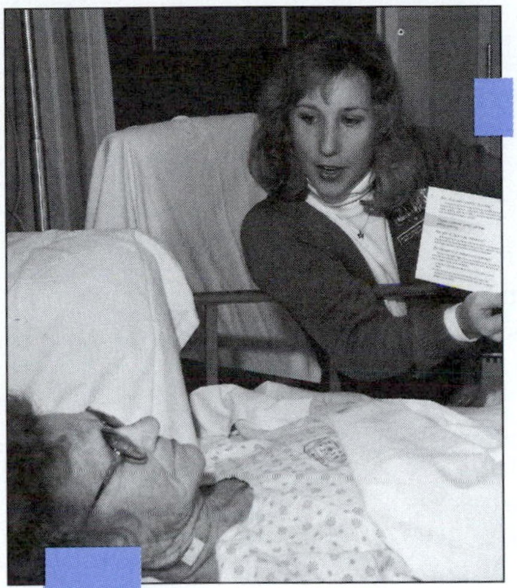

25

Objectives

After completing this chapter, you should be able to:

1. Outline the processes of digestion, absorption, and metabolism for the major nutrients.
2. Define good nutrition, describing in detail how to evaluate a diet.
3. Discuss the roles of hunger, thirst, and appetite in diet.
4. Discuss the role of sociocultural factors in dietary intake.
5. Identify the various ways in which diets may need to be modified because of illness.
6. Outline the data to be collected for nutritional assessment.
7. Explain nursing diagnoses that may be related to nutritional needs.
8. Describe nursing interventions related to maintaining adequate nutrition.
9. Describe nursing approaches to inadequate nutrition, obesity, nausea and vomiting, tube feeding, and parenteral nutrition.

Study Terms

air embolus
anabolism
anorexia
anthropometric measurements
antiemetic drugs
appetite
bolus feeding
carbohydrates
catabolism
elemental formula
enteral feedings
exchange menus
fats
fiber
fluid overload
gastrostomy tube
hunger
hyperalimentation
hyperglycemia
kosher food
macronutrients
malnutrition
metabolic water
micronutrients
minerals
obesity
osmolality
parenteral nutrition
preformed water
projectile vomiting
protein reserve
proteins
Recommended Dietary Allowances (RDA)
trace elements
tube feeding
lactovegetarian
ovolactovegetarian
vitamins

Ellis, Nowlis: Nursing: A Human Needs Approach, 5th ed. © 1994 J.B. Lippincott Company

Outline

Food and water are among human beings' most basic needs. A person cannot go without water for more than a few days; the body soon becomes unable to function. One can survive somewhat longer without food because the body can consume its own stores of fat and protein to provide for its most essential functions. But this supply is limited, and soon the body can no longer function at all.

Even those who nursed in antiquity, without education or an understanding of disease processes, were aware of the value of nourishing food. Through trial and error, they found some foods more helpful than others in restoring health. They also recognized that, in certain illnesses, some foods are better tolerated than others. They were aware of the invalids' need for fluids, and most invalid foods were in liquid or semiliquid form. Many nineteenth century home-nursing manuals focused mainly on the preparation of special broths and other foods for the sick person.

In today's society, a much more scientific background for understanding nutritional needs exists. Information is available about specific needs of the body in specific phases of growth and development as well as about needs related to disease and illness. The more one knows about nutrition, the more one can recognize the complexity of nutritional needs and the importance of maintaining a varied well-balanced diet. Nurses are often in a unique position to help people understand how nutrition can help keep them healthy, as well as to assist them in regaining health.

Basic Nutrients

In the broadest sense, *good nutrition* consists of eating foods that provide all the nutrients needed by the body in amounts adequate for energy, maintenance, repair, replacement of tissue, and—in the young—growth. It also involves avoiding an excessive amount of any nutrient that can damage the body.

As understanding of body physiology and of foods has grown, the definition of good nutrition has expanded. Researchers now recognize as essential a wide variety of nutrients and are beginning to ascertain the optimum amount of each needed for good health.

Carbohydrates

Carbohydrates are the starches and sugars in the diet. Each gram of a carbohydrate provides 4 kilocalories. All fruits and vegetables have some carbohydrate content, but cereal grain products are the major source. Carbohydrates have roughly the same caloric value as proteins, but because carbohydrates require less extensive metabolism, they are available more quickly for energy. Because many low-cost readily available foods are primarily carbohydrates, a majority of the calories in most diets come from carbohydrates. Most primarily carbohydrate foods also contain needed vitamins and minerals and even some plant proteins. The only exceptions are refined simple sugars, which do not have other food value. Providing additional carbohydrate is a way of increasing calorie level to meet the special requirements of growth or unusual activity. Carbohydrate intake exceeding current need is converted in limited amounts to glycogen (an animal starch) for storage in the liver. Excess carbohydrate is converted to fat for long-term storage.

Each society in the world has traditionally based its diet on some staple form of carbohydrate. In much of Asia, rice has been the staple carbohydrate. In some parts of China, noodles form the basis of the diet. In Mexico and Central America, corn has served as the staple carbohydrate. In most of Europe and the United States, bread and potatoes have been the staple carbohydrates, although in Italy various forms of pasta have fulfilled that role. In large areas of Africa, the yam has been the basis of the traditional diet. Diets are now changing across the world; people are showing a tendency to accept the Western diet along with Western technology, which has created nutritional problems for some people. The traditional diet has usually been based on an unrefined carbohydrate product that was also rich in other nutrients. Processed "modern" food may lack these other nutrients, and the individual may not have sufficient income to add other foods to the diet to supply the needed nutrients.

Complex carbohydrates such as those found in whole grains have a wide variety of nutritional advantages over simple carbohydrates, such as those found in sugars. Complex carbohydrates provide other vitamins and nutrients. Because they take longer to digest, complex carbohydrates tend to be released into the blood more gradually and thus contribute to stable blood sugar levels. The fiber that is part of the food remains in the digestive system and provides many benefits.

Fiber is actually a complex carbohydrate the human digestive system is unable to break down. Therefore, fiber does not provide calories. The need for nondigestible fiber in the diet has been receiving increased attention. Fiber, or roughage, is composed mainly of cellulose and is found in fresh fruits and vegetables and in whole-grain cereal products, both raw and cooked. These fibers increase the bulk of the stool, making it pass along the bowel more easily, helping to prevent constipation. Recent research has demonstrated a higher incidence of certain diseases of the bowel in those who eat highly refined diets lacking fiber. Although the exact relationship of diet to these diseases has not been determined, this finding underlines the need for a diet to be highly varied and restricted only when absolutely necessary.

Other research has shown that persons with a diet high in fiber content have lower *cholesterol* levels than do those whose diet contains less fiber. The explanation is that in the intestine the fiber tends to bind with cholesterol that came from food. Many commercial preparations of fiber in the form of wafers, tablets, and granules can be purchased. Because fibrous fruits, vegetables, and whole grains contain other nutrients as well as fiber, they are by far the best way for a person to augment the diet with fiber.

Digestion

Carbohydrates are broken down through digestion into simple sugars that can be absorbed. Carbohydrate digestion starts in the mouth, where the salivary glands secrete saliva containing the enzyme salivary amylase. However, most of the digestive process occurs in the small intestine through the action of pancreatic amylase. Cooked carbohydrates are more easily digested than raw ones because the cooking breaks down cell walls, allowing the body's enzymes to come more rapidly in contact with the material in the cell.

Absorption

A small amount of some simple sugars can be absorbed by passive diffusion across the cell walls of the small intestine. Most sugar is absorbed through an active transport mechanism in the jejunum and the ileum. Energy is required for this process. The sugars are transported by carriers. Sucrose (table sugar) and galactose (milk sugar) are absorbed rapidly. Fructose (fruit sugar) takes twice as long to be absorbed. Mannose and xylose (complex, large molecule sugars) are poorly absorbed, so they are used in some diet foods to provide sweetening without significant calorie intake. Their use is limited because in large amounts they tend to increase the movement of water into the intestine and create diarrhea. Individuals differ in their susceptibility to this effect.

Metabolism

Glucose is the most important carbohydrate. Other simple sugars are metabolized to glucose by the liver. Transport of glucose into cells is facilitated by the hormone insulin. Within the cell, glucose is used for energy in a complex series of chemical reactions. The brain requires glucose for its function and is especially sensitive to changes in glucose level.

Glucose that is not immediately needed may be converted by the liver into glycogen, a starch product that is stored in the liver and can be rapidly converted back to glucose when needed. Excess glucose can also be used to manufacture fatty acids, which are used in various tissues and hormones and can be stored as body fat. When excess glucose accumulates in the blood, the kidneys can excrete the glucose into the urine. This excretion does not usually take place in the healthy individual. Some individuals have a "low renal threshold" for glucose, meaning that they excrete glucose in the urine at a blood sugar level that would not usually cause that to happen.

Proteins

Proteins are the basic material for building and repairing body tissue. They may also be used for energy through a process in which they are broken into a nitrogen fraction and a carbohydrate fraction. The nitrogen fraction is excreted and the carbohydrate fraction is metabolized in the same manner as dietary carbohydrate. Each gram of protein provides 4 kilocalories.

Proteins are found in large quantities in meat, eggs, fish, and milk products. Some vegetables (especially *legumes* such as dry beans and peas), nuts, and whole grains also contain proteins.

Proteins are composed of *amino acids* or amino acids combined with other substances. Twenty or more amino acids are known. The body manufactures about half of these. We call the ones that the body can produce *nonessential amino acids.* Those the body cannot manufacture and that must be obtained from our diet are called *essential amino acids.* Research reveals that for optimum health, the two types of amino acids must be in relative balance (Jackson, 1983).

Amino acids have a "buffering" property, which can alter the pH of a solution. An amino acid in solution can ionize into either an acid or base, so that it can partially correct a pH imbalance. This is an important reason for supplying amino acids to ill persons.

All animal sources of protein contain all 10 essential amino acids and are called complete proteins. Vegetable proteins typically contain some, but not all, of the essential amino acids and thus are called incomplete proteins. For plant proteins to be used most successfully, they must be combined so that the body is provided with all the essential amino acids in appropriate ratios for effective use. In addition, for the body to substitute the amino acids from different foods for complete proteins, the foods must be eaten at the same time. The body is not able to save amino acids until others needed become available. Instead, those amino acids that cannot be used are broken down to be used for their carbohydrate fraction. Examples of effective plant protein combinations are peanut butter combined with whole wheat bread and a corn tortilla combined with beans. Another way to make effective use of plant protein is by combining a small amount of animal protein with the plant protein to provide adequate amino acids. An example of this is putting a small amount of meat in a dish of beans.

Proteins are generally the most expensive nutrient. Animals are costly to raise, and a large amount of waste occurs in processing the animal for consumption; therefore, individuals with serious economic problems may experience their first nutritional problem in protein deficiency.

Although protein needs may rise because of illness or injury, you will find that some people have exaggerated views of how much protein is required for health. When money is limited, it is satisfactory to consume only the essential quantity of protein, deriving additional calories from carbohydrates. Proteins do have an additional value when calorie control is necessary in that their slow digestion and metabolism make for long-sustained calorie availability, and this may decrease hunger.

Digestion

To be absorbed, proteins must be broken down into amino acids. This process begins in the stomach, where pepsin and pepsinogen act on some proteins to break bonds between amino acids. The pancreatic enzymes trypsinogen, chymotrypsinogen, and carboxypeptidase act in the small intestine. Also in the small intestine are trypsin, chymotrypsin, and aminopeptidase. Each of these enzymes acts on a different protein bond.

Heating proteins splits some bonds within the protein, thus facilitating digestion. Heating also destroys some naturally occurring enzyme inhibitors, making the protein more digestible. However, excessive heating may create new bonds that are resistant to enzyme activity. This phenomenon is usually significant only if the diet contains low amounts of protein so that even a small loss affects the amount of protein available. Plant proteins tend to be harder for the body to digest than animal protein, and thus the actual amount of available protein tends to be lower. Eggs are almost completely digestible. Meat proteins are slightly less digestible. Meat requires a lengthy time to be digested and therefore contributes to feelings of satiety. These factors become important when one is planning diets for people with health problems.

Absorption

Amino acids are absorbed in the first portion of the small intestine. Some move into the circulation by passive diffusion. Some move through active transport on carriers. Certain amino acids seem to attach to carriers more readily than others and therefore are absorbed more rapidly.

Metabolism

Amino acids are used within individual cells to manufacture cell components. The liver uses amino acids to manufacture proteins, such as albumin, that are needed by the entire body. The production of protein components by the body is called **anabolism**. For anabolism to occur, all the needed amino acids must be present in adequate amounts at the same time.

Proteins within the body are constantly being broken down in a process called **catabolism**. In the healthy individual, a constant balance between anabolism and catabolism is maintained so that tissues remain intact. When anabolism is occurring more rapidly than catabolism, as it is during growth, and the intake of protein is greater than the loss of nitrogen, the body is said to be in *positive nitrogen balance*. When catabolism is occurring more rapidly than anabolism and the excretion of nitrogen is greater than the intake of protein, the body is in *negative nitrogen balance*. Protein anabolism is affected by the overall health of the person, by the presence of certain hormones (especially steroids, androgens, growth hormone, thyroid hormone, and insulin), and by the adequacy of caloric intake.

Protein that is not needed for tissue building may be available in certain tissues in limited amounts in the form of **protein reserve**. However, most amino acids that are not needed immediately are metabolized in the liver. The nitrogen fraction is removed and excreted by the kidneys. The remainder is used by the body in its carbohydrate pathways. This is why ingestion of protein beyond what is needed for tissue building can contribute to fat production.

Fats

Fats are the most concentrated source of food energy. Each gram of fat provides 9 kilocalories. Fats are building blocks for certain hormones and for nerve tissue. In addition, some stored fat provides cushioning for organs, insulation under the skin to protect the individual from extremes of temperature, and a reserve source of calories in case of food deprivation. Fats also transport some essential vitamins into the system during digestion and are important in the transport of these vitamins to sites where they are used.

There are three types of fats: saturated, which have hydrogen ions attached to all carbon rings; monounsaturated, which have one carbon ring without a hydrogen ion; and polyunsaturated, which have many carbon rings without hydrogen ions. This distinction is significant because the body uses these different types of fats differently. Saturated fats are found in animal fat sources such as butter and red meat and in palm and coconut oils. Polyunsaturated fats are found in vegetable fat sources such as corn, safflower, and canola oils. Monosaturated fats are found in peanut and olive oils.

Within the body, fats occur as simple lipids, also called triglycerides, and as compound lipids. There are several groups of compound lipids. The glycolipids are found primarily in nervous tissue. Glycolipids contain carbohydrate and protein along with triglyceride. The phospholipids contain phosphoric acid and nitrogen along with triglyceride. The lipoproteins contain triglyceride and protein. The lipoprotein group has two major subgroups. The low-density lipoproteins (LDL) are the main carrier for cholesterol in the blood and are implicated in the origins of atherosclerosis, a disorder in which plaques form in arteries, decreasing blood flow and contributing to a wide variety of illnesses such as heart attacks and strokes. High-density lipoproteins (HDL), the second subgroup, appear to carry cholesterol to the liver for excretion and seem to reduce the incidence of atherosclerosis.

The exact roles of these two types of lipoproteins are still under investigation. However, the dietary intake of large amounts of saturated fats tends to raise the level of LDLs, and the intake of polyunsaturated fats tends to lower the levels of both LDLs and HDLs. The intake of monounsaturated fats appears to lower the LDL levels without affecting the HDL level.

One fatty acid, linoleic acid, is necessary to the body and cannot be synthesized. Therefore, linoleic acid is termed an essential fatty acid and must be present in the diet. Linoleic acid is found in large quantities in polyunsaturated fats and in much smaller quantities in other fats. This is another reason for recommending a diet with polyunsaturated fats.

Digestion

Fats are digested in the small intestine. The presence of fat in the material entering the duodenum has an effect on how fast the stomach empties. The more fat, the more slowly the stomach empties, so as to release the high-fat material into the small intestine gradually. This slowing of stomach emptying is the basis for the high satiety value of fats in the diet.

Bile enters the small intestine from the gallbladder when fat stimulates the release of cholecystokinin, a hormone that causes the gallbladder to contract. The bile stimulates peristalsis and neutralizes the acidity of the material from the stomach, creating a better environment for enzymes of the small intestine. Bile also emulsifies fat (*ie*, breaks it into small particles that digest more easily) and lowers the surface tension of the fat droplets so that the enzymes can act more effectively. Lipases, the enzymes for fat digestion, are secreted in both the pancreas and the small intestine itself. During digestion, fats are broken up into small fat molecules.

Fats in liquid form tend to be digested more readily than solid ones. Fats that are combined with other foods generally are easier to digest than large fat particles not mixed with other foods. Fats from milk tend to be digested easily. Fried foods are digested more slowly because the fat on the outer surface must be digested before the enzymes can work on the foodstuff itself. Young children and the elderly are more likely than others to have difficulty with fat digestion.

Absorption

The small fat molecules created by digestion form a complex with bile salts, creating a water-soluble, microscopic particle that can enter the cell membrane of the small intestine. Some fats are absorbed by pinocytosis, a process in which the fat is engulfed by a cell and then released on the other side of the membrane. Most absorption occurs in the jejunum. The cells of the mucous membrane in the jejunum also synthesize complex fat molecules from simple fats absorbed. These complex molecules are then released into the circulation.

Metabolism

The liver is the major location of fat metabolism. There, fats are synthesized to meet body needs. Fats are then used by cells to form needed body components. All cells can also use fats for energy. The oxidation of fats for energy creates ketones, acid substances, which are then further metabolized. If large amounts of fat are being used for energy, as by an individual on a low-carbohydrate, weight reduction diet or by a diabetic without sufficient insulin to facilitate glucose use, ketones are produced more rapidly than they can be metabolized. This rapid production results in an excess of acid products and changes the body's acid–base balance (see Chapter 30).

Minerals

There are 22 different **minerals** known to be needed by the body. Seven are present in the body in fairly large quantities and are termed **macronutrients**. They are calcium, chloride, magnesium, phosphorus, potassium, sodium, and sulfur. Knowledge of the uses of these minerals has been available for some time. The other minerals are termed **micronutrients** or **trace elements** and are present in the body in extremely small quantities. The actual functions of some of the rarer micronutrients have only recently been identified. The micronutrients for which there are known uses are iron, copper, manganese, fluoride, iodine, chromium, selenium, molybdenum, and zinc (Table 25-1).

Minerals are present in almost all foods. Specific foods are recommended to provide specific amounts of those minerals known to be needed, such as iron and calcium. Other minerals, such as sodium and potassium,

Table 25–1. Principal Uses of Minerals in the Body

Mineral	Function
Calcium	Constituent of bones and teeth Muscle contraction Blood clotting
Chlorine	Predominant anion of extracellular fluid Regulation of osmotic pressure
Chromium	Glucose metabolism
Copper	Essential to red blood cells
Fluorine	Resistance to dental caries Deposition of bone calcium
Iodine	Constituent of thyroid hormone
Iron	Constituent of hemoglobin
Magnesium	Constituent of bone Transfer of water into and out of cells
Molybdenum	Essential component of an enzyme that helps produce uric acid
Phosphorus	Constituent of bone and teeth Cell multiplication Activation of some enzymes and vitamins Acid–base balance Carbohydrate metabolism
Potassium	Carbohydrate metabolism Conduction of nerve impulses Muscle contraction Major constituent of intracellular fluid
Selenium	Essential component of enzyme that protects red blood cells
Sodium	Major constituent of extracellular fluid Fluid balance Muscle and nerve irritability
Sulfur	Constituent of protein structure of cells Constituent of bile, saliva, and insulin
Zinc	Synthesis of insulin Synthesis of cell protein Part of many enzymes Normal growth

are known to be present in adequate quantities in foods recommended for other reasons, so a specific recommendation for dietary intake is not given. Many of the rarer minerals are known to accompany other needed nutrients: copper, for example, is found in foods that contain iron. The standard dietary recommendation continues to be for people to eat a variety of foods to increase the likelihood that all micronutrients will be present in the diet.

Excessive amounts of any of the minerals are toxic to the body. Although most are excreted rapidly if ingested in excess, a few create life-threatening toxicities at relatively low levels. The kidneys must be healthy for any excretion to be effective. Some minerals, such as iron, are conserved by the body, and mechanisms do not exist for excreting excessive amounts rapidly. Many people take iron supplements, but this is not always wise. Unless a deficiency is present an excess of iron can develop. An overdose of iron tablets can easily create toxicity in a small child. The use of mineral supplements is potentially hazardous and should be carefully monitored.

Digestion and Absorption

The body does not digest minerals; therefore, they must be ingested in forms that the body is able to absorb directly. It is important to learn not only what minerals are in food, but whether those minerals are in absorbable forms. This is also true of any dietary supplements. An example is calcium. The form of calcium in milk, calcium lactate, is well absorbed, but the form of calcium in spinach, calcium oxalate, is poorly absorbed.

Minerals are absorbed through the walls of the small intestine. Both simple diffusion and active transport, a process in which the cell wall uses energy to move a substance across itself, are used for absorption. The active transport mechanisms become more important when an increased need exists in the body or when a mineral is insufficient in the diet. In such a case, increased activity of the active transport system increases absorption. Hormones play an important role in regulating the active transport mechanisms.

Absorption may be further affected by the contents of the digestive system. Iron is best absorbed in an acid environment such as naturally occurs in the stomach. Certain organic compounds such as phytic acid, found in the outer layer of cereal grains, and oxalic acid, found in spinach, inhibit the absorption of calcium. Other interactions may occur between specific minerals and other foods that researchers are unaware of at this time. However, when diets are well balanced with a plentiful supply of nutrients, these digestive system factors are not usually important. They become important when dietary supplies of the minerals are limited.

Metabolism

Minerals are used in many different ways by the body. Some minerals are essential components of hormones, cells, or tissues such as iodine in thyroid hormone, iron in the hemoglobin, and calcium in bones and teeth. Others are essential to certain chemical processes or cell functions such as potassium's role in electrical conduction within nerve cells and sodium's role in water balance.

Vitamins

Vitamins are minute organic substances essential to body processes. The list of them is still growing, as more are discovered. Vitamins are found in a variety of foods. Fat-soluble vitamins are stored by the body, allowing for intake to fluctuate. The majority of vitamins, however, are water-soluble, and must be ingested daily because amounts not currently needed are rapidly excreted. A balanced diet is the best source of vitamins. The routine use of vitamin supplements is not necessary for individuals in good health.

Many people are concerned about the adequacy of the vitamin supply in modern processed foods. It is true that some vitamins are destroyed by processing methods and others tend to change when products age. Fresh fruits and vegetables continue to be the best sources of many vitamins. However, processed foods do contain vitamins, and a diet containing a plentiful supply of canned or processed fruits and vegetables will certainly be better than one that does not contain fruits and vegetables at all because fresh ones are not available or are too costly. Processing of foods has made a variety of foods available year round at a price the majority of people can afford. Thus, the availability of processing has tended to improve the diet of most people. Processing has also rendered the diet safer because processing destroys many food borne microorganisms.

Digestion and Absorption

The digestion of vitamins involves breaking them into smaller molecules that can be effectively absorbed. Some absorption of vitamins takes place by simple diffusion, but active transport systems are important in ensuring adequate intake. Fat-soluble vitamins are absorbed by the same active transport mechanisms that bring fats into the body. Water-soluble vitamins have a wide variety of active transport mechanisms. For example, the intrinsic factor that is secreted in the stomach facilitates the absorption of vitamin B_{12}. Without the intrinsic factor, the body is not able to absorb adequate vitamin B_{12} from the diet, and a deficiency disease results.

Metabolism

Vitamins are essential to a great many life processes. In fact, their name came from the identification of amines that were essential to life. When additional substances were discovered that were not amines, the *e* was dropped and the word became vitamin.

Water

Water is really the basic nutrient. All body processes occur in the presence of a fluid medium. The human body is approximately 50% to 70% water. The regular intake of water is more important for survival than the intake of any other nutrient. The bodies of infants consist proportionately of more water than those of people of other ages. As people grow older, the proportion of body weight that is water is gradually reduced.

The body takes in the greatest percentage of its water through the digestive system in the form of fluid intake. In the adult this fluid intake usually amounts to between 1,200 and 1,500 ml daily, although 1,900 ml is often recommended as an optimum intake. Water is also ingested as a part of most foods. Intake of this water, termed **preformed water**, usually amounts to 500 to 900 ml daily. In addition, water is produced as an end product of oxidation. The adult produces approximately 250 ml of **metabolic water** daily. Thus, the total water available to the body is 1,950 to 2,650 ml/day. The figure 2,400 ml is often used to simplify computing needs.

The demand for water increases when water losses increase because of profuse sweating, vomiting, diarrhea, or preexisting dehydration. Although the body is able to accommodate a lower intake or a higher need by concentrating the urine and conserving water, such concentration increases the demand on the kidneys and is not the optimal way to cope with the problem. Water balance is discussed more completely in Chapter 30.

Food Additives

Food additives are chemicals or substances added to food for one of four purposes. Each of these purposes is linked in some way to the policies of the Food and Drug Administration (FDA). Additives are used for enrichment, fortification, restoration, and nutrification.

Foods that are *enriched* have substances that would not have naturally occurred added to the product. Enrichment is done to provide a needed nutrient that may be deficient in the diet of large numbers of people. The FDA determines which products can be enriched and in what manner. The term enriched cannot be used unless FDA guidelines are followed. The label on such enriched products must list the ingredients. One example is some breads and grains enriched with iron and the B vitamins. Another example is the addition of iodine to salt to prevent iodine deficiency.

Foods that are *fortified* contain additional nutrients that are the same as those already in the product. Milk and cheese are often fortified by adding vitamins A and D that are already present to some degree. Depending on state laws, fortification can be regulated or nonregulated.

The *restoration* of foods means that because some nutrients are lost in the processing, their previous nutritive value is restored by the replacement of those lost nutrients. Often vitamins that have been lost in the process of milling wheat are added to bread. Restorative substances are added to some canned products before marketing. By regulation, the labels of these products must list those substances that have been restored.

Nutrification is the addition of products that do not

actually enrich the food but contribute another nutritive substance. The most recent example is fiber, added to food products. The FDA requires that the label list the added products.

Nonnutritive additives may also be used if not detrimental to health. A common additive that has no nutritive value is color, which is added so that the product is more attractive. The FDA has found that most of these cosmetic food colors are safe, but a few have been restricted from use because of evidence that they can be harmful to consumers.

Additives intended to preserve food are also used. Two of the most common preservatives are nitrite or nitrate salts. Some persons have adverse reactions to these substances, so foods in the United States must be clearly labeled if these salts are added. Monosodium glutamate (MSG), bacon, and some wines contain these additives.

Sulfites, which are chemical salts in solution, have been added by restaurants to salad greens and other fresh vegetables to retain their color and retard deterioration. Small amounts of sulfites are naturally present in wine. Additional sulfites are also added to some wines as preservatives. Sulfites used as additives are harmless to most people. However, an increasing number of people have been identified as allergic to these salts. Symptoms range from headache and mild nausea to serious vascular or respiratory collapse that can lead to death. In some states, consumers must be warned either on a menu or label that sulfites are being used. In a few states, there are moves to totally ban the use of added sulfites in food and beverages.

Pesticides have recently been under surveillance as unintended "food additives." They may cling to vegetables and fruits so that if the product is not sufficiently washed, they can be consumed. Some types of pesticides are absorbed through the roots into the plant and therefore are not removed by washing. The use of these is usually prohibited on food crops.

Antibiotics and steroids used in animal feeds to prevent disease or promote growth can leave residues in the meat. The effect of these substances on people is not clear, but concerns have been raised and more limits are being placed on this practice.

Hui (1985) calls the additive issue a "question of trade-offs." Certainly, additives have been useful. Iron deficiency anemias and rickets have been prevented by adding iron to baby cereals and adding vitamin D to milk. Additives also are helpful when nutrients and fiber are added to otherwise deficient products. Preservation additives make transport and longer storage time practical, thereby lowering food costs. However, whether additives are capable of producing cancer and other diseases in human beings remains a question. Much more research is needed to resolve these important questions and to increase consumer protection. The controversy on additives continues to rage.

Recommended Diet

Several different approaches can be used to establish a diet that provides for all the necessary nutrients in the proper amounts. Recent research reveals that individual variations in need may be much greater than was previously thought. The universal value of milk long went undisputed because of the predominantly European background of most Americans. Evidence now exists that many people, primarily of Asian and African origin, do not have the digestive enzymes necessary to use milk properly after the age of 3 or 4 years. For these people, milk is actually harmful, causing gas, diarrhea, and digestive upsets. Thus, the concept of good nutrition is constantly being modified in light of the latest knowledge.

Recommended Dietary Allowances

The Food and Nutrition Board of the National Research Council has established a standard called the **Recommended Dietary Allowance (RDA)** for most nutrients. As research has accumulated, these recommendations have been revised. The most recent revision was in 1989. Different recommendations are made for different age levels and, after age 10, for males and females. There are also special recommendations for pregnant women and nursing mothers. The exact recommendations may be found in Table 25-2. They are very generous, providing for considerable variance among individuals and for changes in needs due to minor illness. They do not, however, allow for needs caused by major illness or trauma. Recommendations are given for all nutrients for which sufficient research data exist to establish need. Thus, there are no recommendations for nutrients needed in very small amounts or those for which the exact need has not yet been established.

Other Dietary Standards

The Canadian government has established a set of nutritional standards called the Canadian RNI (Recommended Nutrient Intake). These are similar to the RDA. The RDA standard may not be attainable by low-income persons or those who live in parts of the world where food supplies are limited. *Minimum daily requirements* have been established by some official groups, but because these standards do not take individual variations into consideration, they are of limited value in determining optimum diet. However, they may be useful in eval-

Table 25–2. Recommended Dietary Allowances (RDA)—1989

	Weight		*Height*																				
Age (ys)	**(kg)**	**(lb)**	**(cm)**	**(inches)**	**(g) Protein**	**(μg RE) Vitamin A**	**(μg) Vitamin D**	**(mg α-TE) Vitamin E**	**(μg) Vitamin K**	**(mg) Vitamin C**	**(mg) Thiamin**	**(mg) Riboflavin**	**(mg NE) Niacin**	**(mg)Vitamin B_6**	**(μg) Folate**	**(μg) Vitamin B_{12}**	**(mg) Calcium**	**(mg) Phosphorus**	**(mg) Magnesium**	**(mg) Iron**	**(mg) Zinc**	**(μg) Iodine**	**(μg) Selenium**
Infants																							
0.0–0.5	6	13	60	24	13	375	7.5	3	5	30	0.3	0.4	5	0.3	25	0.3	400	300	40	6	5	40	10
0.5–1.0	9	20	71	28	14	375	10	4	10	35	0.4	0.5	6	0.6	35	0.5	600	500	60	10	5	50	15
Children																							
1–3	13	29	90	35	16	400	10	6	15	40	0.7	0.8	9	1.0	50	0.7	800	800	80	10	10	70	20
4–6	20	44	112	44	24	500	10	7	20	45	0.9	1.1	12	1.1	75	1.0	800	800	120	10	10	90	20
7–10	28	62	132	52	28	700	10	7	30	45	1.0	1.2	13	1.4	100	1.4	800	800	170	10	10	120	30
Males																							
11–14	45	99	157	62	45	1,000	10	10	45	50	1.3	1.5	17	1.7	150	2.0	1,200	1,200	270	12	15	150	40
15–18	66	145	176	69	59	1,000	10	10	65	60	1.5	1.8	20	2.0	200	2.0	1,200	1,200	400	12	15	150	50
19–24	72	160	177	70	58	1,000	10	10	70	60	1.5	1.7	19	2.0	200	2.0	1,200	1,200	350	10	15	150	70
25–50	79	174	176	70	63	1,000	5	10	80	60	1.5	1.7	19	2.0	200	2.0	800	800	350	10	15	150	70
51+	77	170	173	68	63	1,000	5	10	80	60	1.2	1.4	15	2.0	200	2.0	800	800	350	10	15	150	70
Females																							
11–14	46	101	157	62	46	800	10	8	45	50	1.1	1.3	15	1.4	150	2.0	1,200	1,200	280	15	12	150	45
15–18	55	120	163	64	44	800	10	8	55	60	1.1	1.3	15	1.5	180	2.0	1,200	1,200	300	15	12	150	50
19–24	58	128	164	65	46	800	10	8	60	60	1.1	1.3	15	1.6	180	2.0	1,200	1,200	280	15	12	150	55
25–50	63	138	163	64	50	800	5	8	65	60	1.1	1.3	15	1.6	180	2.0	800	800	280	15	12	150	55
51+	65	143	160	63	50	800	5	8	65	60	1.0	1.2	13	1.6	180	2.0	800	800	280	10	12	150	55
Pregnant					60	800	10	10	65	70	1.5	1.6	17	2.2	400	2.2	1,200	1,200	320	30	15	175	65
Lactating																							
1st 6 mo					65	1,300	10	12	65	95	1.6	1.8	20	2.1	280	2.6	1,200	1,200	355	15	19	200	75
2nd 6 mo					62	1,200	10	11	65	90	1.6	1.7	20	2.1	260	2.6	1,200	1,200	340	15	16	200	75

These allowances, expressed as average daily intakes over time, are intended to provide for individual variations among most normal people who live in the United States under usual environmental stresses. Diets should be based on a variety of common foods to provide other nutrients for which human requirements have been less well defined.
Source: National Academy of Sciences: Committee on Dietary Allowances, *Recommended Dietary Allowances*. 10th edition. Washington, D.C.: National Academy Press, 1989.

uating diets for the purpose of establishing gross deficiency or malnutrition.

Public Education in Nutrition

Over the years nutritionists at the Department of Agriculture have devised a variety of ways to help the general public plan healthy diets. These have included a basic meal plan, dietary goals, and general dietary guidelines.

A simple way to plan meals that supply a sound diet was first published in the United States in 1917. Through many revisions that featured "Basic Seven" and "Basic Four" food groups, these guides served the public well (Fig. 25-1). However, all of these guides were based on the prevailing Euro-American dietary pattern. The basic four divided foods into a meat group, a milk group, a bread and grain group, and a vegetable and fruit group. Although this was helpful for many people, meal patterns that do not conform to the pattern may be nutritious and supply all the RDA.

Since 1977, various government agencies have published dietary recommendations for the general public. The most recent of these publications was the National

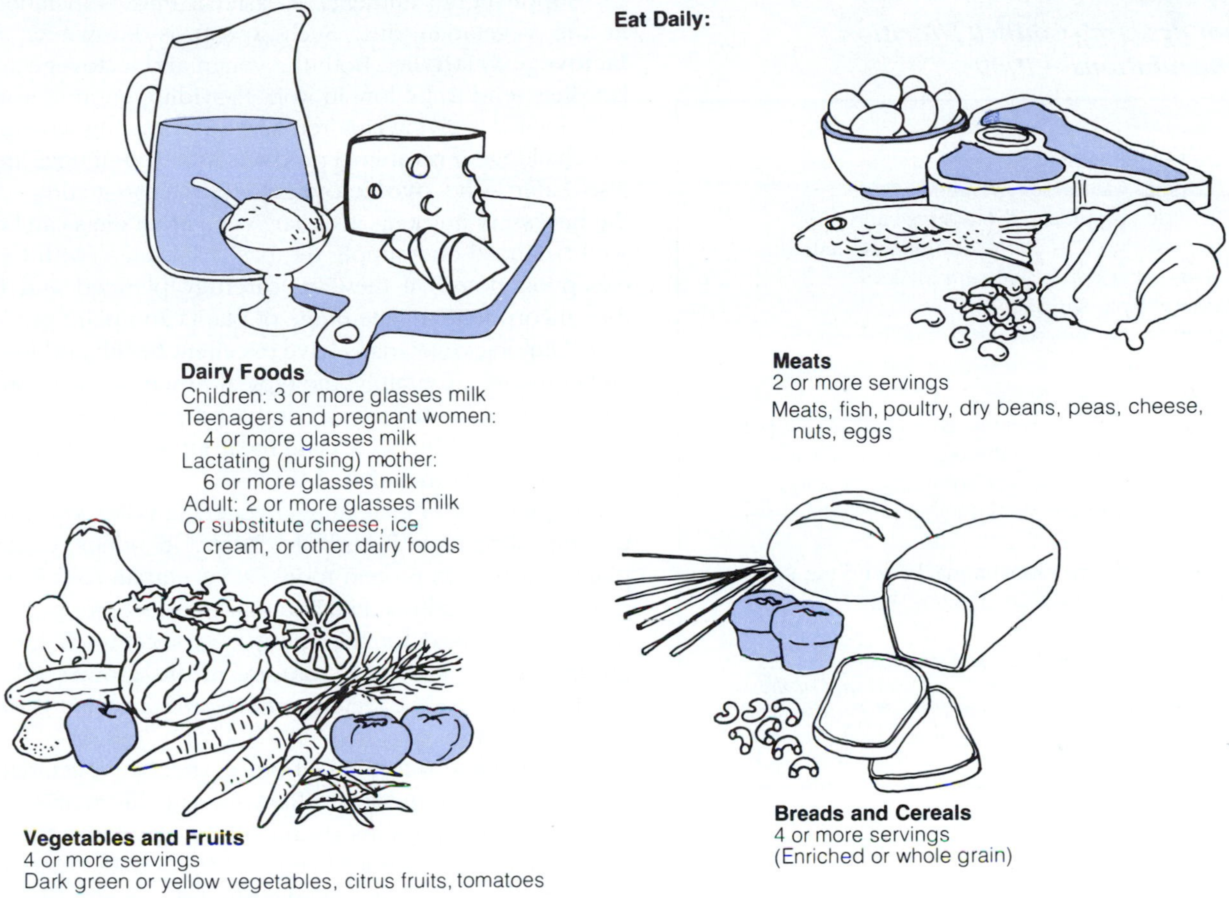

Eat Daily:
Dairy Foods
Children: 3 or more glasses milk
Teenagers and pregnant women: 4 or more glasses milk
Lactating (nursing) mother: 6 or more glasses milk
Adult: 2 or more glasses milk
Or substitute cheese, ice cream, or other dairy foods
Meats
2 or more servings
Meats, fish, poultry, dry beans, peas, cheese, nuts, eggs
Vegetables and Fruits
4 or more servings
Dark green or yellow vegetables, citrus fruits, tomatoes
Breads and Cereals
4 or more servings
(Enriched or whole grain)

Figure 25-1. The four basic food groups.

Research Council's *Diet and Health: Implications for Reducing Chronic Disease Risk.* These recommendations were based on *The Surgeon General's Report on Nutrition and Health* (1988) and include the recommendations discussed in Display 25-1.

Eating Right Pyramid

A new nutrition teaching aid for the general public was released by the Department of Agriculture in 1992. This teaching aid, the Eating Right Pyramid shown in Figure 25-2, was designed to show graphically the information contained in the 1989 recommendations.

The pyramid depicts the general relationship of quantities of different foods in the diet as well as the kinds of foods that constitute a particular food group. The base is shown as complex carbohydrates including bread, rice, cereal, and pasta. These form the basis of a sound diet and should be the largest quantity with 6 to 11 servings per day. At the next level are the vegetable group with 3 to 5 servings per day and the fruit group with 2 to 4 servings a day. The third level shows the milk, yogurt, and cheese group and the meat, poultry, fish, dry beans, eggs, and nuts group, each with 2 to 3 servings a day. The last level is the fats, oils, and sweets group which is labeled "use sparingly."

Controversy occurred over the choice of leveling and the lesser role of meat and milk products. However, research demonstrated that the pyramid clearly communicated the basic concepts of nutrition to the general public. Even children seemed to grasp the relative size of the food groups in the diet and the fact that carbohydrate foods are basic. In addition, the pyramid appears more adaptable to differing cultural diet patterns than does the basic four pattern previously used for public education. Display 25-2 provides clarification concerning what serving size translates to in terms of ounces, cups, and so on of common foods.

Vegetarian Diet Standards

Interest in *vegetarian* diets is widespread, for a combination of religious, economic, and philosophical reasons. The vegetarian diet that includes only plant products is termed the *vegan* diet. The vegan diet is deficient in vitamin B_{12} because there is no plant source of that

Display 25–1
National Research Council Nutrition Recommendations—1989

1. Eat a wide variety of foods.
2. Maintain ideal body weight.
3. Include complex carbohydrates and fiber.
4. Maintain protein intake at moderate amounts.
5. Maintain adequate calcium intake.
6. Limit simple sugars.
7. Limit fats to 30% or less of total calories.
8. Limit cholesterol to less than 300 mg daily.
9. Limit salt.
10. If alcohol is used (its use is not recommended) then limit alcohol to the equivalent of less than one ounce of pure alcohol in a single day. Pregnant women should avoid alcoholic beverages.
11. The use of any supplements beyond the RDA for nutrients is not recommended.

Source: National Research Council, Committee on Diet and Health, Food and Nutrition Board. *Diet and Health: Implications for Reducing Chronic Disease Risk.* Washington, D.C.: National Academy of Sciences, 1989.

vitamin. Vegans are encouraged to take supplemental vitamins. In developing countries, such as India, where vegan diets are common, food and water supplies contain large quantities of bacteria. It is the presence of these bacteria that provide vitamin B_{12} for the vegan diet in these cultures.

Supplying all nutrients is easier if milk is included in the vegetarian diet. Such a diet is known as a **lactovegetarian** diet. Both the vegan and lactovegetarian diets tend to be low in iron. Providing enough iron and zinc for growing children and menstruating women is a challenge if no animal products are used. If eggs are also eaten—the **ovolactovegetarian** diet—getting all the necessary nutrients is easier. Vegetarian diets can be well balanced and supply the basic nutrients (with the exception noted) if they are carefully planned and if they incorporate a wide range of plants and plant products. Lifelong vegetarians have excellent health and longevity records. Certainly, the typical American diet contains more meat than is needed, and protein intake is not jeopardized by decreasing meat intake if other protein sources are included in the diet.

In planning or evaluating a vegetarian diet, you can use the Eating Right Pyramid because it identifies certain plant products as protein foods. A vegetarian four food group plan includes a milk and milk product group (soy milk can be used for this group); a protein-rich food group (cheese, eggs, and tofu are in this group); a legumes, fruits, and vegetables group; and a whole grain cereals group.

If you have questions about a specific vegetarian diet, you should check the RDA for specific nutrients. Many vegetable proteins are incomplete proteins; these are eaten in combinations that provide complete protein in the meal, a technique called mutual supplementation. However, some vegetable proteins such as those found in potatoes and rice are complete proteins. The most important factor for vegetarians is the inclusion of a wide variety of plant food sources to obtain optimum nutrition.

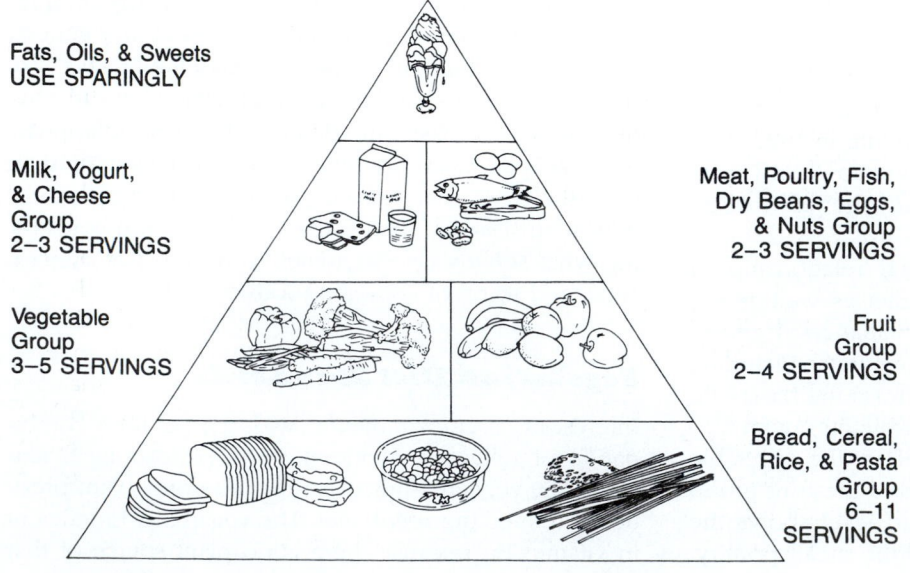

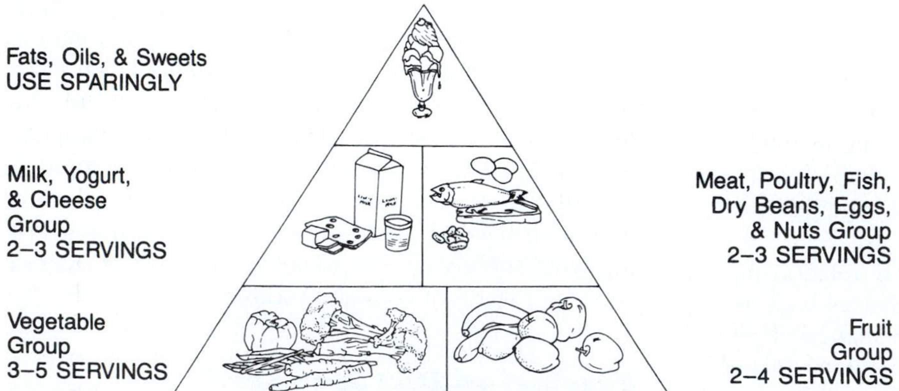

Figure 25-2. The food guide pyramid. From Dudek SG: Nutrition Handbook for Nursing Practice, 2nd ed. JB Lippincott, 1993, as adapted from USDA (prepared by Human Nutrition Information Service), USDA's Food Guide Pyramid. Home and Garden Bulletin Number 249, Hyattsville, MD, 1992.

Display 25–2
Understanding Serving Size

Bread, Cereal, Rice, & Pasta

6–11 servings recommended*
Examples of one serving:
- 1 slice of bread
- 1 oz. of ready-to-eat cereal
- ½ cup of cooked cereal, rice, or pasta
- 3 or 4 small plain crackers

Vegetables

3–5 servings recommended*
Examples of one serving:
- 1 cup raw leafy vegetables
- ½ cup of other vegetables, cooked or chopped raw
- ¾ cup of vegetable juice

Fruits

2–4 servings recommended*
Examples of one serving:
- 1 medium apple, banana, or orange
- ½ cup of chopped, cooked, or canned fruit
- ¾ cup of fruit juice

Milk, Yogurt, and Cheese

2–3 servings recommended*
Examples of one serving:
- 1 cup of milk or yogurt
- 1½ oz. of natural cheese
- 2 oz. of process cheese

Meat, Poultry, Fish, Dry Beans, Eggs, Nuts

2–3 servings recommended*
Examples of one serving:
- 2–3 oz. of cooked lean meat, poultry, or fish (1 ounce is the size of a match box, 3 ounces are the size of a deck of cards. The total daily recommendation equals 4–9 oz.)
- 1 cup of cooked dry beans, 2 eggs, or 4 tablespoons of peanut butter (½ of those amounts equals 1 oz. of lean meat)

*Note: The greater number of servings provides more calories as well as additional other nutrients for those whose needs are larger. The lower number of servings provides fewer calories and somewhat lower levels of nutrients for those whose needs are not as great.

Some people are striving to eat a diet that does not require as much use of natural resources as the traditional American diet. Such a diet uses many more grains and vegetable protein sources and usually omits red meat because of the large amount of grain needed to prepare cattle and hogs for market consumption. However, fish and poultry are usually included, so this diet is not a strictly vegetarian diet although some refer to it as such. This approach to food consumption is discussed in detail in *Diet for a Small Planet* (Lappe, 1984).

Diet for Disease Prevention

People in all areas of life are manifesting increased interest in health practices that prevent disease. Diet clearly is one factor in the development of cardiovascular disease. Diets high in cholesterol and saturated fats lead to high blood cholesterol levels in some individuals. Because the individual response to these foods may not be manifested until late in life, the general recommendation from the American Heart Association and others concerned with preventing cardiovascular disease has been that all individuals limit their intake of all fats in general and of saturated fats and cholesterol in particular.

Excessive intake of salt has been linked to hypertension in some individuals. Although moderation of salt intake is generally recommended, no clear evidence indicates that this will prevent the development of hypertension. In those with currently existing hypertension, reduction in salt intake may facilitate blood pressure control.

Avoiding additives and contaminants in food has been discussed previously. Although much of the research has used animal models and high doses of additives and it is difficult to translate these data into specific recommendations for human beings, it appears that significant pesticide or drug residue should be avoided. Whether minute quantities can be effectively cleared by the body or whether their effects are cumulative is still not clearly determined.

Various individuals have advocated the use of a

wide variety of vitamins in large doses to prevent and treat disease. Much of the evidence of their effectiveness is anecdotal, that is, individuals report that they have benefited. Large scale studies in which subjects did not know whether or not they were receiving the vitamin or an inert substance have not supported the value of this practice for the general public. If individuals believe that they are benefiting from such use of vitamins, then they should be supported in their individual health practices. There is a danger if individuals take large enough doses to create toxic effects. This is more likely for children than for adults.

The National Institutes of Health recently released research data that support dietary measures to prevent colon cancer. The recommended diet is low in fat, contains sufficient fiber, and in addition, includes the use of cruciferous vegetables. These include broccoli, cauliflower, kale, and others in this family of strongly flavored vegetables. They all contain a substance that appears to inhibit the development of cancer in the bowel.

Calcium provides the basic structure for bone density and strength. Current information indicates that women throughout their lives should maintain high levels of calcium intake to enter midlife and menopause with maximum bone density. This helps to protect against osteoporosis, a disease in which bone density is progressively lost as the person ages, and protects against the fractures that result from falls of people whose bones are so affected.

Fluid Intake

Dietary guides in general do not mention fluid intake as part of the basic diet. Thirst is ordinarily a good guide to the body's need for water. With minimal sweating and physical activity and a low-solute diet, an adult requires approximately 1,500 ml of additional fluid in each 24-hour period. The recommended amount of water is 1,900 ml. Infants and children need approximately 1.5 ml of fluid per kilocalorie of food intake. Some references figure fluid needs based on body weight, calculating total fluid needs at 50 ml for each kilogram of body weight. The 50 ml includes the fluid intake, the preformed water, and the metabolic water.

If there are no contraindications to increased fluid intake, a nurse can initiate planning to increase fluid intake for therapeutic purposes, such as for fever, urinary tract infection, or profuse perspiration.

Water may also be *limited* for therapeutic purposes. If the excretory processes are not working adequately, as in kidney disease, or if the heart is not circulating blood adequately, limiting fluid intake to less than the usual amount may be necessary. The exact amount of limitation is determined by a physician.

Special Therapeutic Diets

Illness generally increases nutritional needs. Healing requires greater numbers of calories, more protein, and more vitamins and minerals than does maintenance of health. A fever raises the metabolic rate and increases the body's caloric requirements. Certain illnesses, such as hyperthyroidism, also increase metabolism, which in turn increases the number of calories needed by the body.

When a person is ill, appetite is often adversely affected. Food is less appealing, and fatigue may make eating an effort. Many illnesses cause unpleasant odors or tastes in the mouth, decreasing the desire for food. Furthermore, in some illnesses, specific nutrients are not digested or metabolized in the normal way, necessitating special modifications of the diet. You will need to check the diet manual for your facility for specific dietary recommendations.

Modification of Diet Texture

The simplest modification of diet involves the *form* or *texture* of the food served. A general diet in which all foods are chopped is of special value to those without teeth, those whose dentures fit poorly, making chewing difficult, and those with very carious teeth. It is usually also possible to order all foods pureed for the person who cannot manage solid foods at all. The nurse often recognizes a need for this type of dietary modification and is generally free to order it. The physician may also order such dietary changes. In facilities where only the physician may order dietary modifications, the nurse provides the relevant information to the physician and requests that an order for a change in form be written.

Modification of Dietary Content

Other dietary modifications involve the *content* of the diet. Such diets may be ordered for many different reasons. The physician orders alterations in diet content.

Liquid Diets

Liquid diets are ordered for those whose digestive systems will not tolerate solids and for those with severe mouth problems. A liquid diet is often ordered for the postoperative patient who has been exposed to anesthesia and may also not have normal intestinal peristalsis. The patient may be given only ice chips at first and then may progress to one of the two types of liquid diets: clear liquid and full liquid.

Clear Liquid Diet. In the clear liquid diet, only those items that are liquid at room temperature and through which light will shine are allowed. The liquids allowed usually include clear broth, tea, apple juice, gelatin, and water. In some facilities grape juice and coffee (if not contraindicated for other reasons) are added. The clear liquid diet is not nutritionally adequate, and most hospitals have a policy that it is not used for more than 3 days without nutritional supplements.

Full Liquid Diet. The full liquid diet contains soups made with pureed vegetables and meats, milk products, and pureed fruits in drinks and in gelatin, in addition to the items allowed on the clear liquid diet. Because everything is naturally liquid or cooked and pureed, the full liquid diet is easy to digest and requires minimal energy for eating. A well planned, full liquid diet can provide all essential nutrients. Commercially prepared liquid supplements may also be used in a full liquid diet. These liquid dietary products may also be added to a diet to increase calories and other nutrients.

Soft Diet

In the soft diet the food is chopped or pureed. Foods that might produce gas or be difficult to digest are omitted. The soft diet is nutritionally adequate although it may not have enough fiber for effective bowel function. A mechanical soft or edentulous diet provides all foods in a form suitable for a person without teeth.

Progressive Diets

The phrase "progressive diet" is used when an individual is to move gradually from a clear liquid diet to a full liquid diet to a soft diet to a general diet. This progression is often ordered when a patient has not been eating for a period of time and the physician believes it advisable to make sure the digestive system can cope with simple foods before adding more complex ones. When the progressive diet is ordered, the nurse is responsible for evaluating the patient's response to the diet and advancing the patient to the next level if he or she is free of adverse effects and appears able to manage more foods.

Sodium-Restricted Diet

Sodium-restricted diets are also called low-sodium diets; often they are used to prevent or treat edema of the tissues. Low-sodium diets are ordered with a variety of levels of sodium intake. In some facilities the sodium level is specified in grams or milligrams, and in others it is specified in milliequivalents (see Chapter 30 for an explanation of these terms). At the lowest level, special no-sodium foods are used to keep the sodium level low. At the other end of the scale is the diet that simply specifies no added salt. For the patient on this diet, salt would be omitted from the tray, and obviously salty foods would not be served (Table 25-3).

Low-Saturated Fat/Low-Cholesterol Diet

The low-saturated fat/low-cholesterol diet is sometimes called a cardiac diet. In this diet special attention is paid to substituting polyunsaturated fats for saturated fats, limiting the total amount of fat, and limiting the amount of cholesterol. The purpose of this diet is to decrease the blood cholesterol level in the hope that lowering it will decrease the development of atherosclerosis and subsequent coronary artery disease.

Low-Calorie Diets

Low-calorie diets are ordered to prevent weight gain or to bring about weight loss. The calorie level provided is based on the needs of the individual and the rate at which weight loss is desired. It is usually not wise for a person to try to lose weight after suffering from an illness. If a person wishes to control weight, a diet plan that prevents weight gain in the hospital should promote weight loss at home, where the patient has a greater activity level. Some individuals are hospitalized with serious obesity and restrictive diets may be ordered for them.

Lactose-Restricted Diets

Lactose is the form of sugar found in milk. The enzyme lactase is necessary for digestion of this sugar. When the person does not secrete lactase, undigested lactose passes into the large bowel, where bacterial action on the sugar creates bloating, loose stools, and cramping. A lactase deficiency may occur as a person ages. Lactase deficiency is also common in adults of African and Asian background. Lactase-deficient individuals need to restrict milk and milk products. Some can tolerate limited amounts of lactose; others need to severely restrict their intake to avoid gastrointestinal distress. Persons with

Table 25–3. Levels of Sodium-Restricted Diets

Sodium in Grams	mEq	Restricted Level
3–4	130–175	Mild, no added salt (NAS). Often used with outpatients
2,000 mg	87	Moderate, a common diet that is ordered in the facility
1,000 mg	43	Strict, used only under supervision
500 mg	22	Severe, rarely used, only in facility

lactase deficiency may be able to drink milk to which *acidophilus* has been added. Acidophilus provides the enzyme necessary for digestion of lactose. Yogurt and other cultured products may be tolerated because the lactose has been digested beforehand by the bacterial culture in the food. Lactase tablets to ingest with food and lactase liquid to add directly to milk are available without prescription and some individuals choose to use these rather than avoid milk products.

Diabetic Diets

The diabetic diet involves a specific proportion of carbohydrates, fats, and proteins spread over the day in a method planned to achieve a stable blood sugar level. The diet may be ordered as an "ADA diet," which is the standard American Diabetic Association (ADA) plan. The ADA diet is designed to fit the common eating pattern in the United States and provide nutrients in the desired proportions for the average diabetic person. The specific calorie level for the individual is designated by the ordering physician. Thus, the order might read, "1,500-calorie ADA diet." Another way of ordering the diabetic diet is to specify the grams of protein, carbohydrate, and fat desired and the proportion of calories to be served at each meal. The diet order in this instance might read, "Diabetic diet 65/200/50; $\frac{1}{3}$, $\frac{1}{3}$, $\frac{1}{3}$." This means that the diet should contain 65 g protein, 200 g carbohydrate, and 50 g fat with one-third of the calories served at each meal.

Tube Feeding Formulas

Some individuals must be fed liquids through a tube inserted into the digestive tract. Commercially prepared liquid formulas are used for the tube feedings. All contain carbohydrate, protein, and fat and have vitamins and minerals that provide a complete nutritional diet. Most standard tube feeding formulas contain 1 calorie/ml, although some are designed to have a higher calorie density for the person who is severely calorie deficient. Each brand has a specific protein source and a specific type of fat. A person might have problems with one formula and tolerate another because of these differences in content. The **osmolality** (number of particles per milliliter of formula) also affects the response. A formula with a higher osmolality than body fluids will cause fluid to move into the digestive system and create frequent liquid stools.

Another type of formula is the **elemental formula**. This type of formula is composed of nutrients that can be absorbed without digestion. These can provide nutrients for the person whose digestive processes are not functional but whose absorptive areas are still functional. Elemental feedings leave no residue to be eliminated by the large intestine and thus rest the bowel.

Parenteral Nutrition

Parenteral nutrition, a method of providing nutrients intravenously, is also called **hyperalimentation**. In conventional intravenous fluids, which will be discussed in Chapter 30, 5% dextrose is the source of calories. This solution provides approximately 170 calories in 1,000 ml, which is not adequate for nutritional needs. When a patient cannot take oral food and fluids for a prolonged period, healing may be severely compromised by a lack of nutrients. In parenteral nutrition, all types of nutrients are given intravenously. Total parenteral nutrition (TPN) provides all needed nutrients and calories by the parenteral route. Partial parenteral nutrition provides additional nutrients intravenously but not in amounts necessary to meet all needs.

Dextrose may be given in concentrations of 10% to 20%. In these concentrations, dextrose irritates the veins and causes them to sclerose (become inflamed and close because of scarring). Therefore, a large central vein with a high blood flow in which the solution can disperse rapidly—most commonly the subclavian vein—is used for administration of high concentrations of dextrose. Peripheral vessels may be used for the lower concentrations given for partial nutrition.

Protein may be given in the form of simple amino acids or simple proteins. If extremely dilute, the amino acids may sometimes be given in peripheral veins. Proteins and amino acids in higher concentrations must be given in a large vein with a high blood flow.

Lipids in a special emulsified form may also be given intravenously. The lipids are less irritating and are sometimes given in a peripheral vein. Vitamins, minerals, and trace elements are added to the feedings in amounts determined by the physician. These may be given either peripherally or in central veins.

Other Special Diets

Diets may be modified in a great many other ways. For example, potassium and phosphates may be restricted for the person with kidney disease. Certain foods may be restricted for a person with an allergy. A food that an individual is unable to digest or to metabolize may be omitted. Special modifications are seen less often than the therapeutic diets discussed above. The dietitian in the hospital is an excellent resource in regard to unique special diets.

Modifications for Personal Preferences

Individuals may ask to have a modification of the standard facility diet because of personal preferences. A person might, for example, request a vegetarian diet or a kosher diet. When a person has a severe problem with lack of appetite, an attempt may be made to provide special foods that the person finds appealing. Most hospitals do provide a menu for food selection so that people can have foods they prefer. Long-term care facilities rarely provide choices for menu selection because of the added cost.

Sociocultural Influences on Diet

Culture

Each person grows up in a unique culture composed of the family and the larger community. This cultural background determines what the person perceives as good food and what he or she perceives as not edible (Fig. 25-3). The culture also influences what is seen as appropriate quantity of intake. In a society in which little food is available, meals may be simple, composed of the same staples throughout the day. For a person who grew up in such a society, making food choices in an American supermarket could be distressing. In a family in which large meals are the norm, an individual will tend to grow up eating large amounts of food whether or not the food is needed. A familial trait of obesity may be evident in such a family.

All societies impose values on food, making some foods more acceptable or desirable than others. Pureed foods are regarded as infant foods in the United States, as is milk in some African nations. Other foods, such as lobster and caviar, are accorded prestige or status. Food that is familiar and typical of one's family or social group may arouse feelings of warmth and belonging. For example, a person from a traditional German background may derive feelings of security and comfort from eating dishes like sauerbraten and veal stew with dumplings because they are reminiscent of the comfort and security of the home. During illness, what is familiar may be a remedy in itself. For this reason, one person will prefer chicken soup when ill, whereas another considers tea the perfect remedy. The feelings associated with a given food may render it tolerable to the digestive system when nothing else is acceptable.

Some foods, though nutritious, are simply not acceptable in certain cultures. In fact, cultural aversion to a food can be so great as to cause nausea and vomiting. Fish eyes elicit this response from many people brought up in Western cultures, although they are nutritious and considered a delicacy in Asia. The most extreme manifestation of cultural aversion is a taboo or forbidden food, such as pork for Orthodox Jews and devout Muslims.

The patterns of meals are also cultural in origin. American travelers to Europe find that breakfast is coffee and a roll in one country, a large and hearty meal in another. The main meal may be eaten at noon, at 6:00 PM, or at 10:00 PM. People in the United States are accustomed to three meals a day, whereas in England a fourth small meal called tea is served in the late afternoon. People become used to a given meal pattern and tend to become hungry at regular times.

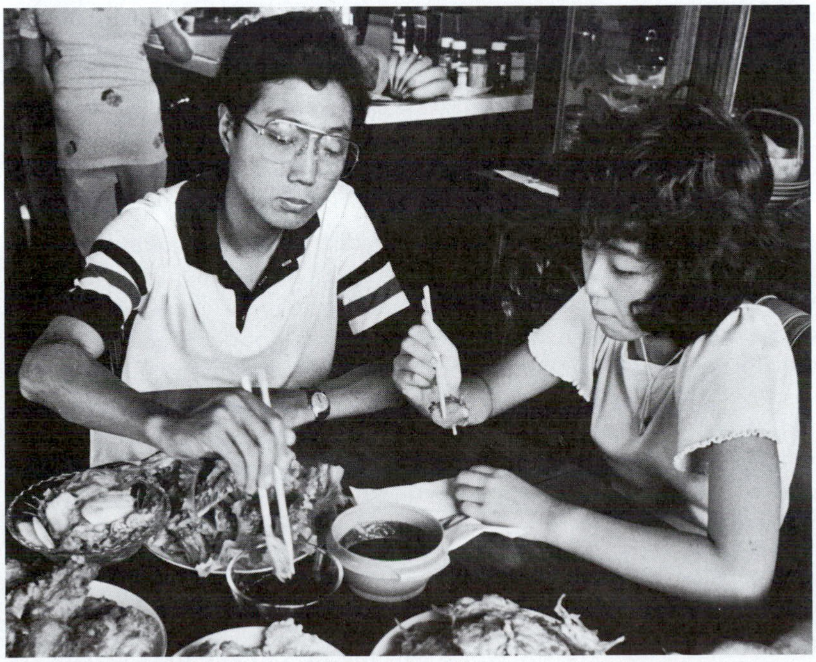

Figure 25-3. Culture affects people's eating habits.

Economic Factors

The cost determines food choices for many people. This obviously applies to the extremely poor, who have difficulty buying any food, but it applies to others as well. People who can afford a high-meat diet may eat more saturated fats and cholesterol than is recommended. Those who have a limited food budget may need to plan much more carefully to make sure that the food dollars available purchase the best possible nutrition. Cheaper foods may also have many calories and contribute to problems of overweight. Severe economic deprivation usually restricts the quantity of food available, which can result in serious weight loss and inadequate growth and development in children.

Geographic Location

People in different geographic locations often have different food habits. Part of the difference may be related to the foods grown or raised in the area. In an area with large fruit orchards, fresh fruit may be plentiful and inexpensive and so be a part of the diet of even the poorest individual. If all fruits are shipped from a distance and are expensive, fresh fruits will not be a part of the general population's usual diet. Where goats are raised, goat milk and goat meat may be dietary staples.

In certain locations, meal patterns have become common because most of the people have a similar cultural background. Meal habits may also arise out of the predominant occupation in an area. If most of the people are in agriculture and live and work in the same locale, the largest meal may be eaten in the middle of the day. On the other hand, if most people work far from where they live, the midday meal may be a small one, with the main meal eaten in the evening when everyone is home.

Religion

Some religions have dietary rules that are an aspect of religious observance. Orthodox Jewish law, for example, requires that all foods be obtained, prepared, and served according to specific rules. Food that conforms to these orthodox Jewish dietary rules is called **kosher food**. Table 25-4 presents an overview of the kosher diet. Hospitals in areas where there are many Orthodox Jews may be equipped to provide kosher food. If you work in such a setting, you will need to be familiar with the rules for serving kosher food. If such food is not available, the Orthodox Jew will usually eat nonkosher food as long as foods specifically prohibited by Jewish law are omitted. Such a person might be expected to eat poorly while hospitalized because of emotional aversion to nonkosher food. Some Christians omit certain foods from their diets during the Lenten (pre-Easter) season. Some Roman Catholics still omit meat on Friday even though the practice is no longer required by the Church. Such customs may usually be set aside during periods of illness, but some people prefer to maintain them regardless of circumstances. The individual's wishes are of primary significance.

Adherents of many Eastern religions, such as Hinduism and Buddhism, are vegetarian. To eat flesh is so repugnant to them that even suggesting they do so may cause them to be ill. Many Seventh Day Adventists are also vegetarian.

World Hunger

North America is indeed blessed with less hunger among its population compared to other parts of the world. Even so, nutritional deficiencies and actual starvation remain major concerns of social programs in the United States. Thirty to 50% of Americans, across all socioeconomic levels, are found to be undernourished or in a state of malnutrition. This situation is due in part to the fact that an estimated 30% of meals are eaten outside the home and so-called fast food constitutes 60% of American diets (Pender, 1987). Another important factor is the increase in numbers of families afflicted with unemployment and poverty in our nation. Many of the families affected include young children or elderly adults who are particularly vulnerable to the effects of a less than nutritious diet.

School lunch programs have ensured at least one balanced meal per day for many young persons, although they do not solve the ongoing problem of malnutrition in this age group. Many schools, especially in inner cities, have added breakfast programs to further support the nutritional needs of students. Day care centers are eligible for food subsidies when they serve low-income clients. Congregate meals are provided for the elderly in some communities.

The federal government provides nutritional aid to some individuals through the allocation of food stamps. Food stamps, which are distributed in booklets bearing specific dollar amounts on each coupon, may be used to purchase only food originating in the United States. Allocations are made on the basis of declared household gross income. This figure has changed over the years but remains below the poverty level. An additional requirement to receive food stamps is that the individual have a fixed home and cooking facilities. The number of participants has risen steadily along with unemployment.

Worldwide hunger continues to overwhelm the resources available for assistance. Just how many of the world's population are in a state of starvation is unclear. In 1992, the world saw photos of thousands starving to

Table 25–4. Kosher Diet Pattern

Food groups	Foods Allowed	Foods Omitted
Milk or milk products	All dairy products *Note:* Milk or milk products are kept separate from meals with meat.	*Note:* Not served at the same meal as meat
Milk or milk products	They are never served together nor on the same set of dishes. Milk and milk products may be taken just before a meal containing meat but not for 6 h afterwards. Cheeses are considered milk products and used as such.	
Fruit and fruit juices	All are *neutral foods.* *Note:* Neutral foods may be served at any time and with either meat or milk products.	
Vegetables and vegetable juices	All are *neutral foods.* May be served at any time and with either meat or milk products	
Potato or substitute	All are neutral foods unless contains a milk product; then it is considered a dairy food.	
Breads and cereals	All are neutral foods unless contain a milk product: then food is considered a dairy food.	
Meat or meat alternates	Forequarter only of animals with split hoof that chew a cud such as: Cattle, sheep, goats, deer Fish with fins and scales are a neutral food.	Hindquarters of any animal; pork, rabbit Shellfish, frogs, catfish, eel, porpoise, turtle, shark, octopus, snake

death in Somalia. Eastern Europeans faced starvation as civil war destroyed commerce and made it impossible to get food to cities. Periodic flooding in Bangladesh brings news of huge numbers without basic foodstuffs. The Presidential Commission on World Hunger in 1980 declared that "while many of us look for an exercise that will help us burn excess calories, many in the world go to sleep hungry." This hunger may not lead to death, but rather manifests itself in impaired growth and development in children and low levels of general health. A striking example is the problem of protein deficiencies among the infants and small children of sub-Saharan Africa where prolonged drought has severely restricted food supplies. Because the brain needs high levels of protein for development, it is feared that even though many of these children may survive (some do not), mental retardation can be a major lifelong health problem. Central to the problem of world hunger is poverty, which is hard to solve because it is "rooted in political, economic, and social realities" (Hui, 1985, p. 11).

Nurses are caring people, and it is essential that we recognize the economic and nutritional problems of the world, for they are, indeed, also health problems. As many of us travel and work in other parts of the world, we will be confronted with problems of hunger and can become involved in small but important ways.

Many of the people we take care of in this country will be among the impoverished. Others will lack information regarding healthful diets. We can become advocates for those who need diet information by supporting educational programs on nutrition. For those who are economically less fortunate than ourselves, we can individually or by group action support programs focused on providing better nutrition to all.

Factors That Influence Food Intake

Hunger

Hunger is the physical sensation of discomfort caused by an empty stomach. Hunger also seems to be affected by some poorly understood central nervous system mechanisms, and such factors as blood sugar level may play a part in the sensation of hunger. The hunger sensation is probably regulated by the hypothalamus. After prolonged food deprivation, as during a deliberate fast or a food shortage, hunger disappears. The person will be listless and without energy but will not feel active hunger pangs.

Appetite

Appetite, the desire to eat, is affected by both physical and emotional factors. Appetite may be felt for food in general or may be limited to a specific food or group of foods and may cause the person to eat far more than the body actually needs. Lack of appetite is called **anorexia**.

The demands of growth usually result in increased appetite and intake of food in children. Conversely, when growth slows or stops for a period, children's appetites usually decrease. This decrease is sometimes a concern to parents who do not understand the relationship between growth and appetite. In fact, some parents mistakenly believe that a large food intake will increase growth. This is true only if food is being restored to a child whose growth has been held back by food deprivation. Parents often become concerned when a 2-year-old with a tremendous appetite turns into a 3-year-old who seems to "pick at" food. At the age of 3, growth usually slows. When growth speeds up again, the appetite returns. The enormous appetite of the rapidly growing adolescent boy is legendary.

Physical activity will usually increase appetite to provide the needed calories. Although decreasing physical activity will usually decrease appetite, this is not universally true. People may become more sedentary in a gradual fashion and not experience any change in appetite. Also, increasing activity does not usually increase the appetite as much as it increases calorie expenditure, which is why exercise is beneficial in a weight reduction program.

A person who is extremely large will usually have a larger appetite than a person who is small because of the needs of the body for nutrients. The small person needs less food for the same level of activity.

Emotional factors affect appetite profoundly. Some people respond to stressors of all kinds by increasing their intake. Others respond in exactly the opposite way, by slowing food intake. Such responses to stressors tend to be lifelong.

Thirst

Thirst is a sensation experienced in the mouth and throat when fluids are needed. Eating foods, particularly if they are dry, stimulates thirst. This is particularly true of salty or bitter foods. On the other hand, many believe that consuming certain liquids stimulates the appetite. An alcoholic beverage taken before a meal tends to stimulate the appetite.

Patients are occasionally placed on fluid restrictions because of some medical condition. When this happens, it is hard for the patient and the nurse to help assuage thirst. Rinsing the mouth and sucking hard candy can be useful, but feelings of thirst, to some degree, persist.

Early Family Influences

Some persons continue to eat the foods that were frequently served to them as children, rejecting new selections. Many persons in midlife never had the opportunity to try such foods as sauerbraten, sushi, tortillas, or tofu as youngsters, so they find these items unpalatable even in later years. Others enjoy such foods as a new experience in eating. Studies have shown, however, that early food preferences of the family have a marked influence on adult selection of food.

Personal Preference

Everyone has likes and dislikes with regard to food. Given the variety of foods available in the United States, it should be possible to plan nutritionally adequate diets composed only of foods a person likes. When people's likes and dislikes are considered in planning meals, they are more likely to eat well. However, extreme and numerous dislikes may interfere with good nutrition, especially when a special diet is needed.

Emotional Attitudes

Some people have strong feelings about food in general. Food is often used to reward children, and the resulting attitudes persist into adulthood. When food is withheld, for example, one may feel punished. Or one may want to reward oneself for enduring illness by eating favorite foods, even when they are contraindicated. The person responsible for withholding desired foods may be seen as antagonistic and punishing.

Being fed or having to eat what is typically considered baby food may make a person feel dependent and inadequate and may result in anger toward the person who provides such food. Recognizing the emotional importance of food will enable you to identify these problems when they occur and to plan effective action. Intervention is based on skills of therapeutic interaction (see Chapter 13).

Health Status

Anorexia (loss of appetite) is common when one is feeling ill. Loss of appetite is frequently equated with illness. Structural problems such as those of the esophagus, stomach, and intestines can make normal meal intake impossible until the condition is corrected, often with surgical intervention. Some drugs, such as those used against cancer, can cause anorexia, nausea, or vomiting. After surgery, a person may have a temporary feeling that food is unattractive. Sometimes only fluids or soft food items can be tolerated. Hospital food is sometimes as unfamiliar as is the environment, two situations that are not conducive to eating well.

Assessment

Assessment of nutritional status involves both assessment of the person's physical status and review of the dietary intake. Because the physical changes caused by nutritional deficits may also arise from a variety of disease states, physical status must be correlated with information about dietary intake. Information regarding current needs, ability to eat, and knowledge of correct diet are all essential aspects of nutritional assessment. A nutritionist may be consulted for assistance with nutritional assessment and planning.

A special emphasis on nutritional assessment of the elderly is being promoted through the Nutrition Screening Initiative. This multidisciplinary effort includes a tool for self-assessment of nutritional status that can be used in ambulatory care settings, home care, or even a senior center. A low score on this tool triggers a referral to a health care professional for more comprehensive assessment. A screening tool for health professionals to use as a primary assessment tool is called the Level I Screen (see Appendix F). A Level II Screen includes laboratory studies.

Interview

To make a comprehensive nutritional assessment, your interview regarding nutrition will include a dietary history, current needs, current intake, ability to eat, and level of knowledge. If you are in a situation in which this comprehensive assessment is not possible, you will have to determine which portions are essential for that individual patient.

Dietary History

Thorough nutritional assessment requires gathering the patient's *dietary history*—information on the usual meal pattern, types of foods usually eaten, types of foods avoided or omitted, and food preferences. This information will enable you to ascertain whether or not the patient maintains a sound diet at home. It will also help you plan a present and future diet that will be most acceptable and involve the least disruption in the patient's pattern of living. Information on the patient's sociocultural group and its attitudes and preferences with regard to food can also be helpful in diet planning.

As you interview the person, you will also be assessing the person's attitudes about diet. The attitude or state of mind will greatly influence the person's interest in and willingness to participate in a dietary plan. A person with serious mental health problems may not be able to tolerate the added stress of major change until adequate psychological support is available.

Current Needs

Assessment of nutrition also involves consideration of current needs. What are the requirements at this age? Is the person growing? Are special needs created by tissue repair and healing? Is the person underweight and in need of weight gain, or overweight and in need of weight reduction?

Current Intake

You will need to gather information about what a patient is currently eating and drinking to compare with the current needs. Almost all charts have a place to record each meal and the approximate amount eaten ($\frac{1}{3}$, $\frac{1}{2}$, or all). If more detailed knowledge is needed, it might be appropriate to design a special chart to record everything the patient eats. This chart is usually analyzed by

Nursing Issues and Trends: *Nutrition Screening Initiative*

Although nutritional state impacts all aspects of an individual's health, a thorough nutritional screening has not been a routine part of health assessment. Elderly individuals are at special risk for inadequate nutrition due to a variety of factors that may include low income, decreased taste sensation, lack of social contacts, tooth and mouth disorders, and other illnesses. The Nutrition Screening Initiative, a document that supports adequate nutritional screening for elderly persons, is being promoted and supported by a wide variety of health-related organizations. The information being disseminated with this initiative includes a variety of screening tools for assessing nutritional status. The goal is improved health status for our nation's elderly persons.

the nutritionist to determine calorie count, patterns of eating, and the patient's food likes and dislikes.

Measuring all fluids ingested may be important to assessment. In such cases, output must also be measured so the two can be compared. Intake measured includes all oral fluids, foods that would be liquid at body temperature (such as gelatin desserts and ice cream), intravenous fluids, and irrigating fluids that are not returned. Output measured includes urine, liquid stool, and all drainage. Profuse perspiration is also noted. See Module 15, Intake and Output, for directions on measuring "I&O" (intake and output).

Ability to Eat

Consideration of the patient's physical ability to eat is especially important in nutritional assessment. A wide variety of factors, ranging from muscle strength and hand coordination to discomfort in the mouth, may affect ability to eat. Some common problems faced by hospitalized people are immobilization in a position that does not allow easy eating or swallowing, restraint or immobilization of the dominant hand with an intravenous line, and extreme physical fatigue and weakness. Paralysis of one hand and arm sometimes occurs in patients who have suffered cerebrovascular accidents (strokes). After the basic aspects of nutritional status have been examined, special needs related to specific diseases—including information on the diet ordered by the physician—are considered.

Level of Knowledge

Another important aspect of nutritional assessment is determination of the extent of the patient's knowledge about nutrition. Does the patient know what constitutes a good diet? Does the person know where to seek information about nutrition? If a special diet is indicated, does the patient understand the diet and its purpose? Does the patient have enough depth of understanding to make appropriate modifications for such circumstances as eating out or attending a party? This information is needed to plan adequately for intervention.

Physical Assessment

Hair should be shiny and firm, not dry and dull or sparse. Changes in the color of the hair may occur in some states of malnutrition. Skin should be smooth and healthy. Loss of skin color or dark areas over the cheeks and under the eyes indicate nutritional deficits. Excessive dryness, scaling, red swollen areas, and excessive bleeding may all indicate nutritional deficits. Eyes should be bright, clear, and shiny with no sores or prominent blood vessels. Pale conjunctivae, excessive redness or a dull appearance of the eyes, or dryness of eye membranes may indicate nutritional deficits. Lips should be moist and smooth. Swollen chapped lips or fissures at the corners of the mouth are a sign of problems. Fingernails should be firm and pink, not brittle or ridged.

The tongue should be deep red, not bright red; it should have a slightly irregular surface, not be smooth or swollen or deeply fissured. Gums should be smooth, not swollen, and should not bleed easily. The gums should be tight around the teeth, not receded away from the tooth surfaces. Teeth should not have cavities and should not be discolored.

A person should have good muscle tone and be able to engage in activities of daily living (ADLs) without discomfort. Problems are indicated by weak, flaccid muscles or lack of muscle tissue. Bones should be straight and firm. Abnormal structures of bones, especially beading on ribs, knock knees, and bowed legs, may be indicators of malnutrition. In an infant the fontanel may be delayed in closing, or the skull bones may be thin and soft.

Malnutrition may cause the heart rate to be persistently high (over 100 in an adult) with an abnormal rhythm. Blood pressure may be elevated. Neurologic reflexes may be decreased. The person may lack a sense of position and be unable to perceive vibrations. People may feel abnormal sensations such as burning or tingling in the extremities with some nutritional deficits. The person may be irritable and confused.

Measurement of height, weight, and body fat are termed **anthropometric measurements**. The height and weight of children are plotted on a graph that has normal growth patterns already plotted on it. The central curve demonstrates the mean (average) growth pattern. In addition, one standard deviation above and below the mean are shown. Most children with good nutrition will fall within one standard deviation on each side of the norm. However, family and genetic characteristics should be considered along with the chart. An Asian child from a family of small people may be perfectly healthy and yet be far below the norm as defined by the standard chart. The pattern of the child's growth is also important. A child that starts at the bottom of the chart and continues in that pattern is likely to be demonstrating normal growth. However, you should be concerned if a child who has been at the mean begins falling below the mean.

Height and weight of adults are often measured against norms on various charts to establish whether the body weight is appropriate for the individual. A body mass index may be determined through the use of a nomogram. A body mass index of over 27 or below 22 should be referred to a physician for evaluation (see Appendix F). In general, men weigh more than women of the same height because they have a higher percentage of muscle tissue and different bone structure. The general bone structure of the individual should also be considered. Those with a light, fine bone structure will weigh less than those with a heavy, broad bone structure. An individual with a large percentage of muscle tissue in the body will appear overweight according to the chart because muscle tissue is heavy.

The real concern is whether the body has excessive fat tissue, not simply too much weight. Special methods are used to measure body fat. One is to measure a skin fold over the triceps muscle approximately halfway between the acromion process and the elbow. Skin fold measurements may also be done below the scapulae. Women in general have a thicker skin fold. This is because the subcutaneous fat layer is usually greater in women. The skin fold can be measured with calipers. The standard male skin fold is 12.5 mm, and the standard female skin fold is 16.5 mm (Blackburn, 1981). A measurement more than 10% to 20% over the standard indicates excess body fat.

Gain or loss of weight may also be a concern. If an individual has gained or lost 10 pounds or more in the last six months without intending to, a thorough investigation of the situation is needed. A physician referral may be appropriate.

Laboratory Studies

When nutritional status is a serious concern, a variety of laboratory studies may be ordered by the physician for assessment. Muscle tissue produces creatinine at a predictable, constant rate. If the kidneys are functioning normally, this product is excreted in a steady pattern. Therefore, measurement of the creatinine excreted in the urine in 24 hours can be related to the person's height to calculate the amount of muscle tissue in the body.

Serum albumin level relates to the lean body mass and may therefore be valuable in determining the presence of adequate protein. Serum albumin below 3.5g/dL indicates a potential problem. Low Serum cholesterol, below 160 mg/dL may indicate poor nutrition and inadequate fat intake. The serum level of most minerals can be measured, giving specific information about whether a nutrient is present in adequate amounts. The adequacy of some nutrients is checked by indirect measures. For example, iron is an essential component of hemoglobin in red blood cells; a low hemoglobin level may suggest an inadequate intake of iron. (See Chapter 29 regarding hemoglobin.) Although some sources are widely promoting hair analysis as a method of evaluating nutritional needs, no scientific evidence has established that hair consistently and accurately reflects nutritional status. Any laboratory study is used only in conjunction with a total assessment because many other factors in addition to diet may affect the results of most of these tests.

Nursing Diagnosis

The nursing diagnoses related to nutrition can involve problems related to eating habits or ability to obtain or prepare food or problems such as difficulty in handling, chewing, swallowing, or digesting food. Some nutri-

Nursing Diagnoses Related to Nutrition

Altered Comfort: Nausea and vomiting related to
- drug therapy
- inadequate peristalsis

Altered Nutrition: Less than Body Requirements related to
- chewing or swallowing difficulties
- anorexia, nausea, or vomiting
- specific disease process
- inability to afford adequate diet

Altered Nutrition: More than Body Requirements related to
- imbalance of intake versus activity expenditure
- sedentary lifestyle
- binge eating
- self-medicating with high-dose vitamins

Altered Nutrition: Less than Body Requirements of Iron related to
- low iron in dietary pattern

Altered Nutrition: Less than Body Requirements of Calcium related to
- dislike of milk and milk products
- intolerance of milk and milk products

High Risk for Altered Nutrition: Less than Body Requirements related to
- growth
- pregnancy
- lactation
- anorexia

High Risk for Altered Nutrition: More than Body Requirements related to
- change in lifestyle

High Risk for Aspiration

Knowledge Deficit concerning
- normal nutritional needs
- special dietary needs

Self-care Deficit: Inability to feed self related to
- fatigue and weakness
- poor neuromuscular control
- inadequate vision
- paralysis on right side

tional problems are related to medication use. For example, poor appetite is a side effect of some common heart medications. Increased appetite is caused by other medications. The following paragraphs describe the nursing diagnoses you will commonly deal with in the care setting.

Self-care Deficit: Feeding

The diagnosis Self-care Deficit: Feeding is a nutritional as well as an activity problem. If not assisted, the patient will develop nutritional deficits. The person who has a motor or neurologic disability may lack the coordination and control necessary for self-feeding. Others are unable to feed themselves because of excessive fatigue and weakness. The confused or disoriented person may lack the focus to eat enough to meet basic needs.

High Risk for Aspiration

Individuals with neuromuscular control problems may develop difficulty with swallowing. As this swallowing difficulty progresses, the patient is in danger of aspirating foods and especially liquids into the lungs. Aspirated material is often the cause of serious pneumonia. Whenever a patient appears to have difficulty swallowing or coughs and chokes frequently when taking food or fluids, a swallowing assessment is needed. This might be done by a speech therapist or a clinical nurse specialist in rehabilitation. If some swallowing ability is present, nursing care can focus on preventing aspiration.

Altered Nutrition: Less Than Body Requirements

Malnutrition is literally "bad" nutrition, the opposite of good nutrition. Malnutrition has two components. The first is lack of adequate calories to meet the body's needs, which results in weight loss, decreased resistance to infection, inhibited healing, and general malaise (lack of energy). Second, malnutrition is characterized by insufficient quantities of some essential nutrients, which can occur even when calories are adequate and the person is of normal weight or even obese. Lack of nutrients may produce deficiency diseases such as scurvy, which arises from a lack of vitamin C.

The North American Nursing Diagnosis Association (NANDA) has identified one general nursing diagnosis related to nutrition, Altered Nutrition. This diagnosis is subdivided into two aspects: Less Than Body Requirements and More Than Body Requirements. Each of these has further subdivisions based on different etiologies. These diagnoses are more helpful when the specific nutrient lacking or in excess is identified. For example, a diagnosis of Less Than Body Requirements of Iron is a different concern from Less Than Body Requirements of Calories. Both an intake that is less than body requirements and one that is more than body requirements can be risk states as well as actual problems (see sample Nursing Care Plan for Altered Nutrition: Less Than Body Requirements).

Earlier in this chapter, we discussed the national and global issue of malnutrition and mentioned the importance of health teaching. There may be a general lack of knowledge about nutrition. Poor budgeting may add to the problem. For example, many people believe that meat is needed and purchase it in large quantities, forgoing other more nutritious foods. Red meat is high in fat and calories. In fact, the RDA for protein can be met with modest amounts of meat or with inexpensive foods such as grains and legumes. Low-income people are often not aware of the assistance programs available to them.

Altered Nutrition: More Than Body Requirements

Obesity is usually defined as body weight of 15% or more above the ideal weight for height, body build, and age. (Occasionally 20% is considered the baseline for obesity.) Another way of defining obesity is to calculate the percentage of body weight accounted for by fat. This may be done with precision by the complex process of weighing in water, or it may be estimated by using calipers to pinch and measure subcutaneous fat. In women, 25% to 30% of body weight is typically fat; men have more muscle and bone mass and thus usually only 14% fat. Higher percentages indicate excess fat.

Obesity is not necessarily synonymous with overweight, which is a matter of individual perception. In modern industrial societies, the fashion ideal for women tends to be a slim figure. Thus, a woman might perceive herself as overweight in light of fashion without being obese or at risk of health problems associated with obesity.

Being obese is a chronic problem. It has been estimated that from 20% to 50% of adults in our country are considered obese, and some who are severely obese may actually die earlier than they would have if they had not been obese (Stewart and Brook, 1983). Obesity poses a variety of health hazards.

The immediate cause of all obesity is intake of more calories than the body can use, these excess calories then being stored as fat. The underlying causes may be more diverse. Some people need fewer calories than the norm and thus gain weight on an ordinary dietary intake. This group includes people with hormonal deficiencies that reduce metabolic rate as well as others whose normal metabolism appears to be efficient. Another reason for needing fewer calories is a lower-than-

Nursing Care Plan
Sample Nursing Care Plan for Altered Nutrition: Less than Body Requirements

Nursing Diagnosis	Altered Nutrition: Less than Body Requirements, related to anorexia secondary to recent chemotherapy **Supportive data:** States "Nothing looks good to me." Eats only a few bites of each meal. Weight 105 lb. Height 5 ft. 7 in.
Desired Patient Outcomes	**Short term:** 1. Expresses interest in food. 2. Eats everything on tray. 3. Gains weight steadily, approximately 2 lb/week. **Long term:** Weight 130 lb.

Nursing Action	**Rationale**
1. Have dietitian meet with patient to ascertain likes and dislikes.	The dietician is the health professional with the greatest knowledge and skill relative to both the foods that are appropriate in specific diets and the resources of the institution.
2. Ask dietitian to provide very small meals with between-meal snacks.	Small, frequent meals provide adequate nutrition without overwhelming an individual at any one time.
3. Schedule all procedures as far from meals as possible.	Unpleasant or tiring procedures may depress appetite.
4. Before each meal check room to make sure environment is clean and pleasant.	The immediate environment affects appetite.
5. Whenever possible, arrange for family to eat with the patient.	Socializing is a part of regular meal patterns for most individuals and therefore tends to enhance appetite.

usual activity level. People with sedentary jobs, those who dislike sports, and those whose lives do not include any regular physical exertion may become obese for this reason (see sample Nursing Care Plan for Altered Nutrition: More Than Body Requirements).

In the developed countries, excessive intake of calories is most often the reason for obesity. The pattern of excessive dietary intake is reinforced socially: most social occasions include food and caloric beverages, and Americans consume large quantities of simple sugar in desserts, snacks, and beverages. Advertising promotes keen interest in and desire for food unrelated to actual needs. Some people habitually overeat for psychological reasons: food may represent security and love or be a defense against the need to relate to others.

Obesity does seem to characterize some families more than others. This pattern may be influenced by heredity, acquired eating habits, or the psychological meanings attached to food in a particular family—factors that cannot be effectively separated.

The development of fat cells in infancy and early childhood is being studied in relationship to obesity. It is known that individuals who are obese as infants are more likely to be obese as adults, and those who were

Nursing Care Plan
Sample Nursing Care Plan for Altered Nutrition: More than Body Requirements

Nursing Diagnosis

Altered Nutrition: More than Body Requirements related to sedentary lifestyle

Supportive data:

Weight 155 lb.

Height 5 ft. 2 in.

Desired weight for height 120 lb.

Minimal walking or physical activity.

Desired Patient Outcomes

Short term (each week):

1. Plans own menus for weight reduction.
2. Eats only those foods allowed on diet plan.
3. Exercises 30 min daily.
4. Demonstrates some weight loss at each visit.

Long term (by 16 weeks):

Weight is 120 lb.

Nursing Action	Rationale
1. Provide written materials on weight reduction.	Written materials provide an ongoing reference for the patient.
2. Review general meal plan and how to adapt menus.	Verbal input provides an additional avenue for learning. Personal interaction provides an opportunity for the patient to ask questions and clarify information.
3. Plan exercise program with patient according to interest.	Regular exercise enhances weight loss. Individuals are more likely to continue an exercise program that they enjoy.
4. Encourage patient to keep diet diary.	A diet diary provides regular feedback to an individual of their progress in maintaining a special diet.
5. Review diet diary and exercise at each visit.	Review of the diet and exercise patterns provides information for possible reteaching if needed.
6. Weigh at each visit.	Regular weighing provides feedback on progress in weight loss.
7. Give positive feedback for all achievements. Do not dwell on "failures."	Actions receiving positive reinforcement are more likely to be sustained. Negative feedback may undermine self-esteem.

obese as infants have a greater number of fat cells as adults.

As people age, they are more likely than before to become obese, usually because of decreased activity levels. Changes in metabolic patterns associated with aging may also have a contributory effect.

Altered Comfort: Nausea and Vomiting

Nausea is the subjective feeling that one might vomit. Discomfort is often localized in the stomach and back of the throat. Increased salivation, headache, and general malaise may accompany the nausea. Vomiting usually but not always follows nausea.

Vomiting is the forceful ejection of the contents of the stomach. Severe vomiting may be accompanied by reverse peristalsis, which brings material from far down in the intestine up to the stomach for expulsion. The force expelling the vomitus may be great enough to eject it several feet from the mouth; this phenomenon is called **projectile vomiting**.

Nausea and vomiting may be problems in comfort when they are present for a short period of time. If they continue or are severe, they then lead to an inability to meet nutritional needs and the nursing diagnosis might be Altered Nutrition: Less Than Body Requirements related to nausea and vomiting. Although this diagnosis is not approved by NANDA, the category of altered comfort is part of the taxonomy and the problem is one that nurses identify and treat.

Knowledge Deficit Concerning Nutrition

Knowledge Deficit related to special diet and Knowledge Deficit related to normal nutrition are both important nursing diagnoses. A major concern in all nutrition is to help the person establish an adequate knowledge base to manage nutrition independently. Often normal nutrition must be taught before you can teach about a special diet.

Planning and Implementation

As you plan for nursing interventions, you must first determine what the desired outcomes are. Long-term aims may be for the patient to achieve the ideal body weight (which should be identified specifically for the individual). However, short-term outcomes are usually essential in the area of nutrition. Short-term outcomes may be related to the specific nutritional intake of each day or even each meal that includes an appropriate diet for the person based on needs for maintenance of health, healing, growth, or other current demands. Nursing interventions are important in preventing nutritional problems as well as in helping to resolve current problems. Here, we will review some of the general actions you can take to promote adequate nutrition for the patient.

Health Teaching

The need for health teaching about nutrition-related problems is common. When you have determined through assessment that dietary teaching is needed, your task is to combine your knowledge of nutrition with your knowledge of health teaching (Chapter 16) in planning your instructional approach (Fig. 25-4). You may find it necessary to teach the patient about normal nutrition before you can teach about special diets.

Health teaching in response to poor nutrition must be done with sensitivity and care. It is important not to undermine the self-esteem of a family that is already struggling with other difficulties. In planning with them to achieve a better diet, consider their cultural and ethnic food preferences, access to stores and transportation, and individual likes and dislikes. Sometimes you may need to make a referral to a social worker or some other person who can help with the family's income problems. If help with budgeting is needed, consumer credit counseling services provide this service without charge. (These organizations should be differentiated from commercial credit counseling agencies.) You can find ways to teach about appropriate nutrition that will help enhance people's self-esteem and pride in their ability to care for themselves and their families.

Stimulating the Patient's Appetite

Environmental factors are important in promoting appetite. Control of odors and unpleasant sights is often difficult in the hospital, but any efforts in this direction that

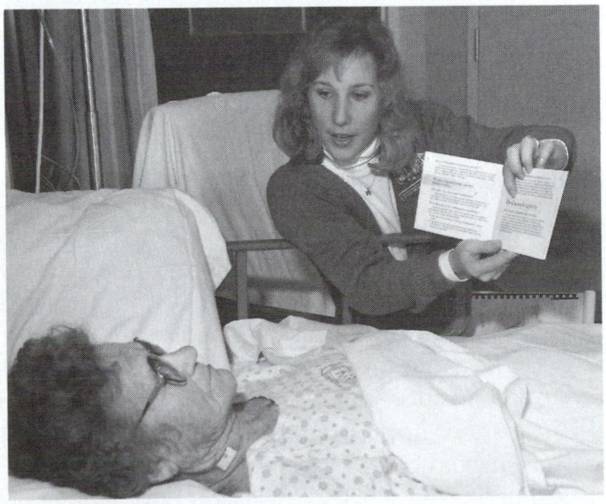

Figure 25-4. Health teaching is an important part of nutritional intervention.

Nursing Research: *Implications for Practice*

Beresford, S.A., Farmer, E.M., Feingold, L., Graves, K.L., Sumner, S.K., and Baker, R.M. "Evaluation of a self-help dietary intervention in a primary care setting." *American Journal of Public Health* 82 (1): 79–84, January, 1992.

Nurses in primary care settings introduced self-help materials designed to encourage individuals to reduce fat consumption and increase fiber consumption. The individuals who received this intervention were compared in terms of dietary fat and fiber consumption with a control group who had not received these self-help materials. There were significant small but consistent changes associated with the self-help materials. Although other factors may also have influenced these individuals, this study supported the use of self-help materials as one intervention to improve dietary patterns.

can be taken may help the patient retain a minimal appetite or regain a lost appetite. Removing soiled linen, opening a window, or using air freshener may be appropriate nursing actions in such a situation.

Personal comfort can promote appetite and may be enhanced by bathing, washing the hands and face, straightening the bed, giving pain medications, or in myriad other ways.

Stressful events tend to decrease appetite and should be avoided immediately before meals are served. Many pieces of equipment found in a hospital (such as those used for venipuncture) are stress producing to observe and removing them from the patient's presence during meals will decrease anxiety.

Most people interact with family and friends at mealtimes. If visitors can stay during the meal, or even order a tray and eat with the patient, a more congenial mealtime atmosphere is created. Sometimes several patients can sit together to visit during a meal, or a staff member might sit with a patient for a few minutes to make the meal a special event. Company is especially helpful when the meal itself is less than tasty because of the omission of seasonings or salt: the interaction replaces the bland food as the focus of attention.

Positioning the Patient for Eating

People who are ill often have special needs with regard to the eating process itself. Positioning is one factor that may make eating a problem. It is easiest to eat in a sitting position, with the food placed directly in front in one's line of vision; this position helps to prevent aspiration. If this position can be maintained, be sure to position the patient appropriately before the meal. If this position is impossible, the nearest approximation of it is most desirable. The weak or disabled person may need pillows or other supports on each side and under the arms to maintain correct posture for eating. If the patient is not permitted to sit up, a side-lying position may be used for meals.

Helping the Patient Eat

Feeding a patient is sometimes necessitated by muscle and joint disability that prevents movement, neurologic involvement that prevents muscle function, or extreme weakness. Many patients are able to feed themselves partially if the nurse helps with difficult tasks. Sometimes a patient can manage finger foods, such as bread and butter, but must be fed foods requiring more dexterity, such as soup. If weak vision is the problem, a description of the items on the tray and their location may enable the patient to eat without help.

People usually use both hands to feed themselves, the dominant hand performing the most skilled tasks. If only one hand is available, the patient will have great difficulty with such tasks as opening a milk carton. If only the nondominant hand is available, even one-handed tasks may require more dexterity than that hand possesses. Planning placement of intravenous equipment and turning the patient so that the dominant hand is free for eating can prevent this problem. You may have to offer to perform some tasks, such as opening a milk carton or cutting meat. However, patients should always be asked whether they want help, what kind of help they want, and how such help is to be given. Independence in eating fosters self-esteem and should be encouraged.

In patients with difficulty in swallowing, foods that are easier to swallow should be included in the diet: soft foods, thickened liquids (such as milk shakes), and foods with cold or hot temperatures that stimulate the mouth and throat. Foods that are difficult to swallow include those that are dry or hard, clear liquids (such as water), and sticky foods.

Special feeding devices and methods are often used to help patients maintain independence in eating. The advisability of use of such equipment—which includes utensils with shaped handles, devices to keep a plate or dish in place, and special straws—needs to be evaluated carefully for each individual. One person may appreciate such an aid, whereas another may prefer to eat more slowly and with greater difficulty using conventional utensils.

Because maximum independence increases the patient's self-esteem, time and effort expended toward this end are well spent. Module 9, Feeding Adult Patients, provides more information on this topic.

Increasing Oral Fluid Intake

Many ill people need to consume large quantities of fluid to allow for excretion of excess waste products or to combat fever. The physician may thus order *force fluids.* This order means not that you literally force the patient to drink, but that you exert maximum effort to encourage the patient to consume fluids. Simply reminding the patient to drink frequently may be all that is needed.

Because patients are likely to consume more of fluids they enjoy, it is worthwhile to take time to learn likes and dislikes and to order what the patient prefers. Because people are more likely to reach desired goals if they receive feedback on their progress, you might design a method of recording intake or graphing it on a wall chart. Furthermore, behaviors that are reinforced tend to be repeated. Thus praise or even marks on a chart for ingesting certain amounts of fluid may have the effect of increasing intake. Setting a specific goal for the 24-hour period and ascertaining when fluid should be taken will help the nursing staff to organize its efforts. If the goal is 3,000 ml/24 hr, a realistic plan acknowledges that the patient sleeps during the night shift and therefore will usually take less than 200 ml if offered fluids only when awakened in the morning. If medications are given during the night, fluid intake at these times may be encouraged. The plan might provide for 2,000 ml to be taken between 7:00 AM and 3:00 PM. That period of time includes two meals and two snacks, and if the patient also drinks fluids between meals, the goal can be reached. If the mechanics of drinking are a problem, special straws and cups are available to assist the patient.

Limiting Fluids

A physician may occasionally order that fluids be limited. Fluids are often withheld for short periods before procedures that require general anesthesia or slight dehydration as well as when disease necessitates restriction of fluids. Lack of fluids is trying for the patient, and careful planning with the patient is needed to space the allowable intake throughout the day and to provide for fluid to accompany oral medications. The patient will also need support from others to tolerate fluid deprivation. When the limitation is severe, close supervision may be necessary: it is difficult to maintain self-control when one's thirst is extreme. Ice chips often serve to minimize the desire for fluid and provide greater relief than the same amount of water; but remember that they, too, must be counted as intake. Allowing responsible patients to perform mouth care and to rinse the mouth may promote a feeling of well-being during this time. If a patient cannot be expected to refrain from drinking fluid while performing mouth care, you may moisten the lips and provide mouth care for the patient.

Supporting Weight Management

A goal for weight loss should be realistic, and it should be set jointly by the nurse and the patient. It is often helpful to set short-term goals as well as an overall long-term goal; a single ultimate goal can be discouraging.

Certain diet plans have been more successful than others. Some diets are monotonous in that the same food (grapefruit is an example) is consumed over an extended period of time. Other diets are expensive to maintain. Of serious concern is the fact that some people may try ineffective and even dangerous approaches to losing weight.

An effective weight control program has two major components: planning actual food intake and helping the person stay on the prescribed diet. Let us first examine the wide variety of ways to plan intake, all of which have had some success.

Calorie counting relies on looking up the caloric value of foods and choosing a diet the total number of calories of which is within the guidelines. The emphasis is on maintaining a nutritious and balanced diet. Although this method works well, it is time consuming and involves careful planning and figuring, and some people find it tedious.

Carbohydrate counting is performed to limit calories from carbohydrates, on the assumption that the high satiety value of the fat and protein eaten in place of carbohydrates will naturally limit their intake. This approach can be effective, but some people gain the mistaken impression that protein foods cannot contribute to obesity. *Ketogenic diets* are those that limit carbohydrates so severely that the body becomes depleted of glucose. For the body to get the energy it needs for basic functioning, it must burn fat in large quantities. Because the body is not equipped to burn fat rapidly, the metabolism is incomplete, producing ketone bodies as waste products. These ketone bodies are acidic in nature and therefore cause a mild metabolic acidosis (see Chapter 30). Although such diets promote quick weight loss, even their proponents recommend limiting them to 7 or 14 days. There is controversy over whether mild metabolic acidosis is dangerous for the well person. Medical supervision is essential when one is undertaking this type of diet.

Exchange menus consist of a basic diet plan that specifies a given number of servings of several types of food—meat, bread or bread substitutes, low-calorie vegetables, high-calorie vegetables, fruits, and milk products—and provides lists of foods that are calorically interchangeable and can be used to fulfill the diet's specifications. This approach has the advantage of greater simplicity than direct calorie counting. Although less exact, it is adequate.

Liquid protein diets, which are commercially prepared, have been promoted as the solution to serious weight control problems. After using the original of these products and sustaining major weight losses, some people died suddenly. The exact cause of death has not been determined, but liquid protein diets are now available only as part of medically supervised programs that provide special monitoring of fluid and electrolytes and cardiac status.

Liquid diets containing a variety of nutrients owe their popularity to the assumption that a liquid diet must have fewer calories than a diet containing solids. However, a liquid diet's caloric value depends on the types of liquids allowed. When the liquids allowed consist primarily of vegetable juices, with some fruit juices and broths, such a diet may indeed be low calorie, but these liquid diets are rarely well balanced and should be used with caution. Commercially prepared liquid diets are available that contain balanced nutrients. These are often used for a limited number of meals with some meals including low-calorie foods.

The second major aspect of weight control is promoting adherence to the prescribed diet. Many different approaches have been used. Group support has proven successful. Behavior modification is often used to help obese people establish new eating habits. The hypothesis underlying this approach is that overeating is learned behavior and one can thus learn not to overeat. Free foods—that is, foods that have few or no calories and may be eaten in unlimited quantities—are often used to help people stay on a diet. Artificially sweetened beverages are popular free foods, but recent reports about the health hazards of artificial sweeteners have led some people to limit their intake of them. Others believe the risk is small compared with the risk of obesity. Caffeinated beverages, such as coffee, tea, and diet colas, do not contain calories, but they may stimulate appetite and thus may be counterproductive for those trying to lose weight.

Starvation has been used to enforce weight loss in some severely obese people. No food at all is allowed (though the person may have water). However, starvation causes the body to break down muscle stores as well as fat and is therefore not recommended.

Sometimes medications have been prescribed by physicians as part of weight loss programs. Amphetamines have the effect of decreasing appetite. However, amphetamines have such side effects as insomnia, irritability, nervousness, and drug dependence. There have been instances of hormones, such as thyroid hormone, being given for weight loss, but by upsetting the body's own hormonal balance, this regimen may create long-term problems. Over-the-counter drugs that purport to decrease appetite may also have side effects. In general, medications are not recommended for weight loss.

Another aspect of weight control is increasing activity level (Table 25-5). If a person's activity level is low, an increase in exercise may help weight loss occur more rapidly. Paradoxically, increased activity may also help decrease appetite in the person who has been overeating. Exercise is discussed more completely in Chapter 23.

Whatever plan is pursued, it must be one the obese person feels comfortable with and is determined to follow. An encouraging and supportive approach is usually more helpful than a critical attitude. When lapses from the diet occur (and they usually do), the person needs reassurance that one slip does not mean failure. Each pound lost should be treated as a significant accomplishment. Slow, gradual weight loss is much more likely to be permanent; drastic, rapid weight loss is more often followed by regaining all the lost weight plus additional pounds.

Administering Tube Feedings

When an individual is unable to eat, the physician may decide that feeding liquids through a tube directly into the stomach or small intestine is necessary to provide adequate nutrition. These feedings are referred to as **tube feedings** or **enteral feedings** and are administered by the nurse. Four different types of tubes are used for this process: the nasogastric feeding tube, the gastrostomy tube, the esophagostomy tube, and the jejunostomy tube.

The nasogastric tube is inserted through the nose to the nasopharynx, and then through the esophagus to the stomach. Although any nasogastric tube may be used for feeding, most commonly, small-diameter silicone rubber tubes are used because they cause less irri-

Table 25–5. Average Calories Expended with Activity

Activity	Calories per Minute	Activity	Calories per minute
Archery	2.8	Mopping floor	4.8
Badminton (singles)	6.0	Mountain climbing	9.5
Basketball	12.0	Music playing (piano)	3.2
Bowling	3.2	Paddleball	10.7
Canoeing (15-min mile)	7.0	Racquetball	10.7
Carpet cleaning	3.5	Roller skating	11.2
Cleaning	4.2	Rope skipping (80 turns/min)	11.3
Climbing hills	9.5	Running (6-min mile)	16.2
(with 10-lb load)	10.1	Scrubbing floors	12.0
Cooking	3.5	Sitting quietly	1.7
Cross-country skiing	14.0	Skin diving (vigorous)	12.0
Cycling (5-min mile)	10.6	Soccer	12.0
Drawing (standing)	1.8	Social dancing	6.0
Eating	1.7	Softball or baseball	7.2
Field hockey	9.0	Square and round dancing	7.0
Food shopping	4.5	Squash	10.7
Gardening	3.8	Standing quietly	1.7
raking	5.4	Swimming (50 yards/min)	9.1
Golf (foursome—cart)	3.8	Table tennis	5.6
Golf (foursome—carrying the clubs)	6.0	Tennis (singles)	6.0
Gymnastics	4.6	Tennis (doubles)	4.0
Handball	10.9	Tetherball	4.6
Horseback riding (trot)	8.0	Trampolining	5.6
Ironing	2.7	Typing	1.8
Jogging (8-min mile)	12.6	Volleyball (6 players)	3.6
Judo	12.0	Volleyball (2 players)	9.2
Knitting/sewing	1.8	Walking (17-min mile)	5.4
Lying at ease	1.5		

tation to nose and throat tissue and the cardiac sphincter of the stomach closes more tightly around them. Many feeding tubes are now passed through the stomach into the duodenum in an effort to decrease the potential for regurgitation of feedings that results in aspiration into the lungs. The nurse inserts a nasogastric feeding tube (see Module 45, Nasogastric Intubation).

The other two types of tubes are used only for long-term tube feedings and must be placed with surgical procedures. The **gastrostomy tube**, which is used for persons who have had strokes and neurologic damage, is placed through the abdominal wall directly into the stomach. Most gastrostomies are now placed in a procedure called a *percutaneous endoscopic gastrostomy* (PEG). In this procedure, an endoscope is passed into the stomach to guide the placement of the tube from the abdominal wall. The tube thus inserted is referred to as a *PEG tube.*

The esophagostomy tube, which is used less frequently, is placed above the clavicle, beside the trachea, and directly into the esophagus from where it is passed into the stomach. The tract through which it passes heals, and the end of the tubing can be clamped and secured under clothing. The esophagostomy tube is especially valuable for the person who will return to active life and wishes to be able to administer tube feedings without partially disrobing to gain access to a gastrostomy tube. This is most common for the individual who has had radical surgery of the mouth, chin, or upper neck or a disease that makes the esophagus nonfunctional.

The jejunostomy tube is also placed surgically through the abdominal wall. It is usually placed during a surgical procedure involving the stomach and duodenum and allows feedings to be given while the stomach and duodenum are healing.

Tube feedings may given as a continuous drip or they may be given in large amount at specified times (**bolus feedings**). Often the feedings are given initially as a continuous drip, and then bolus feedings are gradually begun when the person has adjusted to the liquid diet. Bolus feedings have the advantage of being more like eating regular meals, but if the stomach is not emptying adequately, they may contribute to regurgitation and aspiration.

Additional water must always be given with tube

feedings to meet the body's needs. The exact amount may be determined by the physician. The water also cleanses the tube so that the feeding material does not remain in the tube, where it could serve as a growth medium for microbes.

Directions for giving tube feedings appear in Module 29, Tube Feeding. However, remember that the tube feeding is a meal, not a medical treatment. If the patient is aware of the surroundings, a pleasant atmosphere will increase the flow of digestive juices and enhance digestion. You should take care that the container used for the tube feeding is attractive and that an effort is made to let the patient know that this is indeed a meal.

Certain dangers are associated with nasogastric tube feedings. If the tube is malpositioned, fluid could be deposited in the nasopharynx, allowing aspiration into the lungs to occur. Excessive pressure may cause gastric irritation, gas, and reflex vomiting. Administering the feeding too rapidly may also precipitate vomiting. Allowing air into the tube will cause distention and discomfort and possibly vomiting. Food is ordinarily moderated in temperature in the mouth and esophagus before it reaches the stomach. Temperature extremes can irritate the gastric mucosa, so it is essential that the formula be of moderate temperature before instillation. Any procedure for nasogastric tube feeding should consider tube placement, prevention of air ingestion, the temperature of the fluid, and the force and speed of the fluid as it enters the stomach.

Patients receiving tube feedings frequently experience diarrhea. This phenomenon has been attributed to a variety of factors, including bacterial contamination, too concentrated a solution, inappropriate temperature, the unfamiliar consistency, and lack of fiber. Bacterial contamination can be prevented by careful attention to technique in caring for the equipment and the feeding itself. If care is taken with regard to the other possible causes of diarrhea, the patient usually adjusts to the concentration and consistency of the formula. Some new commercial formulas are designed to minimize diarrhea through attention to osmolarity, eliminating lactose, or providing soluble fiber.

Potential Complications Related to Tube Feedings

Potential complication: displacement of feeding tube

Potential complication: gastric irritation

Nursing Diagnoses Related to Tube Feedings

Diarrhea related to
- bacterial contamination
- high concentration of formula
- lactose intolerance
- unfamiliar consistency

High Risk for Aspiration related to
- malposition of feeding tube
- regurgitation

Altered Comfort: Gas and distention related to instillation of air with feeding

Administering Parenteral Nutrition

The nurse caring for the patient receiving parenteral nutrition assumes responsibility for maintaining the intravenous line and access, preventing complications, and monitoring for early signs of the complications that may occur. Potential complications of parenteral nutrition are many and potentially serious. Module 58, Parenteral Nutrition, provides detailed information regarding procedures for administering parenteral nutrition. Here we will discuss the major potential complications.

Infection, either at the site of administration or systemic (affecting the whole body), is the most common complication. To prevent infection, most facilities have established a strict routine for care of the access site. This regimen usually includes a cleaning procedure and special care in dressing changes. In addition, giving medications into the parenteral nutrition line is discouraged unless there is no alternative. Each needle puncture of the line increases the potential for contamination. Tubings and solutions are changed on a rigid schedule so that organisms will not have time to reproduce if contamination occurs.

Fluid overload, which strains the heart and may cause respiratory distress, can occur if the fluid is given at too rapid a rate. For this reason, a special intravenous pump that measures the flow rate and monitors the line is usually used.

Potential Complications Related to Parenteral Nutrition

Potential complication: air embolus

Potential complication: allergic reactions

Potential complication: fluid overload

Potential complication: infection

Potential complication: hyperglycemia

Hyperglycemia (high blood sugar) may occur if dextrose is given more rapidly than the body can use it. Urine may be checked for the presence of glucose to determine whether blood glucose is so elevated that the kidneys are excreting the sugar. It is sometimes necessary for the physician to order the administration of the hormone insulin to facilitate use of the glucose.

An **air embolus** is an air bubble that moves into the bloodstream and to the heart, where it causes a severe compromise in circulation and possibly death. At the tip of an intravenous catheter in a large central vein, a negative pressure may develop, especially when the person inspires. This negative pressure could pull an air bubble directly into the circulation. To prevent this problem, nurses must carefully use the prescribed technique when changing tubing or opening the line for any reason.

Allergic reactions to the protein in the parenteral nutrition solution are not common but have occurred. This may be manifested as a skin rash or in more serious situations as respiratory distress. If allergic reactions to the protein occur, the fluid must be discontinued. Another brand or type of nutritional solution may be substituted if the physician determines that the allergy is specific and would not occur with a different brand that contained a different protein source.

Despite the potential complications, some patients who cannot take oral foods are now being discharged and are receiving TPN at home. With careful teaching, patients and their families can become very skillful at this type of care.

Evaluation

Desired outcomes for nutritional programs often involve the patient's commitment to making a change and the patient's knowledge of the specific diet needed. Outcomes related to correcting underlying problems are usually long term in nature. When you evaluate your nursing interventions related to nutrition, it becomes especially important to have short-term outcomes. Changes in overall nutritional status do not happen rapidly, and if the only outcomes you have identified are those that represent resolution of the problem, you and the patient may become discouraged. Short-term outcomes may represent changes in intake for a single day or even a single meal. A short-term outcome related to adherence to a special diet may be that the person express an intention to try the new diet. Reaching short-term outcomes that represent milestones along the path may be important in encouraging the patient and family.

Long-term outcomes may relate to the nutritional status and changes in the signs and symptoms that indicated the presence of a problem. It is helpful to review the long-term outcomes from time to time to make sure that they remain appropriate and useful. Sometimes it becomes apparent that a desired long-term outcome was not appropriate to the specific person and needs to be revised. This revision does not represent failure, but rather an openness and willingness to be flexible. Achieving a long-term outcome related to improved nutritional status not only solves a current problem but also provides a foundation for ongoing health maintenance.

Nursing Care Study
An Obese Child

Martha Brown, RN, was working in a well-child clinic, where she assisted with the screening of children and counseling for health maintenance. Observing the first child for the morning, 6-year-old Billy, she noted that he appeared plump and had trouble bending over to pick up a toy he had dropped on the floor. She greeted the mother and introduced herself to Billy.

As part of the standard well-child examination, Ms. Brown weighed and measured Billy. His weight was far above the norms for his height on the growth chart. Interviewing the mother, she asked carefully about Billy's eating habits and was told that Billy was always a good eater and liked to eat snacks too. Questioned further, the mother reported that Billy liked potato chips and pop for snacks and also ate many of her homemade cookies.

Ms. Brown asked the mother if she had noticed that Billy was quite heavy for his height. Ms. Brown pointed out his place on the growth chart and explained what the graph meant. The mother answered that she had thought about it but figured that Billy "would outgrow being fat." Ms. Brown explained that this was a common assumption, but children who were overweight were likely to be overweight as adults. She also pointed out that being overweight compromised Billy's ability to participate in games and sports as well as his acceptance by other children.

(*continued*)

Nursing Care Study (continued)
An Obese Child

MOTHER: "I suppose I should see if he could lose some weight, shouldn't I?"

MS. BROWN: "It would be good for Billy's health."

MOTHER: "Would I have to put him on a diet? He wouldn't like not being able to eat. I'd have a cranky kid on my hands."

MS. BROWN: "The clinic has a special diet you could use. But it's planned so that there are things available for snacks and so the children on it don't have to be hungry. Would you like to look it over?"

MOTHER: "Sure."

Ms. Brown obtained the printed explanation of the diet and sat down to talk with the mother about it. As they discussed the diet, Billy's mother became more positive about her ability to use it for Billy. The diet considered carrying school lunches and substituted fruits and vegetables for high-calorie snacks. Information was also included on how to involve children in more active play.

Ms. Brown encouraged the mother to try the diet and to call if she encountered problems. She set up an appointment for Billy to be checked again the following month. Ms. Brown encouraged the mother to try to involve Billy in the plan and perhaps to offer Billy some nonfood rewards such as special activities for exercising and staying on the diet.

After Billy and his mother had left, Ms. Brown reviewed what she had done. She had obtained information about Billy's eating habits as well as his current height and weight. She had provided information to the mother, who had in turn acknowledged that a problem existed. The mother had been encouraged to make a personal decision to put Billy on a diet. Ms. Brown had performed health teaching about the diet itself and methods of helping Billy stick to the diet. An appointment had been made for follow-up and evaluation. Ms. Brown felt pleased with her efforts.

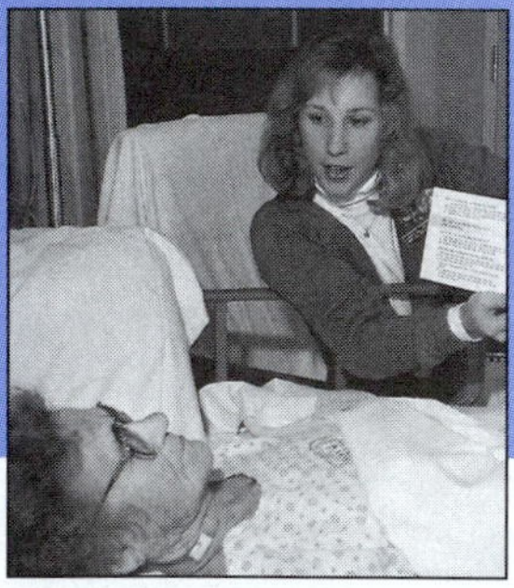

Key Points

- The basic nutrients are carbohydrates, fats, proteins, minerals, vitamins, and water, and each provides something specific that is needed for maintenance and growth of body tissue or for energy.
- Digestion and absorption both affect the amount of the nutrient available for metabolism.
- Methods used to determine the appropriate dietary intake to meet the body's needs include the Recommended Dietary Allowances (RDA) and the Eating Right Pyramid.
- When a person is ill, the diet is often modified to provide adequate nutrition in a form that is more easily digested.
- The types of food eaten are affected by culture, religion, personal preference, emotional attitudes, economic factors, and geographic location.
- Food intake is determined by hunger, thirst, and appetite.
- Assessment of nutritional status is complex and should include the following: history, physical examination, anthropometric measurement, and laboratory studies.
- The nursing diagnoses related to nutrition have a variety of etiologies, which should be stated in specific terms to identify the problem clearly.
- In planning interventions for the patient with a nursing diagnosis related to nutrition, you might consider scheduling care before meals to make the person more comfortable and to stimulate appetite. Short-term goals are important in the planning of care for nutritional problems because they often require a change in long-standing habits.
- Health teaching is an important part of nursing intervention in regard to nutritional concerns. Other interventions include assisting the person in eating, increasing fluids, limiting fluid intake, and supporting weight management.
- Many different approaches to weight control are used. Those that attack both the behavior of overeating and the feelings about food through group support seem to be the most effective.
- Tube feedings and parenteral nutrition may be ordered by the physician for patients who are unable

to eat in the normal way, and the nurse must be alert to the potential complications of these methods of feeding.

- In evaluating the effectiveness of nursing care for nutritional problems, both short-term and long-term goals need to be considered. Short-term goals are likely to be the most successful.

Study Questions

1. How many kilocalories are in 1 g protein? 1 g fat? 1 g carbohydrate?
2. How might the location of protein digestion be important when an individual experiences dysfunction of the gastrointestinal system?
3. What is the significance of whether blood lipids are found as high-density lipoproteins or low-density lipoproteins?
4. What is the purpose of the Recommended Dietary Allowances?
5. How might you use the Eating Right Pyramid in patient care?
6. What special problems does a vegetarian diet pose and how might those problems be resolved?
7. List and define the three main determinants of food intake.
8. How does culture affect diet?
9. In what way do emotional feelings affect food intake?
10. What dietary modifications must be ordered by the physician, and what ones can be ordered by the nurse?
11. What is a progressive diet and when might it be used?
12. Outline the data to be included in a complete nutritional assessment.
13. List actions that can be taken to stimulate appetite.
14. Explain at least three approaches to weight control.
15. List potential complications associated with tube feeding.
16. List potential complications associated with parenteral nutrition.

Critical Thinking Activities

1. Record your own diet for 24 hours. Compare it to your RDA and to the Eating Right Pyramid. Evaluate your diet in relationship to your nutritional needs.
2. Keep track of your own fluid intake for 24 hours. Devise a plan to increase your in take to 3,000 ml/day. Be specific in regard to types of fluids, amounts of fluids, and timing of intake.
3. Plan and conduct a nutritional assessment for a patient in the clinical area identify whether the person has any nutritional deficits.
4. Assess a patient to determine his or her level of knowledge about "normal nutrition." If any learning needs are apparent, plan health teaching to meet those needs. After consulting with a clinical instructor, carry out your health teaching plan.

Relevant Sections in Modules for Basic Nursing Skills

References and Readings

American Institute for Cancer Research. *Dietary Guidelines To Lower Cancer Risk.* Washington, D.C.: Author, 1982.

Bobel, L. M. "Nutritional Implications in the Patient with Pressure Sores." *Nursing Clinics of North America* 22, 2 (June 1987): 379–390.

Brentin, L., and Sich, A. "Caring for the Morbidly Obese." *American Journal of Nursing* 91, 8 (August 1991): 40–43.

Cerrato, P. "Nursing the Mind: Assessing Your Patient's Diet." 54, 1 (January 1991): 60–63.

Chernoff, R. "Physiologic Aging and Nutritional Status." *Nutrition In Clinical Practice* 5, 1 (February 1990): 8–13.

Collingsworth, R., and Boyle, K. "Nutritional Assessment of the Elderly." *Journal of Gerontological Nursing* 15, (January 1989): 17–21.

Crocker, K. S., Gerber, F., and Sherer, J. "Metabolism of Carbohydrate, Protein, and Fat." *Nursing Clinics of North America* 18, 1 (March 1983): 3–28.

Curtas, S., Chapman, G., and Megurd, M. "Evaluation of Nutritional Status." *Nursing Clinics of North America* 24, 2 (June 1989): 301–313.

DiIorio, C., and Price, M. E. "Swallowing : An Assessment and Practice Guide." *American Journal of Nursing* 90, 7 (July 1990): 38–41.

Dwyer, J. T. "Screening Older Americans' Nutritional Health: Current Practices, Future Possibilities." Washington, DC: Nutrition Screening Initiative, 1991.

Eisenberg, P. "Enteral Nutrition: Indications, Formulas, and Delivery Techniques." *Nursing Clinics of North America* 24, 2 (June 1989): 315–338.

Goodwin, J. S. "The Association Between Nutritional Status and Cognitive Functioning in a Healthy Elderly Population." *Journal of the American Medical Association* 249, 21 (June 1983): 2917–2921.

Heins, J. M., Wylie-Rosett, J., and Davis, S. G. "The New Look in Diabetic Diets." *American Journal of Nursing* 87, 2 (February 1987): 196–198.

Holmes, R., Macchiano, K., Jangiani, S. S., et al. "Combatting Pressure Sores—Nutritionally." *American Journal of Nursing* 87, 10 (October 1987): 1301–1303.

Hui, Y. H. *Principles and Issues in Nutrition.* Monterey, Calif.: Wadsworth, 1985.

Jackson, A. A. "Aminoacids: Essential and Non-essential." *The Lancet* (May 7, 1983): 1034–1039.

Johndrew, P. D. "Making Your Patient and His Family Feel at Home With T.P.N." *Nursing '88* 18, 10 (October 1988): 65–69.

Kennedy-Caldwell, C., and Hanson, M. E. "Metabolism of Vitamins and Trace Minerals." *Nursing Clinics of North America* 18, 1 (March 1983): 29–46.

Lappe, F. M. *Diet for a Small Planet.* 10th Anniversary Edition, New York: Ballantine, 1982.

Meehan, M. "Nursing Diagnosis: Potential for Aspiration." *RN* 55, 1 (January, 1992): 30–34.

National Research Council, Committee on Diet and Health, Food and Nutrition Board. *Diet and Health: Implications for Reducing Chronic Disease Risk.* Washington, D.C.: National Academy of Sciences, 1989.

National Research Council, Committee on Dietary Allowances, Food and Nutrition Board. *Recommended Dietary Allowances.* 10th edition. Washington, D.C.: National Academy of Sciences, 1989.

"Nurses' Quick Guide to Nutritional Disorders." *Nursing '83* 13 (April 1983): 56–57.

"Nutrition as Factor X in Pressure Sores." *American Journal of Nursing* 88, 2 (February 1988): 156.

Pender, N. J. *Health Promotion in Nursing Practice.* 2nd edition. Norwalk, Conn.: Appleton-Lange, 1987.

Seller, B. "Strengthening Nutrition Care In Hospitals." *Nutrition In Clinical Practice* 4, 4 (April 1989): 123–124.

Senate Select Committee on Nutrition and Health. *Dietary Goals for the United States.* 2nd edition. Washington, D.C.: US Government Printing Office. 1977.

Starkey, J. F., Jefferson, P. A., and Kirby, D.F. "Taking care of Percutaneous Endoscopic Gastrostomy (PEG)." *American Journal of Nursing* 88, 1 (January 1988): 42–45.

Stewart, A. L. and Brook, R. H. "Effects of Being Overweight." *American Journal of Public Health* 73:2 (February, 1983): 171–177.

Surgeon General's Report on Nutrition and Health: Summary and Recommendations. DHHS (PHS) Publication No. 88-50211, Washington, D.C.: U.S. Government Printing Office, 1988.

U.S. Department of Health and Human Services. *Diet, Nutrition, and Cancer Prevention: A Guide To Food Choices.* Pub. No. 87-2878. Washington, D.C.: National Institutes of Health, 1987.

Walden, R. "The Relationship Of Dietary Supplemental Calcium Intake to Bone Loss and Osteoporosis." *Journal of the American Dietetic Association* 89, (1989): 397–400.

Worthington, P., and Wagner, B. "Total Parenteral Nutrition: Advances In Nutrition Support." *Nursing Clinics of North America* 24, 2 (June 1989): 355–371.

Bowel Elimination

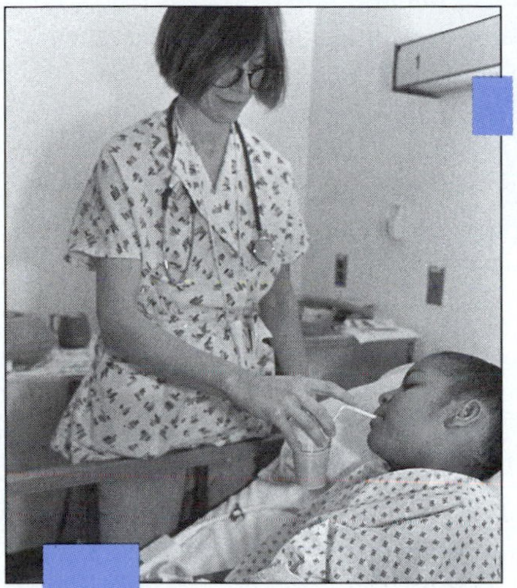

26

Objectives

After completing this chapter, you should be able to:

1. Name and describe the organs of the gastrointestinal system.
2. List the normal and abnormal characteristics of fecal material.
3. Discuss the factors that affect defecation.
4. Name and describe the various radiographic and imagery procedures used to diagnose intestinal problems.
5. Discuss the method of assessment for bowel elimination.
6. Describe appropriate nursing diagnoses for patients with problems of bowel elimination.
7. Discuss nursing actions appropriate for persons with bowel problems.
8. Explain the use of outcomes in evaluating bowel function.
9. List rehabilitation measures that can be used for persons with long-term problems related to bowel elimination.

Study Terms

bolus
chyme
colitis
colostomy
colonoscopy
endoscopy
esophagogastroduodenoscopy (EGD)
flatus
gastrocolic reflex
guaiac
ileostomy
impaction
occult blood
paralytic ileus
proctoscopy
sigmoidoscopy
steatorrhea
Valsalva maneuver

Outline

Ellis, Nowlis: Nursing: A Human Needs Approach, 5th ed. © 1994 J.B. Lippincott Company

The elimination of the waste products of digestion is a basic need of all human beings. In our society, bowel elimination is a private matter for the individual, and discussing it with others embarrasses some people. However, the topic engenders much interest; one need only listen to the radio or watch television to be reminded that "regularity" is considered highly desirable and "irregularity" is regarded as a problem. Most well individuals develop a regular pattern of bowel function although the frequency of bowel movements varies among individuals. Many factors influence regularity of normal bowel elimination. Those who are ill may view problems with the bowel as an indicator that something is wrong with the body even though the bowel problem may not be at all related to the pathology of the illness.

Nurses should both understand the patient's need for privacy to facilitate normal elimination and recognize the anxiety that problems of bowel elimination can cause. Nurses should support and comfort patients with problems, as well as develop proficiency regarding health teaching and know the appropriate procedures and medications, so that problems with defecation can be relieved.

The Gastrointestinal System

The function of the gastrointestinal system is to break down food products so that nutrients and fluid can be absorbed by the body. Those parts of food products that cannot be broken down or absorbed are then converted into solid wastes, which are collected in the intestinal tract before they are excreted as feces. Although this system includes several interrelated components, we will consider only the major parts, all of which are composed primarily of smooth muscle (Fig. 26-1). Impairment of any section can cause elimination problems.

After food or fluids have been taken into the mouth, they pass downward through a collapsible tube called the *esophagus,* through the lower gastroesophageal sphincter (called the *cardiac sphincter*), and into the stomach. The *stomach* lies slightly to the left in the upper portion of the abdominal cavity, under the liver and diaphragm. The stomach can hold up to 1,500 ml when full. When it is highly distended with food, breathing patterns may be altered due to pressure on the diaphragm.

The stomach mechanically breaks down food particles through a churning action and secretes several digestive enzymes. The main secretion is hydrochloric acid, which can cause an acidity level in the stomach of as low as 1.

The stomach does not absorb dietary nutrients except for small amounts of highly lipid-soluble substances and minimal amounts of alcohol and some drugs (Guyton, p 479, 1992). The gastric *antrum,* the long, lower curved mucosal lining of the stomach, secretes several enzymes, including gastrin, which aids breakdown of substances and aids absorption (see Chapter 25).

The emptying time for the stomach varies depending on the composition of the contents and the feedback system stemming from the stretching of the mucosa. The *pylorus* is the lowest pouchlike structure of the stomach and through the degree of contraction, the pylorus plays an important part in monitoring the emptying of gastric contents. The partially digested food particles that are

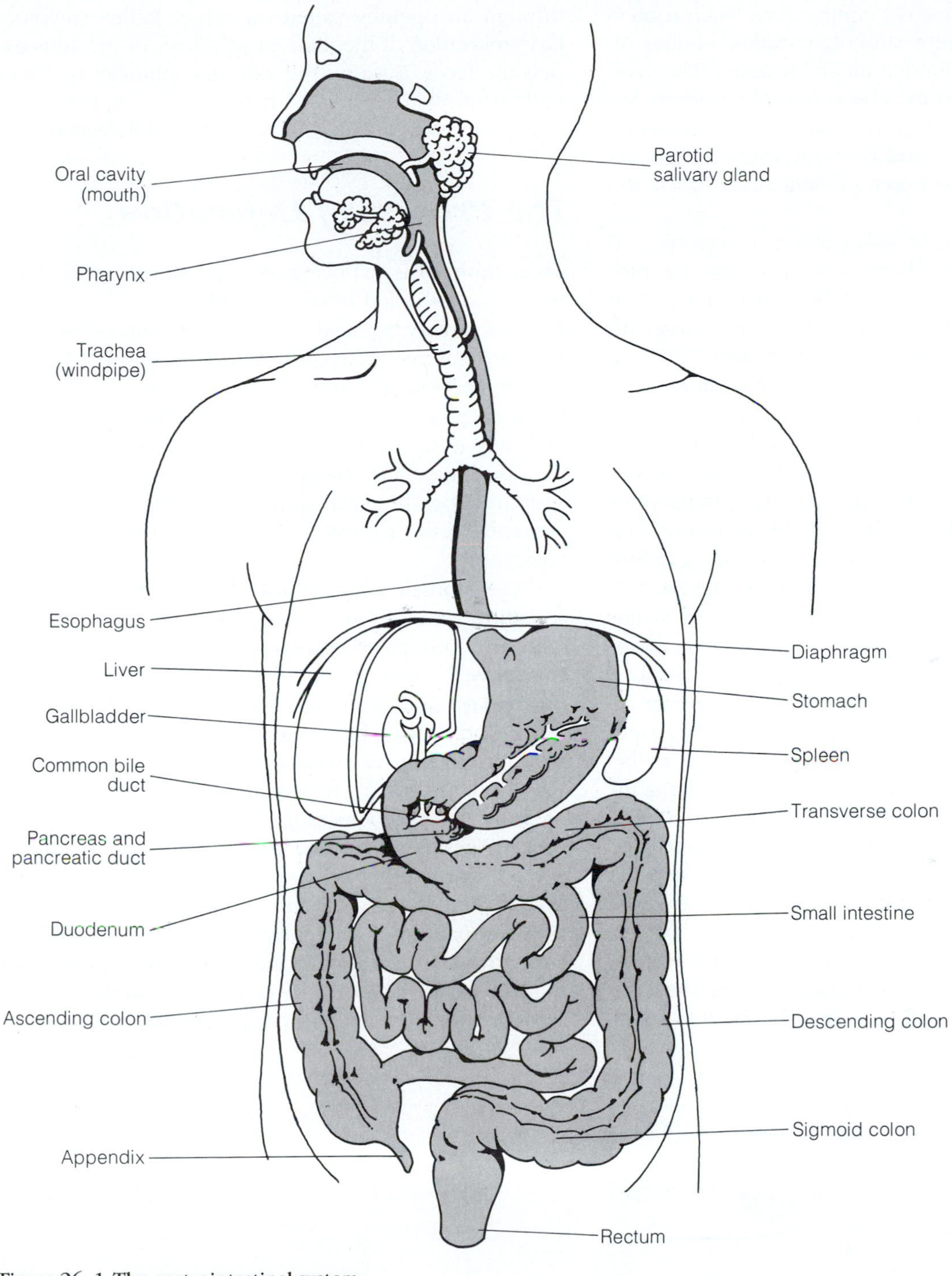

Figure 26-1. The gastrointestinal system.

mixed with the gastric secretions pass downward through the pyloric valve into the first portion of the small intestine.

The *small intestine* is a coiled tubular loop of bowel some 20 feet in length; it is composed of three parts: the *duodenum*, the *jejunum*, and the *ileum*. The duodenum is approximately 11 inches in length. The jejunum is about 8 feet in length and the ileum is 12 feet long. By the time food reaches the small intestine from the stomach it has a consistency that can be described as "gruel-like" and is called **chyme**. The small intestine has both mixing and propulsive contractions, which become stronger when food is present in the stomach. The process of stimulating intestinal contractions when food is consumed is called the gastroenteric reflex. Further digestion occurs in the duodenum and jejunum. The main function of the ileum is the absorption of nutrients. Another function of the small intestine is to absorb water from the ingested food and from enzymes. This structure absorbs 80% of the water, passing along 20% to the large intestine.

The *large intestine*, or *colon*, stores, transports, and expels waste products. These waste products are propelled along the intestinal tract by a wavelike action called *peristalsis* (Fig. 26-2). The colon has a larger diameter than the small intestine, a little over 2 inches, and is only 5 to 6 feet in length. The first portion of the large intestine is the *cecum*, a short pouchlike structure that attaches to the second part, or colon (the same term is applied to the large segment alone and to the entire large intestine). The colon ascends, transverses (crosses), and then descends, and the corresponding parts are known, respectively, as the ascending colon, transverse colon, and descending colon. In the ascending colon, additional water is absorbed. The most important function of this segment is the absorption of sodium and chloride for the maintenance of electrolyte balance. There are also bacteria present, known as colon bacilli, which through bacterial action, form such important nutrients as vitamins K and B_{12} as well as thiamine and riboflavin. The lower portion of the large intestine is the *sigmoid*, which is somewhat flexed and stores feces until expulsion. The sigmoid colon attaches to the rectum. Because much of the water has been absorbed from the small intestine, the feces in the lower colon are now normally soft but formed.

The massive movement of feces into the *rectum* from the colon by means of peristalsis stimulates the receptors in the walls of the rectum. The *rectum*, a vascular, muscular structure, expels feces out of the body through an opening called the *anus*. Reflex (involuntary) relaxation of the internal sphincter of the anus expels the feces. Because the external sphincter is voluntarily controlled, the person may strain to expel feces or relax to inhibit the sphincter to withhold defecation.

The Process of Defecation

Defecation is the expulsion of solid wastes in the form of *feces*, also called *stool*. Defecation is both voluntary and involuntary because of the mechanisms of the internal and external sphincters. The parasympathetic nervous system carries the rectal sensation of fullness to the sacral area of the spinal cord and stimulates peristalsis and muscle tone. The sympathetic nervous system has the opposing effect. The alternating effects of these two systems allow the rectal sphincter to relax and the fecal contents of the rectum and large intestine (bowel) to pass.

The normal position for defecation is sitting or squatting with the body tilted slightly forward. Persons who are constipated sometimes perform the **Valsalva maneuver**, which is done holding the breath, pushing downward, and grunting. Although this can facilitate defecation, it can be dangerous for those with high blood pressure or fragile vessels. Performing the Valsalva maneuver increases intracranial and intraocular pressure, which could cause vessels to rupture in susceptible people. If rupture occurs within the brain, the person can suffer serious complications, such as a stroke. Bleeding into the vitreous of the eye can cause visual impairment. Voluntary control can also be exerted to delay defecation. Some neuromuscular diseases prevent partial or total bowel control leading to fecal incontinence. However, developmentally, neuromuscu-

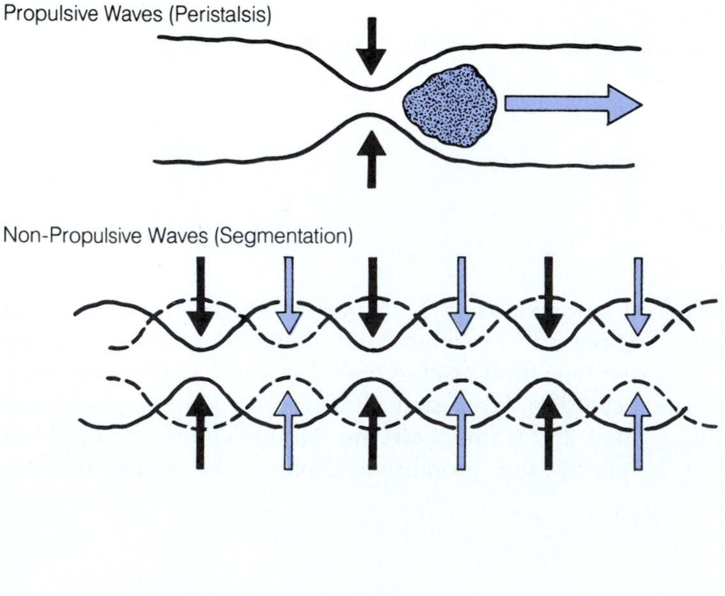

Figure 26-2. Propulsive and nonpropulsive waves in the intestine.

lar maturity, which occurs by age 3, allows most children to have control of bowel function (Murray and Zentner, 1989).

Normal Characteristics of Fecal Material

Unlike urine, fecal material is not sterile; it contains bacteria that make up the normal flora of the intestinal tract. Knowing the characteristics of the feces, like those of the urine, can help in assessment of the patient's state of homeostasis.

The *consistency* of fecal material is normally soft but formed. It contains approximately three parts of water to one part of waste material. The water content determines the firmness of the stool. Patients who have fever or are dehydrated may have less water in the stool, causing the stool to be hard. It is important to know the characteristics of normal fecal material to be able to identify patient problems when making assessments (Fig. 26-3).

The *color* of feces is usually variations of brown, the color caused by bilirubin in the form of bile salts excreted by the liver. The intake of iron preparations can give the feces a black appearance; the black color is undigested iron because only a portion of an oral iron preparation is absorbed from the digestive tract. Foods can also influence color. Green vegetables may lend a green tint to the stool, and beets give feces a reddish color.

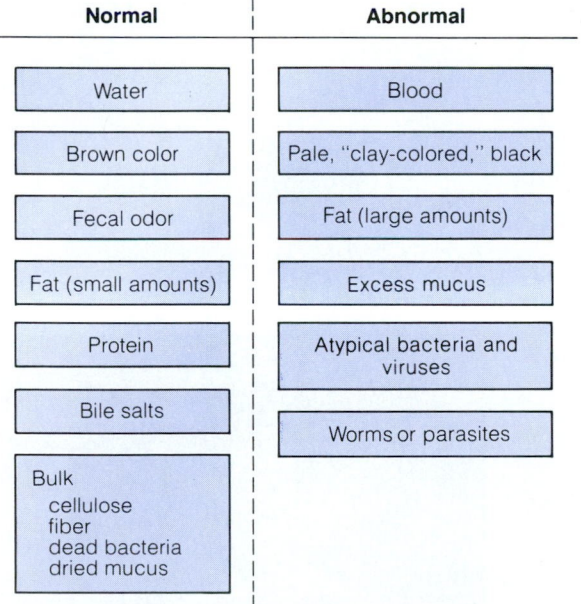

Normal	Abnormal
Water	Blood
Brown color	Pale, "clay-colored," black
Fecal odor	Fat (large amounts)
Fat (small amounts)	Excess mucus
Protein	Atypical bacteria and viruses
Bile salts	Worms or parasites
Bulk cellulose fiber dead bacteria dried mucus	

Figure 26-3. Normal and abnormal components of feces.

The characteristic *odor* of feces is unpleasant and is produced by the by-products of bacterial action. Odors vary with different individuals depending on the amount and type of bacteria present and the food ingested.

Undigested *fat and protein* normally appear in small amounts in the feces. When the diet is high in fat or protein content, the feces will contain more of that component.

Flatulence is the presence of excessive gas in the bowel. **Flatus** refers to the gas itself. A certain amount of gas in the intestines is normal. The most common causes are swallowing air and ingesting gas-forming foods such as cabbage and beans. Some individuals form intestinal gas from other more specific food products. The action of intestinal bacteria on food residue within the digestive tract produces the gas. The small intestine has the ability to absorb gas. If flatulence is a concern, it can be managed by eliminating foods that cause gas. Changing position and increasing activity can help in expelling the gas through the anus.

Basically, intestinal gas comes from three sources: swallowed air, gas created by bacterial action, and gas that passes into the intestinal tract from the blood by diffusion. Some medications such as the bulk laxatives can cause excessive gas by this action in the bowel.

Bulk—the waste product of digestion—is composed primarily of cellulose and fiber. Approximately one-third of the solid waste portion of feces is bulk. Dead bacteria and sloughed off epithelial cells are also present.

Abnormal Components of Fecal Material

The presence of *blood* in feces is abnormal. However, if a person eats a large quality of rare, red meat, the feces may be slightly blood tinged, meaning that undigested blood from the meat is being normally eliminated. Sometimes the blood cannot be seen in this situation so that it is called occult or hidden. Other than this situation, the presence of bright red, fresh blood indicates bleeding low in the intestinal tract. Old (coagulated) blood, which appears black, may have come from a source high in the intestinal tract and gone through the process of digestion.

Feces of an *abnormal color* may indicate disease. Pale "clay-colored" stools occur when bile salts are not being excreted into the intestine by the liver. Dark stools may be caused by increased bilirubin due to liver impairment. Assessment should be made of any stool that has a different color than brown.

Excessive gas in the stomach or intestinal tract is considered abnormal because it can cause symptoms and pressure on tissues. When this happens, the patient is said to be distended. If gas is not relieved in the stomach by eructation (belching), it can pass downward into the intestines. There, it is expelled through the anus.

Postoperative patients often complain of "gas pains." Either the manipulation of the intestines during surgery or any decreased motility of the bowel from medications or lack of exercise can lead to gas build-up in these situations.

Certain diseases impair the ability to absorb dietary fat. When this occurs, the fecal material contains large amounts of undigested *fat*, resulting in a condition called **steatorrhea**. Steatorrhea is caused by malabsorption of fats so that large amounts of fat are contained in the feces. Such stools have a foul odor, are "frothy," and have an oily, fatty appearance. The malabsorption that gives rise to steatorrhea can result from such diseases as sprue. Sprue can be a tropical disease. It can also be nontropical and is called celiac disease. Children with celiac disease have an intolerance for gluten and require special diets (see Chapter 25). Inflammation of the colon, **colitis**, is characterized by the presence of large amounts of *mucus* in the feces. The mucus is caused by inflammation of the bowel. Colitis is often accompanied by diarrhea and cramping.

In cases of intestinal infection, *atypical bacteria or viruses* can be found in the fecal matter. These organisms are not of the variety that make up the normal flora of the intestinal tract. Finally, the warmth and nourishment provided by the intestinal environment invite infestation if a person is exposed to parasites or worms. Many of these organisms can be seen without the aid of a microscope. People in many countries throughout the world are infested with parasites or worms and because of long-term exposure, tolerate this infestation to some degree. With the opportunity for more worldwide travel, more persons in North America will become infected.

Factors Affecting Defecation

A variety of factors affect defecation; they may be negative or positive. Through health teaching, nurses can assist the patient in achieving bowel activity as near normal as is possible.

Age

Most children voluntarily control defecation by the end of the third year. Bowel control usually precedes urinary control, primarily because the urge for defecation is stronger so that the child can more easily anticipate bowel elimination (Whaley and Wong, 1993). However, toilet training is not a simple matter. Dynamics between the toddler and the parents may create a psychological conflict so that the youngster gains a control factor in adjusting to the process.

Peristalsis is increasingly active through the years of childhood and early adulthood, so diarrhea is more likely to be a problem during these years than is constipation. Because defecation patterns are individual, the number of stools within a day or week may vary from person to person. Some adults consider one regular bowel movement per day as normal, whereas others may have a bowel movement only every 3 days. If the person is eating normally and appears and feels well, the bowel pattern is one of only individual variation. Another age-related factor is that many older adults have been raised in a era that equated regularity with well-being. Many of these individuals were "dosed" with laxatives unnecessarily, leading to a lifelong dependence on these preparations. Older adults may also have more problems with elimination because of a lack of dietary fiber, inactivity, and decreased muscle strength.

Pregnancy

The pressure placed on the rectum by the increasing size of the fetus often causes temporary problems with constipation. For a short period after delivery, this may continue to be a concern. A related problem for the pregnant women is that straining at stool can produce hemorrhoids, which decrease in size after delivery but may be permanent. Harsh laxatives should not be taken during pregnancy because of the risk of starting premature labor in some women.

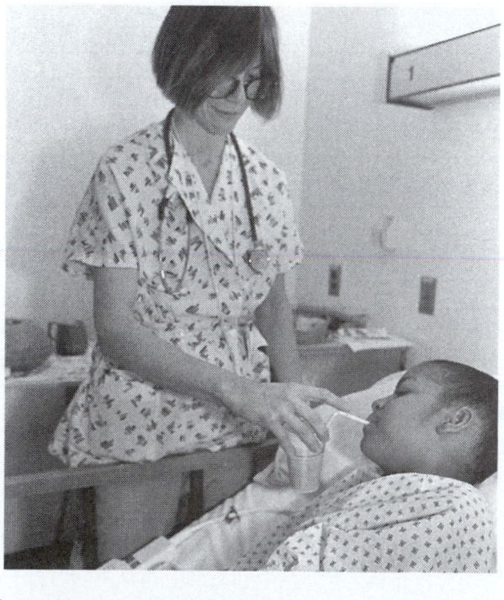

Figure 26-4. Sufficient fluid intake is necessary for proper elimination.

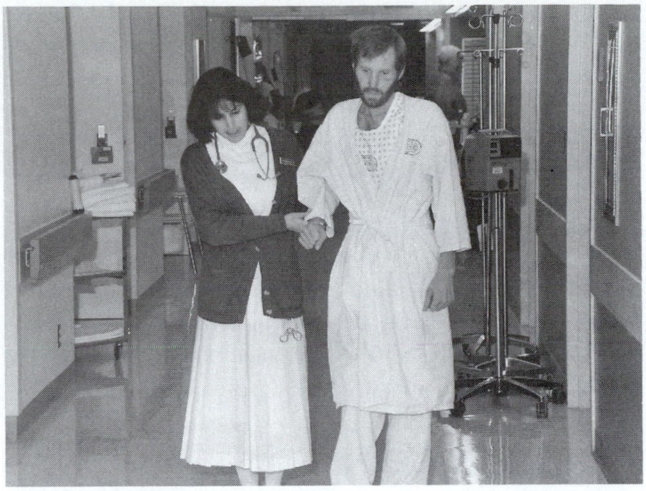

Figure 26-5. Early ambulation after surgery promotes return of normal elimination.

Fluid Intake

Because fecal waste material contains so much water, any decrease in fluid intake or body fluid will cause dryness or hardening of the stool, which makes it difficult to pass. Dehydration can be caused by fever, persistent vomiting, excessive diaphoresis, or bleeding, which depletes the body of fluids so that the stool hardens. The small intestine continues its function of removing water from chyme so that unless fluid is replaced by an increase in the patient's fluid intake, constipation results. Each adult should drink at least 2,000 ml of fluid per day for proper elimination (Fig. 26-4).

Exercise

The amount and type of exercise has a direct effect on bowel function. With exercise, not only does general muscle tone improve but the intestinal muscle layers maintain their elasticity, which encourages peristalsis to take place. When patients are on bed rest or when people have a sedentary lifestyle, they are at risk for poor bowel function.

For some individuals, activity or exercise immediately increases peristalsis so that exercise has an immediate effect on the bowel, causing defecation. Regular bowel habits may include eating a meal and then taking a walk before bowel elimination.

Early ambulation for postoperative patients also promotes regaining effective bowel elimination (Fig. 26-5). An exercise program should be set up for ambulatory patients as well as for bed patients. Bed patients can be taught to perform bed exercises which, although limited in value, are effective in helping regularity for the immobile person.

Diet

Fecal elimination is directly related to diet (Fig. 26-6). Lack of fiber, which characterizes bland or liquid diets, usually causes diarrhea because the substances ingested pass through the intestinal tract rapidly. Certain patients develop constipation because of stagnation of the waste material in the tract. Fiber can be obtained in the diet by including sufficient amounts of raw and cooked vegetables and fruits as well as whole-grain cereal products. Cooked fruits, such as prunes, peaches, or apricots, have long been a part of the diet of many older people. They have recently been added, along with raisins and nuts, to many dry prepared cereals eaten by younger people and will both add bulk to the diet and maintain adequate bowel elimination. Current studies in nutrition substantiate the importance of fiber in the diet because the benefits of increased fiber content for regular bowel elimination are clear.

Gastrocolic Reflex

Closely allied with diet or food intake is the body's natural stimulus for defecation, the **gastrocolic reflex**. After a meal, when the walls of the stomach are "stretched," there is a reflex stimulation for the bowel to empty. The normal individual feels the urge to defecate. This mechanism makes the period after consuming a meal the best time to plan defecation. In addition, knowing about the gastrocolic reflex is helpful in providing for patients' elimination needs. Many persons find the time after breakfast best for this purpose. In

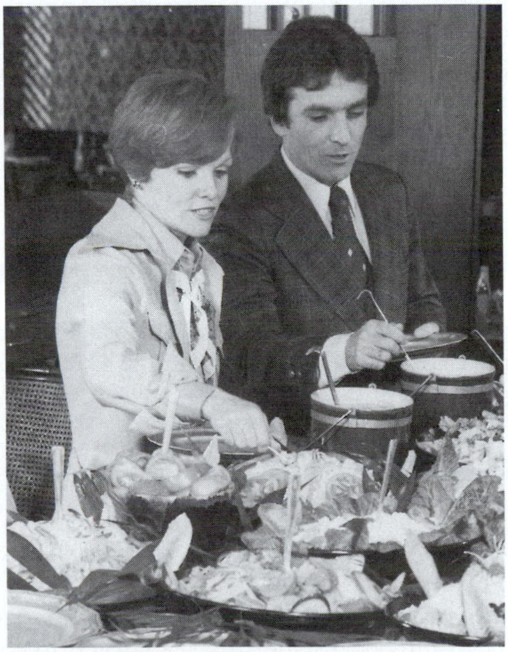

Figure 26-6. Regular elimination is directly related to diet.

addition, the gastrocolic reflex should be taken into consideration when planning bowel rehabilitation for the disabled client. The use of *suppositories* or rectal stimulation is more effective if used in conjunction with this body reflex.

Medications

The effects of drugs on the ability to defecate and on stool consistency have long been known. Some drugs, such as the antibiotics, may cause diarrhea in certain individuals because these drugs not only destroy harmful organisms within the body, but they also destroy the normal bacteria present in the bowel.

Other medications, such as the psychotropic drugs, iron preparations, and some commonly used medications for pain, such as codeine and morphine, can cause constipation. Occasionally, the effect of a drug on defecation cannot be predicted because of individual idiosyncracy to a particular preparation. Your knowledge of the side effects of cathartics, laxatives, and antidiarrheal drugs will help you identify patient problems arising from the administration of these agents.

Bowel Habits

Many people find that the greatest problem for normal bowel functioning is lack of time. In a busy society with many demands, it is often difficult to find sufficient time for elimination. Bowel habits should be attended to on a regular schedule, often after a meal to take advantage of the gastrocolic reflex. Ideally, there should be uninterrupted time to allow the bowel to function spontaneously. For the patient in the hospital, the lack of privacy, the close proximity of others, and interruption for care adversely affect elimination. These interruptions of usual bowel habits are often complicated by having to take bowel-altering medications, poor intake of fiber, lack of activity, and the anxiety or depression experienced because of illness.

Unnatural positions like sitting on a bedpan can also be an obstacle to normal defecation. The best posture for defecation is sitting in a slightly bent position on a toilet with the ability to perform the Valsalva maneuver unless the medical condition contraindicates this action.

Emotions

As we mentioned previously, stress and the emotions can directly affect defecation. Although the effect of the emotions on bowel function is not simple, it has been suggested that overstimulation of the parasympathetic nervous system because of stress results in diarrhea; excessive stimulation of the sympathetic nervous system results in constipation. Studies show that both chronic and acute constipation and diarrhea are some times caused by emotional factors.

Common Disorders Affecting Bowel Elimination

Although several conditions of the bowel require medical treatment, the need for medical intervention may depend on the severity of the condition. Some of these conditions require surgery.

Paralytic Ileus

A medical condition that interferes with normal defecation is paralytic ileus. This is really an uncommon complication that can occur after surgery. **Paralytic ileus** is an abnormal loss of bowel motility. It is most common following surgery and believed to be related to the handling of the intestines during the surgical procedure. Normally, for 12 to 24 hours after surgery, there may be no evidence of bowel sounds, but these should resume spontaneously. Paralytic ileus may also be caused by some drugs and severe shock. The patient with paralytic ileus may experience lack of bowel tones, distention, fever, and electrolyte imbalance. The nurse must notify the physician when this condition is detected because medical intervention is needed. If used for a nursing care plan, it is written as Potential complication: paralytic ileus.

Hemorrhoids

Hemorrhoids are engorged veins that can be outside (external) or inside (internal) the anus. They are intermittently painful and may cause itching or bleeding.

The cause may be long-term straining at stool or pregnancy, which causes additional pressure on the area. In jobs that require sitting for long periods of time, hemorrhoids can occur due to venous stasis in the area. Occasionally, individuals can have a familial tendency for hemorrhoids to occur.

Intestinal Disease and Obstruction

Several other medical conditions can alter patterns of elimination. Because intestinal disease problems and obstruction are medical diagnoses, your nursing diagnoses will be collaborative, listing those concerns that result from the medical diagnosis.

Tumors within the intestinal passage can narrow the passage, interfere with defecation, and cause bleeding. Structural conditions such as loss of tone in the intestinal wall and partial or complete obstruction interfere with the passage of solid waste products. Damage to the brain or spinal cord can interrupt nerve impulses, causing either fecal retention or fecal diversion. Also, neuromuscular diseases can interfere with normal elimination patterns. Inflammatory or infectious conditions, various types of colitis, and the presence of parasites can change intestinal function.

When a portion of the intestine is diseased, it is sometimes necessary for the patient to have a resection in which a part of the intestine is surgically removed. If the rectum is removed, a *fecal diversion* must be devised so that the feces can be expelled. This procedure is called a **colostomy** because after the colon or the rectum is removed, a portion of the colon is brought to the abdominal surface and a stoma is constructed for the passage of feces. If the colon is also not able to function or is removed, the ileum may be brought to the surface forming an **ileostomy**. Stool from an ileostomy is usually more liquid and its movement is more constant than normal because less water has been absorbed from this segment. Feces from a colostomy has a more solid consistency, so that the patient can gain some control over defecation, which facilitates ease of management. With fecal diversion, skin care and health teaching are important responsibilities of the nurse. For more about care of the person with a fecal diversion, consult Module 38, Ostomy Care.

Assessment

Many factors enter into assessment of defecation; the information gathered is both subjective and objective.

Review of the Record

The patient's record will give you information on the current illness and the history of any other elimination problems in the past. The patient's current *diagnosis* is also crucial to assessment. Past or present abdominal or pelvic surgery has a direct effect on defecation because of the mechanical manipulation of the intestinal structures. For example, a patient with ulcerative colitis is observed and assessed for the frequency and character of stools and for intestinal bleeding.

Potential Complications for Bowel Elimination

Potential complication: paralytic ileus

Potential complication: gastrointestinal bleeding

You should also know the patient's *medication orders*. Patients in the hospital often have standing orders for a laxative or an antidiarrheal drug to be provided at the discretion of the nurse, depending on the patient's problem.

Interview

A private interview with the patient is helpful in determining subjective data. The following information should be obtained:

1. When was the last bowel movement and was it normal or abnormal?
2. What is the usual frequency of bowel movements?
3. What bowel problems have existed in the past, if any?
4. Has there been any illness that affected bowel patterns or any intestinal surgery performed?
5. Have laxatives been taken, and if so, what kind and how often?
6. What type of diet has been helpful in promoting bowel elimination?
7. How much exercise does the patient participate in on a regular basis and is any relationship noted between exercise and bowel elimination?
8. Have there been changes in bowel elimination or recent problems?
9. How does the patient perceive current bowel functioning effectiveness?

Physical Assessment

Objective data are also important in that they can either validate the patient's perceptions or add new information. Several factors should be considered in objective assessment of defecation.

The patient's *level of activity* is important because a patient who is immobilized or on bed rest is prone to constipation. Lack of exercise diminishes the tone of the intestinal wall.

You will often be able to directly observe the *characteristics of stool*. Reviewing the earlier section on normal and abnormal contents of feces is helpful in this part of assessment. Stools are usually described as small, moderate or medium, or large, although you may want a more explicit description in some cases. To describe consistency, terms such as formed, semiformed, and liquid are used. Unusual odor or color, such as green, yellow, or clay colored, should be noted when they occur. Occasionally, a stool requires such special terms as frothy, or mucoid (containing unusually large amounts of mucus). You would also observe stools for any unusual or foreign substances.

An important assessment procedure is for you to

listen for the presence or absence of bowel sounds, also called *bowel tones* (BT) in all four quadrants of the abdomen. With the umbilicus as a center of two imaginary lines, listen through a stethoscope over each of the quadrants. Audible "gurgling" sounds should be heard, which means that peristalsis is occurring. If no sounds can be heard or you hear only diminished sounds, a medical disorder may be present and your assessment should be reported.

Diagnostic Testing

A variety of procedures can be ordered by the physician to identify abnormalities of the upper or lower intestinal tract. You should be aware of what tests your patients are having, the significance of those tests, and any necessary nursing actions. Some of these procedures use x-ray or scanning devices; others involve direct visualization through scopes.

Stool Specimens

One important task of the nurse is the collection of stool specimens for purposes of examination of the feces. Examination of stool specimens in the laboratory is an adjunct to diagnosis of a patient's medical status. Tests for the presence of visible *blood* in the stool or **occult blood** (hidden or invisible) in the stool can be done using one of a variety of commercial preparations. Although the resin **guaiac** is no longer contained in many of these preparations, the test for blood in the feces is still commonly referred to as the "guaiac" test. This test is performed by the nurse on the unit. Tests for parasites require that the stool specimens be sent to the laboratory promptly or kept warm so that any parasites present will be viable and observable. Stool cultures reveal the presence or absence of unusual bacteria. It is the nurse's responsibility to see that stool specimens are collected and cared for properly (see Module 18, Collecting Specimens).

Tests Using Radiography or Imagery

Upper Gastrointestinal X-ray (UGI). This test is carried out after the patient swallows a *barium* sulfate solution. The barium, because it is radiopaque, can be seen by x-ray. Strictures, tumors, bleeding, and ulcer formation are some of the conditions that can be detected with upper gastrointestinal inspection. Barium has a tendency to harden in the intestinal tract. To avoid hardening, the person is given cathartics after the examination to facilitate elimination of the barium to prevent constipation.

Lower Gastrointestinal X-ray (LGI). This x-ray examination of the colon is also referred to as the barium enema. The entire colon can be visualized. Strictures, obstruction, diverticuli, and tumors can be detected. Cathartics are also given to rid the body of the barium and prevent constipation.

Computed Axial Tomography (CAT). Using a computerized x-ray, this procedure is considered noninvasive unless a dye is injected for improved visualization. When serious intestinal illness is considered a possibility, the physician may order a CAT scan for a portion of the intestinal tract. This is an expensive procedure but helpful in identifying strictures, obstructions, and the presence of growths.

Magnetic Resonance Imaging (MRI). Another scanning procedure that can be used to observe the gastrointestinal tract is the MRI, which creates a magnetic field around the patient so that a special process can produce a detailed outline of the structures being studied. MRI is not used as commonly as is the CAT scanner for intestinal problems. However, it is helpful in identifying extension of tumor masses within the intestinal system.

Tests Using Direct Visualization of the Intestinal Tract

Observation into any orifice by use of a tube is considered **endoscopy**. One kind of endoscopy is the **esophagogastroduodenoscopy** (**EGD**). This test is an examination of the esophagus, stomach, and duodenum using a scope. During the examination, the person is watched carefully for respiratory difficulties or laryngospasm, a potentially serious complication of the procedure. After the test, the patient may have a mildly sore throat and will have to eat a soft diet for a short period of time.

Direct visualization of the colon is accomplished by performing a colonoscopy. The colonoscopy is increasingly replacing the LGI x-ray. **Colonoscopy** is a procedure in which the physician passes a fiberoptic scope through the entire colon with the patient mildly sedated. Although this test is time consuming for the physician, it provides a view of all segments of the colon for identification of any possible pathology. Lesions of many types can be seen, biopsies secured, and simple resections performed.

The sigmoidoscopy is carried out after the lower bowel contents have been evacuated. This procedure is usually done without sedation. **Sigmoidoscopy** makes use of a shorter scope than the one used with colonoscopy to examine the sigmoid portion of the colon. This test is limited in its application.

Proctoscopy is a procedure for examining the rectum using a lighted scope. The data this procedure can gather are limited so that this test is rarely used. Other procedures such as sigmoidoscopy and colonoscopy are of much greater value for diagnostic purposes.

Nursing Diagnosis

Alteration in Elimination is an approved NANDA category. However, Carpenito (1992) states that this is often a much too broad category for clinical use. Some nurses include the specific system in the category for clarification so that the nursing diagnosis becomes Alteration in Bowel Elimination and then, the specific problem such as constipation and the etiology are added. An etiology statement adds specificity to the diagnosis of constipation. The condition might be due to bed rest or side effects of medications. Another example—Alteration in Bowel Elimination: Constipation related to pain medications—would clearly state the patient's problem.

Bowel Incontinence

Bowel Incontinence is an approved nursing diagnosis that means that the patient has thc inability to control defecation. Although the term does not describe the characteristics of the stool, it is usually more liquid than solid in consistency. A variety of physical conditions can cause this problem. Most common are stroke, spinal cord injury, and other conditions that interfere with the function of the nerves that partially control defecation. Severe mental disorders may also be a cause of the nursing diagnosis of bowel incontinence. Whatever the circumstances, this loss of control leading to involuntary expulsion of feces can be extremely upsetting and embarrassing to the patient.

Constipation

Constipation is one of the most common nursing diagnoses of the intestinal system when there is retention of fecal material within the rectum. This condition is not a disease. There are several parameters for identifying a patient's constipation.

It may be characterized merely by a hardening of the fecal material, which interferes with easy passage or by the lack of stool for a prolonged period due to the build-up of feces in the rectum. It is important to keep in mind the person's usual pattern of defecation. For example, when patients usually defecate daily, an absence of stool for several days for them represents constipation; if persons defecate less frequently, more days must elapse before they consider themselves constipated. A nursing diagnosis should only be written if the constipation is perceived as a problem.

Many nurses are concerned when patients do not have regular bowel movements after surgery, disregarding the fact that these patients may have had surgical preparation that included evacuation of bowel contents, and they may have been on a nothing-by-mouth (NPO) status and have not been eating regularly for several days. In this situation, there simply is not sufficient food or bulk to form fecal contents and it is understandable that the patient is not having bowel movements.

Constipation may also be caused by inactivity. It may also be caused by dietary factors such as inadequate fluids and fiber.

Constipation is also the side effect of many commonly used pain medications given to patients experiencing pain.

Patients with an *intermittent constipation* report having hard, difficult-to-pass stools at intervals, with normal or diarrheal stools in between. This condition is most often related to neuromuscular disease, emotional tension, the intake of various foods, or to spastic colon. If this condition persists for any length of time, a physician should be consulted.

Impaction is a different and more severe condition than constipation: a fecal **bolus**, or rounded stone-hard stool, becomes lodged in the lower bowel and cannot be passed. Although impaction most frequently afflicts the elderly patient, it can occur in a person of any age, particularly in those immobilized.

The patient may have frequent small amounts of liquid stool because of seepage around the irritation of the hard stool mass. To assess for an impaction in the lower bowel, you can put on a clean glove and insert a lubricated finger into the rectum, feeling for and possibly breaking up and removing an impaction. When the impaction is high in the bowel, removal is not possible. A high impaction will usually eventually move downward, where it can be felt and removed. Although impaction is not an approved NANDA nursing diagnosis, it is a problem that nurses identify and treat. It both alters the pattern of elimination and can cause pain so a nursing diagnosis related to impaction is appropriate.

Nursing Diagnoses Related to Defecation

- High Risk for Constipation related to immobilization
- Pain related to retention of intestinal gas
- Constipation
- Diarrhea
- Bowel Incontinence
- Pain: Abdominal related to constipation
- Diarrhea related to the patient's expressed feelings of stress
- Self-toileting Deficit related to extreme fatigue and weakness

Diarrhea

Diarrhea is the frequent and involuntary passage of unformed or liquid stool that can become so profuse that the frequency of defecation becomes intolerable. The most common causes of diarrhea are infection, various food items, and emotional stress. Diarrhea is a particularly troublesome and serious complication for some persons with acquired immunodeficiency syndrome, who report up to 40 bowel movements a day.

Fluid Volume Deficit

The patient with profound, unrelenting diarrhea who cannot drink adequate fluids to offset the fluid loss may develop fluid volume deficit. A nursing diagnosis of High Risk for Fluid Volume Deficit would be appropriate for the person with diarrhea so that measures can be taken to prevent this situation from occurring.

Impaired Skin Integrity

Impaired Skin Integrity is often present in those with diarrhea, because of excoriation, or redness and irritation, of the skin in the rectal area. Breaks in the skin around the anus can lead to pain and infection.

Pain

Pain related to bowel elimination problems may occur. For example, Abdominal Pain related to retained flatus is a nursing diagnosis that would suggest specific nursing actions that could relieve the discomfort. Pain may also be related to cramping that occurs in conjunction with either constipation or diarrhea. Other bowel conditions can cause pain. The most common nursing diagnosis related to *hemorrhoids* is Altered Comfort: Pain related to the presence of hemorrhoids. There may also be diagnoses related to interference in defecation, primarily because the person may delay defecation out of fear of pain.

Other Nursing Diagnoses

Many other nursing diagnoses might be present for patient problems of the intestinal system. Psychological problems can also be incorporated into nursing diagnoses. Some people may be hesitant to ambulate, knowing it will promote elimination, because they fear they may urgently need to use the bathroom.

The patient experiencing constipation may be quite anxious, which further complicates the problem. The person with severe diarrhea may have a problem with fatigue and altered rest and sleep. Following a thorough assessment, many of the nursing diagnoses for defecation problems can also include risk states.

Planning and Implementation

Regardless of the specific nursing diagnosis or risk state, it is imperative that appropriate outcome criteria be established on which evaluation of the plan can be made. The outcome criteria may emphasize prevention of bowel problems or the restoration of the person's usual normal bowel pattern.

As a nurse, you will encounter a variety of types of intestinal dysfunction. By far the most common are constipation and diarrhea. It is not unusual for a patient to experience alternating episodes of constipation and diarrhea during an illness. The nurse must vary nursing actions in response to the immediate situation.

Environment Conducive to Elimination

Your plan of care should allow the patient sufficient time and privacy for bowel elimination. The many interruptions that occur in the hospital setting are not conducive to regular bowel habits. The patient may have to forgo the urge for defecation because a test or procedure has been planned at that time. The nurse can sometimes schedule or delay an interruption so that the patient can fulfill elimination needs. Above all, providing time and privacy are the most important nursing actions to facilitate adequate bowel elimination.

Nursing Actions for Preventing and Treating Constipation

Changes in Daily Living

Preventing and correcting constipation may only involve persons' making simple changes in their lives. Regular exercise, maintaining a high fluid intake, and increasing bulk in the diet are effective for most individuals. Stress reduction is also effective in preventing constipation. Decreasing anxiety and depression is particularly important because bowel function is so closely related to emotional factors. Depression can cause constipation, whereas anxiety can cause bouts of diarrhea. Most patients understandably have some degree of anxiety about being ill and the hospital environment so that normal defecation becomes difficult (see sample Nursing Care Plan Related to Constipation).

Administration of Laxatives

A common means of managing constipation is through the use of *cathartics* or *laxatives*. Many people buy over-the-counter products that they use on a continuing basis. Unless specially prescribed by the physician,

Nursing Care Plan
Sample Nursing Care Plan Related to Constipation

Nursing Diagnosis

Constipation related to bed rest, insufficient oral fluid intake, and lack of fiber in diet

Supportive data:

51-year-old woman.

Admitted with chest pain on bed rest, now on bathroom privileges.

Has not had a bowel movement since admission 3 days ago.

History of constipation.

Fluid intake averages 1,400 ml in 24 h.

Eats few fresh fruits and vegetables.

Desired Patient Outcomes

Short term:

For patient to have a soft formed stool within 24 h.

For patient to have a bowel movement every 1 to 2 days while in hospital.

Long term:

For constipation to disappear.

Regular bowel movements every 1 to 2 days.

Nursing Action	Rationale
1. Obtain an order for a small volume enema.	A small volume enema is effective in removing feces from the colon and is more comfortable for the patient than is a large volume enema.
2. Teach patient regarding increasing fluids and eating more foods with fiber.	Because fiber absorbs water which softens feces and increases its bulk, fluid must be increased so that this absorption process can take place. Patient knowledge will increase compliance.
3. Increase oral fluids to at least 2,500 ml in 24 h.	The basic fluid recommendation is 1,500–1,900 ml/24 hrs. 2,500 ml provides extra fluid to combat hard or dry stools.
4. Consult nutritionist for increased fiber content in diet.	Nutritionist may provide ways for increasing fiber in the diet which are acceptable and individualized for the patient.
5. Encourage patient to use bathroom after breakfast for defecation each morning.	The gastrocolic reflex causes normal emptying of the colon to occur after meals. More fecal material is contained in the colon after the sleeping hours than at other times in the day.
6. Discuss with physician possible use of stool softener during hospitalization.	The use of stool softeners aids fecal water absorption.

laxatives should be used only infrequently as the principal treatment for constipation because of their habit-forming and irritating characteristics. If this use can be avoided by improving the fluid and fiber content of the diet, it is best to do so, because the intestine becomes dependent on the laxative and, over time, ceases to respond as well, often causing the person to move on to using a stronger agent. Sometimes, when persons in such a situation enter a health care facility, the physician will write an order for them to take or be given their "laxative of choice."

Some general guidelines for treatment are that if the patient who is eating does not have a normal stool within the usual time period for that patient, an ordered laxative is administered. NANDA's defining characteristic is less than three times per week.

The terms *cathartic* and *laxative* are often used interchangeably. However, cathartics have a more intense effect than do laxatives. Both groups of agents treat constipation by causing evacuation of feces from the bowel. Cathartics and laxatives are grouped into four general categories according to the nature of their action: saline cathartics, irritant cathartics, emollient laxatives, and bulk-forming laxatives.

Saline cathartics are sodium, potassium, or magnesium salts. These salts cause the bowel to retain more water, which makes the feces more liquid and increases peristalsis.

Irritant cathartics, through contact with the mucosa, set up an irritation that stimulates peristalsis of the smooth muscle. Because the movement and peristalsis can be active, this group of cathartics can cause cramping and diarrhea with some individuals.

Emollient laxatives are also called stool softeners. They are effective with the kinds of constipation problems experienced by older persons and those who have decreased activity following surgery. Their use also prevents straining at stool. Basically, emollient laxatives soften the consistency of the stool and allow easier passage.

Bulk-forming laxatives are usually natural products, primarily polysaccharides and cellulose. They combine with the water in the intestine to increase bulk. The increase in fecal bulk increases the peristalsis and hastens evacuation.

Keeping the stool soft to avoid straining is the best prevention and treatment of hemorrhoids. This may be done through diet or through stool-softening medications. Some persons who have hemorrhoids use ointments that provide an anesthetic effect. These commercial products can make the person more comfortable, but they do not correct the condition. When patients in the hospital experience pain caused by the presence of hemorrhoids, the application of heat and medications ordered by the physician are often used to relieve the symptoms. If bleeding occurs or the pain and swelling is not resolved with conservative measures, surgical removal may become necessary.

Administration of Enemas

If a patient is constipated and does not have a normal stool for 4 to 5 days, an enema may be needed. There is sometimes a standing order for an enema or an order should be obtained. If the constipation is temporary or uncomplicated, you may administer one of the prepackaged, disposable enema preparations. A small-volume enema of tap water or saline can be used to correct temporary constipation. Soap water enemas were commonly used at one time but are now rarely given because the soap irritates the bowel tissue.

If the patient has an impaction, an oil-retention enema is frequently administered to soften the hardened feces and lubricate the intestinal wall. This facilitates passage of the feces. After the oil-retention enema, a

Nursing Issues and Trends: *The Excessive Use of Laxatives*

Commercial promotion in the media stresses the importance of "being regular" which not only raises the awareness of people about the importance of daily bowel elimination but can also raise anxiety. Studies reveal that normal bowel habits of individuals vary greatly but there continues to be emphasis on daily elimination. This may require taking over-the-counter laxatives on a regular basis. It is also true that the majority of laxatives purchased in this country are purchased by those of advanced age whose past life may have included the frequent taking of laxatives. Other options for the treatment of constipation should be recognized. These include maintaining a fiber-rich diet, an adequate fluid intake, regular exercise, and reducing stress. Including these as part of life may make the use of laxatives, if necessary, more appropriate or greatly decrease their use.

cleansing enema may be ordered. If this procedure is not successful, the impaction may need to be broken up and removed with a gloved, lubricated finger.

In the hospital, if the presence of gas causes pain or the person becomes distended, a return-flow enema is sometimes administered to remove gas. Ambulation also helps the person to pass the gas through the anus. For patients who cannot control defecation, either partially or completely because of age or illness, the nurse can provide help in several ways. Assisting the patient to the toilet after meals if possible promotes elimination, as does a diet containing adequate fiber and fluid. Always

Nursing Care Plan
Sample Nursing Care Plan Related to Diarrhea

Nursing Diagnosis

Diarrhea related to gastroenteritis

Supportive data:

31-year-old man.

Admitted with gastroenteritis, symptoms of nausea, and diarrhea.

No longer nauseated, but having five to six liquid stools in 24 h.

Desired Patient Outcomes

Short term:

For liquid stools to be no more than two in 24 h.

For stools to become more formed.

Long term:

For diarrhea to disappear.

For patient to resume normal pattern of one formed stool per day.

Nursing Action	Rationale
1. Allow patient to select from bland diet foods that are appetizing to him.	Bland foods cause less intestinal irritation and thus, decrease peristalsis. Allowing patient to select appetizing bland foods improves appetite and gives patient a sense of participation in care.
2. Encourage increase in fluid intake to 3,000 ml/24 h.	Fluid intake must be increased to replace fluids lost through the intestinal tract. It is essential to maintain the body's water and electrolyte balance.
3. Encourage patient to rest throughout day.	Diarrhea causes decrease in energy so that increased rest is necessary to maintain normal function.
4. Provide quiet environment.	A quiet environment which has few distractions promotes rest and relaxes bowel.
5. Decrease brisk activity until diarrhea subsides.	Avoiding brisk exercise will decrease intestinal peristalsis.
6. Administer medication ordered to be given after each stool.	Antidiarrheal medications slow intestinal motility, decreasing frequent emptying of the colon.
7. Cleanse buttocks and perineal area after each bowel movement.	Thorough cleansing of the buttocks and perineal area after each defecation prevents skin breakdown from exposure to irritating fecal contents.
8. Reassure patient that problem is expected to be short term.	Most diarrhea can be adequately treated. Reassuring the patient can alleviate anxiety and depression.

treating the patient with respect and never belittling incompetencies in elimination is important (see Module 28, Administering Enemas).

Nursing Actions for Preventing or Treating Diarrhea

Some patients with infections or anxiety develop diarrhea. Administering ordered antibiotics for infections, encouraging rest, reducing foods with bulk, and providing adequate fluids are all nursing actions that may prevent the occurrence of diarrhea (see sample Nursing Care Plan Related to Diarrhea). Reducing stress, which will decrease anxiety, also helps certain individuals to avoid diarrhea.

Maintenance of Fluid Balance

Replacing body fluid that is lost is essential in the treatment of diarrhea. A great deal of body fluid can be lost in a short period of time, with the result that the person can become dehydrated and have changes in electrolyte balance. This upsetting situation can also cause generalized weakness, loss of appetite, and nausea. Patients with diarrhea should have lost fluids replaced and adequate rest periods provided. Your plan of care will have to fulfill these needs. Immediate action must be taken with small infants and the elderly who have diarrhea because of the decreased ability of these persons to withstand alterations in fluid and electrolyte balance. Oral rehydration that includes both water and electrolytes is necessary. Broth and fruit juices may provide this. In developing countries, these oral fluids are commonly mixed from packets of electrolytes and boiled water. In developed countries, commercial products such as Pedialyte are used for oral rehydrating of infants and children. If the patient is unable to increase fluid intake orally during periods of extreme diarrhea, an intravenous infusion may be ordered by the physician.

Protection of the Skin

Special nursing actions should be taken to protect the skin of the patient who has diarrhea. After each bowel movement, the skin must be thoroughly washed with gentle soap and water. After careful drying, a non–water-soluble protective ointment should be applied to protect the skin from contact with liquid feces. The skin can also be impaired around a bowel diversion when seepage from the stoma causes irritation. Commercial products that may be used to protect the skin under an appliance and around a stoma are available.

Administration of Antidiarrheals

Prescription medications are often given to treat diarrhea by reducing intestinal peristalsis. A variety of antidiarrheal over-the-counter drugs are available. Because many travelers contact diarrhea when exposed to food and water in other countries, the purchase of these products has greatly increased as travel has become more common.

In the hospital, the physician may write a standing order for the patient who develops diarrhea. Most prescription and over-the-counter antidiarrheal medications are derivatives of either bismuth or loperamide (Immodium). You should be aware of some possible side effects of these drugs. The person may experience dry mouth, fever, abdominal cramping, or loss of appetite. Fluid intake should remain high when these medications are taken (Table 26-1).

Health Teaching

An important responsibility for the nurse related to the maintenance of normal bowel elimination is health teaching. Some general health teaching guidelines for all patients include getting regular exercise, eating diets that contain fiber, having sufficient fluid intake, and decreasing stress.

For patients who have had bowel surgery, following orders for special diets and providing sufficient rest along with periods of ambulation will aid in reestablishing regular bowel habits. An understanding and encouraging attitude on your part will also be of great benefit to the patient.

If a bowel diversion procedure has been performed, you will want to consult a module text or procedure manual to gain special knowledge concerning ways to teach self-care to the patient. Health teaching these procedures should only be carried out when the patient is psychologically ready to accept changes in body image and actively participate in care. Sometimes, you may be teaching a family member who will be caring for the patient after discharge.

Initiation of Bowel Rehabilitation

Many disabled persons experience long-term bowel elimination problems. The rehabilitation nurse is expert in designing a plan of care that integrates bowel rehabilitation. These same principles can be used in assisting any individual with a chronic bowel problem.

Involuntary defecation may characterize patients suffering from chronic illness, particularly of a neurologic nature. The paraplegic patient—who is capable of little or no sensation or movement in the lower portion of the body—can often neither feel nor control bowel movements. However, bowel rehabilitation, sometimes called bowel training, is usually successful. The person who has had a stroke may be restored to self-care for elimination.

Table 26–1. Cathartics and Laxatives

Agent	Dosage Form	Trade Names	Adult Dose	Pediatric Dose	Site of Action*	Approximate Time Required for Action (h)
Contact Cathartics						
Castor oil	Liquid	Emulsoil, Neolid, Purge	15–30 mL	<2 yr: 1–5 mL; 2–12 yr: 5–15 mL	Small intestines	2–6
Phenolphthalein	Tablets/liquid	Ex-Lax, Correctol, Phenolax, Feen-a-Mint	30–195 mg	<2 yr: Avoid 2–6 yr: 15–30 mg <6 yr: 30–60 mg	Colon	6–8
Bisacodyl	Tablets	Cenalax, Deficol, Dulcolax	10–15 mg	>6 yr: 5–10 mg	Colon	6–10
Senna	Tablets	Senexan, Senekot, Senolax	2 tablets	>60 lbs: 1 tablet	Colon	6–10
	Granules	Senekot, Black-Draught	1/4–1 tsp†	See label†		
	Syrup	Casafru, Senekot	5–15 mL†	See label†		
	Liquid/powder	X-Prep	Preradiologic: 75 mL or 22.5 g	1/8–1/2 adult dose		
Cascara sagrada	Tablets		325–650 mg	Avoid	Colon	6–8
	Aromatic fluid extract		5 mL	1/4–1/2 adult dose		
	Fluid extract		1 mL	1/4–1/2 adult dose		
Danthron	Solid/liquid	Modane, Dorbane	37.5–150 mg	<12 yr: Avoid	Colon	8
Saline Cathartics						
Magnesium hydroxide (milk of magnesia, M.O.M.)	Liquid	Phillips Milk of Magnesia, others	15–30 mL	0.5 mL/kg/dose	Small and large intestines	0.5–3
Magnesium citrate (citrate of magnesia)	Liquid	Citroma, Citro-Nesia	240 mL	5 mL/kg/dose	Small and large intestines	0.5–3
Magnesium sulfate (Epsom salts)	Powder		15 g	0.25 g/kg/dose	Small and large intestines	0.5–3
Sodium phosphate and sodium biphosphate	Liquid	Phospho-Soda	20–40 mL	5–15 mL	Small and large intestines	0.5–3
Bulk-Forming Laxatives						
Methylcellulose	Powder/liquid	Cologel, Maltsuprex	1–2 tbsp once or twice daily	1/2–2 tbsp daily	Small and large intestines	12–72
Psyllium	Flakes/granules	Mucilose, Siblin	1–2 tsp with fluid twice daily	See label.	Small and large intestines	12–72
	Powder	Metamucil, Perdiem, Hydrocil	1 rounded tsp one to three times daily	>6 yr: 1 level tsp daily		

(continued)

Table 26–1. Cathartics and Laxatives *(continued)*

Agent	Dosage Form	Trade Names	Adult Dose	Pediatric Dose	Site of Action*	Approximate Time Required for Action (h)
Emollient Laxatives and Stool Softeners						
Mineral oil	Liquid	Nujol, Agoral, Petrogalar	5–30 mL	5–10 mL	Colon	6–8
Docusate sodium (dioctyl sodium sulfosuccinate, Dss)	Tablets/capsules/liquid	Colace, Doxinate, Comfolax, Colax	50–240 mg	<3 yrs: 10–40 mg; 3–6 yrs: 20–60 mg; 6–12 yrs: 40–120 mg	Small and large intestine	12–72
Docusate calcium (dioctyl calcium sulfosuccinate)	Capsules	Surfak, Surfac, Pro-Cal-Sof	240 mg	50–150 mg	Small and large intestine	12–72
Docusate potassium	Capsules	Dialose, Kasof	100–300 mg	Avoid	Small and large intestine	12–72
Polaxamer 188	Capsules	Alaxin	480 mg	240–480 mg	Small and large intestine	12–72
Suppositories and Enemas						
Bisacodyl	Suppository	Dulcolax, Cenalax, Theralax	10 mg	5 mg	Colon	0.5–1
Senna	Suppository	Senokot	One	One-half	Colon	0.5–2
CO_2-releasing	Suppository	Ceo-Two	One	Avoid	Colon	0.5–2
Glycerin	Suppository/rectal liquid	Fleet Babylax	One	1 or 4 mL liquid	Colon	0.5–2
Sodium phosphate and sodium biphosphate	Enema	Fleet	118 mL	60 mL	Colon	0.5–2
Bisacodyl	Enema	Fleet Bisacodyl, Clysodrast	One package	Avoid	Colon	0.5–1
Docusate potassium and benzocaine	Enema	Therevac	3.9 g	Avoid	Colon	0.5–8
Mineral oil	Enema	Fleet Mineral Oil	120 mL	30–60 mL	Colon	0.5–8
Miscellaneous and Combinations						
Polycarbophil	Tablets	Mitrolan	1 g four times daily	3–6 yr: 500 mg twice daily; 6–12 yr: 500 mg tid	Small and large intestine	12–72
Lactulose	Syrup	Chronolac	15–60 mL	Avoid	Small and large intestine	24–48
Docusate plus casanthranol	Capsules/tablets/liquids	Peri-Colace, Diothron, Stimulax, Dialose-Plus	1–2 tablets or capsules; 7.5–30 mL†	See label†	Small and large intestine and colon	8–24
Docusate plus danthron	Capsules/tablets	Unilax, Modane Plus, Doxidan, Dorbantyl	1–2 tablets or capsules; 7.5–30 mL†	See label†	Small and large intestine and colon	8–24

*All agents except the bulk laxatives are absorbed to some extent.
†Varies by preparation; follow label directions.

Nursing Research: Implications for Practice

Schmelzer, M. "Effectiveness of Wheat Bran in Preventing Constipation of Hospitalized Orthopedic Surgery Patients." *Orthopedic Nursing* 9,6 (November–December 1990): 55–59.

Sixteen orthopedic surgery patients were randomly selected to determine if the addition of wheat bran to the diet would decrease the occurrence of constipation. The comparison of this group with a control group proved positive. The patients who ingested wheat bran had a lower incidence of constipation as evidenced by more stools and less need for laxative use.

Bowel rehabilitation requires the patient's understanding and cooperation, even though the program is initiated by the nurse with coordination by the physician. The patient is given extra fluids, often prune juice, with the morning meal. Approximately 30 minutes after breakfast, a glycerin suppository is inserted into the rectum. The action of the medication causes peristalsis to begin shortly thereafter, and the patient is placed on the commode or bedpan to defecate.

Bowel rehabilitation sometimes uses the technique of digital stimulation. Shortly after the suppository is inserted and before defecation occurs, the nurse, wearing a clean lubricated glove, inserts the middle finger into the rectum to stimulate peristalsis. Another method is to give a small-volume enema after the morning meal. The frequency of the procedure is then gradually decreased until the enema is no longer needed. Regardless of the method used, the desired outcome is to cause the bowel to empty of its own volition at approximately the same time each day.

Evaluation

The general desired outcome is that the patient's elimination problem will not worsen and, ideally, be resolved. In addition, outcome criteria specific to the problem should have been developed earlier. The patient who had chronic constipation may have had daily bowel movements since initiation of bran in the diet as part of the plan. With other patients, the evaluation may be that the problem is less prominent but still present. For example, a chronically constipated patient may have established a normal pattern with only two enemas per week when there had previously been four. Outcome criteria may relate to the patient's knowledge base. In this situation, the patient should be able to describe any contributing factors if they are known and understand the plan of treatment. To obtain the desired outcomes with defecation problems, revision of the care plan is often necessary because several or a combination of actions may have to be tried before improvement occurs.

Nursing Care Study
A Patient with Constipation

Mr. Jensen is 88 years old and was recently admitted to the chronic care facility where Judy Gomez is a nursing student. Ms. Gomez's assignment is to develop a nursing care plan on a patient's primary need. She notices, while caring for Mr. Jensen, that he is preoccupied with bowel function and asks several times to be assisted to the bathroom. Each time he is unable to defecate. He refuses to go to morning activities because be might want to go back to the bathroom. She decides to collect data to determine whether a problem with constipation is present.

The nursing history reports that Mr. Jensen had been living alone and eating prepared meals only sporadically; his diet has been insufficient. He states that he has had hard, difficult-to-pass bowel movements every 3 to 4 days and has frequent abdominal distention with pain. She determines that he does have constipation and that the desired outcome would be for Mr. Jensen to have regular, more normal stools.

The student notices that the physician has written an order for glycerine suppositories qod, PRN. Ms. Gomez consults her resources and learns that increased fiber in the diet, extra fluids, and exercise are the best measures to combat constipation.

(continued)

Nursing Care Study (continued)
A Patient with Constipation

With the dietitian, the head nurse, and the patient, she completes her plan:

1. One tablespoon bran over warm cereal each morning.
2. Prune juice with breakfast.
3. Use of the bathroom one-half hour after breakfast.
4. Extra juices and fluids at midmorning and midafternoon.
5. Attendance at the morning exercise program and ambulation with assistance each afternoon and evening.
6. A glycerine suppository if defecation does not occur in 2 days.

When Ms. Gomez assures Mr. Jensen that this plan represents a positive step toward solving his problem and that he can play an active role in it, he eagerly accepts it. At the end of the fourth day, Ms. Gomez writes that her plan is partially successful because only one suppository has had to be given. By day 8, Mr. Jensen is having bowel movements regularly after breakfast. The distention and pain have disappeared. The plan becomes a permanent part of the patient's routine.

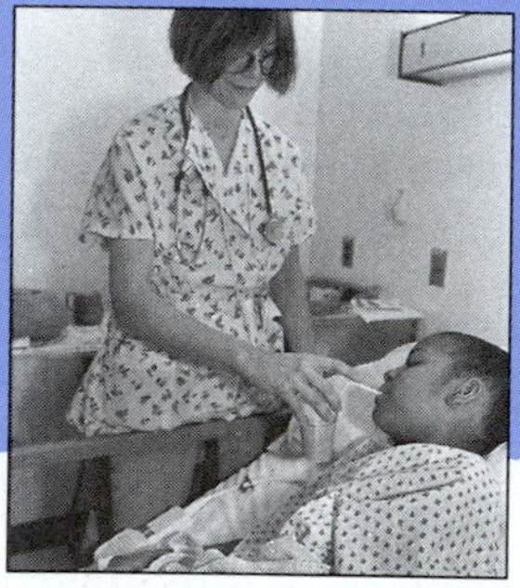

Key Points

- The need for normal bowel patterns of elimination is a basic one.
- The gastrointestinal system consists of the stomach, the small intestine, the large intestine, the rectum, and the anus. Defecation is the expulsion of solid wastes and, like urination, is both voluntary and involuntary.
- Normal feces have an unpleasant odor, are brown in color, and largely cellulose and fiber in content, with small amounts of fat and protein. The percentage of water in feces greatly affects defecation function.
- Abnormal components of the feces include blood, excessive mucus, and gas as well as parasites and worms.
- Nurses collect stool specimens for examination. Sending specimens to the laboratory promptly is a responsibility of the nurse.
- Tests and procedures used to identify pathology of the gastrointestinal tract include radiographic examination using contrast media, direct visualization with a fiberoptic scope, CAT scans, and MRI.
- Many physical and psychological factors affect the ability to defecate normally, including age, fluid intake, exercise, medications, emotions, and bowel habits.
- Altered functions related to defecation include constipation, diarrhea, fecal impaction, incontinence, steatorrhea, flatulence, hemorrhoids, and paralytic ileus.
- When disease or obstruction of the intestinal tract is present, a fecal diversion is sometimes necessary. Caring for the stoma and maintaining the skin around the stoma is an important nursing task.
- Assessment related to bowel elimination includes the patient's subjective data along with the nurse's observations. Nursing diagnoses include risk states and factors that alter function. Planning that allows time and privacy is essential. Nursing actions may include health teaching and administration of medications for the treatment of constipation or diarrhea.
- The patient with long-term bowel dysfunction may require a bowel rehabilitation program to manage function. Evaluation involves determining whether there has been resolution or amelioration of the patient's bowel elimination problem.

Study Questions

1. Briefly explain the process of defecation.
2. Name at least four abnormal components of fecal material.
3. What is the gastrocolic reflex and how does it help or hinder defecation?

4. Name three commonly used tests to detect disease of the gastrointestinal tract.
5. If you were teaching a patient about normal bowel function, what essential areas might you cover?
6. What are two of the most common defecation deficits and who is most at risk?
7. How does exercise promote normal bowel elimination?
8. List nursing actions that would be included in a rehabilitation setting for a patient with bowel problems.

Critical Thinking Activities

1. Visit a pharmacy and make a list of several of the over-the-counter anti-constipation and anti-diarrheal medications that are available. Compare the side effects of these preparations and identify how you could health teach a patient who chooses self-medication about these side effects.
2. Examine the method of recording bowel function in your facility. Is this method sufficient and accurate? Is the nursing staff conscientiously documenting this data and if not, why not?
3. Identify the different ways the emotions of individuals affect bowel elimination. Include aspects of nervous system control.
4. Write a care plan for an elderly patient who experiences ongoing constipation. Identify the nursing actions that you could take to alleviate the problem.

Relevant Sections in Modules for Basic Nursing Skills

Volume 1 Module
Assisting with Elimination and Perineal Care 10
Inspection, Palpation, Auscultation, and Percussion 13
Intake and Output 15
Collecting Specimens 18
Performing Common Laboratory Tests 20
Administering Enemas 28
Volume 2 Module
Ostomy Care 38
Nasogastric Intubation 45

References and Readings

Alterescu, K. B. "Colostomy." *Nursing Clinics of North America* 22, 2 (June 1987): 281–289.

Bass, L. "More Fiber—Less Constipation." *American Journal of Nursing* 77 (February 1977): 254–255.

Becker, K. L., and Stevens, S. A. "Performing In-Depth Abdominal Assessment." *Nursing '88* 18, 6 (June 1988): 59–63.

Broadwell, D. C. "Peristomal Skin Integrity." *Nursing Clinics of North America* 22, 2 (June 1987): 321–332.

Carpenito, L. J. *Nursing Diagnosis: Application to Clinical Practice.* 4th edition. Philadelphia: J. B. Lippincott, 1992.

Davis, A., Nagelhout, M. J., Hoban, M., and Barnard, B. "Bowel Management: A Quality Assurance Approach to Upgrading Programs." *Journal of Gerontological Nursing* 12, 5 (May 1986): 13–17.

Ellickson, E. B. "Bowel Management Plan for the Homebound Elderly." *Journal of Gerontological Nursing* 14, 1 (January 1988): 16–19.

Erickson, P. J. "Ostomies: The Art of Pouching." *Nursing Clinics of North America* 22, 2 (June 1987): 311–320.

Garcia, R. M., "Relationship Between Falls and Patient Attempts to Solve Elimination Needs." *Nursing Management* 19, 7 (July 1988): 80–82.

Guyton, A. C. *Human Physiology and Mechanisms of Disease.* 5th edition. Philadelphia: W. B. Saunders, 1992.

Henry, M. "Fecal Incontinence." *Nursing Times* (August 17, 1983): 61–62.

Long, L. "Ileostomy Care: Overcoming the Obstacles." *Nursing '91* 21, 10 (October 1991): 73–75.

Murray, R. and Zentner, J. *Nursing Assessment and Health Promotion Strategies through the Life Span.* 4th ed. Englewood NJ: Prentice Hall, 1989.

Motta, G. J. "Life Span Changes: Implications for Colostomy Care." *Nursing Clinics of North America* 22, 2 (June 1987): 333–339.

Renkers, J. "GI Endoscopy: Managing the Full Scope of Care." *Nursing '93*. 23, 6 (June 1993): 50–55.

Rideout, B. W. "The Patient with an Ileostomy: Nursing Management and Patient Education." *Nursing Clinics of North America* 22, 2 (June 1987): 253–262.

Rowland, M. A. "When Drug Therapy Causes Diarrhea." *RN* 52, 12 (December 1989): 32–35.

Smeltzer, S. C., and Bare, B. G. *Brunner and Suddarth's Textbook of Medical-Surgical Nursing.* 7th edition. Philadelphia: J. B. Lippincott, 1992.

Smith, C. "Assessing Bowel Sounds—More Than Just Listening." *Nursing '88* 18, 2 (February 1988): 42–43.

Venn, M. R., Taft, L., Carpentier, B, Applebaugh, G. "The Influence of Timing and Suppository Use on Efficiency and Effectiveness of Bowel Training after a Stroke." *Rehabilitation Nursing* 17, 3 (May-June 1992): 116–121.

Wade, B. E. "Colostomy Patients: Psychological Adjustment to 10 Weeks and 1 Year After Surgery in Districts Which Employed Stoma Care Nurses and in Districts Which Did Not." *Journal of Advanced Nursing* 15, 11 (November 1990): 1297–1304.

Whaley, L. F., and Wong, D. L. *Essentials of Pediatric Nursing.* 4th ed. St. Louis: C. V. Mosby, 1993.

Urinary Elimination

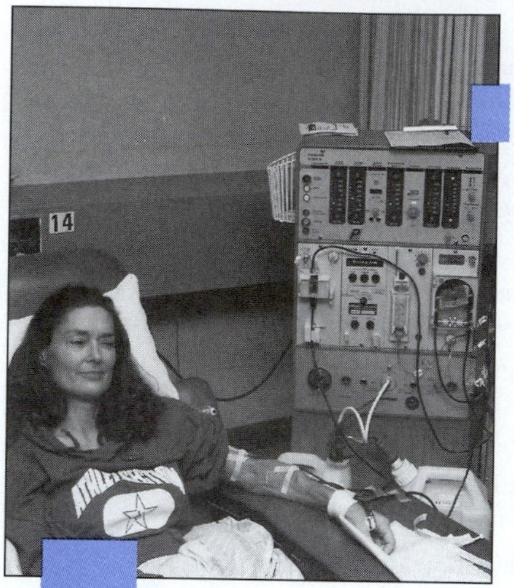

27

Objectives

After completing this chapter, you should be able to:

1. Name the organs of the urinary system.
2. List the normal and abnormal characteristics of urine.
3. Discuss the factors that affect urination.
4. List the kinds of diagnostic tests used to determine the adequacy of urinary function.
5. Discuss how assessment for urinary function is made through the use of subjective and objective data, including observation of intake and output and collection of urine specimens.
6. Identify nursing diagnoses for patients both at risk of and actually experiencing urinary problems.
7. Discuss nursing actions appropriate for persons with urinary problems.
8. Outline a rehabilitation plan for the patient with long-term incontinence.

Study Terms

albuminuria
anuria
bacteriuria
casts
Crede's method
dysuria
enuresis
glucosuria
glycosuria
hematuria
micturition
neurogenic bladder
nocturia
oliguria
polyuria
proteinuria
pyuria
renal calculi
stretch reflex
uricosurics
urimeter
urinary diversion
urinary suppression

Outline

The Urinary System

The Process of Urination

Normal Characteristics of Urine
Abnormal Components of Urine

Factors Affecting Urination

Age
Pregnancy
Fluid Intake
Exercise
Medications
Urinary Habits
Stress and Emotions

Common Disorders Affecting Urinary Elimination

Urinary Problems Related to Other Systems
Urinary Problems Related to Structure
Urinary Diversion
Replacements for Kidney Function

Ellis, Nowlis: Nursing: A Human Needs Approach, 5th ed. © 1994 J.B. Lippincott Company

Another basic need of all human beings is the ability to eliminate wastes and excess water from the body in the form of urine. Many factors can influence the ability to urinate. In this country, urination is considered a private matter and the ability to contain urine sufficiently is important, so that when wetting occurs, it can be upsetting and embarrassing to the person. When people are ill, normal patterns of urination may be altered. Some patients require the insertion of a urinary catheter to manage urinary elimination.

Nurses should recognize the psychological as well as the physiologic implications of urinary elimination. Privacy should be provided so that this sensitive matter can become comfortable for the patient. However, nurses should understand the importance of this body system and learn ways of monitoring and maintaining adequate urinary elimination.

The Urinary System

The urinary system consists of the kidneys, ureters, bladder, and urethra. This system promotes homeostasis by means of its delicate filtration process: substances needed by the body are filtered by the kidneys and reabsorbed back into the blood, whereas those not needed are excreted in the urine (Fig. 27-1).

The two *kidneys* are located posteriorly outside the peritoneum (the membrane lining the abdominal cavity), just above the waistline, and are suspended by connective tissue. Each kidney measures approximately 3 inches by 4 inches and is bean shaped.

Kidney tissue is composed of tiny units called *nephrons*, intricate structures of convoluted tubes and blood vessels that can filter the blood and excrete urine. An almost unbelievable amount of blood is estimated to pass through each kidney every minute—more than 125 ml. This fact is important to us when we care for patients who have blood loss or those who have decreased renal circulation for other reasons.

The kidneys perform several vital functions. First, they excrete toxins and metabolic wastes. Second, they maintain normal electrolyte levels within the body by retaining needed elements such as sodium ions and excreting unneeded or excessive amounts of sodium and other elements. Third, the kidneys regulate the body's pH by responding to the pH of the blood. If, for example, the pH of the blood is too high, the tubules decrease their ion exchange mechanism to correct this imbalance. Last, the kidneys, through a complicated process related to glomerulofiltration, maintain the body's fluid balance.

Each day 190 liters of fluid is filtered, and 189 liters is reabsorbed. Each nephron has its own collecting tu-

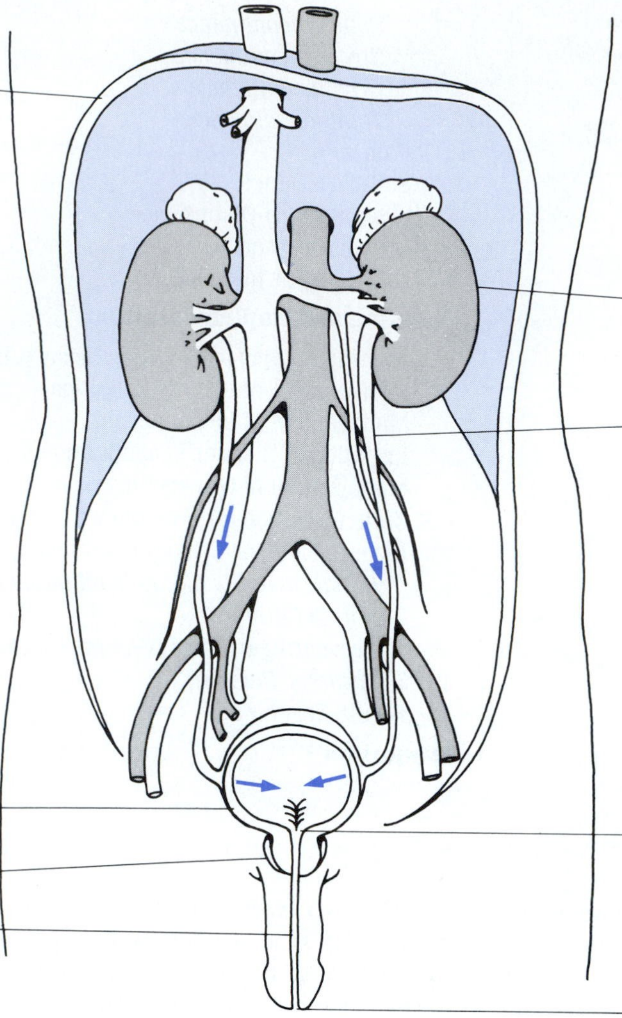

Figure 27-1. The urinary system (male).

bule, which carries minute droplets of urine into the pelvis of the kidney. Urine drains from the kidney pelvis in response to certain pressures and, because of gravity, passes into the ureter.

Leading downward from each kidney is a *ureter*, a tube 10 to 12 inches in length. The ureters are slender, ranging from $\frac{1}{16}$ to $\frac{1}{2}$ inch at the point of attachment to the kidney. A peristaltic (wavelike) action causes urine to pass downward into the urinary bladder, and a mucous membrane fold prevents backward flow of urine into the ureter.

The urinary *bladder* stores the urine in a sterile environment. The bladder lies behind the symphysis pubis, the bony joint in the anterior pubic area. There are three openings on the posterior floor of the bladder: two from the ascending ureters and a descending one for the urethra. When the bladder is full of urine, the bladder's outline can be felt in the lower abdomen. The highly elastic walls of the bladder are made up of layers of smooth muscle fibers, which together comprise the detrusor muscle.

The bladder normally holds about 500 ml of urine before emptying, but has been known to retain up to 2,000 ml. The average adult excretes approximately 1,600 to 2,000 ml of urine in 24 hours.

The *urethral meatus* is the external opening of the *urethra*. The length of the urethra, which is a slender tube, depends on whether the person is a male or female. In the female, it is $1\frac{1}{2}$ inches in length and passes behind the pubic bone anterior to the vagina. In the male, the urethra is approximately 8 inches long and threads through the prostate gland before entering and passing through the penis.

The Process of Urination

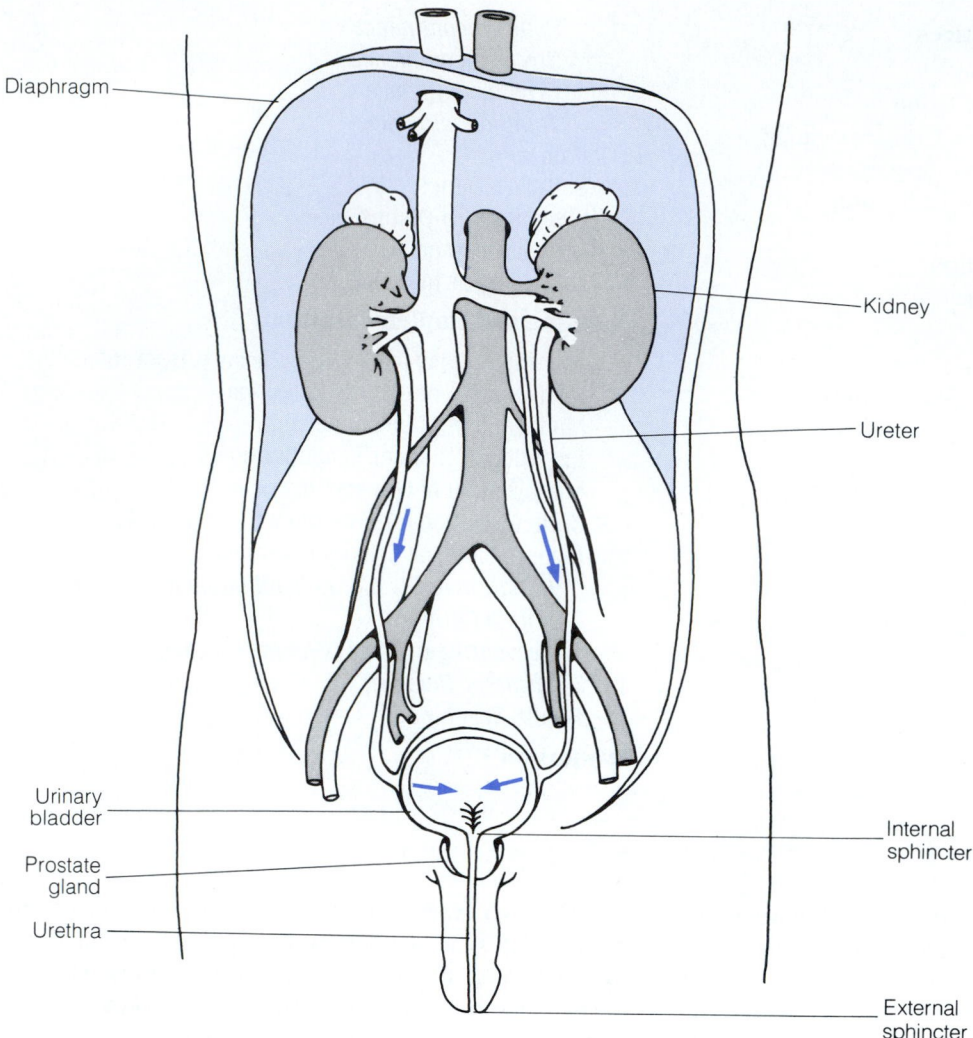

Fluid containing waste products is excreted from the body through the urinary system. Urine is approximately 95% water and 5% nitrogenous wastes from protein metabolism, diluted toxins, and mineral salts. It is normally sterile. To identify abnormal characteristics of urine for purposes of assessment, you should be familiar with urine's normal state.

Voiding, or **micturition**, occurs through what is called the **stretch reflex**. When the bladder fills with urine and the stretch or tension on the wall reaches a threshold unique to the individual, sensory impulses, carried by the nerves of the parasympathetic system, are sent to the sacral portion of the spinal cord. Parasympathetic motor nerves then carry impulses back to the walls of the bladder, setting up contractions in the detrusor muscle. These contractions begin to relax the internal *sphincter,* which is just below the neck of the bladder, signaling to the person the need to void. A second phase of micturition is voluntary because the external sphincter, or urethral meatus, through which urine is finally excreted, is controlled by the cortex or higher centers of the brain. A person can postpone voiding for some time after the internal sphincter relaxes, although there may be some discomfort. A child learns to control urination by about age 3.

Normal Characteristics of Urine

The normal *color* of urine can be described as varying between shades of pale yellow (dilute), straw (less dilute), and amber (concentrated). These differences in coloration are normal and usually are the result of differences in urine concentration. Certain foods and drugs can also affect color. For example, beets give a reddish tinge to the urine. Some drugs turn the urine blue, some brown, and others orange.

Clarity of urine is another characteristic. Urine should be clear or transparent. Allowed to stand, however, it may develop cloudiness because of precipitation of phosphates and urates (salts) and bacterial growth. Some drugs, such as the sulfonamides, may give a hazy appearance to the urine.

A faint *aromatic odor* is normally present in urine. If allowed to stand, urine will give off the odor of ammonia because of the formation of ammonia salts. Some foods, such as asparagus, and some drugs, such as high dosages of thiamine, give the urine a distinctive odor that is considered normal.

The *pH* is a measure of the acidity or alkalinity of a solution. Neutral pH is 7; usually the urine is slightly acid (about 6), although it may vary from 4.8 to 7.5. The intake of certain foods may change the pH of the urine. For example, vegetarian diets can cause the urine to be slightly alkaline.

The pH of urine is usually measured on the nursing unit with a dip stick, a litmus-impregnated plastic strip (see Module 20, Performing Common Laboratory Tests).

The *specific gravity,* or concentration of wastes, in urine is measured with a hydrometer, consisting of a glass bulb on a stem. When the glass bulb device floats freely in a small container of urine, the device registers a number depending on the level of flotation. The hydrometer operates by displacement: the more particles in the urine, the higher the instrument floats. Normal specific gravity of urine is approximately 1.010 to 1.025, which compares the weight of urine against the weight of distilled water.

Abnormal Components of Urine

In cases of infection, *bacteria* can be found in the urine. The term for this condition is **bacteriuria**. A specimen of urine can be sent to the laboratory, where the organisms are grown in a culture for purposes of identification.

Blood in the urine is abnormal. Bleeding occurring anywhere in the urinary tract may be detected in the urine. The presence of blood in the urine is called *hematuria.* **Occult blood** (hidden blood) is blood in the urine that is not observable except by testing. You should always consider menstrual flow as a possible source of **hematuria** in female patients of childbearing age.

Casts are small hardened dish-shaped mucous particles that are "cast" in the tubules and discarded in the urine. It is not unusual to find a limited number of casts in urine that is otherwise normal in character. Such a condition is not considered harmful.

Sugar is not normally found in urine. A finding of *glucose* in the urine may be attributable to an abnormally high intake of sugar or to infectious, metabolic, or inflammatory diseases. The presence of abnormally high sugar in the urine is called **glycosuria** or **glucosuria**.

Although small amounts of protein are sometimes present in otherwise normal urine, amounts large enough to measure are considered abnormal. Protein in the urine can be indicative of bleeding, infection, or inflammation. This condition is called **proteinuria** or **albuminuria**.

The presence of *pus* in the urine, called **pyuria**, indicates the presence in the body of a highly infectious process. The person will probably have other signs and symptoms of infection, such as fever, flank or back pain, and difficulty or pain when voiding.

Stones can originate in the bladder or the kidney and are called **renal calculi**. They are formed from various kinds of salts that precipitate out of the urine. Smaller stones, regardless of their origin and resembling sand, may pass out of the body in the urine. Bladder stones may reside in the bladder for long periods of time but can cause inflammation. It is not uncommon for larger calculi to lodge in the pelvis of the kidney or in the ureters, causing severe pain and inflammation. Stones sometimes have to be surgically removed. Figure 27-2 presents the normal and abnormal components of urine.

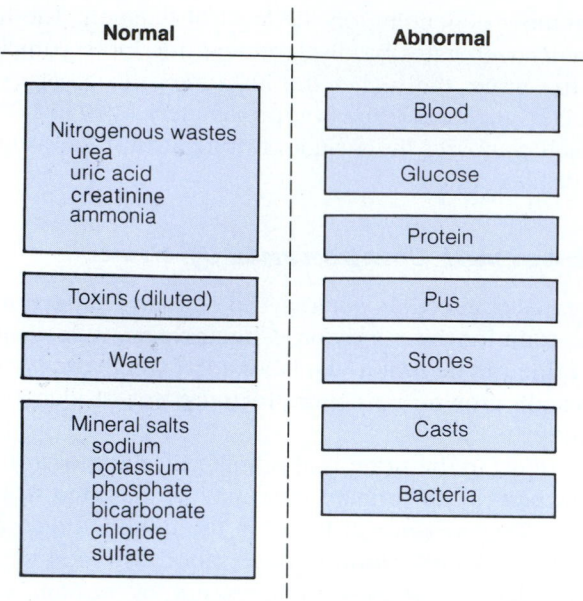

Normal	Abnormal
Nitrogenous wastes: urea, uric acid, creatinine, ammonia	Blood
	Glucose
	Protein
Toxins (diluted)	Pus
Water	Stones
Mineral salts: sodium, potassium, phosphate, bicarbonate, chloride, sulfate	Casts
	Bacteria

Figure 27-2. Normal and abnormal components of urine.

Factors Affecting Urination

Several factors affect urine production and excretion, including age, fluid intake, exercise, medications, stress and emotions, and urinary habits.

Age

In children, bladder control is more complex than is bowel control because maturation of the needed neurologic reflexes comes later. Control is usually achieved between the ages of $2\frac{1}{2}$ and $3\frac{1}{2}$ (Murray and Zentner, 1989). The child may have urinary control in the daytime before control during the sleeping hours when awareness is lessened. **Enuresis** (bedwetting) may occur in children who are sound sleepers, those who drink large amounts of fluid before going to bed, or those who have small bladders. Enuresis should disappear by age 5 to 6.

Young and middle-aged adults usually have adequate bladder control. The physical and psychological conditions that affect urination are discussed later in this chapter.

Older adults may have a variety of problems leading to faulty control of urination. Physically, they may be less agile, and therefore they may have more difficulty reaching toilet facilities in time to urinate. Inadequate fluid intake may decrease urine flow. Neurologic changes, as well as changes in the organs of micturition, such as relaxed bladder muscles and decreased sphincter control, can lead to dribbling or incontinence in some people. **Nocturia** (excessive urination at night) can disturb sleep (see Chapter 24).

Pregnancy

During pregnancy, the increasing weight of the uterus places pressure on the urinary structures. The woman may experience urgency and frequency of urination over the months of gestation. Glucosuria may also be present because of the increase in glomerular filtration. Ureters become dilated during the early months of pregnancy, probably related to increased amounts of progesterone. Later, the ureters are compressed, which may lead to incomplete emptying of the bladder, placing the woman at risk for bladder infections.

Fluid Intake

The amount of fluid ingested directly influences urinary quantity and flow. Water is used by all body systems as a medium to facilitate elimination of waste products. Water is also a medium for digestion, and the saliva and gastric juices contain large amounts of water and enzymes. Normally, most persons drink 1,200 to 1,500 ml of fluid daily for optimal elimination. Some people drink as much as 2,000 ml daily. Fluids are lost through insensible loss as well as through kidney action. (Insensible loss is the large amount of water we lose through the lungs by exhaling and through the moisture of the skin; see Chapter 30).

The type of fluid consumed also affects the quantity of urine produced. Fluids that contain alcohol increase production of urine because antidiuretic hormone (ADH) release is inhibited (Fig. 27-3). Caffeine in coffee, tea, and cocoa also increases urinary elimination.

You would expect that any patient who cannot take

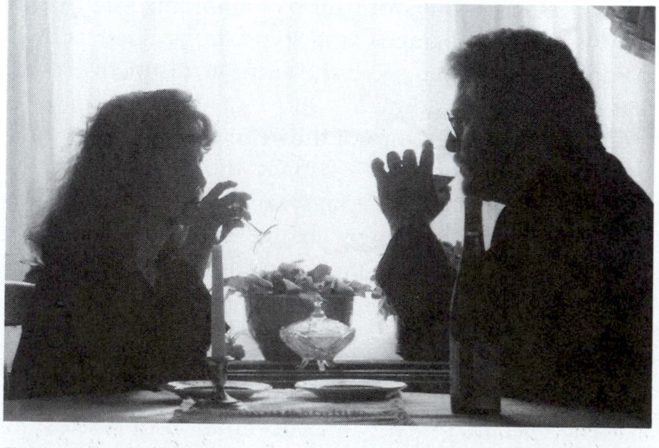

Figure 27-3. Fluids that contain alcohol increase the production of urine.

in fluids for one reason or another would have decreased urinary flow. For example, patients placed on NPO (nothing-by-mouth) status would have less output unless they receive intravenous fluids. Barring medical reasons for not doing so, one should encourage patients to take in sufficient fluids to maintain urine production of 1,500 ml in 24 hours.

Exercise

General toning of the muscles through exercise helps elimination. The bladder and abdominal muscles all facilitate emptying of the bladder. When ill persons feel well enough to increase their activity, urinary elimination often improves.

Medications

Several groups of medications affect urination. *Diuretics* decrease reabsorption within the kidney tubules, thus increasing urinary output. Some patients on diuretics think that because drugs are being taken to get rid of water, drinking should be decreased. This is not true. The drugs are most effective when the patient continues to take adequate fluids. Some pain medications decrease urine production.

Drugs that facilitate emptying the bladder are a group called the *cholinergics*. Used for urinary retention, these medications stimulate the release of acetylcholine from the parasympathetic nerves that initiate contraction of the bladder. Bethanechol chloride (Urecholine) is one example. These drugs may cause the patient to urinate often, which can interfere with the daily routine.

Another group that can cause urinary frequency as a side effect are the **uricosurics**, drugs that block reabsorption of uric acid within the tubule. In turn, this allows for lowering the uric acid levels in the blood. One example is probenecid (Benemid).

A number of urinary tract antiseptics are used to rid the urine of bacteria. Although these are concentrated within the urinary tract, they may not change urinary function, but they kill the bacteria as a component of the urine. All require high levels of fluid intake to prevent crystallization within the kidney. Some change the color of the urine. One example is Azo Gantrisin, which is a combination of sulfisoxazole, a bacteriostatic agent, and phenazopyridine, a urinary antiseptic that turns the urine orange. Health teaching is essential when patients are taking these drugs.

Although many other drugs may not alter urination, they can change the color of the urine. Unless the patient is told of this fact ahead of time, the result can generate fear that something is wrong. Examples of such drugs are methylene blue derivatives, which turn the urine blue green; phenytoin (Dilantin), which gives the urine a reddish color; and some phenothiazines, such as chlorpromazine (Thorazine), which darken the urine.

Urinary Habits

Urinary habits begin within the culture and the family. In most Western societies, privacy is a requirement. Children learn early to close the bathroom door when urinating. Not only is privacy important but time is a factor in thoroughly emptying the bladder. Because of anatomy, girls sit and boys stand to urinate. Hospitalization can disrupt normal urinary habits by interfering with privacy, normal position, and sufficient time to urinate. Some adults find themselves unable to urinate if privacy and their normal voiding position are not possible.

Stress and Emotions

As a student you are aware that you may have the urge to void just as the time for an important examination approaches. Persons in a health care facility frequently feel great stress caused by the strange environment and health concerns. It is not unusual for patients to experience urgency or frequency when situations are stressful. Extreme fear may actually cause sudden involuntary urination.

Common Disorders Affecting Urinary Elimination

Basic knowledge of any underlying medical urinary problem of the patient is important for the nurse who is gathering data. Medical urinary problems may have accompanying nursing diagnoses. Nursing interventions can then be based on these diagnoses.

Urinary Problems Related to Other Systems

Because all the systems of the body are interrelated, disturbances of other systems can cause urinary problems. Localized problems can also occur in specific parts of the urinary tract, such as the kidneys, ureters, bladder, or urethra. An example of urinary dysfunction caused by another system is **neurogenic bladder**, which occurs when the bladder does not empty because of a lesion or injury of the nervous system.

A number of other systemic factors can cause urinary problems. Heart disease and complications of the circulation cause urinary disturbances because of the decreased flow of blood to the kidneys. Without sufficient blood to process, the body retains fluid and substances, and the kidney tissue may be damaged. The patient may show signs of electrolyte imbalance, such as muscle weakness, lassitude, and even confusion. Fluid is also retained in the tissue, resulting in edema, most commonly in the lower part of the sacrum and the ankles. Hormonal factors can also cause problems. Because certain hormones, such as aldosterone, have a regulatory effect on the kidneys, a disturbance of the pituitary or adrenal glands that produce those hormones can cause urinary disturbance.

Severe dehydration, regardless of cause, may bring about serious kidney problems because of the decreased circulation to the organs. Any overwhelming generalized trauma to the body has a systemic effect, causing kidney dysfunction. Generalized infection brings elevated temperatures that deplete body fluids, affecting kidney function. Loss of muscle tone, often seen in the elderly and in patients suffering disease of the muscular system, may bring about an inability to exercise muscular control over urination. Conditions of the central nervous system and spinal cord may also directly influence urinary efficiency through interruption of innervation. The interplay between urinary function and other systems can greatly complicate assessment.

Urinary Problems Related to Structure

The anatomic differences between males and females make for some differences in the prevalence of specific problems. The female is more prone to infection than the male because of the relative shortness of the urethra. The male may, however, be more susceptible to obstruction: because the *prostate* gland surrounds the male urethra, any hypertrophy (swelling) of this gland will cause some degree of obstruction. The male is more vulnerable to trauma of the urethra because of its external position.

As for localized factors, *obstruction* may occur anywhere within the urinary system. Abnormal cell growth, benign or malignant, may occur in the kidney, ureters, bladder, or urethra. Stones can also form, causing obstruction. Localized trauma may be evident in the form of bruising, hemorrhaging, or swelling of localized parts of the system. Although the mucous membranes of the body usually protect against pathogens, microorganisms can travel upward along the surface of the mucous membrane lining of the urinary tract and spread infection. This is the reason sterile technique is essential when you perform procedures that involve the urinary system.

Urinary Diversion

When the urinary bladder is diseased and must be surgically removed, a **urinary diversion** is devised. This diversion can be accomplished in one of two ways. First, after the bladder is removed, the two ureters can be anastomosed (sutured together so that one opens into the other) and the free end brought to the anterior abdominal wall to form a stoma (opening) for the emptying of urine onto the skin. This procedure is called a cutaneous ureterostomy. A second procedure is called an ileal conduit or ileal loop. In this procedure, a portion of the ileum is separated from the intestinal tract and formed into a passageway leading to the abdominal skin surface as a stoma. The ureters are attached to this ileal loop and urine drains from the stoma. The choice of a device to catch and hold the urine is important so that leaking and skin breakdown do not occur. This requires that some kind of external pouch (usually called an appliance) be used to collect the urine as it flows from the stoma.

A newer procedure is the continent urostomy, or Kock pouch, named after the surgeon who first constructed it. After the diseased bladder is removed, an approximately 26-inch length of the ileum is resected to form a false, or pseudo, bladder. The ureters are implanted into this section. Instead of the usual stoma, a nipple valve that remains closed is constructed out of the ileum tissue and a stoma to the skin is made. To drain the pouch, the patient inserts a clean catheter and drains the urine four to six times per day (Brogna and Lakaszawski, 1988). This procedure has a considerable number of advantages over the more traditional ileal conduit procedure. The patient is continent and does not need appliances. Sexual activity is not interrupted except for resolution of any psychological problems that may arise. No adaptations need to be made regarding special clothing, activity, diet, or travel. Responsibilities of the nurse in caring for the patient with a urinary diversion will be discussed under the section on nursing actions.

Replacements for Kidney Function

When complete renal (kidney) failure occurs, a number of procedures replicate kidney function; these are called *dialysis* procedures (Fig. 27-4). Several dialysis methods are currently in use, and research is continuing to refine them and decrease complications. One is *hemodialysis,* which is circulation of the patient's blood through a filtering "kidney" machine. The blood may be drawn and returned through an arteriovenous shunt, which is a synthetic U-tube connector usually inserted between an artery and a vein, just above the inner wrist. Some long-term dialysis patients have a fistula that is the surgical

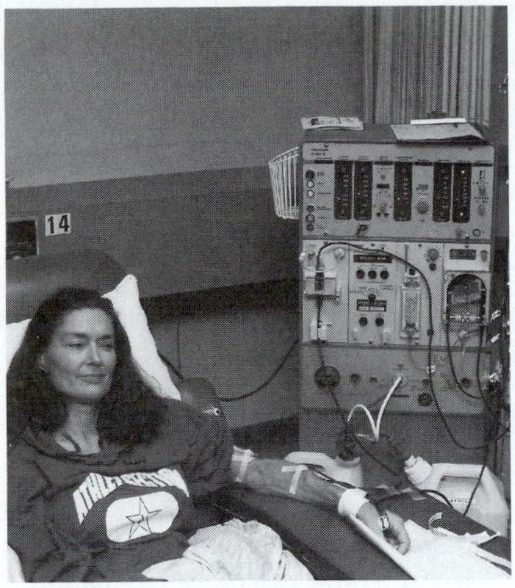

Figure 27-4. Dialysis has become a lifesaving procedure for many people in renal failure.

anastomosis (connection) of an artery and a vein that fulfills the shunting purpose. The semipermeable membranes of the machine allow waste products to diffuse out of the blood into special dialysis solution. The patient's blood pressure must be constantly monitored during the procedure.

Because hemodialysis is increasingly being performed on nursing units, you should be aware that the access arm must never be used to draw blood, start an intravenous infusion, or take blood pressure measurements. The vascular access must be protected from any compromise or injury.

A second dialysis method is *peritoneal dialysis*, whereby carefully measured amounts of a special dialyzing solution are introduced into and withdrawn intermittently from the peritoneal cavity through a small incision and cannula. Waste products diffuse from the blood in the fluid and then are removed when the fluid is withdrawn.

Home and ambulatory dialysis procedures are becoming more prominent treatment modes as techniques improve, freeing patients from the need to spend hours each week in the hospital for the purpose of dialysis. Both hemodialysis and conventional peritoneal dialysis may be done at home. *Continuous ambulatory peritoneal dialysis* (CAPD), first used in 1980, is a method whereby the person, with an indwelling peritoneal catheter, instills the sterile dialyzing solution in the abdomen, allows it to "dwell" (remain in the abdomen) so that the particle exchange can take place, and then drains off and discards the solution. This procedure is done three to six times during the waking hours. The health teaching and support of people for whom this method is appropriate and who choose to do their own dialysis is an exciting new challenge for the nurse.

Diagnostic Tests and Procedures

A variety of tests and procedures are related to urinary function. An important part of assessment is determining if the patient has had or is to have any diagnostic tests or procedures. Some are measurements or examination of the urine. Others measure the amounts of various waste products in the blood or urine. X-rays are also performed, with or without a contrast material. Biopsies (which obtain tissue samples) are another way to diagnose abnormalities of the urinary system. Although many of these occur in other departments of the hospital or the laboratory, you will be participating in preparing the patient for these tests.

You may be performing simple urine tests on the nursing unit such as those which identify abnormal characteristics. You should be aware of any urinary tests ordered for the patient and the reasons they were ordered.

Testing the Process of Urination

Urodynamics tests may be ordered. A specialist in urologic medicine usually orders these tests performed when patients have a neurologic or other medical problem that affects urination. Through a series of complicated tests using highly sensitive measuring equipment, the actual flow of urine through the tract can be observed, measured, and evaluated.

Measurement and Collection of Urine

Intake and output is a measurement kept by the nursing staff, listing and then computing the 24-hour fluid intake and output of the patient. The figures should approximate each other. When intake is normal but urinary output is low, the patient may have been dehydrated and simply be replacing body fluid or may have some type of illness. Placing the patient on "intake and output" can be either a medical or nursing order (see Module 15, Intake and Output).

Urine specimens are often collected by the nurse for a variety of tests that may be performed on the nursing unit or in the laboratory. A urine specimen may be collected at the discretion of the nurse for measuring glucose, pH, or specific gravity or ordered by the physician for the purpose of determining a medical diagnosis or identifying improvement in a medical problem. Although the procedures for collecting these specimens are outlined in Module 18, Collecting Specimens, some important points should be mentioned in this chapter.

Methods Used for Collecting a Urine Specimen

Some hospitals always collect a urine specimen for testing when a patient is admitted. Each type of test requires an appropriately collected specimen. A urine specimen may be generally obtained in three ways; a voided specimen, a clean-catch specimen, or from a catheter.

The *voided specimen* is usually obtained when a routine urinalysis is desired, as in a general physical examination. Urine collected this way may contain a number of organisms that have been "washed" into the specimen from the meatus so that it is not as accurate for examination as that gathered by other methods.

A *clean-catch specimen* is most frequently used for a culture to check for the presence of infection of the urinary tract. Clean-catch means that you or the patient clean the urinary meatus with soap and water before a specimen is caught in midstream. A specimen obtained this way is less contaminated with organisms than a voided specimen. For most routine urine cultures, a clean-catch specimen is sufficiently clean.

A *catheterized specimen* is obtained by the insertion of a small tube or catheter through the urethra into the bladder. Catheterization provides a sterile urine specimen. Medications for treatment and dyes for diagnostic tests may also be instilled through a catheter. It is unwise to catheterize the patient for the sole reason of obtaining a urine specimen because of the possibility of introducing organisms into the sterile environment of the bladder with the passage of the catheter. You must also consider the patient's discomfort, inconvenience, and expense. If a catheter is already in place, a specimen can be withdrawn from the catheter itself without interrupting the system, and thus sterility is maintained. Usually a physician will not order a catheter inserted for the purpose of obtaining a urine specimen unless the patient has a serious kidney disease, is acutely ill, or is unresponsive.

Frequency of Collecting Urine Specimens

The admission urine specimen or one used for physical examination is usually collected as a single voided specimen. At other times, specimens are required on a serial basis for specific diagnostic tests. The term used for this is fractionals. The timing of the collection of these specimens is important. For patients whose urine may contain glucose, such as diabetics or those on parenteral nutrition, the policy of the facility will determine the individual schedule to be followed.

For some tests such as the urine creatinine clearance test mentioned below, a 24-hour specimen is collected by saving all urine for that period of time. For accuracy, the patient is asked to void to empty the bladder. This urine is discarded. All urine is then saved for the next 24 hours. At the end of that time, the patient is again asked to empty the bladder completely. This urine is added to the collecting container, and the entire specimen is sent to the lab. If a voiding is inadvertently discarded, you should call the laboratory and explain the circumstances. If precise measurement is not required for that patient's medical condition, the laboratory is sometimes able to recalibrate the procedure to allow for this loss. This in no way suggests that the collecting of urine specimens should be done in less than a responsible manner.

The Nurse's Responsibility for Collecting Urine Specimens

Whatever method is used to obtain a urine specimen, the nurse is responsible for seeing that the specimen is labeled according to the policy of the facility. All specimens are collected wearing clean gloves, and specimens are placed in an unleakable plastic bag before being transported to the laboratory. These actions are taken to protect staff and laboratory personnel. A urine specimen should either be sent to the laboratory reasonably promptly or refrigerated to prevent its character from changing as it stands.

Direct Testing of Urinary Function

Urinary analysis (*UA*) is a common test in which the urine is tested in the laboratory for normal and abnormal characteristics. The urine sent for examination can be obtained in a number of ways.

The *culture and sensitivity test* (*C&S*) examines the urine for microorganisms. The microbes are grown in a culture and then exposed to various antiseptic medications to determine which might be the most effective for treatment. This test is sometimes done in conjunction with the urinalysis.

The *creatinine clearance* test, which requires a 24-hour specimen, measures the amount of creatinine, the nitrogenous waste product of skeletal muscle, in the urine. If the substance is not "cleared" in the urine, kidney disease may be indicated.

Testing for the presence of *glucose or ketones* in the urine may be done to determine whether there is an increased blood level of these substances. The tests are done on the unit by the nursing staff using various reagents. Usually, however, the blood is tested directly to obtain a more accurate measurement of these substances.

Indirect Testing of Urinary Function

The measurement of the serum (blood) *electrolytes* tells the physician a great deal about the kidney's ability to maintain the body's balance of these components. Although other conditions can certainly cause a disruption in the electrolyte balance, renal function can be one factor.

The *BUN* is a test that measures the amount of *blood urea nitrogen* in a sample of blood. It determines if nitrogenous wastes are being sufficiently eliminated or are collecting in the blood. An elevation (a rise in the normal amount) may signify problems with renal function, although dehydration may cause a mild elevation in a person's BUN. Normal values are approximately 10 to 20 mg/100 ml.

A *serum creatinine* test measuring the creatinine in the blood can be done with or separate from the urine creatinine clearance test. When performing a serum creatinine test, a blood sample is drawn and sent to the laboratory, where the creatinine level is measured. Creatinine is a stable product of muscle metabolism that is normally kept at a low level in the blood by kidney excretion. An increased level usually indicates kidney dysfunction.

X-rays and Imagery

An x-ray of the *kidney, ureter, and bladder* (*KUB*) shows the general outline of these structures but does not indicate a great deal about their functioning. They are used primarily to complete a series of other tests or for determining the presence and relationship of one structure to an other. They are also ordered to identify injury to organs of the urinary system.

An *intravenous pyelogram* (*IVP*) requires an injection into the circulatory system of a radiopaque contrast material. The dye normally makes the person feel warm, and the face flushes. These side effects should be explained beforehand so that the patient will not become alarmed. As the dye is excreted by the kidneys, x-rays are taken at short intervals so that the urinary process can be observed.

A *kidney scan* involves the instillation of a radioisotope into the circulatory system. After a brief waiting period, the kidneys and surrounding structures are scanned to see the uptake of the isotope. The procedure is noninvasive and safe for the patient.

Computed axial tomography (*CAT*) scan can be useful in diagnosing urinary problems. As with other systems, a dye may be used so that you should consult a resource regarding this procedure.

Although it is an expensive procedure and has other disadvantages, *magnetic resonance imaging* (*MRI*) is sometimes performed. Through the use of a special magnetic field, an image can be made of the organs of the urinary system.

After mild sedation, a *cystoscopy* can be performed by the insertion of a fiberoptic cystoscope through the urethra. When sterile water is instilled, the interior walls of the bladder can be observed. Bleeding, infection, and bladder tumors can be detected. The patient must be observed after the test for bleeding, retention, and indications of bladder trauma.

At the same time as the cystoscopy, *ureteral catheters*, which are much smaller than those used for bladder catheterization, can be passed through the cystoscope into the ureters, up to the kidney pelvis. This allows visualization as well as the retrieval of cells for examination.

Biopsies

Biopsies of tissue from various locations can be done to identify histologic changes that signify diseases of this system. The kidney is usually biopsied percutaneously. This means that a large-bore needle is inserted through the anesthetized skin, and a small amount of tissue is withdrawn for examination.

Assessment

Review of the Record

Urinary problems are common with hospitalized people. It is important to know the patient's *condition* and *diagnosis* as well as how the patient perceives the problem. The female patient with an infection of the vagina can readily develop an infection of the bladder as well because of the close proximity of the organs. The male patient with an enlarged prostate may have difficulty voiding. Any surgical patient who is to spend a relatively long period under anesthesia should be assessed afterward for urinary retention. If the patient has been admitted for a urinary problem, you should have knowledge of this condition and may consult a text to gain more information.

Changes in fluid intake, the presence of fever, which can dehydrate the patient, and infection can all alter urinary function. Also, anxiety, stress, and depression, as well as altered states of awareness, can have an impact on the ability to urinate normally. The record will also assist you in identifying persons who may be at risk for problems. For example, persons who have had recurrent kidney stones or urinary tract infection as well as those immobilized are at risk.

Information regarding both the medications that the patient has been taking as an outpatient and those ordered within the facility are important for assessment. Many older persons take diuretics so that you should assess for adequate oral fluid intake as well as potassium replacement.

Interview

During an interview with the patient, you will want to ask about the patient's usual urinary habits and the problems applicable to the patient's diagnosis. A patient who trusts the nurse is more likely to discuss urinary problems. If the patient does not volunteer information, the nurse might, without embarrassment, ask one or two direct questions. The following information should be gathered.

1. How much does the patient exercise?
2. What is the person's usual fluid intake?
3. Has the patient ever had or is the person having any difficulty with urination? Urgency or frequency? (These problems are described below.)
4. Has there been any concern about the amount or color of the urine?
5. Are there foods or fluids that affect urination?
6. Has the patient ever experienced pain with urination?
7. Does the person void at night and if so, how often?

Physical Assessment

Not only are subjective data important but your physical assessment will add valuable information. Several areas need to be assessed.

Measurement of Intake and Output

One of the first items to consider is the amount of urine excreted compared to the amount of fluid ingested. For a person who is not in the health care setting or a patient whose intake and output are not being recorded, simply questioning the patient may elicit baseline information. How much does the patient drink and what might affect this amount? For example, salty or bitter condiments or foods can cause thirst and, therefore, increase fluid intake. What factors might influence output? Some fluids such as coffee, wine, and beer are diuretic and stimulate the production of urine.

For the patient on intake and output recording, the total intake of fluid must be calculated, including fluids in the diet, any intravenous fluid, blood, and any irrigating solution that is not returned. Output includes not only urine but vomitus and drainage. Severe diaphoresis (perspiration) or diarrhea should also be considered. For instructions on measuring intake and output, see Module 15, Intake and Output.

Amount of Urine

It is important to determine the amount of urine being excreted. You should know the terms used to describe amounts of urine for your assessment.

The terms **anuria** and **urinary suppression** both refer to the same condition, total absence of formation of urine by the kidneys. No output will be observed and the patient will not feel distended because there is no urine in the bladder. Complete kidney shutdown (a commonly used phrase) is sometimes called *renal failure.*

Oliguria is scanty formation of urine by the kidneys, which may occur in patients suffering from dehydration or blood loss. The healthy adult kidneys secrete approximately 50 ml/hr. As a general guideline for assessment, any amount less than 30 ml/hr is considered insufficient to eliminate body waste, and output below 10 ml/hr is considered likely to lead to damage to the kidney itself. When a seriously ill patient has a catheter, you may use a special device called a **urimeter**, which measures urine in a small calibrated cylinder as it flows through the tubing before entering the collection bag. For accurate assessment, you may need to measure the urine every hour.

Polyuria is the secretion of an excessive amount of urine. A patient who consistently excretes more than 2,000 ml of urine in 24 hours might be said to have polyuria. Although often simply a result of high fluid intake, this condition also characterizes hormonal disturbances. Both diabetes mellitus (a disease of carbohydrate metabolism) and diabetes insipidus (a pituitary disorder) cause polyuria.

Discomfort With Urination

Dysuria can mean either difficulty urinating or pain on urination (micturition). Strictures (narrowing) of the urethra and infection of the urinary tract are causative factors.

A burning sensation accompanying urination is one type of dysuria. Because it is a common occurrence, the more specific term *burning* is typically used. Infection is the most frequent cause of burning when urinating.

Timing and Control of Urination

Several conditions involve the time of urination. *Frequency* is the need or desire to void at more frequent intervals than usual. Each voiding may produce as little as 50 ml. Neuromuscular diseases, pressure on the bladder, stress, or infection of the urinary tract can cause frequency.

Nocturia is urination during the night, either voluntary or involuntary. Involuntary urination during sleep is called *enuresis.* We have discussed enuresis in children as a possible delay in maturation. Common causes of nocturia in adults are infection and high fluid intake during the evening. In the elderly, nocturia is often caused by diminished bladder tone or control of the sphincter.

Urinary *retention* is the holding of urine within the bladder due to an inability to void. This condition often occurs in the patient whose urinary system is obstructed, as well as in the postoperative patient as an effect of anesthesia or local trauma. If a patient fails to void within 8 to 10 hours after surgery, particularly if a hydrating intravenous infusion is in place, you should consult the physician, who may order catheterization. Palpating with care over the bladder area will indicate the extent of retention.

Urgency, which often accompanies frequency, is the inability to postpone urination. The diminished sphincter control of some elderly people and some women who have borne a number of children leads to urgency, as do stress and infection.

Difficulty in starting the stream of urine when the desire to void is present is called *hesitancy.* Another condition related to this is called *start and stop.* This means that the patient has difficulty starting the stream of urine and trouble stopping the flow. Men with enlargement of the prostate frequently report this problem.

Urinary incontinence, or involuntary micturition, is not a simple problem. It has variants: inability to hold urine in the bladder at all is called complete incontinence; partial incontinence is occasional or infrequent inability to retain urine in the bladder. Complete urinary incontinence causes dribbling, which is particularly stressful to the individual. Incontinence calls for special nursing actions, discussed later in the chapter.

Stress incontinence refers to the leakage of urine when one is coughing, sneezing, or laughing and is caused by the relaxed state of the perineal and gluteal muscles. This leakage is more common in middle-aged women who have borne children. Both women and men can experience stress incontinence when lifting heavy objects. Exercises, called Kegel exercises, tighten and relax these groups of muscles and are sometimes helpful in correcting this type of incontinence.

Nursing Diagnosis

Several approved nursing diagnoses are specific to problems of urination. These pertain to changes in patterns of urinary elimination. Other pertinent nursing diagnoses reflect additional problems that may occur.

Urinary Retention

The category for many problems of urinary elimination is Altered Patterns of Urinary Elimination. For clarification, you should identify the specific problem such as retention, urgency, or incontinence.

For example, if *retention* is the problem, it could be related to exposure to anesthesia or to mechanical obstruction. Retention is a real or high risk problem based on your objective and subjective assessment data. Knowing whether your patient is at risk for retention is essential. Accurate observation of the postoperative patient until chances for retention are no longer a concern is important (see the sample Nursing Care Plan Related to Urinary Retention).

Incontinence

Incontinence is the inability to control urinary elimination. If incontinence is the problem, you will specify whether it is functional, reflex, stress, total, or urge incontinence. The U.S. Department of Health and Human Services' Agency for Health Care Policy and Research has developed a monitoring tool that can be used for people in hospitals or nursing homes to monitor the presence and control of incontinence (Fig. 27-5). Keeping such a record can often lead to identification of the etiology of the incontinence. Adding the etiology, such as neurologic deficits or altered mentation, for example, further increases its usefulness as a diagnosis.

Functional Incontinence

Functional incontinence can be related to advancing age. The person is unable to reach the toilet facilities in time to urinate normally. Other factors for delay in reaching the toilet may be limited cognitive, sensory, or physical status. It may also be an environmental barrier such as the location of the chair or bed in relation to the toilet. Outcome criteria include recognition of the problem by the person and care providers. Another desired outcome is adaptation of the environment to facilitate easy use of the toileting facilities.

Reflex Incontinence

Reflex incontinence is loss of urinary elimination control related to spinal cord damage. The injury can innervate involuntary reflexes that cause spontaneous urination without voluntary control. The desired outcomes include an awareness on the part of the person regarding dryness and learning techniques through a teaching program for "triggering" reflex voiding. Reflex incontinence can be a permanent condition unless interventions are undertaken.

Urge Incontinence

Urge incontinence occurs when the person feels a forceful urge to void and is unable to voluntarily hold back the flow. Both children and older adults may be affected due to small or incompetent bladders. Infections, the performance of diagnostic procedures, and conditions of the nervous system are other causes of urge incontinence. The desired outcomes are to identify the cause of decrease the incidence of incontinence.

Total Incontinence

Total incontinence means that the person continuously has episodes of involuntary loss of urine. Total incontinence can be related to age, infection, or congen-

Nursing Care Plan

Sample Nursing Care Plan Related to Urinary Retention

Nursing Diagnosis

Urinary Retention related to exposure to anesthesia during surgery

Supportive data:

47-year-old man.

Hernia repaired this AM.

Has not voided since surgery (12 h).

States, "I feel like I have to go but I just can't start the flow."

Bladder distended two finger-breadths above symphysis pubis.

Desired Patient Outcomes

Short term:

Patient voids voluntarily. If not, the bladder is emptied by catheterization within the next 2 h.

Long term:

No further episodes of retention.

Nursing Action	Rationale
1. Assess the patient's intake, including intravenous fluids.	Amount of urine produced will depend upon the total intake of fluids.
2. Gently palpate over the bladder for signs of distention.	A distended bladder can be palpated above the symphysis.
3. Provide privacy.	The social norm is for privacy during urination. The patient may be more likely to void if uninterrupted and unobserved.
4. Have the patient try voiding into a urinal.	Providing an accessible receptacle for the male patient may bring about the urge to urinate.
5. If not successful, obtain an order for patient to stand by bed to void.	Standing is the usual male position for urination. Approximating the normal position may assist the patient to urinate. A physician's order is needed to protect the nurse for liability issues if this is the policy of the facility.
6. Run water in room while patient attempts to void.	The sound of running water often causes the person to begin to urinate.
7. If not successful, catheterize as per postop order.	Distention can be uncomfortable and may even injure the bladder, therefore, catheterization may be necessary.

INSTRUCTIONS: EACH TIME THE PATIENT IS CHECKED:

1) Mark one of the circles in the BLADDER section at the hour closest to the time the patient is checked.
2) Make an X in the BOWEL section if the patient has had an incontinent or normal bowel movement.

• (slashed) = Incontinent, small amount	∅ = Dry	**X** = Incontinence BOWEL
● (slashed) = Incontinent, large amount	△ (slashed) = Voided correctly	**X** = Normal BOWEL

PATIENT NAME ______________ ROOM # ______ DATE ______

	BLADDER			BOWEL			
	INCONTINENCE OF URINE	DRY	VOIDED CORRECTLY	INCONTINENCE X	NORMAL X	INITIALS	**COMMENTS**
12 am	• ●	○	△ cc ___				
1	• ●	s	△ cc ___				
2	• ●	s	△ cc ___				
3	• ●	s	△ cc ___				
4	• ●	s	△ cc ___				
5	• ●	s	△ cc ___				
6	• ●	s	△ cc ___				
7	• ●	s	△ cc ___				
8	• ●	s	△ cc ___				
9	• ●	s	△ cc ___				
10	• ●	s	△ cc ___				
11	• ●	s	△ cc ___				
12 pm	• ●	s	△ cc ___				
1	• ●	s	△ cc ___				
2	• ●	s	△ cc ___				
3	• ●	s	△ cc ___				
4	• ●	s	△ cc ___				
5	• ●	s	△ cc ___				
6	• ●	s	△ cc ___				
7	• ●	s	△ cc ___				
8	• ●	s	△ cc ___				
9	• ●	s	△ cc ___				
10	• ●	s	△ cc ___				
11	• ●	s	△ cc ___				
TOTALS:							

Figure 27-5. Incontinence monitoring record for hospital and nursing home residents. From Urinary Incontinence Guideline Panel. *Urinary Incontinence in Adults: Clinical Practice Guideline.* AHCPR Pub. No. 92-0038, Rockville, MD: Agency for Health Care Policy and Research, Public Health Service, US Department of Health and Human Services, March 1992.

ital or neuromuscular conditions. This is stressful for the patient and the family. Desired outcomes include identifying the cause and finding ways to reduce or eliminate the periods of incontinence.

Pain

Pain of the urinary tract can occur from infection, injury, or obstruction. The person who has a kidney stone that obstructs urinary flow and causes spasm of a ureter may have severe, spasmodic pain. Pain can also be caused by a diagnostic or urinary procedure. An example is Pain: Bladder spasms related to cystoscopy. Pain may occur only on urination and may be described as a burning pain. Low abdominal discomfort also occurs with some bladder disorders.

Self-care Deficit

Self-care Deficit: Toileting is another nursing diagnosis that is appropriate for some patients. This nursing diagnosis describes the inability to independently perform the functions needed for urinary elimination.

A patient who has extreme fatigue and weakness or altered level of consciousness may be unable to ask for assistance with toileting. Older persons may have phys-

Nursing Diagnoses Related to Urination

Urinary Retention related to
- Exposure to anesthsia
- Mechanical obstruction
- Functional incontinence
- Reflex incontinence
- Stress incontinence
- Urge incontinence
- Total incontinence

Pain: Bladder spasms related to irritation of cystoscopy

Self-care Deficit: Toileting related to extreme fatigue

Sleep Pattern Disturbance related to nocturia

Low Self-esteem related to long-term incontinence

High Risk for Infection related to presence of indwelling catheter

ical conditions such as arthritis that limit mobility and prevent their normal use of toilet facilities. In some of these situations, if assistance is delayed, incontinence may occur.

Sleep Pattern Disturbance

Sleep Pattern Disturbance: Deprivation related to nocturia is another nursing diagnosis of importance. For persons with nocturia, the necessity of having to urinate frequently during the night can cause sleep pattern disturbance. If this is the case, the nursing diagnosis focuses on that specific problem and elimination is stated as the etiology. The resolution of this kind of problem will consider actions centered around urinary function.

Low Self-esteem

Persons who have long-term problems of incontinence, whether total or partial, may develop low self-esteem. Episodes of incontinence may interfere with ability to participate in activities or hold a job. People may consider themselves unclean and be fearful of interacting socially.

High Risk for Infection

Nursing diagnosis often focuses on identifying patients at risk of problems. Because the sterile urinary tract opens into the perineal area, as well as other factors, many patients with urinary conditions are at high risk for infection.

Incontinence is a problem that may lead to high risk for urinary tract infection. The presence of an indwelling catheter also places the individual at risk for urinary tract infection. A diagnosis stating that the patient is at risk for infection reminds the nurse that special observations and actions must be taken to ensure the patient remains infection free.

Planning and Implementation

Whatever the patient's problem, the desired patient outcome is for the person to recognize deficits that are present and to participate in the plan of care. The goal is to reestablish urinary function at a level that is as normal as possible.

Because urinary problems cause the patient not only physical pain but also embarrassment and anxiety, a confident and accepting attitude on your part can be of the utmost value in comforting the patient.

Nursing Actions for Treating Urinary Tract Infections

If the patient has an infection, fluids should be increased. The patient may need the fluid intake increased to as high as 3,000 to 4,000 ml in 24 hours. The plan of care is more effective if the patient helps in planning. If nausea is not present, the patient may tell you what fluids are preferred. Usually, the greatest percentage of fluid is given during the daytime hours with less fluid intake during the late afternoon and evening so that the need to urinate does not interfere with rest.

You may be required to administer special medications for pain or infection. Knowledge of these specific drugs will allow you to inform the patient about their actions and uses. Most urinary medications require adequate fluid intake.

Management of Urinary Retention

Urinary retention may be temporary, as in patients who have been exposed to anesthesia, or it may be longstanding in patients who have neuromuscular disease. For any patient, feeling the need to void or having a full bladder and being unable to urinate voluntarily is distressing.

When retention is transient, the nurse can take several actions. First, the patient will benefit from privacy and an unhurried attitude on the part of the nurse. Adequate fluid intake is essential because sufficient urine must be present before the bladder reflex is activated. Only when the bladder contains at least 300 ml is the desire to eliminate usually activated. Placing the patient's hands in a pan of warm water, pouring warm water over the perineum, running tap water within the patient's hearing, or putting pressure on one side of the urinary meatus may facilitate voiding. Men who experience retention can sometimes void if they are allowed to stand, thus assuming the usual voiding position. If none of these measures is successful, the physician may order catheterization.

When the condition is long-term, as, for example, with those in rehabilitation programs, the **Crede's method** may be used. This method involves exerting manual pressure on the bladder to promote elimination of urine. There is some reason to believe that this maneuver should be avoided in those with short-term problems because it does not allow the bladder wall to stretch and relax naturally and may damage the internal or external sphincter.

When appropriate, the physician may order that patients be catheterized every 4 to 8 hours to decompress the bladder. This approach is called "in and out catheterization." If meticulous sterile technique is used, these patients have fewer urinary tract infections than those with indwelling catheters. Before discharge from the hospital, some patients are taught to self-catheterize. With practice, patients become very skillful at self-catheterization, which effectively deals with their retention problem.

Management of Incontinence

Care of incontinent patients in the hospital or in the long-term care setting requires special nursing actions. However, nurses should encourage nursing actions other than catheterization to treat incontinence. These actions include providing frequent opportunities for toileting. For some patients who are physically and psychologically impaired, actions may include assisting the patient to the bathroom or placing the patient on the commode or bedpan on a regular basis throughout the day. The patient must also be checked frequently to determine if wetting has occurred. If the patient is wet, immediate skin care is essential to avoid skin breakdown. Some patients may have to wear protective undergarments, which should be changed promptly if wetting occurs. External catheters that attach to the leg to collect urine are available for incontinent men. If the patient is unable to participate in a bladder rehabilitation program, you can implement the same actions for that person that you would plan for the less impaired patient.

Patients vary in the degree of urinary control present. The attitude that nothing can be done for incontinence is defeatist and not useful to the patient or family. A variety of aids and medical intervention may improve this condition and help the individual regain a higher quality of life.

It is only fair to state that the degree of regaining continence also varies with the individual and medical status. Midlife women may have a surgical procedure performed that corrects certain urinary structural positions and helps the individual gain urinary control. Other people with intermittent and partial urinary problems may choose to use one of the many garment protective products now commercially available. Although their use may not be the chosen solution for some individuals and their families, it must be recognized that being freed from the fear of an accident and gaining a renewed feeling of being socially acceptable are impor-

Nursing Issues and Trends: *Living with Urinary Incontinence*

It has been estimated that approximately 10 million people in the United States have some degree of urinary incontinence, not all of them elders. The fact that this problem has been so widely recognized commercially with the promotion of waterproof undergarments is a statement in itself of increased awareness and acceptance of the problem by the public. The availability of these items has "freed" many of those affected so that they can resume social interaction and be less hesitant to join in activities of the community. Even though the availability of these products may offer a partial solution, many cases of incontinence are treatable. The Department of Health and Human Services has studied the research on this wide-ranging problem and recommended participation by those with incontinence in regional programs specializing in bladder rehabilitation. Nurses can encourage public education so people with urinary incontinence will participate in programs to seek more long-standing solutions which will maximize their lives.

tant. We will discuss regaining bladder control in the section on rehabilitation.

Initiation of Bladder Rehabilitation

As more persons in our society reach advanced age, the problem of urinary incontinence has increased. Incontinence is the primary reason elders are admitted to long-term care facilities by families who are unprepared to care for such a problem. Decrease in mentation is another main reason older persons are admitted to long-term care. In many situations, incontinence is directly related to decreased mental status, which only compounds the problem. An action plan should be written by the nurse for all incontinent patients, regardless of their impairment (see sample Nursing Care Plan Related to Urinary Incontinence).

Although incontinence usually has a physiologic

Nursing Care Plan

Sample Nursing Care Plan Related to Urinary Incontinence

Nursing Diagnosis

Urinary incontinence related to age and mildly confused state

Supportive data:

82-year-old woman.

Incontinent of urine two to three times per shift.

Expresses surprise and shame when this occurs.

States, "I don't know where the bathroom is."

Desired Patient Outcomes

Short term:

Incontinence to occur not more than one time each shift.

Patient explains measures she can take to maintain continence.

Long term:

No episodes of incontinence.

Nursing Action	Rationale
1. Spend time with patient to carefully explain plan.	Spending time with the patient and explaining the plan denotes interest on the part of the nurse and fosters compliance.
2. Remind the patient of the location of the bathroom and assure her that you will assist in taking her there.	Making sure that the patient knows the location of the bathroom and assuring her that she has assistance will encourage her to use the toilet when she has the urge to urinate.
3. Provide television or books for diversion.	Diversion promotes relaxation.
4. Encourage fluid intake to 2,600 ml/day.	Increasing fluids hydrates the patient and produces enough urine to stimulate the bladder to empty every two hours per plan.
5. Take patient to the bathroom on even hours on day and evening shifts and encourage her to take enough time to empty bladder.	Assisting the patient to the bathroom every two hours during the day and evening shifts provides the opportunity to urinate and avoid incontinence.
6. Praise her for voiding on toilet. Do not blame her for incidents of incontinence.	Praise reinforces desired behavior. Blame hinders the occurrence of desired behavior.
7. Record progress on flow sheet.	Documentation of progress allows the health care team to actively participate and continue the plan.

basis, it also has overtones of dependency. With older patients, getting up out of bed, dressing in their own clothing, and being offered bathroom accommodations on a regular schedule can often reverse a trend toward incontinence. This is especially important for the older person with decreased mental status. Health teaching is an important part of a bladder rehabilitation program in assisting persons to manage incontinence. As in any other health teaching, there must be a cooperative effort on the part of both patient and nurse if at all possible. The nurse should explain the program and the desired outcomes to the patient. Patients who fully understand that the goal is more normal functioning of the bladder usually become highly motivated. Increased fluid intake to as high as 2,000 ml daily is essential. The patient is encouraged to retain the urine as long as possible or at least up to 2 hours or longer. Use of the bathroom toilet to void is preferred because it most approximates what is normal. A man may be more successful in voiding if encouraged to stand. Positioning, of course, is contingent on the patient's physical condition.

Voidings are spaced increasingly far apart from the duration that can initially be tolerated. The stretching–relaxing sequence of this process reinstates bladder muscle tone, eventually affording the patient more voluntary control.

Because incontinent persons have a greater risk for infection, assessment and management of infection become essential parts of the plan of care. Health teaching or carrying out meticulous personal hygiene so that the urinary meatus is cleaned after every exposure to urine helps prevent infection.

If the patient has a fever, discomfort on urination, or scant or cloudy urine, the presence of infection should be considered. Some older patients may have infection without symptoms other than incontinence. Other older patients may have symptoms of urinary tract infection such as vomiting, diarrhea, and abdominal or lower back pain (Pritchard, 1988). You can increase fluids and notify the physician of your observations.

Nurses in the community and working both in the hospital and long-term care are important in health teaching, exploring alternatives in care, and most of all, changing attitudes. Many nurses have a difficult time caring for the incontinent patient.

Whether the patient has difficulty voiding or controlling voiding, the nurse's attitude is crucial. Understandably, patients tend to be noticeably embarrassed and upset over such a situation, and the nurse should exhibit a sympathetic attitude.

Fortunately, the action of immediate catheterization with placement of an indwelling catheter is decreasing and nurses are learning newer techniques for management of incontinence.

Management of Urinary Diversion

Urinary diversion creates responsibilities for the nurse. Health teaching is essential so that the patient can care for the appliance and skin. Patients who have undergone urinary diversion are at risk for infection of the urinary tract and skin breakdown. Thus, the nurse must constantly carry out skin assessment and give meticulous care to the stoma. For specific instructions on the care of patients with urinary diversion, consult Module 38, Ostomy Care.

Catheterization for Retention, Incontinence, or Urinary Diversion

Performing catheterization in a manner that provides for the safety of the patient is a nursing responsibility. It must be done correctly so as not to injure the patient. Also, because of the risk of infection, the nurse must maintain sterility at all times. For instructions on per-

Nursing Research: *Implications for Practice*

Bristoll, S. et al. "The Mythical Danger of Rapid Urinary Drainage." *American Journal of Nursing 89*, 3 (March 1989): 344–345.

Six patients with bladders containing 1,000 ml of urine or more and with an order for catheterization were studied. The bladders of one-half the patients were completely drained using a single-phase method, which drained all urine present within the bladder. The bladders of the other patients were drained using a clamp/release technique. The pulse rates and blood pressures of all patients wre monitored during the procedures, and urine samples were obtained and examined for the presence of blood. This small study presented no evidence to support the myth that complete, one-phase bladder drainage causes changes in the patient's vital functions and is hazardous. This supports results of earlier studies.

forming catheterization, refer to Module 39, Catheterization.

When a patient's retention of urine or inability to empty the bladder completely is thought to be only temporary, *intermittent catheterization* may be performed. This means that a straight catheter (one without a balloon) is inserted by the nurse to drain the bladder. Intermittent catheterization to check for residual urine can also be done after a patient voids if the possibility exists that the bladder is not completely emptying. Each time the patient is catheterized, the same standards of sterility and safety must be maintained.

Intermittent self-catheterization is a procedure that allows the person to be free of a permanent indwelling catheter. Intermittent self-catheterization is used primarily by patients with spinal cord injuries or those who have a neurologic deficit that does not allow the bladder to empty normally.

The person is taught to introduce the catheter, using clean technique, and drain the bladder at regular intervals throughout the day. The goal is to obtain approximately 300 ml with each procedure. During the night, when the person usually does not perform self-catheterization, a protective undergarment may be worn to prevent leakage. It is easier for a man to perform self-catheterization than for a woman because of the visual accessibility of the male organs. Nurses teach women how to perform self-catheterization by using a mirror technique to identify the site properly and to insert the catheter.

Indwelling catheterization is performed for both retention and incontinence. Indwelling catheters may be left in place to continually drain urine from the bladder of patients who have had surgery and cannot void voluntarily or for those who are incontinent. Patients who are catheterized for any reason have an increased risk for urinary tract infection, but those with an indwelling catheter are at high risk for infection. Ruge (1987) suggests several ways to avoid infection. First, as long as the catheter can be kept patent (unobstructed), the smaller the size (14 or 16 French), the better. A large catheter can cause bladder irritation and leakage of urine and can encourage infection. Second, routine hygienic care of the meatus is sufficient if carried out once a day, as recommended by the Centers for Disease Control and Prevention. Studies have also shown that the use of ointments at the meatus is not helpful, and because they coat the tissue around the meatus, they may, in fact, actually promote infection. Last, Ruge suggests that catheters should remain in place for as short a time as possible. "After five days, the risk for infection is high." The catheter should also be changed only when it is no longer patent, for each time the catheter is changed, there is a chance of introducing bacteria that can cause infection.

Initiation of Bladder Rehabilitation for the Patient With a Catheter

When a patient has an indwelling catheter, a bladder rehabilitation program can be initiated to help the bladder return to normal functioning after the catheter has been discontinued. The goal is to restore the normal elasticity of the bladder for proper emptying. A physician may order a "clamp and release" routine before the catheter is removed, which means that the catheter is clamped for a period of time and then released so that the bladder empties. The rationale is that the alternate stretching and relaxing of the bladder walls simulates normal bladder wall functioning and helps maintain or restore tone. At first, the conscious patient may be able to tolerate clamping for only 30 minutes at a time. The duration of clamping is gradually increased until the patient can tolerate it for 2 hours. After removal of the catheter, the bladder rehabilitation program continues in the same manner.

The unconscious patient who has an indwelling catheter may also be placed on such a program. One word of caution: if the patient is unconscious and cannot voice discomfort, the nurse must be scrupulously conscientious about releasing the catheter clamp at the designated time. The bladder can be seriously injured if proper drainage does not occur.

Prevention of Urinary Tract Infections After Catheter Removal

The patient who has had an indwelling catheter is in need of health teaching when it is removed. It is unusual for a patient who has an indwelling catheter for a long time to be completely free of urinary tract infection. For this reason, the importance of consuming large amounts of fluid before, during, and after the insertion of an indwelling catheter is stressed. A high fluid intake flushes the system and prevents the pooling of urine in the bladder so that it acts as a reservoir for the growth of microorganisms. It is sometimes recommended that the patient drink cranberry juice, which tends to render the urine more acid, discouraging the growth of pathogens. Although the fluid in cranberry juice cocktail is a pleasant method to increase fluid intake, the small amount of cranberry juice in the mixture has proven insufficient to change the pH of the urine. The patient may be warned that a mild burning sensation might occur initially on urination after the catheter has been removed. The patient should also notify the nurse when voluntary voiding first occurs so that it can be determined if the quantity of urine is sufficient to indicate that the bladder is completely emptied.

Health Teaching

All individuals should be taught principles of healthy living that lead to adequate urinary elimination. These principles incorporate good general hygiene as well as concern for other systems of the body. Adequate fluid intake provides the water needed for more efficient filtration. Adequate nutrition is essential to prevent and overcome infection as well as build tissue. Exercise stimulates output, and rest provides for needed relaxation of the body.

All patients undergoing catheterization are taught the importance of knowing the signs and symptoms of urinary tract infection (Fig. 27-6). Prophylactic antibiotics are occasionally given to susceptible persons or those who have experienced frequent bouts of urinary tract infection.

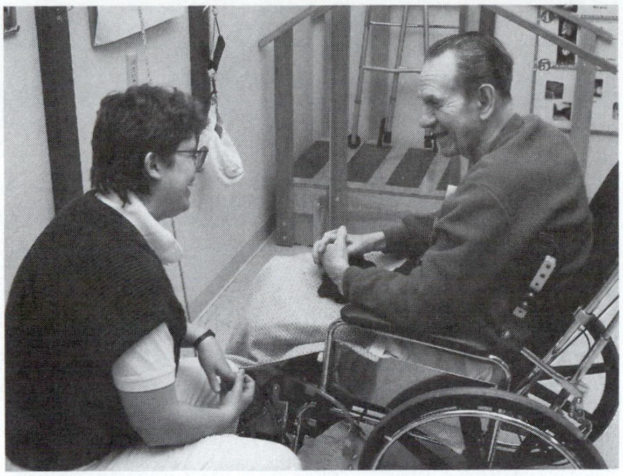

Figure 27-6. Health teaching is essential for the patient who will perform self-catheterization.

Evaluation

Evaluation of urinary function entails reviewing the goals and outcome criteria established earlier in the process. For the patient with a nursing diagnosis related to urination, the evaluation may be that the patient no longer has a problem; for example, measured urinary output may be within normal limits. Alternatively, the patient may have a decrease in a problem. The patient may no longer report burning on urination. You must also keep in mind that evaluation may reveal no evidence of a positive outcome because of underlying problems. For example, a patient may still be unable to assist with the performance of toileting because fatigue and weakness are still present. Perhaps for this patient, the appropriate desired outcome is that incontinence is prevented through the nurse providing assistance with toileting. Evaluation, as we have discussed, often necessitates revision of the care plan.

Nursing Care Study
A Patient with Urinary Incontinence

Mrs. Juarez is a 76-year-old woman who has been in the chronic care facility for 2 months. Her family placed her there when they felt they could no longer care for her. One problem was her incontinence several times a day, which caused hygiene and skin complications.

Alan Prosser, the nursing student, decided to review the care plan and add any information he had gathered. He noticed that Mrs. Juarez seemed withdrawn and refused to attend any activities available to residents. When he met her daughter later that afternoon, he shared his concerns with her regarding her mother's behavior. With some embarrassment, the daughter, Mrs. Wilson, revealed that it was probably because her mother wet herself sometimes. Alan decided to make this his priority problem for the resident, obtain further data, and read up on bladder training.

When Mrs. Juarez refused to attend a group the next day to plan for an outing, Alan touched her hand and asked if there was some reason why she would not like to go. Looking down, Mrs. Juarez said she liked to be near the bathroom. Alan did not encourage her to say more but said he understood. He said that she had a great deal to offer the other residents and asked if he and she could get together later in the day to devise a plan that would let her be comfortable getting out with the group. Mrs. Juarez hesitated for a moment but agreed to talk about it with Alan.

Alan designed a plan and presented it for Mrs. Juarez's approval:

1. Before the next morning group session, she would limit her morning beverages to juice and one cup of decaffeinated coffee.
2. After using the bathroom, she would wear a protective undergarment in case she had an "accident."

(continued)

Nursing Care Study (continued)
A Patient with Urinary Incontinence

3. Alan would also be attending the group meeting and after 1½ hours, he would help Mrs. Juarez to the bathroom. This was the usual time for a tea break, so her absence would not be unduly noticed.
4. During the day, he or another staff person would assist Mrs. Juarez to the bathroom every 1½ hours, extending this period when she could manage a longer interval.

By the end of the first week, Mrs. Juarez was a regular member of the morning planning group and enjoying the interaction even more than Alan did. She was still wearing her undergarments but planned not to use them the following week since she had not had an "accident" and, on one occasion, had gone 2½ hours without the urge to void. Mrs. Wilson validated the remarkable change in her mother when she told Alan that she looked forward to getting her mother out sometime the following weekend for a drive.

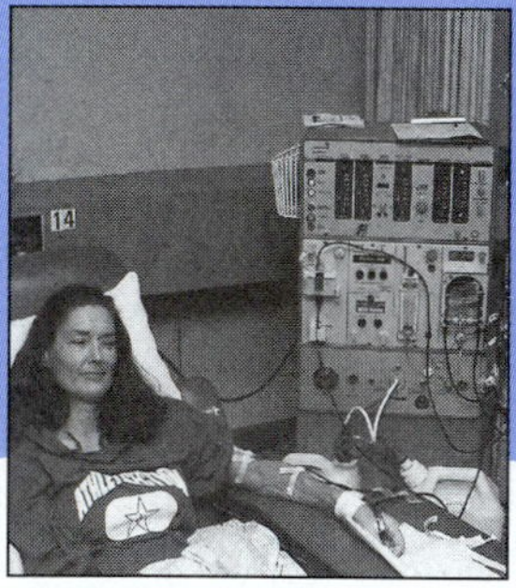

Key Points

- Adequate urinary function is an essential need of all persons to eliminate excess body fluid and nitrogenous wastes.
- In American society, urination is a private matter, a fact that nurses need to keep in mind when approaching the patient concerning urinary problems.
- The urinary system consists of the kidneys, ureters, bladder, and urethra.
- The process of elimination is both voluntary and involuntary, and the urine that is voided has a characteristic color, pH, odor, and specific gravity.
- Abnormal components of urine include bacteria, blood, casts (small numbers are not harmful), glucose, protein, pus, and stones.
- Factors affecting urination include age, fluid intake, exercise, medications, stress and anxiety, and urinary habits.
- Intake and output measurement and collection of urine specimens are nursing responsibilities.
- Urine specimens can be obtained by a number of means, including voiding, clean-catch, by catheterization, and from an indwelling catheter.
- There are intersystem and structural medical problems that can cause urinary dysfunction, some of which may require the use of urinary diversion or dialysis.
- Important areas for urinary assessment are amount of urine produced, evidence of discomfort when voiding, time, and control of urination.
- Urinary retention, incontinence, and pain are some of the nursing diagnoses applicable to problems of urinary function.
- Common problems associated with urinary elimination include frequency, hesitancy, nocturia, and urgency.
- Planning and implementation for urinary problems focus on both reinstating normal patterns of urination and preventing urinary tract infection.
- Ongoing evaluation is important in the nursing care for problems of urinary elimination, and success in meeting desired outcomes may need to be measured in small increments.
- Urinary incontinence is one of the main reasons persons of advanced age are admitted to the long-term care facility. For the patient with long-term urinary management problems, a bladder rehabilitation program that is appropriate for the individual is in order.
- When the patient can participate in the plan of care, health teaching is vital. The plan may include a toileting schedule, an increase in fluid intake, rest, exercise, and meticulous perineal hygiene.

Study Questions

1. Name the four major organs of the urinary system.
2. Briefly explain how urination occurs.

3. Name at least four abnormal components of urine.
4. Describe the usual patterns of urinary elimination for different ages of life: the toddler, young adult, middle adult, and older adult.
5. How does the level of fluid intake effect urination?
6. What does measurement of 1.021 for specific gravity of urine mean?
7. What is the primary danger to the patient being catheterized, and how might this danger be avoided?
8. How does structure relate to urinary problems?
9. Discuss two methods used for urinary diversion.
10. Explain how waste products are removed through the three types of dialysis procedures.
11. List the general principles of health teaching the patient with urinary problems.
12. How would you interact with a granddaughter who is discouraged concerning the incontinence of her grandmother in the long term care setting?

Critical Thinking Activities

1. Familiarize yourself with the intake and output procedures in your health care facility. Is the record complete? Relate this information to the health status of three patients in terms of fluid and electrolyte balance.
2. Identify the different ways emotions of individuals effect urinary elimination. Include aspects of nervous system control.
3. What nursing diagnoses might be appropriate for the patient with nocturia. Write the nursing actions with rationale for each diagnosis identified.
4. Invite a home dialysis nurse to a small group of students. Prepare a list of questions regarding the type of clients served, the health teaching needed, the problems encountered, and the funding of the program.

Relevant Sections in Modules for Basic Nursing Skills

Volume 1 Module
- Assisting with Elimination and Perineal Care 10
- Intake and Output 15
- Collecting Specimens 18
- Performing Common Laboratory Tests 20

Volume 2 Module
- Ostomy Care 38
- Catheterization 39
- Irrigations: Bladder, Catheter, Ear, Eye, Nasogastric Tube, Vaginal, Wound 48

References and Readings

Adams, F. "How Much do Elders Drink?" *Geriatric Nursing* 9, 4 (April 1988): 218–221.

Bielski, M. "Symposium on Infection Control: Preventing Infection in the Catheterized Patient." *Nursing Clinics of North America* 15, 4 (December 1980): 703–713.

Birdsall, C. "How Do You Teach Female Self-Catheterization?" *American Journal of Nursing* 85, 11 (November 1985): 1226.

Brogna, L, and Lakaszawski, M. L. "The Continent Urostomy." *American Journal of Nursing* 86, 2 (February 1986): 160–163.

Carpenito, L. J. *Nursing Diagnosis: Application to Clinical Practice.* 4th edition. Philadelphia: J. B. Lippincott, 1992.

Cheater, F. "Attitudes Toward Urinary Incontinence." *Nursing Standard* 5, 26 (March 1991): 23, 25–27.

Colley, W. "Continence: The Colley Model." *Nursing Times* 87, 7 (February 1991): 13–19.

Conti, M. T., and Eutropius, L. "Preventing UTI's: What Works?" *American Journal of Nursing* 87, 3 (March 1987): 307–309.

Dowd, T. T. "Discovering Older Women's Experience of Urinary Incontinence." *Research in Nursing and Health* 14, 3 (June 1991): 179–186.

Gaspar, P. M. "What Determines How Much Patients Drink?" *Geriatric Nursing* 9, 4 (April 1988): 221–224.

Hahn, K. "Think Twice About Urinary Incontinence." *Nursing '88* 18, 1 (January 1988): 65–67.

Hollingsworth, M. B. "Urinary Incontinence." *Journal of Urological Nursing* 9, 1 (April-June 1990): 869–882.

McKeever, M. P. "An Investigation of Recognized Incontinence Within a Health Authority." *Journal of Advanced Nursing* 15, 10 (October 1990): 1197–1207.

McConnell, E. A. "Assessing the Bladder." *Nursing '85* 15, 11 (November 1985): 44–46.

McCormick, K. A., Newman, D. K., Colling, J., Person, B. D. "Urinary Incontinence in Adults." *American Journal of Nursing* 92, 10 (October 1992): 75–88.

Murray, R. B., and Zentner, J. P. *Nursing Assessment and Health Promotion Strategies Through the Life Span.* Englewood Cliffs, N.J.: Prentice-Hall, 1989.

Newman, D. K., Lynch, K., Smith, D. A., Cell, P. "Restoring Urinary Continence." *American Journal of Nursing* 91, 1 (January 1991): 28–34.

Palmer, M. H. "Urinary Incontinence." *Nursing Clinics of North America* 25, 4 (December 1990): 919–934.

Palmer, M. H. "Detecting Urinary Incontinence in Older Adults During Hospitalization." *Applied Nursing Research.* 5, 4 (November 1992): 174–180.

Perry, J. D., and Hullett, L. T. "The Role of Home Trainers in Kegel's Exercise Program for the Treatment of Incontinence." *Ostomy Wound Management* 30 (September-October 1990): 46–48, 50–51, 53–57.

Petillo, M. H. "The Patient with a Urinary Stoma: Nursing Management and Patient Education." *Nursing Clinics of North America* 22, 2 (June 1987): 263–279.

Pieper, B., Cleland, V., Johnson, D. E., O'Reilly, J. I. "Inventing Urine Incontinence Devices for Women." *Image* 21, 4 (Winter 1989): 205–209.

Powers, I., and Williams, D. "Urinary Incontinence: Helping a Patient Regain Control." *Nursing '92* 22, 12 (December 1992): 46–47.

Pritchard, V. "Geriatric Infections: The Urinary Tract." *RN* 51, 5 (May 1988): 36–38.

Ruge, C. A. "Catheter Related UTIs: What's the Best Way to Prevent Them?" *Nursing '87* 17, 12 (December 1987): 50–51.

Stark, J. L. "Urinary Tract Assessment." *Nursing '88* 18, 7 (July 1988): 57–58.

Strangio, L. "Peritoneal Dialysis Made Easy." *Nursing '88* 18, 1 (January 1988): 43–46.

Tester, K. "Changing Time. . . Association of Continence Advisors." *Nursing Times* 87, 14 (April 3–9, 1991): 70.

Toth, J. M. "When Your Patient Faces a Urostomy." *RN* 48, 11 (November 1985): 50–55.

Urinary Incontinence in Adults: Clinical Practice Guidelines. Agency for Health Care Policy and Research. U.S. Department of Health and Human Services. Pub. No. 92-0038, 1992.

Wanich, C. K., and Reilly, N. J. "Incontinence Care Products: Non Surgical of Management of Urinary Incontinence." *Ostomy Wound Management* 34 (May-June 1991): 45–46.

Wilson, M. F. "Bladder Training for the Chronically Ill." *Nursing '88* 18, 1 (January 1988): 43–46.

Oxygenation

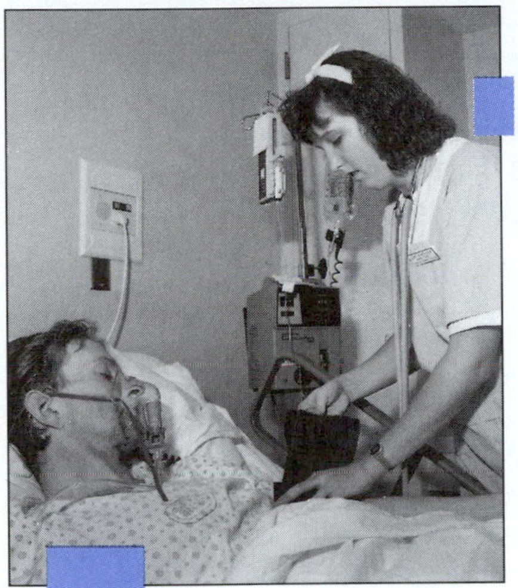

28

Objectives

After completing this chapter, you should be able to:

1. Describe briefly the respiratory system and the process of oxygenation.
2. Explain the terms used to describe lung volumes and capacities and blood gases, and state the norms for each.
3. Describe the various lung clearance mechanisms.
4. Explain the relationship of respiration to acid–base balance.
5. Describe normal respiration with regard to rate, depth, rhythm, breathing sounds, lungs sounds, and comfort.
6. Discuss factors that affect oxygenation.
7. Outline appropriate respiratory assessment.
8. List common nursing diagnoses related to oxygenation and nursing interventions appropriate for each.
9. Discuss specific nursing actions that can be used for a wide variety of patient problems.
10. Describe briefly ways that health teaching and participation in community programs can help prevent respiratory disease.

Study Terms

adventitious sounds
apnea
atelectasis
Biot's respirations
bradypnea
Cheyne-Stokes respirations
cough suppressant
crackles
cyanosis
dyspnea
eupnea
expectorant
expiratory reserve
external respiration
functional residual capacity
gurgles
Heimlich maneuver
hemoglobin saturation
hiccoughs
"huff" cough
hyperpnea
hyperventilation
hypoventilation
hypoxemia
hypoxia
inspiratory capacity
inspiratory reserve
intermittent positive pressure breathing (IPPB)
Kussmaul's respirations
nebulization
orthopnea
orthopneic position
pleural rub
postural drainage
pulmonary embolus
productive cough
quad cough
residual volume

Ellis, Nowlis: Nursing: A Human Needs Approach, 5th ed. © 1994 J.B. Lippincott Company

respiratory acidosis
respiratory alkalosis
retractions
sighing
singultus
sputum
stridor
tachypnea
tidal volume
total lung capacity
tracheostomy
vital capacity
wheezing

Outline

All body cells need oxygen for survival. Oxygen depletion can rapidly cause death of organs and body parts or the death of the individual. For this reason, the respiratory system may be the most important system of the body. Its function is oxygenation through respiration, which is an intricate exchange of two gases, oxygen and carbon dioxide. The acid–base balance of the body is maintained by the appropriate loss of carbon dioxide brought about by respiration.

The Respiratory System

The purpose of the respiratory system is to provide for the exchange of oxygen, which is essential to the metabolism of all body cells, and carbon dioxide, which is given off by the cells. The system is composed of a series of interconnected passages through which air is able to enter and exit (Fig. 28-1).

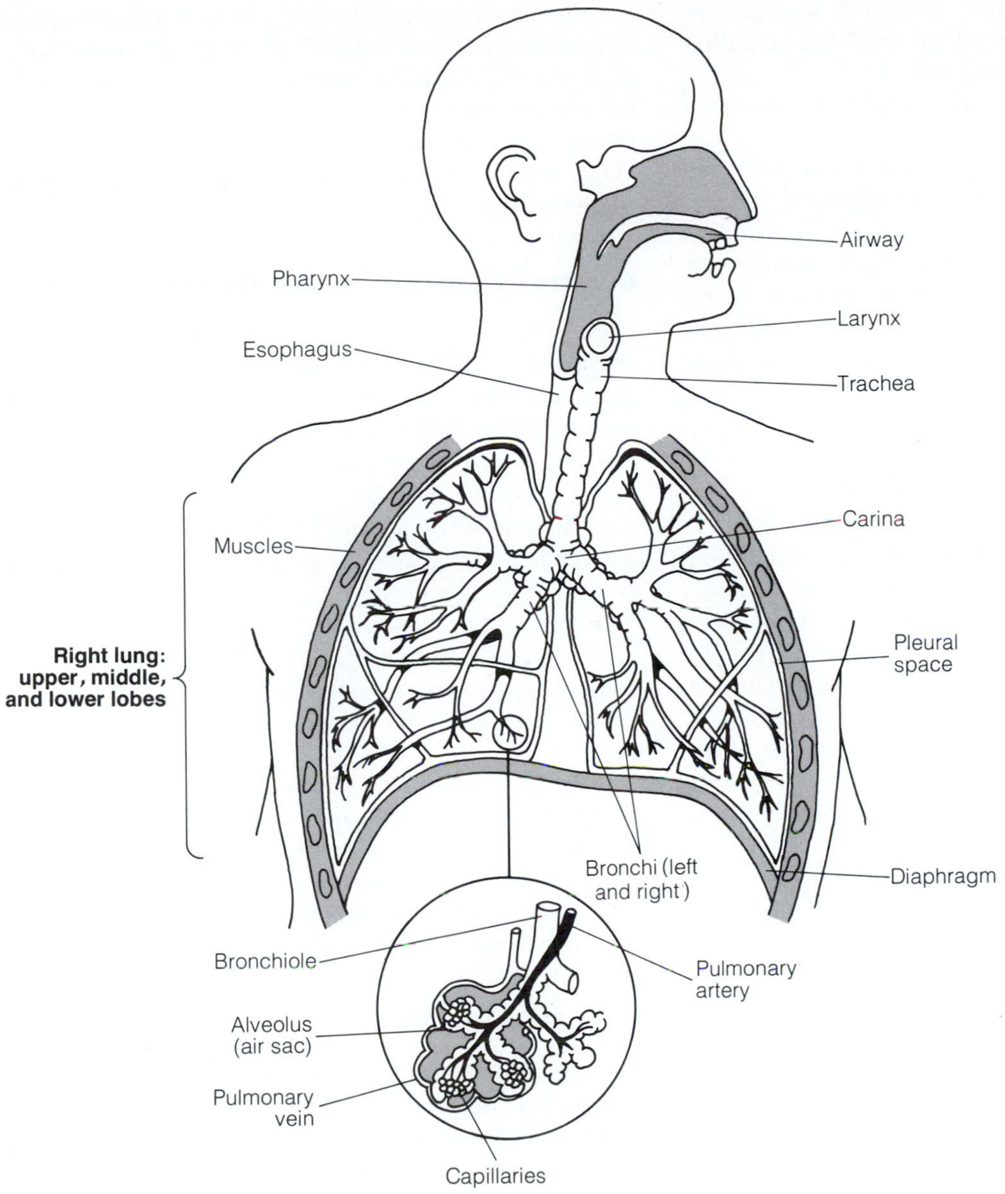

Figure 28-1. The respiratory system.

Air enters the body through the *nose*, where the air is warmed and particles are filtered out. The air then flows through the *pharynx* into the *larynx*, or voice box. From there, the air moves downward to the trachea.

The *trachea* is a tube, composed of a number of horseshoe-shaped cartilaginous rings, leading from the larynx to the bronchi. The trachea branches into two main *bronchi*, also composed of cartilaginous rings. One leads to each lung, right and left. They are the "pipes" through which air enters the lungs. The right bronchus is larger and straighter than the left. Branching off the bronchi are the smaller bronchioles, which form a network of passages through which the air reaches large portions of lung tissue. The muscular walls of the bronchioles can constrict to decrease the air flow or relax to increase it.

The *lungs* are two cone-shaped structures, one on the left side and one on the right side of the chest. They differ slightly in shape; the left is more concave to allow room for the heart. The lungs have lobes to allow for greater surface exposure to the inspired air. The left lung has two lobes: upper and lower. The right lung has three lobes: superior, middle, and inferior. The round-pointed top of each lung is called the *apex*; the lower flattened portion is called the *base*.

The *bronchi* then continue to branch in a pattern often referred to as "the bronchial tree" because their structure resembles an inverted tree.

After many subdivisions, the bronchioles are connected to millions of *alveoli* by the alveolar ducts. The alveoli are highly vascular air sacs surrounded by a thin single-layer membrane through which gases can diffuse. It is in the alveoli that the exchange of gases occurs.

The *diaphragm* is a broad, flat, elastic muscle that stretches across and seals off the lower thoracic cavity, enclosing the lungs. It maintains pressure, facilitating the movement of gases, and is innervated by the phrenic nerve.

The Process of Ventilation

Ventilation is the process by which air is taken into the lungs, where gas exchange can take place, and then expelled from the lungs to rid the body of excess carbon dioxide. The process of ventilation is subject to a variety of physiologic control mechanisms. These mechanisms adapt the ventilation process to changing demands within the body. The control mechanisms consist of receptors, located throughout the body, that are able to stimulate centers in the brain. The centers in the brain then stimulate the function of the muscles of respiration, which results in inspiration and expiration.

Peripheral Receptors

Centers that receive stimuli and respond by stimulating respiratory centers in the brain are found in several different locations.

Chemoreceptors are receptors located in the aorta and carotid bodies that are stimulated by a rise in carbon dioxide. When stimulated, they signal the brain to change the respiratory rate. When the carbon dioxide level falls, respirations slow. When the carbon dioxide level rises, respirations increase. These chemoreceptors also respond to low oxygen level. When the oxygen level falls severely, the receptors respond by a reflex stimulation of inspiration. This mechanism is not normally used and becomes important when the carbon dioxide response is absent.

In the aortic arch, the internal carotid arteries and the carotid sinuses are *baroreceptors* (pressure receptors) that respond to arterial blood pressure. When blood pressure rises, a reflex slows respirations. When blood pressure decreases, the reflex increases the rate and depth of respirations.

The *proprioceptors* in the muscles respond to increases in activity by stimulating increased respirations. Thus, respiration increases before adverse changes in blood gas levels occur.

Stretch receptors and *compression receptors* respond to the filling and emptying of the lungs. When the lungs fill to the usual tidal volume, receptors in them send to the respiratory center impulses that inhibit further inspiration. When air has been expired, the lungs are deflated and the receptors are inhibited, and inspiration occurs again.

Control Centers in the Brain

The respiratory center in the medulla is sensitive to hydrogen ion concentration (acidity) and the carbon dioxide level of the arterial blood. When levels rise, the receptors in the medulla respond by increasing respiratory rate and depth. Oxygen level also affects the respiratory center in the medulla, but it is a secondary stimulus.

The *pneumotaxic center* in the pons makes respirations even and regular. It responds to impulses from the inspiratory center in the medulla and provides a feedback mechanism that inhibits inspiration.

The *apneustic center* in the lower pons can create gasping breaths (apneusis) when other centers are no longer functioning. Its role in normal respiration is not clear.

The cerebral cortex provides voluntary control over respirations to a limited extent. You can consciously increase depth and rate of respirations. You can also decrease respirations. However, if you attempt to decrease respirations too greatly, the natural control mechanisms take over to provide for respirations.

Respiratory Muscles

The muscles that create respiration are the *intercostal muscles* and the diaphragm. The muscles of the abdomen also assist in ventilation. Other muscles, in the neck and chest, act as accessory muscles for respiration. They are stimulated from the control centers in the brain. As the changes in respiration create changes in the environment of the sensors, the stimulation of the control areas changes through a system of negative feedback.

Inspiration

Inspiration is the breathing-in phase of ventilation; normally lasting 1 to 2 seconds, it is half the length of expiration. It is accomplished primarily by the diaphragm. At rest, the diaphragm is curved upward toward the lungs. When it contracts, it moves downward. This downward movement increases the capacity of the thoracic cavity, creates a negative pressure in the chest, and air enters the lungs. The abdominal muscles can assist with inspiration by relaxing, thus making it easier for the diaphragm to displace the abdominal contents.

When an increase in volume of ventilation is

needed, additional muscles may be used. The external intercostal muscles can facilitate inspiration by increasing the diameter of the chest. Although this effect is not a major factor in ordinary ventilation, it may contribute significantly to increasing ventilation at times of high demand.

The muscles of the neck, the jaw, and the nares (nostrils) are not usually involved in breathing. When **hypoxemia** (low blood level of oxygen) exists, these muscles may be added to increase air movement. If you notice that these muscles are being used in a patient's respiration, you should recognize that this indicates **hypoxia** (low oxygen to body tissues), and intervention is needed to assist oxygenation.

Expiration

Normal *expiration* lasts approximately 1 to 4 seconds. It is a passive process that does not require energy. The lung and chest tissues are elastic; after being stretched for inspiration, they will recoil to their former shape when the inspiratory muscles relax. When demand is great, the intercostal muscles and the abdominal muscles can work actively to enhance expiration. This action uses energy. Changes in the elastic properties of the lung tissue that occur as a result of disease may alter the character of normal expiration, requiring that energy be used for routine expiration. When energy must be used on a routine basis for expiration, more oxygen is used and less energy is available for other activities.

Lung Volumes and Capacities

Understanding the terminology that describes the volume of air that the lungs can hold is helpful in understanding how ventilation can alter to meet changing needs. **Total lung capacity** is the total potential amount of air that the lungs can hold. It can be broken down into two segments: the residual volume and the vital capacity. The **residual volume** is the air that cannot be expelled from the lungs. The amount of residual volume cannot be directly measured but must be calculated, using other measurements. The residual air keeps the lungs from totally collapsing at the end of an expiration. The **vital capacity** is the total amount of air that can be moved in or out by the person's efforts.

The **functional residual capacity** is the amount of air that is left in the lungs after a normal respiration. The difference between the functional residual capacity and the residual capacity is called the **expiratory reserve**, which is the air that can be expelled with effort.

The **inspiratory capacity** is the maximum amount of air that can be breathed in after a normal expiration. The **tidal volume** is the amount of air that is breathed in and out in a regular breath. The difference between the inspiratory capacity and the tidal volume is called the **inspiratory reserve**.

Table 28-1 and Figure 28-2 illustrate how these volumes relate to one another and how they reflect the respiratory pattern.

Oxygen–Carbon Dioxide Exchange

The air that enters the lungs is approximately 20% oxygen. In the respiratory bronchioles and the alveoli, the capillaries are separated from the air only by the capillary wall and thin lung tissue. Oxygen from the air and carbon dioxide from the blood are both able to diffuse across these membranes. All gas exchange occurs across these membranes. The rest of the respiratory system is merely a passage to transport air to the respiratory bronchioles and the alveoli. This space where gas exchange

Table 28–1. Norms for Lung Volumes and Capacities

Measurement	Adult Male*	Adult Female
Total Lung Capacity	5,800 ml	4,600 ml
Residual volume	1,200 ml	1,000 ml
Vital capacity	4,600 ml	3,600 ml
Inspiratory Capacity	3,500 ml	2,800 ml
Tidal volume	500 ml	400 ml
Inspiratory reserve	3,000 ml	2,400 ml
Functional Residual Capacity	2,300 ml	1,800 ml
Expiratory reserve	1,100 ml	900 ml
Residual volume	1,200 ml	1,000 ml

*Guyton, A.C. *Human Physiology and Mechanisms of Disease.* (5th ed.) Philadelphia: W.B. Saunders, 1992.

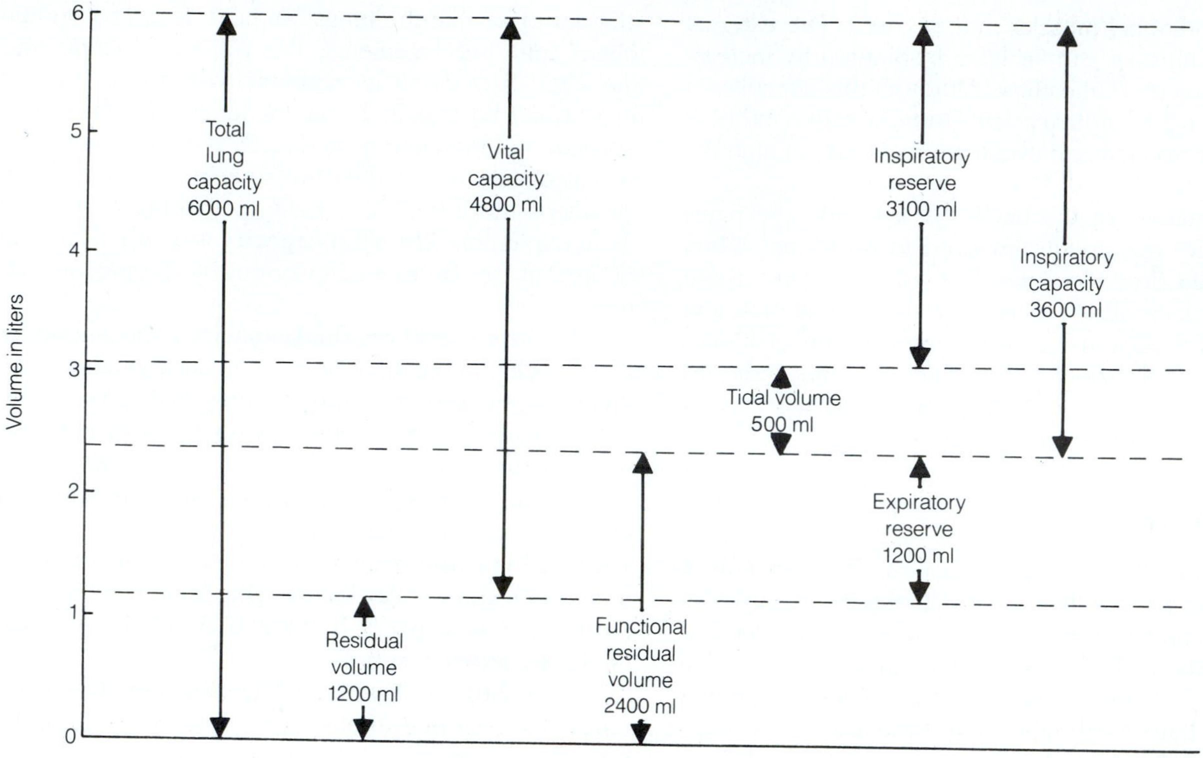

Figure 28-2. Lung volumes and capacities.

does not occur is called *dead air space.* It includes the nose, pharynx, trachea, main bronchi, and bronchioles.

Oxygen is transported in the bloodstream from the lungs to the cells both as a dissolved gas and attached to hemoglobin molecules as oxyhemoglobin. Carbon dioxide is transported as a dissolved gas and, when it is attached to the hemoglobin molecule as it makes its return journey from the cells to the lungs, as carboxyhemoglobin. Additional carbon dioxide is carried in compounds in the blood. These compounds are buffers and most contribute to the overall base content of the blood. The measurement of total carbon dioxide content is a measure of these compounds and reflects base available for the acid–base balance.

Gas exchange also takes place at the cellular level in the form of *internal respiration.* The same *diffusion* process occurs except that at the cellular level oxygen leaves the blood and carbon dioxide enters it.

The major *blood gases* are carbon dioxide and oxygen. These two gases are measured in terms of the partial pressure exerted by the gas dissolved in the blood expressed in millimeters of mercury. The symbol for partial pressure of arterial oxygen is PaO_2. Although you may see this written without the "a" as PO_2, it is preferable to add the "a," which indicates arterial blood, because the figures are different for venous blood. The symbol for partial pressure of arterial carbon dioxide is $PaCO_2$. For arterial blood gases, normal values are PaO_2, 80 to 100 mm Hg; $PaCO_2$, 35 to 45 mm Hg. For venous blood, the values are P_vO_2, 35 to 40 mm Hg; P_vCO_2, 45 mm Hg.

In many facilities, the respiratory therapy department is responsible for drawing arterial blood to measure blood gas content. In others, the laboratory is responsible. In some hospitals drawing arterial blood is a nursing procedure. The radial artery is located by palpation. After cleansing, a long, thin-gauged needle is inserted straight downward until bright red blood appears in the barrel. After a sufficient amount has been collected, the needle is withdrawn and firm pressure must be applied for 5 minutes to prevent bleeding from the artery. Some degree of pain accompanies insertion of the needle, and applying ice a few minutes before the procedure can be helpful. A heel stick is usually done in newborns and small infants because the radial artery is too small to enter. Because this method produces capillary blood, however, the values will be lower than those for arterial blood and higher than those for venous blood; they are usually evaluated in light of the individual infant's circulatory status. The pH of the blood is always reported with blood gases. Hemoglobin saturation may be also be reported with blood gases.

Hemoglobin saturation is a measure of the oxygen-carrying status of hemoglobin and is expressed as a percentage. The normal hemoglobin saturation of arterial blood is 95% to 100%. When hemoglobin saturation falls below 85%, the level of dissolved oxygen falls rapidly, because the hemoglobin molecule releases oxygen more slowly when it is less than 85% saturated. Hemoglobin saturation can be measured by drawing arterial blood, but it is more frequently measured by a noninvasive technique called *pulse oximetry*.

Lung Clearance Mechanisms

Inhaled air always contains particulate matter and microorganisms. These substances do not usually create problems for the individual because the lungs have an excellent set of mechanisms for clearing unwanted material.

Filtration in the nose is the first of the respiratory clearance mechanisms. The nose contains hairs that filter out large dust particles. The effectiveness of the filtering mechanism becomes apparent when large amounts of dust are in the air.

Mucous production is an important factor in protecting the respiratory system. Mucus is secreted by glands in the membranes throughout the respiratory system. Small particles are trapped in the mucus. Mucus thereby both protects the tissue from the particle and provides a medium for removal. Any irritation of the respiratory tissue will increase the production of mucus. This is a protective mechanism but may create difficulties when the production outstrips the lung clearance mechanisms.

Ciliary action is the next factor in lung clearance. Tiny cilia throughout the bronchial tree are continuously active in propelling mucus toward the upper airway. Smoke paralyzes cilia in the lungs, thus inhibiting lung clearance. Cilia may also be damaged by disease processes. Once mucus is in higher airways, cough may be activated to remove large quantities. Effective cough clears large quantities of mucus.

The alveoli have no cilia. There, *macrophages* engulf particles to remove and destroy them. The particles are disposed of via the lymphatic system. The mucus then moves to an area where cough may effectively remove it.

When the *position* of the body is changed, mucus (with its particulate load) moves in the lung as a result of gravity. Because of the branching nature of the lungs, almost any position will cause some lung segments to drain. As the position is changed, different segments are able to drain.

Coughing is a mechanism to protect the lungs from aspiration of foreign material in the upper airway and to clear material from the lower airway. For optimum cough to occur, first there must be deep inspiration; the glottis is closed, expiratory muscles contract, forcefully building up pressure in the chest; then the glottis is opened, expelling material from the airway. Cough may be caused by stimulation of receptors in the upper airway (trachea and pharynx) or those in the lower airway (larynx and bronchi). Irritant gases (such as smoke), fluids, touch, and particles in the air may all stimulate these receptors. Hard coughing may raise intracerebral and intraocular pressures and are sometimes contraindicated. Hard coughing in the absence of secretions may cause collapse of some alveoli.

Effects of Respiration on Acid–Base Balance

The *pH,* or acidity–alkalinity balance, of arterial blood must remain within an extremely narrow range—7.4 or a few hundredths below or above—for the body to function optimally. Thus, arterial blood is slightly alkaline. Any factor that alters this level produces a state of either acidosis or alkalosis in the body. One such factor is respiration.

Acid–base balance is discussed more fully in Chapter 30. You will also study it in more detail in your medical–surgical nursing course. We will confine ourselves here to a general overview of acid–base balance as it relates to respiration (Fig. 28-3).

Respiratory Acidosis

When a patient is **hypoventilating** (breathing shallowly) for any reason, excess carbon dioxide is retained. This carbon dioxide is converted to carbonic acid in the circulating blood, causing the pH of the blood to fall as the partial pressure of carbon dioxide in the arterial blood ($PaCO_2$) rises. **Respiratory acidosis** can occur in patients with central nervous system depression, with certain types of drug overdose, and with pulmonary disease that prevents full ventilation.

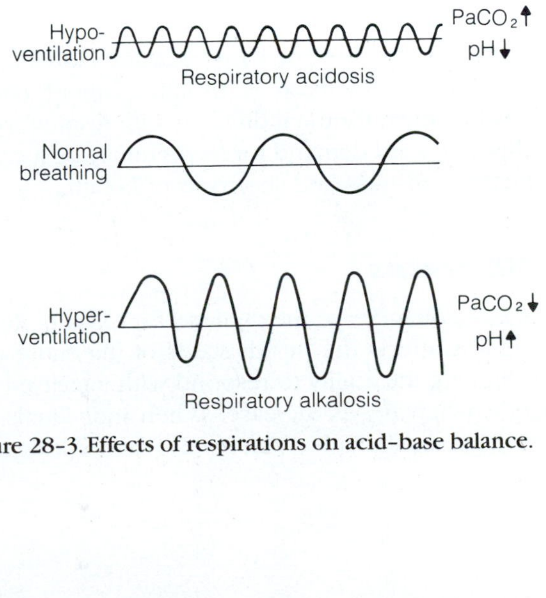

Figure 28-3. Effects of respirations on acid-base balance.

Respiratory Alkalosis

Conversely, when a patient is **hyperventilating** (breathing very deeply and rapidly), excessive amounts of carbon dioxide are exhaled. The lowered level of carbonic acid in the blood causes the pH to rise and may eventually lead to **respiratory alkalosis**. Hyperventilation may accompany fever or anxiety.

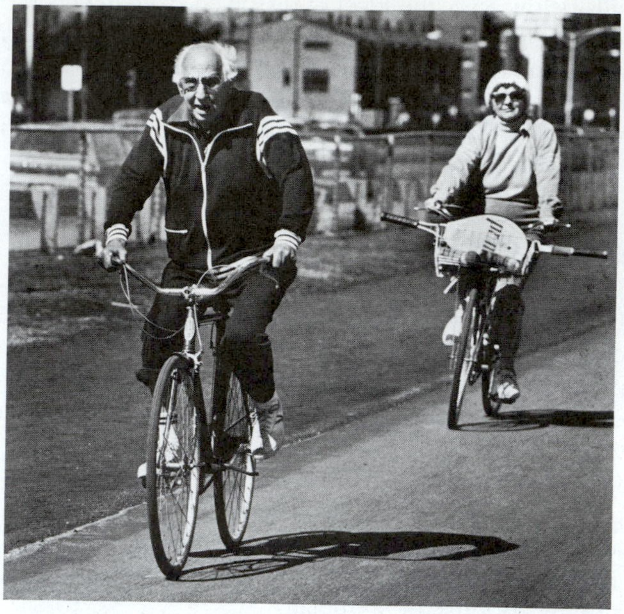

Figure 28-4. Activity increases the body's need for oxygen.

Factors Affecting Oxygenation

Many different factors affect the process of oxygenation. Some of the major ones are activity, emotions, health status, the environment, and smoking.

Activity

Activity increases the body's need for oxygen and sets in motion a variety of mechanisms to increase the rate and depth of respirations. The increased rate and depth of breathing associated with activity are valuable to the lungs themselves. Alveoli are opened up, secretions that may have accumulated are stimulated to move, and gas exchange is enhanced.

The actual amount by which one can increase one's oxygen supply depends on conditioning as well as basic physical health. Conditioning strengthens all muscles, including those of respiration, making them better able to work hard. Conditioning is also critical to the functioning of the heart in circulating the oxygen throughout the body (see Chapter 29). For the individual with respiratory illness, activity must be carefully balanced with the ability of the lungs to respond to increased oxygen demand. The positive effects of activity on respiratory status are also considered (Fig. 28-4).

Emotions

Strong emotions increase the heart rate, blood pressure, and muscle tension. These all require more oxygen, so the respiratory rate also increases. For the individual in good health, this increase is usually without consequences; however, for the individual with respiratory illness, this increased demand for oxygen may be a significant factor in distress and shortness of breath.

Health Status

Any illness may increase the demand for oxygen. Respiratory illness affects the health status of the entire person by limiting the ability to respond with increased oxygenation when needs increase. When individuals are ill, they may also have less energy available for ventilation. Thus, respiratory status is an important factor in any illness.

The health of the cardiovascular system is important to oxygenation. The blood must be circulated throughout the lungs for the exchange of gases and then circulated to the organs of the body to provide oxygen for tissue function. When the heart does not function adequately, or if the blood contains inadequate hemoglobin to carry oxygen (a condition called anemia), the person will not be able to adapt to increased activity and may suffer dyspnea on exertion (DOE) and shortness of breath.

Disease of the respiratory tract itself is often a cause of problems with oxygenation. Although disease in the upper airway may not decrease a person's ability to oxygenate, disease in the lower respiratory tract almost always affects oxygenation.

Environment

An environment free of pollution and containing adequate oxygen is essential for effective oxygenation. Oxygen is decreased in higher altitudes, and in such areas many individuals find that they cannot engage in strenuous activities.

Air quality is an increasing concern, especially in many urban areas. Pollutants in the air not only cause direct damage to fragile lung tissue causing chronic lung disease, they can also decrease the effectiveness of gas exchange. As levels of carbon dioxide and carbon monoxide rise in the atmosphere, their levels increase in the body.

The combination of motor vehicle exhaust, industrial exhausts, and exhaust from home heating plants (especially those that burn wood or other solid fuels) combine to create poor air quality that is known to cause difficulty for everyone, especially for those with respiratory disease.

Air pollution in indoor environments is also a concern. Industrial plants have historically been known to create hazards. Asbestos was not recognized as hazardous in manufacturing in the 1940s and 1950s, and individuals who worked with asbestos in those years may develop chronic lung disease now. Currently, asbestos is also significant because it remains in many buildings where it was used for sound deadening and fire protection. Asbestos in some of those buildings is now being removed under careful environmental precautions. This again has its difficulties. In some instances, asbestos removal creates more hazards in the air than leaving it sealed within the structure. The debate on the best method to eliminate this problem continues.

Large office buildings are coming under scrutiny for the air recirculating systems that they use in their heating and ventilating systems. These systems may concentrate mold spores, gases given off by curing paints and plastics, and a variety of other contaminants. Concern is being expressed that the quality of the air being circulated has not been adequately evaluated and the health of workers may be at risk. Indoor air quality may also be poor in homes that are heavily insulated and so tightly constructed that little exchange of air occurs. You may expect to continue to read about indoor air quality and methods for maintaining that quality.

Smoking

Smoking is a major health hazard for society. Fielding (1985) reported that smoking is responsible for 30% of cardiovascular deaths, 30% to 40% of cancer deaths, and 62,000 deaths from respiratory disease in the United States each year. In addition to deaths, smoking causes innumerable lost days of work, much discomfort, and great expense because of respiratory illness.

Illness related to smoking is not confined to the smoker. Recent studies have shown that sidestream (second-hand) smoke (that which is emitted from burning cigarettes in the room) also has deleterious effects on respiratory health (U.S. National Research Council, 1986). In a long-term study, nonsmoking wives of smokers were found to be 34% more likely to develop lung cancer than nonsmoking wives of nonsmoking men (Telch et al., 1982). When pregnant women smoke, the noxious effects are seen in the fetus, with low birth weight being a typical outcome (U.S. Department of Health and Human Services, 1980). Children who reside in homes with a smoker have more frequent respiratory illnesses.

Most individuals who smoke began in adolescence. The reasons for beginning to smoke are complex, but those most frequently cited are peer pressure, desire to appear mature and adult, curiosity, role modeling, and rebellion. The maintenance of smoking as a behavior is related to addiction to nicotine, behavioral habits, stress management, and cues in the environment.

The most effective attack on smoking would be to urge individuals not to begin smoking. The American Lung Association, the American Heart Association, and the American Cancer Society all have programs, public service announcements, and posters aimed at the adolescent age group. Although these programs may be effective, they often fail to reach young people who have dropped out of school or to move those who are in rebellion against adults.

Although some individuals successfully quit smoking independently, many find the assistance of a stop-smoking program valuable. Such programs use a wide variety of techniques, from behavior modification to hypnotism to nicotine chewing gum or patches. The Department of Health and Human Services has published a review and evaluation of the various stop-smoking programs (Schwartz, 1987) that you might find valuable as a resource.

Nursing Issues and Trends: *Smoking In Public Places*

As more and more evidence accumulates that smoking affects not only the smoker but also the bystander who breathes smoke in the air, pressure has grown to limit smoking in public places. Many hospitals and schools have become total nonsmoking environments. Restaurants increasingly provide separate smoking and nonsmoking sections. Workers are asking that smoking in the workplace be curtailed. In some states these practices are mandated by law, but in others there is considerable opposition to any limitation on the rights of smokers.

As a health professional, you may assist individuals to recognize that smoking is harmful to their health status and to select a method for stopping smoking that is most appropriate for the individual. Even when initial attempts to stop smoking are unsuccessful, subsequent attempts may be successful. Therefore, it is important to not ignore the problem because someone has smoked for a long period of time. Nurses who smoke are modeling inappropriate health behavior and may be reluctant to suggest to a client health practices that they themselves are not willing to adopt. Thus, smoking by the nurse may interfere with providing high quality nursing care as well as result in personal health problems.

Body Temperature

An increased body temperature increases metabolic processes and therefore increases oxygen needs. The person with a fever experiences an increased respiratory rate. If oxygenation is marginal, the onset of fever may result in inadequate oxygenation. Conversely, lowered body temperature decreases metabolic activity and decreases oxygen need. This principle may be used therapeutically and body temperature may be deliberately reduced in some surgeries to lower overall metabolic demands.

Assessment

Accurate assessment of the entire level of oxygenation requires attention to careful interviewing, physical examination, and understanding of special laboratory and diagnostic tests.

Interview

When interviewing an individual in regard to oxygenation, you must be alert to indications of respiratory distress. If a person is having difficulty breathing, it is inappropriate to ask the usual open-ended questions (see Chapter 13). Ask key questions that can be answered by yes or no to conserve the person's oxygen supply (Display 28-1).

Display 28–1
Suggested Interview Questions Related to Oxygenation

Current Symptoms

1. Are you having any breathing problems now? If so, describe them to me. How long have you had these problems?
2. Is it uncomfortable when you breathe?
3. What seems to increase your breathing problem?
4. Are there measures that help you to breathe more easily?
5. Have your breathing problems interfered with your ability to do the things you want to do? In what way?
6. Do you cough up sputum (phlegm)? How often? How much? What color is it?

Chronic Symptoms

1. Have you had respiratory or breathing problems in the past? If so, describe them to me. How often have these recurred?
2. How did those episodes compare with what you are experiencing now?
3. What was your doctor's diagnosis at the time you had these problems?

Smoking History

1. Do you smoke currently? If so, what do you smoke: cigarettes, cigars, pipe?
2. How much do you smoke in a usual day?
3. When did you first start smoking?
4. Have you ever tried to stop smoking? Tell me what happened?
5. Are you interested in trying to stop smoking now?

Current Symptoms

You will need to know what symptoms of respiratory illness are currently present and how long they have been present. This information may be important for you in planning care to decrease symptoms or in teaching the patient how to prevent symptoms from becoming worse.

Normal respirations occur without noticeable effort. The individual does not feel fatigued by the work of breathing nor uncomfortable while breathing. **Dyspnea** is the condition in which the individual experiences the need to exert effort to breathe and has difficulty maintaining adequate ventilation. Dyspnea is a subjective sensation and may be experienced by an individual before respiratory effort is visible. If dyspnea is felt only when the person increases activity, it is referred to as dyspnea on exertion (DOE). Some individuals severely curtail activity because of the DOE.

You will need to determine whether there is discomfort associated with breathing. In normal painless breathing, called **eupnea**, the person is almost unaware of breathing effort. Discomfort associated with respiration may include pain on inspiration or on expiration, discomfort from excessive coughing, or tightness in the chest. Other specific things to check for include the presence of cough, wheezing, and excessive respiratory secretions.

You should also determine how position changes affect respirations. Difficulty breathing associated with lying down is called **orthopnea**. The person with orthopnea will be most comfortable sitting up because this position allows for the greatest lung expansion. Orthopnea may be identified when a patient tells you that he or she prefers to sleep with at least two pillows or frequently sleeps in a favorite recliner. When this information is shared, you should follow with a discussion of why this makes a difference in comfort to determine if orthopnea is present.

You will need to ask about the sequence of events in the present illness. Was there a precipitating event? How long has the person been feeling ill? These facts will help you to plan appropriate care for the present illness.

Chronic Symptoms

Even if the patient has no current symptoms, you will ask about chronic symptoms that have recurred in the past. The same symptoms that may be currently present may have occurred previously. Is there a history of respiratory disease? If so, what kind? When did disease occur in the past? Were problems then similar to or different from the current problem?

Smoking History

You will gain more accurate information about smoking history if you ask in a way that does not create guilt feelings about smoking. Be straightforward, matter of fact, and nonjudgmental. You need to ascertain what was smoked (cigarettes, cigars, or pipe), how long the person has smoked, and the quantity smoked per day. The number of packs of cigarettes per day is multiplied by the number of years the person smoked to arrive at a statement of pack-years of smoking. This figure is often used to judge the potential for chronic lung disease.

Physical Assessment

Physical assessment will include observing the respirations, auscultating the lungs, and looking for evidence of adequate oxygenation in other body system (Fig. 28-5).

Assessment of Respirations

Module 16, Temperature, Pulse, and Respiration, provides complete instructions on how to time respirations accurately. Here we will briefly review some main points.

Rate. The first task in respiratory assessment is to measure the rate of respiration. A single cycle of inspiration and expiration is counted as one respiration. It is usually easiest to count inspirations. Because it is difficult for a patient to maintain a normal breathing pattern knowing he or she is being watched, the nurse often counts by resting the patient's arm across the chest with the nurse's hand in place as if feeling for the pulse. The risings of the chest can thus be felt and counted. Beginning at zero will make for a more accurate count. Count for a full 30 seconds. If the respirations are irregular, however, it may be desirable to count for a full minute. The respiratory rate is highest in the newborn—35 to 40 respirations per minute—and gradually decreases, reaching the adult level of 14 to 20 respirations in the adolescent.

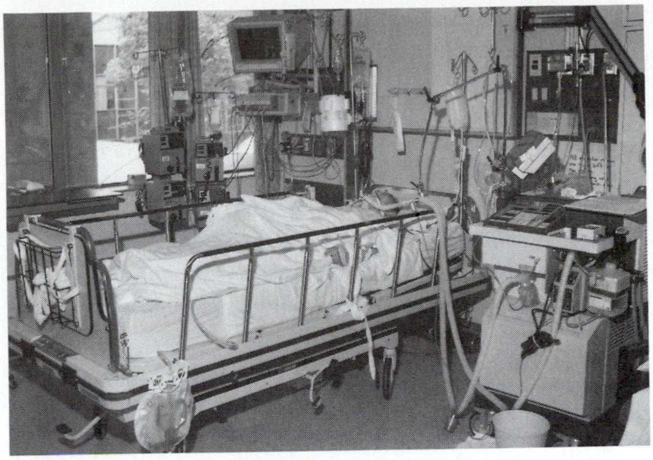

Figure 28-5. Respiratory assessment and treatment are important parts of the care for the critically ill.

Respiratory rate is increased by activity, fever, anxiety, and all the factors that affect the pulse rate. Many health problems create rises in respiratory rate; others cause the rate to decrease. Very rapid respiration is called **tachypnea**. Unusually slow respiration is called **bradypnea**. Absence of respiration is called **apnea**.

Depth. The extent to which the whole lung is involved in respiration is called the depth of respiration. A shallow respiration is characterized by minimal chest movement and thus minimal air exchange. A deep respiration is one in which the rib cage is fully expanded and the diaphragm descends to create maximum lung capacity. Shallow respirations are not effective, even at a rapid rate, because they produce air movement in the physiologic dead space, where no gas exchange with the blood can occur, and inadequate air movement in the alveoli, where gas exchange does take place. Sighing and yawning are automatic mechanisms to increase ventilation by forcing deep breaths. In addition to the lack of oxygen exchange, hypoventilation—shallow respiration—causes secretions to accumulate and alveoli to collapse. This problem, common to immobilized and postoperative patients, can be combated by encouraging movement, deep breathing, and coughing up of secretions.

Rhythm. Healthy respirations are characterized by a regular rhythm of expirations twice as long as inspirations (a 1:2 inspiration–expiration ratio). Irregularities in rhythm may indicate the presence of illness. **Cheyne-Stokes respirations** consist of very deep respirations (**hyperpnea**) and rapid respirations (tachypnea) at the beginning of the cycle, gradually tapering off to the point of cessation (apnea), and then gradually becoming deep and rapid again. They usually indicate that the patient is in very critical condition.

Biot's respirations resemble Cheyne-Stokes respirations except that the respirations between the episodes of apnea appear normal. Certain references may describe this term in slightly different ways. In assessing rhythm, always check for yourself; never rely entirely on someone else to monitor for potentially serious signs. **Kussmaul's respirations** are deep and rapid respirations. Their extreme depth resembles that of blowing and gasping.

Audible breathing sounds. Assessment of sounds occurring while the person is breathing can be helpful in determining pulmonary status. Some abnormalities in breath sounds are easily discerned without a stethoscope merely by standing near the patient in a quiet room.

Wheezing is a clearly audible whistling sound particularly characteristic of the patient suffering from asthma. It can also be present with other respiratory conditions. *Snoring* is a breath sound normal in deep sleep but possibly indicative of coma in the neurologic patient. The child with croup may make a crowing sound called **stridor**; this sound is a result of laryngospasm (a narrowing or even closing of the passage through the larynx caused by spasm of the laryngeal muscles). Laryngospasm may also occur as a serious complication of second-stage anesthesia.

Sighing, **hiccoughs** (**singultus**), and *yawning* are all familiar breath sounds: sighing can be a sign of anxiety, hiccoughs frequently occur after anesthesia, and yawning can indicate narcolepsy (a sleep disorder).

Auscultation. Listening to lung sounds through a stethoscope is auscultation. Several standard technical terms are used to describe lung sounds. However, research has suggested that the use of ordinary descriptive words promotes accuracy and minimizes the subjectivity of listening. In normal lung sounds, air can be heard moving clearly and smoothly. Expiration is audible for a shorter time than inspiration, although it lasts longer. **Adventitious** is a general adjective used for any abnormality, commonly used in the negative; that is, the nurse might record, "no adventitious sounds heard." Try to characterize the sound you hear as descriptively as possible. You might say, for example, "a soft rustling" or "a loud crackling."

Crackles (previously called *rales*) are crackling or bubbling sounds made by air moving through moisture or secretions in the bronchioles or lungs. **Gurgles** (previously referred to as *rhonchi*) are lower pitched and drier sounding than rales. *Wheezes* sound very much like the sound made by a toy whistle. Some whistling sounds are interrupted and some continuous. They may occur during inspiration, during expiration, or both. **Pleural rub** is a distinct grating or rubbing sound as the pleurae rub together; *friction rub* is another term used for this sound.

The skills needed for listening to lung sounds are described in Module 13, Inspection, Palpation, Auscultation, and Percussion.

Appearance of respiration. Normal respiration is even, with little chest movement. The abdomen moves in and out regularly. As demand increases, abdominal movement becomes greater, and the chest movement becomes pronounced. If an individual has difficulty with breathing, accessory muscles such as the neck muscles and those around the trachea, mouth, and nose begin to work. With severe respiratory distress, the intercostal muscles may retract (pull inward) between the ribs on inspiration. There may also be **retractions** in the supraclavicular space and beneath the sternum. When retractions are seen, they are designated by their location: supraclavicular, substernal, or intercostal. The trachea may move downward with each inspiration. This movement is called *tracheal tug*. The nares may flare with each inspiration, and the cheeks and the area under the chin may move.

Color of Skin and Mucous Membrane

Well-oxygenated blood gives a bright pink color to white skin, nailbeds, and mucous membranes. Those with darker pigmented skin have a rosy undertone from the oxyhemoglobin of well-oxygenated blood. When blood is poorly oxygenated, it contains unoxygenated hemoglobin and has a darker hue and thus imparts a dusky hue to the tissue. This change is more apparent in light skin, but may be apparent even in dark-skinned individuals to those who are familiar with their usual skin tone (see Chapter 22). Severe oxygen deprivation creates a condition termed **cyanosis**, in which the tissue turns a dark bluish color. This condition is evident in conjunctiva, mucous membranes, and nailbeds of all people, regardless of their skin color.

Sputum Assessment

Sputum is predominantly composed of mucus, epithelial cells, and microorganisms. It is usually tenacious in consistency. The quantity of sputum may be described as small, moderate, or large. Sputum in large quantities is abnormal and may indicate disease or irritation of the airways. Sputum that becomes thick and tenacious is hard to cough up and may block air passages. Normal sputum is clear, white, and slightly frothy from air bubbles. Infection will cause sputum to be opaque and have a different color, such as yellow or green tinge. Some disease processes may cause sputum to be red tinged, indicating that it contains blood. Descriptive words that may be appropriate to use are thick, clear, frothy, and stringy. Normal sputum is almost odorless. Sputum with a foul odor usually indicates infection.

Cough Assessment

The cough center, located in the medulla, is activated by any threat of obstruction of the respiratory tract. Cough is an important protective mechanism and remains active even during sleep. A foreign body, such as dust, will activate the cough reflex as will the presence of secretions. When the movement of secretions can be heard during a cough it is called a moist cough. Irritation of the trachea or bronchi may cause cough in the absence of any substance that needs to be removed. This is termed a dry cough. In the patient with respiratory problems, such as an infection with irritation or the build-up of secretions, coughing may be long and persistent causing further irritation to respiratory passages and fatigue. Cough is described as **productive** or **nonproductive**, depending on whether or not the patient is coughing up and expectorating (spitting) sputum. When a patient has a productive cough, you should assess the character of the sputum being expectorated.

Simply to say that the patient is coughing does not provide enough information on which to base action. Consider the persistence of the cough and when it occurs. It is common for cough to be more pronounced on arising because secretions have accumulated during the night when the person is in the horizontal position. Describe the sound of the cough and whether or not it is productive.

Laboratory and Diagnostic Tests

Arterial blood gas measurements may be ordered by the physician. The PaO_2 and the $PaCO_2$ are both measured. The arterial pH is also reported when blood gases are drawn. Measures of the combining power of carbon dioxide and of the bicarbonate level may be used to evaluate acid–base status.

Hemoglobin saturation may be measured with a simple device called a *pulse oximeter* that uses an external probe attached to a fingertip or ear lobe. The pulse oximeter uses light reflectance from capillary hemoglobin to determine the percent of oxygen saturation in the hemoglobin. Because this measure may be done at the bedside and is noninvasive, it is widely used to determine response to treatment. The device is attached, turned on, and the hemoglobin saturation read from the dial.

The hemoglobin and hematocrit are studied to determine whether the blood has adequate oxygen-carrying capacity. In patients with chronic respiratory disease or those who normally live at high altitudes, these may be elevated as the body attempts to compensate for the respiratory problem or decreased atmospheric oxygen by increasing the oxygen-carrying capacity.

The chest x-ray is the most common diagnostic test used for respiratory illness. An x-ray may be done from an anterior to posterior (AP) view or from the side (a lateral view). The x-ray can reveal areas in which the lung is not expanded, as well as growths and other disease processes in the lung. The radiologist writes a report explaining what has been identified in the x-ray. The computed axial tomography (CAT) scan is a form of x-ray imaging that may provide additional information regarding soft tissues in the chest. Magnetic resonance imaging (MRI) uses a different technology to identify structural and tissue changes. MRI provides excellent imaging but is still costly and not suitable for a patient who must be constantly monitored or who cannot lie still. The perfusion lung scan is used to study the pattern of uptake by the lungs of a radio isotope injected intravenously. This reveals abnormalities in circulation as well as abnormal growths.

Nursing Diagnosis

Several nursing diagnoses specifically address the problems found in those with alterations in respiratory function.

Activity Intolerance Related to Respiratory Dysfunction

People who experience shortness of breath and distress when attempting desired activity may have a diagnosis of Activity Intolerance related to the respiratory disease state. This nursing diagnosis is discussed in Chapter 23 on activity. When the etiology is respiratory dysfunction, nursing intervention focuses on arranging the activity to fit in with the lung function. Both the intensity and the duration of the activity must be decreased so that the activity is within the oxygenating capacity of the lungs. You may need to use oxygen that has been ordered on a PRN (when necessary) basis by the physician to assist an individual in functioning with comfort. Instructions

Nursing Diagnosis Related to Oxygenation

Activity Intolerance related to respiratory dysfunction

Altered Comfort related to cough

Altered Respiratory Function* related to
- immobility
- smoking
- respiratory dysfunction

Impaired Gas Exchange related to respiratory dysfunction

Ineffective Airway Clearance related to:
- excessive respiratory secretions
- lack of gag reflex
- paralysis of respiratory muscles

Ineffective Breathing Pattern: Hyperventilation related to anxiety

Ineffective Breathing Pattern: Hypoventilation related to:
- anesthetic
- narcotic analgesics
- painful surgical site

*Carpenito, L. *Nursing Diagnosis: Application To Clinical Practice.* 4th edition. Philadelphia: J. B. Lippincott, 1992.

on the use of oxygen are found in Module 40, Administering Oxygen. If dyspnea is related to activity, to avoid increasing distress to the person, you must be careful not to add activities to the care plan without planning rest periods and careful evaluation of response to the new activity.

Altered Respiratory Function

The nursing diagnosis Altered Respiratory Function appeared in an early list of nursing diagnoses drawn up by the original National Conference Group. During the 1982 National Conference, it was made a general category, and other more specific problems became subgroups under it. However, Carpenito (1992) argues convincingly that there are situations in which a more specific problem is not yet present, but there is a serious concern about respiratory function. She identifies three etiologies that create this problem: immobility, smoking, and chronic allergy. In these general situations, the nursing interventions focus on actions that will prevent more specific problems from occurring. You will want to determine whether in your setting this general category is being used as a nursing diagnosis.

Potential Complications Involving Oxygenation

Potential complication: atelectasis

Potential complication: hypoxemia

Potential complication: pneumothorax

Potential complication: pulmonary edema

Potential complication: tracheobronchial constriction

Altered Comfort Related to Cough

Altered comfort is a general category in the NANDA taxonomy and is not currently listed as a specific nursing diagnosis. However, this is another instance where the use of a more general category may be more accurate than the specific diagnosis in the category. Altered Comfort related to cough can occur in a variety of ways. Coughing can cause the throat to become sore and irritated. Discomfort may also be related to exhaustion from a nonproductive cough.

Impaired Gas Exchange

Impaired Gas Exchange becomes the diagnosis when the exchange of oxygen and carbon dioxide in the lungs is inadequate. It is most often the result of disease processes in the lung itself. This disease may be an acute illness in which secretions fill alveoli, preventing air exchange, or a chronic illness in which there has been destruction of lung tissue.

Impaired Gas Exchange may also be the diagnosis when the supply of hemoglobin is inadequate to carry oxygen in the blood or when blood supply to a section of the lungs has been blocked by a blood clot (**pulmonary embolus**). In these situations, there is adequate oxygen in the alveoli, but the ability to carry the oxygen from the lungs to the tissues is impaired. The person will exhibit ongoing shortness of breath and (dyspnea) on exertion. There may be inability to breathe in any position other than an upright one (*orthopnea*). Various body organs may function less effectively because they do not have an adequate oxygen supply. Muscles may be weak and chronically fatigued. Alertness may be impaired because of decreased oxygen to the brain. There may be evidence of cyanosis in capillary beds of the fingernails, mucous membranes, and lips, indicating inadequately oxygenated blood; this, however, is a late sign of hypoxemia.

Other nursing diagnoses may accompany this diagnosis and would need to be approached separately. Accompanying diagnoses commonly relate to inadequate nutrition, constipation, and lack of knowledge regarding self-care.

Ineffective Airway Clearance

Ineffective Airway Clearance may be the diagnosis because a deficient cough reflex prevents the person from clearing any kind of foreign matter from the airway. Ineffective Airway Clearance may also be the diagnosis if the person experiences pain or discomfort when attempting to clear the airway (*eg*, because of a surgical incision). Because of the discomfort, the person will not try to clear the airway. Fatigue and weakness may also contribute to the diagnosis of Ineffective Airway Clearance.

When airway clearance is ineffective, secretions will be heard in lung fields on auscultation. Another indication of this diagnosis is that the person gags and chokes when saliva or any liquid is in the mouth.

Ineffective Breathing Patterns

An Ineffective Breathing Pattern diagnosis may arise from either hypoventilation or hyperventilation. When individuals are anxious or upset, they may hyperventilate. In hyperventilation respirations become extremely deep and rapid. Inspirations and expirations are of approximately the same length. The result is the release of too much carbon dioxide, creating respiratory alkalosis. The person may feel numbness and tingling in extremities or sensations of dizziness and faintness.

In hypoventilation respirations become shallow and slow, and some areas of the lungs never inflate. On auscultation some areas of the lungs may be silent. Hypoventilation results in decreased ventilation and oxygenation is impaired. Hypoventilation often occurs when a person is recovering from anesthesia or is sedated. It may also be the result of pain. For example, chest or abdominal surgery may cause an individual to hypoventilate because deep breathing causes movement in the incisional area and increases pain.

Knowledge Deficit

The person with an acute or chronic respiratory problem may need to carry out basic care measures or even a complex treatment plan. The nurse must identify what the patient knows and compare this with the various self-care needs that are present. Another area of deficit may regard knowledge of health promotion measures, such as smoking cessation or avoiding air pollutants. The patient may not understand the role that these factors play in the development or exacerbation of chronic respiratory disease.

Anxiety Related to Oxygenation Problems

The need for oxygen is a primary need of all people. When one is deprived of oxygen, even briefly, survival is profoundly threatened. Try holding your breath for just a few moments; you will probably begin to experience the fear that accompanies a delay in resumption of breathing. The patient who has difficulty breathing or getting enough air for comfort can experience anxiety to the point of panic if the situation is not relieved.

Individuals in whom oxygenation is impaired may also suffer from a physiologically induced anxiety. When the brain is not receiving adequate oxygen, feelings of anxiety arise (see Chapter 34).

Ineffective Management of Therapeutic Regimen

Therapeutic regimens for persons with major respiratory disorders may be complex and require time and attention to many details. The inability to manage this regimen may be related to a variety of factors other than knowledge deficit. The regimen may require time that the person feels is not available. This may be a particular concern for a family with a child who has a respiratory disorder. If parents work and time is limited this may pose many problems. Other factors may also be a concern. Careful assessment of individuals and their ability to manage what has been prescribed will help you determine whether this problem is present.

Planning and Implementation

To determine appropriate desired outcomes in relationship to respiratory problems, you will need to look carefully at your baseline data. What specific areas of function were you hoping to improve? Then consider how much improvement is realistic. For example, if you were caring for a patient who was short of breath, you might conclude that the best outcome would be absence of shortness of breath and normal respirations. However, if this person has chronic lung disease, it may be that respirations will never be normal. What, then, can you realistically hope for as an outcome? Perhaps shortness of breath could be decreased to the point where a patient can eat all of the food served at a meal. Another possible outcome would be for shortness of breath to be decreased to the point where the person is able to bathe himself or herself. These outcomes indicate movement toward a more independent and functional lifestyle.

You might also write outcomes that relate to specific abnormalities heard on auscultation of the lungs. For example, if you heard lung sounds indicating the presence of secretions in the base of the right lung, your

Nursing Care Plan
Sample Nursing Care Plan Related to Oxygenation

Nursing Diagnosis

Impaired Gas Exchange related to retained secretions and fluid infiltrates in the lungs

Supportive data:

Respiratory rate 26.

Lungs have bilateral rales in lower lobes.

Chest x-ray report states fluid infiltrates throughout lungs.

States feels short of breath and fatigued.

Shortness of breath becomes more apparent when patient ambulates to bathroom or in room.

Desired Patient Outcomes

Short term:

Patient states feels less fatigued and less short of breath.

Long term:

Lungs clear to auscultation. Patient resumes self-care without shortness of breath.

Nursing Action	Rationale
1. Use long tubing for oxygen.	Long tubing allows the patient to receive oxygen while moving about the room, thus supporting oxygenation as activity and demand increase.
2. Encourage patient to use PRN oxygen whenever getting up and increasing activity.	Activity increases the body's need for oxygen.
3. Teach effective deep-breathing and coughing technique.	Effective deep breathing expands all alveoli providing more effective gas exchange. Correct coughing clears secretions from airways to facilitate ventilation.
4. Remind patient to practice deep breathing every hour while awake.	Frequent deep breathing will counteract the hypoventilation and potential atelectasis that may result from immobility.
5. Space activities with rest periods to avoid increased shortness of breath.	When oxygenation is limited, activity restriction prevents oxygen demand from exceeding oxygen supply.

desired outcome might be that there be no secretions in the right lung and that the right lung be clear on auscultation.

If the person is at risk for respiratory complications of immobility or surgery, outcomes might relate to the patient's independent actions designed to prevent complications. Goals might be that the patient independently use the incentive spirometer 10 times each hour and that the lungs remain clear on auscultation. The more specific your desired patient outcomes, the more accurate and exact your evaluation will be.

In the paragraphs that follow, we present an overview of the nursing actions that relate to almost all problems of oxygenation (see the sample Nursing Care Plan Related to Oxygenation).

Positioning for Effective Ventilation

The upright position results in the ability to increase lung expansion because the abdominal contents move away from the diaphragm, enabling the lungs to move further downward. This upright position, called the **orthopneic position**, is the position of preference for most individuals with breathing difficulties. The person

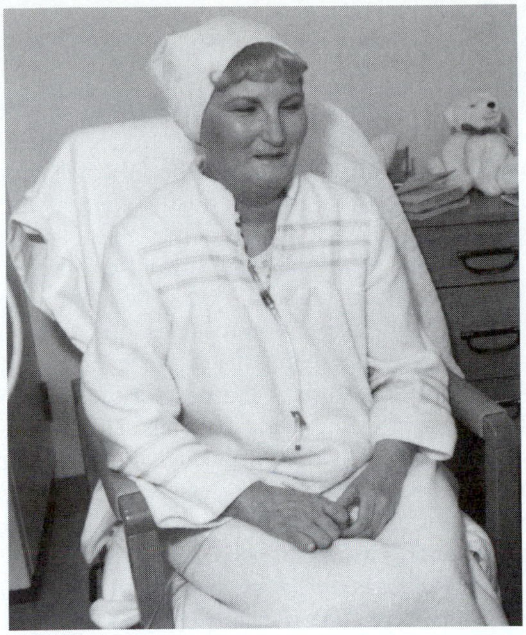

Figure 28-6. Change of position can help facilitate oxygenation.

who cannot breathe adequately unless in an upright position is said to be orthopneic. Sometimes sitting upright is facilitated by placing a table in front of the patient so that he or she can lean forward, resting weight on the arms. This position facilitates the use of abdominal and shoulder girdle muscles to increase expiration and is especially useful to the person with chronic lung disease, who has difficulty with expiration and trapping of air in the alveoli, because of restriction of the airways.

Change of position is also valuable to the individual with respiratory problems (Fig. 28-6). Changing position facilitates the drainage of mucous secretions through gravity. The structure of the lungs is such that different alveoli drain in each position. As secretions drain from alveoli and terminal bronchioles, they enter larger airways, where the cough may more effectively remove them. In addition, changes in position encourage the expansion of different alveoli, resulting in more effective oxygenation.

Occasionally a patient finds a position in which it is comfortable to breathe and resists suggestions to change position. This is a problem because of the overall effects on the lungs and because of potential effects on skin integrity.

Balancing Activity and Rest

Remember that activity is important for overall health and the functioning of the digestive system, elimination, and circulation. For the person with respiratory disease, activity is particularly important in promoting drainage from the lungs and greater lung expansion. Therefore, although pulmonary problems limit the oxygen available for use by vital tissues, it is desirable to include activity if at all possible. The key is balancing the activity with the patient's oxygen availability. The patient will usually tolerate some activity if it is interspersed with rest periods. Also, the type of activity should be selected carefully in light of the limited reserves of the person. Using a commode at the bedside for toileting usually requires less energy than does using a bedpan. A shower taken seated in a chair may use less energy than the efforts involved in bathing in bed. Ambulating for a short distance in the room may be possible if a long tubing to the oxygen is used, but may have adverse consequences if oxygen is removed to allow for activity. The patient's/client's preference for how limited energy is to be used is also important. One individual may wish to rest to be able to visit with family members and use the available energy in talking. Another would rather use the available energy in self-care. These individual preferences must be considered as plans are made for balancing activity and rest.

Nursing Research: *Implications for Practice*

Tyler, D. O., Winslow, E. H., Clark, A. P., & White, K. M. "Effects of a 1-Minute Backrub on Mixed Venous Oxygen Saturation and Heart Rate in Critically Ill Patients." *Heart and Lung* Supplement 19, 5 (September 1990): 562–565.

Venous oxygen saturation and heart rate responses were measured in critically ill patients before and at 4-minute intervals after a 1-minute backrub. There was a statistically significant change in both the oxygen saturation (which decreased) and the heart rate (which increased). However, although statistically significant, the changes were small and did not represent a clinically significant change. The researchers concluded that the traditional backrub, which provides a comforting touch, was a minor stimulus. However, because there is variability in the responses of patients, the individual patient needs to be carefully assessed in regard to oxygen saturation and heart rate after any change in activity.

Providing Oral Care

Oral care is important for the patient with respiratory problems. Mouth breathing causes the build-up of crusts, accompanied by *halitosis* (unpleasant mouth odor). This in turn may affect appetite and nutritional status.

Maintaining Hydration

Encourage the patient with respiratory problems to drink more fluids than usual. Fluids help liquefy secretions, making them easier to move upward and out of the congested lungs. Although it has been said that the patient should desist from ingesting milk products because they tend to increase the production of secretions, no scientific evidence supports this contention. Patients should be encouraged to identify their own responses to foods and fluids and modify their behavior based on that.

Humidification—increasing the amount of water vapor in the air—helps tissue stay moist and lessens irritation. For this reason, adding moisture to the room air has long been a treatment for respiratory difficulty. A humidity tent is commonly used with children who have croup. A portable misting device is used with adults. Some humidifiers are designed to deliver cool mist and others provide warm mist. Some combine the mist with oxygen. Hot steam devices require particular attention to safety, especially if the patient is a child.

Nebulization is a type of humidification in which small particles of moisture are dispersed into the air with a hand-held device containing water or medication. It is either manually operated or attached to a ventilating machine. Unless the patient can breathe only through the mouth from the nebulizer, a plastic nose clamp is applied. Then all the mist or medication will be inhaled into the respiratory tract.

Coaching Regarding Breathing Pattern

When someone is hyperventilating, careful coaching to restore breathing to a slower rate with expiration twice as long as inspiration will help to restore the normal breathing pattern. It may also be necessary for the person to breathe into a paper bag to rebreathe the carbon dioxide expelled and thus conserve the body's carbon dioxide. This rebreathing will change the blood pH and restore normal acid–base balance.

Promoting Lung Expansion

Full lung expansion results in more effective oxygenation. A variety of different measures are used to promote lung expansion. Actively breathing deeply 10 times each hour will significantly improve ventilation. Various devices to encourage deep breathing, such as the incentive spirometer, may be of assistance.

Deep breathing causes bronchodilatation and increases the ventilation of the lungs. In deep breathing, the patient is encouraged to breathe in slowly through the nose, allowing the abdomen to expand as the diaphragm moves downward, and the chest to expand also. The patient is then asked to hold the breath momentarily and then breathe out slowly through the mouth, making the expiration twice as long as the inspiration. The nurse may place his or her hands lightly on the person's abdomen or at the base of the ribs to note whether chest movement is occurring. This action also helps to cue the individual about what should happen when doing deep-breathing exercises. Breathing deeply in this manner will help to expand all the alveoli in the lungs, preventing **atelectasis** (collapse of alveoli). This in turn facilitates gas exchange as each alveolus is filled. Deep breaths, repeated 10 times every hour, are a frequent recommendation for those on bed rest or those who have had surgery. Doing this maintains a pattern of good lung expansion and oxygenation. Deep breathing is valuable to all patients and is not contraindicated because of any medical condition.

When deep breathing is especially important, the physician may order a device called an *incentive spirometer* (IS) to encourage deep breathing. There are many different types available, ranging from simple plastic tubes with a ball that is raised in the tube by inspiratory effort and that provides visual feedback of the volume of inspiration to complex electronic machines that measure the volume inspired, count the number of uses, and provide flashing lights as feedback signals to successful use. *Blow bottles* are used to encourage sustained expiratory effort and may be used for those who have had air trapping in the alveoli. Directions for using these devices may be found in Module 41, Respiratory Care Procedures.

Intermittent positive pressure breathing (IPPB) is a mechanical device used to help inflate the lungs more fully in the individual who is unable to deep breathe independently. IPPB can be used postoperatively to prevent respiratory problems or as a treatment for any patient who cannot fully expand the lungs and who has or may develop atelectasis, a condition in which a number of alveolar sacs have collapsed, thus preventing adequate oxygenation. Because the air is delivered to the lungs under positive pressure, all the alveoli are more fully inflated. The machine can be set to deliver a precise volume of air, to deliver air until a preset pressure is reached in the lungs, or to deliver air for a preset amount of time. In some facilities, IPPB is performed by the respiratory therapist; in others, it is a nursing function. The procedure is ordered by the physician, usually to be administered for about 15 minutes several times a day.

If pain from a surgical incision or an injury such as fractured ribs is contributing to hypoventilation, measures such as splinting may be of assistance in supporting deep breathing. Adequate pain control also is essential to help the person breathe effectively.

Promoting Airway Clearance

Nursing interventions to promote airway clearance are aimed at increasing the effectiveness of the cough in clearing the airway when possible. *Coughing* is used for those whom you have identified as having secretions that need to be moved out of the airways for ventilation to be effective. Forceful coughing in those with no secretions to be removed may result in the collapse of some alveoli and may thus decrease gas exchange. It may also result in fatigue and chest discomfort. Coughing is never done without deep breathing, although deep breathing may be done without coughing. For some individuals, there is medical contraindication to forceful coughing. The pressure that is raised inside the chest while the glottis is closed may have adverse effects on persons with certain cardiac and neurologic diseases.

If pain or discomfort is responsible for the problem, you may need to relieve pain before airway clearance can become effective (see Chapter 32). When pain is from a surgical incision, splinting the incision may allow the person to cough effectively. Splinting is holding the area over the incision so that it does not pull and increase pain when the person is coughing. Splinting may be done by holding a pillow over the incision or by firmly pressing the hands against the incision. Some patients may be able to splint the incision independently if taught how. Others may need someone else to splint for them.

The **"huff" cough** is like a regular cough except that it is done with the glottis open. High pressures are not achieved in the chest, but it appears that this type of cough facilitates peripheral airway clearance without the adverse effects of a hard deep cough. This cough may be appropriate for the individual who has secretions but for whom the forceful cough with closed glottis that significantly raises intrathoracic pressure is contraindicated.

The **quad cough** is so named because it was developed for the use of quadriplegic patients (those paralyzed in all four extremities). The quad cough is also used to assist individuals with weak or ineffective muscle action to enable them to raise secretions. When the person coughs, the nurse applies pressure with the hand on the abdomen with an upward and inward motion, thus increasing the pressure for expulsion of secretions.

If the patient cannot raise and expectorate secretions effectively through coughing and breathing is hampered, the patient may have to be suctioned. Suctioning is carried out with the use of either a portable suction machine or a wall suction unit. A catheter is connected to the suction source and, using sterile technique, inserted through the nose or mouth (nasally or oropharyngeally) downward into the pharynx to remove secretions emerging from the bronchi. Because the respiratory tract is susceptible to infection, asepsis should always be maintained. For the patient in acute distress, a **tracheostomy**—a surgical opening into the trachea that bypasses upper airway obstruction—may have to be performed to allow for direct removal of secretions by suction. These techniques are described in Module 42, Oral and Nasopharyngeal Suctioning, and Module 43, Tracheostomy Care and Suctioning.

When the cough reflex is absent, interventions are designed to prevent aspiration. To prevent aspiration the person is positioned on the side or with the head turned to the side so that any substance in the mouth will drain out and not obstruct the airway. When substances are blocking the airway, they may be removed through suctioning. Large objects that have been aspirated may be removed using abdominal thrust (the **Heimlich maneuver**) or chest thrust techniques (see Module 32, Emergency Resuscitation Procedures).

Administering Cough Medications

Cough medications are typically administered by the nurse in accordance with the physician's prescription. These medications, often given PRN, should be used with discretion. There are several categories of such drugs.

Cough suppressants suppress cough by depressing the cough center in the medulla. This is especially useful if the cough is creating discomfort or interfering with sleep. If you want your patient to rid the lungs of excessive secretions by coughing, the use of these drugs would be inappropriate and, indeed, harmful to the patient.

Expectorants are drugs that promote cough and expectoration. They are used for patients who have audible secretions but little cough activity. Increased fluid intake will also thin secretions and assist with expectoration.

A number of nonprescription cough preparations basically soothe the pharynx or upper respiratory tract. These preparations may be adequate for the patient who describes the cause of the cough as "a tickle in my throat" if the patient does not need to raise secretions and a dry cough is interfering with sleep or activity.

Many cough medications, particularly those used to soothe the throat, are elixirs containing sugar. Keep the sugar content in mind if the patient is a diabetic on sugar restriction. Water is not given immediately after such an elixir because water tends to wash away the soothing effect.

Antihistamines depress the production of secretions and may thus lessen the patient's need to cough to expel sputum.

Administering Oxygen

The physician usually orders the amount of oxygen and the route of administration. The amount of oxygen is measured in either liters per minute (L/min) of oxygen flow or percentage of oxygen in the inspired air. The newer ventilating equipment is able to deliver the precise percentage of oxygen desired. The physician may also indicate the desired level of hemoglobin saturation and direct that oxygen delivery be adjusted to maintain this level.

Too much oxygen can be not only harmful but also potentially fatal to some patients. The patient who has had long-term pulmonary compromise with serious breathing problems has adjusted to an abnormally high $PaCO_2$ in the blood (see Figure 28–3) because of changes in lung structure causing impaired gas exchange. In such a patient, lack of oxygen rather than increased carbon dioxide is actually the stimulus for breathing; it is the trigger mechanism to the medulla for respiration. Giving this particular patient high concentrations of oxygen thus eliminates the trigger for respiration, and acute respiratory failure may result. Although this is fortunately an uncommon occurrence, the nurse should always be extremely cautious in delivering oxygen to patients in this category. Generally speaking, oxygen at 1 to 2 L/min is safe for these patients.

There are other dangers in oxygen administration. Very high levels of oxygen are detrimental to the fragile lung tissue and may stimulate changes in the lung tissue that actually decrease ability of oxygen to diffuse across the membrane.

Additionally, oxygen is not in itself combustible or explosive, but it greatly accelerates burning. Signs should be posted prohibiting smoking near oxygen, and any equipment or objects that could produce sparks should be removed.

Oxygen may come from a central reservoir and be piped into individual patient units, or it may come from a tank. Whatever its source, oxygen is administered by the same techniques. Oxygen may be delivered by mask, catheter, cannula, or tent. For long-term oxygen therapy, a catheter may be surgically inserted directly into the trachea just above the clavicle. This is called a transtracheal oxygen catheter.

The oxygen mask is used primarily for short-term or emergency consumption. Masks are efficient in delivering precise levels of oxygen (Fig. 28-7). Catheters are irritating to the nose and uncomfortable for the patient and thus used infrequently. The nasal cannula is used most commonly because it has prongs that fit the nostrils and is much more comfortable than other devices. Even if the patient mouth breathes with the cannula in place, the oxygen is breathed through the mouth because oxygen is heavier than air. Air flows in front of the mouth as well as into the nostrils and significantly increases the percentage of oxygen in the air inspired into the lungs. Patients receiving nasal oxygen need nasal care to remove accumulated secretions and prevent irritation of nasal tissue. Tents are expensive and difficult to clean, and require high concentrations of oxygen to maintain ordered levels and therefore have been almost completely superseded by other oxygen delivery methods. Because the transtracheal oxygen catheter uses less oxygen and can be covered with clothing, helping the person to maintain a more "normal" appearance, it is increasing in use for those with chronic lung disease who need continuous oxygen.

Although usually a physician orders the amount of oxygen and method of administration, it may become necessary for you to initiate the administration of oxygen to a patient if you assess a threat to patient safety or extreme discomfort. After starting the oxygen, immediately consult with the physician for further instructions. For the specifics of oxygen administration, see Module 40, Administering Oxygen.

Some patients keep portable oxygen in the home. This may be used only with activity, only during the night, or constantly. Through the use of oxygen many individuals are able to extend their capacity for the ac-

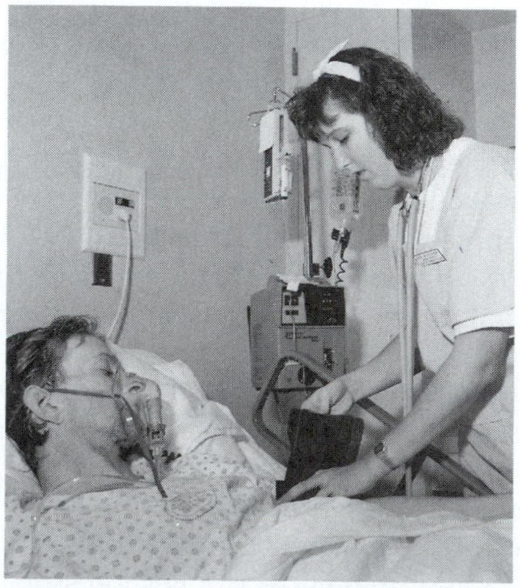

Figure 28–7. This man is receiving moisturized oxygen by mask.

tivities of daily living. Small, light-weight, portable oxygen containers that can be carried by a shoulder strap are now available and have greatly increased the ability of some individuals to engage in a fulfilling life.

Chest Physical Therapy

Chest physical therapy includes postural drainage, percussion, and vibration of the chest. **Postural drainage** is a procedure to bring about drainage of secretions from various lung segments by placing the patient in different positions. Gravity will drain secretions from a segment if it is positioned higher than the rest of the chest. Before the treatment, bronchodilating drugs are sometimes given by inhalation to further promote drainage. While the patient is in the prescribed position, the nurse may perform percussion (tapping) over the chest area to loosen secretions. Vibration is vibrating the external chest wall for the same purpose. Both percussion and vibration may be done with the hands or with small battery-powered devices. Directions for performing postural drainage, vibration, and percussion may be found in Module 41, Respiratory Care Procedures.

Alleviating Anxiety

When you are with a patient who is experiencing respiratory distress, any appropriate actions you take to help the patient breathe more effectively will also provide assurance that help is possible. Touching or holding the patient's hand indicates that you are near, are aware of what the patient is experiencing, and can help. Asking the patient to try to relax and conserve energy is helpful if you remain and assist with this process. Coaching in deep breathing enhances relaxation and may calm the patient. Avoid prolonged verbal interaction for anxiety reduction. By increasing oxygen demand this can increase anxiety. If family or friends are visiting, it is sometimes necessary to discuss the importance of not trying to engage the patient in conversation. Their quiet presence can be reassuring and supportive.

Health Teaching

As health care providers, nurses are in a position to teach by example and by sharing knowledge. Health maintenance and prevention of illness are two of the most important subjects of health teaching.

Because poor posture and obesity can both cause difficulty in breathing, nurses should encourage correct posture and weight control. The federal government has amassed clear evidence that cigarette smoking and air pollution are among the causative agents of lung cancer and serious pulmonary disease. Clearly, nurses should not smoke and should encourage others to not smoke. National and regional programs to minimize air pollution merit the support of health care personnel. The American Lung Association offers respiratory patients and their families a wide variety of services.

People afflicted with respiratory problems may have to revise their patterns of daily living. Avoiding pollutants in the air, such as smoke, is essential. An individual may need to learn greater assertiveness in regard to others' smoking. Conserving energy for important tasks may prove necessary. Therefore, part of your teaching may be centered around helping the patient examine what is most important in life. Avoiding individuals with respiratory infections will also be necessary. Again this may require assertiveness in interpersonal relationships.

Specific techniques for self-care such as the deep-breathing and coughing exercise and postural drainage previously discussed may be taught. Individuals with chronic respiratory illness may need to learn to manage their own oxygen therapy, nebulizers, and medication regimens. Through effective management they may be able to prevent serious exacerbations of their disease and maintain a higher quality of life.

Encouraging Immunization

Influenza vaccination is available each fall to combat the viral strains expected during the "flu season." Individuals with chronic respiratory disease, chronic heart disease, and those over age 65 are specially targeted to receive this preventive therapy. Health care providers are also at higher risk of contracting influenza and should be immunized. Nurses can be effective in teaching about the importance of influenza immunization.

Pneumococcal pneumonia is especially serious for the elderly. A vaccine is available and recommended for all those age 65 and older. This one-time immunization prevents this illness which has been fatal to some elderly individuals.

Maintaining Mechanical Ventilation

A number of complicated ventilators are used to aid or sustain respiration for the critically ill patient. These ventilators use positive pressure to inflate the lungs. They can be set to meet the individual needs of a particular patient with regard to rate and depth of respirations, as well as the concentration of oxygen needed at a given time. Close monitoring of the blood gases or hemoglobin saturation allows constant assessment and readjustment of the ventilator. Operating ventilators requires a high level of nursing expertise. Although at one time ventilators were only found in intensive care settings, some individuals are now maintained on ventilators in the home and in long-term care settings. Information on maintaining the patient on a ventilator will be found in a medical–surgical nursing text.

Coordinating With Respiratory Therapy

Most large hospitals have departments devoted to the care and treatment of patients with respiratory problems. The personnel of these departments may hold associate or baccalaureate degrees or may have received on-the-job training. Some are called respiratory therapists and some inhalation therapists. There is a designation called the Registered Respiratory Technician (RRT) that requires meeting national standards. This is not required in all states. Depending on the facility, these caregivers may perform all respiratory care, including health teaching, or may share such responsibility with nurses. Wherever you practice, it will be your responsibility to coordinate care with the respiratory therapist to ensure that the patient's care remains of the highest quality.

Evaluation

When evaluating outcomes for the individual with respiratory problems, you will need to collect data in the same way you did for initial assessment. You will need to count respirations, determine depth of respirations, auscultate lungs, and percuss the chest. You will also need to interview the patient in regard to feelings of shortness of breath, cough, or difficulty in breathing. Laboratory data or oximetry may also be essential for effective evaluation.

These data will then be compared both with the initial assessment and with the desired outcomes you previously identified. You will need to judge whether or not the patient has made progress in moving toward the desired outcomes. If no progress has been made, you will need to determine whether plans need to be revised or whether more time is needed. Ongoing evaluation is important to making effective adjustments in treatment plans.

Nursing Care Study
A Patient with Emphysema

Edna Donner, RN, left the nursing station to help transfer the new admission from the stretcher to her bed. She knew that Mrs. Alder, aged 51, had *emphysema,* a condition characterized by loss of alveolar tissue leading to inefficient oxygenation. An oxygen mask was in place, with 3 liters of oxygen per minute running. Mrs. Alder was attempting to pull off the mask and was moving her head from side to side as she cried out, "Oh, please, please, somebody help me!"

Mrs. Donner made a quick assessment. The mask seemed to be complicating matters, giving Mrs. Alder the sense of being suffocated. The transfer to the bed appeared to have taxed Mrs. Alder's energy reserves, and she lay back, restless but exhausted. Her color was slightly dusky.

A plan formed in Mrs. Donner's head. With words of assurance and explanation as to what she was doing and why, she held Mrs. Alder's hand as she raised the bed with the electric control. She then placed a pillow under Mrs. Alder's shoulders and head so as to elevate the thorax. A nursing assistant who entered the room to take Mrs. Alder's vital signs was sent to obtain a nasal cannula with prongs. As soon as it arrived, Mrs. Donner, continuing to reassure the patient, changed the oxygen from the mask to the prongs. Mrs. Alder's head-twisting movements stopped. Mrs. Donner quietly spoke to Mrs. Alder: "Try to breathe more deeply and evenly now. Concentrate on your muscles, and feel them begin to relax. Notice how much more easily you are able to breathe now." Mrs. Donner repeated this message over and over, until Mrs. Alder became calm and relaxed and her duskiness disappeared. An hour later, as Mrs. Donner again sat with Mrs. Alder, Mrs. Alder said, "Thank you, I really thought I was going to die until you helped me breathe."

Back at the nursing station, Mrs. Donner noticed the blank nursing history form. She had forgotten all about it during Mrs. Alder's crisis. "Well," she thought, "that will just have to wait."

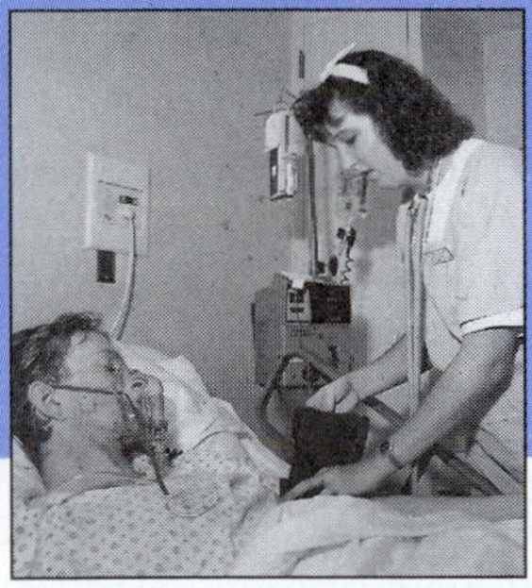

Key Points

- The respiratory system is divided into two major sections. The upper respiratory system includes the nose and pharynx down to the epiglottis. The lower respiratory system includes the larynx, the trachea, the bronchi, the lungs, and all of the lung parts, that is, the terminal bronchioles and alveoli. The diaphragm, although part of the musculoskeletal system, is important in lung function.
- The process of ventilation is complex and involves receptors that are located in the aorta, carotid bodies, chest, muscles, and lungs. These receptors respond to various stimuli and in turn stimulate the respiratory centers in the brain. The primary respiratory center is in the medulla, and there are additional centers in the pons and in the lower pons.
- Lung volumes and capacities are measurements of the quantity of air that the lungs contain or are able to move and are used to identify respiratory abnormalities.
- Oxygen and carbon dioxide exchange is the major function of the lungs. To prevent the entry of particles and microbes, the lungs have an effective set of lung clearance mechanisms. The exchange of carbon dioxide also affects acid–base balance within the body.
- Assessment of oxygenation includes interview questions related to current symptoms, past respiratory diseases, and smoking history. In checking respirations, the nurse notes rate, depth, rhythm, audible respiratory sounds, lung sounds, and the appearance of respirations. Other factors to consider are color of the skin and mucous membranes, presence and appearance of sputum, and the presence of cough. Laboratory studies of blood gases, pH, and hemoglobin saturation and diagnostic studies such as chest x-rays can provide specialized information.
- Nursing diagnoses related to oxygenation include Activity Intolerance related to respiratory disease, Altered Respiratory Function, and Discomfort related to cough. Impaired Gas Exchange, Ineffective Airway Clearance, and Ineffective Breathing Patterns are other common nursing diagnoses.
- Nursing interventions include proper positioning to facilitate breathing, administration of oxygen, providing oral care, maintaining fluid balance, suctioning, humidification, deep breathing, and coughing, and postural drainage may all help to make airways clear and breathing more effective. IPPB is used in specialized situations at the physician's order. Providing for rest and health teaching may be an integral part of many of these nursing actions. Encouraging immunization prevents illness in susceptible groups. Allaying psychological discomfort is a challenging part of intervention.
- Evaluation requires that the nurse identify the desired outcomes based on the underlying problems and also be realistic about the patient's potential.

Study Questions

1. What is the function of chemoreceptors in the aorta and the carotid body?
2. How does the respiratory center in the medulla control respiration?
3. Describe the process of expiration.
4. What is tidal volume?
5. What is residual volume?
6. What are the norms for arterial carbon dioxide and arterial oxygen levels?
7. Describe six aspects of lung clearance.
8. Explain how hyperventilation causes respiratory alkalosis.
9. How is a figure for pack-years of cigarette smoking computed?
10. Describe a normal respiratory cycle.
11. How can you assess for cyanosis in a person with dark skin?
12. Explain criteria for identifying activity intolerance.
13. Describe appropriate actions for the patient with activity intolerance.
14. Why is oxygen not administered at high levels to persons with chronic lung disease?
15. How does the patient's underlying condition affect the writing of outcome criteria?

Critical Thinking Activities

1. In the clinical facility, visit the respiratory therapy department. If possible, have a respiratory therapist demonstrate the types of care provided. Identify actions you could take to coordinate care with respiratory therapy in this setting.

2. Identify a patient in the clinical area who has a respiratory problem. Write out your complete assessment, nursing diagnoses, and plan for supporting respiratory function.
3. Check your facility's policy regarding the level of autonomy nurses have in initiating oxygen therapy. Construct a theoretical situation that demonstrates a need for the nurse to initiate oxygen therapy.

Relevant Sections in Modules for Basic Nursing Skills

References and Readings

Carpenito, L. J. *Nursing Diagnosis: Application to Clinical Practice.* 4th edition. Philadelphia: J. B. Lippincott, 1992.

Carroll, P. "Safe Suctioning." *Nursing '89* 19, 9 (September 1989): 48–51.

Carroll, P. "Good Nursing Gets COPD Patients Out of Hospitals." *RN* (July 1989): 24–28.

Felton, C. L. "Hypoxemia and Oral Temperatures." *American Journal of Nursing* 78 (January 1978): 56–57.

Fielding, J. E. "Smoking: Health Effects and Control." Part 2. *New England Journal of Medicine* 313 (August 19, 1985): 555–561.

Finesilver, C. "Respiratory Assessment." *RN* 55, 2 (February 1992): 22–30.

Graas, S. "Thermometer Sites and Oxygen." *American Journal of Nursing* 74 (October 1974): 1862–1863.

Hanley, M. V., and Tyler, M. L. "Ineffective Airway Clearance Related to Airway Infection." *Nursing Clinics of North America* 22, 1 (March 1987): 135–150.

Hopp, L. J., and Williams, M. "Ineffective Breathing Pattern Related to Decreased Lung Expansion." *Nursing Clinics of North America* 22, 1 (March 1987): 193–206.

Kim, M. J., and Larson, J. L. "Ineffective Airway Clearance and Ineffective Breathing Patterns: Theoretical and Research Base for Nursing Practice." *Nursing Clinics of North America* 22, 1 (March 1987): 125–134.

Lareau, S., and Larson, J. L. "Ineffective Breathing Pattern Related to Airflow Limitation." *Nursing Clinics of North America* 22, 1 (March 1987): 179–192.

Larson, J. L., and Kim, M. J.. "Ineffective Breathing Pattern Related to Respiratory Muscle Fatigue." *Nursing Clinics of North America* 22, 1 (March 1987): 225–248.

McNaull, F. W. "Tobaccoism in America." *American Journal of Nursing* 87, 11 (November 1987): 1430–1432.

Mechner, F. "Patient Assessment: Examination of the Chest and Lungs." *American Journal of Nursing* 76 (September 1976): 1–23.

Meehan, M. "Nursing Dx: Potential for Aspiration." *RN* 55, 1 (January 1992): 30–35.

Mims, B. "Interpreting ABGs." *RN* 54, 3 (March 1991): 42–46.

Price, S. A., and Wilson, L. M. *Pathophysiology: Clinical Concepts of Disease Processes.* 3rd edition. New York: McGraw-Hill, 1990.

Rokosky, J. S. "Assessment of the Individual with Altered Respiratory Function." *Nursing Clinics of North America* 16, 2 (June 1981): 195–209.

Schwartz, J. L. *Review and Evaluation of Smoking Cessation Methods.* National Institutes of Health, Pub. No. 87-2940. Washington, D.C.: U.S. Government Printing Office, April 1987.

Shekleton, M. E., and Nield, M. "Ineffective Airway Clearance Related to Artificial Airway." *Nursing Clinics of North America* 22, 1 (March 1987): 167–178.

Smoking and Health: A Report of the Surgeon General. U.S. Department of Health, Education and Welfare, Pub. No. 79-50066. Washington, D.C.: U.S. Government Printing Office, 1979.

Smoking and Its Effects on Health: A Report of WHO Expert Committee. World Health Organization Technical Report Series, No. 568, World Health Organization, 1975.

Spearing, C., and Cornell, D. "Incentive Spirometry: Inspiring Your Patient to Breathe Deeply." *Nursing '87* 17, 9 (September 1987): 50–51.

Spyr, J., and Preach, M. "Pulse Oximetry." *RN* 53, 5 (May 1990): 38–45.

Telch, M. J. et al. "Long-term Follow-up of a Pilot Project on Smoking Prevention with Adolescents." *Journal of Behavioral Medicine* 5 (March 1982): 1–8.

U.S. Department of Health and Human Services. *The Health Consequences of Smoking for Women: A Report of the Surgeon General.* Rockville, Md.: USDHHS, 1980.

U.S. National Research Council. *Environmental Tobacco Smoke: Measuring Exposures and Assessing Health Effects.* Washington, D.C.: National Academy Press, 1986.

Wesmiller, S. W., Hoffman, L. A., and Wiseman, M. "Understanding Transtracheal Oxygen Delivery." *Nursing '89* 19, 12 (December, 1989): 43–47.

Circulation

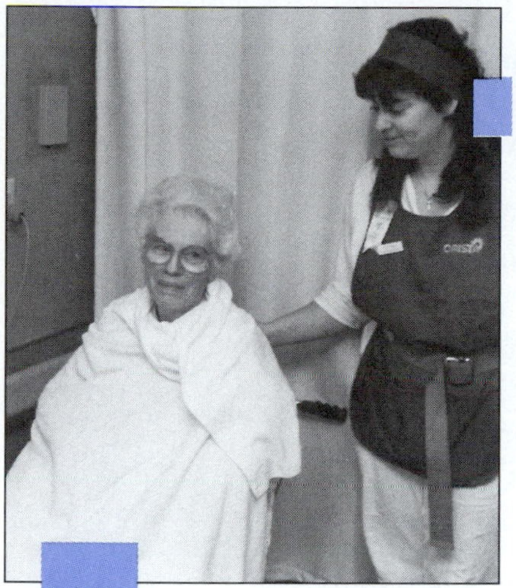

29

Objectives

After completing this chapter, you should be able to:

1. Discuss briefly the function of the heart, blood vessels, and blood.
2. List lifestyle modifications that will contribute to the maintenance of cardiovascular health.
3. Describe an appropriate exercise program for cardiovascular conditioning.
4. Outline information necessary for basic circulation assessmcnt.
5. Define the terms used to report on pulse and blood pressure.
6. List common nursing diagnoses related to circulation.
7. Describe appropriate nursing interventions for supporting effective circulation.
8. Explain the processes involved in basic life support.

Study Terms

apical pulse
ascites
blood pressure
bradycardia
central venous pressure (CVP)
complete blood count (CBC)
cyanosis
diastolic pressure
differential white blood count
edema
hematocrit
Korotkoff's sound
peripheral arterial insufficiency
peripheral venous insufficiency
point of maximal impulse (PMI)
postural blood pressure
postural hypotension
pulse
pulse deficit
pulse pressure
pulse rate
pulse rhythm
pulse strength
systolic pressure
tachycardia

Outline

The Circulatory System

Heart
Vessels
Blood
  Red Blood Cells
  White Blood Cells
  Platelets
  Blood Typing

Factors Affecting Cardiovascular Health

Prudent Diet
Eliminating Cigarette Smoking
Stress Management
Regular Physical Activity
  Types of Exercise
  Frequency of Exercise
  Intensity of Exercise

Ellis, Nowlis: Nursing: A Human Needs Approach, 5th ed. © 1994 J.B. Lippincott Company

Circulation of the blood brings oxygen and needed nutrients to cells so that life functions may proceed. In addition, adequate circulation is necessary to remove waste products from the tissue. Various tissues have different specific needs for circulation. Central nervous system tissue will not survive for much longer than 5 minutes if deprived of circulation. Central organs are able to survive for longer periods of time but may still suffer irreversible damage when circulation is interrupted. Peripheral tissues may survive longest with interruption in blood supply. An extremity severed from the body may be reattached a number of hours later if the extremity is kept cool so that metabolic demands are lowered until reattachment so that the tissues can survive. (Of course, other factors such as the extent of tissue damage are also important.) However, there is a physiologic limit on how long tissue can survive without circulation, so adequate circulation to every body part remains a basic need.

The Circulatory System

The circulatory system is composed of the heart, which pumps blood throughout the system; the vessels, which carry the blood; and the body fluid, composed of blood and other body liquids, which carries oxygen, nutrients, and wastes to appropriate parts of the body (Fig. 29-1).

Heart

The heart is a muscular organ located in the middle of the chest. The wide upper end is called the *base*. The more pointed lower end, called the *apex*, extends toward the left in the chest. The heart is contained in a membranous sac called the pericardium. The muscle layer of the heart is the myocardium. The lining of the heart is the endocardium. The central space in the center of the chest occupied by the heart, great vessels, and trachea is called the mediastinum.

The heart has four chambers. The left and right atria both receive blood into the heart; the left from the pulmonary vein, which comes directly from the lungs, and the right from the great vessels, which come from the rest of the body. The right and left ventricles are strong pumps, which propel the blood forward in the system. The right ventricle pumps blood to the lungs, and the left ventricle pumps blood to the rest of the body.

Valves are present between the atria and corresponding ventricles and at the entrance to the great arteries from each ventricle. The valves prevent blood from flowing backward when the ventricles contract.

Cardiac rate and rhythm are controlled by autonomic nerves and also by a conduction system intrinsic to the heart muscle itself. For further explanation of the functioning of the heart, consult a physiology text.

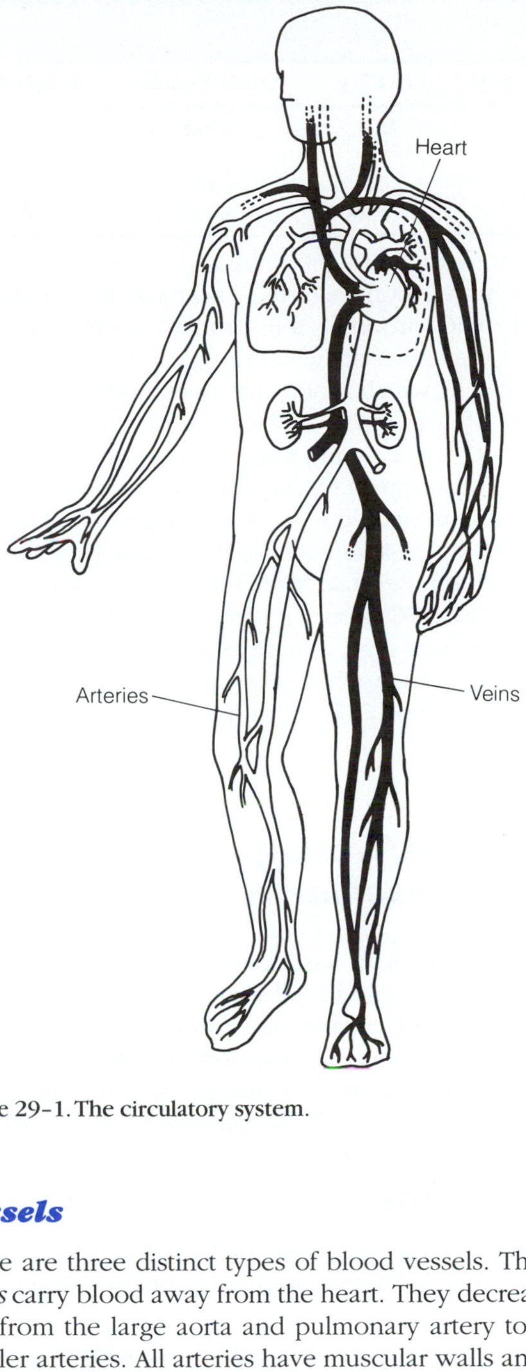

Figure 29-1. The circulatory system.

Vessels

There are three distinct types of blood vessels. The *arteries* carry blood away from the heart. They decrease in size from the large aorta and pulmonary artery to ever smaller arteries. All arteries have muscular walls and are able to constrict.

Capillaries are located at the end of the arteries and join them with the veins. Capillaries extend to each body cell and have thin permeable walls. It is through the capillaries that all exchange of oxygen, nutrients, and wastes occurs. The permeability of the capillary walls varies with the stimulation of various body chemicals and in response to toxins.

Veins return blood to the heart. Tiny in the periphery of the body, the veins gradually become larger and larger as they near the heart. There is, of course, no pump propelling blood through the veins, as there is at the starting point of the arteries. Blood flows through them in response to several forces: the pressure of more blood entering from the arterial end, the pumping action of skeletal muscles around the veins, and changes exerted by gravity when the position of the body is changed. Valves in the veins prevent blood from flowing backward and maintain flow toward the heart.

Blood

Blood is a complex body fluid. Its basis is *plasma*, which is composed of water, chemicals, and circulating proteins. In addition, a variety of specific blood cells are suspended in the plasma. Let us look at some of the important components of blood. The normal amounts of each component are listed in Table 29-1.

Red Blood Cells

Red blood cells (RBCs), also called *erythrocytes*, contain *hemoglobin*, an iron-based compound that gives blood its oxygen-carrying capacity. A person's RBC count specifies the number of RBCs per 100 ml (deciliter) of blood. The norms for women are lower than those for men because of blood loss through menstruation. Scarcity of RBCs may indicate bleeding or a deficit in the body's ability to produce RBCs.

Hemoglobin is measured in terms of the weight of the hemoglobin contained in the RBCs in 100 ml of blood. Hemoglobin will, of course, be reduced if the number of RBCs is low. It is also reduced if there is a deficiency of iron in the diet, which results in inadequate hemoglobin production, and if various disease processes such as anemia are present.

Hematocrit, the percentage of the whole blood accounted for by RBCs, is measured in terms of volume per 100 ml. Hematocrit is lowered by the same factors that lower hemoglobin and RBC count and by the presence of excessive fluid in the body. Dehydration increases hematocrit.

Hemoglobin and hematocrit are both high at birth if the mother is well nourished. Over the first 3 months of life, they gradually decrease. During childhood, hemo-

Table 29–1. Complete Blood Count (CBC) Norms for Adult Men and Women

Test	Men	Women
Hemoglobin	14.5–16.5 g/100 ml	13–15.5 g/100 ml
Hematocrit	45% (43%–50%)	40% (40%–45%)
Erythrocytes (RBC)	4.3–5.5 × 10^6/mm^3	4.5–6 × 10^6/mm^3
Leukocytes (WBC)	5,000–10,000 mm^3	5,000–10,000 mm^3

Table 29–2. Hemoglobin and Hematocrit

		2 wk	3 mo	6 mo–6 y	7–12 y	Adult Female	Adult Male
Hemoglobin g/100 ml	*Mean*	16.5	12.0	12.0	13.0	14.0	16.0
	Range	13.0–20.0	9.5–14.5	10.5–14.0	11.0–16.0	12.0–16.0	14.0–18.0
Hematocrit %	*Mean*	50	36	37	38	42	47
	Range	42–66	31–41	33–42	34–40	37–47	42–52

globin and hematocrit are normally maintained at a lower level than in the adult (Table 29-2).

White Blood Cells

White blood cells (WBCs), or *leukocytes*, contain and destroy anything that is a threat to the body. The several types of WBCs have specific functions. WBCs are able to move under their own power.

The WBC count is measured in terms of the number of cells per 100 ml of blood. A **differential white blood count** (often called a diff) is a further analysis of the leukocytes that differentiates cells of each type and gives the percentage of each. Consult a physiology text for a complete discussion of the differing functions of the various types of WBCs.

Platelets

The third major type of blood cell is the *platelet* (also called *thrombocyte*), which initiates the formation of blood clots. Whenever an injury or irregularity occurs in the lining of a blood vessel, the platelets adhere to the edges of the injury and begin the clotting process. The normal platelet count is approximately 150,000 to $300{,}000/mm^3$.

Blood Typing

Protein substances called *antigens* may be attached to the RBCs. Although there are several groups of these antigens, the two of common clinical significance are the ABO group and the Rh group.

The ABO group includes two different antigens, A and B. The person whose RBCs carry only the A antigen has type A blood. If the RBCs carry only the B antigen, the blood is type B. If the RBCs carry both A and B antigens, the blood is type AB. If the blood cells carry neither antigen, the blood is type O. Type O is the most common blood type.

The Rh group consists of only one antigen, the Rh factor. If the RBCs contain this factor, the blood is termed Rh positive; if not, it is Rh negative. The majority of individuals are Rh positive.

A person is capable of producing antibodies against any antigen that person's own blood does not carry. Thus, a person with type A Rh-negative blood would be capable of producing antibodies against type B blood and against any Rh-positive blood. In the event of a blood transfusion, exactly matching the recipient's blood type prevents the production of antibodies against unfamiliar antigens. However, there are several instances in which blood that does not exactly match can be safely transfused. This is the case, for example, if the blood given simply does not contain any antigens capable of causing a reaction. Rh-negative blood can be given both to people who are Rh negative and to those who are Rh positive because it contains no antigen in the Rh group. Because type O does not contain any antigen in the ABO group, it can be given to people with any ABO blood type, as long as Rh-positive blood is not given to a person whose blood is Rh negative. Thus a person with type O Rh-negative blood is called a "universal donor."

Factors Affecting Cardiovascular Health

The American Heart Association (AHA) has identified a variety of ways in which people without existing heart or blood vessel disease can lessen their risk of heart disease. These recommendations involve changes in diet, smoking habits, and activity, which need to become part of the individual's lifestyle to be effective.

Prudent Diet

The prudent diet recommended by AHA is one that is low in cholesterol, saturated fats, and salt and does not contain excessive calories (AHA, 1980). This diet will help to decrease atherosclerosis (a condition in which plaque forms in the arteries), high blood pressure (associated with high salt intake), and excess weight (the consequence of excessive calories). These diet factors were discussed in Chapter 25. AHA has many pamphlets available giving specific suggestions for implementing such a diet (AHA, 1986).

Eliminating Cigarette Smoking

Cigarettes contain nicotine, which causes arteries to constrict. When arteries are constricted, the heart works harder in circulating the blood. At the same time, the heart's own blood supply is decreased because the arteries in the heart are also constricted. Smoking also decreases the ability of the lungs to oxygenate the blood, making it necessary for the heart to expend greater effort to provide adequate oxygen to the body. Numerous programs have been established to assist those who wish to quit smoking. For many, this is a difficult task, but it has rewards. AHA has strongly recommended that individuals interested in cardiovascular health not smoke (AHA, 1986).

Stress Management

Psychological factors play a part in cardiovascular disease although their effect on an individual cannot be directly measured. AHA recommends that individuals acknowledge this factor and try to control life stress (see Chapter 6).

Regular Physical Activity

The AHA Committee on Exercise stated that "regular, vigorous exercise enhances the quality of life by increasing the physical capability for work and play" (AHA, 1972). In 1991 they published standards to be used to evaluate exercise and exercise tolerance (AHA, 1991). Exercise is recommended only as a part of a total lifestyle management program.

Appropriate exercise for the person with existing heart or blood vessel disease should be determined by the physician. A variety of tests may need to be made before a specific prescription for exercise may be safely made. Any sedentary person who is in the age group at risk of undetected heart disease (over 45 for men and past menopause for women) should consult with a physician before beginning an exercise program (Fig. 29-2).

For the healthy person or one who has routinely been physically active, some general guidelines have been established for exercise. These guidelines relate to the type of exercise and the frequency, intensity, and duration of activity (AHA, 1991).

Types of Exercise

To provide for cardiorespiratory conditioning, the exercise must produce a sustained increase in metabolic, respiratory, and cardiovascular function (Display 29-1). Exercises that do this are called aerobic exercises. Examples are vigorous walking, running, swimming, rope jumping, and some calisthenics. Some active sports provide aerobic exercise, but many provide only for bursts of activity and therefore are not as useful for conditioning. Competitive activities are not recommended for the beginner because the inadequately conditioned individual may be tempted to overdo, causing injury. Choosing activities that are pleasurable to the individual is recommended because it increases the likelihood of continuing the exercise program. Including exercise in the normal pattern of daily activity by walking instead of driving, climbing stairs instead of using the elevator, and gardening will contribute to overall fitness. For older individuals, more moderate types of exercise such as walking and swimming are generally preferable to high intensity activities such as running unless they have maintained a high level of fitness on a continuing basis.

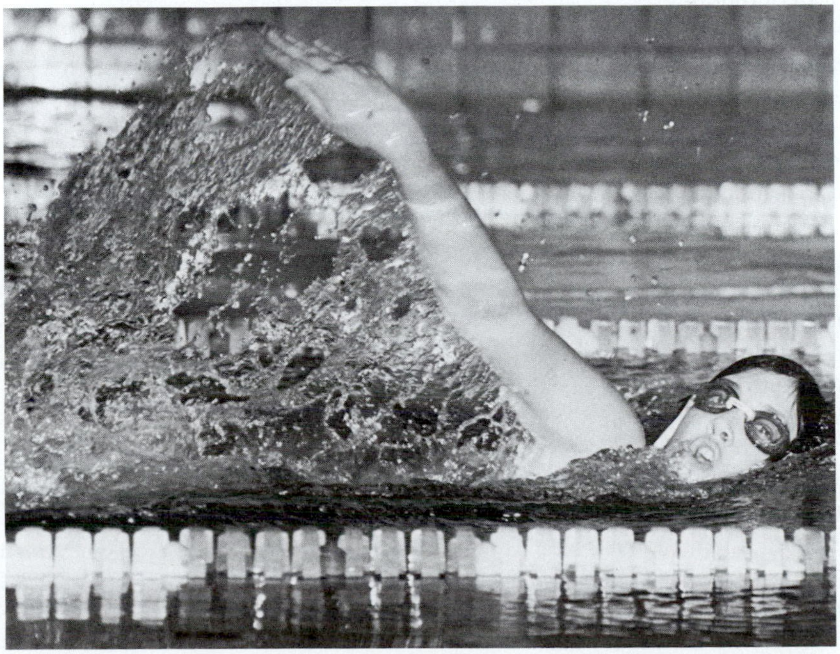

Figure 29-2. Swimming is one aerobic exercise that provides for cardiovascular conditioning.

Display 29–1

Suggested Activities for Cardiovascular Conditioning

Aerobic dance	Roller-skating
Bicycling	Rowing
Calisthenics	Running
Ice-skating	Skiing
Jogging	Swimming
Jumping rope	Walking

Frequency of Exercise

Ideally, an exercise program would be based on daily exercise, but this is not a realistic possibility for many people. AHA has determined that *cardiovascular conditioning* can take place if exercise is conducted three times a week on nonconsecutive days. After cardiovascular fitness has been achieved, it can be maintained with sessions at least twice a week on nonconsecutive days although three times a week is recommended. To maintain fitness, one must make a lifetime commitment to exercise (AHA, 1991).

Intensity of Exercise

The intensity of the dynamic phase of exercise can be measured by many complicated laboratory tests. However, the test most commonly recommended is checking the pulse. The intensity needed to produce cardiovascular conditioning varies among individuals. In addition the intensity needed for conditioning varies with the length of time you exercise. A lesser intensity of exercise requires a greater length of exercise time for conditioning. However, the general recommendation is that the pulse rate must reach at least 60% of peak heart rate. During the conditioning phase, while the person is working toward a conditioned level, the pulse should reach 70% to 85% of the peak heart rate for best conditioning effect. Those who are older or not in condition may start out only reaching 60% to 70%. Once conditioning has been achieved, the pulse may then be allowed to reach 85% of peak heart rate. However, this is not essential. For most individuals, continuing to reach 70% to 75% of peak heart rate will provide a satisfactory level of conditioning that supports ongoing health.

Although peak heart rate may be tested in an exercise laboratory, the healthy individual may use a table of predicted maximal heart rates as a standard. Another alternative is to use a table of target heart rates during exercise. This table eliminates the need to figure a percentage, but is less precise (Tables 29-3 and 29-4).

Another approach to measuring intensity of effort is for the individual to indicate a personal perceived exertion level as very, very light, very light, fairly light, somewhat hard, hard, very hard, and very, very hard (Pollock and Willmore, 1990). A person exercising somewhat hard or hard is accomplishing conditioning and is probably not exceeding safe levels of cardiovascular stress. (Remember that these are guidelines for healthy people.)

Table 29–3. Average Maximum Heart Rates During Exercise

Age	Target Zone 60%–75% (beats/min)	Average Maximum Heart Rates During Exercise
20	120–150	200
25	117–146	195
30	114–142	190
35	111–138	185
40	108–135	180
45	105–131	175
50	102–127	170
55	99–123	165
60	96–120	160
65	93–116	155
70	90–113	150

Data from *Exercise and Your Heart*. Dallas: American Heart Association, 1984, p. 17.

Duration of Exercise

Exercise sessions of 15 to 20 minutes of 70% to 85% intensity can provide conditioning although more rapid conditioning will occur with longer sessions. However,

Table 29–4. Safe Heart Rate Ranges During Exercise*

Age	Beats/Min	Beats/10 Seconds
10–20	156–168	26–28
21–30	150–162	25–27
31–40	144–150	24–25
41–50	138–144	23–24
51–60	126–138	21–23
61–70	120–126	20–21
71+	108–120	18–20

*These are normal ranges for people who do not have cardiovascular disease or who are not taking medication that may tend to falsely lower their heart rate.

Table adapted from information provided by the American Medical Association. © American Medical Association. Reprinted with permission from *The Staying Well Personal Fitness Diary*, p. 10. © 1983 Blue Cross and Blue Shield Association. All rights reserved.

longer sessions at high intensity have greater potential for causing soreness, severe muscle fatigue, or even injury when the person is not yet conditioned. Longer sessions of less intense activity can also provide conditioning. A gradual approach to exercise does not create discomfort and is more likely to be followed.

In the standard conditioning pattern, each exercise session should start with 5 to 10 minutes of warm-up activity. This period of loosening and warming of muscles helps to prevent injuries. The warm-up is followed by a 15- to 30-minute period of dynamic exercise for conditioning. The session is concluded with a 5- to 10-minute cool-down phase. The cool-down phase is essential to prevent an unstable circulatory state during recovery from the dynamic phase (AHA, 1991).

Those who choose a less intense activity (*ie,* the heart rate not reach more than 60%–70% of the peak heart) will need the same pattern beginning with warm-up, engaging in a longer period of dynamic activity, and ending with a cool-down.

General Guidelines for Conditioning Exercise

In addition to monitoring the pulse, AHA (1991) has suggested the following general guidelines for exercising.

1. Exercise only when feeling well.
2. Do not exercise vigorously soon after eating.
3. Adjust exercise to the weather.
4. Slow down for hills.
5. Wear proper clothing and shoes.
6. Understand personal limitations.
7. Select appropriate exercise.
8. Start slowly and progress gradually.
9. Watch for these signs and modify exercise to lesser intensity or decreased time if they occur:
   a. Inability to finish planned exercise
   b. Inability to converse during the activity
   c. Faintness or nausea
   d. Chronic fatigue
   e. Sleeplessness
   f. Aches and pain in joints
10. Be alert for the following symptoms; stop exercising immediately; contact your physician if they occur:
    a. Discomfort in upper body, chest, arm, neck, or jaw
    b. Appearance of signs of vasoconstriction, such as pale or clammy skin
    c. Progressive drop in heart rate as exercise continues
    d. Irregular pulse rate
    e. Faintness
    f. Shortness of breath that is uncomfortable, prevents talking, is characterized by wheezing, or takes more than 5 minutes for recovery of breathing
    e. Discomfort in bones or joints that persists

Common Disorders Affecting Circulation

Cardiovascular diseases are one of the major health threats for individuals in midlife and beyond. Although the death rate for cardiovascular disease has dropped 51% since 1950, cardiovascular disease affects more than one in four Americans (AHA, 1991). Three common cardiovascular problems that require collaborative action by the nurse are peripheral venous stasis, hypertension, and decreased cardiac output.

Peripheral Venous Stasis and Thrombophlebitis

Peripheral venous stasis refers to blood pooling in the large veins of the lower extremities. This condition is most frequently a consequence of immobility. You can identify the person who is not ambulating or not moving the legs while in bed. The major concern is that spontaneous clots might form in the deep veins (thrombosis), become inflamed (thrombophlebitis), and break loose and travel to the lungs (pulmonary embolus). This may be prevented by regular leg exercises.

Another approach to prevention of thrombus formation is the prescription of anticoagulant drugs. These drugs decrease the ability of the body to respond rapidly with clot formation. It is possible to provide a low dosage of these drugs that does not place the patient at risk for bleeding but does decrease the potential for spontaneous formation of clots in veins. If such drugs are prescribed, you will be responsible for a thorough understanding of the individual drug and its potential hazards.

High Blood Pressure

High blood pressure has been linked with an increase in such life-threatening disorders as stroke and heart attack. A major thrust of disease prevention has been the early identification of high blood pressure and the institution of treatment to manage this condition. The nurse is often involved in screening programs to detect asymptomatic high blood pressure. When blood pressure is found to be elevated, the person is then referred to a primary health care provider for further evaluation and treatment.

When the person being treated for high blood pressure enters the hospital, the nurse may be the one to identify that this underlying problem exists. Often this occurs because the nurse recognizes that routine medications taken at home are for the treatment of high blood pressure. This reinforces the importance of carefully checking the purpose of each medication the patient takes.

The use of intravenous fluids, pain medications, and a wide variety of other treatments may affect blood pressure management. The nurse will work collaboratively with the physician to determine when medications should be given and how the problem should be managed while treatment for another problem is being given.

Assessment

Assessment of circulatory status is an essential aspect of basic assessment. To assess circulatory status correctly, you must master a considerable body of knowledge as well as skills. Specific directions for performing these skills are found in the specific modules listed at the end of this chapter.

Interview

Basic interviewing will help you determine whether or not an individual has cardiovascular risk factors. Also you will need to identify whether symptoms of current problems are present.

Cardiovascular Risk Factors

Identifying specific cardiovascular risk factors in an individual's life will help you plan for health teaching. This includes the person's current dietary pattern and whether it conforms to the prudent diet pattern recommended, smoking habits, exercise pattern, and ways of managing stress.

Although not all of these items may be pertinent to an initial interview, their importance remains. Often people will assume that their current lifestyle patterns are not a health problem if no health professional has ever taken the time to discuss them. Sometimes this discussion is more pertinent to discharge planning from a hospital and may be especially appropriate in the home care setting.

Response to Activity

Activity tolerance refers to the ability to engage in activity without experiencing discomfort and shortness of breath. The amount of activity that can be tolerated without adverse changes in pulse, blood pressure, or feelings of well-being is significant. Cardiac difficulties are a major cause of *activity intolerance* in the ill person; the heart is unable to circulate blood adequately to meet cell needs.

Fatigue level is assessed by comparing the degree of fatigue experienced with that expected in response to a given activity. In other words, after strenuous activity fatigue is expected; fatigue induced by ordinary activities of daily living (ADLs) may indicate cardiac problems. Because fatigue may also result from respiratory difficulties, it is only a general indicator of potential problems.

Chest Discomfort

Any history of discomfort in the chest that may also radiate to the jaw or left arm is an indicator of potential cardiovascular disease and should be brought to the physician's attention. Whenever discomfort is reported, you will need to obtain a thorough description that includes the circumstances under which it occurred, where it was felt, the severity, the progression (did it get worse, stay the same, or get better gradually), what relieved it, what made it worse, and whether it was treated medically at the time. This provides you with a broad picture of the problem and will be of value to decision-making by the physician.

Peripheral Vascular Concerns

The patient may also have concerns in regard to circulation in the extremities, reporting distended veins,

Nursing Issues and Trends: *Reducing Cardiac Risk In Children*

Most people think middle-aged adults should take action to reduce cardiac risk factors, but few think about reducing these same risk factors in children. However, lifetime habits of diet and exercise begin in childhood. Children need active exercise to help them grow and develop, but this same exercise also helps them maintain appropriate weight and cardiovascular conditioning. A diet low in both saturated fat and total fat will help to prevent atherosclerosis which can begin very early in life. A healthy life style can be for all of life. Could it be that a larger portion of our educational efforts in regard to preventing heart disease need to be directed at families with young children?

a history of thrombophlebitis, or a pattern of swelling and aching at the end of the day. Some individuals may report that activity creates pain in the extremities. These all indicate that poor circulation may be present.

Physical Examination

The physical examination related to circulation includes measuring the pulse and blood pressure. It will include an examination of the skin and mucous membranes, the extremities, and indicators of peripheral circulation.

Pulse

The **pulse** is a shock wave produced within the artery as the heart beats. It can be felt as an increase in the size of the artery each time the heart contracts. Counting the pulse rate (beats/min) is an indirect means of counting the heart rate. Although present in every artery, the pulse is counted at points where a large artery passes close to the surface near a bone and can be easily palpated.

Counting the pulse. For reasons of convenience and accessibility, the pulse is most commonly counted at the radial artery in the wrist. The pulse may be counted at other points for specific reasons. If the wrist is inaccessible because of a cast or intravenous line, another site would be used. If the radial pulse is weak and hard to find, as in a critically ill person or a small infant, a stronger pulse such as the carotid or the apical pulse might be used. To assess arterial circulation to a specific part of the body, you use the pulse point just proximal to that part. A Doppler ultrasound stethoscope, which is an instrument that uses sound waves to detect blood moving in the artery, may be used to check for very faint pulses or those not palpable.

It has been variously recommended that pulses be counted for 15, 30, and 60 seconds. At least one study (Jones, 1967) found that the shortest duration is the most accurate for regular pulses, probably because it allows for fewer counting errors. Irregular pulses may need to be counted for 60 seconds to compensate for irregularities over time. Apical pulses (direct heart rate) are also usually counted for a full minute. Because all manually counted pulses deviate somewhat from direct readings taken by an electrocardiogram (ECG), the pulse rate should be considered approximate. If gross abnormalities are found, the pulse should be rechecked. An effort should be made to use a consistent technique so that trends and changes may be noted. It is advisable to check the policy of a facility when you begin working there so that your technique will be consistent with that of others who are checking a patient's pulse rate. One source of counting error can be avoided by beginning the count at 0 instead of 1 so that you are counting the beats that actually occur within a given period. For a patient whose condition is such that even small changes in rate and rhythm are serious, an electronic monitoring system is used.

Electronic pulse counters are now in limited use. Some function by sensing pulse in the ear lobe, others by sensing the pulse in the tip of a finger. The accuracy of these devices makes it possible to identify even slight changes in pulse rate and to keep a record of patterns in the pulse rate. Cardiac monitors, which maintain a continuous surveillance of the heart's action, also monitor heart rate (see Module 16, Temperature, Pulse, and Respiration, for complete directions on counting the pulse.)

Apical pulse. Heart rate may also be counted directly over the apex of the heart by using a stethoscope. The heart rate counted in this way is called the **apical pulse**. The apex of the heart is usually located on the left side of the chest at the fifth interspace between the ribs, directly below the arch of the clavicle. This is called the **point of maximal impulse (PMI)**.

In the elderly person with an enlarged heart, the apex may be farther to the left and lower. In the infant or young child, it is usually located closer to the midline and higher. You may need to listen at a number of spots throughout the general area to identify the site where the beat is heard most clearly. In children and those who are thin the PMI can be palpated through the chest wall.

If the pulse is regular, counting for 15 seconds will provide an accurate rate. However, the apical pulse must be counted for a full minute before the administration of drugs, such as digitalis products, that are given to treat abnormal rhythms and those that may create abnormal rhythms as a side effect. Such a drug may be held and the physician consulted if the rate is too slow or too fast or new dysrhythmias have developed.

Pulse deficit. On occasion, some heartbeats are so weak that the waves they produce in the artery cannot be felt in the periphery. In such a case, the heart rate counted at the apex will be greater than the peripheral pulse. The difference between the apical and radial pulse rates, measured simultaneously, is called the **pulse deficit**. The pulse deficit represents the number of weak, ineffective beats per minute.

Pulse rates. Pulse rates vary greatly and are affected by such factors as activity, eating, emotional tension, drugs, and illness. Mild to moderate activity usually raises the rate 20 to 30 beats/min. In the healthy individual, the rate will return to normal within 2 minutes after such activity is discontinued. Age is also an important determinant of pulse rate: pulse rate is very rapid in the infant—120 to 140 beats/min—and decreases throughout life to approximately 80 beats/min in the adolescent and adult (Table 29-5).

Consistent strenuous exercise will cause the heart to enlarge and to beat more slowly and forcefully. Thus, a normal resting pulse rate for an athlete may be 50 to 60

Table 29–5. Resting Heart Rates

Age	Average	Lower Limits of Normal	Upper Limits of Normal
Newborn	120	70	160
1–12 mo	110	80	140
1–5 y	95	80	110
5–10 y	85	70	100
10–15 y	75	55	90

Modified from Kelminson, L. and Nora, J. Heart and great vessels. In *Current Pediatric Diagnosis and Treatment,* 2nd edition,: edited by C. H. Kempe, Los Altos, Calif.: Lange Medical Publishers, 1972, p. 277.

beats/min. An adult pulse rate below 60 beats/min is referred to as **bradycardia**, and a pulse rate that is above 100 is called **tachycardia**. Because these are relative terms, the heart rate itself is a more accurate way of characterizing heart function.

Pulse rhythm. It is also important to observe the **pulse rhythm**. A normal pulse has a regular beat. When the beat is irregular, the specific type of irregularity should be noted because it may be of diagnostic significance. For example, double beats (bigeminy) may occur, either occasionally or at frequent regular intervals. The rate may vary from rapid to slow and back, or beats maybe skipped. Any such pattern needs to be recorded.

Pulse strength. Pulse strength may be weak, thready, or strong; a pulse may also be said to be bounding. The strength of the pulse reflects the strength of the heart contraction. When no cardiac pathology exists, strength may not be recorded on the patient record; when there is cardiac pathology or an abnormality, pulse strength should be included in the chart.

Heart Sounds

The sounds heard when listening to the heart are termed the *heart sounds*. The normal sounds are those created by closure of the valves. These are usually described as the "lub-dup" heart sounds and are officially termed S_1 and S_2. S_1 occurs when the atrioventricular (AV) valves close. S_2 occurs when the semilunar valves leading from the ventricles into the great arteries close. The sounds are actually caused by the vibration of the taut valves along with the adjacent blood, walls of the heart, and the major vessels around the heart.

When other sounds are heard, they represent other cardiac events. Extra heart sounds, clicks, and murmurs (whooshing sounds) may all be heard and may represent pathology. At a beginning level, you will be asked to identify S_1 and S_2 and describe any other sounds you hear. Note at what point in the cycle the abnormal or extra sounds are heard (before the S_1, between the S_1 and S_2, after the S_2). The differentiation of heart sounds is beyond the scope of this text.

Blood Pressure

The pressure of the circulating blood is a significant indication of the effectiveness of heart action and of the adequacy of the blood supply to the tissue. The term **blood pressure** usually refers to arterial pressure measured in millimeters of mercury. However, the pressure in the largest veins—central venous pressure (CVP)—and pressure in the pulmonary artery are also important indicators of circulatory efficiency.

Measuring blood pressure. An indirect measure of blood pressure taken with a sphygmomanometer (blood pressure cuff) and a stethoscope is commonly performed over the brachial artery at the elbow. It is also possible (although not commonly done) to measure blood pressure over the popliteal artery behind the knee, using a large cuff on the thigh. The principle underlying indirect measurement is as follows. Blood flowing through healthy arteries does not make sounds audible through a stethoscope. But when the flow of blood in the artery is occluded by external pressure and the pressure is then reduced until the heart is again able to pump blood through the artery past the point of occlusion, a sharp sound called **Korotkoff's sound** is produced with each contraction. The pressure at which the blood is first able to push past the point of occlusion and make a sound is equal to the **systolic pressure**, or the maximum pressure exerted by the heart during a contraction.

True **diastolic pressure** is the lowest pressure maintained in the artery between heart contractions. The proper means of indirect measurement of this pressure has been the subject of some difference of opinion. As the pressure applied by the blood pressure cuff continues to decrease after the first sounds are heard, a change or "muffling" of the sounds occurs. This is referred to as the first diastolic sound. Then, as the pressure decreases more, the sound disappears entirely. This is referred to as the second diastolic sound. Direct measures of blood pressure reveal that neither of these points, the muffling or the cessation of sound, is consistent with true diastolic pressure. In healthy arteries, the true diastolic pressure is usually 10 mm below the muffling and coincides with the cessation of sound. At present, AHA (1987) recommends that a blood pressure reading consist of two figures in most instances: 1) the first sounds heard; and 2) the muffling of sound (first diastolic) for children, or the cessation of sound (second diastolic) for adults. However, in arteries diseased through atherosclerosis, the sound may continue to be heard far below the true diastolic because of turbulence in the vessel. If sounds are heard until the pressure in the cuff falls to near 0 mm Hg, then the muffling sound should be recorded as the second sound and the 0 recorded as a third sound. Some facilities routinely record all three sounds for all patients. If the muffling is not heard, then a dash is drawn at the second number (Fig. 29-3). Module 17, Blood Pressure, presents specific directions for measuring blood pressure.

Blood pressure measurements are sometimes made by people with minimal training, and there are many possibilities for error in selection of cuff size, hearing, and reading of the instrument. When a gross abnormality is reported, it is wise for the nurse to recheck the measurement.

Various new electronic machines for the indirect measurement of blood pressure are being used in some settings. A blood pressure cuff is placed on the patient's arm. The machine is then set to take the blood pressure at precise intervals. Alarms can be set to notify the nurse if the blood pressure is over or under a predetermined figure. Many of these machines maintain a record of blood pressures taken so they can be reviewed and entered on the patient's chart if appropriate.

Direct measurement of arterial blood pressure is ordinarily performed in special care units or the operating room. A special catheter must be inserted into an artery, and equipment that permits direct readings of blood pressure is then attached.

Blood pressure levels. Blood pressure is lowest in the newborn—approximately 40/20—and gradually increases to the adult level—approximately 120/80—during adolescence (Table 29-6). Statistically, blood pressure rises as the individual grows older. However, recent evidence suggests that this phenomenon may be due not to aging but to decreasing physical activity. Those who maintain regular physical activity and do not gain excessive weight are less apt to experience increases in blood pressure with aging. As is true of all other body measures, there are wide individual variations in blood pressure. The usual range for adults is 110–140/60–90. Pressures above 150 systolic and/or 90 diastolic are labeled *hypertensive*. A systolic pressure below 100 is labeled *hypotensive*. Such judgments must not be made, however, without gathering baseline data on the individual to determine whether the blood pressure reading represents the person's usual blood pressure or is an isolated instance.

Factors affecting blood pressure. Many factors affect blood pressure. Activity, drugs, anxiety, anger, joy,

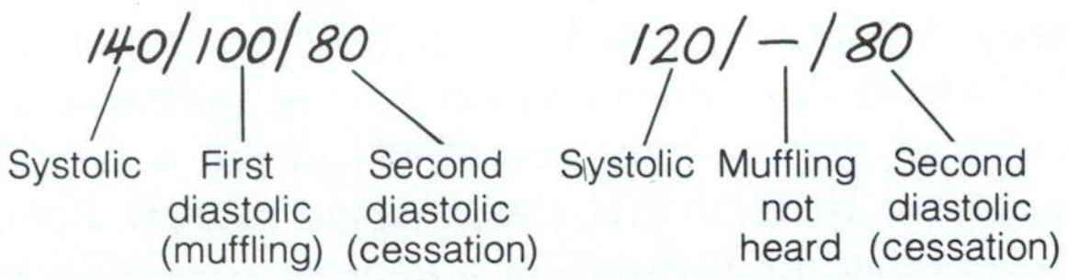

Figure 29-3. Recording blood pressure readings.

Table 29-6. 50th Percentile Values for Blood Pressure

Age	Systolic Pressure	Diastolic Pressure
0–6 mo	80	45
3 y	95	64
5 y	97	65
10 y	110	70
15 y	116	70

Adapted from Mitchell, S. and others. "The Pediatrician and Hypertension." (Commentary) *Pediatrics 56* (July 1975):3.

or any strong emotion can cause a sharp rise in blood pressure. Anything that dilates blood vessels or causes blood loss will result in a fall in blood pressure. The pattern of rising or falling blood pressure is important to the diagnosis of many pathologic conditions.

If the circulatory system is functioning correctly, there will be relatively little difference in blood pressure when body position changes. However, illness and certain medications render the system unable to make the rapid changes required to maintain consistent blood pressure in the face of position change. In these instances, the blood pressure will be lower sitting than lying, and still lower standing. This condition is called **postural hypotension**. When postural hypotension is suspected because of the patient's problems or when it might occur as a side effect of medications, postural blood pressures are often ordered. These are described below.

Frequency of blood pressure measurement. When changes are noted in blood pressure, when medications are given that alter blood pressure, and after some procedures and surgery, measurements may be taken at frequent intervals, for some patients as often as every 5 minutes. Every 4-hour blood pressure measurement is not uncommon for the extremely ill person. For other patients, such as those in rehabilitation, blood pressure may not be measured after an admission screening. The physician may make a decision on the frequency of blood pressure checks, but it is the nurse's responsibility to recognize any situation that demands closer monitoring and to act independently as necessary (Fig. 29-4).

Postural blood pressures. Postural blood pressure measurement is checking the blood pressure while the person is in different positions. The usual sequence is lying, sitting, and standing. The purpose of this is to determine whether the circulatory system is adapting adequately to changes in position.

The blood pressure cuff is left in place while the person changes position. Approximately 3 minutes elapses between measurements to allow the blood pres-

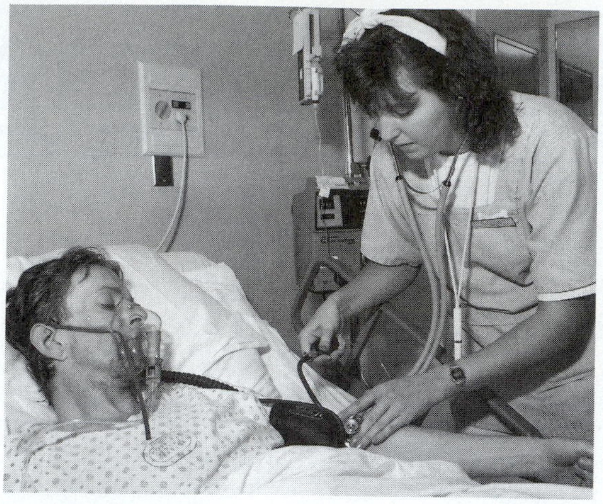

Figure 29-4. Taking the blood pressure is an important component of circulatory assessment.

sure to adjust. A difference of 15 mm Hg in the systolic blood pressure and a slight drop or rise of 10 mm Hg in the diastolic blood pressure is considered within the normal range. Of particular concern is a greater than normal drop in blood pressure. This indicates that the circulatory system is not adjusting adequately, and the person is in danger of dizziness and falls because of decreased cerebral tissue perfusion.

The pulse is also taken when postural blood pressures are measured. The pulse rate normally rises approximately 5 to 15 beats when the individual moves from lying to sitting to standing. This is part of the process of adaptation. If the pulse rate fails to increase, this lack also indicates a problem in the responsiveness of the circulatory system.

Pulse pressure. Another important diagnostic indicator is the difference between the systolic and the diastolic readings, which is called the **pulse pressure**. An increasing pulse pressure may indicate a serious problem, such as an increase in intracranial pressure (pressure on the brain). Average pulse pressure is 40 mm Hg. A pulse pressure of greater than 60 mm Hg is considered elevated.

Central venous pressure. Central venous pressure (CVP) is the pressure present in the superior and inferior vena cavae just outside of the heart. It can be measured by a catheter inserted into a large peripheral vein and threaded into a large central vein. This catheter is kept open by an intravenous drip or by heparinization. Direct measurement of the pressure may be taken with a special manometer. Normal CVP is 5 to 10 cm water. Low values indicate a low blood volume; a high value indicates that the circulating volume is increased and the heart is overloaded with fluid to pump. Measuring CVP is an advanced technique. More detailed information on the procedure is available in several of the references listed at the end of this chapter.

Central venous pressure may be estimated by examining the internal jugular veins in the neck. These veins are normally filled when the person lies flat; they empty as the head is raised. They are expected to be empty by the time the head is at a 30° elevation. If the internal jugular veins are not empty, the pulsations in the vein can be observed. The vertical height of the pulsations above the sternal angle is measured in centimeters. A measurement of greater than 3 to 4 cm is considered elevated. Both the angle of the head of the bed (15–30°) and the number of centimeters above the sternal angle are recorded.

Skin Color and Temperature

The color and temperature of the skin are indicators of circulation. It is possible to identify both lack of circulation and lack of oxygenation in the circulating blood by observing skin color. With good circulation, the extremities are warm and the presence of bright red oxygenated blood in the capillaries lends color to the skin. White skin has a pink tone, and darker skin has a reddish or warm overtone. A variety of abnormalities may be seen.

Pallor. *Pallor* is paleness of the skin caused by a lack of blood supply to a given area. Pallor signifies that the area is receiving neither oxygenated nor unoxygenated blood. Pallor makes the skin of a white person look extremely white. The skin of a black- or brown-skinned person will lack healthy reddish overtones but will not have the bluish gray over tones characteristic of cyanosis. Again, the areas without pigment most clearly manifest a lack of circulation: the conjunctiva, mucous membranes, and nailbeds will lack their normal healthy pink color.

Cyanosis. Cyanosis is a bluish gray skin color caused by the presence of inadequately oxygenated blood. Easily identified in a person with white skin, it appears as a blue or gray overtone to darker skin. Where cyanosis is suspected, examination of the conjunctiva of the eyes, mucous membranes, and nailbeds will indicate the amount of cyanosis present; because these body parts have relatively little pigment, their color derives from the blood itself.

Fluid Retention

Inadequate cardiac function is a major cause of fluid retention, which most commonly takes the form of **edema**, fluid retained in the interstitial spaces between cells. Edema may be identified by the puffiness and swelling of tissues, most commonly in the dependent areas of the body, that is, the legs and sacrum. Edema so severe that the pressure of a finger leaves an indentation is called *pitting edema*. Degrees of edema may be further characterized as 1+ (slight), 2+ (moderate amount), 3+ (large amount), and 4+ (marked or severe). This is not a precise scale. Measuring the circumference of a swollen extremity gives a more exact observation from which to determine whether the edema is increasing or decreasing. To be sure that all subsequent measurements are taken at the same level, an indelible mark is made on the skin.

The liver may become swollen and distended from fluid retention. Instead of feeling firm and semisolid to palpation, a "boggy" liver is palpable below the margin of the ribs and feels spongy.

Fluid retention may also be identified by an increase in the size of the abdomen from fluid retained in the peritoneal cavity, a condition called **ascites**. Ascites may be accurately identified by measuring abdominal girth daily. Just as with the extremity, a mark is usually made on the abdomen to ensure that subsequent measurements are made at precisely the same location.

Sometimes fluid is retained in the lungs. This condition, called pulmonary edema, is characterized by difficulty in breathing, *orthopnea* (the need to sit up to breathe), and frothy white sputum. Pulmonary edema may be a serious threat to life and is treated by the physician.

Total fluid retention may be measured by weighing the person daily (Fig. 29-5). Weighing for this purpose must be done consistently. Usually the person is weighed before breakfast and after emptying the bladder. If possible, the same type of garment should be worn and the same scale used consistently. Each kilogram of body weight added or lost through fluid equals 1 liter of fluid (1 kg is approximately 2.2 lb).

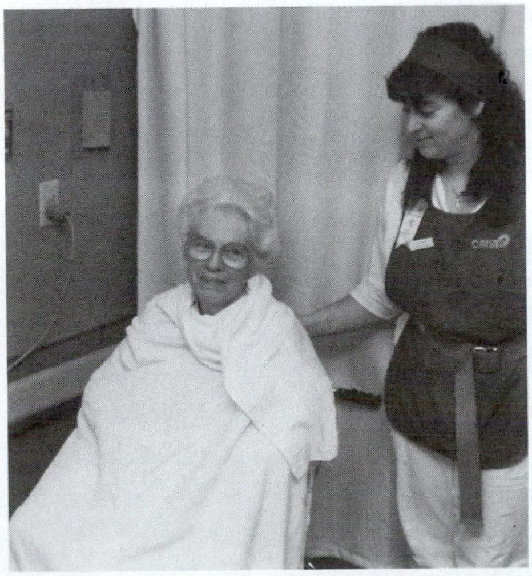

Figure 29-5. Fluid retention may be assessed by weighting the patient daily.

Measuring intake and output on a regular basis will allow you to determine when the total intake is greater than the total output, thus indicating that fluid may have been retained. This observation is subject to error through the failure to record some intake and output, estimates that must be made for incontinence, the difficulty in judging the precise volume of fluids in common beverage containers, and the differences in fluid losses other than urine. Fluid intake will also be greater than output when the patient started out with a deficit. In general, fluid balance must be evaluated over a period of not less than 24 hours and preferably over several days.

Peripheral Circulation

Both venous and arterial peripheral circulation are assessed. There are important differences in the information you will need to gather for each.

Peripheral arterial assessment. Check the peripheral pulses of the extremity. Comparing the peripheral pulses to the central pulses in terms of strength and rhythm will reveal how much circulation is reaching that particular extremity. When the peripheral pulse is extremely weak, a Doppler ultrasound stethoscope described previously may be needed to detect the pulse.

Compare the color and temperature of opposite extremities. Because color and temperature both reflect the blood flow, this will reveal differences in circulation. An extremity with inadequate arterial flow will usually be pale and cold.

Look at the skin condition. Skin with inadequate arterial circulation tends to be smooth, shiny, and hairless. There may also be evidence of unhealed abrasions because healing is slowed if circulation is deficient. The person may complain of itching; skin with poor circulation often itches.

Peripheral arterial insufficiency causes pain when activity begins to demand more oxygen for the muscles than the inadequate circulation can provide. With a chronic problem, pain may occur gradually. With acute arterial circulation blockage, pain is immediately very severe.

Peripheral venous assessment. When **peripheral venous insufficiency** occurs, the presence of unoxygenated blood tends to give the extremity a dark, mottled color. Swelling of the extremity results from the inability of the tissue to get rid of excess fluid. Veins may become distended and appear tortuous on the surface.

Inflammation of a deep vein is usually accompanied by pain, redness, and swelling over the area of inflammation. Deep vein inflammation that is not yet visible will often cause pain to occur in the calf when the foot is dorsiflexed, stretching the vein. This symptom is called a positive Homan's sign.

Laboratory and Diagnostic Tests

The laboratory and diagnostic tests commonly included for assessment of circulation include the complete blood count and the electrocardiogram.

Complete Blood Count

A **complete blood count** (**CBC**) is frequently done when a person is admitted to a hospital. It is also a component of many physical examinations. The CBC consists of a RBC count, a WBC count, and a measurement of hemoglobin and hematocrit. Table 29-1 lists norms for each.

Electrocardiogram

The ECG provides a recording of the electrical conduction pattern of the heart. At this level of education, you are not expected to interpret the study directly, but merely to read the interpretation made by the physician. This will show problems in rate and rhythm that will adversely affect cardiac output. When critical cardiac complications are a risk, a continuous monitoring system is attached to the patient to identify abnormalities immediately. The patient with continuous cardiac monitoring will usually be in a special care unit where the nurses have had education in understanding the monitor readings and in responding to emergencies.

Nursing Diagnosis

Nursing diagnoses that you might identify may be related to the effect of decreased cardiac performance on a variety of functional areas as well as cognitive and psychosocial responses to the circulatory problem.

Activity Intolerance

A nursing diagnosis of Activity Intolerance is most often related to a sedentary lifestyle. The person does not have a diagnosis of cardiovascular disease but becomes short of breath and tires rapidly when attempting vigorous activity. This person can be helped to plan a program of cardiovascular conditioning. If the person has poor cardiovascular conditioning related to disease, the physician should be consulted regarding any exercise plan.

Altered Peripheral Tissue Perfusion

Decreased peripheral tissue perfusion is a lack of arterial circulation and is identified by the pale appearance and coolness of the extremities and the absence or weakness of peripheral pulses. The nurse cannot change the arterial insufficiency, but should plan goals relative to safety. For this reason, some believe that the most useful nursing diagnosis is High Risk for Impaired Tissue Integrity related to decreased peripheral tissue perfusion. Inadequate arterial circulation is a special concern for people with the medical diagnosis of diabetes.

Nursing Diagnoses Related to Circulation

Activity Intolerance related to
- poor cardiovascular conditioning
- cardiovascular dysfunction

Altered Peripheral Tissue Perfusion related to
- immobilization
- pressure sites/constriction
- vascular disorders

Pain: Chest, related to lack of oxygen to myocardium

Decreased Cardiac Output related to cardiovascular dysfunction

High Risk for Altered Skin Integrity related to decreased peripheral tissue perfusion

Fluid Volume Excess related to decreased cardiac output

Anxiety related to lack of knowledge concerning circulatory disorder

Knowledge Deficit related to cardiovascular health

Decreased Cardiac Output

Decreased Cardiac Output has been identified as a nursing diagnosis by the North American Nursing Diagnosis Association (NANDA). However, at the beginning level, this is primarily a collaborative problem that will be identified by a physician and treated collaboratively. This diagnosis is related to various types of cardiovascular dysfunction. It may be present when there are abnor-

Potential Complications Related to Circulation

Potential complication: compartmental syndrome
Potential complication: deep vein thrombosis
Potential complication: decreased cardiac output
Potential complication: dysrhythmia
Potential complication: hypovolemic shock
Potential complication: pulmonary edema
Potential complication: pulmonary embolism

mal rhythms, when the heart muscle itself is failing, or when there is inadequate oxygen supply to the heart muscle. Characteristics that help to define this nursing diagnosis include low blood pressure, rapid pulse, shortness of breath, chest pain, cyanosis, fatigability, low urine output, dizziness when attempting activity, and fluid retention. Not all of these need be present. This diagnosis would not commonly be made by a student at a beginning level, but might be made by one who has studied theory relative to cardiac pathophysiology.

Knowledge Deficit

Many people lack basic knowledge on how to maintain health. Teaching about health maintenance is an important nursing responsibility. You will already have assessed the individual's knowledge level to arrive at this nursing diagnosis, so your teaching plan can be individualized.

Other Nursing Diagnoses

Patients with circulatory problems may also have a wide variety of other nursing diagnoses. Anxiety is not uncommon because circulatory problems are seen as serious. Information on identifying and managing anxiety is presented in Chapter 34. A diagnosis of Fluid Volume Excess may be made if the heart is unable to pump effectively (see Chapter 30). Ineffective Management of the Therapeutic Regimen might be present in the individual with chronic cardiac disease who does not manage prescriptions for self care effectively.

Planning and Implementation

Outcome criteria must be developed for the individual with specific problems related to circulation. The desired outcome need not indicate an expectation that the problem will no longer exist. Rather, outcomes should be written to emphasize current comfort and activity tolerance. The absence of complications should also be mentioned in the outcome criteria. For even the severely compromised patient, nursing actions can make a significant difference in overall feelings of well-being. Often improvement will be gradual; therefore, short-term as well as long-term outcome criteria need to be identified.

Understanding underlying disease pathophysiology will assist you in identifying appropriate desired outcomes for the person with circulatory problems. If the person has long-standing compromised arterial circulation in the lower extremities, your outcomes will focus on preventing discomfort and complications of the impaired circulation. If, however, this is a new or temporary problem in the lower extremities, outcomes might reasonably be improvements in circulation.

As you develop a nursing care plan for any of the preceding nursing diagnoses, you will need to provide specific details for actions (see sample Nursing Care Plan Related to Cardiac Dysfunction). Statements such as "good foot care" and "reduce activity" do not help others to structure their care for the patient's optimum benefit. A plan for foot care should carefully spell out each step. This approach can then be taught to the patient consistently as well as be carried out consistently in the hospital setting. Describing the precise way in which activity is to be curtailed and what activity is to be encouraged is essential. The plan for activity may need to be changed frequently as the person improves.

Health Teaching

For the person in good health, the nurse may teach about cardiovascular health and assist the person to set up a regular exercise program. The nurse may also serve as a resource, recommending programs in the community that might help the individual. To do this, you have to acquaint yourself with community resources. Common resources include the YMCA, YWCA, YMHA, park department recreation programs, and community college community service programs. Your local AHA office may be able to recommend resources. Many commercial exercise programs are available also.

All programs should be carefully screened before you recommend them. Questions you might wish to ask include:

1. What are the qualifications of the instructors?
2. How does the program consider individual differences and needs?
3. Are the participants taught to monitor their own progress?
4. Does the program fit AHA recommendations in regard to type of activity, frequency, duration, and intensity?
5. Do the instructors have a plan for emergency care of an individual who has an untoward response to activity?
6. What is the cost of the program?

For the person with a cardiovascular disorder, health teaching will focus on understanding of the disorder and managing self-care in a way that maximizes ability to function and minimizes symptoms. The patient may need instruction on special diet, an exercise plan prescribed by the physician, or medications. For some of these patients, the treatment plan will require lifestyle modification and may mean continued use of medications to support cardiac function. Special attention to helping the individual accept the need for these changes

Nursing Care Plan

Sample Nursing Care Plan Related to Cardiac Dysfunction

Nursing Diagnosis

Activity intolerance related to imbalance between oxygen supply and demand.

Supportive data:

Shortness of breath upon exertion

Verbal reports of fatigue and weakness

Murmur heard over aortic valve area

Abnormal heart rate in response to activity

Cardiac dysrhythmias

Desired Patient Outcomes

Short term:

Patient can manage self-care activities without experiencing symptoms

Long term:

Patient can manage activities of daily living without experiencing symptoms

Heart rate between 60 and 85

Nursing Action	Rationale
1. Keep head of bed elevated	Raised upper body allows full lung expansion and facilitates gas exchange
2. Schedule daily care activities to allow time for rest periods	Rest periods allow patient to conserve energy for activities of daily living
3. Promote a calm environment to decrease anxiety	Anxiety puts stress on the heart and diverts energy from productive activities
4. Gradually increase activity within the limits prescribed by the physician	Small increments in activity allow the nurse to monitor the patient's response
5. Take vital signs q.i.d.	Monitoring vital signs provides feedback about the patient's level of tolerance for activity
6. Encourage patient to use PRN oxygen at all times	↑ Oxygen in inspired air ↑ Potential gas exchange and blood oxygen content, resulting in less shortness of breath

and incorporate them into an acceptable lifestyle will help to support effective compliance.

Balancing Activity and Rest

To balance activity and rest, all ADLs are examined, and alterations are made in areas where changes are most acceptable to the patient. For example, in nutrition, large meals with lots of chewing and many fats require more energy for processing. Frequent smaller meals that are low in fat and soft in texture require less energy. Struggling on and off a bedpan generally takes more energy than using the bedside commode, so the commode would be chosen for assisting with bowel function.

Self-care activities would be examined, and some performed by the nurse. The person might feel more comfortable and less anxious if allowed to wash his or her own perineal area, but be too exhausted by the effort to bathe the entire torso, much less the legs. The list of progressively increasing activity levels in Table 29-7 can be used in determining the appropriate overall level of activity.

Rest may be interspersed with activities so that the

Nursing Research: Implications for Practice

Kison, C. "Health Beliefs and Compliance of Cardiac Patients." *Applied Nursing Research* 5 (4): 181–185, November, 1992.

Health beliefs and compliance with treatment recommendations were studied in thirty-one people who had sustained a major cardiac event (heart attack, heart surgery, or other serious cardiac problem). These individuals had high compliance with taking their medications and having their checkups. Those who were still smoking reported more barriers to and fewer benefits from checkups. Those who believed that checkups were beneficial were more likely to comply with dietary instructions. The college-educated subjects reported more benefits to checkups and were more likely to comply with exercise. This study supported the theory that health beliefs are an important factor in compliance. Nurses should assess for health beliefs as they work to help individuals maintain or improve their health.

person does not become overly tired. An amount of activity that is overwhelming if done in a block of time may be manageable if completed in small increments throughout the day. The person who is being discharged may be helped to plan for activity and rest balance at home, spreading ADLs out and managing self-care effectively.

The position used when resting may be important both for comfort and for effective cardiac function. A sitting position, well supported, demands the least work from the heart. Even a slight elevation of the head of the bed may allow a person with cardiac problems to rest more comfortably. Lying flat often creates shortness of breath and discomfort.

Maintaining Fluid Balance

Because excess fluids in the body may overload the heart and because a heart that is not functioning may cause fluid to be retained, attention to fluid balance is often essential. Ongoing monitoring of intake and output, daily weights, and evidence of edema will be im-

Table 29–7. Cardiac Activity Levels

Level		
1	Complete bed rest Bedside commode	May turn self, watch TV, wash own face and hands, brush own teeth. Will be given complete bed bath and will be shaved.
2	Dangle on side of bed with feet supported Assisted pivot transfer to chair bid to tid as tolerated	As above plus self-grooming, shaving, combing own hair
3	Unassisted transfer to chair tid to qid as tolerated. BRP for BM only. Walk in room 1–2 min bid as tolerated	As above plus bathing self except for back and feet
4	Full bathroom privilege. Up in chair as tolerated. Walk in room as desired	As above plus standing at sink to groom or shave Sitting to dress self
5	Walk in hall 2 min each time up	Sitting shower with assistance for back and feet
6	Walk in hall 5 min each time up	Full standing shower
7	Walk in hall as desired. If stairs at home, walk up and down one flight of stairs slowly once a day.	Full standing shower

Courtesy Swedish Medical Center, Seattle, Washington.

portant. Sodium causes fluid to be retained within the body. Therefore, sodium intake may be limited to prevent fluid retention. See Chapter 30 for more information on prevention and treatment of fluid volume excess.

Promoting Venous Return

To promote venous return, you can institute a program of active exercising of the legs. Active range-of-motion exercises in which venous flow is increased by the position of the legs relative to gravity as well as by the action of the muscles are the most successful in promoting venous return. When active range of motion is contraindicated, isometric exercises of the legs are used to promote venous return. The quadriceps muscles are tightened, held for a count of four, and then relaxed. The gluteal and posterior thigh muscles are tightened and relaxed in the same manner. The calves are then exercised through calf-pumping, in which the toe is alternatively dorsiflexed and plantar-flexed (see Module 24, Range-of-Motion Exercises). Passive range-of-motion exercises may also be used. They are less effective than active exercise because there is no pumping action of muscles around the veins. However, gravity does have some effect in increasing venous return.

The physician may prescribe elastic stockings that support veins and decrease stasis. Another device that may be used when a patient is at high risk for venous stasis and thrombosis is a set of inflatable stockings that use alternating pressure to increase venous return. These devices require careful attention to skin care of the legs. You will also need to ensure that improper placement has not caused them to cut off venous return rather that support venous return (see Module 26, Applying Bandages and Binders).

Preventing Peripheral Tissue Injury

Your intervention for any person with compromised peripheral circulation will be directed at preventing injuries to the extremities and teaching the person how to safeguard against injuries and tissue breakdown. The patient should wear shoes at all times to protect against bruising and cuts. Clean stockings, preferably cotton, should be worn daily to decrease the chance of developing a fungal infection (athlete's foot) or of creating blisters on the feet. Careful attention should be paid to the fit of shoes to prevent blisters and corns. Each day the person should carefully wash and dry the feet and inspect them for injuries. This helps to keep tissue healthy and ensures that care can be sought immediately for any problem. The importance of seeking medical care for even minor injuries is a crucial point to teach. With inadequate arterial circulation, healing tends to be delayed, and medical help may prevent more serious problems from developing. Toenails should be trimmed straight across to prevent ingrown nails at the corners. Nails should not be trimmed so short that there is danger of injuring the tissue under the nail. A podiatrist, a specialist in foot care, may be consulted for care of problems with nails and corns.

Another aspect of intervention is helping the person to manage an activity pattern. This person may experience excessive muscle fatigue and even pain when activity outstrips the ability of the circulatory system to provide oxygen. If activity is divided into small increments with rest periods interspersed, the person may be able to do more without distress because the tissue has time to recover before additional demands are placed on it.

Encouraging Cardiac Rehabilitation

An individual who has a major cardiac disorder may be a candidate for a comprehensive cardiac rehabilitation program. These programs involve an interdisciplinary team usually consisting of a nurse, a physical therapist, and a physician. Others, such as the nutritionist, may also provide assistance to this core team. The focus is on helping the individual to engage in a conditioning program that will result in a better quality of life and a decrease in adverse symptoms. Exercise is carefully planned to provide a gradually increasing load that promotes conditioning without danger to the heart. Education is a central aspect of the program to enable the patient to manage his or her own health maintenance activities.

Evaluation

Evaluation of circulatory status requires that you gather data as a baseline and then continue to gather data as you implement your planned actions. Evaluation must be concurrent, that is, taking place as you work with the patient. At any time it may be necessary to discontinue the planned actions because of the patient's untoward response. Along with desired outcomes, you must carry in your mind indicators that would help you to recognize adverse responses and an alternative plan for coping with complications.

As you identify the patient's responses, you will compare them with the desired outcomes that were initially determined. Identifying whether the patient is beginning to make progress will be as important as identifying the ultimate achievement of desired outcomes. You will also review the actions you have taken to determine whether your plan needs revision or whether it should continue as initiated.

Basic Life Support

The National Conference on Standards for Cardiopulmonary Resuscitation (CPR) and Emergency Cardiac Care has recommended that all medical and allied health personnel be trained in techniques of basic life support. These techniques include 1) recognition of airway obstruction, 2) recognition of respiratory arrest and cardiac arrest, and 3) ability to perform *cardiopulmonary resuscitation* (*CPR*), which includes rescue breathing and *external cardiac massage.* Patients with underlying circulatory pathology are those who are most likely to need your prompt intervention with basic life support, but any individual may have a sudden adverse response that demands immediate attention.

It is necessary for *all* health care personnel to be so prepared because resuscitation cannot wait for the arrival of special personnel; resuscitation must begin as soon as the need is discovered. Many communities have established extensive programs to teach basic CPR skills to as many citizens as possible. Basic life support is not an exclusively medical skill (Fig. 29-6).

Once basic life support is instituted, a team trained to perform advanced cardiac life support (ACLS) is summoned to continue care. In the hospital this may be referred to as a "Code Team," because the need for the ACLS team was traditionally announced over the public address system through a code to avoid alarming the general public. In many facilities the ACLS team now carries individual pagers so a general announcement is not needed.

To standardize techniques of CPR, a national task force formulated "Standards for Cardiopulmonary Resuscitation (CPR) and Emergency Cardiac Care," which were published in a supplement to the *Journal of the American Medical Association.* These standards were revised in 1986 (Albarron-Sotelo, Flint, and Kelly) and further refined in 1990 (Sotelo, Flint, and Kelly). Although no training in CPR is adequate unless it provides both a theoretical understanding of the process and manikins on which to practice one's skills, we shall review some basic concepts here.

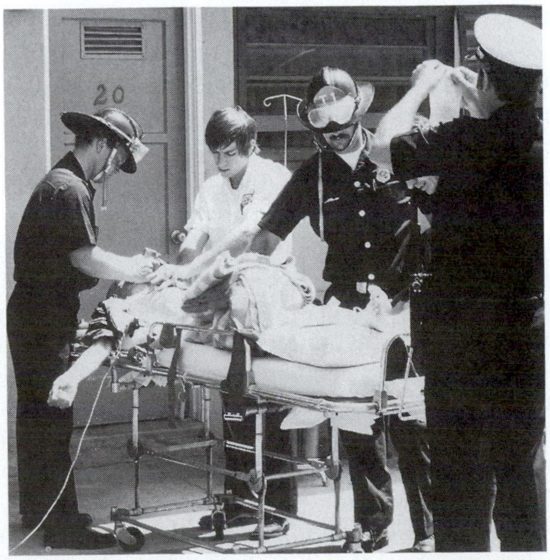

Figure 29-6. Emergency life support may be performed in many different settings.

Recognizing the Need for Life Support

Because all basic life support measures have the potential to injure the victim, a clear determination of need must be made before they are undertaken. The criterion for determining the need for respiratory support is absence of breathing. Absence of breathing is determined by observing for chest movement and feeling for air movement through the mouth and nose. Sometimes chest movement can be felt when it cannot be seen.

The criterion for determining the need for cardiac support is absence of heart action. Absence of heart action is determined by checking for pulse in the carotid arteries. Peripheral pulses are not checked because they may be too weak to be detected even though the heart is still beating. Checking for dilated pupils is not recommended as a means of checking for circulation to the brain. Fixed and dilated pupils may indicate anoxia of the brain but are not used as a criterion for the initiation of action.

Administering Emergency Life Support

The actions that constitute emergency life support are most easily remembered as the ABCs: 1) airway, 2) breathing, and 3) circulation.

The airway is checked and, if necessary, cleared, and positioned to maintain patency (open passage). Then rescue breathing (*mouth-to-mouth resuscitation*) is begun. After rescue breathing has been started, circulation is restored by means of external cardiac massage. This process is performed most efficiently by two people but may be accomplished by one.

Your nursing education program or the hospital where you have laboratory practice may train you in emergency life support. Alternatively, such training is available from some fire departments, the Red Cross, and local AHA chapters. It is your responsibility to acquire these emergency skills and review them as often as necessary to maintain your proficiency. The directions in Module 32, Emergency Resuscitation Procedures, conform to AHA recommendations.

Nursing Care Study
A Patient with Decreased Peripheral Tissue Perfusion in the Lower Extremities

Mrs. Rebecca Berkowitz was a 72-year-old widow admitted for newly diagnosed diabetes mellitus. Her diabetes was to be controlled by diet. As part of her admission examination, Susan Cartland, RN, did a complete cardiovascular assessment. She paid special attention to peripheral circulation because she knew that vascular insufficiency is a common concern for those with diabetes.

In her assessment she identified that the popliteal pulses were very weak. The pedal pulse on the right was faint but consistently palpable. The pedal pulse on the left was not always palpable and was faint when present. The skin over the lower legs appeared smooth and hairless. The skin color was pink, but the legs were cold to the touch. Mrs. Berkowitz stated that she usually had cold feet. However, she had never experienced pain in the lower extremities when walking. No abrasions were seen on the legs or feet. The toenails were in need of trimming.

Susan determined that Mrs. Berkowitz had decreased peripheral tissue perfusion related to arterial insufficiency secondary to diabetes mellitus. She reviewed her knowledge of ways of improving circulation and preventing complications. She decided that the desired outcome of care was that Mrs. Berkowitz understand her circulatory problem and care for her feet independently. The long-term desired outcome was that Mrs. Berkowitz not develop injuries or lesions on her legs and feet and that she be able to continue with her present level of activity. Specific outcome criteria were: Mrs. Berkowitz 1) will describe the symptoms and cause of arterial insufficiency, 2) will list those actions she can take to care for her feet, 3) will remain free of any complications of arterial insufficiency, and 4) will maintain self-care, personal home maintenance, and the ability to walk without developing leg pain.

Susan decided that the care plan needed to include patient teaching in regard to care of the feet and prevention of injury to the feet and legs. Mrs. Berkowitz would also need to be taught why care of her feet was important. As she sat down to write the nursing care plan, Susan began to review all of those specific actions she felt would be appropriate to institute for this patient.

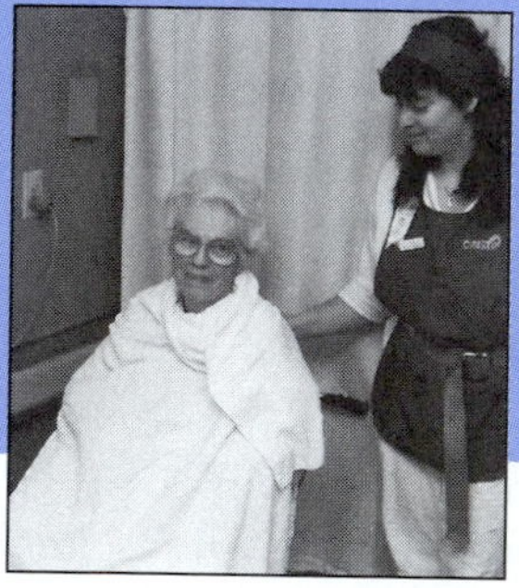

Key Points

- The circulatory system is composed of the heart, the blood vessels (arteries, veins, and capillaries), and the blood itself. The blood circulates in a consistent pattern as a result of the pumping action of the heart.
- The blood returns to the heart because of the contraction of muscles around the veins and the one-way valves within the veins.
- The blood is composed of red blood cells, white blood cells, and platelets. Blood typing is a method of determining certain characteristics of the red blood cells that are significant when transfusions are given.
- Cardiovascular health may be maintained by eating a prudent diet in which saturated fats, salt, and cholesterol are restricted; eliminating cigarette smoking; engaging in regular physical activity; and adequately managing stress. Physical activity should be monitored in relationship to frequency, duration, and intensity. Aerobic activities are effective in cardiovascular conditioning.
- Basic circulatory assessment includes checking the pulse for rate, rhythm, and strength; measuring the blood pressure; checking skin color and temperature; checking venous and arterial peripheral circulation; and looking for such problems as fluid retention, activity intolerance, and fatigue.
- Nursing diagnoses in the area of circulatory function include Knowledge Deficit related to cardiovascular health maintenance, Activity Intolerance related to poor cardiovascular conditioning, Decreased Peripheral Tissue Perfusion, Decreased Cardiac Out-

put, and Anxiety related to lack of knowledge concerning circulatory disorder. Each of these requires that you look carefully at the patient's current status and underlying health problems to determine realistic patient outcomes.

- Nursing interventions for problems related to circulation include health teaching, balancing activity and rest, maintaining fluid balance, promoting venous return, preventing peripheral tissue injury, encouraging cardiac rehabilitation, and administering basic life support.
- Basic life support is a skill appropriate for all members of the community. It provides the skills necessary to act decisively in a situation in which there is sudden loss of cardiac function or cessation of breathing. Basic life support is instituted and maintained until an advanced life support team arrives to take over care.
- Because the circulatory system is complex, circulatory assessment and intervention demand great depth of knowledge on the part of the nurse. The introductory material in this chapter should help you to organize your thinking and actions. Alertness is crucial so that you can identify impending problems before they become severe.

Study Questions

1. Explain the three principal recommendations of AHA in regard to altering lifestyle to improve cardiovascular health and discuss the barriers to effective lifestyle change in regard to these factors.
2. Which groups of people should consult a physician before beginning an exercise program? If asked, how would you provide this information to an individual who should not be exercising without seeing a physician?
3. What are AHA guidelines in regard to intensity, frequency, and duration of exercise for cardiovascular conditioning?
4. Under what circumstances should the apical pulse rather than a peripheral pulse be checked?
5. How does blood pressure change as one grows older?
6. Discuss three factors that may cause blood pressure to rise and the implications of these factors for health teaching.
7. How does skin color differ when venous circulation is impaired as opposed to when arterial circulation is impaired?
8. What is the focus of nursing action for the patient with a decreased cardiac output?
9. What three techniques are included in basic life support?

Critical Thinking Activities

1. Take your own pulse. Run in place or do some other physical activity for five minutes. Take your pulse again. Then take your pulse every thirty seconds and determine how quickly it returns to normal.
   a) Compare these data to what you know of norms. Then evaluate your own cardiovascular health considering the general risk factors and your pulse data.
   b) In your clinical group, discuss what occurred for each of you when you were doing the activity in #1. Together make a chart of your before and after pulse rates. Calculate a group average and discuss the factors within your clinical group that might affect the group average.
2. Participate in a blood pressure screening clinic sponsored by an organization such as the American Heart Association. While there keep records of the blood pressure, gender, and approximate age of each individual you screen. Calculate the incidence of high blood pressure and compare the incidence in your sample with the incidence given in a health care reference. If these differ, analyze your sample and suggest reasons they might differ from national statistics.
3. On a clinical unit, take and record the blood pressures of a group of patients. From the patients' records obtain the medical diagnosis and age for each of these patients. Using this information evaluate the significance of the blood pressures you have measured.

Relevant Sections in Modules for Basic Nursing Skills

Volume 1 Module

Inspection, Palpation, Auscultation, and Percussion 13
Intake and Output 15
Temperature, Pulse, and Respiration 16
Blood Pressure 17
Emergency Resuscitation Procedures 32

References and Readings

Albarron-Sotelo, R., Flint, L. S., and Kelly, K. J. (Eds.). *Instructor's Manual For Basic Life Support.* Dallas: American Heart Association, 1987.

American Heart Association. *Dietary Guidelines for Health American Adults.* Dallas: AHA, 1986.

———. *Exercise Standards: A Statement For Health Professionals.* Dallas: AHA, 1991.

———. *Heart and Stoke Facts.* Dallas: AHA, 1992.

———. *Public Policy on Smoking and Health: Toward a Smoke-Free Generation by the Year 2000.* Dallas: AHA, 1986.

———. *Rationale of the Diet-Heart Statement of the American Heart Association.* Dallas: AHA, 1982.

———. *Recommendations for Human Blood Pressure Determination by Sphygmomanometers.* 5th edition. Dallas: AHA, 1987.

———. *Risk Factors in Coronary Disease: A Statement for Physicians.* Dallas: AHA, 1980.

Beaumont, E. "Product Survey: Blood Pressure Equipment." *Nursing '75* 5 (January 1975): 56–62.

Cantwell, J. D. "Exercise and Coronary Heart Disease: Role in Primary Prevention." *Heart and Lung* 13 (January 1984): 6–13.

Doyle, J. E. "All Leg Ulcers Are Not Alike: Managing and Preventing Arterial and Venous Ulcers." *Nursing '83* 13 (January 1983): 58–63.

Ehrhardt, B. S., and Graham, M. "Pulse Oximetry: An Easy Way To Check Oxygen Saturation." *Nursing '90* 20, 3 (March 1990): 50–54.

Eorgan, P. A., and Greer, J. L. "Cough CPR: A Consideration for High-Risk Cardiac Patient Discharge Teaching." *Critical Care Nurse* 12, 6 (August 1992): 21–27.

Gehring, P. E. "Vascular Assessment." *RN* 55, 1 (January 1992): 40–45.

Hackett, C. "Limbering Up Your Neurovascular Assessment Technique." *Nursing '83* 13 (March 1983): 40–43.

Handerhan, B. "How to Measure Jugular Venous Distention." *Nursing '87* 17, 9 (September 1987): 48–49.

Hargest, T. S. "Start Your Count with Zero." *American Journal of Nursing* 74 (May 1974): 887–889.

Hill, M. N., and Grim, C. M. "How to Take a Precise BP." *American Journal of Nursing* 91, 2 (February 1991): 38–42.

Hudson, B. "Sharpen Your Vascular Assessment Skills with the Doppler Ultrasound Stethoscope." *Nursing '83* 13 (May 1983): 54–56.

Jones, M. *Accuracy of Pulse Rate Counted for 15, 30, and 60 Seconds.* Master's Thesis, University of Washington, 1967.

McAdams, R. C., and McClure, K. "Hypovolemia: How to Stop It." *RN* 49, 12 (December 1986): 38–42.

Pollack, M. L., and Wilmore, J. H. *Exercise in Health and Disease: Evaluation and Prescription for Prevention and Rehabilitation.* 2nd edition. Philadelphia: W. B. Saunders, 1990.

Saunders, P. "CPR in a Small Hospital." *American Journal of Nursing* 89, 6 (June 1989): 812–815.

Sonnesso, G. "Are You Ready To Use Pulse Oximetry?" *Nursing '91* 21, 8 (August 1991): 60–64.

Sotelo, R. A., Flint, L. S., and Kelly, K. J. *Health Care Providers Manual for Basic Life Support.* Dallas: American Heart Association, 1990.

Sparks, C. "Peripheral Pulses." *American Journal of Nursing* 75 (July 1975): 1132–1133.

"Standards and Guidelines for Cardiopulmonary Resuscitation (CPR) and Emergency Cardiac Care (ECC)." *Journal of the American Medical Association* 255 (June 1986): 2843–2984.

Stright, P. A., and Soukup, S. M. "How To Hear It Right: Evaluating and Choosing a Stethoscope." *American Journal of Nursing* 77 (September 1977): 1477–1479.

Fluid and Electrolyte Balance

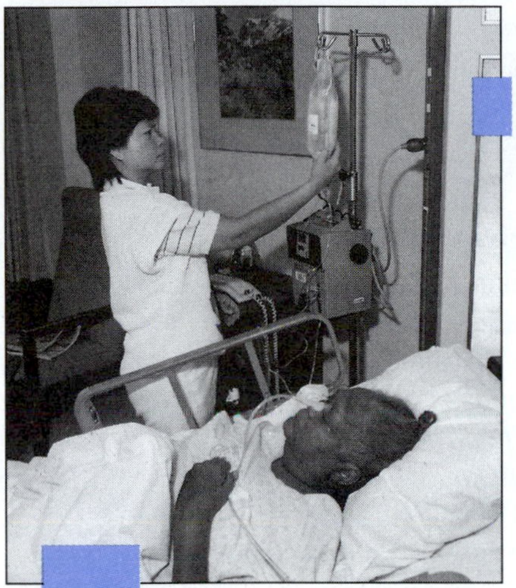

30

Objectives

After completing this chapter, you should be able to:

1. Define the three basic fluid compartments within the body.
2. Explain how fluid and electrolytes move between these fluid compartments.
3. Discuss the control mechanisms for fluid and electrolyte balance.
4. Define and describe the major types of fluid and electrolyte imbalances.
5. Explain acid–base balance and the principal factors responsible for its control.
6. Define and describe the four major acid–base imbalances.
7. List data necessary for basic assessment of fluid and electrolyte and acid–base balance.
8. Explain the major nursing diagnoses related to fluid and electrolyte balance.
9. Identify actions that the nurse can take to maintain fluid and electrolyte balance.
10. Outline the nurse's role in fluid therapy.
11. Explain the potential complications of blood and blood product administration.

Study Terms

acid–base balance
acidosis
alkalosis
balanced solution
colloidal osmotic pressure (COP)
combining power
Davenport nomogram
electrolytes
extracellular fluid
filtration pressure
fluid volume deficit
fluid volume excess
hemolytic reaction
hydrostatic pressure
hypercalcemia
hyperkalemia
hypernatremia
hypertonic fluid
hypocalcemia
hypokalemia
hyponatremia
hypotonic fluid
intracellular fluid
isotonic fluid
metabolic acidosis
metabolic alkalosis
milliosmole (mOsm)
osmolality
osmoles
replacement solution
respiratory acidosis
respiratory alkalosis
tonicity

Outline

Water is found in all body tissue. It is the major component of all cells as well as of body fluids. As you will note in Figure 30-1, water accounts for an even greater percentage of body weight in infants than in adults. For this reason, infants and children are more susceptible than adults to problems arising from water deficit.

Electrolytes are chemicals that, when dissolved in water, dissociate (divide) into charged particles called *ions.* The presence of electrolytes enables a solution to conduct electricity. Those ions carrying a positive charge are called *cations* and those carrying a negative charge are called *anions.* The number and types of electrolytes in all the body fluids are critical to the body's biochemical processes.

Body Fluid Compartments

The fluid compartment inside the cell is termed the intracellular fluid compartment. **Intracellular fluid** has the fairly precise composition necessary for the effective functioning of the cells (Fig. 30-2). The major cation of the intracellular fluid is potassium, and the major anion is phosphate.

The fluid compartment outside the cell is termed the extracellular fluid compartment. **Extracellular fluid** is further subdivided into the *plasma* (the circulating fluid) and the *interstitial fluid* (the fluid between the cells). The composition of the extracellular fluid is not as critical to the body as that of the intracellular fluid. It tends to fluctuate in response to food and fluid intake throughout the day. Norms are usually given for fasting levels. The body will also alter the extracellular composition to maintain the composition of the intracellular fluid.

Maintaining Fluid and Electrolyte Balance

Fluid and electrolyte balance is maintained by a complex set of mechanisms through which both fluids and electrolytes are moved back and forth between the var-

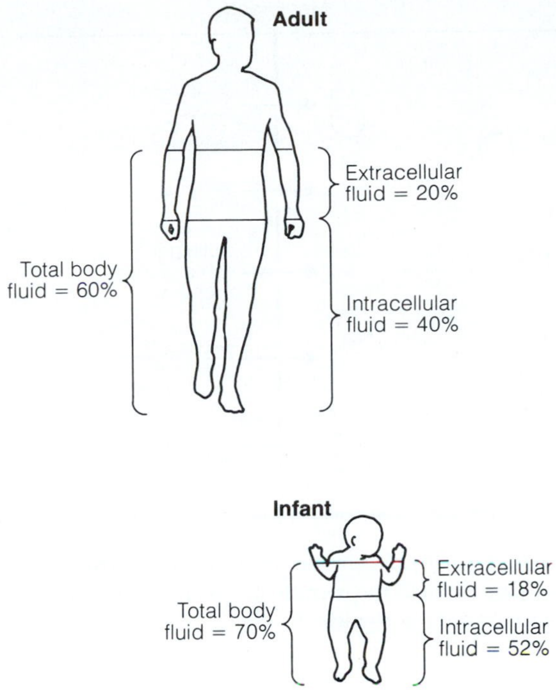

Figure 30-1. Body water compared to total weight.

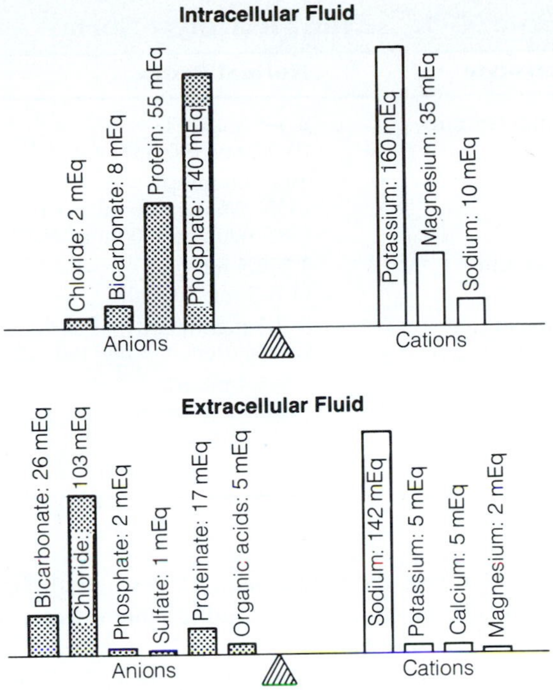

Figure 30-2. Chemical composition of the body.

ious fluid compartments. These mechanisms are controlled by hormones and blood pressure.

Movement of Electrolytes

Electrolytes move from one fluid compartment to another in two ways. The first process, *diffusion*, is movement of substances from areas of greater concentration to areas of lesser concentration (Fig. 30-3). This process tends to equalize concentration of the electrolytes in all fluid compartments.

Electrolytes are also moved across cell membranes by a process called *active transport*. Active transport is an energy-requiring process of living cell membranes capable of moving electrolytes in the direction needed for optimum cell function, regardless of the concentrations on either side. The active transport system of the cell membrane serves to maintain the difference in composition between the extracellular and intracellular fluids (Table 30-1).

Movement of Water

Two processes move water across membranes. The first is *filtration*: pressure in the arteries creates pressure in the arteriole end of the capillary, which in turn forces fluid through the capillary wall. This pressure is called **filtration pressure** (FP) or **hydrostatic pressure** (HSP).

The second process responsible for water movement is *osmosis*, a special type of diffusion involving water movement through a membrane rather than the movement of dissolved substances. For osmosis to occur, the fluid on one side of the membrane must contain more water and fewer particles than the fluid on the other side. Water then moves from the area where the fluid contains relatively more water and fewer particles

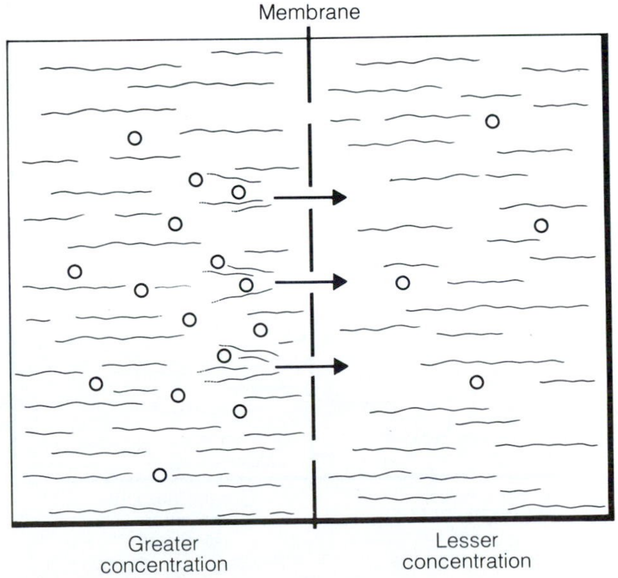

Figure 30-3. Diffusion of electrolytes. Dissolved substances move from an area of greater to an area of lesser concentration.

Table 30–1. Serum Electrolyte Norms

Electrolyte	Normal Range
Calcium (serum)	4.5–5.5 mEq/L (9–11 mg/100 ml)
Chloride	100–106 mEq/L (355–376 mg/100 ml as Cl) (585–620 mg/100 ml as NaCl)
Magnesium	1.5–2.5 mEq/L (1.8–3 mg/100 ml)
Phosphate (inorganic)	3–4.5 mg/100 ml (in children, 4–7 mg/100 ml)
Potassium	3.5–5.4 mEq/L (14–20 mg/100 ml)
Sodium	136–145 mEq/L 313–334 mg/100 ml)

to the area where the fluid contains less water and more particles (Fig. 30-4). Osmosis tends to move water until the concentration of the fluid is uniform on both sides of the membrane. The osmotic pressure caused by the presence of *colloids* (large particles that are unable to diffuse through the membrane) is called **colloidal osmotic pressure** (**COP**; Fig. 30-5). The presence of serum albumin is particularly important to the COP of the blood. Electrolytes can also cause osmosis of water to occur.

At the arterial end of the capillary, filtration pressure tends to push fluid into the interstitial tissue. However,

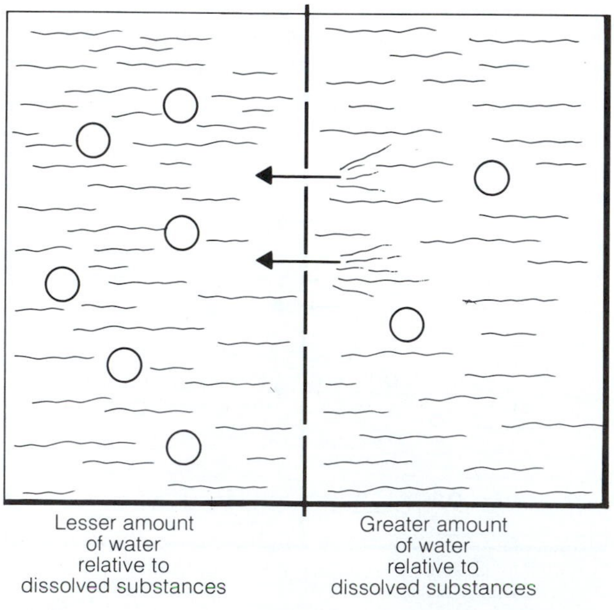

Figure 30-4. Osmosis of water. Water moves from an area of relatively more water and fewer dissolved substances to an area of less water and more dissolved substances.

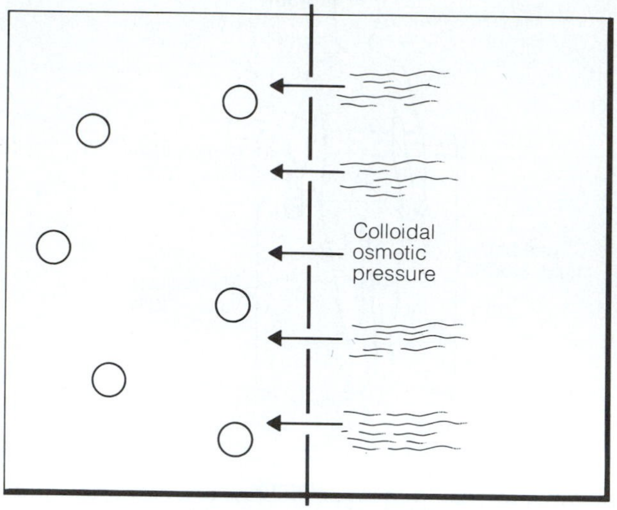

Figure 30-5. Colloidal osmotic pressure. Large particles that cannot pass through the membrane create colloidal osmotic pressure toward the particles.

at the venous end of the capillary, filtration pressure is diminished and therefore the COP of the blood tends to move fluid back into the vessel. This process helps to maintain a constant exchange of fluid between the blood and the interstitial fluid (Fig. 30-6).

Control Mechanisms for Fluid and Electrolyte Balance

The body has a number of different mechanisms that alter fluid and electrolyte balance. Blood pressure is critical because all filtration begins with the pressure in the circulating blood. Changes in blood pressure will create changes in fluid and electrolyte balance.

Blood proteins constitute one of the major dissolved substances in the blood that cause water to move into the capillary from the interstitial space by means of COP. Any disease (such as liver disease) that affects the body's production of proteins or any condition (such as protein starvation) that affects the amount of protein available to the body will affect fluid balance.

The kidneys are able to reabsorb selectively both water and electrolytes according to the body's needs. This process is regulated by a variety of hormonal controls. The *antidiuretic hormone* (*ADH*) released by the posterior pituitary causes the kidney to reabsorb water. *Aldosterone*, which is secreted by the adrenal cortex, causes sodium and water to be retained by the body. These hormonal control mechanisms respond to blood pressure changes and other changes in fluid and electrolyte balance in the body. Because of the pivotal role of the kidneys, diseases of the kidney often create problems of fluid and electrolyte balance. Other hormones

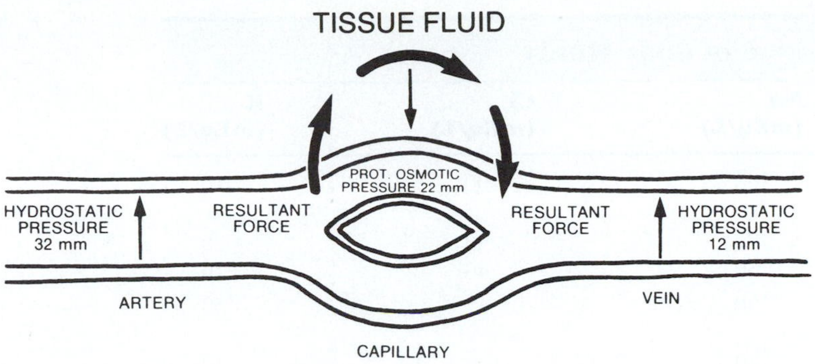

Figure 30–6. Because protein plasma colloidal osmotic pressure is constant at 22 mm Hg and blood pressure is 32 mm Hg at the arterial end of the capillary and 12 mm Hg at the venous end of the capillary, the net effect is for fluid to flow out of the capillary on the arterial end and into the capillary on the venous end.

affect specific electrolytes; for example, the parathyroid hormone regulates calcium.

Measuring Electrolytes

Each of the three commonly used ways of measuring electrolytes provides a different type of information.

The weight of electrolytes is measured metrically, usually in milligrams. When electrolytes are given orally as drugs, they are often measured by weight. In fluids, the number of milligrams per 100 milliliters (mg/100 ml) is most often used as a basis for comparison (Table 30-2).

The **combining power** of electrolytes is a measure of the number of charges present, either positive or negative; it is expressed in *milliequivalents (mEq)*. Electrolytes in most fluids, including intravenous fluids, are measured in milliequivalents per liter (mEq/L). One milliequivalent of any cation (positively charged particle) will combine with one milliequivalent of any anion (negatively charged particle).

The number of particles of an electrolyte in a solution, called its **osmolality** or **tonicity**, determines the movement of body water through osmosis; osmolality is usually measured in **osmoles** per liter (Osm/L) or **milliosmoles** per liter (mOsm/L). Body fluid under normal conditions has an osmolality of approximately 300 mOsm/L. A fluid with the same osmolality as body fluid is an **isotonic fluid**. One with fewer particles and thus a lower osmolality is a **hypotonic fluid**. One with more particles and thus a higher osmolality is a **hypertonic fluid**. Fluids administered intravenously are usually isotonic to prevent potentially harmful movement of body water across cell membranes.

Table 30–2. Weights and Combining Powers of Some Electrolytes

	Weight (mg/100 ml)	Combining Power (mEq/100 ml)
Sodium (Na^+)	3266	142
Potassium (K^+)	195	5
Calcium (Ca^+)	100	5
Bicarbonate (HCO_3^-)	1546	26
Chlorine (Cl^-)	3605	103

Common Fluid and Electrolyte Imbalances

Fluid and electrolyte problems are often complex and may involve multiple abnormalities (Table 30-3). For purposes of clarity, we will discuss the most common of such problems as they would appear in isolation from other problems.

Potassium Imbalances

Potassium is the major intracellular electrolyte. Potassium must be replaced daily because it is responsible for both skeletal and heart muscle action. Serum potassium is normally 3.5 to 5.5 mEq/L (Table 30-4).

Hypokalemia

Potassium deficiency—in which serum potassium is below 3.5 mEq/L—is known as **hypokalemia**. The most common causes of hypokalemia are the use of diuretic drugs (which cause potassium excretion) and the loss of large amounts of gastrointestinal secretion through suction or diarrhea. If potassium is not replaced by medication or by foods high in potassium, a deficit may appear.

Because potassium is critical to muscle function, many of the early symptoms of hypokalemia involve lack of muscle function. Fatigue, weakness, and lack of appetite may occur. Given the importance of potassium in the functioning of the heart muscle, arrhythmias can arise. An electrocardiogram (ECG) will reveal characteristic signs, which include a flattened T wave and a de-

Table 30–3. Electrolyte Content of Body Fluids

	Na (mEq/L)	Cl (mEq/L)	K (mEq/L)
Bile	140	100	10
Colostomy			
New cecostomy	80	50	20
Transverse colostomy	50	40	10
Diarrhea	60	45	30
Gastric fluid			
pH <4	60	100	10
pH >4	100	100	10
Ileostomy			
Recent	130	110	20
Adapted	50	60	10
Pancreatic juice	140	75	10
Small bowel fluids	100	100	20

pressed ST segment. (You will learn about ECG patterns when you study cardiac disease.)

When hypokalemia is identified, the physician will order replacement of potassium by means of intravenous fluids containing potassium or oral potassium supplements.

Hyperkalemia

Hyperkalemia, or potassium excess, is defined as serum potassium level above 5.6 mEq/L. Potassium excess occurs most commonly in patients being given potassium replacements in larger amounts than necessary, those whose intravenous fluids containing potassium run too rapidly, and those who continue taking a potassium replacement when a diuretic has been discontinued. Potassium excess also occurs in those with kidney failure.

The most common symptoms are irritability, nausea, and diarrhea. If hyperkalemia continues, cardiac arrhythmias (peaked T waves on the ECG) may occur. Severe potassium excess can lead to muscle paralysis and cardiac standstill.

Potassium excess is usually treated by restricting potassium intake and allowing the body to restore balance. An oral medication that causes potassium to be excreted into the intestines may be given. An enema solution that exchanges sodium for potassium through the bowel mucosa may be given. In severe instances, kidney dialysis may be used to reduce potassium levels rapidly.

Calcium Imbalances

Most of the body's calcium is stored in the bones. The 1% found in the serum is partly bound to protein and partly ionized. Calcium plays a major role in nerve function and muscle contraction. The normal serum calcium level is approximately 4.5 mEq/L (9–11 mg/100 ml).

Hypocalcemia

Hypocalcemia, or calcium deficit (serum calcium level below 4.5 mEq/L), is most commonly attributable to disturbance in the parathyroid gland or to renal failure. Inadequate vitamin D, acute pancreatitis, and the infusion of large quantities of citrated blood may also cause hypocalcemia. Tingling of the fingers and extremities is followed by muscle cramping and spasm, and, in extreme cases, grand mal seizures (see Chapter 31).

In cases of mild calcium deficit, the physician may order extra calcium taken as tablets. In acute calcium deficit, intravenous calcium in the form of calcium gluconate is usually ordered.

Table 30–4. Laboratory Values for Common Electrolyte Disturbances

Electrolyte	Dangerously Low	Normal	Dangerously High
Calcium	<6 mg/100 ml	9–11 mg/100 ml	>14 mg/100 ml
Potassium	<2.5 mEq/L	3.5–5.5 mEq/L	>6.5 mEq/L
Sodium	<110 mEq/L	136–145 mEq/L	>170 mEq/L

Hypercalcemia

Hypercalcemia, or calcium excess (serum calcium level above 5.8 mEq/L), is uncommon. It occurs when the parathyroid glands are oversecreting, when intravenous calcium is given in excessive quantities, or when bone is broken down rapidly, as in advanced bone cancer. Muscles become hypotonic. Hypotonicity in muscles of respiration may cause serious oxygenation problems; hypotonic skeletal muscles cause weakness and may contribute to falls. Over a longer term, hypercalcemia can bring about renal stones composed of calcium salts, bone changes and bone pain, and coma. The physician may order injections of the hormone calcitonin to help deposit calcium in bone. As a palliative measure, dialysis may be undertaken to remove excess serum calcium. Reducing calcium intake may be of value in some instances.

Sodium Imbalances

Sodium is the major electrolyte in the extracellular fluid. Normal serum sodium concentration is 135 to 145 mEq/L. Because sodium is the major electrolyte responsible for body water movement, it is difficult to distinguish excesses or deficits of sodium from excesses or deficits of water. For example, when serum sodium content is low, the true problem may be not a deficit of sodium but an excess of water in the body. Let us look first at genuine disturbances in the sodium level, keeping in mind that they are less common than disturbances in fluid balance, which we shall discuss next.

Hyponatremia

Hyponatremia, or sodium deficit (serum sodium level below 135 mEq/L), occurs when the loss of sodium is greater than the corresponding loss of water. This may occur when a person perspires excessively, because perspiration has a high sodium concentration, or when diuretics are used vigorously and excessive amounts of sodium are excreted. In rare instances, hyponatremia occurs because of excessive water intake, either oral or intravenous.

A person suffering from sodium deficit may have abdominal cramps, diarrhea, and feelings of anxiety. In extreme instances, seizures may occur and death may follow.

People who work in hot environments and perspire profusely should be encouraged to eat salty foods. In some instances, salt tablets may be taken for replacement. Intravenous solutions containing sodium may be given to people who are acutely ill.

Hypernatremia

Hypernatremia, or sodium excess, is a serum sodium level above 147 mEq/L. A true excess of sodium that is not a result of changes in body water is rare, but may result from excessive ingestion of salt tablets or of seawater in cases of near-drowning. Hypernatremia causes severe nausea and vomiting. Urine output is decreased in an attempt to conserve body water to dilute the sodium. Effects on central nervous system tissue are manifested by agitation, hyperactivity, and sometimes convulsions. Temperature may rise, and death can result.

Hypernatremia is treated by providing large amounts of water, orally or intravenously, which the body uses to dilute the sodium and promote its excretion by the kidneys.

Fluid Imbalances

Fluid imbalances take two general forms. If the total volume of body fluid is abnormal but its composition is normal, the body functions better than if both volume and composition are abnormal.

Fluid Volume Excess

Fluid volume excess is a condition in which there is a greater volume of fluid in the circulatory system than can be managed effectively by the body. Fluid volume excess can result from the administration of excessive amounts of intravenous fluids and from certain disease states. The neck veins will be distended when the head is elevated above 45° because the circulatory system is overloaded. Pulse and respirations may be rapid. The pulse may be full and bounding, and the blood pressure may be elevated. (Module 13, Inspection, Palpation, Auscultation, and Percussion, demonstrates how to check neck veins for distention.)

The body will begin to store the excess fluid in the tissues to shift the load away from the circulating plasma so that the heart does not become overloaded. One of the places where fluid begins to accumulate first is the base of the lungs because the tissue in that area is characterized by an extensive network of fine capillaries, allowing fluid to move out of the vessels, and the tissue itself is open and does not resist the entry of fluid. This condition is a form of pulmonary edema and can be identified by shortness of breath, orthopnea, and moisture heard on auscultation.

Slowly occurring fluid volume excess may be caused by a variety of illnesses and situations, including congestive heart failure, excessive administration of adrenal cortical hormones, and renal disease. In such cases the symptoms set in slowly and the circulatory system may not be overloaded. There may be weight gain, edema of tissues, puffy eyelids, shortness of breath, and a bounding pulse.

When the fluid volume is high, the laboratory report will reveal below-normal hematocrit, hemoglobin, and red blood cell (RBC) count values because of an abnormal amount of fluid relative to the cells. Although electrolytes are being retained, there may initially be a low serum sodium level because the body retains water faster than it retains sodium. As the condition progresses, electrolyte concentrations will return to normal: the total body content of all electrolytes will be elevated along with the total body water.

Treatment is aimed at correcting the underlying cause of the fluid disturbance. Diuretics may be ordered. If large amounts of fluid have accumulated in the pleural space, restricting breathing, a thoracentesis may be done. If large amounts of fluid have accumulated in the peritoneal cavity, causing severe distress, a paracentesis may be done. In each of these procedures, a large needle is introduced into the cavity to withdraw the fluid. These procedures are avoided if at all possible because they result in the loss of plasma proteins and electrolytes as well as excess fluids. Furthermore, unless the underlying cause has been corrected, fluid will again begin to accumulate.

Fluid Volume Deficit

Fluid volume deficit is characterized by a deficit of both water and electrolytes. The remaining body fluid is of approximately normal content in terms of electrolytes.

Such a deficit occurs when a person does not drink fluids or when loss of fluids is greater than intake, as in cases of high fever, diaphoresis (excessive perspiration), or burns. At first the extracellular fluid may be hypertonic, but the water is quickly moved out of the cells to establish equilibrium and the body excretes electrolytes to establish the proper level.

The skin and mucous membranes are usually dry, and there may be acute weight loss (a loss of up to 5% of body weight in the adult is considered a moderate loss). There may be longitudinal wrinkles in the tongue. Urine output will be decreased or, in severe cases, absent. Urine will appear concentrated and have a high specific gravity. The pulse rate may be rapid. Laboratory findings will reveal normal electrolyte values. The hematocrit, hemoglobin, and RBC count will all be high as a result of hemoconcentration (concentration of blood cells). The person may experience thirst, nausea, or dizziness. Treatment is to provide both fluids and electrolytes so that the body can restore fluid balance. This may be accomplished by oral feeding of water, broth, or soups or by parenteral administration of intravenous fluids.

Maintaining Acid–Base Balance (pH)

The **acid–base balance**, a specialized kind of electrolyte balance, is the correct balance of hydrogen ions with bicarbonate ions in the body fluids. As the concentration of hydrogen ions in a fluid increases, that fluid becomes more acidic. As the concentration decreases, it becomes more alkaline (basic). Degrees of *alkalinity* and *acidity* are measured on a scale from 1 to 14 called a *pH scale.* (For more information on this scale, consult a chemistry text.) On the pH scale, 7.0 is neutral. Numbers above 7.0 indicate a lower concentration of hydrogen ions and thus a more alkaline or basic solution; numbers below 7.0 indicate a greater concentration of hydrogen ions and thus a more acidic solution.

All body fluids are normally basic in pH. The normal pH for arterial blood is 7.45; for venous blood, it is 7.35. The usual norms given for blood pH are 7.35 to 7.45. Any body pH below these norms is called **acidosis**. (Strictly speaking, it is only a relative acidosis because body pH remains above 7.0 and thus remains alkaline.) Any pH above 7.45 is referred to as **alkalosis**, signifying that the body is relatively more alkaline than normal.

The body has many sets of buffers that maintain acid–base balance. A *buffer* is a chemical compound that can combine with a strong acid to make it weaker and with a strong base to make it weaker.

Protein is important to the body's system of buffers. It is always present, flexible, and capable of handling large quantities of acid or base products. Hemoglobin also serves as a buffer although not a major one. It too tends to be stable, and problems associated with hemoglobin buffering are rare. The phosphate buffering systems are active, especially within the cells; these systems can be disturbed by certain poisons but are not of common clinical concern.

The two mechanisms of the greatest clinical concern are the base bicarbonate system (often called the metabolic system) and the carbon dioxide system (often called the respiratory system). These two mechanisms act in relationship to each other.

Essentially, the body is able to maintain acid–base balance when the ratio of bicarbonate and carbon dioxide is 20:1—that is, when there is 20 times as much bicarbonate as carbon dioxide (Fig. 30-7). The bicarbonate ion can be produced by the kidney when needed, though this response is not immediate. Carbon dioxide, which dissociates (divides) in solution to form carbonic

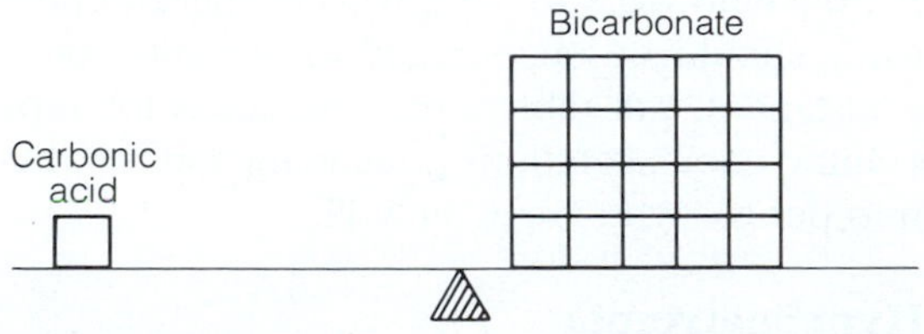

Figure 30-7. Acid-base balance. Appropriate acid-base balance requires a 20:1 ratio of base bicarbonate to carbonic acid.

acid and water, results from cellular oxidation. Constant elimination of carbon dioxide by the lungs maintains the balance.

Common Acid–Base Imbalances

Acid–base imbalances are analyzed in two different ways: by whether the respiratory mechanism (carbon dioxide level) or the metabolic mechanism (base bicarbonate level) is responsible for the problem and secondly by whether the change is in the direction of greater acidity or great alkalinity. Table 30-5 lists laboratory values for common acid–base imbalances.

Base Bicarbonate Imbalances

Base bicarbonate imbalances are also called metabolic imbalances. They result from an excess or deficit of bicarbonate.

Metabolic Acidosis (Base Bicarbonate Deficit)

In **metabolic acidosis**, the body produces acid end products of metabolism (which must be buffered by base bicarbonate) in quantities so great as to exhaust the body's supply of base bicarbonate. This results in an acid excess and base bicarbonate deficit.

The first step in assessment is to identify patients at risk of metabolic acidosis. Such people include those in shock (because producing energy without adequate oxygen creates more acid end products) and those who use excessive amounts of fat for energy (people on rigid high-protein diets and diabetics with inadequate insulin to use carbohydrates), because excessive acid end products result from large-scale fat metabolism.

Observation should focus on identifying the effects of low pH: disorientation, drowsiness, stupor, and eventual coma. Respirations may become deep and rapid as the body tries to compensate for the lack of bicarbonate by eliminating carbon dioxide, which is also in solution.

Laboratory values will show a plasma pH of less than 7.35. The plasma bicarbonate level will be less than 25 mEq/L in the adult and less than 20 mEq/L in the child. Urine pH may be less than 6.0. $PaCO_2$ is within normal limits.

Intervention by the physician is aimed at correcting the underlying metabolic cause of the problem. Temporary treatment with intravenous bicarbonate is common in cases of severe shock and cardiac arrest.

Metabolic Alkalosis (Base Bicarbonate Excess)

In **metabolic alkalosis**, the body has more base bicarbonate than is needed to buffer carbon dioxide and other acid end products. Base bicarbonate itself may be increased, or anions that balance base bicarbonate, such as chloride, may be decreased, causing a relative increase in bicarbonate.

Particularly at risk are people who are losing large amounts of acid (such as gastric or biliary secretions) from the body, those who take large amounts of bicarbonate of soda for relief of stomach distress, and those with impaired kidney function who drink carbonated beverages in large quantities.

Observation may reveal shallow respirations, as the body seeks to conserve carbon dioxide for its acidifying effect. The muscles will be hypertonic, and tetany and muscle spasms might occur. In severe cases, generalized seizures could occur.

Laboratory findings reveal a plasma pH of greater than 7.45. The plasma bicarbonate level will be greater than 29 mEq/L in the adult and will be greater than 24 mEq/L in the child. When there is a primary bicarbonate excess, both the plasma chloride and the plasma potassium tend to be decreased as the body makes compensatory shifts in electrolytes. Urine pH will be greater than 7.0. $PaCO_2$ is within normal limits.

Table 30–5. Laboratory Values in Common Acid–Base Imbalances

Imbalance	Plasma pH	Plasma Bicarbonate	$PaCO_2$	Urine pH
Metabolic acidosis (base bicarbonate deficit)	<7.35 (low)	<25 mEq/L (low)	35–45 mm Hg (normal)	<6.0 (low)
Metabolic alkalosis (base bicarbonate excess)	>7.45 (high)	>29 mEq/L (high)	35–45 mm Hg (normal)	>7.0 (high)
Respiratory acidosis (carbonic acid excess)	<7.35 (low)	22–26 mEq/L (norm) or >29 mEq/L (high)	50 mm Hg (high)	<6.0 (low)
Respiratory alkalosis (carbonic acid deficit)	<7.45 (high)	22–26 mEq/L (normal)	30 mm Hg (low)	>7.0 (high)

Intervention is directed at correcting the cause of loss of acid, if possible. Vomiting, for example, might be controlled. Fluid and electrolytes would be replaced to offset losses and enable the body to restore homeostasis.

Carbonic Acid Imbalances

Carbonic acid imbalances are also called respiratory imbalances. They result from an excess of or deficit in carbonic acid.

Respiratory Acidosis (Carbonic Acid Excess)

In **respiratory acidosis**, the level of carbon dioxide rises, most frequently because of a breathing difficulty such as obstructive lung disease. Respiratory acidosis may or may not be associated with hypoxia (lack of oxygen).

Patients at risk are those with ventilation problems, particularly those with respiratory diseases that interfere with exchanges of carbon dioxide and oxygen. Also at risk is the person who has taken or been given excessive narcotics, causing hypoventilation.

Observation may reveal shallow respirations. Initial disorientation, if unchecked, may progress to stupor, coma, and even death. Should hypoxia also be present, its symptoms may intermingle with those of acidosis (see Chapter 28).

Laboratory values reveal a plasma pH below 7.35. The $PaCO_2$ will be greater than 50 mm Hg. Urine pH will be less than 6.0. Bicarbonate concentration may also be elevated, as the body tries unsuccessfully to compensate for the excess acid. The bicarbonate level may be greater than 29 mEq/L in the adult; it may also be within normal limits.

Intervention to remedy the respiratory problem is needed. This might involve breathing exercises to encourage expiration of carbon dioxide or use of mechanical breathing devices, such as intermittent positive pressure breathing devices, to facilitate air exchange. Medications to help remove secretions blocking the respiratory passages may be needed.

Respiratory Alkalosis (Carbonic Acid Deficit)

In **respiratory alkalosis**, the person breathes out excessive amounts of carbon dioxide, leaving the bicarbonate unbalanced. In an effort to adjust, the body decreases the amount of ionized calcium.

Those at risk include patients on ventilating machines that cause excessive expiration because they are set incorrectly. Those who hyperventilate when anxious or hysterical are common victims of respiratory alkalosis.

Many of the symptoms relate to the decrease in ionized calcium. Such a person might complain of headache, dizziness, faintness, tingling, and abnormal sensations in the lips and the extremities. Tetany (muscle rigidity), muscle spasms, and minor seizures might occur.

Laboratory values include a plasma pH above 7.45 and a urine pH greater than 7.0. Plasma $PaCO_2$ will be low. Plasma bicarbonate will be normal, 22 to 26 mEq/L.

Treatment, usually simple, is aimed at changing the respiratory pattern. If the person is on a breathing device, the settings are corrected. If the person is hyperventilating, efforts are made to slow the respiratory pattern. The person may be encouraged to breathe into a paper bag to rebreathe the same air and increase the carbon dioxide level. Symptoms usually disappear rapidly.

Assessment

Although there are many kinds of fluid and electrolyte (including acid–base) problems, basic assessment can be approached in a uniform way. You will need to focus on three areas: identification of patients at risk of problems through history taking, physical assessment of the patient by observation of key parameters that are related to cell function, and review of laboratory reports.

History: Identification of Patients at Risk

Several categories of patients are at particular risk of fluid and electrolyte problems. Any patient who is not receiving any intake is at risk. If fluids and electrolytes are not replaced, the body may quickly become unable to maintain homeostasis (Display 30-1).

Taking note of all fluid intake is part of the assessment for risk of fluid and electrolyte imbalance. A patient receiving any type of intravenous fluid is also at risk. Introducing fluids and electrolytes directly into the

Display 30–1

Related Factors in Fluid and Electrolyte Imbalance

1. No intake
2. Receipt of intravenous fluids
3. Excessive loss of body secretions
4. Frequent irrigations
5. Disease affecting the liver or kidney or hormone production
6. Receipt of medications that affect fluid and electrolyte balance (diuretics, adrenocorticosteroids, potassium replacements)

circulatory system bypasses the gastrointestinal system, which normally selects those items needed by the body. It is possible to provide fluids and electrolytes faster than the body is able to use them, which can cause serious and even life-threatening problems.

Any person who is experiencing excessive loss of body secretions is at risk. Gastrointestinal secretions can be lost through vomiting, applying suction, or diarrhea. Excessive perspiration due to heat or fever, wound drainage, or moisture lost from the surface of a large burn can also result in dangerous loss of fluids.

Patients undergoing frequent irrigations of a body cavity are also at risk. The irrigation process can cause electrolytes to move across the walls of the organ being irrigated into the fluid. When the irrigating fluid is removed, electrolytes are removed with it.

People with diseases involving the organs that regulate or control fluid and electrolyte balance are at risk. Diseases of the liver and kidneys are particularly problematic, as are conditions that affect hormonal function. Some diseases alter metabolic or respiratory patterns. These increase risk of acid–base imbalance. Those with chronic respiratory disease are at risk of respiratory acidosis, and those with diabetes are at risk of metabolic acidosis.

Another general group of people at risk are those receiving medications that affect fluid and electrolyte balance. Most prominent among these medications are the diuretics, which cause the body to excrete excess fluid and also various electrolytes.

Physical Assessment

Six general categories of direct observations will provide evidence of fluid and electrolyte balance. Assessing these parameters will not reveal the nature of the problem, only that a problem exists (Display 30-2).

Display 30–2
Signs and Symptoms of Fluid and Electrolyte Imbalance

1. Intake and output imbalance
2. Changes in alertness or mental capacity
3. Changes in muscle tone
4. Changes in respirations unrelated to activity
5. Changes in cardiac rate and rhythm
6. Alterations in the fluid present in the tissue
   a. Rapid weight gain
   b. Visible edema or ascites
   c. Poor skin turgor
   d. Pulmonary edema

Intake and output balance is indirect evidence of fluid balance. All fluids taken in and output from all sources must be carefully recorded. Intake and output are balanced when the amounts over several days are approximately equal. A short period of time is not adequate to reveal whether intake and output are balanced because the body makes adjustments over time and the bladder is capable of holding up to 500 ml of urine. When intake and output are not balanced, a thorough assessment is necessary to determine the nature of the problem. For example, if the person entered the hospital after several days of vomiting at home, output might be considerably less than intake because the body is restoring lost fluid. If output is less than intake, the body may be retaining excessive fluid; in such a circumstance, it is appropriate to check for edema. Because intake and output balance is so basic, it is common practice in many hospitals to put all patients identified as being at risk on intake-and-output recording. An alert nurse will independently decide to record fluid intake and output, without waiting for an order from a physician, if the patient is identified as being at high risk.

Changes in alertness or mental capacity may be caused by electrolyte imbalance. When such changes as disorientation, depression, and even coma (see Chapter 31) or their opposites—apprehension, hyperexcitability, and delirium—occur rapidly without known neurologic disease, you should be alert to the possibility of electrolyte imbalance. Neurologic tissue is particularly sensitive to electrolyte concentrations.

Changes in muscle tone may also reveal electrolyte abnormalities because electrolyte balance affects the ability of muscle to contract. Muscles may become weak, hypotonic, and even atonic; alternatively, they may become hypertonic, with cramping, tetany, or tremors.

Changes in respiration that are unrelated to activity are another cue. When respirations become rapid and deep in the absence of strenuous exercise, or when they become excessively shallow, abnormalities in some key electrolytes may be present or impending.

Changes in cardiac rate and rhythm that are not due to heart disease may be caused by electrolyte changes. This reaction is most easily discerned when the person is on a cardiac monitoring device, which allows for precise recordings of the heart's conduction. It can sometimes be detected by auscultation of abnormal heart rhythms.

Finally, *alterations in the fluid present in the tissue* suggest possible fluid imbalance. You will need to check for *skin turgor* (firmness or fullness). Poor skin turgor, manifested in slow recovery from a pinch, may indicate lack of fluid. The eyes may be dull and lack luster. When fluid deficit is severe, the eyeball itself may lack firmness when palpated. The presence of excessive fluid, in the form of *edema, ascites,* or *pulmonary edema,* has been described previously. *Daily weight* may be checked to identify fluid retention. Observations for fluid retention are described in detail in Chapter 29.

Laboratory Tests

Measurement of serum electrolytes is essential to determining electrolyte and fluid balance. Although laboratory reports specify the serum level, not the intracellular level, of electrolytes, they may indicate what is occurring in the cell also. When fluid and electrolyte imbalances are suspected, the physician will usually order serum electrolytes tested. In some facilities, a nurse with appropriate education may also order a specific electrolyte checked. Each laboratory publishes a list of the norms for that laboratory based on the specific laboratory methods used. These norms may vary slightly from one facility to another. The norms in Tables 30-2, 30-4, and 30-5 are general, and you will need to compare them with those of the facility in which you work.

The **Davenport nomogram** is a graph that can be used to plot laboratory values and thus determine the acid–base state (Fig. 30-8). The patient's pH and bicarbonate are the two values plotted. The bicarbonate value is located on the vertical axis, and the plasma pH on the horizontal axis. Each of these points is extended into a straight line across the graph, and the point where the two lines intersect represents the person's current status.

Often the body is able to make adjustments in balance that compensate for a deficit or excess and thereby preserve the body's pH. If so, the condition is known as a compensated acid–base balance problem. It is possible, for example, to have a compensated metabolic acidosis or a compensated respiratory acidosis. This is presented in the nomogram.

Nursing Diagnosis

The specific signs and symptoms of severe fluid volume abnormalities were discussed above. The North American Nursing Diagnosis Association (NANDA) has approved two nursing diagnoses regarding fluid and electrolyte balance—Fluid Volume Deficit and Fluid Volume Excess.

Fluid Volume Deficit

Fluid volume deficit was described above in light of all of the fluid and electrolyte imbalances that might occur. The NANDA definition encompasses fluid deficits in vascular, cellular, or intracellular fluid compartments. Although in some instances because of its severity, fluid volume deficit must be treated as a collaborative problem requiring medical intervention, in other cases it can be treated as a nursing diagnosis. This is true when a person is having a high level of fluid loss occurring through excessive perspiration, diarrhea, or vomiting that can be treated by the oral administration of fluids. To determine whether the problem is appropriately one for independent nursing intervention, you will examine the patient's ability to respond, ability to take oral fluids, and the extent of the problem. When the person is able to respond to instruction, take oral fluids, and the problem is not so severe as to need immediate change, then independent nursing responses are appropriate. When the person is not able to respond to teaching, cannot take oral fluids, or the situation is so severe as to require

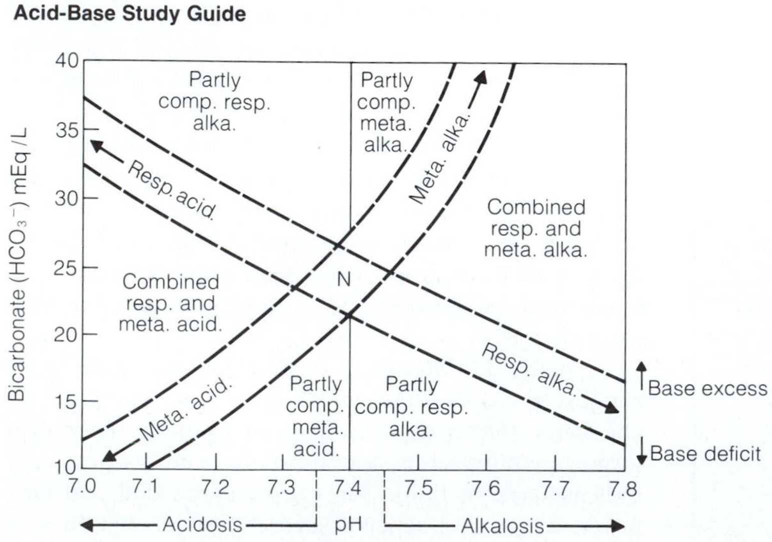

Figure 30-8. The Davenport nomogram. Locate the pH on the horizontal axis and the bicarbonate on the vertical axis and note where the lines cross to determine the acid-base balance. (Courtesy of Jones Medical Instrument Co., Oakbrook, IL, and Dr. J. D. Hackney.)

Nursing Diagnoses Related to Fluid and Electrolyte Balance

Fluid Volume Deficit

High Risk for Fluid Volume Deficit

Fluid Volume Excess

High Risk for Fluid Volume Excess

Altered Oral Mucous Membranes related to fluid volume deficit

Altered Thought Processes related to electrolyte disturbances

Fatigue related to electrolyte imbalance

Impaired Skin Integrity related to edema

immediate changes, then fluid volume deficit should be treated collaboratively with the physician.

Fluid Volume Excess

Fluid volume excess was also described above in the section on fluid imbalances. It is defined as a state in which the person experiences fluid retention and edema. Fluid Volume Excess can be an independently managed nursing diagnosis when it can be managed by limiting sodium intake to prevent fluid retention and by resting with feet elevated above heart level to promote kidney excretion of fluid. Limiting sodium limits the amount of fluid that can be retained because the sodium retains fluid in the tissues. Lying down and elevating the feet promotes venous return to the heart, increases the cardiac output to the kidneys, and thus results in greater fluid excretion by the kidneys. This mechanism depends on having a heart that functions well enough to meet the increased demand. If fluid overload occurs from rapid intravenous infusion, the rate of infusion must be greatly reduced to give the kidneys an opportunity to excrete the excess fluid. When the problem is greater or the heart is unable to increase its load to excrete fluid, fluid volume excess must be managed with the physician as a collaborative problem. The physician may then order diuretic drugs to increase the rate of fluid excretion.

Potential Complication Related to Electrolyte Balance

Potential complication: hypokalemia

Potential complication: hyperkalemia

Potential complication: hypocalcemia

Potential complication: hypercalcemia

Potential complication: hyponatremia

Potential complication: hypernatremia

Potential Complications Related to Acid–Base Balance

Potential complication: respiratory acidosis

Potential complication: respiratory alkalosis

Potential complication: metabolic acidosis

Potential complication: metabolic alkalosis

High Risk States

High risk states for fluid imbalances, either fluid volume excess or deficit, are other problems that you should identify. For some of these high risk states, nurses can implement preventive actions. For others, nurses will monitor and then notify the physician as quickly as possible when the problem occurs.

The diagnosis of High Risk for Fluid Volume Deficit is pertinent to situations in which the person is currently losing fluids rapidly and not replacing them or in which the person is not taking fluids even when loss is not high. The diagnosis of High Risk for Fluid Volume Excess may be present in individuals receiving large volumes of intravenous fluids, those with cardiac, renal, or hepatic disease, and in women during pregnancy.

Other Relevant Nursing Diagnoses

The patient with a fluid and electrolyte problem may also have related nursing diagnoses. Knowledge Deficit related to managing fluid volume and sodium needs may be important if the person must have the information to manage fluid status independently. When there are large amounts of edema, circulation to the skin is more limited and tissue is stretched resulting in High Risk for Impaired Skin Integrity. The underlying disorder causing the fluid excess may also create Activity Intolerance. Impaired Gas Exchange may be the diagnosis if fluid is accumulating in the lungs and interferes with the diffusion of oxygen from the alveoli into the capillary blood. Complete information about these nursing diagnoses was discussed previously.

Planning and Implementation

Under Assessment, we discussed situations in which the individual is at risk of fluid and electrolyte and acid–base imbalances. The most desirable outcome for any situation in which the patient is at risk for fluid and electrolyte imbalance is that the imbalance not occur and that electrolytes stay at appropriate levels and fluid status remain balanced. Problems can often be prevented by careful nursing actions.

An additional outcome criterion might relate to the early notification of the physician when these conditions occur because they usually require medical intervention for correction. The nurse then has a role in the treatment modalities that are prescribed.

Desired outcomes for patients with identified fluid and electrolyte problems include meeting identified quantities for intake and output amount. The resolution of fluid excess would be seen by the weight returning to close to the baseline or "dry" weight and the absence of edema. Establishing normal values for electrolytes may be an appropriate outcome for the person with an electrolyte disturbance. When a patient is expected to have an ongoing concern regarding fluid and electrolyte

Nursing Care Plan
Sample Nursing Care Plan Related to Fluid and Electrolyte Balance

Nursing Diagnosis

High Risk for Fluid Volume Deficit related to diarrhea

Supporting data:

Has had liquid watery stools every hour for last 8 h.

States feels exhausted and weak.

Anorexia but no nausea or vomiting.

Desired Patient Outcomes

No fluid volume deficit as evidenced by:

1. Urine clear and dilute.
2. Skin turgor firm.
3. Mucous membranes moist.

Nursing Action	**Rationale**
1. Measure intake and output and daily weight.	Intake and output and daily weights both provide data basic to early detection of fluid imbalances.
2. Air out room and use deodorizer as necessary to keep room pleasant.	Unpleasant odors depress appetite and oral intake of food and fluids.
3. Explain reason why fluid intake is important. Emphasize value of "Gatorade."	Understanding of the rationale for prescribed actions increases compliance. "Gatorade" provides calories, fluid, and electrolytes, all of which are lost in diarrhea.
4. Keep fluids at bedside. Check every hour to see that fluid is present and fresh.	Intake of fluids is increased when they are readily available. Fresh fluids are more palatable and therefore more likely to be ingested by the ill person.
5. Encourage sips of fluid frequently. Try to reach intake equal to output.	Large volumes in the stomach stimulate the gastrocolic reflex and increase diarrhea but small amounts of fluids do not create this effect. Frequent small sips can provide an appropriate intake of fluids. Intake equal to output represents fluid balance.

status, desired outcomes might reflect the person's knowledge of self-care management. This might include verbalizing self-assessment, understanding of any prescribed medications, and ability to manage diet and fluids as recommended.

As planning is done, you need to keep in mind both the nursing diagnoses that you will be able to recognize and treat and the potential complications that you will identify and refer to a physician for collaborative intervention (see sample Nursing Care Plan Related to Fluid and Electrolyte Balance).

Providing Appropriate Oral Intake

When you monitor patients for fluid and electrolyte imbalances, you must constantly weigh your information to decide when you can take action through providing food and fluids and when the physician must be informed of the data. Timely referral to a physician of those problems that need medical intervention is important for patient safety.

Sodium excesses and deficits are primarily seen as problems with fluid balance. In profuse perspiration, excess quantities of sodium are lost. These may be replaced through ingestion of salty fluids such as broth or salty foods along with water.

When a *fluid deficit* is present, nursing actions are designed to conserve the body fluids and to replace fluids. Fluids are replaced by providing oral fluids in a palatable form and encouraging fluid intake. Fluids that also contain electrolytes, such as broth and fruit juices, provide the essential ingredients for the body to replace fluids and needed electrolytes. When the problem is severe, it must be referred to the physician, who may order intravenous fluids.

When a *fluid excess* is present, nursing actions are designed to limit intake of fluids to a moderate level. Provided fluids are apportioned throughout the day to maintain comfort and prevent excessive thirst. For individuals with fluid excess, a diet that is restricted in sodium is often prescribed because sodium retains fluid in the tissues. Ensuring that the diet served is correct and helping the patient with food choices will assist in compliance with sodium restriction. A major responsibility of the nurse is teaching the patient about the diet and how to plan for the level of sodium restriction that will be needed. The various sodium-restricted diets were described in Chapter 25.

Many diuretics cause *excessive loss of potassium.* Providing potassium-rich foods and teaching the patient for whom these drugs are prescribed to include potassium-rich foods in the diet can prevent this problem. When the drug prescribed creates very high risk, the physician often prescribes an oral potassium supplement. The patient must be taught the purpose of this medication and how it relates to the diuretic being taken.

When an actual *deficit of potassium* through diuretic therapy or other mechanisms does occur, prompt intervention by the physician in ordering potassium replacements is necessary because cardiac dysfunction may result from potassium imbalance. This may be done with additional oral supplements or may be accomplished through fluid therapy as discussed below.

Those who are taking potassium replacement are at risk of *potassium excess* if they should stop taking the diuretic. It also is possible for excess potassium to be present if the person inadvertently takes too much of the prescribed potassium product. Again, careful patient teaching is the best preventive action.

When parathyroid tumors are present, abnormalities of calcium metabolism may occur. A *calcium excess* could create renal stones as well as muscle weakness and cardiac dysfunction. A high fluid intake can help to prevent the precipitation of calcium in the urinary system. A decrease in dietary calcium helps to keep levels low. Again, symptoms of excess would need to be reported promptly for treatment by the physician.

Nursing Issues and Trends: *Treating Infant Diarrhea*

In developing countries infants with diarrhea are treated with special glucose and electrolyte solutions that are mixed from an inexpensive powder and boiled water. This rehydration solution is given orally, spoon by spoon if necessary. Oral rehydration has been responsible for saving countless infants all over the world. In the United States this inexpensive mix is not available. Oral solutions to treat infant diarrhea are sold as premixed formula at a high cost. The majority of infants treated for severe dehydration from diarrhea are hospitalized and treated with intravenous fluids. Those familiar with the international work in treating infant diarrhea have questioned whether "high tech" and "high cost" always constitute the best care.

Addressing Related Concerns

The parathyroids control calcium balance. If surgery is performed on the parathyroids and one or more of the glands is removed, the person is at risk of *calcium deficit.* There are no preventive measures available, but treatment is needed before the deficit becomes severe enough to cause seizures. Therefore, the physician is notified at the earliest symptom of calcium deficit.

The person with chronic lung disease is at risk of *respiratory acidosis* if expiration is inadequate and carbon dioxide is being retained. Coaching this person in correct breathing techniques with expiration twice as long as inspiration can facilitate carbon dioxide exhalation. Pursed-lips expiration maintains a slight pressure in the respiratory tract during expiration and prevents premature collapse of airways, which can trap carbon dioxide in alveoli. The person who is anxious can be coached to slow respirations and maintain the appropriate inspiration–expiration ratio so that respiratory alkalosis from excessive carbon dioxide loss does not occur.

Metabolic acidosis may occur in the person with kidney disease. The diseased kidney may not be able to produce bicarbonate to buffer the carbon dioxide in the system. Although the nurse is unable to institute preventive actions, early identification of symptoms will allow the physician to begin treatment promptly.

A problem with skin integrity often compromises a fluid volume excess. Edematous tissue breaks down more easily than healthy tissue and then requires extra care.

Nursing Care Plan

Sample Nursing Care Plan Related to Patient with Intravenous Therapy

Nursing Diagnosis

High Risk for Fluid Volume Excess related to intravenous therapy and history of decreased cardiac output

Supportive data:

81-year-old woman.

Currently NPO.

Receiving 2,000 ml of fluid per 24 h.

Hospitalized for heart failure last year.

Currently taking digoxin.

Desired Patient Outcomes

No fluid volume excess as evidenced by:

1. No distention of neck veins or delayed emptying of hand veins.
2. No fluid detectable on auscultation of lungs.
3. No peripheral edema.

Nursing Action	Rationale
1. Measure intake and output.	Intake and output provide data basic to early detection of fluid imbalances.
2. Weigh daily.	Daily weights provide data basic to early detection of fluid imbalances.
3. Use IV controller to maintain prescribed IV rate of 83 ml/h consistently.	An IV controller provides for precise control of the rate of administration of fluids.
4. Check for neck vein distention, hand vein emptying, and auscultate lungs bid 0900 & 2100.	Neck vein distention, delayed hand vein emptying, and fluid heard on auscultation of the lungs are early indicators of circulatory overload.

Providing Fluid Therapy

Intravenous fluids are given in many different circumstances. Although ordering the fluid therapy is the physician's responsibility, you need to understand its purposes to monitor what is happening to the patient (see sample Nursing Care Plan Related to Patient With Intravenous Therapy).

Types of Solutions

There are many types of solutions. Although each manufacturer has different names for the different types, they can be identified by looking at the contents of the solution (Display 30-3).

The primary purpose of *hydrating solutions* is to provide water. These solutions contain water and either a carbohydrate or sodium chloride; they do not contain any other electrolytes. The most common hydrating solutions are 5% dextrose in water and 0.9% sodium chloride (normal saline). Hydrating solutions may be used to determine whether kidney function is adequate to allow for rapid replacement of fluids containing electrolytes. When the adequacy of kidney function is in question, a large volume of fluid is given over a period of 45 minutes. If kidney function is adequate, the patient will void (or urine will be drained out of the catheter).

Hydrating solutions are also used as diluents for intravenous drugs or to keep an intravenous line open at a slow rate to be available for medications or other solutions when ordered.

Balanced solutions are those containing water, a carbohydrate for basic calorie needs (to prevent muscle tissue wasting), and basic electrolytes. The electrolytes included are sodium, potassium, and magnesium as cations and chloride, lactate, and phosphate as anions. The expectation is that the person's own kidneys will sort, select, and reject electrolytes as needed. Lactated Ringer's solution is a common electrolyte solution that contains sodium, chloride, potassium, calcium, and lactate in the same concentrations as plasma. Dextrose may be added to Ringer's solution to provide calories.

For maintenance when there is no oral intake, a total amount of 1,500 ml/m^2 of body surface area is given in each 24-hour period.

If a moderate deficit exists, the person will need the maintenance amount plus an additional 2,400 ml/24 hr for each square meter of body surface area. A moderate deficit is defined as a weight loss of 5% in an adult and up to 10% in a child.

If a severe deficit exists, the person will need the maintenance amount plus 3,000 ml/24 hr for each square meter of body surface area. A severe deficit is defined as a weight loss of over 5% in an adult and over 10% in a child.

Balanced solutions are useful for 80% to 90% of patients. They are not used for severely burned persons, those with kidney damage, or those with certain hormonal diseases.

Replacement solutions are used to replace concurrent losses of water and electrolytes in abnormal amounts. The solution used must resemble what is being lost.

Losses due to intestinal suction, vomiting, enterostomy (an intestinal opening) drainage, and diarrhea are replaced with solutions containing additional chloride, in the form of ammonium chloride or calcium chloride, but no additional sodium. This formula matches the electrolyte concentration of the secretions being lost. Lactated Ringer's solution is often used for this purpose, but because the basic formula for lactated Ringer's does not contain adequate potassium, extra potassium is often added. Acidifying or alkalinizing solutions may be used to help correct acid–base imbalances.

Replacement solutions are given in addition to needed maintenance solutions in amounts equal to what is being lost. It is common practice to alternate administering the replacement solution and the maintenance solution.

Solutions used to provide for basic nutrition include those with a high percentage of dextrose; protein hydrolysates or amino acids; and fat emulsions such as Intralipid. The administration of parenteral nutrition was discussed in Chapter 25.

Ethanol (ethyl alcohol) may also be given intravenously to provide calories. One gram of alcohol yields six to eight calories and is used first by the body, sparing glucose for use by the brain. If sedation is desired, a 5% solution of alcohol may be given at a rate of 200 to 300

Display 30–3
Commonly Used Parenteral Fluids

Hydrating Solutions

Normal saline (NS)	0.9% NaCl
Half normal saline (½ NS)	0.45% NaCl
Fourth normal saline (¼ NS)	0.22% NaCl
Dextrose in water (D_5W)	5.0% Dextrose

Dextrose in saline
(may be in any concentration of saline D_5NS, D_5 ½ NS, D_5 ¼ NS)

Maintenance Solutions

Lactated Ringer's (LR)
Contains Na, K, Ca, Cl, and lactate (which is metabolized to bicarbonate) in roughly the same concentration as plasma.
Dextrose in lactated Ringer's (DLR)

ml/hr for an adult. Be careful to give it slowly enough not to cause inebriation.

Water-soluble vitamins are added to intravenous fluids when the patient will be without oral intake for 3 or more days. These vitamins provide the body with essential compounds necessary for metabolic processes.

Volume expanders are solutions containing large molecules that will tend to increase osmotic pressure and thus maintain the volume of fluid inside the vessels. Volume expanders are used when fluid losses have been massive, as in severe burns or hemorrhage. Volume expanders may also be used to provide proteins the body is unable to manufacture because of liver disease. The most commonly used volume expanders are plasma, human serum albumin (both prepared from whole blood), and dextran, a product with large carbohydrate molecules. When volume expanders are used, you must be very attentive to the possibility of circulatory overload (fluid volume excess).

Monitoring Fluid Therapy

To prevent fluid volume disturbances, intravenous fluids must be monitored with extreme care. Rates of flow should be supervised carefully. A patient receiving fluid therapy requires assessment initially and monitoring on an ongoing basis to identify problems early and to ensure that the system continues to function correctly (Fig. 30-9).

Checking the physician's order for fluid therapy is essential to initial assessment. You will need to know the type of fluid ordered, any additives, and the rate of administration.

Checking the nursing care plan or card index will reveal whether the fluid ordered is the initial fluid or one of a series. You will need to find out where the intravenous line is located and any special information about the system being used, such as whether or not a heparin lock is present.

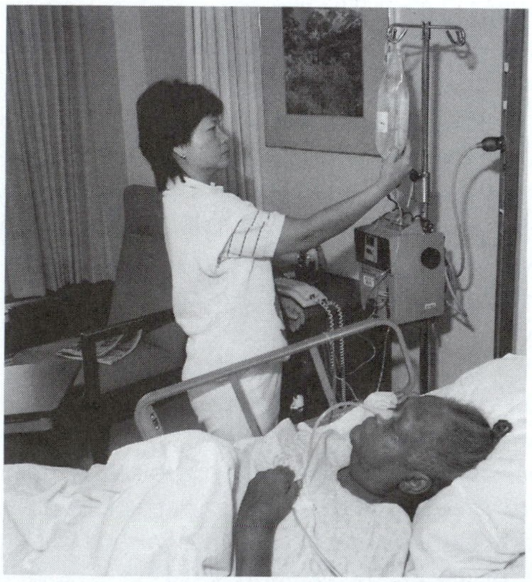

Figure 30-9. The patient receiving fluid therapy requires ongoing assessment.

Display 30–4
Monitoring Fluid Therapy

Initial Assessment

Check physician's order
Check nursing record
Check patient:
- Site appearance
- Fluid container, type of fluid, and volume remaining
- Flow rate

Hourly Monitoring

Check patient:
- Site appearance
- Fluid container, type of fluid, and volume remaining
- Flow rate

Checking the patient involves examining the site of the infusion, comparing the rate of administration with the desired rate, and verifying that the correct fluid is being administered. You will want to watch for abnormalities at the site; redness and heat, for example, might indicate phlebitis (inflammation of the vein), and cold swelling might indicate infiltration (leakage of the fluid into the tissue around the vein).

After the initial assessment, it is not necessary to recheck the physician's order or the nurse's records each time the intravenous line is monitored. The intravenous line itself and the patient should be checked hourly in routine situations and more frequently when the condition of the patient is more serious (Display 30-4).

Regulating the Rate of Flow

The physician may specify the rate of flow in a variety of ways. Often the 1,000-ml container is used as a standard, and the duration is varied (6 hours, 8 hours, 10 hours, and so on) to provide for the appropriate volume in each 24-hour period. Such an order might read "1000 ml D5NS, run 10 hours." Some physicians order fluids in milliliters per hour. This type of order would read "D5NS run at 60 ml/hr until further orders." Still others order the total fluid to be run in a 24-hour period. In this case the order might read "3,000 ml D5NS over next 24 hours." The rate of flow is important because it is possible to give too little to meet the patient's needs or so much that the circulatory system is overloaded. When electrolytes—especially potassium—have been added, circulatory overload is of particular concern.

An intravenous infusion is regulated by adjusting the flow in the tubing in terms of drops per minute. You must therefore be able to translate the physician's order as written into a drops-per-minute figure. Intravenous tubings are not standardized. Each manufacturer has established its own standard for the number of drops delivered per milliliter. After checking the package for this information, you may use the following formula to figure drops per minute:

$$\frac{\text{drops per ml of equipment} \times \text{no. of ml ordered}}{\substack{\text{time to run in min} \\ (\text{no. of hrs to run} \times 60\text{ min})}} = \text{drops/min}$$

Intravenous flow controllers or pumps may also be used to regulate intravenous fluid administration. A controller relies on gravity for flow and monitors the rate of flow. Some brands require that the rate be set in drops per minute and others require that it be set in milliliters per hour. Controllers maintain a constant rate, although the volume per hour may not be precise. The volume delivered is within an acceptable range of accuracy, however. Most controllers are less expensive than pumps and therefore are used when rate of flow must be kept constant but precision in volume is not critical. The controller might be used when fluids with electrolytes or other additives are being given. The concentration of these electrolytes is low enough that the kidneys will readily maintain balance if the rate is constant and a difference of a few milliliters per hour in volume would not be critical to the person.

Intravenous pumps use positive pressure to deliver a precisely measured volume of intravenous fluid per hour. Intravenous pumps are used when precision of volume as well as rate of flow is critical. This might be true for solutions containing drugs, parenteral nutrition solutions, or for replacement fluids in the infant, young child, or critically ill person.

When an intravenous pump or controller that delivers fluid in milliliters per hour is used, the following formula will enable you to set the pump correctly:

$$\frac{\text{ml of fluid order}}{\text{number of hours to run}} = \text{ml/hour}$$

Sometimes a bottle of intravenous fluid is marked with the approximate level the fluid should reach at specified times to provide the amount ordered. This is a helpful aid in maintaining a general overview of fluid administration but is unsatisfactory as the only method of checking the rate. If the intravenous infusion is behind schedule, it may be tempting to increase the rate to catch up, without regard to how fast the fluid is being administered during the catch-up period. As a general guideline, 2 ml/min is a moderate flow rate for a *healthy adult*, 1 ml/min is a slow rate, and 3 ml/min is a rapid rate. If you must readjust an infusion, consider the person's age, size, and cardiovascular status to determine a safe speed.

Changing the Fluid Container

In most situations the fluid bottles or containers are changed frequently to add more fluid. However, when the intravenous is being run very slowly to keep the vein open, a container could potentially hang for a long period. The Centers for Disease Control and Prevention (CDC) recommend that, to minimize the potential for infection, no bottle hang for more than 24 hours.

Changing the Tubing and Dressing

The CDC recommend that the tubing be changed every 48 hours to lessen the potential for local inflammation of the vein and for infusing contaminated solution although some facilities have extended this time based on their studies of complication in their own facility. The dressing over the intravenous site may be changed at that time. An iodine-based or antibiotic ointment (depending on the policy of the facility) is applied to the needle entry site, and a new sterile dressing is applied over the site.

Changing the Infusion Site

The CDC suggested that changing the peripheral site every 72 hours would decrease the potential for phlebitis. In patients who have poor veins that offer relatively few peripheral sites, the access site may be left in place until a problem is detected, at which time the site is changed. This approach makes early detection of problems important. Central venous lines are left in for longer periods of time. The maximum time depends on the type of venous access device being used. Rigid intravenous catheters have the shortest life span. Some silicone rubber catheters are designed for long-term use that may stretch weeks, months, or in the case of some surgically implanted devices, years.

Administering Blood and Blood Products

Blood and blood products have many important medical uses and are frequently used in therapy. You should be familiar with the different types of blood products, the assessment and monitoring needed, and the specific details of how to administer each type. Whole blood, packed RBCs, platelets, human serum albumin, plasma, plasma protein fraction, and clotting factors are the products commonly administered (see Module 57, Administering Blood and Blood Products). Although adverse reactions to blood transfusions are not common, they can be serious and you need to understand them.

Potential Complications of Blood or Blood Products

A wide variety of complications can occur as a result of blood transfusions. These are outlined in detail below.

Potassium excess may occur from the administration of stored blood because it is subject to RBC breakdown as it ages. As RBCs are broken down, their potassium is released into the plasma. Old blood may have a very high potassium level. Although not a problem for a person with adequate kidney function, this circumstance may cause problems for people with kidney disorders and those already having difficulties with potassium balance. The adverse symptoms presented are the same as those of any other potassium excess as discussed above. If such symptoms appear, the transfusion ought to be stopped until the physician decides on a course of action. It may then be restarted slowly. In rare instances, rapid administration of citrated blood may cause a calcium deficit due to the ability of the citrate to combine with the serum calcium. If blood is given no faster than 1 unit in 30 minutes, this will not be a problem. More rapid administration is indicated only in severe hemorrhage. The symptoms are the same as those of ordinary hypocalcemia discussed previously. Treatment is to administer intravenous calcium compounds; the administration of blood may be continued.

The administration of whole blood to a person who has an adequate volume of blood may overload the circulatory system. Because the blood contains proteins and cells, the fluid cannot be moved into the interstitial spaces with ease and will thus accumulate, especially in the lungs. *Circulatory overload* is also a hazard if the patient has an existing cardiac problem; in such cases, packed RBCs are usually administered. If circulatory overload occurs, the transfusion is slowed. Diuretics may be required to remove the excess fluid.

Serum hepatitis is a viral disease transmitted from an individual blood donor to the recipient. To guard against serum hepatitis, a careful history must be taken before blood is taken from a donor. However, people who have had undiagnosed hepatitis may not be screened out, and donors who are paid for their blood may deliberately give false histories. Blood is screened in the laboratory for hepatitis B to protect blood recipients. The disease may appear at any time from 6 weeks to 6 months after the transfusion of affected blood. Consult a medical–surgical text for information on symptoms and care. Hepatitis may be transmitted by whole blood, packed RBCs, and plasma.

Pyrogenic reactions, which are characterized by a fever, chills, and headache, are relatively common in people who receive blood. Attributable to sensitivity to white blood cells or platelets in the blood, pyrogenic reactions become increasingly common the more transfusions the individual receives and usually occur after at least 250 ml blood or blood product has been administered. The pyrogenic reaction may also be a result of contamination of the blood or equipment. If the reaction is due to bacterial contamination, the symptoms are much more severe and may include nausea, vomiting, and diarrhea. A shock reaction may occur with gram-negative bacterial contamination. If the pyrogenic reaction is mild, aspirin or acetaminophen may be ordered and the transfusion continued by the physician. If it is severe, the transfusion is stopped.

Hemolytic reaction, the most serious of all adverse transfusion reactions, is caused by incompatibility of types of RBCs. In a hemolytic reaction, RBCs are rapidly hemolyzed (broken down) and the reaction is due to the effects of these products on the body. This type of reaction usually occurs in about the time it takes to administer the first 100 ml blood but may take place more quickly. Symptoms include flank pain (from the RBC breakdown products precipitating in the kidney), dark urine (from the excretion of the hemolyzed RBCs), constriction in the chest (from the precipitation of hemolyzed RBCs in the lungs), a feeling of fullness in the head, rapid respirations and rapid heart rate (from stress and lack of oxygen), fever, and chills. Later, jaundice

Potential Complications Related to Blood Transfusion

Potential complication: potassium excess related to multiple transfusions

Potential complication: hypocalcemia related to rapid administration of citrated blood

Potential complication: circulatory overload related to inability to manage volume and osmotic load

Potential complication: pyrogenic reaction related to white cell and/or platelet sensitivity

Potential complication: hemolytic reaction related to incompatibility of red blood cells

Potential complication: allergic response related to sensitivity to foreign proteins in blood administered

The following are now rare in countries where the blood supply is adequately tested, but may be seen in those transfused before blood testing was instituted.

Potential complication: serum hepatitis related to hepatitis-contaminated blood transfusion received more than 6 weeks but less than 6 months previously

Potential complication: AIDS related to HIV-contaminated blood transfusion will set in if a large quantity of blood has hemolyzed. Death may result from damage to the renal tubules. It is crucial that the blood be stopped immediately when a hemolytic reaction is suspected.

Allergic reactions may include outbreaks of hives, itching, and flushing. Respiratory allergic response, with shortness of breath and bronchospasm, is rare. Symptoms may occur after 125 ml has been infused or even after the entire transfusion is completed. Antihistamines are given, and if the reaction is mild the blood may be continued by the physician. Severe reactions require that the blood be stopped; in some cases adrenocorticosteroids may also be given.

Acquired immunodeficiency syndrome (AIDS) is caused by the human immunodeficiency virus (HIV). This virus is transmitted in blood and body fluids. Blood supplies are protected by a two-pronged approach. First, donors are screened and those who are in the high risk groups for the disease (gay men, those who have had any sexual contacts with gay men, intravenous drug users and their sexual partners, individuals with multiple sexual partners, and those who have had sexual relations with a prostitute) are not permitted to donate. In those blood centers where donors are not paid for their donations, this screening is successful in protecting the blood supply. Second, all blood is tested for the antibodies to HIV. Blood that tests positive (indicating that the donor has contracted the HIV virus) is destroyed. Most blood centers also have a program to inform donors of positive test results and counsel them in regard to this information. Many blood centers have individuals who donate frequently; this factor adds additional safety because repeated testing has continued to demonstrate its freedom from both HIV and hepatitis B.

Although the above safeguards have made the blood supply safe, it is not possible to guarantee absolutely that all blood is free of the HIV virus. There is a period of time between infection with the virus (the time when the virus enters the body) and the development of antibodies. If an individual were newly infected and did not admit to high risk behavior, it is possible that a contaminated unit of blood would be donated. The current estimate is that the chance of this occurring is quite low. Most experts consider this risk to be negligible in the face of the reasons blood transfusions are given in today's health care system. Since the information about HIV transmission became generally available, physicians have drastically curtailed the use of transfusions. This may slow recovery, but has long-term safety.

Research into methods of detecting the virus itself rather than detecting antibodies to the virus and into methods of treating blood to destroy any possible virus is now being carried out. Success in these methods could guarantee the safety of blood.

Maintaining Safety in Administration of Blood and Blood Products

A primary concern for the nurse is the maintenance of safety when administering blood and blood products. Clear identification of both the patient and the product, correct use of the right equipment, and careful monitoring are all required. Specific techniques are discussed in Module 57, Administering Blood and Blood Products.

Evaluation

When evaluating outcomes for fluid and electrolyte concerns, you will need to again collect data regarding the patient's current fluid status. You will observe for function and appearance and check laboratory values. Then you will compare the results with your desired outcomes. Has the problem for which the patient was at high risk been avoided? Have the potential complications been prevented? How is the patient responding to the plan you have designed? Your concern is identifying whether the patient is now in a state of fluid and electrolyte balance and whether the risks have been avoided. These adjustments may create problems of their own if the fluid and electrolyte status has returned to a normal state too rapidly for the other processes to make necessary changes. Actions may have to be adjusted for rate of change as well as for the direction and amount of change.

As you evaluate the patient's status, you will also be evaluating the actions that have been taken and the rate at which the patient is returning to a state of balance. One concern in fluid and electrolyte problems is that the return to balance must occur slowly enough that the body is able to make effective changes in all the homeostatic processes. When the imbalance occurs, the body makes many adjustments to support homeostasis and these must be reversed.

Desired outcomes for patients with identified fluid and electrolyte problems include meeting identified values for intake and output amount. The resolution of fluid excess would be seen by the weight returning to close to the baseline or "dry" weight and the absence of edema. Establishing normal values for electrolytes may be an appropriate outcome for the person with an electrolyte disturbance. When a patient is expected to have an ongoing concern regarding fluid and electrolyte status, desired outcomes might reflect the person's knowledge of self-care management. This might include verbalizing self-assessment, understanding of any prescribed medications, and ability to manage diet and fluids as recommended.

Nursing Care Study
A Patient with Electrolyte Imbalance

Mrs. Eileen Merslake, RN, the team leader, was at the desk when a nursing assistant approached her. "Mrs. Merslake, I just can't get Miss Stapleton to wake up enough to eat any lunch." Mrs. Merslake replied, "I'll go and check on her right away."

As Mrs. Merslake walked down the hall, she reviewed what she knew about Miss Stapleton, an 82-year-old woman who lived independently in a large home. She had been admitted 4 days before with a diagnosis of congestive heart failure. Although Miss Stapleton had been very short of breath and fatigued on admission, she had been completely alert and oriented. She had had severe fluid retention and had immediately been started on diuretics and medications for her heart problem. Mrs. Merslake remembered that the night nurse had commented in the morning report that Miss Stapleton had lost 16 lb in 4 days, her breathing was back to normal, she had slept all night, and she was progressing well.

When she arrived at the patient's room, Mrs. Merslake found that it was almost impossible to rouse Miss Stapleton enough to speak. She seemed somewhat confused, could not grasp anything firmly, and was slumped in the armchair. On the basis of all the information she had, Mrs. Merslake hypothesized that the patient might well have a low potassium level because of the rapid loss of fluids and electrolytes through the use of diuretics.

The team leader was aware that she could have a blood chemistry run on a blood specimen that had already been drawn; the physician had ordered a fasting blood sugar measurement that morning. Mrs. Merslake telephoned the lab and asked them to run a potassium level on the specimen. The lab called back with a report of a serum potassium level of 3.26 mEq/L, clearly very low. Mrs. Merslake then called the physician. Whe the physician called back, she reported the patient's condition, reminding the physician of the medications being given, especially the diuretic, the fluid lost over the past 4 days, and the current laboratory report on potassium level.

The physician reduced Miss Stapleton's diuretic dosage by half and ordered an oral potassium supplement to be given stat. Mrs. Merslake implemented these medical orders immediately. She also added this problem to the patient's nursing care plan and wrote nursing directives for observations to be made over the next 48 hours to evaluate the patient's response to the treatment.

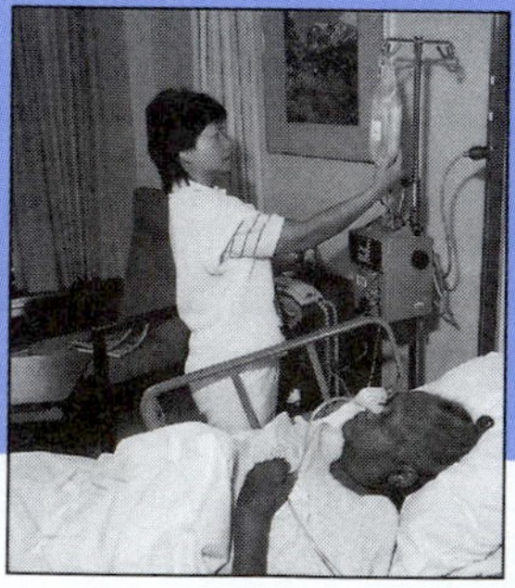

Key Points

- The proper fluid and electrolyte composition of the body's fluids is critical to effective functioning.
- Water is found in all cells and accounts for a high percentage of body weight. Within the body, fluid is found in three compartments: the intracellular, the interstitial, and the plasma or circulating fluid.
- Electrolytes move from one compartment to another by diffusion and active transport and water moves by osmosis and filtration. Using these mechanisms, the body maintains the appropriate levels of fluids and electrolytes in each compartment.
- Fluid and electrolyte balance is controlled by the blood pressure and by hormones that affect kidney function and other key body mechanisms.
- Electrolytes may be measured in terms of their weight (milligrams), their combining power (milliequivalents), and their osmolality (milliosmoles).
- Hypokalemia is a potassium deficit that especially affects muscle function.
- Hyperkalemia is a potassium excess that may occur when potassium replacement has been too vigorous. Excess potassium causes diarrhea, nausea, and irritability and may alter cardiac function.
- Hypocalcemia is a calcium deficit that can result in muscle twitching and seizures. Parathyroid disease, pancreatitis, and some cancers also cause hypocalcemia.
- Hypercalcemia is a calcium excess that can result in muscles that become hypotonic and respiratory distress.

- Hyponatremia, that is, sodium deficit, may result from excessive perspiration.
- Hypernatremia, sodium excess, may occur from ingestion of salt tablets or seawater.
- Fluid volume excess may be identified by symptoms indicating too much fluid in the circulating volume or by symptoms indicating too much fluid in the interstitial spaces.
- In fluid volume deficit, there may be inadequate fluid in the cells as well as in the interstitial spaces and in the circulating volume.
- Acidosis is indicated by a pH below 7.35; alkalosis is indicated by a pH above 7.45.
- The body maintains appropriate pH by a system of buffers. The buffers protein, hemoglobin, and phosphate are rarely associated with problems. The base bicarbonate and the carbon dioxide systems are the most clinically significant.
- Metabolic acidosis is a base bicarbonate deficit, and metabolic alkalosis is a base bicarbonate excess.
- Respiratory acidosis is a carbonic acid excess, and respiratory alkalosis is a carbonic acid deficit.
- Assessment of fluid and electrolyte and acid–base balance requires that you first identify those patients who are at risk. Then, you make direct observations of intake and output balance, changes in alertness or mental capacity, changes in muscle tone, changes in respiration, changes in cardiac rate and rhythm, and alterations in the fluid present in the body. Laboratory tests are also valuable.
- Fluid volume excess and fluid volume deficit are the two NANDA-approved nursing diagnoses.
- There are many situations in which a high risk state for imbalance is present. Nursing actions may help prevent the imbalances from developing. In addition, the risk states require careful nursing observation so that abnormalities can be reported promptly to the physician for treatment.
- Nursing interventions include health teaching and providing oral fluids that meet the patient's needs. Fluid therapy is ordered by the physician. Hydrating solutions, balanced solutions, replacement solutions, nutritional solutions, and volume expanders may be used.
- Nursing assessment is important throughout fluid therapy. The intravenous line must be cared for correctly to prevent complications.
- Blood and blood products are used to provide needed components for effective physiologic function. Whenever possible, individual components are used instead of whole blood.
- Nurses need to be vigilant about potential adverse responses to the administration of blood and blood products. Although these are not common, they are very serious when they do occur.
- As the nurse evaluates the patient's response, he or she will be looking at the current status in relationship to the desired outcomes that were established.

Study Questions

1. When a person has edema, which fluid compartment contains the excess fluid volume?
2. When a person has circulatory overload, which fluid compartment contains the excess fluid volume?
3. Describe the processes by which fluid and electrolytes move between the fluid compartments?
4. If a person has an increase in the secretion of aldosterone, what would be the effect on fluid balance?
5. How would a drop in a patient's blood pressure affect fluid balance?
6. How would an accumulation of carbon dioxide in the blood affect a patient's acid–base balance?
7. What diseases might create acid–base imbalances?
8. How would you assess for acid–base imbalance?
9. What patients are at risk for hypokalemia?
10. How can you assess for fluid volume deficit?
11. How might you prevent the potential complications of fluid therapy?
12. How might you prevent the potential complications of blood transfusions?

Critical Thinking Activities

1. At your facility, check the intravenous fluids routinely used on the unit. Write down the exact contents of the three most commonly used ones.
2. Check the laboratory report forms for blood chemistry. Identify the norms listed for the blood electrolytes discussed in the chapter.
3. For a patient for whom you are caring, assess for fluid and electrolyte balance.
4. Check the packages for intravenous fluid and blood administration in your facility to ascertain the number of drops per milliliter delivered by the sets.
5. Check the blood administration procedure for your facility.
6. Arrange to spend time with an RN who is monitoring intravenous therapy.

Relevant Sections in Modules for Basic Nursing Skills

Volume 1 Module
Inspection, Palpation, Auscultation, and Percussion 13

References and Readings

Butler, S. "Current Trends in Autologous Transfusions." *RN* 52, 11 (November 1989): 44–66.

Chenevy, B. "Overview of Fluids and Electrolytes." *Nursing Clinics of North America* 22, 4 (December 1987): 749–760.

Feldstein, A. "Detect Phlebitis and Infiltration Before They Harm Your Patient." *Nursing '86* 16, 1 (January 1986): 44–47.

Girard, N. J., Morgan, R. G., and Orr, M. D. "Autologous Salvage of Blood." *AORN Journal* 47, 2 (February 1988): 492–503.

Intravenous Nurses Society. *Intravenous Nursing Standards of Practice.* Belmont, Mass.: IVS, 1990.

Irwin, M. "Encourage Oral Intake—Yes, But How?" *American Journal of Nursing* 87, 1 (January 1987): 100–106.

Klass, K. "Troubleshooting Central Line Complications." *Nursing '87* 17, 11 (November 1987): 58–61.

Lenox, A. C. "I.V. Therapy: Reducing the Risk of Infection." *Nursing '90* 20, 3 (March 1990): 60–61.

Lowery, S. J., and Ash, S. R. "Diminishing the Risk of IV Potassium Chloride." *Nursing '88* 18, 6 (June 1988): 64.

McConnell, E. A. "Administering Blood Therapy Safely." *Nursing '92* 22, 8 (August 1992): 91.

McConnell, E. A. "Preventing Air Embolism in Patients with Central Venous Catheters." *Nursing Life* 6, 2 (March-April 1986): 47.

Metheny, N. M. *Fluid and Electrolyte Balance: Nursing Considerations.* 2nd edition. Philadelphia: J. B. Lippincott, 1991.

Peck, N. L. "Action Stat! Blood Transfusion Reaction." *Nursing '87* 17, 9 (September 1987): 33.

Persons, C. B. "Preventing Infection from Intravascular Devices." *Nursing '87* 17, 4 (April 1987): 75, 77–78.

Poyas, A. S. "Assessment and Nursing Diagnosis in Fluid and Electrolyte Disorders." *Nursing Clinics of North America* 22, 4 (December 1987): 773–784.

Schwartz, M. W. "Potassium Imbalances." *American Journal of Nursing* 87 (1987): 1292–1298.

Viall, C. D. "Your Complete Guide to Central Venous Catheters." *Nursing '90* 20, 2 (February 1990): 34–41.

Walpert, N. "An Orderly Look at Calcium Metabolism Disorders." *Nursing '90* 20, 7 (July 1990): 60–64.

Witek-Janusek, L. "Metabolic Acidosis: Pathophysiology, Signs, Symptoms." *Nursing '90* 20, 7 (July 1990): 52–53.

York, K. "The Lungs and Fluid and Electrolyte and Acid-Base Balance." *Nursing Clinics of North America* 22, 4 (December 1987): 805–814.

Cognition and Sensory Perception

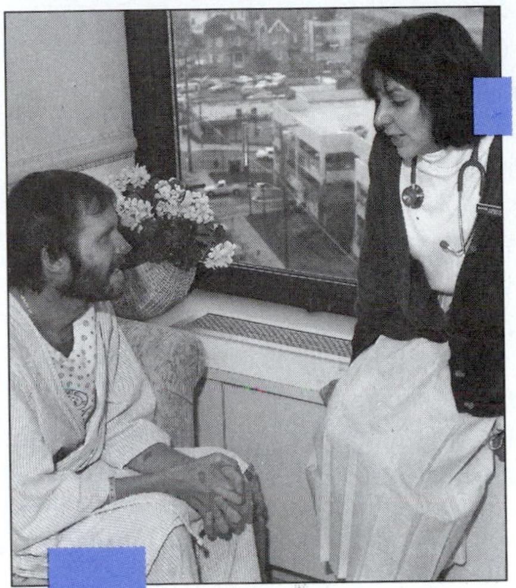

31

Objectives

After completing this chapter, you should be able to:

1. Name the four major parts of the nervous system and the general function of each.
2. Describe data you would gather in each of the areas of sensory function and cognition.
3. Identify nursing diagnoses that are common in the patient with sensory or cognitive impairment.
4. Focusing on the areas of sensation and cognition, outline the nursing actions that would be appropriate for a patient with the nursing diagnoses identified.
5. Discuss the importance of evaluation of cognition and sensory perception as it pertains to the patient and the nurse.
6. Describe the role of the interdisciplinary team in care of persons with sensory or cognitive impairment.
7. Name factors that can contribute to nurses' experiencing sensory disturbance.
8. List ways in which nurses can offset sensory disturbance they may experience.

Study Terms

aphasia
cognition
level of awareness
perception
sensation
sensory deprivation
sensory overload

Outline

The Nervous System

The Brain
The Spinal Cord
The Autonomic Nervous System
Sensory Receptors
  Eye
  Ear
  Touch
  Smell
  Taste

Common Functions Controlled by the Nervous System

Sensation
Perception
Cognition

Common Disorders Affecting Sensory Perception

Visual Impairment
Hearing Impairment
Sensory Disturbances
  Sensory Deprivation

The need for an effective means to perceive the environment is fundamental to being able to function. Sensory perception is so much a part of all of our lives that we often do not even realize how much it forms a foundation for every action. In addition to perceiving the world, we also must be able to process information to meet our needs.

To understand sensory and perceptual disturbances, one must first be aware of the difference between sensation and perception. "Sensation is the physical energy, and perception the subjective experience" (Crow, 1981). **Sensation** originates with a particular stimulus, which is conveyed by the neurons to the thalamus, where the neurons synapse, or connect, with other neurons; they then connect with the parietal lobe of the brain. **Perception** is the way in which each person individually organizes and consciously interprets these sensations. Disturbances can occur with either the process of sensing or that of perception. **Cognition** is the way people think, learn, and make judgments.

The Nervous System

Anatomically, the nervous system can be subdivided into two large entities: the *central nervous system (CNS)* and the *peripheral nervous system (PNS)*. The CNS is composed of the central organs for neurologic control—the brain and spinal cord; the PNS consists of all other structures and nerves. You might think of the brain as a computer that has remote and recent memory. The computer brain both sends and receives messages and coordinates the complex operation of the body (Fig. 31-1).

The Brain

The *brain*, the most vital and vulnerable of all the organs of the body, is encased in a bony structure called the *cranium*. The brain is an active organ that needs oxygen, glucose, electrolytes, and water in precisely the correct proportions for it to function properly. Although the brain is only 2% of body weight, it requires 20% of the body's oxygen supply.

The three main portions of the brain—the *cerebrum*, *brain stem*, and *cerebellum*—are covered with three fiberlike coverings: the dura mater (outer), arachnoid (middle), and the pia mater (inner). These coverings also enclose the spinal cord.

The *cortex* is the thin outer gray matter layer of the cerebrum, where awareness, cognition, and emotions reside. Other parts of the brain control and regulate vital functions such as temperature, respiration, and heart rate. Speech, sight, hearing, taste, touch, and smell are also central to the brain. Movement is controlled by op-

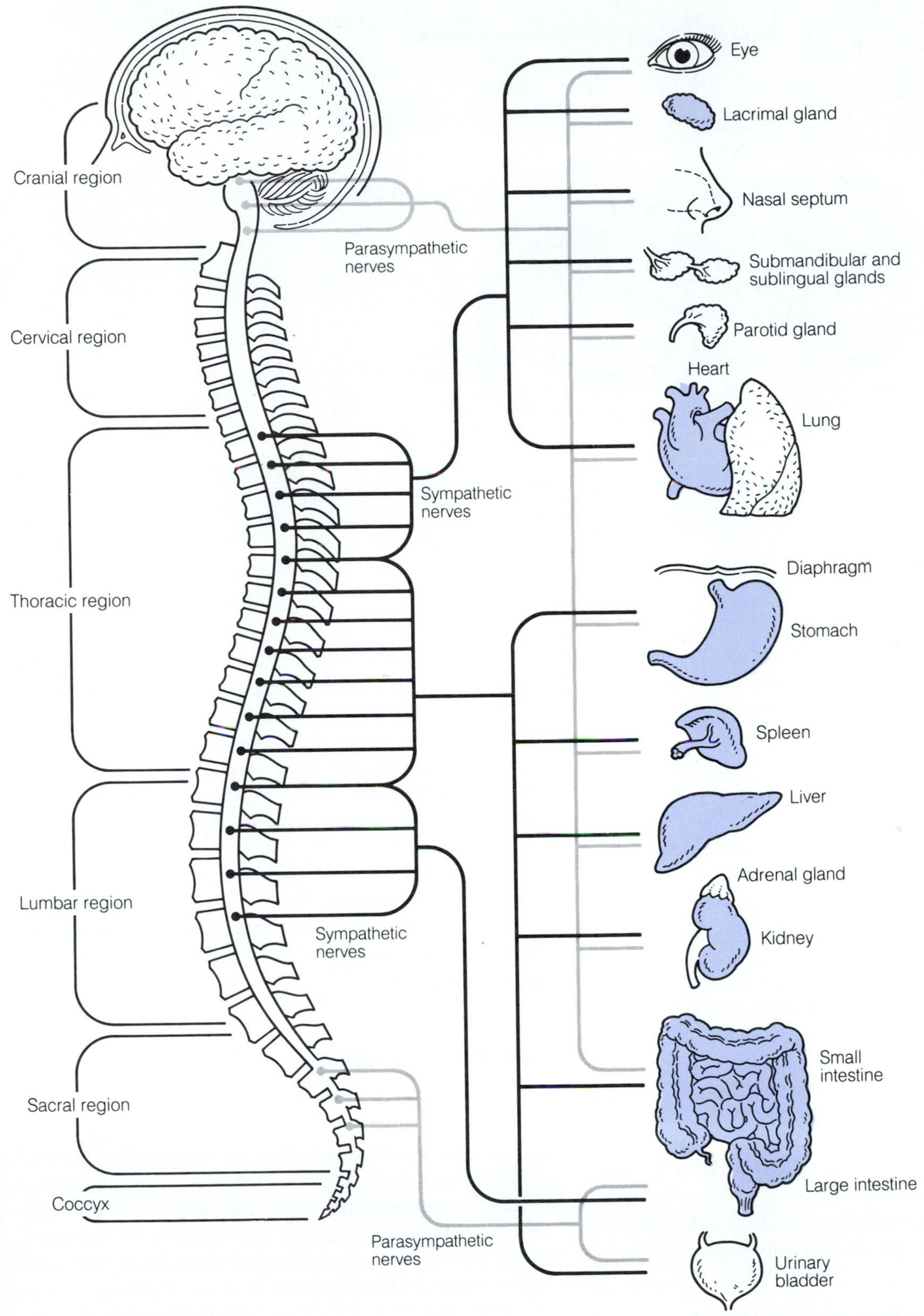

Figure 31-1. The nervous system.

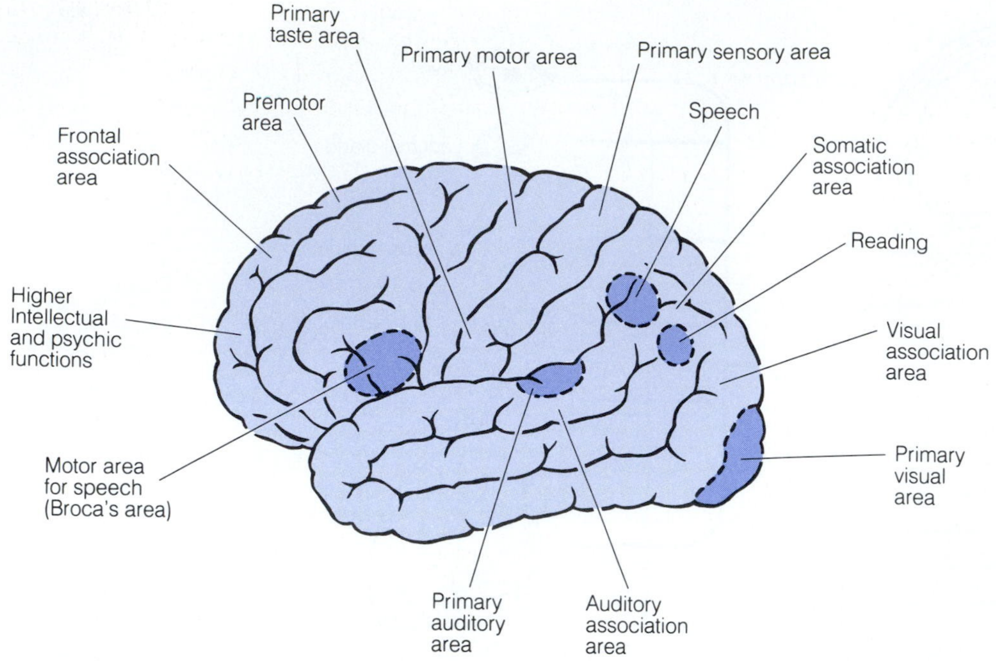

Figure 31-1. (Continued)

posing sides of the brain in most people. For example, the left-sided movement of the body is controlled by the right side of the brain. The cerebellum provides coordination of movement.

The Spinal Cord

The spinal cord, protected by the bony vertebrae that compose the spinal column, carries messages to and from the brain. It carries both *motor impulses*, having to do with movement, and *sensory impulses*, having to do with sensation.

Because it can carry both types of messages, the spinal cord is the reflex center for the body. It has the ability to act as a protective mechanism in warning the cortex of threat and signaling muscular response to avoid injury (see Chapter 32). Surrounding and bathing the brain and spinal cord in the adult is approximately 150 ml of cerebrospinal fluid (CSF). This fluid is normally colorless and sterile. The CSF provides a constant pressure on these vital structures. Measuring the pressure of the CSF and identifying its components can help with the diagnosis of disease and injury of the CNS.

The Autonomic Nervous System

The *autonomic nervous system* is the involuntary part of our nervous system. We are not conscious of its functioning. Composed of *motor neurons* (nerve cells), it carries impulses from the CNS to the heart muscle and the smooth muscle tissue of blood vessels and hollow organs, and it also controls the secretions of glands.

The autonomic nervous system is further subdivided into two parts: the *sympathetic nervous system* and the *parasympathetic nervous system*. Distinguished only by function, the nerves of each part act in opposition to each other. For example, stimulation of the sympathetic branch increases the rate and strength of the heart beat, whereas stimulation of the parasympathetic branch decreases both. Similarly, sympathetic stimulation of neurons to the stomach will decrease gastric secretions, and parasympathetic stimulation will increase gastric secretions.

Sensory Receptors

All over the body are millions of *sensory receptors* that register sensations and elicit reflexes (involuntary responses to stimuli). Changes in the external and internal environment cause these receptors to respond so that bodily adjustments are made that restore or maintain homeostasis. On a cold day, for example, the receptors in the skin register the sensation of coldness and send this message to the thalamus, a mass of gray matter in the inner portion of the brain, which interprets the sensation. A message is then sent, by way of the motor neurons, to the musculature and skin. The result is shivering, the body's attempt to generate heat.

Sensory input refers to all the messages and impressions transmitted to the brain by any of the five senses.

The five senses—vision, hearing, smell, touch, and taste—are essential in providing sensory input. Sights, sounds, tastes, odors, and the sensations of temperature and texture all constitute input. During one's waking hours, thousands of these stimuli are registered in one's consciousness, where they are not only received but also interpreted and sometimes acted on. These messages are received in a repetitive, "rapid-fire" manner, but they are perceived in a smooth-flowing pattern. For example, a symphony is a series of sounds—high and low, short and prolonged but perceived as an overall pattern. Without appropriate sensory input, a person can become disoriented and out of touch with reality and lose the ability to interact with others.

Sensory input is received in a number of ways, both through senses and by receptors within the body. There are three categories: exteroceptors, which are situated on the body's surface for reception of stimuli from the environment, and visceroceptors and proprioceptors, which are internal. The five senses are the exteroceptors: sight, hearing, smell, touch, and taste. These receptors receive stimuli, including temperature and moisture from the environment.

The visceroceptors, which are located in blood vessel walls, the intestines, and other organs, convey changes such as internal pressure and pain to the brain where perceptions (interpretations) occur. The proprioceptors are centered in the muscles and joints and the inner ear. Their function is to help a person sense the position of the various body parts. For example, you can fairly easily put on a coat in the dark because your proprioception tells you the location of your hands and arms when you cannot see them.

Eye

The anatomy and physiology of the *eye* are complex (Fig. 31-2). The eyeball is protected by being recessed into a bony compartment. The outer transparent covering of the eyeball is called the cornea. The tough white portion just beneath the cornea is the sclera, and the pigmented portion is the iris. The choroid layer, which lies just under the sclera, supplies oxygen to the eyes through its vast network of blood vessels and produces aqueous humor. The third, or innermost, layer of the outer eye is the retina, which is made of nerve tissues that comprise the receptors for visual input. The ends of the dendrites of these receptor cells are classified by shape as either rods or cones. The rods provide mainly night vision, and the cones receive daylight images and color. In an opening in the center of the iris is the lens

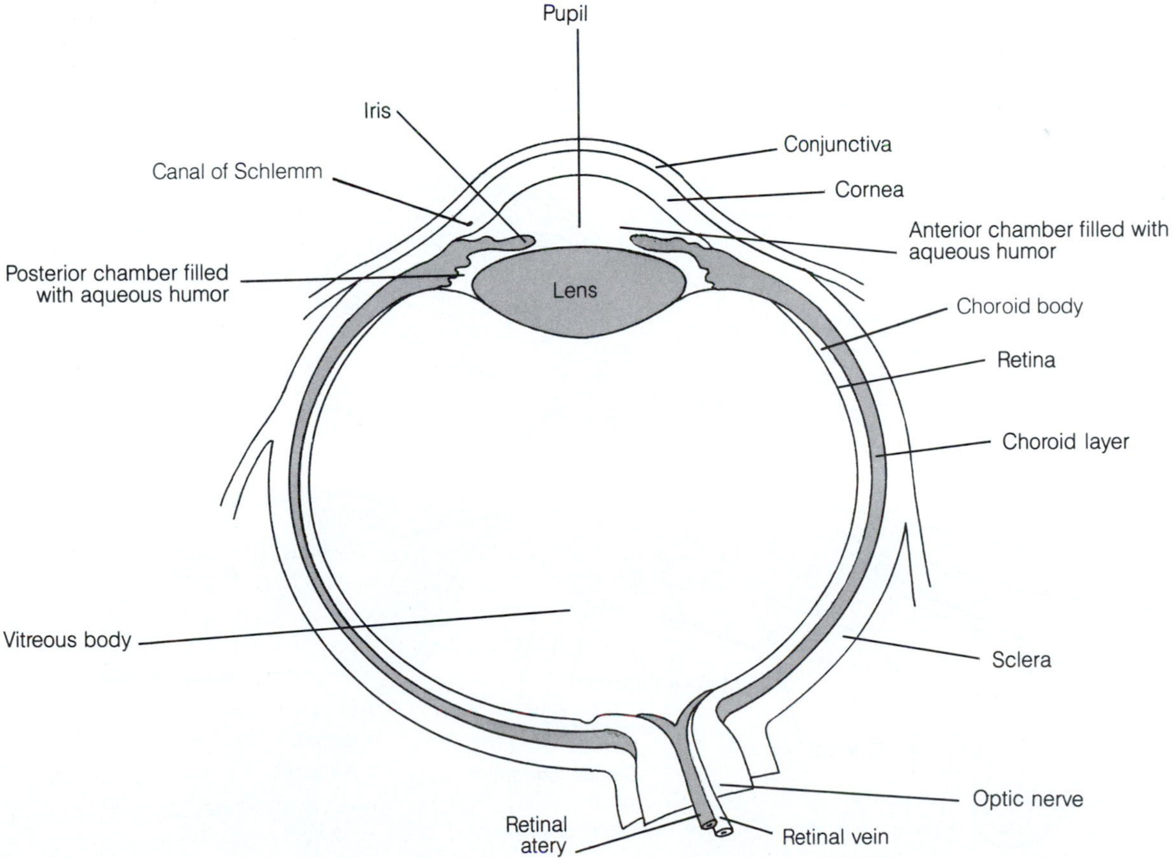

Figure 31-2. Cross section of the left eye.

of the eye, through which pass the images. The opening in front of the lens is called the pupil.

In front of and around the lens is a chamber filled with a clear fluid called the aqueous humor. Posterior to the lens is a much larger chamber filled with a more gelatinous fluid substance called the vitreous humor, the purpose of which is to exert enough inner pressure to prevent the structure of the eye from collapsing. Through a complex system of optic reception by the retina, the optic nerve, located in the posterior portion of the eye ball, transmits visual images. An important point with respect to potential sensory disturbance is the fact that each eye provides images of both the right visual field (what is seen on the right) and the left visual field (what is seen on the left). These images are carried to a point within the brain, the optic chiasma, where the nasal optic fibers cross. This structural phenomenon explains why a person with certain optic nerve deficits in one eye may have impaired sight in both fields rather than total loss of sight in one.

Ear

To better understand the process of hearing, we will briefly discuss the structure and function of the *ear* (Fig. 31-3). Located on each side of the head for maximum reception, the ears are composed of three parts: the outer, middle, and inner ear. The outer ear is the visible trumpetlike cartilage. It is connected to the middle ear by a slightly curved canal. At the end of the canal is the tympanic membrane, or eardrum.

Within the middle ear and surrounded by the temporal bone are three ossicles (small bones), which take their names from their shapes. The malleus (hammer) is attached to the eardrum, the incus (anvil) is attached to the malleus, and the stapes (stirrup) is attached to the incus. The stapes fits precisely into a small membranous structure called the oval window. In the temporal bone there are multiple air spaces for resonance, making up what is called the mastoid area of the middle ear. The middle ear is connected to the pharynx by a tubelike passageway called the eustachian tube, which provides equal pressure within the ear.

The inner ear, or labyrinth, has many parts. The main structure gets its name "cochlea" meaning snail shell, from its spiral shape. Above the cochlea are the three semicircular canals. Some contain hair cells for reception, and others contain a lymphlike fluid.

Stretching the full length of the base of the cochlea is the ear's sensory organ, the organ of Corti. It is within the organ of Corti that hair cells receive sound and transmit it to the brain. Auditory input in the form of sound waves is transmitted from the outer ear, setting up a vibration in the tympanic membrane. The attached malleus also vibrates. Because the three ossicles are at-

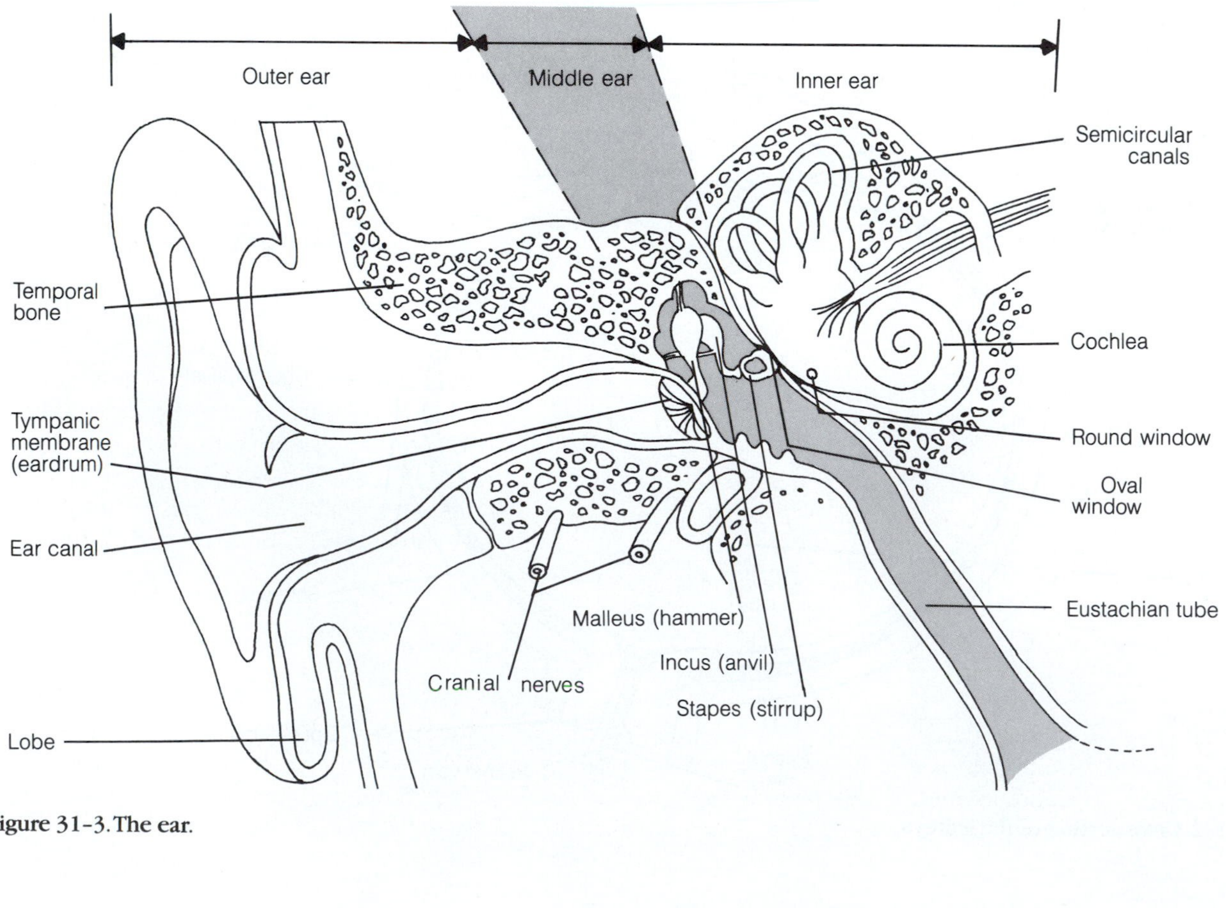

Figure 31-3. The ear.

tached to one another on one end, the incus also moves, causing the stapes to strike the oval window. The fluid on the other side of the window carries the sound waves to the sensing organ, the organ of Corti. Synapsing at locations within the medulla, pons, midbrain, and thalamus, the sound finally reaches the auditory center in the temporal lobe of the brain, where perceptions are made of the input.

Touch

Sensations of *touch* are transmitted by way of sensory neurons on the skin to areas in the spinal cord, or brain stem. After synapsing (connecting with other neurons), the impulses are carried to various parts of the cortex of the brain for interpretation or perception of the stimuli. Receptors may respond differentially to sharp and dull touch. Firm pressure and light touch are also different.

Smell

Structurally much simpler than the eyes and ears, the *nose* consists mainly of the outer portion made up of cartilage that concentrates scents. Persons "sniff" to intensify odors because the first cranial nerves, or sensing organs of the nose lie in the upper portion of the nasal cavity. The ends of these receptors, called the olfactory bulbs, convey smells to the olfactory center in the cortex of the brain for interpretation or perception. These sensing organs fatigue easily, explaining why odors seem to disappear after lengthy exposure times. Touch, pain, itch, and tickle are each carried by different neurons.

Taste

Taste or *gustatory input* is received through the taste buds, which are located on the tongue and the roof of the mouth. These receptors are stimulated by chemical components found in varying amounts in different substances. Taste is either sweet, sour, salty, or bitter. Although some tastes appear to be none of these, they are, in fact, combinations of the four.

Common Functions Controlled by the Nervous System

The nervous system "orchestrates" or coordinates the vital functions of the body. Three of the more important functions of the nervous system are sensation, perception, and cognition.

Sensation

The millions of sensory receptors all over the external surface of the body and in mucous membranes are highly sensitive to changes in the environment. These receptors send messages to the CNS. Within the spinal cord these sensory perceptions from the periphery may be immediately routed to appropriate locations. If, for example, the fingers should touch a hot kettle, a reflex arc within the spinal cord is activated and they are immediately drawn away. The position of the body in space and of the various body parts is constantly monitored by the areas in lower brain that includes the medulla, pons, mesencephalon, amygdala, and hypothalamus. The body responds with coordinated movements that keep the person standing or make walking movements coordinated. Lower brain centers are also responsible for the coordination of such activities as swallowing.

Perception

Perception is the development of an awareness of something within the environment. Perception is a complex phenomenon that begins with the stimulus from the sensory receptor, but involves the processing of that stimulus within the brain. According to Guyton (1992), the brain simply discards as unimportant or irrelevant 99% of the sensory input it receives. The brain selectively passes on sensory data as a part of its integrative function. Strong sensory signals are most likely to be communicated within the brain. The brain will also communicate sensory signals that relate to meaningful stimuli. One of the simplest examples of this is your heightened awareness of people driving cars that are of the same make and model as the new car you just purchased (Fig. 31-4).

Another part of perception is the ability of the brain to sort stimuli into patterns that are meaningful. Because of this ability, you may see a portion of a face and immediately perceive what the whole face would look like. This same ability may cause an individual to perceive something different than what is there. When an individual sees a movement out of the corner of the eye and responds as if a person were there, that may be because the brain "filled in" the details. The brain can also convert distorted or nonmeaningful stimuli into a meaningful pattern. If a person puts on prism glasses that invert all visual stimuli, after a period of time the brain will convert these stimuli into patterns that allow the person to perceive objects in their correct relationships.

Cognition

Cognition, also called mentation, which is controlled by the cortex of the brain, refers to intellectual functioning, that is, the ability to think, recall events, calculate numbers, and solve problems. Cognition also involves more indepth thinking such as the ability to formulate and

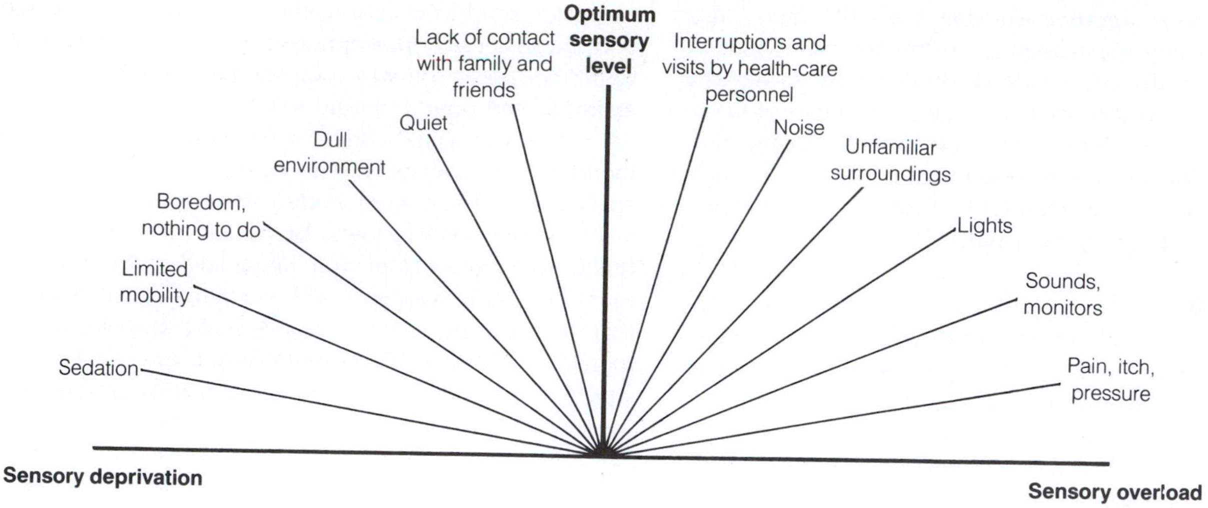

Figure 31-4. The continuum of sensory input.

move toward goals. Abstraction and creativity are other important parts of mentation.

Awareness is the ability to respond to sensory input. **Level of awareness** is the degree to which a person is aware of the surroundings. Part of cognition is to be alert and aware of one's surroundings and therefore able to respond. Normally people are alert and aware of their surroundings.

Another aspect of cognition is *orientation*, which is the person's awareness of the environment in relationship to specific aspects of person, place, and time. Person refers to an understanding both of who he or she is, and who others in the environment are. Orientation to place is the ability to identify current location, such as a hospital in a specific city. Orientation to time is the ability to understand the day and date and might be further expanded to an understanding of the time of day.

There may be a considerable discrepancy between awareness and orientation. A person can be alert and interested in the surroundings and responsive to interpersonal relationships and, at the same time, be disoriented as to person, place, or time. For example, a patient may sit in the dayroom and play cards skillfully and animatedly, all the while recounting numerous telephone calls from the president requesting help with international affairs. Such a patient is considered to have a normal level of awareness while being obviously disoriented.

Common Disorders Affecting Sensory Perception

Several diseases disturb sensory perception because they cause damage to the nerve endings. Among these diseases are diabetes, alcoholism, and multiple sclerosis. Because such disturbances follow the irregular distribution of nerves normal to the body, the affected areas are often uneven or patchy.

Disturbances in sensation most often afflict the extremities, but may also involve the face or trunk. When assessing, ask the patient to describe the disorder. You should know the following terms. *Paresthesia* is distorted skin sensation, such as itching, tingling, crawling, or prickling. A term for decreased sensation is *hypesthesia*. *Hyperesthesia* is increased sensation. Decreased perception of pain is *hypalgesia*, and heightened perception of pain is *hyperalgesia*. Controlled by the nervous system and critical to human function are the five senses: vision, hearing, smelling, touching (tactile), and taste.

Visual Impairment

People can be totally blind or have a visual defect that may range from mild to moderate visual impairment. Many disorders can affect sight. Some people retain central vision while others retain only peripheral vision. Head injury and brain tumors, depending on their location, can affect the CNS so that blindness occurs. Diabetes and degeneration of the macula in advanced years affects the vascular system of the eyes or the integrity of vessels. A common condition in the older adult is *presbyopia*, difficulty in the eyes' accommodating to the distances of objects.

People who were born blind appear to function well using their other senses to compensate. For those who have always relied on sight, however, the adjustment to blindness can be extremely difficult.

Hearing Impairment

Hearing impairments are of two general groups. The first are disorders that prevent normal transmission of sound due to abnormalities of the cochlea or auditory nerve. This category is often referred to as nerve deafness. Congenital conditions and tumors of the auditory nerve can cause this type of deafness. Head trauma can also cause this kind of deafness. The second category of hearing impairment is referred to as conduction deafness, which is common in older adults.

Hearing loss affects those in all phases of the life span, from birth (loss caused by congenital abnormality) through childhood (usually from infections involving the ear) and on into later life (as a result of nerve changes), when hearing loss occurs more frequently than blindness.

Sensory Disturbances

When sensory input is nonmeaningful or of an inappropriate amount, an individual may experience a sensory disturbance.

Sensory Deprivation

Sensory deprivation results from a lower level of sensory input than the individual needs for optimal functioning. Studies show that normal people experimentally subjected to as low a level of sensory input as possible experience irritability, inability to think clearly, perceptual distortion, and changes in brain wave pattern (Bexton, Heron, and Scott, 1954). That such symptoms occurred even though the subjects were consciously participating in an experiment on sensory deprivation suggests that sensorially deprived persons have little control over their reactions.

Sensory Overload

Sensory overload occurs when an individual receives more sensory stimuli during a given period than can be tolerated. It is usually a combination of auditory, visual, and tactile stimuli that overtaxes the patient's sensory receiving mechanism. Overstimulation can disturb perception. The cortex of the brain has difficulty assigning a meaning to each impulse because so many impulses are being received almost simultaneously. Touching a patient at a time of sensory overload may add to the overload to such an extent that it is disturbing rather than comforting. The persistent barrage of input produces symptoms similar to those of sensory deprivation.

Sensory Overload in Nursing

Sensory disturbance does not happen exclusively to patients in the hospital. As a student, you can adjust sensory input to meet your own needs by changing the environment or moving elsewhere. If you want to increase input while studying, you may listen to music. If the phone rings repeatedly, the family or others return home, or street noises become obtrusive, you may take refuge in the library, where the environment is more subdued and input is decreased. However, some people whose professions do not allow them to adjust their environments may suffer from sensory disturbance. Night-duty nurses, computer programmers, miners, and people who work in windowless rooms have been reported to suffer from the effects of sensory deprivation due to monotony and lack of sensory stimuli. Control tower operators in busy airports have sensory overload because of the input produced by aircraft traffic, monitoring equipment, and radio interchange with pilots.

Nurses who work in particularly busy and stressful areas of the hospital, such as the emergency room and intensive care unit, often feel the effects of sensory overload, notable irritability, and undue fatigue. However, it is becoming apparent that sensory overload is not confined to nurses working in these specialty areas. Nurses on any unit are at risk of long periods of sensory overload. The many daily interpersonal interactions that are necessary and the many types of equipment that must be operated substantially contribute to feelings of sensory overload. The stress of nursing, which focuses on repeated and sometimes critical decision-making, adds to overload. The burnout syndrome so widely described is forcing some nurses to quit bedside nursing and its overload potential.

Nurses can take many positive steps when they determine that chronic sensory overload is interfering with their work. Brown (1983) suggests that nurses pursue, in their free time, activities that "bend" the mind in creative ways. Some ideas are classes, art, music, or anything else that is creative and enjoyable. It has been suggested that claiming burnout may be a way of avoiding dealing with work problems that are contributing to sensory overload. Johnson (1982) recommends mutual discussion of problems among coworkers and in groups to reduce burnout from professional overload. Each nurse must develop individual ways of reducing and managing overload so that the care offered to patients remains of the highest quality.

Common Disorders Affecting Cognition

A variety of problems may cause alterations in cognition. Some of these are temporary and others are long term and even permanent.

Delirium

Some disorders such as high fever or toxic conditions can cause a rapidly occurring, temporary, short-term cognitive alteration called delirium. Situations such as low oxygen levels or abnormal fluid and electrolyte levels can also adversely affect the brain and cause delirium. The physiologic disruption affects the ability of the brain to function appropriately. The individual may become confused and disoriented. This may be accompanied by agitation and severe anxiety. A central characteristic of delirium is that it resolves when the condition causing the alteration is resolved.

The patient with delirium may have visual, auditory, or olfactory *hallucinations*, which are perceptions of sights, sounds, or smells that are not present. *Illusions* are misinterpretations of real sights, sounds, or smells, such as perceiving a shadow on the wall as a cat. *Delusions* are faulty thinking patterns. For example, the patient may think she is the mayor of the city.

Dementia

Cognitive impairment may also be based on more serious damage to brain tissue that is slowly developing and may be a permanent disorder called dementia. Dementia is characterized by impairment of memory, judgment, abstract thinking, and changes in personality. Alzheimer's disease is an example of a degenerative process that occurs in the brain tissue. Dementia may also be caused by circulatory impairment in the brain.

Altered Level of Awareness

Depending on the type of disorder, the patient may have different and changing levels of awareness. Generally there are five levels identified. At the level of *consciousness*, one is awake, alert, able to talk, and responsive to all appropriate verbal, visual, tactile, and auditory stimuli. The second level of awareness is *lethargy* or *somnolence*. The person is sleepy and appears to be dozing much of the time. The normal sleeping person can be awakened by stimuli and will respond appropriately. The lethargic person may not respond to your touch or voice. At the third level, *stupor*, the person is so sleepy that continual input is necessary to maintain wakefulness. You may have to repeatedly touch the person or call out the name more than once. The person's conversation may be confused or unclear. At the fourth level of awareness, *light coma* or *semicoma*, the patient no longer responds to verbal stimuli but may move spontaneously in response to physical stimuli. You may notice restlessness in response to discomfort such as from hunger or a wet bed. In *deep coma*, the fifth level, the patient is totally unresponsive to any stimuli except severe pain. There is no voluntary movement, and many of the protective reflexes, such as gagging, blinking, and coughing, may be lost. The very seriously ill patient in deep *coma* may progress to a state of *decerebration*, which is partial or total interruption of the connection between the spinal tracts and the brain. On assessment, these persons are unable to respond to stimuli.

As the patient's level of consciousness changes, you can determine what stimuli he or she responds to and what the patient is aware of. Specific details are much more useful, for example, the word "stupor," which may mean different things to different nurses.

Assessment

Because many of the functions of the body are regulated and controlled by the nervous system, it is important to understand what comprises each function so that you can focus your assessment process. Identification of a deficit does not necessarily mean there is a problem. A problem only arises when the deficit adversely affects the patient's pattern of daily living. Because the nervous system is complicated, for our purposes, we will discuss nursing process in relation to the following functions: cognition and sensory function.

Interview

The most useful interview is one during which you interact with the patient and the family. Sometimes, this is not possible because cognitive impairment may interfere with appropriate responses. On the other hand, if the impairment is one of sensory perception, the patient will be the one who is most able to describe the problem and its impact on daily life. An interview also provides an opportunity to find out about patients' feelings. Emotionally healthy persons have and show feelings about the events in their lives and the environment in which they live. The following are suggestions that you may choose to ask during the interview:

1. Has there been a similar problem at present or in the past with others in the family?
2. How would the person or family describe the problem?
3. How long has the problem been present and is its cause known?
4. How does the problem affect daily living?
5. Are there things that have been done which appear to improve the problem or solve factors that interfere with daily living?
6. Have any resources been used, either in the facility or in the community?
7. Tell us how we might help.

The interview gives the nurse valuable information and allows the patient and family to review the illness or disability together in a sharing environment.

Physical Assessment

Because the problems in these areas are so numerous and diverse, the nurse is compelled to assess the particular area that is of concern. It may be more difficult to assess cognitive impairment than it is to assess sensory concerns such as visual or hearing impairment.

Assessment of Cognitive Function

A mental status examination (MSE) is a comprehensive approach to assessing cognitive function. This includes both descriptive parameters and parameters that require active testing of the individual, beginning with the more basic testing of person, place, and time. This means that you assess whether the patient is oriented in terms of *person* (who he or she is), *place* (present location), and *time* (the general time of day, month, and year). When this information is recorded, the notation "Oriented × 3" means that the patient is oriented in all three spheres—person, place, and time. You then can assess higher level functioning, ending with judgment questions.

The nurse should consider the feelings of those being questioned and be sensitive to the fact that some can become anxious if they are unable to answer appropriately. The elderly may become angry because they see it as an indication that we think they are "crazy" or are "losing it." If the patient is assessed as confused, it is important to be specific about the type. For example, a patient may know his name and where he is but have no idea of the year; any variation is possible in a confused state. You must be cautious when gathering such information, for assertions that sound confused may not be so. For example, an elderly patient in an acute care facility stated that she was dictating a book about Indians in Montana. Although she was severely handicapped and had come to the facility from a nursing home where she had resided for some time, she had indeed been writing such a book and was not confused. Another patient stated that he had walked to a town 50 miles away the night before, when the nurses knew he had been in bed. This was clear evidence of confusion. Assessment should carefully describe any delusions rather than state that the patient has delusions.

A comprehensive MSE takes considerable time and because it is reported as a detailed narrative, it is sometimes not suited to situations where a brief preliminary assessment of cognitive status is needed. It is also more difficult for different observers to be sure that they are judging behavior in exactly the same manner. Therefore, short, quantified mental status assessment tools have been developed to provide a rapid method of assessment and a numeric score that allows for ease of comparing an individual's status as it changes over time. The two most commonly used are the Folstein Mini-Mental Status Questionnaire (Folstein and Rovner, 1987; Fig. 31-5) and the Short, Portable Mental Status Questionnaire, SPMSQ (Pfeiffer, E, 1975).

Assessment of Sensory Function

Although the physician uses a variety of techniques to test sensory integrity, the best data may be the patient's subjective description.

Touch can be assessed through using a variety of objects to touch the skin. You can assess for light touch by touching the skin with a cotton ball, or a tongue depressor may be used to exert more pressure on the skin and test for firm touch. Sharp and dull touch may be differentiated by using a pin point and a blunt object. Assessment should include having patients describe the ability to feel touch in their own words. Some medical conditions such as diabetes and neuromuscular conditions affect touch.

Vision is often assessed through an interview with the patient or family. The wearing of glasses or contact lenses is also assessment data. You may observe the patient's difficulty with vision. To perform a thorough assessment, it is useful to have knowledge of the structure of the eye.

Assessment of vision is a sensitive matter because no one who is sighted can truly understand what it means to lose one's sight—the familiar environment becomes unfamiliar and frightening, and one can no longer see the facial expressions of the people one loves.

Nurses can make assessments of long-standing visual impairments through use of the nursing history. Visually impaired patients can usually describe their disabilities and tell you how you can be of help. Ongoing assessment of visual changes can be made through subjective and objective data.

Techniques to assess *hearing* are similar to those you can use to assess vision. The nursing history will tell you of long-standing problems. Speak to the patient in a normal, well-modulated voice and observe the person's comprehension of what has been said. You may notice that the person is not hearing well on one side or that the hearing loss is generalized. The older patient's hearing loss is usually bilateral (on both sides), but one side will often be better than the other.

The nurse should also assess for the ability to *smell*. The sensations of smell are called *olfactory input*. Some medical conditions diminish the ability to smell. Loss of smell is termed *anosmia*. You can assess for smell by asking the patient to close the eyes and identify the odor of vanilla, cloves, or other familiar household odors.

You may assess *taste* by listening to statements made by the patient about tasting the various components of food or specific tastes such as salty or sweet.

Mini Mental Status Examination

Maximum Score	Patient Score
	Orientation
5	What is the date (ie, day of week, day of month, month, year), season?
5	Where are we: (hospital) (state) (county) (town) (floor)?
	Registration
3	Name three objects, taking 1 s to say each. Then ask the patient to repeat all three. Give 1 point for each correct answer. Then repeat them until patient learns all three. Count trials and record. Number of trials _______
	Attention and Calculation
5	Serial 7s. Give 1 point for each correct answer. Stop after five answers. If subject refuses, ask him to spell "world" backwards.
	Recall
3	Ask the patient to name the three objects cited above. Give 1 point for each correct answer.
	Language and Praxis
2	Point to a pencil and a watch and ask the patient to name them. (2 points)
1	Ask the patient to: Repeat the following: "No ifs, ands, or buts." (1 point)
3	Follow a three-stage command: "Take a paper in your right hand, fold it in half, and put it on the floor." (3 points)
1	Read and obey the following sign: "Close your eyes." (1 point)
1	Write a sentence. (1 point)
1	Copy this design. (1 point)
30 Maximum Score	Patient Total

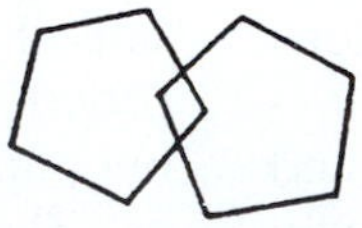

Figure 31-5. Folstein Mini Mental Status Questionnaire. (From Folstein M. F., Rovner, B. W. Mini mental status exam in clinical practice. *Hospital Practice* 22, 1A (1987):99–110.)

Because the nose and mouth are in close proximity, smell and taste affect each other. For example, a common cold may cause one to lose a portion of the ability both to taste and smell.

Assessment of Sensory Input

The level of sensory input is the result of the sum total of all types of sensory stimuli. You will need to observe the environment and identify what the sensory stimuli are in that environment. Examine the lighting. Is it overly bright? Does it change from day to night? Can the patient control the lighting? What is the noise level on the unit? Consider the sounds that are present. Are the sounds loud or soft? Can voices be understood or are there constant sounds of voices that cannot be distinguished? If music is in the environment, consider whether it is the type of music that the individual prefers.

To assess a patient for possible sensory disturbance, you should know something about the sensory level to which the patient is most accustomed and accommodates best. A busy, outgoing, aggressive businessman suddenly placed on strict bed rest in a private room may develop sensory deprivation fairly rapidly. Conversely, a nursing home resident who is transferred to the hospital could develop sensory overload because of a sudden rise in the level of input.

Patients in hospitals are in a captive environment in the sense that they typically have little control over the quantity of input they receive. Because the study of sensory input is relatively new, many patients and health care workers are unaware that certain feelings and symptoms are attributable to sensory disturbances and not directly to the disease process.

The optimal level of sensory input to which a patient can respond appropriately at any given time is greatly influenced by how that person perceives the stimuli. Several factors influence this. The first is *knowledge* of the input. For example, if a strange sound is heard, its source needs to be identified so that it can be integrated and a response made. Knowledge is based on *past experience.* Has the sound been heard before? *Attitude and mental status* also play a part in perception. Input that may be perceived as pleasant at one time and may prove irritating at another because the listener is too fatigued for proper integration to occur. If a person has a serious illness that has altered the level of awareness, even familiar sensory input may be misperceived because of the organic nature of the medical condition. Perception of sensory input may also change because of the level of input desired at a certain time. For example, a patient may have the need to relax and rest, having low sensory input. The administration of medications or the taking of vital signs may intrude on a desired level of input. It is also important to recognize that people usually cope better if high input periods are followed by lower levels of sensory input. When the *sensory level* is perceived as being too high or too low or when perceptions are faulty, sensory and perceptual disturbances can occur. Persons who are ill and in an unfamiliar environment are particularly prone to these problems.

Assessment of the Individual's Response

Assessment for potential or existing problems of sensory disturbance consists of studying the environment in which the patient is placed and the patient's response to that environment. Assess for the presence of symptoms such as irritability and childish responses that may be caused by sensory disturbance. If sensory disturbance becomes severe enough, lack of clarity in thought and illusions can occur. *Illusions* are false perceptions of visible objects. For example, a patient may see a rounded vase of fluffy pussywillows as a bird with a large feathery tail. If sensory disturbance becomes extreme, actual *hallucinations* can develop. A patient who hallucinates sees sights or hears sounds that are not actually there. A thorough assessment of the patient and the situation is necessary to determine whether sensory deprivation or sensory overload is responsible for hallucinations.

The nurse sees such symptoms manifested in the behavior of the patient. Assessment is especially important when patients are immobilized or psychologically less responsive than usual because such patients are often unable to give clear cues as to the source of their discomfort.

Each patient must be assessed as an individual. Irritability and unclear thought do not necessarily mean that a patient has a sensory disturbance. The same symptoms may be caused by such other conditions as generalized infection, electrolyte imbalance, drug intoxication, or the illness itself. Keeping in mind the patient's diagnosis will make your assessment more accurate and complete.

Assessment of Speech

Speech is a complex phenomenon controlled both by the speech center in the cerebral cortex (usually in the left hemisphere for right-handed people and in the right hemisphere for left-handed people) and by motor innervation of the mouth and tongue. **Aphasia** literally means "absence of speech," but usually implies impairment of language function due to brain involvement. *Dysarthria* means interference with enunciation and articulation, usually due to impairment of motor innervation to muscles of speech. A speech therapist should be involved in the assessment and care of the aphasic patient. However, nurses are often the first to assess such a deficit and, as members of the health care team, enter into the ongoing plan of care.

Table 31–1. Levels of Awareness

Level	Behavior	Responsiveness
1. Consciousness	Awake, alert, able to talk	Responsive to all verbal, visual, tactile, and auditory stimuli
2. Lethargy or somnolence	Very sleepy or asleep; able to verbalize when awake	Can be awakened by and will respond appropriately to normal stimuli
3. Stupor	Very sleepy, may fall asleep in the middle of a conversation; able to verbalize when awake	Can be aroused with concerted effort, which may have to be physical as well as verbal; needs constant input to stay awake
4. Light coma or semicoma	No longer responsive to verbal stimuli, difficult to arouse; some spontaneous movement; restlessness in response to discomfort	Responsive to bright lights, light pin prick, discomfort, physical movement
5. Deep coma	Totally unresponsive, many protective reflexes lost; if decerebrate, may emit high-pitched cry, assume opisthotonos position, exhibit disturbance of vital signs	May respond to severely painful stimuli

Assessment for aphasia may involve any of four types of deficits. First, many patients, particularly those suffering strokes, have what is called *expressive aphasia.* These persons have difficulty expressing the correct word for objects although understanding is intact. For example, they may call a chair a television set although they know the difference. Hearing themselves express the incorrect word for objects they know is distressing. This deficit may also extend to written communication.

Receptive aphasia is present when hearing is intact but the patient has difficulty understanding spoken or written words. This type of aphasia interferes greatly with providing care because the patient may have difficulty following directions or participating in decisions.

Amnesic aphasia involves completely forgetting the names of objects, rather than assigning incorrect names. This type of aphasia occurs less frequently than the others. Finally, some unfortunate patients with serious neu-

Table 31–2. Neurologic Assessment

	Normal	Abnormal
Mentation	Alert, aware of surroundings; oriented to person, place and time	Any disorientation, including confusion, hallucinations, illusions, or delusions
Level of awareness	Alert and responsive to the environment	Any alteration in level of awareness; lethargy, stupor, semicoma, or deep coma
Coordination	Hand and finger movement and ambulation free of unsteadiness or tremor	Difficulty using hands or fingers, as to hold objects; unsteady gait; tremor
Muscular strength	Strong, equal grip; legs able to support weight; face symmetrical	Weak grip, difficulty elevating legs, drooping eyelids or drooling mouth
Movement	No evidence of paralysis; able to move all musculature normally	Unable to move one or more extremities or any other muscular area voluntarily
Swallowing	Able to swallow solid foods, liquids, and saliva without difficulty	Unable to swallow solid food and/or liquids without choking
Speech	Speaks clearly and understandably	Unable to speak and/or understand words; may be unable to interpret symbols
Vision	Able to read newspaper or magazine print and see persons and objects, with corrective lenses if necessary	Unable to read newspaper or magazine print and see persons or objects, even with corrective lenses
Hearing	Able to hear and understand normal voice and other sounds with each ear	Unable to hear and understand normal voice and other sounds with one or both ears
Smell	Able to detect the odor of ordinary household items (e.g., vinegar, vanilla)	Unable to detect the odor of ordinary household items (eg, vinegar, vanilla)
Touch	Appropriately sensitive to sensory stimulation	Distorted, increased, or decreased sensation, including pain

Nursing Diagnoses Related to Sensory Perception and Cognition

High Risk for Injury
Altered Thought Processes
Sensory/Perceptual Alterations
Unilateral Neglect
Self-care Deficit (specify bathing/hygiene, feeding, dressing/grooming, toileting)
Impaired Verbal Communication
Social Isolation
Anxiety
Anticipatory Grieving
Dysfunctional Grieving
Altered Health Maintenance
Situational Low Self-esteem
Body Image Disturbance
Sexual Dysfunction
Diversional Activity Deficit

rologic deficit have *global aphasia.* These patients have both expressive and receptive aphasia to some degree and are greatly handicapped in communicating.

When you are assessing the patient, difficulty with speech will be apparent to you. Family members can also add to your data by reporting speech difficulties or changes in speech patterns.

Assessment of Level of Awareness

When assessing sensory input level, making the assessment as specific as possible renders changes in status more noticeable. For example, if a patient who did not previously appear aware of the lowering of a side rail begins to roll about when the rail is let down, this might indicate that the patient's level of awareness has risen and therefore might be regarded as a sign of improvement (Table 31-1).

Specific testing may be used to determine whether an unconscious patient's level of awareness is changing. One technique is to observe the patient for signs of awareness of nearby voices or noise. The patient may, for example, grimace or move about in bed. Calling the patient's name to see if he or she responds is referred to as *name-call* and charted that way. A bit more complex is the *command.* Instruct the patient to do something, such as "move your left leg" or "squeeze my hand," and observe the response. The only requirement is to command something the patient is reasonably capable of doing. Neurologically, one step beyond response to a command is *verbalization.* Depending on the patient's visual acuity, you might ask the color of the ceiling or a bright cup.

Assessment of Neurologic Signs

Neurologic signs, or *neuro signs,* are a set of brief tests of neurologic status performed first for baseline data and then to identify changes of status (Table 31-2). Although there is some variation among facilities, testing neuro signs usually includes checking 1) pulse, respiration, and blood pressure; 2) determining level of awareness; 3) examining pupillary response to light; and 4) testing for muscle strength and control (see Module 13, Inspection, Palpation, Auscultation, and Percussion).

Nursing Diagnosis

A variety of nursing diagnoses related to cogntion or sensory perception occur.

High Risk for Injury

Patient safety is always of first priority when providing care. The variety of problems that can emerge for the patient with cognitive or sensory problems are numerous. Consider the person's impairment when writing the diagnosis and outcome so that the implementation can be focused toward adequate protection.

At High Risk for Injury is also a nursing diagnosis related to decreased mentation or levels of awareness because the person cannot respond to the environment in a way that offers protection. People in this category may range from those with a short attention span and lack of concentration to individuals in a state of coma. The desired outcome for any nursing diagnosis centered around safety is that the patient will remain safe and not experience any untoward incident.

Lack of sensation can lead to *decreased sensitivity* to injury or heat and cold. The nursing diagnosis of High Risk for Injury related to peripheral insensitivity should also have added the specific threat that may occur. This diagnosis would serve to protect the patient.

Altered Thought Processes

The nursing diagnosis Altered Thought Processes is written for the patient who is confused and has a deficit in reality orientation, judgment, or problem solving. To guide implementation, a clearer statement of the exact condition that the patient is experiencing is helpful in determining actions that are appropriate and providing safety for the patient. If the etiology is known, this is also helpful in understanding whether the alteration is long or short term and determining desired outcomes.

Altered thought processes can result from genetic disorders such as developmental delay, maturational disorders that occur in the very old, or situational disorders such as those that occur with profound loss and depression. The nurse's focus on nursing actions may vary depending on the type of alteration.

Sensory/Perceptual Alterations

An important nursing diagnosis approved by the North American Nursing Diagnosis Association (NANDA) for those with deficits of any of the five senses is Sensory/Perceptual Alteration. After this category, specify whether the deficit is visual, auditory, kinesthetic, gustatory, tactile, or olfactory and indicate the etiology. People who are visually or hearing impaired could also have their problems identified under this category.

Although not yet adopted by NANDA, many nurses indicate problems with potential or actual sensory overload or sensory deprivation under this general NANDA category. At High Risk for Sensory Overload (or Deprivation) would be written so that the environmental or personal factor creating high risk is indicated. The nursing diagnosis, then, identifies the person at risk. Actual problems, supported by assessment, must also include the presenting situation causing the patient's signs or symptoms.

Sensory Deprivation

The following discussion refers to the defining characteristics of nursing diagnoses for disturbances in sensory input. In the assessment phase, nurses must identify patients who are at high risk of sensory disturbance. Some are more susceptible than others to sensory deprivation. Using one or more of the three parameters—condition, environment, and symptoms (behavior)—consider several categories of patients for whom you might care. Patients residing in chronic care facilities commonly suffer sensory deprivation, for they may be in bed much of the time and may have roommates who are unable to communicate, infrequent visitors, and contacts with the staff only when care is given. Private rooms, intended to provide for undisturbed rest, may promote deprivation of the senses.

Patients with mild sensory deprivation often complain simply that they are bored. After less than 3 hours of lying in the recumbent position, patients can begin to exhibit signs of sensory deprivation (Downs, 1974). The recumbent position distorts visual images and auditory perception and forces the patient to adapt to a new spatial environment. An understanding of sensory deprivation has resulted in hospital rooms becoming more colorful and visually stimulating.

When a fragile older adult with diminishing senses appears listless and withdrawn, the cause may be insufficient sensory input (Fig. 31-6). Efforts to engage the remaining senses can bring about a remarkable reversal in attitude and behavior, making the person more outgoing and contented.

Patients in isolation are particularly susceptible to sensory deprivation. Patients may be isolated for various medical reasons and with different degrees of stringency. It appears that sensory deprivation is directly related to the degree of isolation imposed. For example, when you care for a patient in strict isolation for meningitis, the patient has little input of you as a person when you wear a gown, a cap over your hair, a mask, gloves, and cloth boots over your shoes. The room is often sparsely furnished to diminish the likelihood of the spread of bacteria. Individuals rely greatly on visual impressions of the people with whom they interact, and to see only people's eyes can be disconcerting.

Sensory Overload

The defining characteristics of the nursing diagnosis of sensory deprivation also apply to the nursing diagnosis of sensory overload. The parameters used for assessment for sensory deprivation are also used for assessment for sensory overload: condition, environment, and symptoms. Is the patient's condition such that he or she needs constant surveillance by sophisticated medical equipment and personnel? This situation demands a multiplicity of stimuli within a small area and can lead to sensory overload. A hospital unit, which is different in appearance, routine, and pace from a private home, can bombard the patient with unfamiliar input. A patient awakened for the measurement of vital signs, disturbed for morning care, and subjected to many tests and procedures will commonly exhibit irritability. Patients who are extremely ill are particularly at high risk. The insertion of tubes or catheters and frequent injections repre-

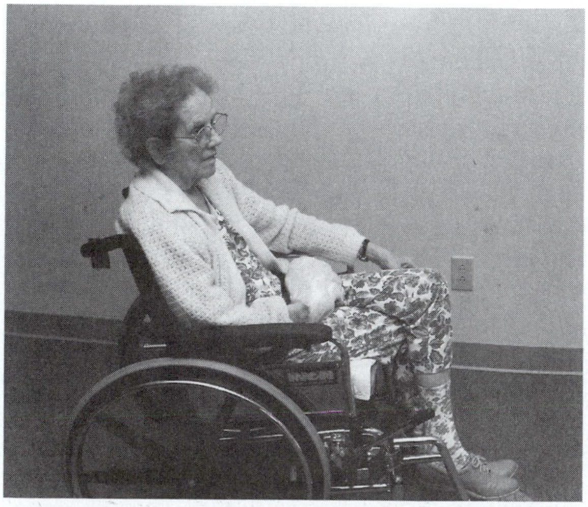

Figure 31-6. A patient at high risk for sensory deprivation.

sent additional input, as well as causing discomfort. Touch, which is valuable to the patient suffering from sensory deprivation, can arouse anxiety in the patient with an overload of stimuli. Constant touching, turning, and testing may raise anxiety to the level of panic.

Unilateral Neglect

The person with a nursing diagnosis of Unilateral Neglect is one who is perceptively unaware or inattentive to one side of the body. A variety of patients have this problem. Some stroke patients have lost sensation to touch over areas on one side of the body. Before some of these people are aware enough to understand that they have suffered a neurologic deficit, they may actively attempt to disown the affected extremity by "throwing" the part from the bed (hemiballismus). Other people with this nursing diagnosis are those with hemianopsia with a visual field defect so that they cannot see to one side.

The patient with Unilateral Neglect as a nursing diagnosis may have other related nursing diagnoses such as self-care deficits or deficiencies in nutrition related to leaving part of the diet on the plate because of the inability to see.

Self-care Deficits

A person may not be able to perform hygiene or other aspects of self-care unaided if cognition is impaired. You would write Self-care Deficit and identify the specific activities that cannot be performed. This might involve feeding, toileting, or hygiene. If all of these functions are impaired the deficit is indicated as total.

Impaired Verbal Communication

Impaired Verbal Communication is a general category approved by NANDA to describe the various speech problems experienced by patients with neurologic involvement. These diagnoses may be written in such a way as to identify how the speech difficulty may be interfering with the person's ability to communicate needs as well as how the speech problem may be causing emotional distress.

Social Isolation

A related nursing diagnosis might be Social Isolation, which reflects feelings of loneliness or the inability to respond to significant others. This is especially likely to occur in those whose ability to communicate with others is impaired by their sensory deficits. The person with a hearing deficit may be severely limited in the ability to interact in a meaningful way with others. In turn, others may find that it is so much effort to communicate that they stop trying and the person is further isolated.

Anxiety

Both anxiety and depression can be present for the person with temporary or long-standing impairments that interfere with quality of life. Anxiety is an approved NANDA nursing diagnosis. Depression may be the etiology for a diagnosis of Ineffective Individual Coping. It is important to recognize that these feelings may be appropriate for those whose lives have been disrupted by disabling illness. You should look carefully at the person's coping abilities before arriving at the conclusion that there is a specific problem. Thorough assessment through establishing a trusting relationship with the patient is crucial before arriving at these diagnoses.

Anticipatory or Dysfunctional Grieving

When a person has lost any of a variety of bodily functions, a grieving process is not only present but necessary for resolution and adaptation. Although Grieving has only recently been approved as a NANDA nursing diagnosis, it is appropriate to use because all health care providers need to recognize the presence of grieving so that they can be supportive and understanding. The nurse must also be sensitive to any problems with this process that interfere with opportunities for personal growth. Again, defining characteristics and outcome criteria are essential to include (see Chapter 41).

Altered Health Maintenance

A diagnosis of Altered Health Maintenance indicates that a person has an inability to identify, manage, or seek out help to maintain health. The individual with sensory or cognitive disturbance may lack the ability to plan for and carry out essential health maintenance activities. A high level of understanding, conceptual processing, and future orientation are necessary precursors to participation in many health-related activities. When planning for patient discharge from a hospital, this is an especially important consideration.

Other Pertinent Nursing Diagnoses

Many other nursing diagnoses are often relevant for care of the person with regulatory or cognitive impairment. Some of these are Self-esteem Disturbance, Body Image Disturbance, Spiritual Distress, and Altered Family Processes. Many nursing diagnoses may have both physiologic and psychological components. Some examples are Sleep Pattern Disturbance, Sexual Dysfunction, and Diversional Activity Deficit. Writing nursing diagnoses for patients with multiple impairments requires a high level of skill and practice on the part of the nurse.

Planning and Implementation

As you plan for the individual with a nursing diagnosis related to cognitive or sensory dysfunction, you will want to consider the appropriate desired outcomes. Disorders of the nervous system may be serious and long standing. Nursing intervention can seldom change the underlying cause. Frequently, the desired outcome is that a person make adaptations or adjustments that can lead to a more acceptable pattern of daily living. Desired outcomes may involve the person's emotional response to the situation as well as behaviors that may change.

You cannot plan for nursing action unless you accurately identify the perceptual or cognitive deficits and their effects on the patient's life. Some people may have more than one deficit. Determining how the problems are perceived by the individual and the family and how they actually interfere with living is essential. Both of these may be addressed when planning. Planning must be specific to the patient and the problem. Understanding some general approaches will assist you to plan effectively.

Providing Care for the Person With Cognitive Impairment

Patients who are confused or disoriented tend to make us uncomfortable. In our everyday lives, we expect people to react to us in rational ways. Some patients recognize and acknowledge their confusion and are upset by it. Telling such patients that you can appreciate how upsetting their confusion must be and assuring them that the confusion is due to their illness elicits a sense of relief in many. It is important to note that we are not considering the severely disturbed psychiatric patient here; the care of such patients requires special knowledge and training.

Cognitive impairment may be temporary and reversible or long standing and irreversible. Identifying the type and length of impairment guides appropriate implementation. For example, when a child is temporarily cognitively impaired by a high fever or injury, providing a safe, comforting environment that includes the parents may be the most important nursing action. Because the condition is temporary, reorienting the child has merit. Adults who have a temporary cognitive impairment or are in the early stages of irreversible impairment may also benefit from comfort measures and reality orientation. When caring for persons with temporary reversible impairment, it may be helpful to include the family with whom the patient relates, play familiar music, display a calendar, and explain unfamiliar objects in the environment. If the patient is not fearful, a gentle touch is an effective way of communicating caring. Distraught and confused patients usually react positively to a quiet, confident attitude on the part of the nurse.

A far different approach may be appropriate when caring for the confused patient with advanced Alzheimer's disease or another irreversible dementia. Attempting to orient this person to reality may be counterproductive, resulting in increasing agitation. In 1966, Feil developed a method called Validation Therapy in which the health care provider "validates" the individual by demonstrating interest and empathy. For example, an older, confused nursing home resident might say, "I have to go home now and fix dinner for my young children!" If the staff person, even with intended kindness

Nursing Research: *Implications for Practice*

Abraham, I. L., Neundorfer, M. M., and Currie, L. J. "Effects of Group Interventions on Cognition and Depression in Nursing Home Residents." *Nursing Research* 41,4 (July-August 1992): 196–202.

Seventy-six older nursing home residents with mild to moderate cognitive impairment and depression were participants in a nurse-led 24-week intervention group. Subjects were assessed for degree of impairment 4 weeks before intervention, at 8 and 20 weeks into the intervention protocol, and 4 weeks after the treatment intervention. Two groups and techniques were used: first, "cognitive behavioral," which focuses on actively exploring attitudes about the self and their effects on social interactions; and second, "visual imagery," which involves deep breathing and relaxation to achieve the ability to imagine restful and interesting "pictures."

Participants in both groups showed significant improvement on cognitive scores 8 weeks after the intervention group experience. The investigators suggest that using these techniques may reduce cognitive impairment in a selected number of nursing home residents.

says, "Oh, no, this is your home now and your children are all grown," the cognitively impaired may become agitated, hostile, and frightened. Using the validation technique, you would instead reply, "You have never told me about your home and when the children were young—could you tell me about that?" This encourages reminiscing, focusing on positive accomplishments, and reinforces the individual's worth as a person. The central principle is to encourage the individual to share life as he or she remembers it and to validate the person's worth. A 1973 study by Feil showed that "denial is the common life-time defense against stress for disoriented old-old (80–100 years) who use fantasy to survive" (Feil, 1989). Nursing intervention should include neither arguing nor agreeing with confused perceptions.

Providing Care for the Person With Sensory Impairment

Loss of any of the *special senses* can be accompanied by a disturbance in body image (see Chapter 35). Implementation must relate directly to assessment. Many patients have been sightless or deaf since birth and have adjusted to living life normally. They enter the facility for other reasons so that your nursing actions revolve around care to meet the special needs of the individual patient. On the other hand, a sudden loss of hearing or sight interferes directly with the person's interaction with others and the environment and causes understandable grief; in such a situation, the ultimate sensitivity is required by the nurse.

Visual Impairment

Planning care of the patient with visual impairment takes a thoughtful and creative approach. The person may manage well within the familiar surroundings of the home or a long-term care setting but have difficulty in the unfamiliar acute care setting. The plan should include learning the spatial arrangement of the hospital and should address hazards that may place the person at risk of injury. The plan should also consider that the patient needs to feel psychologically safe.

Although the needs of sightless patients differ, several things are always necessary when you give care to the blind. On entering the room, immediately identify yourself. This lets the patient know who is there and gives a sense of security. Most visually impaired people welcome touch, and grasping the patient's hand or touching the shoulder is comforting. When an ambulatory blind patient is first admitted, orient the person to the room by explaining where the furniture and bathroom facilities are located while at the same time helping the patient locate each object by touch. Do not change the arrangement of the furniture and arrange food items the same way on the tray at each meal. You might help the patient make selections from the menu because usually it is printed.

Safety must be considered when a blind person is hospitalized. Hot liquids should be set aside to cool to a safe temperature until the patient is ready to drink them. Any smoking behavior should be carefully monitored. Encourage the person to ask for assistance when getting out of bed and ambulating.

The blind person lacks much meaningful stimuli. Music may be a valued diversion. For the patient who reads Braille, many publications can be obtained. The U.S. Library of Congress has an excellent program for the sightless, providing the Bible, books, magazines, recipes, and instructional materials on tape or cassette free of charge; the tape and recording equipment are also provided at no cost. A blind person can also request that any material not already available be recorded on tape or record. Regional counseling services for the blind provide a variety of services, including special thermostats, telephone dialing devices, and many other conveniences for use in the home (Fig. 31-7).

The advent of sudden blindness can be frightening and isolating. It is a time for family and friends to move close to the patient psychologically. The nurse can offer encouragement and support for the maintenance of maximum independence.

Hearing Impairment

The patient who is aware of hearing loss will often tell you how you can be of assistance. "Could you please speak louder? I don't hear well" is a common response. Some persons wear hearing aids. You should be able to care for these devices. The patient who is aware usually does not need assistance in changing batteries. You should learn to do this (a simple procedure) and also know that the aid should not come in contact with water. You should also not allow wax deposits to build up in the hearing chamber of the device. For guidelines on caring for hearing aids, consult a nursing procedure module.

Many of the hearing impaired have learned to lip-read. Some deaf people communicate by means of *signing*—visual language that uses the positions of the hands and fingers to denote letters, words, and phrases.

Planning for care of the patient with a hearing impairment also takes a thoughtful and often creative approach although safety may not be as large an issue as it is with those who are visually impaired. A major concern is planning to meet communication needs. A variety of alternative approaches to meeting communication needs are presented here. You may need to use more than one method to establish effective communication. If one approach does not work, you may wish to try another.

Keep several things in mind when caring for a patient with a hearing deficit. When entering the patient's

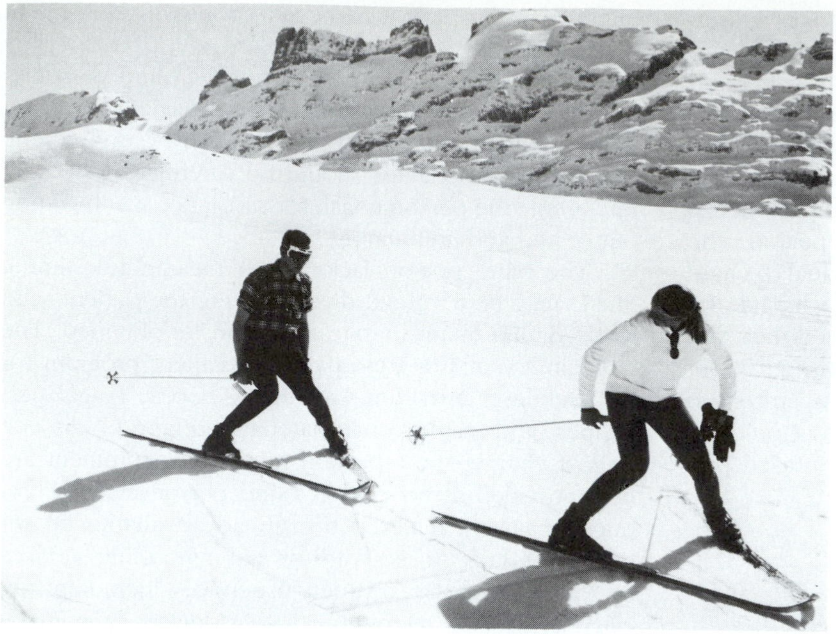

Figure 31-7. The visually handicapped individual may still enjoy active sports such as skiing.

room, come into the person's line of sight immediately so that he or she knows you are there and can identify you. If the patient has some hearing in one ear, stand on that side when you speak. With patients who lip-read, stand or sit directly in front of the patient and speak distinctly but normally. Electronic sound amplification instruments enable some patients to hear better. Write down important communications so that they will not be misunderstood. Use visual aids when performing health teaching. Most large facilities have staff members who know *signing* and will be glad to help you communicate with the hearing impaired. If no such person is on the staff, a call to the local organization for the deaf will locate a resource person. Sign languages vary, and more than one method may be used in your area.

Safety is also a matter of particular concern in dealing with the hearing impaired because deaf people cannot hear alarms or verbal warnings. Fire alarm systems that use bright lights instead of aural alarms are available for use in the home. Many states now have a law that makes it possible for those designated as hearing impaired to have a special telephone device for communication. This device, formerly called a TTY (for teletype), is now referred to as a TDD, which stands for a telecommunication device for the deaf. Both the person sending the message and the person receiving the message must have a TDD. Messages are typed out and received either on a screen or as a printout. This device allows the hearing-impaired person to communicate with another hearing-impaired person as well as with those whose hearing is intact. The device is purchased by the user. The cost of the service to the hearing-impaired person is no greater than that paid for regular telephone service by other customers. The states in which this is in effect levy a small tax on all customers to pay for the difference in costs. These devices are also available in most large hospitals through their telecommunication department, or they can be supplied to the individual patient by the local telephone service company for a fee. The use of computers offers new technology that can assist the hearing impaired.

Providing Care for the Person With Sensory Disturbance

Nursing planning and implementation for sensory disturbance may focus on prevention and intervention. Preventing sensory disturbance is far preferable to intervening once it has occurred. If the patient's condition or environment seems to be a potential cause of sensory disturbance, the nurse may be able to modify one or the other. Changing the environment is usually easier than altering the patient's condition. A variety of specific interventions may be used with sensory disturbance.

Studies show that the input provided to relieve sensory disturbance must be meaningful to the patient. For example, music the patient enjoys stimulates the senses, whereas incidental noise in the hall may be ineffective in relieving symptoms and only produce agitation. Only stimuli interpreted by the individual as serving some purpose represent effective input.

Overcoming Sensory Deprivation

Overcoming sensory deprivation usually requires that additional meaningful stimuli be provided (see sample Nursing Care Plan Related to Sensory Deprivation).

Nursing Care Plan
Sample Nursing Care Plan Related to Sensory Deprivation

Nursing Diagnosis

Sensory/Perceptual Alterations: Sensory deprivation, related to restricted environment

Supportive data:

46-year-old man.

Myocardial infarction 3 days ago.

On cardiac monitor in unit.

States, "This place is beginning to drive me buggy! There is nothing to do."

Occupation: financial planner.

Orders to restrict visitors.

Interests: classical music, travel. Does not enjoy television.

Desired Patient Outcomes

Verbalizes that increased input lessens boredom.

Nursing Action	Rationale
1. Because patient now appears to be stable, consult physician regarding increasing visitors to one person per day in addition to wife.	Visitors provide social contact and stimulation to confined patient.
2. Ask wife to bring cassette player and tapes of music and any books or magazines patient might like to read.	Music and literature provide mental involvement. These are particularly helpful if they have been valued by the patient before hospitalization.
3. Ask wife to bring slides and photographs from recent trip to Greece that patient said he would like to organize and catalogue.	Memories of a recent pleasant vacation offer patient hopes of recovery. Participating in the delayed project of organizing the photos allows patient to feel involved and useful.
4. Reassure patient that his condition is improving and he may be able to move from the unit soon.	Assurance of progress by the nurse fosters hope and decreases anxiety.
5. Suggest that persons at his place of work purchase a music tape rather than send flowers.	By serving as a resource to friends of the patient, they are able to contribute to the patient's well-being.

Every member of the health care team has meaning for the patient in that each helps plan and provide care. It is frequently the nurse who spends the most time with the patient and thus has the best opportunity to offer the patient meaningful input. The nurse presents a visual image, provides auditory input by speaking, and may touch the patient as well. The presence of family and friends is also important to consider. It may be that the hallucinations experienced by some persons suffering extreme deprivation are functional in that they provide input, that is, the creation of hallucinatory images compensates for lack of real input in the environment. When you increase meaningful input, hallucinations usually disappear. The most meaningful input experienced by human beings is personal contact with others. The few people who have dared lone voyages across the ocean have reported severe sensory deprivation and hallucinations, despite the abundance of sensory input provided by the sea, changing weather, and wildlife. They attributed this phenomenon to loss of human contact, a hypothesis that has important implications for nurses.

The significance of touch cannot be overemphasized. The earliest meaningful input in a person's life is from touch. Long before the infant can focus on objects or interpret sounds, stroking and fondling will quiet cries and produce a sense of contentment. Touch continues to be important throughout life. For the patient in the hospital, touch is a means of orientation to the environment, reassurance in stressful situations, and an expression of caring (Fig. 31-8). In adulthood, some people use touch more expressively and more spontaneously than others. Although you may initially have to make a conscious effort to use touch, touching a patient's hand or shoulder while you are speaking soon becomes automatic. It is unusual for a patient to show any objection to this practice. In fact, most find touch a warm, pleasant experience. However, there are always exceptions, so it is essential when providing this kind of sensory input to be perceptive and use touch with discretion.

Another effective source of input is radio or television. Television has the advantage of being visual as well as auditory. If the patient is unable to express a preference, you should choose music or a program that seems suitable for the patient. The family may be of help here. For example, a rock music radio station may be inappropriate for a 76-year-old patient but suitable for a teenager (Fig. 31-9).

Taste is another source of input. If you are selecting a menu for a patient who is unable to do so, you might choose foods characterized by a variety of tastes and consistencies. Taste can be particularly meaningful if a special selection is prepared and brought from home by a family member. A teenager of Italian descent who had been badly injured was beginning to feed himself when his sister brought in a small hot dish of homemade spaghetti. With the initial spoonful he grinned broadly for the first time since his accident.

You should not overlook olfactory stimulation. A friend brought a teenage patient a small box of incense

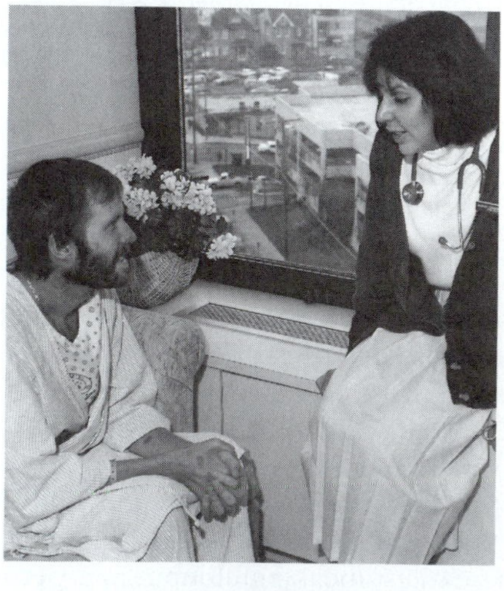

Figure 31-8. Meaningful stimuli prevent sensory deprivation.

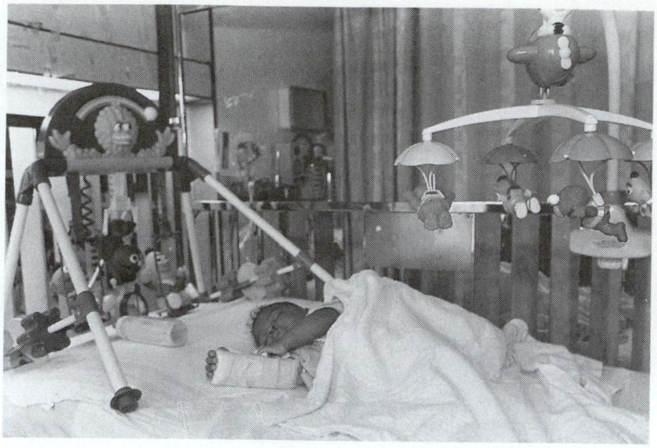

Figure 31-9. Toys and mobiles are appropriate for the sensory-deprived child.

to create an odor the patient associated with home. You might apply mildly scented skin lotions, deodorants, aftershave lotions, or colognes to the patient after a bath.

Relieving Sensory Overload

When you plan to relieve sensory overload, it is always a sound first step to consider sources and levels of sensory input (see sample Nursing Care Plan Related to Sensory Overload). Some of these sources might be eliminated, and input could be timed more satisfactorily. For example, you could plan to perform several procedures at once, allowing the patient periods of low input between periods of care. Input simultaneous with but unrelated to medical procedures can be therapeutic and relieve anxiety. Soft, restful music for limited periods of time has proven effective.

Human beings are social and attach much importance to contact with others. However, contact with too many persons can sensorially overload an individual because of the adjustments required for interpersonal communication. It may be appropriate in some situations to limit visitors to the patient so that interpersonal contacts are decreased.

Any additional stimulus such as pain, itching, or pressure from casts or dressings should be relieved to minimize input. Also measures to assist in relieving stress and anxiety, which compound overload, are helpful (see Chapter 34).

Because a strong component in sensory overload is perceptual disturbance, continuing to make input meaningful for the person is important. Identifying or explaining the reason for unfamiliar sounds can decrease anxiety. For example, if an alarm on monitoring equipment sounds at uncertain intervals, a reasonable explanation of why it does so may reduce the patient's distress. If a short period of discomfort is associated with a

Nursing Care Plan
Sample Nursing Care Plan Related to Sensory Overload

Nursing Diagnosis	Sensory Perceptual Alterations: Sensory overload related to change in environment from chronic care setting to hospital. **Supportive data:** Woman, 79 years old. Resident of chronic care facility last 3 years. Slipped on bathroom floor yesterday and fractured femur. Transferred to hospital for hip pinning.
Desired Patient Outcomes	**Decreased agitation as evidenced by the following behaviors:** Speaks in softer voice, sounding less angry. Verbalizes that she feels more comfortable since change in care.

Nursing Action	Rationale
1. Give care in blocks of time free of interruption.	Giving care in blocks of time eliminates frequent stimulation which can cause more sensory overload.
2. Coordinate visits by respiratory therapy, dietician, and lab with scheduled blocks of nursing care when possible.	Having other departments give therapy at the same time as nursing care confines stimulation to designated time periods and provides time for uninterrupted rest.
3. Play patient's preferred music on radio—likes religious and classical music.	Playing music relaxes and involves patient in a restful, less stimulating environment.
4. Sit with patient twice each shift for conversation and quiet sharing.	Sitting quietly with the patient offers meaningful communication and reassurance.
5. Ask patient's feedback regarding alteration of schedule.	Requesting feedback from patient regarding plan of care promotes a feeling of involvement and increases self-esteem.

procedure, telling the person helps prepare the person to receive the input and accept it perceptually.

Nurses can take numerous actions to help the patient who is having difficulty with sensory and perceptual overload. Revision of the care plan and cooperation of the rest of the health care team may be needed, but the effort is well worthwhile.

Providing Care for the Person With Speech Impairment

The patient who suddenly loses speech often becomes agitated, frustrated, and eventually depressed over the inability to communicate. Such patients respond well to a quiet, organized environment, devoid of confusion. With these patients as well as the others we have discussed, music can be therapeutic because it can be enjoyed without words. Most aphasic patients can hear normally, and shouting is not only unnecessary but upsetting. Unfortunately, some nurses assume that a patient who cannot speak also cannot hear.

Establishing some form of communication is essential to care. You should use whatever works best for the individual patient. If the patient understands simple words, use them but never talk down to the patient. More complex sentences may only confuse the patient. Maintain eye contact and speak slowly and distinctly. If the patient understands symbols, you could make a simple symbol board with pictures of care items and other pertinent objects. Some patients with aphasia, however, cannot recognize symbols and another method of communication must be found. If the patient can write, a "magic slate" or paper and pencil can provide for communication.

The aphasic patient is often seen by a speech therapist for evaluation and treatment. If a patient of yours is in such a program, make it a point to become knowledgeable about the therapy. Consult with the therapist to find out how you can help the patient relearn speech. New computerized programs are becoming more available for use by those with speech impairment. You may wish to refer the patient and family to a resource that has knowledge of this technology.

Providing Care for the Person With Decreased Level of Awareness

Caring for the somnolent, unconscious, or comatose patient requires special skills of assessment and intervention on the part of the nurse. The nurse must not only constantly assess the patient's level of awareness but also attempt to adjust to, supplement, and replace deficiencies that develop in any system of the body.

Nursing actions for the patient with lowered levels of awareness may focus on protecting an area of the body or an extremity from injury or discomfort. A patient who cannot perceive high temperature or pain in a particular body part should never be exposed to heat or sharp objects of any kind. If an arm is involved, for example, injections should not be given there because a resulting reaction or inflammation could escape detection until late because of decreased sensation.

As a patient becomes less aware, the nurse must take increased precautions to guard the patient against injury. Some of these actions center around preventing the patient from falling from the bed or chair, preventing foreign objects from entering the eyes or mouth, and protecting the patient against exposure to unusually hot or cold temperatures. Safety in the environment becomes a priority in planning care (see Module 3, Safety).

Planning also includes continual monitoring of changes in the level of mentation. Because there are constant changes in mentation, your plans may have to be altered. The ability to do this will ensure safety during what may be a critical time for the patient. Ongoing communication with the physician is essential.

All those nursing actions that would be directed toward caring for any patient who is immobilized are included. Most body systems, however, also require special attention. The critically ill unstable patient will probably be in the critical care unit. As a nurse on a general unit or in a long-term care facility, however, you may care for a long-term comatose or unconscious patient. Maintaining the patient's respiratory function is of primary importance. As part of care, you must constantly assess for a patent (open) airway. Keep the patient's head to the side so that secretions can drain and, if vomiting should occur, vomitus will not be aspirated. Most unconscious patients can safely be placed in high Fowler's position and turned from side to side, as well as placed prone, if this is done with utmost care. Change of position helps move secretions and prevent skin breakdown. The unconscious patient may have to be suctioned because the cough reflex may be absent. If a tracheostomy has been performed, tracheostomy suctioning and care will be necessary (see Chapter 28 and Module 43, Tracheostomy Care and Suctioning).

Oral care must be provided carefully. Examine the mouth for loose teeth that may be aspirated and be sure all equipment used is lint free. Use oral care equipment and solutions in such a way that the airway remains unobstructed at all times. Because unconscious patients frequently mouth breathe, frequent oral care is essential.

Optimum nutrition provides the patient the best prospects for recovery. Because the patient cannot voluntarily ingest food, a nasogastric tube can be introduced for the instillation of tube feedings. Enteral feedings provide the patient with a nutritional solution through a small tube passed through the nose and directly into the jejunum. If the intestinal tract cannot absorb nutrients effectively, nutrition by hyperalimentation can be initiated (see Chapter 25).

Skin integrity and musculoskeletal maintenance are essential to keep the patient free of deformity. To some extent, the comatose patient's circulation is always compromised. Any pressure may cause the beginning of a pressure sore. Because the patient cannot report discomfort, you must be aware of positions that may cause undue pressure and change the patient's position completely at least every 2 hours. A nerve palsy (partial paralysis) could develop if a patient is allowed to lie on an arm or hand. Check every position change critically for body alignment. Use trochanter and hand rolls to prevent contracture (see Module 8, Moving the Patient in Bed and Positioning). Frequent massage stimulates circulation and prevents skin breakdown. Monitor water temperatures when bathing closely to prevent burning. The use of heat devices is discouraged for reasons of safety. Range-of-motion exercises are essential to maintain joint mobility in a patient who cannot move voluntarily.

Urinary incontinence is cared for by padding the bed and being conscientious about cleanliness. Some nurses and physicians regard use of the catheter as a safety threat because of the likelihood of infection although some physicians may order a catheter inserted. Good perineal and catheter care helps prevent infection. Monitoring output is crucial. To maintain bladder tone in a patient with a long-term catheter, a clamp-unclamp routine is sometimes used (see Chapter 27). This procedure is controversial because it is possible to forget to unclamp the catheter at the prescribed period (usually every 2 hours), causing damage to the bladder or sphincter through hyperdistention. If this technique is used, a large sign should be placed over the bed to alert the nurse to adhere to the schedule. Intestinal (bowel) incontinence also requires extreme cleanliness for esthetic reasons and to prevent infection.

All unconscious patients need ear care. Wax and foreign bodies should be removed to prevent inflammation. If the patient has suffered a head injury, inspect for the emission of blood or spinal fluid from the nose or ears and report either to the physician immediately.

Eye care is needed to prevent permanent damage. Contact lenses should be removed (for specific techniques, see Module 11, Hygiene). Lenses should be carefully stored or given to the family along with other valuables. If the eyes of unconscious patients remain open, the corneas dry and ulceration can occur. The lids can be kept closed with eye patches; if patches are used, daily inspection is essential to detect any inflammation or infection. Sterile saline can be administered as an eyewash. Eye drops are sometimes prescribed by the physician.

Patients in light coma can experience pain, which may be demonstrated by grimacing, restlessness, or moaning. Repositioning or adjustment of dressings, binders, or appliances may make the patient more comfortable. Pain medications should be used sparingly because they depress the CNS and may compromise respiration.

Side rails should always be raised when the patient is left alone, even for a few moments. Changes in level of awareness sometimes occur swiftly, and a quiet patient can become suddenly agitated and fall from bed.

Even comatose patients benefit from psychological care. Patients who appeared to be in deep coma have, on recovery, reported hearing people and sounds. Hearing remains intact even when other senses are absent. Converse with the patient. The nurse and others should remember not to say anything within the patient's hearing that could be disturbing or undermine the patient's dignity. The patient's level of awareness may be improved by the stimulation of familiar voices and sounds. Encourage the family and others close to the patient to visit and talk to the patient. Play music the patient has been known to enjoy. As you care for the patient, explain what you are going to do, as if the patient were responsive.

Health Teaching

Although the areas of cognitive and sensory perceptual impairment involve a wide variety of disorders and problems, there are some important principles for health teaching the patient, the care provider, and the family. To be effective, the nurse should have carefully assessed the individual and others involved in care regarding their knowledge and willingness to learn.

First, it is essential to emphasize strengths, not weaknesses. Determine the quantity and quality of function that remains so that it can be maintained or maximized to its fullest. The nurse must believe in the ability of the patient to progress and in many situations, to find other strengths that can be developed to meet goals.

Secondly, health teaching the cognitively and perceptually impaired involves the nurse's knowledge of resources. These resources may be within the facility and can be used before discharge or may be community programs that can offer ongoing assistance after the patient has entered a long-term facility or returned home. Health teaching is an important part of the patient's continuity of nursing care.

Evaluation

Effective evaluation of the ever-changing response related to sensation and cognition depends on careful consideration of the established desired outcomes. At times, evaluation is difficult because of the inability to observe subtle changes. This means that ongoing assessment may be needed for accurate evaluation. Some areas of evaluation are clearer than are others. For example, objective data such as body temperature lend themselves to quick and accurate evaluation; the outcome criteria have been met when the patient's temperature is lower and the patient no longer has a fever. More difficult is when the nurse may observe that the patient appears to be more steady when ambulating but needs to validate this observation with the person. Evaluation may also involve identifying the patient's new learning of abilities for coping with the specific loss. The fact that the conclusions you reach in your evaluation of function may guide the physician and the health care team in altering the plan of care creates an added responsibility.

Communicating with the Health Care Team

Communicating with others on the health care team is essential when one is caring for the patient with sensory or cognitive problems. The best approach is interdisciplinary so that the patient has the benefit of the expertise of many members of the health care team. The nursing plan should be written in clear terms, incorporating both the input of others on the team as well as possible referral to disciplines that will help in the rehabilitation of the patient. Some of the people who might be consulted are speech therapy, nutritional support, physical therapy, occupational therapy, and the clergy. Each member of the health care team should add to the flow sheet or notes in the record so that progress can be evaluated. Freeman and Hefferin (1984) state that only by "going back periodically to evaluate the efficacy of your interventions can you help ensure social, emotional and perceptual well-being."

Nursing Care Study
A Patient with Sensory Overload

Maria Palmucci, age 38, is admitted to the acute care unit of the hospital with severe cardiopulmonary problems. Her room is designed for intensive care, the glass on the upper half of the wall contiguous to the hallway permitting close observation by the nursing staff. The room itself is a clutter of equipment, mostly electrical. Lights blink and sounds emanate from the appliances constantly. Oxygen and suction equipment bubbles and gurgles. The ceiling lights are left on night and day to allow the nursing and medical staffs to perform tests, treatments, and procedures. Vital signs are taken hourly, oxygen and intravenous fluids are under constant scrutiny, and the patient is turned frequently. Mrs. Palmucci is becoming increasingly apprehensive.

The condition of the patient is such that almost constant attention and touching are required. Tubes and catheters add to the general confusion experienced by the patient. The environment inflicts a high level of visual, auditory, and tactile input on a continuing basis. A heart-monitoring machine is equipped with an alarm that rings loudly in response to even moderate movement on the part of the patient, as well as to heart irregularity. Mrs. Palmucci's symptoms are apparent in her behavior. Apprehension is fast escalating into panic. Mrs. Palmucci grasps the sheets until her knuckles are white. She hyperventilates (takes rapid, deep breaths), and her eyes appear frightened. At times she pulls at her gown and violently shakes her head. Although it is believed that the loss of REM sleep exaggerates her state of mind, the primary problem is sensory overload.

The nursing care plan is reviewed in assessing the patient's condition and environment. All unnecessary equipment is removed from the room. The ceiling lights are dimmed for long periods of time; only a small, dim wall light is left on. When the nurse is in the room, the shade on the large hallway window is pulled to shut out the sight of busy traffic up and down the hall. The door is kept closed to diminish sound. The heart-monitoring alarm is moved by the hospital's mechanical department so that it rings only at the nurse's station and does not continue to distress the patient. Suction equipment is turned off when not in use. The nurse plans for care to be provided at a few set times so that the patient will not receive constant stimuli. Soft music is played in the unit for short periods of time. The nurse sets aside time to hold Mrs. Palmucci's hand in silence.

Within a short time, Mrs. Palmucci grows quieter and her breathing becomes more regular and efficient. With the improvement in breathing, her cardiac status also improves. The look of fear on her face disappears and her muscles relax.

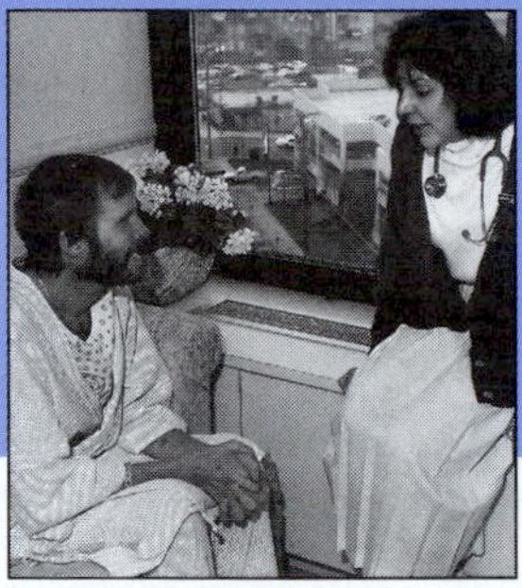

Key Points

- Although the underlying causes of problems of sensory perception may be medical, the manifestations of disturbances require effective, well planned nursing care.
- The nervous system is composed of four main parts: the brain, spinal cord, autonomic nervous system, and sensory receptors. Together, these structures regulate and control cognition (thinking), motor and sensory function, speech, thermoregulation, and level of awareness.
- Cognition, or intellectual function, is often assessed by a nursing interview and the use of a mental status assessment guide.
- Problems with coordination, muscle strength, and movement, all of which are regulated by the nervous system, can present difficulties for the patient in daily living.
- Neurologic deficits, including those of touch and the ability to swallow, can jeopardize safety.
- The need to maintain an optimal sensory and perceptual level is both a physical and a psychological need.
- Sensory input consists of all the messages and impressions received through the five senses by way of the various receptor organs of the body.
- The eyes are the organs of visual input; the purpose of the ears is to receive auditory input. The nose receives olfactory input, or smell, which complements taste ability. Taste, or gustatory input, is mainly received through stimulation of the taste buds on the tongue and the roof of the mouth. Touch, or tactile input, is received through a complicated system in which different mechanisms are used for receiving touch, pain, itch, and tickle.
- Some persons have special sensory deficits such as visual or hearing impairment. When these persons enter the health care setting, nurses must include in the plan of care any special nursing actions appropriate to the individual with the sensory impairment.
- There is an optimal level of input to which any person, including care providers, can respond appropriately and comfortably at any given time. This level is influenced by such factors as normal tolerance for input and understanding of the input that is occurring.
- Persons in health care facilities are subject to fluctuations of sensory level that can lead to disturbances such as sensory deprivation and sensory overload.
- Basic communication is essential to human beings; interference with the power of speech is extremely stressful to patients and to nurses who provide care.
- Patients can suffer one of a number of types of aphasia: expressive aphasia, receptive aphasia, amnesic aphasia, and global aphasia.
- The level of awareness of a person is the relative ability to respond to the environment. In general, there are five levels: total alertness, lethargy, stupor, light coma, and total unconsciousness.
- For patients who are unresponsive, specific nursing actions address the needs of an altered level of awareness, including the basic need for protection.

Study Questions

1. List the four parts of the nervous system and briefly state the function of each.
2. For each of the five senses, give one example of appropriate sensory input for the patient who is in the health care setting.
3. What hazards are present in the hospital setting for the patient who has a sensory impairment?
4. Describe four special nursing actions that are helpful in caring for the patient who is visually impaired.
5. Describe four special nursing actions that are helpful in caring for the patient who has hearing impairment.
6. What is the definition of sensory deprivation?
7. Name three persons who might be at risk for sensory deprivation.
8. What is the definition of sensory overload?
9. Name three persons who might be at risk for sensory overload.
10. Briefly discuss times in your life as a student when you have felt sensorially deprived or overloaded.
11. List activities you do to improve the situation when you have these feelings.
12. Describe the different levels of awareness, from alert to unconscious.

Critical Thinking Activities

1. Visit a long-term care setting and request permission to attend a residents' group. Write a brief report on the cognition and interests of the residents. What

was the purpose of the group and who attended? Were any impairments evident and were these age-related?

2. Identify the nursing diagnoses that might be appropriate for an unconscious patient. Write out nursing actions for each nursing diagnosis. Designate the body system or impairment which will be affected by your action.
3. Examine the Folstein Mental Status Questionnaire What modalities does it test? What are its strengths and limitations of each?

Relevant Sections in Modules for Basic Nursing Skills

Volume I Module

- Moving the Patient in Bed and Positioning 8
- Feeding Adult Patients 9
- Inspection, Palpation, Auscultation, and Percussion 13
- Ambulation: Simple Assisted and Using Cane, Crutches, or Walker 23
- Range-of-Motion Exercises 24

References and Readings

Batt, L. J. "Managing Delirium." *Journal of Psychosocial Nursing* 27, 5 (May 1989): 22–25.

Bender, P. "Deceptive Distress in the Elderly." *American Journal of Nursing* 92, 10 (October 1992): 28–33.

Bell, L. "Rx for Burnout: Vacations With a Difference." *American Journal of Nursing* 92, 10 (October 1992): 52–55.

Bexton, W. H., Heron, W., and Scott, T. H. "Effects of Decreased Variation in the Sensory Environment." *Canadian Journal of Psychology* 8 (June 1954): 70.

Birdsall, C., and Greif, L. "How Do You Manage Extraventricular Drainage?" *American Journal of Nursing* 90, 11 (November 1990): 47–49.

Blacker, J. "Starting the Neurologic Exam." *Patient Care* 17, 16 (September 30, 1983): 75–76.

Brown, D. L. "Burnout or Cop-Out?" *American Journal of Nursing* 83, 7 (July 1983): 1110.

Carpenito, L. J. *Nursing Diagnosis: Application to Clinical Practice.* 4th edition. Philadelphia: J. B. Lippincott, 1992.

Christian, E., Dluhy, N., and O'Neill, R. "Sounds of Silence: Coping with Hearing Loss and Loneliness." *Journal of Gerontological Nursing* 15. 11 (November 1989): 4–9.

Cohen, S. "Programmed Instruction: Sensory Changes in the Elderly." *American Journal of Nursing* 91, 10 (October 1981): 1851-1880.

Crow, R. "Perception." *Nursing* 28, 8 (August 1981): 1205–1211.

Dellasego, C. "Home Health Nurses' Assessment of Cognition." *Applied Nursing Research*. 5, 3 (August 1992): 127–133.

Downs, F. S. "Bed Rest and Sensory Disturbance." *American Journal of Nursing* 74, 3 (March 1974): 434–438.

Fanslow, C. A. "Therapeutic Touch: A Healing Modality Through Life." *Topics in clinical Nursing* 5, 2 (July 1983): 72–79.

Feil, N. *V/F Validation: The Feil Method.* Cleveland: Edward Feil Productions, 1989.

Folstein, M. R., and Rovner, B. W. "Mini-Mental State Exam in Clinical Practice." *Hospital Practice* 22, 1A (January 30, 1987): 99–110.

Freeman, C. C., and Hefferin, E. A. "Are You Out of Touch with Your Patients?" *RN* 47, 4 (April 1984): 51–53.

Guyton, A. C. *Human Physiology and Mechanisms of Disease.* 5th ed. Philadelphia: W. B. Saunders, 1992.

Heron, W. "The Pathology of Boredom." In *Altered States of Awareness.* San Francisco: W. H. Freeman, 1971.

Hickey, J. V. *The Clinical Practice of Neurological and Neurosurgical Nursing.* 3rd edition. Philadelphia: J. B. Lippincott, 1992.

Holden, L. "Hearing Aids: Handle with Care." *Nursing '82* 12, 4 (April 1982): 64–67.

Johnson, S. H. "Burnout's Contagious." *Nursing Management* 13, 2 (February 1982): 34–38.

Kopec, C. A. "Sensory Loss in the Aged: The Role of the Nurse and the Family." *Nursing Clinics of North America* 18, 2 (June 1983): 373–384.

Lower, J. S. "Rapid Neuro Assessment." *American Journal of Nursing* 92, 6 (June 1992): 38–45.

Martin, E. W. "Confusion in the Terminally Ill: Recognition and Management." *Hospice and Palliative Care* (May-June 1990): 20–23.

McCorkle, R. "Effects of Touch on Seriously Ill Patients." *Nursing Research* 23, 2 (March-April 1974): 125–132.

Moore, P. C. "When You Have to Think Small for a Neurological Exam." *RN* 51, 6 (June 1988): 38–43.

Norman, S. "The Pupil Check." *American Journal of Nursing* 82, 4 (April 1982): 588–591.

Pace, K. "Keeping Track of Confused Patients." *Nursing '90* 20, 6 (June 1990): 64.

Pfeiffer, E. "A Short Portable Mental Status Questionnaire for the Assessment of Organic Brain Deficit in Elderly Patients." *Journal of American Geriatric Society*. 18, 10 (October, 1975): 433–441.

Purath, J. "Assessing Headache Pain." *RN* 54, 10 (October 1991): 26–30.

Rainer, J. D., and Hollis, J. "Evaluation of the Comatose Patient." *Journal of Neurological Nursing* 15, 5 (October 1983): 283–286.

Roberts, B. L., and Fitzpatrick, J. J. "Improving Balance: Therapy of Movement . . . Elderly People Receive Vestibular Stimulation Rocking in a Rocking Chair." *Journal of Gerontological Nursing* 9, 3 (March 1983): 150–156.

Webber-Jones, J. "Doomed to Deafness." *American Journal of Nursing* 92, 11 (November 1992): 37–39.

Comfort

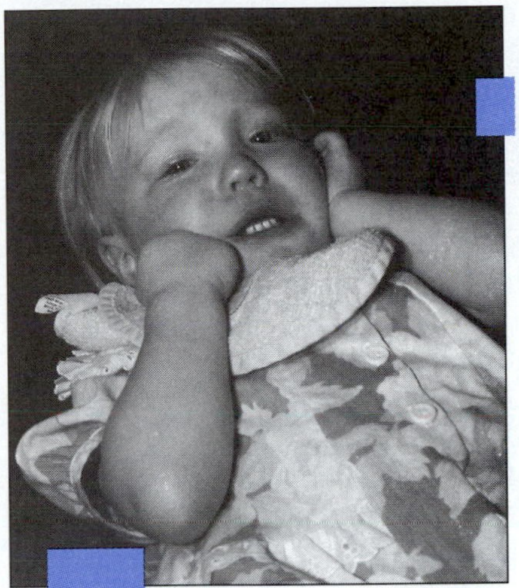

32

Objectives

After completing this chapter, you should be able to:

1. Discuss various definitions of pain.
2. Explain the purpose of pain in the body.
3. Discuss the routes the pain impulse may travel after reaching the spinal cord.
4. Describe the various responses to pain.
5. List data to be gathered when assessing for pain.
6. Describe nonpharmacologic nursing interventions for the relief of pain.
7. Discuss the different drug interventions for the relief of pain.
8. Explain approaches to treatment of chronic pain and terminal pain.

Study Terms

acupuncture
addiction
agonist/antagonist effect
behavior modification
benign pain
chordotomy
chronic pain syndrome
dorsal column stimulator (DCS)
drug abuse
drug dependence
epidural analgesia
gate-control theory
intraventricular analgesia
ischemia
modified Brompton's mixture
nociceptors
pain interpretation
pain receptors
pain threshold
patient-controlled analgesia (PCA)
phantom pain
physical dependence
placebo
referred pain
stoicism
superficial pain
terminal pain
tolerance
transcutaneous electric nerve stimulator (TCS, TNS, TENS)
visceral pain

Outline

Ellis, Nowlis: Nursing: A Human Needs Approach, 5th ed. © 1994 J.B. Lippincott Company

Comfort is a physical state of ease or well-being in which the individual is free to use energy for meeting basic needs and for seeking growth and actualization. As with all other human needs, comfort is not an all-or-none phenomenon. There are relative levels of comfort, and an individual may have some level of discomfort or alteration in the comfort state and still be able to function well.

Comfort may be altered by interference with various needs. In many instances, nausea and vomiting of short duration are not a threat to nutrition, but they are a problem to the individual because of their threat to comfort. Distention and gas in the gastrointestinal system are likewise threats to comfort. These particular problems are discussed in the Chapters 25, 26, and 27. In this chapter, we focus on pain as a threat to the need for comfort.

The Nature of Pain

Pain is an essentially lonely experience. It cannot be shared, and words are inadequate to explain the feeling to someone else. Pain can crowd out the rest of the world, making itself the center and focus of consciousness. Pain is frequently what prompts a person to seek medical care and often continues to be the person's primary concern during treatment. What is pain? What is its purpose? What causes it? What can be done to alleviate pain? Answers to these questions are highly important for nurses.

Pain is a warning system for the body. It signals when tissue damage may occur and thus alerts us to protect ourselves from injury or to care for an injury that has already occurred. Thus, pain is essential to meeting our basic safety needs. Those whose pain sensation is decreased or lacking as a result of a disease or a congenital defect are at risk for injuries and untreated health problems.

However, most people regard pain as a problem, something to be avoided. Once its alarm function has been met, its persistence may make it impossible to carry out ordinary activities of daily living (ADLs) and to meet other basic needs. To explain how pain affects the person, we will first review the definition of pain and then discuss the neurophysiology of pain.

Defining Pain

Pain is a subjective perception of discomfort. There are no effective ways to measure it or detect its presence objectively. McCaffery (1979) provided a widely used and helpful definition when she stated, "Pain is whatever the experiencing person says it is, existing whenever he says it does." Many health care people are uncomfortable with this definition because it puts the diagnosis of the problem in the hands of the patient. It requires that you *believe* what the patient tells you about the pain. As a nurse you need to remind yourself that pain is defined by the person experiencing it.

The beliefs and value systems of health care providers affect their views of pain. Some health professionals wish to identify "real pain" as perception of discomfort resulting from actual or potential tissue injury or damage. Therefore, if tissue injury or damage cannot be demonstrated or is not imminent, they state that "real pain" does not exist (Sternbach, 1978). As we explore the physiology of pain perception, you will see that pain is a complex phenomenon and that whatever the person feeling pain perceives is real.

Another commonly held view is that it is good to endure pain and bad to need help in coping with pain. To encourage patients to endure pain, the nurse with this view would try to help the patient redefine perception and not to define the problem as pain. This nurse might encourage the patient to use terms such as uncomfortable or suggest that the patient is defining the pain as more severe than it really is. Conversely, the nurse for whom pain is upsetting might be unwilling to accept a patient's view that the pain is tolerable or merely discomfort when the nurse expects severe pain to be present. All of these values held by health care providers interfere with effectively assisting the patient. The definition and measurement of pain are subjective, and the person experiencing the sensation is the person who must define and measure it.

Pain Receptors

The **pain receptors** are called **nociceptors**. They are nerve endings for different types of nerve fibers. One type, the A delta fibers, are larger than the others and have a myelin sheath. They transmit sensation rapidly and allow for precise localization of the pain stimulus. There are more A delta fibers in the skin and surface tissues, and thus pain in those tissues can be better localized. When stimulated, A delta fibers are responsible for sharp, pricking types of pain sensation.

A second type of nerve is the C fiber. This very small fiber does not have a myelin sheath. Sensation travels more slowly through this fiber, and localization of sensation is less precise. There are more C fibers in internal structures. When stimulated, C fibers are responsible for dull, burning types of pain sensation. One stimulus is able to produce response in both A delta fibers and C fibers. The pain sensation then has components of both types of stimuli (Porth, 1990).

Many kinds of stimuli can produce response in the nociceptors. The ones most clearly understood are those that are associated with tissue injury. Temperature extremes, sharp pressure, and chemicals liberated from damaged cells can all stimulate these nerve endings.

Ischemia (lack of adequate blood supply to tissues) may, in some instances, cause severe pain in the affected part. Excessive stretching of tissues is a source of much visceral or internal pain, as when the bowel is overstretched or the bladder is excessively distended. *Neurogenic pain* is pain that arises from damaged or injured nerves or nerve roots. Such pain may accompany crushing injury, infection, inflammation, or scarring. Because of the effect on the nerve itself, neurogenic pain may continue long after the initial damaging agent has disappeared.

In muscle tissue, there may be trigger points, which, when pressed, stimulate radiating pain. These trigger points may be asymptomatic or may cause pain problems. They appear to be areas of irritation secondary to changes in microcirculation (Chapman and Bonica, 1985).

Pain Transmission

The A delta fibers and the C fibers transmit the *pain impulse* to the spinal cord. In the spinal cord, these fibers synapse with other nerve fibers. They may synapse directly with a motor (efferent) nerve and create a simple reflex to remove the body part from danger (Fig. 32-1). Some local autonomic responses, such as changes in microcirculation, also occur through reflex arcs.

In the spinal cord, the impulses are transferred to other neurons, which cross the cord to specific tracts where the impulse is then transmitted by the *ascending fibers* within the tract to the brain.

The pathways for pain impulses and the chemical and neuronal factors that affect transmission in the spinal cord are extraordinarily complex and not completely understood at this time. Pain impulses may be decreased, enhanced, or blocked entirely. It also appears that pain impulses may be transmitted on the basis of

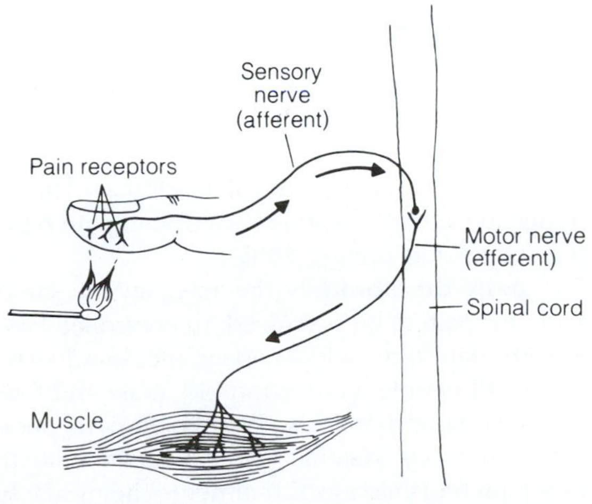

Figure 32-1. First pathway for pain impulses: the simple reflex arc.

what is happening in the cord itself rather than on only nociceptive input.

Some neurons in the spinal cord transmit impulses directly to the thalamus without any intervening synapses. Others form a route that leads to the medulla and the midbrain before going to the thalamus. There are receptor sites in the spinal cord for naturally occurring chemicals called endorphins. When these receptor sites are occupied by endorphins, the transmission of pain impulses is inhibited. The supply of endorphins appears to increase with strenuous exercise and certain other stimuli. It has been hypothesized that some nonmedication pain relief techniques are effective because they stimulate the production of these endorphins.

The **gate-control theory** of pain developed by Melzack and Wall (1965) focuses on the spinal cord as an area where the transmission of pain impulses can be controlled. According to this theory, pain-inhibiting impulses travel down the spinal cord constantly. Therefore, pain impulses must be sufficient to overcome these pain-inhibiting impulses if they are to travel upward to the brain and be perceived. In addition, impulses from peripheral nerves for vibration and touch compete with the pain impulses for ascending fiber transmission. If these other peripheral impulses are sufficiently strong, they will prevent pain impulses from being able to move up the spinal cord. This theory has been valuable in explaining how some types of therapy such as nerve stimulators are effective in pain relief. (These will be discussed later.) Another aspect of the theory is that in some instances the spinal "gate" remains permanently open to pain impulses traveling upward that would ordinarily not be of sufficient intensity to overcome the inhibitory impulses. Exactly why this "gate" remains open is unclear, but it helps to explain why chronic pain may continue when the observable tissue damage is no longer present.

Pain Perception

In the brain, the impulses are received in the thalamus, where *pain perception* takes place. If higher brain centers are removed, a person will still perceive pain but will be unable to localize it—it will be diffuse. The brain stem reticular formation also plays a role in pain perception (Chapman and Bonica, 1985.)

The **pain threshold** is the intensity of stimulus necessary for pain to be perceived. In controlled laboratory studies, pain threshold has been measured as fairly constant in all people, young and old, male and female (Porth, 1991). Endorphins also block pain perception in the central nervous system (CNS) in addition to their effect on pain transmission. Other neurochemicals, such as serotonin, may also be significant in the suppression of pain. Some pain relief therapies such as relaxation and guided imagery act in part by increasing the production of endorphins. Many narcotic drugs used for pain relief block pain perception in the thalamus. Psychological and cognitive factors occurring in the cerebral cortex may also affect pain perception.

Pain Responses

From the thalamus, the impulse moves to several different parts of the brain. Each area is responsible for different responses to the pain impulse.

Physiologic Responses

In the medulla, sympathetic autonomic centers are stimulated (Fig. 32-2). These centers increase perspiration, tearing on the eyes, dilation of the pupils, and blood flow to the brain. The latter increases alertness and causes restlessness. Blood pressure, pulse, and respirations all rise. With continued pain, the sympathetic center may cease responding to the impulses and the physiologic responses to pain may disappear. This is adaptation to the pain.

If the pain impulse is brief but intense, the parasympathetic autonomic centers respond after the sympathetic autonomic centers. The parasympathetic autonomic response causes blood pressure, pulse, and respiration to return to the prepain level. There may also be vomiting and constriction of the pupil.

When severe deep visceral pain occurs, this para-

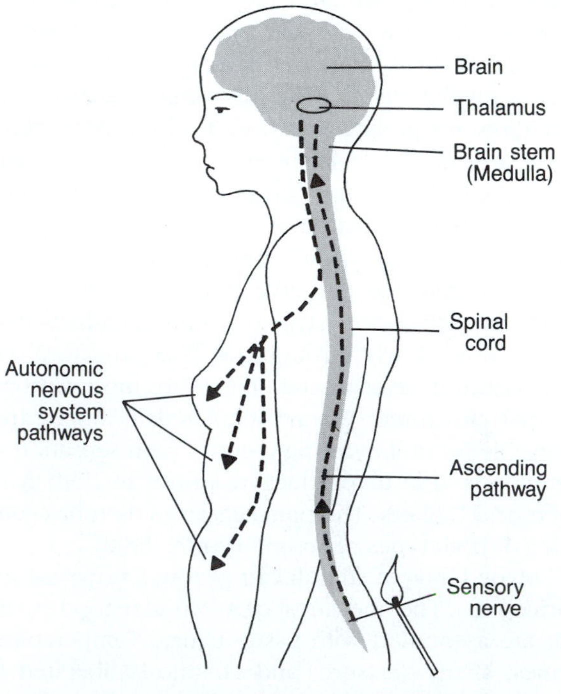

Figure 32-2. Second pathway for pain impulses: to the medulla and autonomic nervous system.

sympathetic response may cause blood pressure to drop below the normal level. This is occasionally seen after surgery. When the pain is treated, blood pressure rises to a normal level. The nurse must be alert to differentiate this situation from shock, in which the blood pressure also falls. A patient in shock would respond adversely to medications used to treat pain.

Motor Responses

Motor activity changes in many ways when an individual is experiencing pain. Frequently, muscles are tense; this muscle tension can become severe enough that it too contributes to pain impulses. Muscles that hold a painful part stable may become fatigued and muscle spasms may occur. When movement increases the pain, the person may hold the body rigid to guard against pain. The postoperative patient, for example, may say, "I'm all right as long as I don't move at all." This rigid posture is often a clue to the presence of pain.

Restlessness may manifest itself as constant motor activity if this does not increase pain. The person may pace the floor, rock the body, or tap the fingers. Such activity discharges some of the accumulated muscle tension.

Responses Determined by the Cerebral Cortex

Identifying the precise location of the pain is the job of the cerebral cortex (Fig. 32-3). Pain in surface areas of the body, **superficial pain**, is usually well localized. Pain in deeper structures is often diffuse and hard to pinpoint. **Visceral** (*internal*) **pain** may be **referred**, that is, felt as originating in organs or areas other than those where the stimulus originated. This occurs because the fibers that transmit the pain impulses from that area are spaced relatively far apart and because in the nonmyelinated fibers impulses are transmitted more widely to other nerve structures in the spinal cord. Referred pain may also *radiate*, that is, spread from a central location to other areas. A familiar example is the pain of a myocardial infarction (heart attack), which often radiates from the chest down the left arm and up into the jaw.

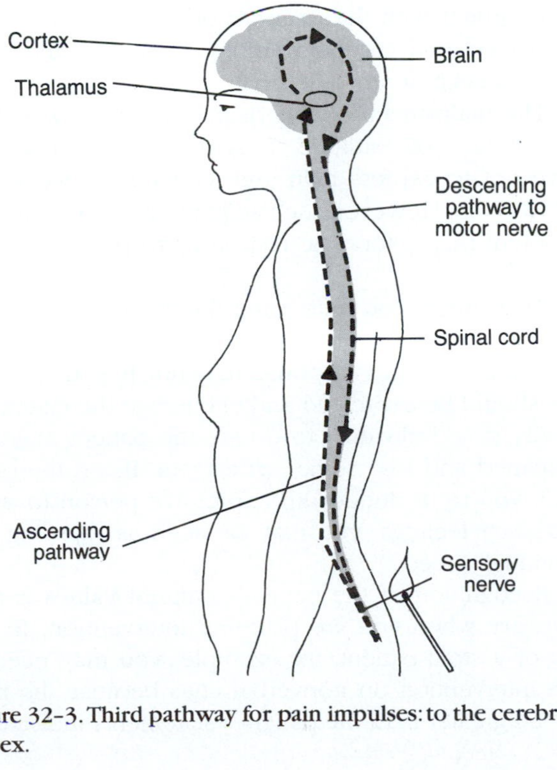

Figure 32-3. Third pathway for pain impulses: to the cerebral cortex.

Pain tolerance refers to the amount of pain that a person is willing to endure. Some individuals have learned to tolerate high levels of pain and to function effectively despite its presence. Other individuals are not able to endure even very low levels of pain. They may take pain medication before a pain is present, when it is expected that pain will occur. In Western society there is often positive value attached to being able to tolerate greater amounts of pain, and there may be negative feelings toward those with a low pain tolerance.

Pain interpretation is a function of the cerebral cortex and refers to identifying the intensity of the pain and ascribing meaning to the pain. The severity and meaning of the pain to the individual affects how that person responds. Anticipation of pain may have a profound effect on the interpretation of pain. The pain may be seen as moderate, but if the person believes the pain indicates something is seriously wrong, the response will be different from that to pain of the same intensity that is seen as not serious. When pain is anticipated, anxiety may be raised, muscle tension increased, and the pain defined as more acute.

Other reactions to pain are determined by the interpretation of the cerebral cortex. Evidence indicates that cognitive and psychological factors interact to affect pain perception. Additionally a given sensation of pain is compared with other experiences of pain and defined with an appropriate term such as sharp, aching, or cramping. Its intensity is classified in light of prior experience as mild, moderate, or severe. It is important to remember that, because pain is a subjective experience, its intensity is rated subjectively. You cannot classify the intensity of someone else's pain. Although you may become highly knowledgeable about the levels of pain that usually accompany given conditions or procedures, each individual's pain is unique.

Interpretations of the type, intensity, and location of the pain are then integrated with feelings about pain, prior experiences of pain, cultural and social attitudes toward pain, ideas about the origin or purpose of this particular pain, and current emotional and physiologic status to produce a *pain reaction.*

If the pain has been experienced before and the person knows exactly what to do about it, pain reaction may be different from that experienced if the pain is entirely unfamiliar. For example, a person who suffers chronic sinus headaches may have a whole regimen of pain-relieving measures, including medications prescribed by a physician, and will thus react differently to sinus pain than to unfamiliar pain of equal intensity in the abdomen.

Because it indicates that something is wrong and interrupts normal life patterns, pain arouses anxiety in many individuals. Anxiety may be manifested in a variety of ways, depending on its severity (see Chapter 34). The severity of the anxiety is not necessarily a function of the severity of the pain. Preexisting anxiety often greatly accentuates reactions to pain. In some cases anxiety is so severe that the individual uses denial as a means of coping. This response may be seen in the heart attack victim who, despite all the evidence, insists the pain can only be heartburn.

Other emotions may also be evoked by pain. Some people feel guilt because they have previously learned to equate pain with punishment; children in pain tend particularly to perceive severe pain as punishment for wrongdoing. For some people, pain may provide a means of relating to others in such a way as to elicit their attention and concern. For them, pain is rewarding. Depression is a common response to chronic pain.

In some situations, pain may be seen as a means to an end. A woman in childbirth may see the pain of labor as worthwhile because it results in the birth of a much-desired child. Adherents of certain religious beliefs see pain as earning merit or favor from God.

When pain seems useless or undeserved, the reaction to it may be anger or increased tension and anxiety. This reaction may characterize the woman delivering an unwanted child or the person who has a body part removed. Such feelings tend generally to exaggerate both the perceived intensity of pain and reaction to pain.

Factors That Affect Response to Pain

The behaviors that occur when pain is present are socially and culturally determined. The young infant responds to pain by withdrawing from the painful stimulus and then crying loudly. If the painful event is over, the young infant can be coaxed quickly to return to prepain behavior. As the person gets older, behaviors become more complex and are less predictable for any given individual. The cerebral cortex is responsible for these complex learned *pain responses* (Display 32-1).

Display 32–1
Factors Affecting Response to Pain

- Cultural background
- Previous experience with pain
- Family pain models
- Responses of others
- Fatigue and energy level
- Age level
- Environment
- Gender

Cultural Background

Different cultures are characterized by different patterns of response to pain. The passive or nonresponsive attitude of members of certain Native American tribes in the face of the most extreme pain has become legendary. Some individuals within these cultures even learned to control autonomic responses to severe pain. This attitude, manifested in many different cultures throughout history, has been named for the Stoics of ancient Greece. **Stoicism**, then, is one way of responding to pain.

Other cultures encourage *expressive responses*, both verbal and nonverbal; to keep one's feelings hidden is considered inappropriate. Such expression may take the form of talking, moaning, praying, or cursing. That verbal and nonverbal expressions of pain are not necessarily congruent with the intensity of the pain stimulus is understood and accepted among people of the same cultural background.

The mainstream of American culture tends to lean toward the stoic attitude. It is considered good and brave not to express pain and, conversely, weak and bad to do so. However, such acquired responses are not so potent that autonomic responses to pain are inhibited.

As a nurse, you must carefully examine your own attitudes toward pain to guard against value judgments of another person's response to pain. If you feel that pain should be expressed and encourage the characteristically stoic individual to do so, the patient may feel demeaned and lose some self-esteem. If, on the other hand, you try to induce an expressive person to withhold such feelings, you may be seen as rejecting the individual's needs.

Recognition of the patient's cultural values is also necessary when you are planning intervention. In the case of a stoic patient, for example, you may need to base intervention on nonverbal cues because the pain may be greater than the patient's statements indicate.

Previous Experience With Pain

Previous experience with pain may greatly affect how an individual responds to current pain. If in previous experiences the person lost control, pain was not relieved, and anxiety was high, a new pain experience is likely to be viewed with excessive anxiety and feelings of loss of control. If in previous experiences the person felt that he or she had gained control over the pain and that there had been adequate support from those around, the person is likely to approach another painful experience with the idea that pain is controllable.

Family Pain Models

Family dynamics and the influence of family pain models may result in individuals' reporting higher frequencies of pain. Edwards and colleagues (1985) found that the more pain models there were in a person's family, the more frequently that person was likely to report pain. They also found that this was more likely for women than for men. They suggested that this pattern might result from learning family methods of coping with stressful interpersonal and environmental events. They further suggested that individuals in families with many complaints of pain might come to the conviction that pain was not under personal control. Another explanation is that there may be inherited physical conditions that lead to increased general pain complaints. Although this study does not provide clear answers, it does provide general information to add to your understanding of pain.

Responses of Others

The person who receives support during pain and feels that others are concerned can often use energy constructively to cope with pain. The person who feels alone or abandoned by others will cope less successfully.

The person in pain sometimes receives secondary gains from others. People who had been indifferent or emotionally distant may become concerned, involved, and caring. The patient may be freed from responsibilities and accountability for actions. For the person whose life has been well adjusted, these secondary gains are not as important as being free of pain. For the person who has not had a satisfactory life adjustment, these secondary gains may provide significant reinforcement of pain-related behaviors. This is one factor in the perpetuation of some chronic pain.

Fatigue and Energy Level

Fatigue makes it much more difficult for a person to tolerate pain. Coping with pain takes energy, and those who have pain find that they tire more quickly and need more rest. Likewise, if rest and sleep are limited, the ability to cope is decreased. Besides making it more difficult to cope emotionally with pain, fatigue may also make it harder to maintain a posture that prevents strain on a painful part or to move in ways that do not stress the painful area. Those in pain do not always recognize the energy used in coping and may become discouraged about their lack of ability to accomplish other tasks.

Age

Actual pain perception appears to be consistent at all ages; however, ability to cope with pain appears to increase as the person ages. Because children do not express their pain, some nurses believe that children experience less pain. Actually children do not express pain because they do not have the communication skills to express what they are feeling, not because they do not feel pain. Children do have an advantage when they do not anticipate pain. In that situation, they may not develop the degree of anxiety an adult would. Infants and young children have little ability to understand the causes of pain and frequently perceive it as outside of their control and totally unpredictable. When a child has had experience with pain, the reaction to a new painful episode may be one of massive fear. As people get older and have experience with pain, they develop coping skills. They also develop philosophical views of why pain occurs and the meaning of pain in life. Some elderly people cope well with high levels of pain on a continuing basis. Of course, not all individuals make this adjustment. Those who are successful in life adjustment in general are more likely to have developed ways of coping with pain.

Environment

A calm and quiet environment that does not create additional stress is important in modifying response to pain. Loud noises, bright lights, and constant activity may deplete the person's energy and create fatigue. However, a bland environment with inadequate sensory stimulation may focus attention on the pain sensation. For example, a person may be able to cope successfully with pain during the day when distractions are present in the environment, but find the pain overwhelming at night when there are no alternative stimuli on which to focus.

Gender

Western society generally gives women permission to express all types of emotions and sensations, including pain. But then their comments are sometimes discounted because of a cultural bias that women overreact to pain. Men are often expected to not express feelings, including feelings of pain. When a man does express pain, the attitude may be that the pain must be very severe for the man to express it. However, if the man is seen as expressing pain too freely, staff members and others may send nonverbal cues that this is not appropriate. McCaffery and colleagues (1992) found that 67% of nurses felt that gender did not affect pain perception, but the other 37% did feel that men and women perceived pain differently. This means that 37% might mistreat pain based on their beliefs about gender differences. They also indicated that doctors are more likely to undertreat pain in women than in men. Recognizing this potential for bias is one of the best ways to prevent it.

The Placebo Effect

A **placebo** is an inert substance administered in place of a pharmacologically active drug. It is considered effective when it has the effect that might be expected from the drug for which it substitutes. Although the effectiveness of placebos is not clearly understood, we do know that *all* treatment is subject to a placebo effect—the effect may be greater than the treatment itself. This phenomenon appears to be related to the atmosphere of trust and confidence in which the treatment is given and the ability of the neuroendocrine system to change body responses.

You will find that interventions for pain are more effective if you accompany them with explanations of their effectiveness and an attitude of certainty that they will indeed help to relieve the patient's pain. This in no way indicates that the pain is not real or is imaginary. It reflects the still poorly understood ability of the brain to alter perception. For some individuals this effect is a major factor affecting response. Other individuals may show no evidence of placebo response. Again, the variability of placebo response is poorly understood.

Occasionally a physician may order an inert substance, usually normal saline for an injection or flavored syrup administered orally, instead of a narcotic in response to a patient's request for pain medication. The purpose of giving a placebo is usually to guard against or treat drug dependence associated with pain relief measures or to determine whether the pain has an organic cause. This approach raises many ethical questions. The patient does have the right to know what treatments are being used, and dishonesty with the patient is considered unethical. In some instances patients have been told that this may be a part of their treatment and they have consented to this procedure. They simply do not know when it will be used.

Every nurse must make an individual decision, on the basis of conscience, with regard to each individual case in which a placebo is ordered. You will want to gather information in regard to what the patient has been told, what consent has been given, and the purpose of the placebo medication before deciding. When you have made your decision, you can act by giving the placebo or by asking not to participate in that aspect of care. Whatever your choice, you should also support the rights of other health care workers to make contrary ethical choices.

In some settings, the patient is informed in advance that a placebo may be used at some point in treatment but that he or she will not be so notified at the time the placebo is administered. The patient is then asked to consent to this mode of treatment. Placebos also prove effective under these circumstances, which eliminate the ethical problem.

Types of Pain

Pain may be either acute or chronic. Chronic or long-term pain may be considered **benign** (not life threatening), **terminal** (when it is from a condition that will lead to death), **chronic pain syndrome** (when objective evidence of continuing tissue damage is not present), or psychogenic pain. **Phantom pain** occurs after removal of a body part.

Acute Pain

Acute pain is pain of short duration. It is what most people think about when they consider pain. Acute pain usually occurs when a tissue injury or potential injury initiates nociceptors. Acute pain is experienced after surgery or with infection, inflammation, and trauma.

Chronic Pain

Chronic pain is of long duration. Pain is usually considered chronic when it has persisted for 3 to 6 months or even longer. There are many variations of chronic pain.

Terminal pain caused by a life-threatening illness such as cancer is often long term. Some prefer to call terminal pain ongoing acute pain because tissue damage is continuing and new nociceptive input is constantly occurring. Because the person is not expected to survive the illness, the treatment of terminal pain should be aimed at providing optimum quality of life. The components of optimum quality of life must be determined by the individual. For example, being alert enough to relate effectively with family and friends may be the most important aspect for one person, who might choose to tolerate a higher intensity of pain in return for clarity of thought processes. For another person, optimum quality of life might be the opportunity to rest in a pain-free state. Physical dependence on pain medications is not a concern for these individuals because they need not become involved in addictive behaviors and increasing dosages may be given as needed. We will discuss addiction later in the chapter.

Another kind of chronic pain is the continuing pain from a non–life-threatening long-term illness such as arthritis. This type of pain has been called *chronic benign pain* by some, although constant pain that disrupts life cannot really be considered very benign. Others have termed this type of pain *recurrent acute pain* because the pain does get worse (exacerbation) and then better (remission). Continuing tissue injury is occurring with this type of pain. Although the pain may be severe, in determining treatment the caregiver must consider that the disease process will continue and that the treatment should not create additional problems for the person.

A third type of chronic pain is found in some individuals after all objective evidence on ongoing tissue injury is gone. Such pain has been called the *chronic pain syndrome.* Low back pain, head pain, and abdominal pain are common chronic pain syndrome problems. The pain may relate to tissue injury that cannot be detected using current methods, or it may relate to physiologic changes in the natural pain control mechanisms and disruptions in the gate-control mechanism. Another strong component may be learned pain behaviors that have overridden non–pain-related behaviors. For some individuals, maladjustment in life may be associated with chronic pain syndrome. This pain is real and should never be considered imaginary.

Health care providers may inadvertently contribute to the development of chronic pain syndromes by their responses to patients with pain. To prevent narcotic addiction, some nurses and physicians are unwilling to provide adequate pain relief. Therefore, the patient is constantly in the position of feeling pain and feeling out of control. The patient then develops many behaviors designed to convince others that the pain is severe or that it really exists and to establish personal control. These behaviors tend to be perpetuated, disrupting life.

A fourth type of chronic pain is *psychogenic or psychosomatic pain*—pain for which there is no history of verifiable tissue injury or other cause of nociceptive input. The pain is related to severe psychological problems. Again, this pain is not imaginary. The person really does hurt. It is only the origin of the pain that is different. This type of pain is rare.

Phantom Pain

Phantom pain is pain perceived in a body part that is no longer present, such as an amputated leg. This phenomenon does not seem to result from stimulation of the sensory nerves because surgery to sever nerves at the spinal level has not always relieved such pain. Phantom pain is not well understood, and research into its cause is continuing. Application of the gate-control theory to this problem suggests the possibility that the pain impulses originate higher in the spinal pathways, at some point where the gate-control mechanism has failed, or in the brain itself. It is important to recognize that phantom pain is not imaginary; the person truly experiences pain.

Phantom pain is initially treated with medication as a self-limiting acute pain. In most instances phantom pains gradually subside and do not recur. When phantom pain persists, it is treated as a chronic pain syndrome.

Assessment

The purpose of assessment in relationship to pain is to formulate a plan for adequate and appropriate pain relief. Although extensive assessment is presented here, judgment as to what assessment information is needed is important. When an individual has just had major surgery, verification that the pain being experienced is the expected postoperative pain may be quickly accomplished, and you may proceed rapidly to planning and intervention. In other instances, extensive information is needed to assist with medical diagnosis as well as for planning nursing intervention. Thus, the first step in assessment for pain is determining what type of situation you are confronting and what data gathering is appropriate.

Interview

It is essential to try to elicit the patient's subjective sensations and description of the pain because pain is so personal and subjective in nature. You will need information on the location, severity (or intensity), and quality (sharp, dull, throbbing, or whatever) of the pain. Display 32-2 lists terms commonly used to describe pain.

Severity may be estimated by asking the patient to identify the level on any of several different scales. Three of the most commonly used with adults are the Simple Descriptive Pain Intensity Scale, the 0 to 10 Nu-

Display 32–2
Terms Used to Describe Pain

Aching	Electric-like	Pounding
Burning	Gnawing	Radiating
Cramping	Heavy	Tearing
Crushing	Intractable	Throbbing
Cutting	Knifelike	Sharp
Dartlike	Lancinating	Shocklike
Dull	Pinching	

meric Pain Intensity Scale (0–5 is used in some settings), and the Visual Analog Scale shown in Figure 32-4. A variety of other scales have been devised for use with children. These include the Poker Chip Tool (Hester, 1986) and the Word-Graphic Rating Scale (Savedra, Tesler, Hozemer, & Ward, 1989). All personnel should use the same scale to be able to track the progress of the pain and the response to treatment. You should also assess pain intensity using the scale both when the patient is at rest and when the patient is engaging in essential activity such as coughing and deep breathing or getting out of bed.

Related factors, such as when the pain began, changes since it began (increasing, decreasing, radiating), and measures that have previously been successful in combating it are also important. Factors that might have precipitated the pain or might be related to it are also significant. For the child, you will need to question both the child and the parent. From the parent you will learn what words the child uses for pain and the responses the parent is seeing. Parents are often attuned to their child's responses. When questioning the child, consider the age and developmental level and use language that the child will understand.

Remember that not all questions are appropriate for every patient. For example, a person who has just had surgery and complains of severe pain should be asked where the pain is located to make sure it is the expected postsurgical pain. If so, it is not necessary to ask further about precipitating factors and related events; they are self-evident. In such an instance, you should proceed rapidly to intervention to relieve the pain (Display 32-3).

Some individuals express themselves better than others with regard to pain. Because pain is a subjective sensation, words are often inadequate to describe it. For some, the effort of talking about the pain they are experiencing is too great for their physical and emotional strength; such individuals should not be pressed to do

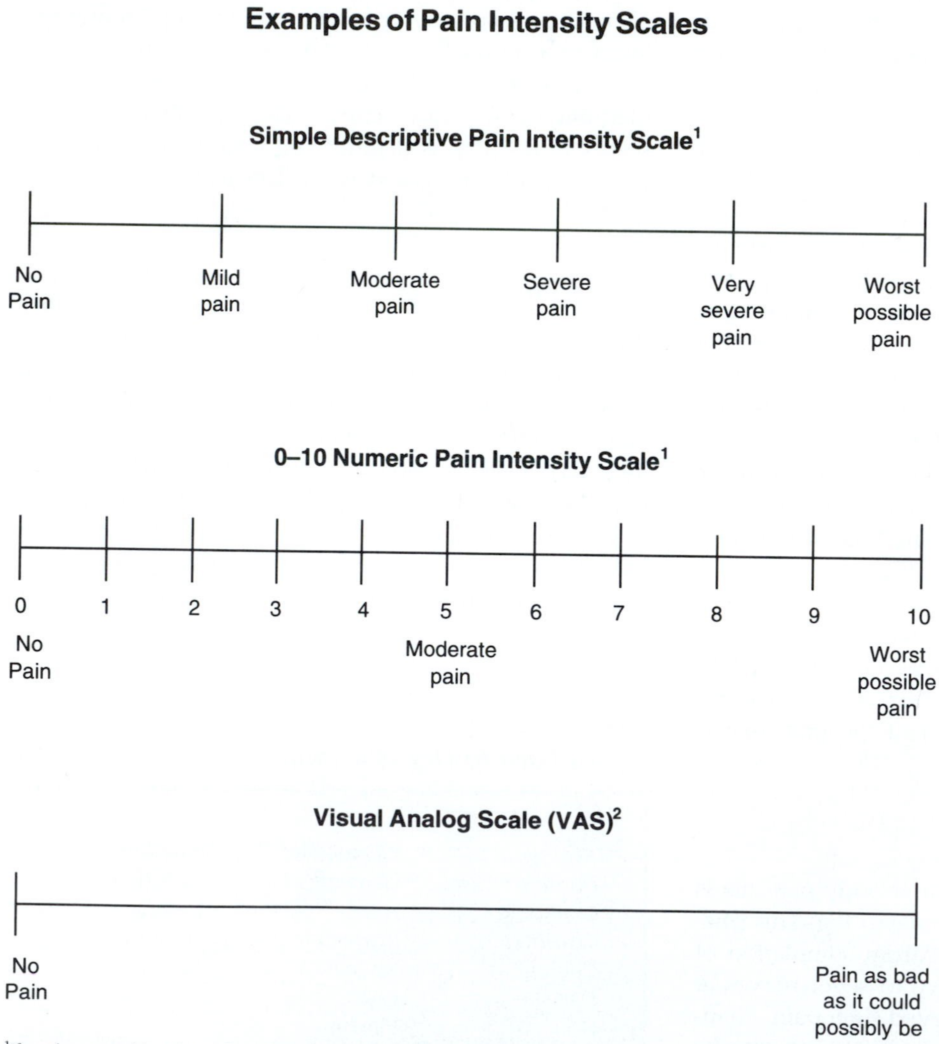

[1]If used as a graphic rating scale, a 10-cm baseline is recommended.

[2]A 10-cm baseline is recommended for VAS scales.

Figure 32-4. Examples of pain intensity scales.

Display 32–3
Questions to Ask Regarding Pain

1. Location

"Point to where it hurts the most."
"Outline the area of pain."
"Describe exactly where you are feeling the pain."
"Does your pain extend from where it starts to other places?"

2. Severity

"Would you describe this pain as mild, moderate, or severe?"
"On a scale of 0 to 10, with 0 being no pain and 10 the worst possible pain, how would you rate your current pain?"
"How does your pain now compare with your pain yesterday?"
"Is it worse during the day or at night or at any other time of the day?"

3. Quality

"Describe for me what your pain feels like."
"Can you describe your pain using words like *sharp* or *dull* or *aching*?"

4. Related Factors

"When did your pain begin?"
"Can you identify anything that caused your pain?"
"Is there anything that tends to make your pain get worse?"
"Has your pain changed in any way since it began?"
"What have you done in the past that relieved your pain?"
"How does position affect your pain?"
"How does activity affect your pain?"

so. Children may not have adequate vocabularies to describe their pain or may use words in their own ways. For example, one 4-year-old repeatedly told the nurse she had a headache. This was duly noted on the chart. Only when a more perceptive nurse asked the child to point to the hurt was it discovered that the pain was in the abdomen. This child called any kind of pain a headache.

Sometimes it is helpful to ask the patient to draw pain, either freehand or using a prepared diagram with symbols to identify types of pain. The visual approach helps the patient to find ways to describe adequately what he or she is feeling.

Figure 32-5 shows a diagram that can be used to assess complex pain. It is most often used when chronic pain is being assessed, but it is also valuable for assessing pain in children.

Physical Assessment

You should carefully observe the patient with regard to pain. Respiration, pulse, skin color, wincing, restlessness, and inability to sleep are important indications of the patient's physical response to pain. The patient's muscles may be tensed, the brow may be furrowed, and a position that relieves stress on the painful part may be maintained. The person may move slowly and carefully to protect the painful site or may resist moving at all. Such nonverbal cues may be the only evidence of pain in the child or the person unable to communicate (Fig. 32-6).

Sometimes objective behaviors do not correlate with the intensity of pain expressed on the scale. A patient may state that the pain is 8 on a 0- to 10-point scale and yet be talking with family and showing no autonomic signs of pain. This does not mean the patient is not really in pain but is more likely to indicate that the person has excellent coping skills (Acute Pain Management Guideline Panel, 1992a). Other patients may deny pain, yet have many objective signs of pain. This may result from denial, fear of treatment methods, or a belief that stoicism is appropriate.

It is sometimes helpful to have patients rate their mood or distress separately from their pain intensity. This may indicate when anxiety needs to be treated as well as pain.

Nursing Diagnosis

A large number of nursing diagnoses relate to pain. Some refer to problems in daily living that result from the pain and others to the pain itself.

Pain

When the pain itself is the concern, the nursing diagnosis would be Pain. The etiology would clearly state the cause of the pain, for example, abdominal surgery on 12/1 or open ulcer on heel. It may be helpful to add a modifier such as acute, chronic, or terminal. The modifier may help in realistic planning for pain relief. The location of the pain may be specified in the original statement, or it may be a part of the etiology. The location is an essential part of the nursing diagnosis. The intensity may also be included as part of the initial statement. You should guard against making a statement about pain intensity based on any measure other than the patient's subjective assessment. It is not uncommon for nurses to underestimate pain if the person's re-

Describing your pain

Select the symbol(s) from the key below that most appropriately describe(s) the pain sensation(s) you feel. Mark the symbols on the figures below in the areas of your body where you feel the sensations. Include all affected areas. Just to complete the picture, please draw in your face.

Name

Date

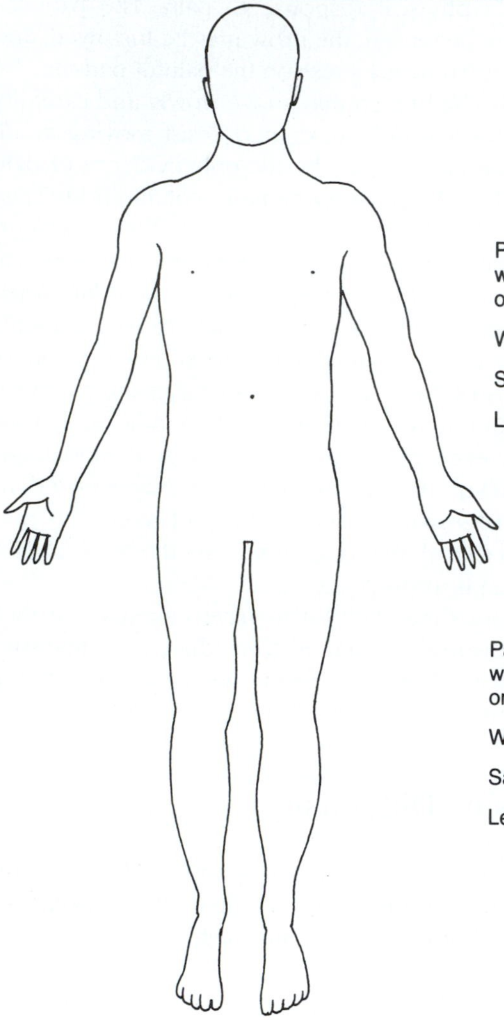

Pain in arm(s) compared with pain in neck (check one):

Worse than____________

Same as____________

Less than____________

Pain in leg(s) compared with pain in back (check one):

Worse than____________

Same as____________

Less than____________

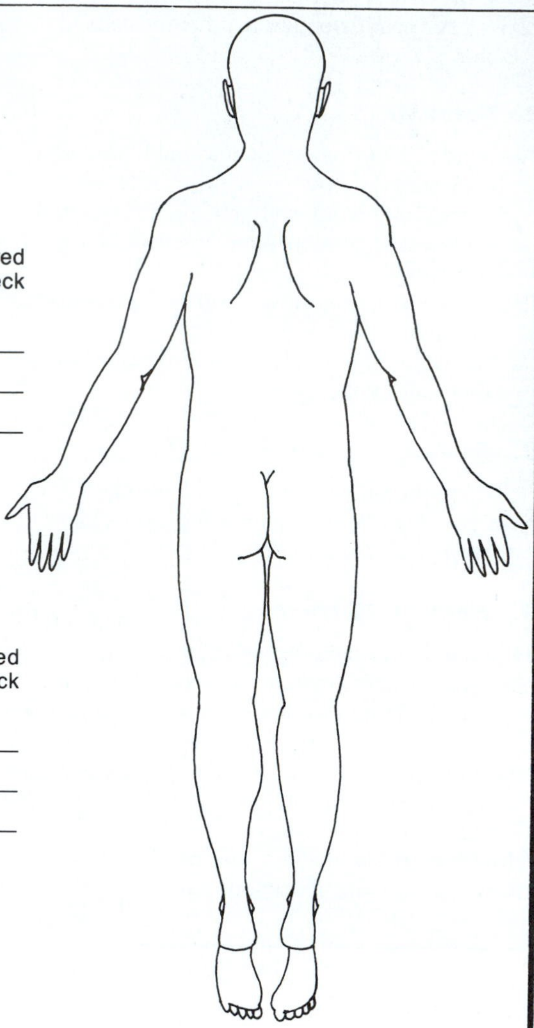

KEY:

Ache	Numbness	Pins and needles	Burning	Stabbing
Λ Λ Λ Λ	= = = =	o o o o	X X X X	/ / / /
Λ Λ Λ Λ	= = = =	o o o o	X X X X	/ / / /
Λ Λ Λ Λ	= = = =	o o o o	X X X X	/ / / /

Figure 32-5. Pain assessment tool. (Reproduced with permission from *Patient Care* magazine, January 30, 1984. Copyright © 1984, Patient Care Communications Inc., Darien, CT. All rights reserved.)

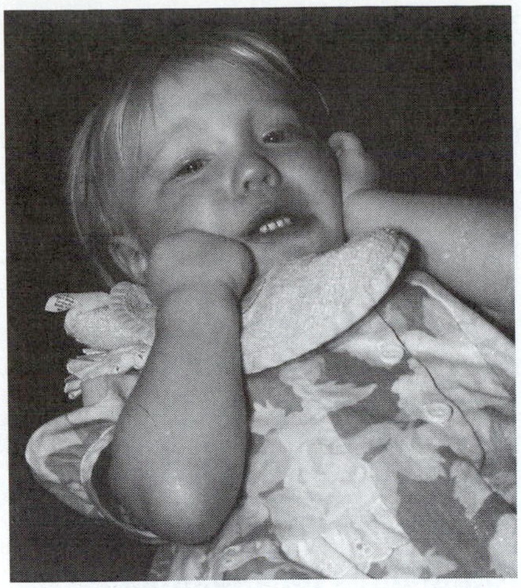

Figure 32-6. Nonverbal clues may indicate the presence of pain.

sponse is different from what the nurse's personal belief system holds to be appropriate.

Knowledge Deficit Related to Pain Management

When a person does not understand the plans for managing pain, he or she is not able to be an active participant. Gaining knowledge may be the first step in regaining control over a life that seemed out of control. The person may need knowledge about the source of the pain, but more important is knowledge about personal strategies for pain management. This includes a need to understand how nonpharmacologic as well as pharmacologic interventions may be used to manage pain effectively.

Impaired Mobility Related to Pain

Often pain limits a person's ability to be physically active, either because the pain is increased by movement or because the pain creates fatigue and lack of energy. Because activity is a basic need, disruption of normal patterns of activity can be a serious concern. You may note that the person is reluctant to move, moves with slowness, or holds a part of the body rigid to prevent movement. In other instances the patient may not be participating in usual activities and may be spending a majority of the time in a chair or in bed.

Nursing Diagnoses Related to Comfort

- Pain
- Knowledge Deficit related to pain management
- Impaired Mobility related to pain
- Anxiety related to acute pain
- Impaired Adjustment related to chronic pain
- Ineffective Individual Coping related to chronic pain
- Hopelessness related to chronic pain
- Powerlessness related to chronic pain

Anxiety Related to Acute Pain

Anxiety is often a response to acute pain, especially when the person has no reference point from which to understand the pain. The anxiety may make pain perception more acute, and the pain thus increases the anxiety. Pain and anxiety often feed on one another in a circular fashion. It is usually not helpful to try to identify which came first. It really does not matter. Instead, actions should be directed at both concerns. See Chapter 34 for suggestions on interventions for anxiety.

Impaired Adjustment Related to Chronic Pain

Impaired adjustment may take many forms. For some people, an impaired adjustment occurs because the individual is unable to engage in leisure activities such as sports. For others it means being unable to adjust to the changes at a job or to the inability to be productive in the home. For still others it means not making the adjustments to limitations on ordinary ADLs. The significant point is that the style is a change from the way the patient would like things to be.

Ineffective Individual Coping Related to Chronic Pain

When the individual is having difficulty meeting other demands of life because of the presence of chronic pain, the nursing diagnosis is Ineffective Coping related to chronic pain. This diagnosis is not usually appropriate for the person with acute pain because that person is not usually expected to be managing other aspects of life and the disruption is temporary.

Hopelessness and Powerlessness Related to Chronic Pain

When pain continues and no clear relief is predicted, a feeling of hopelessness often prevails and the person appears depressed. Sometimes people mistake the quiet withdrawn behavior of the person for an indication that the pain is not present. Rather, the physiologic responses to pain have ceased through a process of accommodation, and acute anxiety is not present because the person has lost hope for relief. Hopelessness is often accompanied by feelings of losing control and powerlessness. The individual does not feel any ability to change or alter personal circumstances. Actions aimed at restoring control and hope for pain relief are appropriate (see Chapter 34).

Other Nursing Diagnoses

Self-care deficits may occur because of the pain. There may be difficulties in ventilation or elimination or other basic needs related to pain. These are outlined in the chapters on the individual topics.

Planning and Implementation

We believe that pain relief is important to well-being and that the desired outcome or goal of pain intervention should be complete elimination of pain (see sample Nursing Care Plan Related to Pain and sample Nursing Care Plan Related to Chronic Pain). Fortunately, this is usually possible. Nurses should not assume that this outcome is not appropriate without consulting with both patient and physician and trying a variety of approaches to pain relief.

When total relief is not possible, then reduction of pain to a level that the client considers acceptable is the desired outcome. To accomplish this, the nurse must work cooperatively with the patient and the patient must understand the goal. Some conflicts between staff members and patients are rooted in differences of goals for pain relief. If the patient expects complete eradication of pain and the nurse is satisfied with pain reduction, then the stage is set for conflict.

Reduction of suffering is also an appropriate desired outcome of pain relief measures. Suffering is the degree to which the person experiences distress, interference with ADLs, and inability to meet life goals. Particularly with chronic pain, the primary desired outcome may be that the person experiences less distress, is able to participate as desired in life activities, is able to sleep or rest, feels less fatigue, and is able to meet personal goals in life.

Philosophical beliefs about pain and its meaning underlie decisions made in regard to initiating treatment of pain. If a nurse believes that most people try to be exact about pain and that complete eradication of pain is important to well-being, plans will differ considerably from those made by a nurse who believes that most people exaggerate pain or that complete eradication of pain is not important. Our belief is that the patient should be the determinant of the goal of pain relief, that is, the person whom the pain most affects and whose life is disrupted by the pain. Based on patient goals, you can work collaboratively with the patient in planning for pain relief.

Interventions can take many forms, depending on such factors as the origin and severity of the pain, the patient's response to it, and medical orders regarding drugs and activity. Intervention may be aimed at 1) eliminating the source or stimulus of pain, 2) preventing the pain receptors from reacting, 3) interrupting the impulse somewhere along the pathway, 4) decreasing perception of pain, or 5) altering the patient's interpretation of and response to the pain. An approach that aims at several aspects of the pain simultaneously may be more effective than intervention directed at only a single aspect. Many individual strategies for pain relief act in more than one way.

General Guidelines for Planning Pain Intervention

The following general guidelines are helpful in planning for pain relief.

Always acknowledge the patient's pain. Remember that pain is present when the patient states that it is and the intensity is what the patient identifies. Having another person acknowledge the pain allows the patient to focus on personal coping strategies rather than on the reactions and responses of those providing care.

Intervene before the pain becomes severe. It is much easier to keep pain at a low level if it never is allowed to get severe. Once pain has become severe, it may take much more vigorous intervention to lessen it again. When acute pain occurs, it is more effective to provide frequent large doses of narcotics initially so that pain is relieved and then reduce the doses as long as the patient states that pain is under control. The patient will often be comfortable with a lower dose when the anxiety and feelings of loss of control are not present. More and more experts are recommending that pain medications be provided to patients in pain on a regular schedule rather than on a PRN basis (Acute Pain Management Guideline Panel, 1992a).

Use a variety of pain relief measures simultaneously. An approach that includes more than one type of intervention is more likely to be effective than using only one because more than one aspect of the pain cycle is being addressed. Even when narcotics are used, pain relief is enhanced, narcotic dosage may be lessened, and side effects may be averted by using other interventions at the same time.

Include those interventions the patient believes to be helpful. The role of the placebo effect, the role of anxiety, and the role of psychological and emotional factors in pain tolerance and pain interpretation support the view that those interventions the patient believes in are more likely to be effective.

Teach the patient to initiate pain control measures independently, whenever possible. Providing the patient

Nursing Care Plan
Sample Nursing Care Plan Related to Pain

Nursing Diagnosis	Pain related to abdominal incision **Supportive data:** First postoperative day after abdominal hysterectomy. Winces and grimaces whenever attempting movement. Expresses reluctance to deep breathe because "it hurts too much." P 94, R 28 and shallow.
Desired Patient Outcomes	Turns and moves in bed. Deep breathes and coughs up secretions. States is comfortable.

Nursing Action	**Rationale**
1. Give ordered IM pain medication q4h.	Regular administration of pain medication maintains the level of pain control and results in better pain relief for the amount of medication administered.
2. Encourage patient to use pillow to splint incision when deep breathing and coughing.	Splinting of an incision prevents the abrupt movement of wound edges that sharply increases pain.
3. Reinforce relaxation techniques taught preoperatively.	Relaxation exercises are effective in decreasing pain perception and serve as an adjunct to pain medication.
4. Remind patient of techniques of moving to decrease strain on abdomen that were taught preoperatively.	Strain on an abdominal incision increases pain. Correct movement techniques prevent strain on the abdominal incision.
5. Give backrub to promote relaxation while waiting for medication to take effect.	Back massage provides distraction from pain, alternative input that competes with pain impulses in the spinal cord, relaxation of tense muscles, and psychological comfort.

with ways to manage pain independently increases feelings of personal control and enhances self-esteem. The patient who feels personal control will be less anxious and this, in turn, will assist with alleviating pain.

Maintain careful records of pain assessment and intervention and evaluate all measures attempted. In noncomplex situations, this may be done as part of a routine flow sheet. When pain is severe, more complex, or being treated with narcotic analgesics, the use of a pain control flow sheet facilitates effective pain management. Figure 32-7 presents an example of a pain management flow sheet.

If pain is not relieved by initial interventions, consult with others and try additional methods. There are many different ways of relieving pain and many different medications available. It is a disservice to the patient/client to give up prematurely.

Basic Nursing Interventions for Pain Control

Nurses have many different measures they can use to assist in pain relief. The first thing to consider is whether the source of pain can be removed. When the source cannot be removed then other measures are necessary. These include distraction, relaxation, guided imagery, comfort measures, physical stimulation, establishing interpersonal relationships, and the use of medications ordered by the physician. These are discussed below. The scientific evidence supporting pain relief measures is outlined in Tables 32-1 and 32-2.

Nursing Care Plan

Sample Nursing Care Plan Related to Chronic Pain

Nursing Diagnosis

Chronic pain related to arthritis in hands

Supportive data:

Has had rheumatoid arthritis for 20 years.

Hands are deformed, with swollen joints.

States hands are too painful to do "anything."

Desired Patient Outcomes

Pain reduced to the place where patient can participate in self-care as evidenced by the following behaviors:

1. Feeds self.
2. Bathes self.
3. States pain is reduced.

Nursing Action	Rationale
1. Give first AM aspirin dose at 6:00 AM with milk.	Aspirin is a non-steroidal anti-inflammatory drug that acts to decrease the inflammation that causes pain and also acts on peripheral nerve receptors. Administering the first dose early allows it to take effect before activity begins. Milk decreases stomach irritation often associated with aspirin.
2. Provide warm water for soaking hands before meals.	Moist heat decreases inflammation and pain and increases joint flexibility in arthritis.
3. Prepare food to decrease stress on hands.	Cutting food, opening milk cartons, and other preparatory tasks can put stress on inflammed joints in the hands thus increasing pain.
4. Make sure patient has utensils with large handles for meals.	Large handles are easier to grasp with stiff or painful joints.
5. Provide shower chair and sponge mitt for her to bathe self.	Showering while seated reduces pressure on lower joints while maintaining usual activities. A shower mitt slips on a hand and does not require grasping with painful joints.
6. Stay with her during activities to assist and provide positive feedback for all independent activities.	Interpersonal relationships reinforce independent actions and provide emotional support.

Eliminating the Source of Pain

Eliminating its cause is certainly the most long-lasting and effective means of dealing with pain. Such actions as removing open safety pins, changing wet bedding, and smoothing wrinkled sheets are all aimed at eliminating the source of pain. For the postsurgical patient who has gas pains, helping the person to expel the gas by administering return-flow enemas or encouraging movement to increase peristalsis is the most effective approach. The nurse who automatically thinks medication when a patient says, "I hurt!" is doing the patient an injustice.

Complex or inaccessible sources of pain are more problematic and may not be subject to nursing intervention to remove the cause. The surgeon must remove painful calluses on the feet or a gallbladder filled with stones to provide long-term relief of pain.

Certain drugs may, by reducing inflammation and swelling of a body part, reduce or eliminate the pain caused by those conditions. When severe muscle

Nursing Issues and Trends: *Inadequate Treatment of Severe Pain*

The inadequate treatment of severe pain is a serious concern in health care. The Agency for Health Care Policy and Research studied the treatment of pain throughout the United States as they prepared their recommendations. They discovered a disturbing incidence of inadequate treatment of severe pain in both children and adults. A variety of factors such as lack of current information about drug effects and side effects, fears regarding addiction and dependence, and attitudes about the role and effect of pain might contribute to this situation. Nurses are in a key role to support the effective treatment of pain and to act as advocates for patients in pain.

spasms are the cause of pain, muscle relaxant drugs will help. Massage can also relieve muscle spasms, especially in the neck and back. When pain is caused by ischemia, measures to increase blood flow may reduce pain. Intervention to remove the source of the pain is the best long-term response to pain and the preferred method of intervention. However, it is not always possible.

Distraction

By preoccupying the attention, distractions can prevent pain from being perceived. If a person with a headache becomes engrossed in a hobby, for example, the head pain may recede from awareness, only to return when the distraction ceases. Pain is not perceived because all cerebral cortex activity is focused elsewhere, and impulses from the thalamus are blocked. When concentration decreases, impulses will be transmitted to the cortex and pain will be noticed. This mechanism is most effective in cases of relatively mild pain. However, if concentration is extreme enough, even severe pain may not be perceived until the distraction is gone. For example, a football player may not realize he is injured until after an important play is completed. Thus, you can sometimes help a person in pain by engaging him or her in an engrossing activity. This approach will not necessarily minimize perception of severe pain that is already present but may increase the patient's comfort.

A wide variety of activities may provide distraction. Visitors, a television program, a book, or anything else the patient is interested in can be effective. For many

USE IN ACCORDANCE WITH PROCEDURE AND PROTOCOL

CIRCLE PAIN TREATMENT MODALITY:

1. PO
2. SUBLINGUAL
3. PATIENT CONTROLLED ANALGESIA (circled)
4. CONTINUOUS IV OPIOID INFUSION
5. TEMPORARY EPIDURAL INTERMITTENT INJECTION
6. PERMANENT EPIDURAL INTERMITTENT INJECTION
7. IM
8. RECTAL
9. CONTINUOUS SUBCUTANEOUS OPIOID INFUSION
10. INTERMITTENT IV OPIOID INJECTION
11. TEMPORARY EPIDURAL CONTINUOUS INFUSION
12. PERMANENT EPIDURAL CONTINUOUS INFUSION

PAIN SCALE:
0 = none
1 = mild
2
3 = moderate
4
5 = severe

SEDATION SCALE:
3 = Awake and responding
2 = Sleeping, but responds to normal voice
1 = Sleeping, but responds to loud voice or movement
0 = Sedated, doesn't respond

DATE	TIME	MED	BAG OR SYRINGE #	ROUTE #	BOLUS	DOSE	PCA DELAY (min)	CONT. RATE or basal	8 hr	BP	P	RR	SEDATION SCALE	PAIN	SKIN ANESTHESIA N=Normal T=Tingling Nb=Numbness A=Absent	SITE CHECK	COMMENTS (e.g., Tubing, filter &/or SQ needle change)	INITIALS
6/26/94	1100	Morphine	#1	IV	2mg	1mg	10	1mg/hr.		118/72	68	16	2	2	N	✓	New tubing	[illegible]
	1200									122/74	74	18	2	3	N	✓	Enc. to	[illegible]
	1300									128/78	86	24	3	4	N	✓	use PCA	[illegible]
	1400									120/72	74	20	2	2	N	✓	Using PCA	[illegible]

Figure 32-7. Pain management flow sheet.

Table 32–1. Scientific Evidence for Nonpharmacologic Interventions to Manage Pain in Adults

Intervention*		Type of Evidence	Comments
Simple Relaxation (begin preoperatively)	Jaw relaxation Progressive muscle relaxation Simple imagery	Ia, IIa, IIb, IV	Effective in reducing mild to moderate pain and as an adjunct to analgesic drugs for severe pain. Use when patients express an interest in relaxation. Requires 3–5 min of staff time for instructions.
	Music	Ib, IIa, IV	Both patient-preferred and "easy listening" music are effective in reducing mild to moderate pain.
Complex Relaxation (begin preoperatively)	Biofeedback	Ib, IIa, IV	Effective in reducing mild to moderate pain and operative site muscle tension. Requires skilled personnel and special equipment.
	Imagery	Ib, IIa, IIb, IV	Effective for reduction of mild to moderate pain. Requires skilled personnel.
Education/ Instruction (begin preoperatively)		Ia, IIa, IIb, IV	Effective for reduction of pain. Should include sensory and procedural information and instruction aimed at reducing activity related pain. Requires 5–15 min of staff time.
TENS		Ia, IIa, III, IV	Effective in reducing pain and improving physical function. Requires skilled personnel and special equipment. May be useful as an adjunct to drug therapy.

*Insufficient scientific evidence is available to provide specific recommendations regarding the use of hypnosis, acupuncture, and other physical modalities for relief of postoperative pain.

Type of Evidence—Key

Ia Evidence obtained from meta-analysis of randomized controlled trials.
Ib Evidence obtained from at least one randomized controlled trial.
IIa Evidence obtained from at least one well-designed controlled study without randomization.
IIb Evidence obtained from at least one other type of well-designed quasi-experimental study.
III Evidence obtained from well-designed nonexperimental descriptive studies, such as comparative studies, correlational studies, and case studies.
IV Evidence obtained from expert committee reports or opinions and/or clinical experiences of respected authorities.

Note: References are available in the *Guideline Report. Acute Pain Management: Operative or Medical Procedures and Trauma.* AHCPR Pub. No. 92–0001. Rockville, Md.: Agency for Health Care Policy and Research, Public Health Service, U.S. Department of Health and Human Services. 1992.

individuals, music is an excellent distraction. This can be especially effective when earphones are used and thus other sources of input are blocked. You need to be careful not to convey the idea that pain from which a person can be distracted is trivial; the importance or strength of the distractor is the primary factor. A patient who is effectively using distraction may lack behavioral indicators of pain, but when asked, is able to describe pain and estimate its severity.

Relaxation Techniques

The relaxation techniques discussed in Chapter 6 may be of value in altering pain perception. Relaxation provides other input to the brain, blocking pain perception. The complex techniques are most effective when learned before pain is present, but some simple relaxation techniques can be taught at the time the pain is present. Once patients learn to use these techniques they can use them independently; however, some individuals do better when they are coached.

Slow rhythmic breathing is perhaps the simplest relaxation technique to teach. You coach the person to breathe slowly and deeply while focusing on feelings of relaxation. Abdominal breathing in which the abdomen rises on inspiration works particularly well. The patient is further encouraged to imagine a place that is calming and relaxing. This technique may be used for only a few seconds for a short procedure or for up to 20 minutes at a time (McCaffery and Beebe, 1989).

Jaw relaxation is another effective relaxation technique. The patient is coached to let the lower jaw drop slightly as though starting a yawn. The tongue rests quietly and the lips soften. The person breathes rhythmically. The patient is encouraged to let the mind drift and not think in words (McCaffery and Beebe, 1989).

Progressive relaxation of the entire body effectively

Table 32–2. Scientific Evidence for Pharmacologic Interventions to Manage Pain in Adults

Intervention*		Type of Evidence	Comments
NSAIDs	Oral (alone)	Ib, IV	Effective for mild to moderate pain. Begin preoperatively. Relatively contraindicated in patients with renal disease and risk of or actual coagulopathy. May mask fever.
	Oral (adjunct to opioid)	Ia, IV	Potentiating effect resulting in opioid sparing. Begin preop. Cautions as above.
	Parenteral (ketorolac)	Ib, IV	Effective for moderate to severe pain. Expensive. Ueful where opiods contraindicated, especially to avoid respiratory depression and sedation. Advance to opioid.
Opioids	Oral	IV	As effective as parenteral in appropriate doses. Use as soon as oral medication tolerated. Route of choice.
	Intramuscular	Ib, IV	Has been the standard parenteral route, but injections painful and absorption unreliable. Hence, avoid this route when possible.
	Subcutaneous	Ib, IV	Preferable to intramuscular for low-volume continuous infusion. Injections painful and absorption unreliable. Avoid this route for long-term repetitive dosing.
	Intravenous	Ib, IV	Parenteral route of choice after major surgery. Suitable for titrated bolus or continuous administration (including PCA), but requires monitoring. Significant risk of respiratory depression with inappropriate dosing.
	PCA (systemic)	Ia, IV	Intravenous or subcutaneous routes recommended. Good, steady level of analgesia. Popular with patients but requires special infusion pumps and staff education. See cautions about opioids above.
	Epidural and intrathecal	Ia, IV	When suitable, provides good analgesia. Significant risk of respiratory depression. sometimes delayed in onset. Requires careful monitoring. Use of infusion pumps requires additional equipment and staff education.
Local Anesthetics	Epidural and intrathecal	Ia, IV	Limited indications. Expensive if infusion pumps used. Effective regional analgesia. Opioid sparing. Addition of opioid to local anesthetic may improve analgesia. Risks of hypotension, weakness, numbness. Use of infusion pump requires additional equipment and staff.
	Peripheral nerve block	Ia, IV	Limited indications and duration of action. Effective regional analgesia. Opioid sparing.

Type of Evidence—Key
Ia Evidence obtained from meta-analysis of randomized controlled trials.
Ib Evidence obtained from at least one randomized controlled trial.
IIa Evidence obtained from at least one well-designed controlled study without randomization.
IIb Evidence obtained from at least one other type of well-designed quasi-experimental study.
III Evidence obtained from well-designed nonexperimental descriptive studies, such as comparative studies, correlational studies, and case studies.
IV Evidence obtained from expert committee reports or opinions and/or clinical experiences of respected authorities.
Note: References are available in the *Guideline Report, Acute Pain Management: Operative or Medical Procedures and Trauma*. AHCPR Pub. No. 92–0001. Rockville, Md.: Agency for Health Care Policy and Research, Public Health Service, U.S. Department of Health and Human Services. 1992.

blocks pain perception. The patient starts by tightening all muscles to feel the tension and then starting with the toes, gradually relaxes each muscle group in term, moving up the body. Slow breathing during this process enhances relaxation.

Biofeedback for relaxation may be used as a mechanism to teach an individual to focus on other body processes, thus blocking pain perception. This technique usually requires an investment in time, an expert instructor, and a mechanical feedback device.

Guided Imagery

Guided imagery, in which the patient visualizes being in a happy or peaceful scene, can be an effective distraction. Guided imagery has been used with much success to help children with cancer manage ongoing pain and endure painful procedures. The patient selects the restful and pleasurable scene. This might be walking by the seashore, sitting by a warm fire on a winter evening, or watching a sunset. The nurse then quietly and slowly helps to describe the scene and encourages the patient to imagine being there. Feelings and sensory impressions are described. To be effective with this technique requires practice.

Comfort Measures

Interpretation of pain may be influenced by comforting measures that counteract the pain impulses. Bathing to remove excess perspiration, combing the hair, or providing a backrub that is soothing to the skin may help decrease the severity of the pain. It is important to find out what the individual regards as soothing because people vary greatly in their choice of comforts.

Cutaneous Stimulation

Massage, pressure, and the application of cold (icing) to the skin have all been found to decrease the transmission of pain impulses. When these techniques cannot be used on the painful site itself, application to the contralateral (opposite side) body part may be effective in relieving pain (McCaffery, 1980). In some facilities, you will need a physician's order to use icing.

Therapeutic touch is a specific therapy in which the touch therapist transmits energy to the patient with the intent of potentiating the healing process. The theoretical basis of therapeutic touch rests on the concept of the human being as an energy field and that energy can be transferred from one person to another. Special training in therapeutic touch is necessary to use the technique effectively (Wright, 1987).

Protecting Pain Receptors From Stimuli

It is sometimes possible to protect the receptors from the source of pain. Examples are putting petroleum jelly on excoriated buttocks to protect the skin from urine and putting a cloth over the eyes to protect them from light. The patient with trigeminal neuralgia, a disorder of the fifth cranial nerve, may use a silk scarf to protect the overly sensitive nerve from air movement that might stimulate it.

Establishing an Interpersonal Relationship

Pain interpretation may also be modified beneficially by an interpersonal process involving the nurse and the patient (see Chapter 13). For example, a person who interprets pain as punishment can be helped to examine and deal with such feelings. This process may, in turn, decrease anxiety about pain, reduce physiologic response to pain, and change the patient's interpretation of the severity of pain. Other interpretations of pain may be dealt with in the same manner. A warm, accepting interpersonal relationship establishes trust and an atmosphere for mutual problem-solving in regard to pain management. It may help to alleviate anxiety and support the individual in effective problem-solving.

Using Pharmacologic Interventions for Pain

A major segment of nursing intervention for pain involves collaborative action with the physician in giving medications for the person in pain. Nonnarcotic medications, narcotic medications, and medications to treat other symptoms are all part of the pharmacologic intervention for pain.

Using Nonnarcotic Medications for Pain Relief

Nonnarcotic analgesics, narcotic agonist–antagonist drugs, antidepressants, antiemetics, and sedatives, are all used for managing pain. Medications are an important part of pain management, but they are much more effective when used in conjunction with nonpharmacologic methods of pain relief. Nurses must work collaboratively with physicians to determine the optimum combination of medications for the individual patient.

You should be familiar with the individual drug being used, its actions, side effects, and usual dosage. The effectiveness of any drug used to treat pain is variable and depends on the type of pain and the individual response to the medication as well as the drug itself. Therefore, suggested dosages must be used as guidelines and patients observed closely for individual response. The Acute Pain Management Guideline Panel has published a list of equianalgesic dosages of pain medications. The reference dose for these charts is 10 mg morphine every 3 to 4 hours by the parenteral route and 30 mg morphine every 3 to 4 hours by the oral route (Table 32-3).

The *nonnarcotic analgesics*, which include the nonsteroidal anti-inflammatory drugs (NSAIDs) such as such as aspirin, acetaminophen (Tylenol, Datril, etc.) and ibuprofen, act at peripheral sites to reduce nociceptor stimulation and through inhibiting prostaglandin synthesis (Coyle, 1987). Most of the nonnarcotic analgesics are given orally. Aspirin is also given rectally and a parenteral NSAID, ketoralac, is now available. They may be used alone for mild to moderate pain or in combination with narcotics for severe pain. Those with anti-inflammatory properties, such as aspirin and the NSAIDs, are especially useful when inflammation is a part of the cause of pain and in bone, joint, and muscle pain.

These drugs differ in their effects on the individual, and therefore identification of the best one in any specific instance is often a matter of trial and error. This also means that the failure of one of these drugs to achieve pain relief should not be used as a reason to eliminate the whole group as ineffective in a particular situation.

Narcotic agonist–antagonist drugs act on the CNS and include such drugs as pentazocine (Talwin) and nalbuphine (Nubain). They have an **agonist effect**, which means they act as narcotics do. Simultaneously,

Table 32–3. Dosing Data for Opioid Analgesics

Drug	Approximate Equianalgesic Oral Dose	Approximate Equianalgesic Parenteral Dose
Opioid Agonist		
Morphine*	30 mg q3–4h (around-the-clock dosing) 60 mg q3–4h (single dose or intermittent dosing)	10 mg q3–4h
Codeine†	130 mg q3–4h	75 mg q3–4h
Hydromophone* (Dilaudid)	7.5 mg q3–4h	1.5 mg q 3–4h
Hydrocodone (in Lorcet, Lortab, Vicodin, others)	30 mg q3–4h	Not available
Levorphanol (Levo-Dromoran)	4 mg q6–8h	2 mg q6–8h
Meperidine (Demerol)	300 mg q2–3h	100 mg q3h
Methadone (Dolophine, others)	20 mg q6–8h	10 mg q6–8h
Oxycodone (Roxicodone, also in Percocet, Percodan, Tylox, others)	30 mg q3–4h	Not available
Oxymorphone* (Numorphan)	Not available	1 mg q3–4h
Opioid Agonist-Antagonist and Partial Agonist		
Buprenorphine (Buprenex)	Not available	0.3–0.4 mg q6–8h
Butorphanol (Stadol)	Not available	2 mg q3–4h
Nalbuphine (Nubain)	Not available	10 mg q3–4h
Pentazocine (Talwin, others)	150 mg q3–4h	60 mg q3–4h

Note: Published tables vary in the suggested doses that are equianalgesic to morphine. Clinical response is the criterion that must be applied for each patient; titration to clinical response is necessary. Because there is not complete cross tolerance among these drugs, it is usually necessary to use a lower than equianalgesic dose when changing drugs and to retitrate to response.
Caution: Recommended doses do not apply to patients with renal or hepatic insufficiency or other conditions affecting drug metabolism and kinetics.
Caution: Doses listed for patients with body weight less than 50 kg cannot be used as initial starting doses in babies less than 6 months of age. Consult the *Clinical Practice Guideline for Acute Pain Management: Operative or Medical Procedures and Trauma* section on management of pain in neonates for recommendations.
Source: Acute Pain Management Guideline Panel. *Acute Pain Management: Operative or Medical Procedures and Trauma: Clinical Practice Guidelines.* AHCPR Pub. No. 92–0032. Rockville, Md.: Agency for Health Care Policy and Research, Public Health Service, U.S. Department of Health and Human Services, 1992.

they have a narcotic **antagonist effect** in that they will reverse the effects of a narcotic already in the body. These drugs will not prevent withdrawal symptoms in the individual who is narcotic dependent. They are effective in some individuals, providing adequate pain relief with minimal sedation. Others respond less well to these drugs and do not receive adequate pain relief.

Ointments containing *topical anesthetic agents* are used to decrease the sensitivity of skin and mucous membrane receptors. Topical anesthetic agents are found in products for hemorrhoids, sunburn, minor skin lesions, and mouth washes. Allergies to these agents are common; therefore, careful assessment of the site is essential when they are used.

Rubbing a *menthol ointment* on the skin produces local stimulation and heat, which relieve pain. Menthol ointment has been most frequently used over joints, but has been long used in the Filipino culture for other types of pain as well. It appears that the stimulation of the ointment competes with the pain for ascending pathways and may serve to block pain perception (McCaffery, 1980).

The use of *antidepressant medications* in the treatment of chronic pain has been a matter of much investigation. These medications may be active in various ways, some of which are still poorly understood. However, the pain relief is often apparent before the drug is effective in changing the person's mood. Their ability to provide pain relief may be related to the effect of the medication on the neurotransmitters that are part of the inhibiting impulses in the spinal column and the brain ("Pain Management," 1984). Thus, the antidepressant may be blocking the transmission of pain impulses.

Antiemetic drugs may be given when nausea is an

accompaniment of pain and contributing to overall discomfort. Antiemetic drugs may also be of assistance when individuals respond to a narcotic with nausea. Although changing the drug given for pain is a preferable action, sometimes this is not possible, and treating the nausea may allow for good pain relief. Tolerance to the nausea effect does occur and therefore for long-term use antiemetics may be needed only initially and then may be discontinued.

Sedatives and tranquilizers do not enhance pain relief itself (although many individuals mistakenly believe that they do). However, when anxiety is a significant accompaniment of pain, these drugs decrease anxiety and therefore may contribute to overall pain relief by breaking the anxiety–pain cycle. Their sedative effects contribute to rest.

Using Narcotic Analgesics for Pain Relief

Narcotic analgesics are a group of drugs that depress the CNS and interfere with pain perception both in the spinal cord and centrally; they also alter pain interpretation in the cerebral cortex. Narcotics encompass a large group of drugs, and although technically some of them are considered equally effective, individual persons do respond differently to different drugs. If one drug is not effective, others should be tried until the most effective one is found.

In certain types of severe pain, narcotics are the preferred method of intervention. They are simple to use, effective, and inexpensive, and adverse effects are usually minimal. Other methods are less reliably effective, and there is no reason to withhold narcotics. Postoperative pain and pain from severe trauma are two of the appropriate instances. Other methods of pain relief may be used as adjuncts in these situations, making the person more comfortable, but narcotics remain the central method of intervention.

One factor that is involved in planning for pain relief is concern for balancing possible adverse effects of narcotics on other body systems with the need for pain control. Narcotic analgesics slow propulsive peristalsis in the digestive system, especially the bowel, creating gas and constipation. They also cloud the sensorium, making the person less alert. Lack of alertness may create safety problems, inability to carry out desired activities, and difficulties in interpersonal relating. These changes may also make it difficult to assess neurologic status. Narcotics also affect the cardiovascular system and may lower blood pressure and cardiac output. Respirations may also be depressed by narcotics; in fact, this is perhaps the most adverse response to narcotics. Planning must consider the overall effects of medications given.

Unfortunately, some nurses believe that these adverse effects are more widespread and severe than they are, making the nurses reluctant to use even usual dosages. An understanding of medications, their appropriate dosages, and the incidence of side effects is essential to effective planning.

A wide variety of methods are used to administer narcotic analgesics. Each method has its advantages and disadvantages. Understanding these is important as you work with physicians in making decisions about narcotic administration. In addition, dosages vary with the same drug depending on the method of administration. Typically, oral doses must be larger than injectable doses, but this is not always true.

The simplest method of giving narcotics is through *oral administration.* Narcotics administered through the oral route take approximately 15 to 30 minutes to be effective. Their absorption time varies from individual to individual. The advantage of the oral route is that patients or families as well as health care workers can administer the drug with ease. The potential for infection and the pain from injections are eliminated.

Many moderate-level narcotics, such as oxycodone, are available only in the oral form. Potent narcotics, such as morphine, are effective orally and are available in oral forms that are slowly released to allow for less frequent dosing. Some narcotics, such as meperidine (Demerol), are poorly absorbed orally and therefore the dosage must be greatly adjusted if the oral form is used.

Oral narcotics, of course, cannot be used for those who cannot take medications by mouth. They are most commonly used when pain is expected to be long term, like cancer pain and other types of terminal pain, or when the patient is progressing away from injectable narcotics to less potent drugs.

Narcotics given by *intramuscular injection* are readily absorbed and quickly effective. The effect lasts for several hours and thus provides ongoing relief. The length of time during which pain is relieved depends on the narcotic used and the ability of the individual to break down and excrete the drug. Although it is conventional to order these drugs on an every-4-hours (q4h) schedule, in reality some drugs such as meperidine (Demerol) are commonly cleared within 3 hours. In the elderly, on the other hand, some drugs may last much longer than 4 hours. Individual assessment of effect is critical.

The injection itself may cause discomfort, and if circulation is impaired, absorption may be delayed. Repeated injections may cause sclerosing (scarring) of the muscle tissue. Scar tissue has poor circulation; therefore, absorption is impaired in those areas. This becomes a problem for those with long-term pain. Intramuscular narcotics are commonly used after surgery or injury when pain is expected to be acute and needs immediate intervention. Antiemetic and tranquilizing drugs may be added to intramuscular narcotics for injection when needed. These drugs do not potentiate the pain relief, but they do add sedation and provide relief for other symptoms such as anxiety, nausea, and vomiting.

Intravenous narcotics are immediately available and provide prompt pain relief. However, adverse effects may also occur rapidly, so careful attention to dosage, proper dilution, rate of administration, and assessment is essential for safety. The intravenous route is preferred in emergency situations and those in which circulation to muscles might be decreased, resulting in delayed absorption of intramuscular injections. Intravenous drugs are also rapidly metabolized; therefore, their effects are short acting. This permits more precise adjustment of dosage to fit the needs and response of the patient than does intramuscular administration.

Maintenance of an intravenous access route is essential if multiple doses will be given. This may be done through an ongoing intravenous fluid infusion or the placement of an injection adaptor plug (heparin lock) in the intravenous access needle (see Module 54, Administering Intravenous Medications). One difficulty with using the intravenous route for routine needs has been the time involved in frequent administration. When medications are needed for long periods, the use of continuous infusions and patient-controlled units (discussed below) overcomes this problem.

The use of pumps that can deliver medications in precise dosages has made the safe continuous intravenous infusion of narcotics possible. The amount of drug is carefully titrated to provide a stable blood level that provides constant pain relief. This method avoids peaks and troughs of pain relief. It has been used most frequently for terminal pain, but has also been successful for short-term pain relief after major surgery or trauma. A careful plan for nursing assessment of pain relief, blood pressure, respirations, sedation, and other side effects through the use of a pain control flow sheet is important.

Patient-controlled analgesia (PCA) is the administration of intravenous narcotics using a special pump with computer controls activated by the patient. The pump can be programmed for a beginning larger dose of narcotic (called the bolus), which establishes a blood level of narcotic. The program may then be set for the maintenance dose that is automatically administered every hour. Sometimes this maintenance level is not used. The third aspect of the computer allows the patient to self-administer a preset dose whenever needed. The interval between these patient-administered doses is controlled by a lockout time (*ie*, a time in which a dose may not be administered). This provides for control of the total amount of narcotic that may be administered. The patient is then taught how to press a control button to obtain pain medication when it is needed. The patient is reassured that overdosage is not possible because both the individual dosage and interval are controlled by the information programmed into the machine.

The PCA pumps place control over pain relief in the hands of the client. Most studies have shown that patients prefer this method: they are able to participate more effectively in self-care, and nurses believe that they are more effective than intermittent nurse-administered medication. Patient use of analgesics is either the same as or less than when narcotics are administered intramuscularly at intervals. Actual pain relief based on patient rating scales may not be improved, but feelings of anxiety and loss of control are lessened, thus contributing to overall well-being (Kleiman, Lipman, Hare, and MacDonald, 1987).

Narcotics may also be administered as *epidural analgesia.* The dura is the covering over the brain and spinal cord. For many years *anesthesia* has been administered by infusing drugs outside the dura for absorption through the dura onto receptors in the spinal cord. Anesthesia completely blocks transmission in the cord, producing both loss of sensation and loss of motor function. Epidural anesthesia is administered only by those with specialized education in the administration of anesthetics.

In recent years techniques have been developed for **epidural analgesia** by administering narcotics into the epidural space for absorption through the dura onto receptor sites in the spinal cord. Narcotics can attach to specific receptors in the spinal cord and thus block the transmission of pain impulses. Minimal amounts of the drug are absorbed and reach the CNS. Thus, CNS depression and sedation are minimized. Autonomic nervous system responses such as hypotension are also minimized (Cousins and Mather, 1984).

Anesthesiologists surgically place the epidural catheter. Temporary catheters are placed for use after surgery or for other short-term situations. Temporary catheters emerge along the spine and are covered with dressings. Long-term catheters are used for cancer or terminal pain. These catheters are tunneled under the tissue to emerge in a location convenient for care.

Preservative-free narcotics are administered in small, widely spaced doses through the catheter. (Preservatives tend to be neurotoxic.) Assessment is still needed for potential adverse effects. Although side effects are less common, response is individual and adverse effects may still occur (see Module 59, Giving Epidural Medications).

Intraventricular analgesia is produced by infusing a narcotic directly into the ventricles of the brain. A reservoir may be surgically implanted under the scalp with a catheter attached that extends into the ventricle of the brain. This is commonly referred to by its inventor's name, the Ommaya reservoir. A variety of therapeutic drugs in addition to narcotics may be administered through this route. Effects of intraventricular narcotics are long lasting, but the risk of respiratory depression is high. This is not a common method of administration of narcotics and has been limited to those who have pain related to cancer in the CNS (Paice, 1987).

Because narcotics do have the potential for tolerance, physical dependence, addiction, and abuse, there are legal controls over their use. The nurse has special responsibilities for accurate recordkeeping and the medications themselves must be kept in locked cabinets to which access is limited.

Tolerance indicates that a drug given in the same dosage has a lessened effect over a period of time or that increasing dosages are needed to provide the same level of effect. Tolerance affects not only desired pain relief but also the occurrence of adverse effects. Thus, for the person who needs ongoing pain relief, dosages can be raised to obtain pain control without creating a greater chance of adverse effects such as respiratory depression. The time for development of tolerance is individual. Tolerance is most frequently seen in the person with cancer or terminal pain. If the drug is available and relief of pain continues to be needed, there is no medical contraindication to raising dosage of certain narcotics, such as morphine, to produce the desired effect. Meperidine (Demerol) is an exception to this. Increasing dosage will produce increased amounts of a metabolite (normeperidine) that causes severe side effects. This drug is usually avoided for terminal pain for this reason.

Physical dependence indicates that physiologic changes have occurred within the body such that adverse symptoms, called withdrawal symptoms (nausea, vomiting, chills, sweats, insomnia, muscle spasms, and a general feeling of illness), will occur if the drug is no longer administered. The emergence of withdrawal symptoms may be prevented by a gradual rather than abrupt discontinuance of narcotics if they have been administered for more than 7 days (Coyle, 1987). Because gradual discontinuance is the usual pattern when pain has been a problem, physical dependence is rarely a concern. It may become a problem when an abrupt change from a narcotic to a nonnarcotic drug is made without gradually decreasing the narcotic, or if a surgical procedure has made narcotics for pain control no longer necessary. In these cases, a plan for gradual withdrawal over several days will eliminate the problem of withdrawal.

When it is necessary to withdraw narcotics from a patient who has been receiving them for a period of time and is still in pain, the task should be approached in a straightforward and direct way. The patient should be informed of the planned reduction in narcotic dosage and of the reasons for this reduction. At no time should the patient's statements of pain be discounted or disbelieved. Remember that pain is what the person says it is. Instead, you should express concern and offer nondrug interventions. You should clearly convey that the drug is not being reduced because the pain is not real, but because long-term use of narcotics is incompatible with a lifestyle of good quality. Your goal will be to find other ways of relieving the pain and ways of helping the person to tolerate pain that cannot be relieved.

Addiction is a complex pattern of behavior that involves both physical dependence and drug-seeking behaviors. Psychological and sociological factors are prominent in the development of addiction. It is rarely a problem when narcotics are administered for pain control. The health care situations in which it becomes a problem are usually those associated with chronic pain syndromes, in which narcotics were used for long periods of time and there were accompanying psychological and sociological problems. Fear of addiction is one reason why pain is sometimes inadequately treated. Both patients and caregivers may have unrealistic fears of addiction. It is important to note that addiction from health care use of narcotics is rare and is not related to short-term use of narcotics for surgery or trauma nor to the long-term use of narcotics for terminal pain. Addiction is not the same as tolerance or **physical dependence**.

Drug abuse refers to the use of drugs for purposes and in a manner other than those for which they were intended. Thus, the use of narcotics for relief of personal stress, for relaxation, or to produce feelings of well-being and euphoria constitutes abuse. Many drugs in addition to narcotics have the potential for abuse. Individuals may abuse prescription narcotics by using them after the problem for which they were prescribed is resolved, by using prescribed drugs more frequently than indicated, or by using drugs prescribed for other persons. The person abusing drugs may or may not initially have tolerance, physical dependence, or addiction. Drug abuse often leads to these problems. Of course, drug abuse may also involve nonprescribed and illegal drugs.

Other Pain Control Measures

As a nurse you will need to participate knowledgeably with the team that may be using other pain control measures. Often your role will be to teach and emotionally support the person who is receiving these other modes of treatment.

Interrupting the Pathways for Pain

Interruption of the pathways for pain is usually the physician's responsibility although nurses performing in expanded roles are also acting in this capacity. A local anesthetic may be injected at a point along the nerve pathway to interrupt the transmission of pain impulses. This is called a *local or regional block.* Injections are most commonly done just proximal to the origin of the pain (as in dental work) or close to the spine.

Pain pathways in the spinal thalamic tracts (a group of nerves in the spinal cord) may be interrupted surgically in certain cases of long-term intractable pain. This procedure, called a **chordotomy**, cannot be guaranteed to be successful because of anatomic variations in the spinal cord, but it has helped immeasurably in certain cases.

The **dorsal column stimulator (DCS)** is an electric stimulation device developed for use in the control of intractable pain. The device is surgically implanted along the spinal column. When activated, it provides an electrical stimulation, felt as a buzzing sensation, which can interrupt a pain impulse and prevent pain perception. The person can activate the DCS when pain begins, thus stopping the pain.

A **transcutaneous electric nerve stimulator (TCS**, **TNS**, or **TENS)** functions in the same manner as a DCS through electrodes attached temporarily to the skin. This device provides an electrical stimulation that interrupts conduction of the pain impulse. TENS units are being used for postoperative pain management as well as for treatment of chronic pain. Careful attention to care of the skin where the electrodes are applied will prevent skin irritation and breakdown. Some peripheral nerve stimulators are being implanted into the tissue to avoid the constant skin irritation experienced with TENS in long-term use.

Hypnosis and Acupuncture

Pain relief from *hypnosis* lasts for the duration of the hypnotic trance and may last longer through the effect of posthypnotic suggestion on pain perception. Although used in some health care settings, hypnosis is not a common method of pain relief. The person using hypnosis must be trained in all aspects of its use. Acupuncture, which has been practiced as a medical art in Asia for hundreds of years, is receiving increasing attention from medical researchers. In **acupuncture**, long slender needles are inserted into specific points on the body. These needles may be twirled, heated, or attached to a mild electrical current. The effect is to provide anesthesia to a given body part. The part anesthetized is not necessarily in close proximity to the entry point of the needle. For example, a point near the base of the thumb may be used to relieve pain in a tooth. Many kinds of surgery are performed in China using only acupuncture to prevent pain, and the process has also been used to treat different types of long-term pain. Understanding of acupuncture is still limited, and there are many theories about how it works. In acupressure, direct pressure instead of needles, is used to provide stimulation to the acupuncture points.

Supporting the Person With Chronic Pain

Chronic pain is pain that persists for weeks, months, or even years. The condition responsible for the pain may be one for which no means of correction is available, such as severe arthritis, or the cause may not be apparent. Narcotic analgesics are not advisable in such cases because they can create dependence and even addiction. This kind of chronic pain may threaten one's occupation, undermine interpersonal relationships, and destroy the fabric of life.

To modify reactions to such pain, a variety of methods have been used. **Behavior modification** techniques that reward non–pain-oriented behavior and ignore pain-oriented behavior are meeting with some success. This approach does not assume that the pain is not real, but it does assume that it is the person's response to pain that disrupts life.

Such techniques are not to be used lightly because they can change a person psychologically as surely as surgery does physically. The patient must be informed about the situation and consulted about the treatment plan and must give informed consent such as would be required for surgery. Success with these techniques depends on a total health team approach.

Another approach is to reduce pain medication gradually while encouraging the person to remain active and involved. Use of a liquid pain medication composed of a syrup and an undisclosed amount of drug allows the amount of the syrup to remain the same while the drug content is gradually reduced. This approach helps prevent psychological reactions to the withdrawal of the drug.

Surgery is an alternative method of pain relief in cases of chronic pain. Although such surgery does not alter motor function, it may adversely affect other sensory perception. The resulting inability to perceive harmful heat and cold may create safety problems. Surgery for pain relief is not always successful.

The various nerve stimulators, such as the TCS, TNS, or TENS, have had their greatest success in treating chronic pain. The stimulator may at first be used continuously; gradually the duration of use is reduced, and eventually the stimulator is turned on only as needed. The final step is to stop using the stimulator altogether. In cases in which use of the stimulator is a permanent necessity, implanted electrodes are used in preference to those that must be attached to the skin. Pain medication is often used as an adjunct to TENS. In many facilities the physical therapist is responsible for maintaining the TENS device.

All of the nonpharmacologic interventions such as distraction, relaxation, self-hypnosis, acupressure, and so forth may be taught as alternative ways to manage chronic pain. These are often quite successful. In addition to pain relief, they also provide the individual with a sense of personal control.

Antidepressant medications may be used for chronic pain. They have a combination of effects that make them particularly suitable for long-term pain. By interfering with the breakdown of certain neurotransmitters that are essential to the maintenance of the spinal control "gate," they help to prevent the transmission of pain impulses. Antidepressants also are effective in combating the depression often present with chronic pain.

Assisting the Person With Terminal Pain

Pain related to a terminal illness, usually called *terminal pain*, requires a different approach to pain management than does acute pain. During the early stages of the illness, through surgeries and treatment, pain may be managed much as it is for acute pain. When the disease is far advanced and there is no expectation of cure, the approach changes.

The patient is encouraged to become an active participant in managing pain. Nondrug pain management techniques are important mechanisms for the patient to maintain personal control. Many drugs used to control pain may cause drowsiness and diminished ability to relate to others or perform tasks. Only the patient can decide whether pain relief or alertness is more desirable. Because terminal pain is not necessarily uniform or always progressively worse, ongoing assessment can lead to more individualized treatment.

To minimize discomfort and promote independence, oral pain medications are used as long as possible. The use of *pain mixtures*—mixtures of drugs in alcohol, water, and flavoring syrup—is common. The drugs in such a mixture usually include a narcotic analgesic and an antianxiety/antiemetic agent. Cocaine has sometimes been added for its mood-elevating effects although some authorities recommend against it. Sometimes other drugs are added. You may hear of *Brompton's mixture*, a mixture with a heroin base used in England. Some facilities in the United States use a mixture they call **modified Brompton's mixture**, which substitutes another narcotic (often methadone or morphine) for the heroin. Phenothiazine is often included to counteract the nausea sometimes induced by oral morphine and for its tranquilizing effect; the alcohol helps prevent the growth of microorganisms in the syrupy base. Medication is given on a regular schedule, not on a PRN basis. This approach is used because the pain is always present, and allowing pain to increase substantially before giving the next dose would be counterproductive. The patient may be allowed to increase or decrease the dose in light of the severity of the pain and the desirability of being alert and active.

With this approach, most patients can be kept relatively pain-free and free of symptoms of drug withdrawal. Although some physiologic drug dependence may be present, it is of minimal concern because there is no expectation that the person can be free of the need for drugs. Because the mixtures are given orally, the patient is saved the prospect of repeated injections. This approach can work only with a person who is conscious and able to take oral fluids. If severe nausea and vomiting are present, those conditions must be controlled before an oral pain mixture can be given.

Some authorities oppose the use of mixtures on the grounds that they make it harder to adjust dosages of individual drugs. Instead, each individual drug may be given separately. In addition, the medication schedule is not adjusted but instead the dosage is adjusted as needed to achieve the desired level of pain relief. Basic

Nursing Research: *Implications for Practice*

Beck, S. L. "The Therapeutic Use of Music for Cancer-Related Pain." *Oncology Nursing Forum* 18, 8 (November–December 1991): 1327–1337.

This researcher studied the therapeutic use of music as an intervention for pain for individuals with cancer who were also receiving scheduled analgesic medications. The sample included 15 outpatients who agreed to participate. The subjects listened to their preference of seven different types of relaxing music. Listening to music resulted in a statistically significant decrease in pain as measured by the McGill Pain Questionnaire. The researcher suggests that music can be used as an independent nursing intervention for pain.

to this approach is the selection of a single drug for pain relief. This drug would be given every 4 hours around the clock, even if it is necessary to wake the patient. Additional drugs (tranquilizers, antiemetics, anti-inflammatories, mood elevators, and the like) can be given as needed on separate schedules. The addition of aspirin or other nonsteroidal anti-inflammatory drugs is often recommended. These drugs may decrease the amount of narcotic needed.

When oral medications are no longer effective, the long-term use of narcotics may be supported by subcutaneous injection pumps, permanent epidural catheters, peripherally inserted central intravenous lines, or surgically implanted central intravenous lines. Intramuscular injection is avoided whenever possible because of the discomfort it causes and the difficulty of giving many injections to the person who has muscle wasting.

Of course, the patient with terminal pain also needs all the other skilled care the nurse is able to provide. Medications must not be viewed as lessening the patient's need for personalized care. Whether it is the small comfort of a simple physical act, such as straightening wrinkled bed clothes, or the immeasurable value of the presence of another human being, the nurse has much to offer the patient with terminal pain (Fig. 32-8).

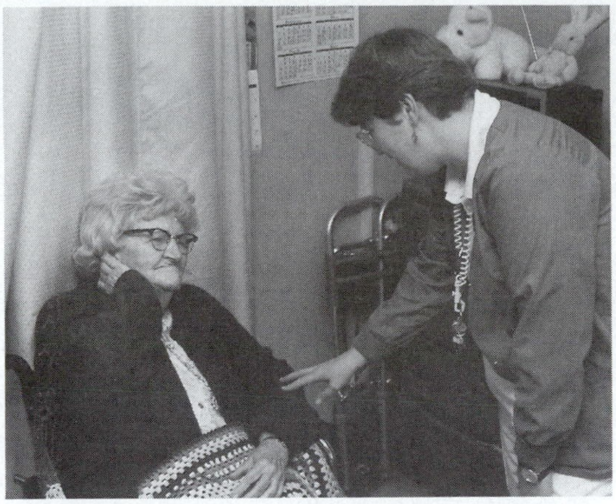

Figure 32-8. The nurse has much to offer the patient with terminal pain.

Evaluation

Evaluation must take place within the context of the desired outcomes that were determined by the patient in conjunction with health care personnel. You must keep in mind what the patient's goals were and what the patient's values are when you begin your evaluation.

The result of nursing intervention to relieve pain must be evaluated at each point in the process of intervention. The most effective way to evaluate pain relief is to ask the patient to evaluate the pain on the same scale used before initiating treatment. The scale should be used both when the patient is resting and when the patient is engaging in essential activity such as walking, deep breathing, or coughing. In addition to the intensity of pain inquire about other parameters. Be specific in your questions. Often the pain will still be present but activity may again be possible, and the patient may feel less distressed by the pain.

Another important way to evaluate pain relief is to observe the patient's behavior. If you identified the presence of pain by assessing nonverbal behavior, look to see if that behavior has changed. Is the facial expression more relaxed? Is the body less tense? Is the patient willing to move about?

To evaluate the effectiveness of a medication accurately, you need to know its expected effect and the time needed for it to work. For example, an injected narcotic might begin to take effect in 10 minutes and reach its maximum effect within half an hour. An oral medication, on the other hand, might not begin to work for 20 to 30 minutes.

If the initial efforts at pain relief do not prove adequate, additional steps may need to be taken to make the patient more comfortable. If you conclude that the medication ordered is not effective, it may be necessary to consult with the physician. Whatever the situation, the patient will benefit from the knowledge that you care about his or her pain and are actively working to alleviate it.

Nursing Care Study
A Patient in Pain

Sue Chou, a nursing student, is assigned on Thursday to care for Mr. Ralph Jarvis, who had had a cholecystectomy (gallbladder removal) on Tuesday morning. Mr. Brown is standing at the nursing station, checking the card index, when the nursing assistant walks up and says, "Mr. Jarvis needs a shot for pain."

Ms. Chou goes to Mr. Jarvis's room to make an assessment before planning intervention. She enters the room, introduces herself, and explains her role, and then asks Mr. Jarvis to describe his pain. Mr. Jarvis says, "It's sharp and all across here," indicating his lower abdomen. Ms. Chou thinks about the surgery, the length of time since the surgery, and the patient's description of the pain, and then says, "Mr. Jarvis, it sounds to me as if you may be having gas pains, which is usual this length of time after surgery, and the location of your pain indicates the same thing. Does this feel like bad "gas" that you have had in the past? Mr. Jarvis responds, "Well, it sure could be." Ms. Chou answers, "Your doctor has ordered a 'return-flow enema' to relieve gas." Ms. Chou then explains the procedure. "I'll give you one right now and we'll see if it helps."

Ms. Chou performs the enema, and a large amount of gas is returned. After the procedure is over, she asks Mr. Jarvis how he feels. Mr. Jarvis replies, "Wow, that did the trick—I feel pretty good. I don't think I need that shot now"

Ms. Chou returns to the nursing station to record the entire process on Mr. Jarvis' chart.

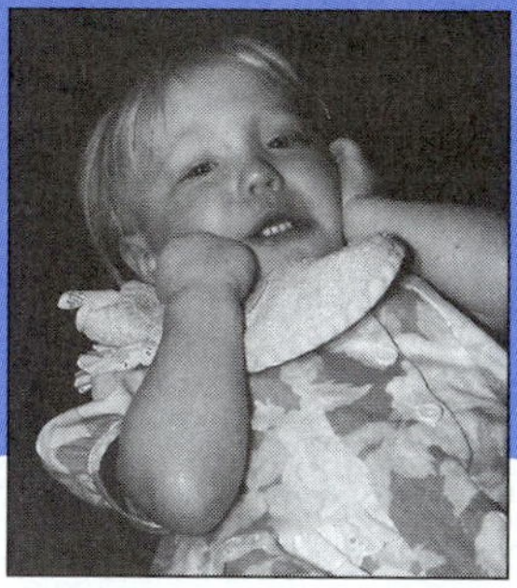

Key Points

- Pain is a subjective experience and must be defined and evaluated by the person experiencing it.
- The pain stimulus is received by nociceptors in the tissue; the pain impulse is transmitted from the nociceptors to the spinal cord and from there upward to the thalamus, where pain is perceived.
- Physiologic and motor responses to pain are determined by lower centers in the brain.
- The cerebral cortex governs interpretation of and reactions to pain.
- An individual's response to pain is affected by cultural background, previous experience with pain, family pain models, responses of others, fatigue and energy level, age, and the environment.
- Acute pain is pain of short duration and is usually associated with surgery, infection, inflammation, and trauma.
- Chronic pain is divided into several types: chronic benign pain occurs with non–life-threatening chronic illnesses; terminal pain occurs with life-threatening illnesses; chronic pain syndrome occurs when the pain perception continues after evidence of nociception is gone; psychogenic pain is caused by severe psychological problems; phantom pain is pain perceived in a body part that is no longer present.
- Assessment for pain includes observation of the person's behavior, interviewing the patient in regard to pain, and integrating the information gained with your understanding of the illness and of pain in general.
- Some of the nursing diagnoses related to the need for comfort are Pain, Ineffective Individual Coping, Impaired Mobility, Anxiety, Knowledge Deficit, Impaired Adjustment, Hopelessness, and Powerlessness.
- Desired outcomes for nursing interventions involving pain include eradication of pain, reduction of pain, or relief of suffering.
- The general guidelines for nursing interventions involving pain include using a variety of pain relief measures, not waiting until pain is severe before intervening, including those interventions the patient believes to be helpful, and continuing to explore new avenues for relief if initial efforts are unsuccessful.

- To combat pain effectively, the members of the health care team must work together.
- Elimination of the source of pain is the most effective intervention strategy.
- Protecting pain receptors from stimuli may be appropriate in some instances.
- Interruption of pain pathways is another method of combating pain.
- Pain perception may be decreased by analgesic administration, hypnosis, distraction, or relaxation techniques.
- Pain interpretation may be modified by narcotics, interpersonal relationships, comfort measures, or the placebo effect.
- For chronic pain, the following measures may be used: surgery, electrical stimulation, and behavior modification.
- The person with terminal pain requires sensitive management and consistent support.
- Evaluation of pain relief measures must include the patient's evaluation as well as objective evidence that the patient is able to participate in activities.

Study Questions

1. What is McCaffery's definition of pain?
2. What is the purpose of pain in the body?
3. What are the responses of the person to pain?
4. Where is pain perceived?
5. What happens to the physiologic responses to pain when pain is long term or chronic?
6. Discuss the factors that affect response to pain?
7. Outline interview questions to be used when assessing for pain.
8. How might you ask a young child about pain?
9. How can the pain impulse be blocked?
10. Explain nonpharmacologic interventions for pain.
11. Describe the various ways that narcotic analgesics may be administered.
12. What is the most common desired outcome for the person with pain?
13. Why is narcotic addiction not a concern for the person with terminal pain?

Critical Thinking Activities

1. Recall an occasion when you experienced pain. List words to describe that pain. In a group meeting, discuss what the words listed mean to each person in the group. Do the words have different meanings to different individuals?
2. Write a brief paper on different cultural groups' attitudes toward pain. Synthesize information from at least three professional references.
3. Prepare a case study of a patient with pain. Include your assessment, planning, implementation, and evaluation.

References and Readings

Acute Pain Management Guideline Panel. *Acute Pain Management: Operative or Medical Procedures and Trauma. Clinical Practice Guideline.* AHCPR Pub. No. 92-0032. Rockville, Md.: Agency for Health Care Policy and Research, Public Health Service, U.S. Department of Health and Human Services, February, 1992a.

———. *Acute Pain Management in Adults: Operative Procedures. Quick Reference Guide for Clinicians.* AHCPR Pub. No. 92-0019. Rockville, Md.: Agency for Health Care Policy and Research, Public Health Service, U.S. Department of Health and Human Services, February, 1992b.

———. *Acute Pain Management in Infants, Children, and Adolescents: Operative and Medical Procedures. Quick Reference Guide for Clinicians.* AHCPR Pub. No. 92-0020. Rockville, Md.: Agency for Health Care Policy and Research, Public Health Service, U.S. Department of Health and Human Services, February, 1992c.

———. *Pain Control After Surgery: A Patient's Guide.* AHCPR Pub. No. 02-0021. Rockville, Md.: Agency for Health Care Policy and Research, Public Health Service, U.S. Department of Health and Human Services, February, 1992d.

American Pain Society. *Principles of Analgesic Use in the Treatment of Acute Pain and Chronic Cancer Pain: A Concise Guide to Medical Practice.* 2nd edition. Skokie, Ill.: American Pain Society, 1989.

American Pain Society, Committee on Quality Assurance Standards. "Standards for Monitoring Quality of Analgesic Treatment of Acute Pain and Cancer Pain." *Oncology Nursing Forum* 17, (1990): 952–954.

Armstrong, M. E. "Acupuncture." *American Journal of Nursing* 72, 9 (September 1972): 1582–1588.

Beyer, J. E., and Levin, C. R. "Issues and Advances in Pain Control in Children." *Nursing Clinics of North America* 22, 3 (September 1987): 661–676.

Bonica, J. J. (Ed.). *The Management of Pain.* Philadelphia: Lea & Febiger, 1990.

Chapman, C. R., and Bonica, J. J. *Chronic Pain.* Kalamazoo, Mich.: The Upjohn Company, 1985.

Cotanch, P. H., Harrison, M., and Roberts, J. "Hypnosis as an Intervention for Pain Control." *Nursing Clinics of North America* 22, 3 (September 1987): 677–704.

Cousins, M., and Mather, L. "Intrathecal and Epidural Administration of Opioids." *Anesthesiology* 61 (September 1984): 276.

Coyle, N. "Analgesics and Pain: Current Concepts." *Nursing Clinics of North America* 22, 3 (September 1987): 727–741.

Edwards, P. W., Zeichner, A., Kuczmierczyk, A. R., and Boczkowski, J. "Familial Pain Models: The Relationship Between Family History of Pain and Current Pain Experience." *Pain* 21, 3 (March 1985): 379–384.

Ferrell, B. R. "Managing Pain with Long-Acting Morphine." *Nursing '91* 21, 10 (October 1991): 34–39.

———. "Pain Management in Elderly People." *Journal of the American Geriatric Society* 39 (1991): 64–73.

Fritz, D. J. "Noninvasive Pain Control Methods Used by Cancer Outpatients." *Oncology Nursing Forum* Suppl. (1988): 108.

Haight, K. "What You Should Know About Epidural Analgesia." *Nursing '87* 17, 9 (September 1987): 58.

Hargreaves, K. M., and Lander, J. "Use of Transcutaneous Electrical Nerve Stimulation for Postoperative Pain." *Nursing Research* 38, (1989): 159–161.

Hecker, B. R., and Albert, L. "Patient-Controlled Analgesia." *Virginia Mason Clinic Bulletin* 41, 3 (Fall 1987): 93–97.

Hensley, J. R. "Continuous SC Morphine for Cancer Pain." *American Journal of Nursing* 91, 3 (March 1991): 98–101.

Holderby, R. A. "Conscious Suggestion: Using Talk to Manage Pain." *Nursing* 11, 5 (May 1981): 44–46.

International Association for the Study of Pain. "Pain Terms: A List With Definitions." *Pain* 6, (June 1979): 24.

Kavanagh, C., and Freeman, R. "Should Children Participate in Burn Care?" *American Journal of Nursing* 84, 5 (May 1984): 601.

Kleiman, R. L., Lipman, A. G., Hare, B. D., and MacDonald, S. "Pain Consult: PCA vs. Regular IM Injections for Severe Postop Pain." *American Journal of Nursing* 87, 11 (November 1987): 1491–1492.

Lisson, E. L. "Ethical Issues Related to Pain Control." *Nursing Clinics of North America* 33, 3 (September 1987): 649–660.

Marzinski, L. R. "The Tragedy of Dementia: Clinically Assessing Pain in the Confused Nonverbal Elderly." *Journal of Gerontological Nursing* 17, 6 (June 1991): 25–28.

McCaffery, M., and Beebe, A. "Giving Meperidine for Pain: Should It Be So Mechanical?" *Nursing '87* 17, 4 (April 1987): 60–66.

———. *Nursing Management of the Patient With Pain,* 2nd ed. Philadelphia: J. B. Lippincott, 1979.

———. "Relieve your Patient's Pain with Noninvasive Techniques." *Nursing '80* 10:12 (December, 1980): 55–57.

———. "A Practical, Postable Chart of Equianalgesic Doses." *Nursing '87* 17, 8 (August 1987): 56–57.

———. "Patient-Controlled Analgesia: More Than a Machine." *Nursing '87* 17, 11 (November 1987): 62–64.

———. *Pain: Clinical Manual For Nursing Practice.* St. Louis: C. V. Mosby, 1989.

McCaffery, M., Ferrell, B. R., and O'Neill-Page, E. "Does Life-Style Affect Your Pain Control Decisions?" *Nursing '92* 22, 4 (April 1992): 58–61.

———. "Patient Age: Does It Affect Your Pain Control Decisions?" *Nursing '91* 21, 9 (September 1991): 44–48.

McGuire, D. B. "Advances in Control of Cancer Pain." *Nursing Clinics of North America* 22, 3 (September 1987): 677–690.

Melzack, R. "The Tragedy of Needless Pain." *Scientific American* 262, 2 (February 1990): 27–33.

Melzack, R., and Wall, P. "Pain Mechanisms: A New Theory." *Science* 150 (November 1965): 970–979.

Paice, J. A. "New Delivery Systems in Pain Management." *Nursing Clinics of North America* 22, 3 (September 1987): 715–726.

"Pain Management: Where We Stand." *Patient Care* 18: 7 (January 30, 1984): 24–27, 30–32, 37–38.

Porth, C. *Pathophysiology: Concepts of Altered Health States.* 3rd edition. Philadelphia: J. B. Lippincott, 1991.

Schultz, N. V. "How Children Perceive Pain." *Nursing Outlook* 19 (May 1971): 670–673.

Sternbach, R. A. Pain: *A Psychophysiological Analysis.* New York: Academic Press, 1978.

Walding, M. F. "Pain, Anxiety, and Powerlessness." *Journal of Advanced Nursing* 16, 4 (April 1991): 388–397.

Wells, N. "Responses to Acute Pain and the Nursing Implications." *Journal of Advances in Nursing Science* 9 (January 1984): 51–58.

World Health Organization. *Cancer Pain Relief and Palliative Care.* WHO Technical Report Series, No. 804, Geneva, Switzerland: WHO, 1990.

Wright, S. M. "Therapeutic Touch in the Management of Pain." *Nursing Clinics of North America* 22, 3 (September 1987): 705–714.

Psychosocial Needs

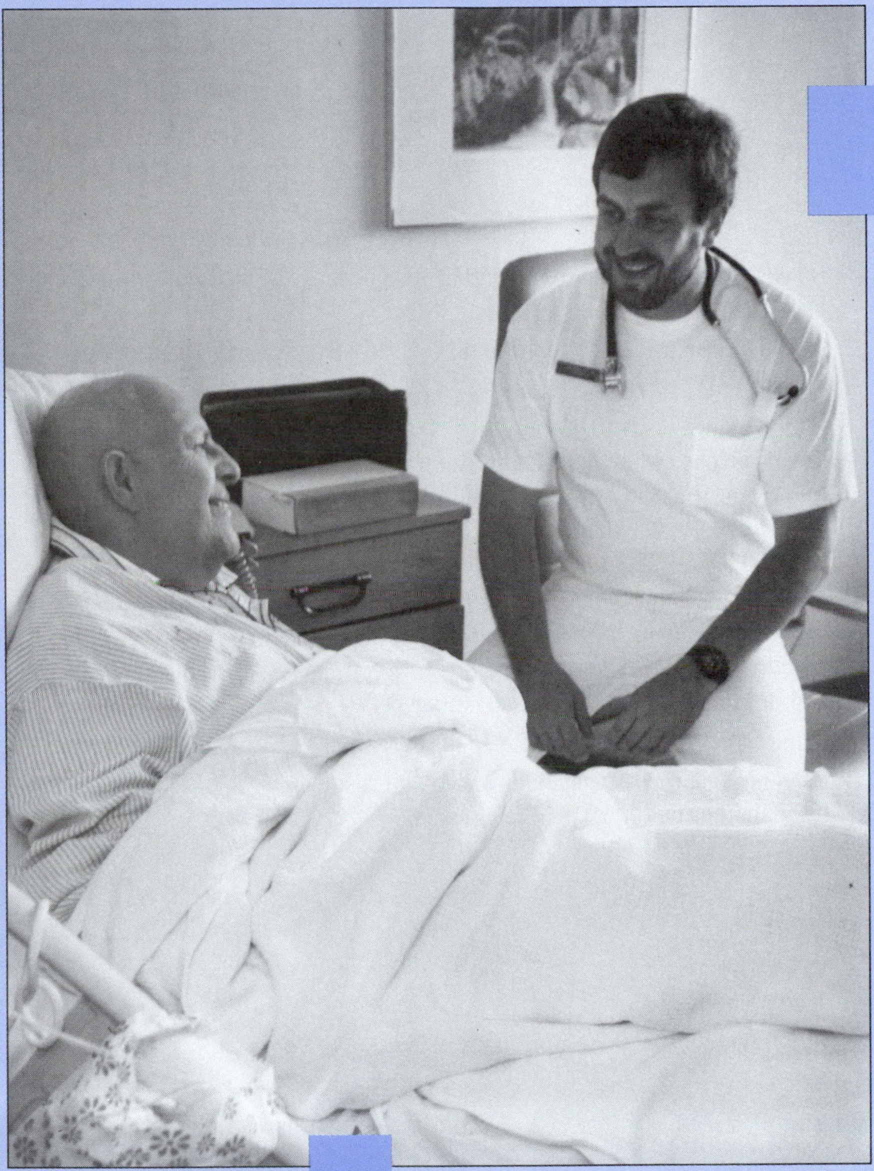

VII

Social, Cultural, and Ethnic Identity

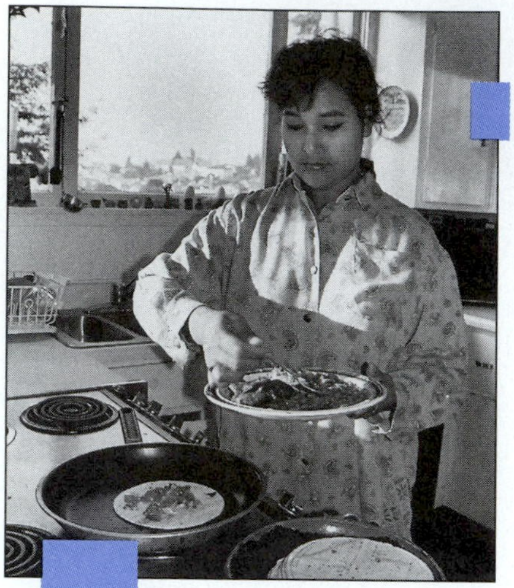

33

Objectives

After completing this chapter, you should be able to:

1. Discuss briefly why nurses should have knowledge of transcultural nursing practice.
2. Identify three areas of understanding essential to sensitive transcultural nursing care.
3. Define ethnocentrism, bias, prejudice, stereotyping, and discrimination.
4. Briefly discuss white Americans, American Indians and Eskimos, Asian Americans, African Americans, and Hispanic Americans in terms of: 1) health care and incidence of disease, 2) family, 3) territoriality, 4) diet, 5) communication, 6) religion and healing, and 7) death and grief.
5. Discuss the unique health needs of women and the ways in which they have been influenced by a changing society.
6. Identify particular health and health care problems experienced by migrants and the socioeconomically disadvantaged.
7. Summarize the general guidelines for care of persons of other cultures.
8. Use nursing process when identifying and resolving problems of the patient from another culture.

Study Terms

bias
brujas
comparable worth
curanderos
discrimination
diverse
ethnocentrism
global community
institutional racism
mal de ojo
minority
moxibustion
prejudice
remedios
stereotyping
territoriality
trigger words

Outline

The Need for Social, Ethnic, and Cultural Identity
Problems of a Diverse Society
Transcultural Nursing
The Nurse in the Setting of Cultural Diversity
Diversity Among Health Care Providers
Health Care and Ethnic Background
Communication
Territoriality
Health Teaching
Diet
Spiritual Beliefs and Healing
Death and Bereavement
Major Cultural and Ethnic Groups
White Americans
  Health Care and Incidence of Disease

Ellis, Nowlis: Nursing: A Human Needs Approach, 5th ed. © 1994 J.B. Lippincott Company

We live in a heterogeneous society composed of a variety of social, cultural, and ethnic groups. Every person has a need for identity, not only as an individual but as a member of a group. This chapter discusses the advent of transcultural nursing and the opportunities and challenges that diversity creates for nurses.

The Need for Social, Ethnic, and Cultural Identity

To be **diverse** means to be varied. The Western world is becoming more diverse. Diversity involves not just being different in race and culture but may include any human attribute or experience. Our differences help us to learn from one another and tend to broaden our personal experiences in life. People who come from smaller social, cultural, and ethnic groups within a country are often referred to as minorities. **Minority** means simply "not the majority," that is, a group that is smaller than the main group. In this chapter, we discuss the nursing care of people who differ in a variety of ways from the majority in our society.

Except for American Indians and Eskimos, the United States and Canada are immigrant nations. By and large, the millions of immigrants North America has received have come willingly, even eagerly, for compelling economic, religious, and political reasons. During the European immigration at the turn of the century, the image arose that our society was a *melting pot*—a place where diverse nationalities and ethnic groups would "melt" into the established population, losing many of their distinguishing features in the process. For some early immigrants, this description is accurate. The fear of being different and the desire to become American and "fit in" to the surrounding social and economic world caused some families to give up their native customs and language. Far more common was a gradual loosening of emotional and cultural ties to the homeland over the course of three or more generations. This pattern has been paralleled by a tendency for newcomers to crowd together in ethnically homogeneous neighborhoods, usually in older urban areas or small rural communities, and for their children or grandchildren to leave the area as soon as they could. Changing patterns in employment opportunities have also contributed to mobility.

Not all immigrants came voluntarily: millions of Africans were brought to our eastern shores as slaves to work the land. Over a century later, millions of Asians landed on our western shores, not precisely as slaves but as ill-paid unskilled laborers brought here to build the nation's vast network of railroads. More recently, large numbers of Hispanics have emigrated to escape severe economic and political hardship in Mexico and Central and South America. Many of these families have found a livelihood as migrant agricultural laborers, primarily but not exclusively in the Southwest.

In general, opportunities have been more limited for, and prejudice more pronounced toward, nonwhite people and others whose physical characteristics distinguish them from the majority population. The dominance of white cultural standards was reflected, particularly early in this century, in the tendency of minority groups to prize those of their people who most nearly conformed to the norms of beauty and behavior of the surrounding culture. Some individuals denied their ethnic backgrounds in efforts to achieve total *assimilation*.

The current resurgence of curiosity about and pride in one's "roots," that is, one's ethnic, cultural, and family *heritage*, may be attributable to increasing acceptance of diversity and cultural differences. People have grown to value their origins, both emotionally and socially.

Problems of a Diverse Society

Ignorance of others' lifestyles and values can arouse suspicion, intolerance, and even fear. The result is perceived competition for jobs and housing, mutual contempt, and sometimes overt clashes.

Ethnocentrism is a belief that one's ethnic group and pattern of behavior are central or superior to those of other groups. People who are different are judged to be wrong or less important. Nurses cannot accept this premise but must deliver care with the understanding that no single social, ethnic, or cultural group is superior to another. Ethnocentrism within our society has led to unfortunate problems that have infringed on human rights.

Bias and **prejudice** are interchangeable terms for adverse attitudes and opinions unsupported by evidence or understanding. Nurses and others who come into frequent and intimate contact with people of backgrounds different from their own must confront and acknowledge their own biases to begin ridding themselves of negative attitudes and behavior. The dominant American culture—to which most nurses belong—prizes equality, practicality, individualism, responsibility for one's own actions, conformity, perseverance, honesty, efficiency, effectiveness, and related values. When this system of beliefs is internalized and then comes into conflict (consciously or unconsciously) with another system of values, prejudice results. Awareness of this process in oneself can lead to significant insights. Often, getting to know another person who has a different belief system, lifestyle, or ethnic heritage helps to minimize prejudice.

Finding commonalities among nurses and their ethnic patients can also help them to get to know one another as individuals. Two persons who each relate to a 3-year-old, care for an older grandfather, or are busy raising teenagers have many life experiences to share.

One should be careful not to make assumptions about an individual or a group without knowledge. Recognizing patients' individuality is essential to providing quality care and establishing relationships. If we allow our prejudices to persist, we will become confined to a narrow outlook, endlessly uncomfortable with whatever differs from the familiar.

Stereotyping is the presumption that an individual member of a group typifies or conforms to the perceived characteristics of the group as a whole. For example, you may think that all American Indians are quiet and never express what they are thinking. In taking a nursing history, then, you might find yourself prodding the patient inappropriately to reveal information or abbreviating the history-taking in the belief that you will not be able to gather sufficient information. The inaccuracy of much stereotyping undermines objective assessment. Stereotyping also narrows our thinking about others. Even more objectionable is the tendency of inaccurate stereotyping that leads to harmful discrimination.

Discrimination is action motivated or influenced by bias, prejudice, or stereotyping. Discriminatory acts may be implied as well as overt. For example, a nurse who repeatedly fails to respond promptly to the call light of a Chicano patient because the nurse believes that Chicanos overreact to illness is discriminating on the basis of stereotyping. If, in the staff dining room, white staff members always sit apart from people of color, their behavior could be construed as discriminatory.

Institutional racism is any pattern of practices on the part of social institutions, including health care facilities, that has tended to promote racism. Consider employment; the practice of filling jobs with individuals recommended by staff members had the effect for many years of perpetuating ethnically homogeneous staffs. The printing of signs, posters, and policies only in English in a hospital where much of the staff or many patients speak another language is a form of racism. In hospitals, ethnic people of color have typically been more numerous in lower-level jobs than in positions with substantial decision-making responsibility. The traditional pattern has been that housekeeping and maintenance were performed by people of color, whereas nursing and management were done by whites. Although this pattern is changing, its existence should be recognized. Active recruitment of minorities will offset its effect, but health care practitioners must also resolve not to participate knowingly in the perpetuation of this or any other type of racism.

Transcultural Nursing

The term global community is particularly relevant for nurses in health care. By **global community** we mean that we are a part of a community that is much more vast than the neighborhood community surrounding us. We are no longer in an isolated environment; we must broaden our vision of who we are within the context of the world and the patients for whom we provide care.

Although *transcultural nursing* has become a nursing specialty since the first national conference on transcultural nursing was held in 1975, the concept of meeting the needs of all patients, regardless of ethnic or cultural orientation, is inherent in all aspects of nursing practice. The goal is to provide individualized nursing care to people of various social, cultural, and ethnic groups to better meet their special needs. Orque and colleagues (1983) call this goal "ethnic nursing care" and define it as "the nurse's effective integration of the patient's ethnic cultural background into her (his) nursing process-based patient care" (p. 7). As more and more ethnic groups become integrated into North American society, the importance of transcultural nursing grows. Leininger (1984) believes that its practice is the greatest and most important challenge for professional nurses today. According to Orque and coworkers, the nurse must not only integrate cultural characteristics into plans for care, but must also identify commonalities shared with patients so that intercultural communication can take place.

Two concepts are basic to an understanding of transcultural nursing—human rights and diversity. The phrase *human rights* has been widely used over the past 15 or 20 years. In most states, the law now reads that there shall be no discrimination on the basis of "race, religion, color, national origin, marital status, sex, age, or handicap." In a broader context, human rights means the right of people to live in harmony, regardless of individual or group differences. Fundamental to the philosophy of nursing is the responsibility to care for all people in an effective and sensitive manner, regardless of their social, cultural, or ethnic origin.

Nurses have sometimes treated patients across an artificial barrier erected by the we/they dichotomy (division). A study by Louie (1983) showed that female registered nurses did not respond favorably toward clients who were culturally different from themselves. Particularly with minority patients, this attitude can threaten quality care. It is time we worked at ridding ourselves of suspicions, ignorance, unfamiliarity, and fears. Leininger (1984) writes that transcultural nursing, which is both humanistic and scientific, is challenging nurses today to reexamine nursing care practices to determine cultural aspects of care.

The Nurse in the Setting of Cultural Diversity

Although each of us, nurses and patients, is different from everyone else, we share common needs to reach our full potential. We need to feel comfortable and safe, physically and psychologically. Adequate cleanliness, nutrition, exercise, and sleep are all parts of feeling well. Productive work, close family ties, and good friends give meaning to life. A strong belief system sustains us. Finally, we need to die with dignity in a way that is appropriate to the life we have led (Display 33-1).

Not long ago it was typical for nurses to practice for a number of years in the same setting, caring only for patients much like themselves. Black patients, for example, were cared for in largely black facilities by black nursing staffs. Many white nurses felt uncomfortable caring for black patients, partly because they were not used to doing so. Just as the ethnic composition of most facilities' providers has changed, so has that of their patients. Patient populations in most large health care facilities are highly diverse, enabling nurses and patients of different backgrounds to learn and care about one another (Fig. 33-1).

When you consider factors that may modify your care of patients from a different ethnic background, you must remember that individuals differ from each other more than groups do. Nevertheless, it will prove enlight-

Display 33–1
Culture and Human Needs

Regardless of my origin or culture, I need:
to feel comfortable and safe within my psychological and physical space.
a home that reflects my individuality.
surroundings that are esthetic.
to find meaning in my natural environment.
nutrition that conforms to my customs and religion.
to be clean and in a state of comfort.
time and energy so that I can have adequate exercise.
quiet and restful sleep and leisure.
productive work.
constantly to learn new things in life.
for others to understand my verbal and nonverbal communication.
respect and dignity.
family love and belonging.
friends who understand me.
a belief system that offers spiritual comfort.
a death appropriate to the life I have lived.

ening to look in a general way at aspects of care that may be affected by the patient's background. Some of these aspects are physical in nature and some psychological.

In every aspect of nursing care, you should consider whether appropriate adaptations related to ethnic background should be made for the patient. The purpose of any such variation in care is to provide what is needed and meaningful to the patient and thus to strengthen the nurse–patient relationship. At the same time, any modification must adhere to the principles of safe and effective care.

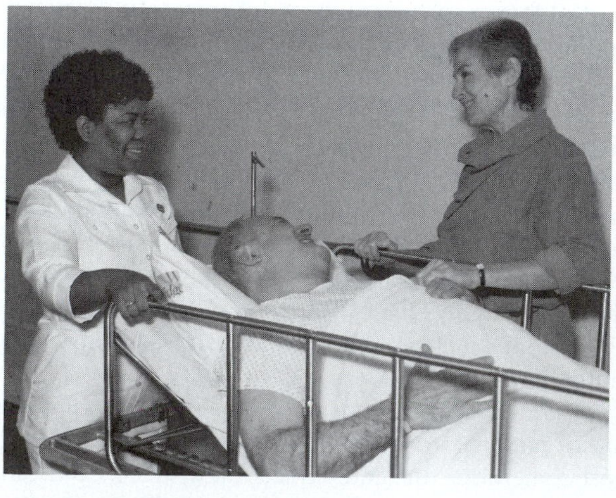

Figure 33-1. Smiles have universal meaning.

Fong (1985) states that sometimes what seems important and rational to the ethnic patient seems senseless to the nurse. This kind of misunderstanding can negatively affect the person's response to health care. She gives several other reasons for the nurse in practice to study cultural differences. Understanding other ethnic groups and cultures helps avoid ethnocentrism (feeling superior to rather than just different from others). Having knowledge of other cultures aids nurses to understand their own group better and patients to view good health as a satisfactory state so that they are more compliant when care is offered.

Diversity Among Health Care Providers

Many nurses, particularly those working in urban health care settings, will be working with health care providers from different cultures. Equal opportunity hiring practices in hospitals and health care agencies are resulting in more social, cultural, and ethnic diversity on their staffs.

Nurses as a group are far more diverse than was the case only a few years ago. Historically, nurses have come primarily from the middle and lower-middle classes of society; most have been white, female, and recent high school graduates. This profile has radically changed with the national increase in community college nursing programs, which have made nursing accessible as a career to substantial numbers of the disadvantaged, minorities, and foreign born. Today, the majority of practicing nurses are from associate degree programs.

Patients may be from the same culture as a nurse on the staff so these patients have a more immediate trust relationship than is possible to establish with a nurse not from that culture. A nurse with a different cultural background can help you understand factors that may be important to that patient. Having the nurse share with you the customs of the culture will result in mutual acceptance and understanding. For example, when a patient from one of the Greek Islands died, the loud wailing of the family was upsetting to the staff who were resistant to providing clear water and cloths requested by the family for washing the body after death. A staff nurse from the same culture explained that this was the custom. The staff was then able to share in this special ritual. This indicates that the presence of health care workers from other cultures is clearly an advantage.

In a world that is much more culturally linked, learning about other cultures provides a treasured opportunity. You can also be helpful to the nurse from another culture by acting as a resource for information that may not be familiar to that person. The word "team building" means that each person on the health care team works together, recognizing a common goal, providing effective care to those who need assistance (see Chapter 2).

Health Care and Ethnic Background

In the United States, the death rate is significantly higher among nonwhites than among whites. In fact, the mortality rate among nonwhites in the United States is almost double the mortality rates in whites (U.S. National Center for Health Statistics, 1992). This difference is a reflection of the different patterns of use and the inequities of the health care system, as well as of differences in general health status.

For environmental and economic reasons, infant mortality is higher among minorities than in the general population. The overall national rate of infants of low birth weight is 6.9%. However, the percentage of white infants of low birth weight is 5.6%; black infants, 13.0%; and other minority groups, 11.5% (Olds, London, and Ladevig, 1992).

Some cultural groups have more members who live in poverty, which leads to generally poor nutrition and sanitation, placing them more at risk for disease. Certain groups seem to have high susceptibility to specific medical conditions, for example, a high incidence of hypertension among black males and *cystic fibrosis* among white children compared with children of other races. A higher incidence of diabetes is found among Hispanics than in other ethnic groups. Tuberculosis is increasing among the disadvantaged as well as among those infected with the virus for acquired immunodeficiency syndrome.

Certain diseases and conditions are more prevalent in certain small population groups. For example, Tay-Sachs disease, an hereditary, terminal neurologic disease of Eastern European Jews, is found exclusively in that single population group. Others occur in many ethnic populations. In general, minority people also suffer from higher incidences of such conditions as hypertension, cirrhosis, respiratory disease, alcoholism, homicide, and suicide.

Communication

Mutual understanding between patient and nurse is paramount in quality nursing care. Any use of language that disrupts your relationship with the patient should be carefully examined. Body language, too, differs from ethnic group to ethnic group. The use of derogatory terms for ethnic groups is inexcusable at any time. Also offensive are such practices as calling minority group patients by their first names without permission, "talking down," or underestimating the patient's skill at English. More subtle, but also distressing to the minority group patient, is the use of so-called **trigger words** or phrases. Trigger words might appear to be innocuous, but they set off negative emotions in certain individuals. Phrases such as "bury the hatchet" suggest that the American Indian is hostile or warlike and may be offensive to the American Indian patient. Phrases such as "cotton-pickin' hands," which refers to the menial labor once done by slaves, may be offensive to African Americans. On the other hand, you need not try to speak like the patient; the effort can prove to be awkward and contrived. It is more important to convey respect.

Recent immigrants often have trouble with idiomatic English. For instance, a patient admitted for mild head trauma reported he had been struck by a ball; a bystander had suddenly yelled, "DUCK!" and he looked around for a duck. Try to choose literal, commonly used, straightforward language—the kind you would appreciate if you were learning a new language (see Chapter 13).

To better provide care for the patient who is not English speaking, you should be aware of the language interpretation services available in your area. Your goal is to attempt to resolve any language barrier. Although nonverbal cues are useful, determining the degree of pain or the more subtle needs of the patient requires a common language or means of communication. One solution may be to use the services of a bilingual family member. However, you must be sure this person understands clearly what you are asking. Medical terms may be unfamiliar and may need to be defined in words the family interpreter would know. Additionally, there is a concern regarding the patient's confidentiality and privacy that might be violated by providing information to a family member.

Some larger facilities have designated staff persons who speak various languages to be available for interpreting. These persons are helpful because they respect confidentiality and also know medical terminology. If you are bilingual, you may wish to volunteer to help with communication. Bilingual students and staff nurses are a welcome addition to hospitals and agencies because of their language abilities in interpretation.

If a staff person cannot be found for interpretation, most large cities have a *language bank* agency sponsored by the American Red Cross and private donations. This agency offers free translation services for health care agencies. When contacting them, it is helpful not only to tell them about the patient's origin but whether their services are needed for an emergency situation or routine interpretation. The interpreter may be useful when the nurse is planning to give health information to the patient. Some hospital libraries have bilingual books available for nurses and other medical personnel.

Territoriality

Territoriality refers to a person's emotional perception of spatial relationships with other individuals. Many colloquial phrases and metaphors attest to the emotional content of proximity and distance between people. Sometimes, phrases such "get off my turf," "I need my own space," or "clear out," indicate a desire to distance the relationship. At other times, there is a need for closeness and other phrases are used, such "we're very close," "let's keep in touch," or "you're part of me." Trust has a great deal to do with territoriality when closeness is wanted.

Territoriality is an issue when caring for any patient, but particularly when dealing with the person from another culture. Members of some groups are made uncomfortable and even anxious if the nurse comes close; others will interpret standing 6 feet away to talk as a sign of unfriendliness or haughtiness. An individual's sense of privacy and of modesty is essentially an aspect of territoriality. Much nursing care may be looked on as an intrusion on privacy, particularly by members of ethnic groups who consider the body sacred or sacrosanct. Some people will consider a daily bath excessive and an unnecessary affront to modesty.

Some cultures consider it unwise to talk in an intimate way about others for fear of causing them harm. This outlook might lead you to characterize certain minority people as closed and secretive unless you understand the patient's perception of safe territory. Finding a way to interact that respects the patient's physical and psychological territoriality is basic to a satisfactory therapeutic relationship. Sensitivity to what makes the patient uncomfortable is essential.

Health Teaching

Some minority group patients will have had little or no experience with health teaching and unpleasant or limited experience in formal education. The role of learner may seem humiliating or may cause role confusion if the nurse is viewed as a deliverer of physical care rather than a teacher. The process may have to be clearly delineated somewhat more specifically than usual. Visual aids are helpful particularly if they use symbols or words familiar to the patient (see Chapter 16).

Diet

The traditional American meat-and-potatoes diet has become less popular with increasing emphasis on eating a more healthy diet. Recognition that diet plays a central role in health has given rise to a variety of diets, such as those that are low fat, low cholesterol, high protein, or high fiber. Furthermore, people are becoming more willing to try the foods of other cultures. Although health providers are accustomed to thinking about variations in diet for health reasons, they may be unfamiliar with thinking about diets in terms of the patient's customs and beliefs (see Chapter 25).

Some people from other cultures assign to foods not just preventive but also curative power. Some popular foods may be totally unappetizing to a patient or taboo from either a cultural or religious standpoint. Many Asian and Hispanic people believe in elaborate systems of "hot" and "cold" foods with a direct relationship to wellness and illness; this belief will be discussed more later. Nurses should elicit information from the family and the patient about dietary practices and their relationship to health and cultural beliefs and seek to incorporate these into dietary planning whenever possible.

Spiritual Beliefs and Healing

In many minority groups, religion has traditionally been an important part of daily life. In particular, religious practice is often viewed as fundamental to the prevention of disease and to healing. Diet, hygiene practices, exercise, rest, and attire may have religious significance. Another outlook shared by people of many backgrounds is the concept of balance: religion is seen as maintaining health by preserving a balance between man and nature. Because spiritual beliefs are so closely intertwined with health care, assessing the minority group patient's spiritual beliefs as they relate to health care is essential. Of course, not all minority group patients belong to a formal religious group.

The person may have a religious leader, whether a minister, priest, chief, shaman, or healer. The family may wish to burn or smoke substances at the bedside as part of a ceremony or to bring in foods forbidden by the patient's diet. The nurse should support and, if necessary, try to gain permission for any religious practice that is meaningful to the patient and not injurious (see Chapter 36).

Death and Bereavement

Some cultures view death much more realistically than does Western society. Particularly if the person's life has been productive, death is viewed as the natural end of existence. Sudden death may be attributed to outside influences, real or supernatural. The hereafter has varying degrees of importance: some see it as redemptive, with heaven or another sacred abode as the desired goal; other groups consider the hereafter a reuniting with one's ancestors.

Burial practices are expressions of *bereavement.* It is important for the nurse to help the family of the deceased prepare the body according to the family's ethnic or religious customs; conformity to tradition helps greatly to resolve grief. Matters of concern may include sitting with the body in the hospital; prayers, chants, and rituals; cleansing and dressing the body; and whether or not all the body parts are to be released to the family for burial. The nurse must determine the family's specific wishes; assumptions are inappropriate. Hospital policies are becoming more accommodating of cultural death rituals (see Chapter 41).

Major Cultural and Ethnic Groups

More than 100 distinct population groups are recognized in the United States. We must limit ourselves to discussing the largest or most visible groups.

Composing by far the largest group in Western society are the whites, or persons considered to be of white skin and not formally aligned with any specific ethnic group of color. These persons total 199,686 million of the 248,710 million persons in our country. Asians and Hispanics constitute by far the most rapidly increasing ethnic groups in the United States (Table 33-1).

Various terms have been used to describe the people in this society who come from ethnic groups with a skin color other than white. The census bureau categorizes these people simply as nonwhite. Because ethnic does not specifically mean those of a different color, the phrase people of color has frequently been used. Some prefer one term over another. Whatever term is used, everyone, including nurses in particular, should recognize that belonging to such a group does not necessarily denote a different national or ethnic lifestyle. It is not uncommon for people of the second and third generations as Americans to be taken for recent immigrants, when actually they may practice few of the traditions of their heritage.

Table 33–1. Population of Major U.S. Ethnic Groups (number in 1000s)

Total U.S. Population	248,710
White	199,686
Black	29,986
Hispanic	22,354
Asian, Pacific Islanders	7,274
American Indian and Eskimos	1,959

Statistical Abstract of the United States. 111th edition. Washington, D.C.: U.S. Bureau of the Census, 1991.

The main ethnic peoples of color in the United States are American Indians and Eskimos, Asian Americans, African Americans, and Hispanic Americans. There is risk in generalizing about any group because doing so may suggest stereotyping. It must be repeated that individuals vary more from one to another than groups do. To assume that every Asian American eats rice or that every African American understands and uses Black English is a disservice to the individual.

The following brief portraits are not meant to be taken as definitive. Using other resources, including the family, and performing thorough individual assessments are the keys to caring for individuals from different cultural backgrounds.

White Americans

The most outstanding characteristic of whites is the degree of diversity within the group itself. It includes persons with a wide spectrum of lifestyles and beliefs. The statements here are generalizations to assist the nonwhite person in understanding certain trends among whites. You must always assess the individual, however, to determine that person's lifestyle and beliefs.

The *historical background*, which is well known, is that these persons are of European descent and include those whose ancestors were early settlers as well as immigrants who passed through Ellis Island in New York City, the great "gateway" for Europeans entering the United States. A commemorative museum has been created at Ellis Island holding memorabilia of those early immigrants. These immigrants tended to be English, Irish, Scottish, Dutch, French, and German. Later immigrants were Scandinavian and Eastern and Southern European. These people emigrated for many reasons, including economic and religious oppression. They also came to take advantage of the economic opportunities promised by a young country.

Health Care and Incidence of Disease

Although access to health care is a national problem for all, whites are in some ways at an advantage. Because they are not identifiable by appearance as belonging to any special ethnic or cultural group, these persons are "mainstreamed" into the more conventional and available resources to care. However, government and private agencies have recently been focusing more attention toward solving the health care crisis in the United States for all citizens. Meanwhile, whites and others who are without sufficient finances but too young to have Medicare often "fall through the cracks" of the health care system.

Whites experience a wide variety of diseases. As a group, they share most conditions that occur in other ethnic groups. They may acquire diseases based on their own family genetic makeup, habits, or living conditions. It is difficult to find distinct patterns of diseases that are specific to this particular culture. An exception is sickle cell anemia, an inherited, severe anemia found primarily in blacks; however, this disease has been documented in a few persons living in areas near the Mediterranean.

Family

White people tend to think of the family primarily as the nuclear or immediate family: parents and children living in the same household. However, those who identify more closely with European backgrounds may have large extended families. There are increasing numbers of nontraditional families, such as unmarried adults of both sexes living together. Single parenting is common. Statistically, the incidence of divorce *and* of marriage is rising, and there appears to be a renewed feeling that the family is of great importance.

Communication

When communicating, most whites are more likely to reflect the area of the country in which they live rather than their hereditary or cultural group. A few newly arrived immigrants have retained speech patterns related to European languages, which give some indication of their native origin. Mainly, however, the language of whites is not indicative of the background group.

Territoriality

The many persons who make up this group have various concepts of territoriality. Many Southern and Eastern Europeans are comfortable with touch and use touch extensively in the most casual contact between members of the same sex as well as between members of the opposite sex. Many Northern Europeans are not as culturally comfortable with the use of touch. The Southern and Eastern Europeans tend to be more communicative about feelings, and the Northern Europeans tend to be more formal and less revealing in interpersonal relationships. Some whites see the home as a private place and expect people to visit only by invitation unless they are part of the family or close friends.

Diet

Diets of whites do vary somewhat according to their heritage, but generally do not reflect heritage as much as do the diets of other groups. For example, although Germans may cook an occasional German item, more often their diets are planned around foods found in conventional supermarkets. The dominant pattern is to eat three meals a day with the largest meal in the evening. The diets of most whites are changing to include more fruits, vegetables, and healthy choices. Many whites are consuming more chicken and seafood than red meat in an effort to decrease cholesterol levels. Pastas and rice are gaining popularity.

Spiritual Beliefs and Healing

Whites have a variety of beliefs about religion and healing. Those who attend religious services are usually members of the larger Protestant denominations or are of the Roman Catholic or Jewish faith. Many whites do not align themselves formally with any organized religious group. However, there appears to be a resurgence of formal religion in the country, although this has not been accurately documented.

Death and Bereavement

Beliefs about death and bereavement follow the many patterns of beliefs held by whites. Although the scattering of cremated ashes has been on the increase nationally, particularly on the West Coast, the majority of whites still prefer burial of the body or cremated ashes in a cemetery. There is more open expression regarding death, but this is not confined to the group.

American Indians and Eskimos

For several years the term Native American was used to describe the American Indian. More accurately, native Americans are all those people who lived in the United States before the settlers arrived. This group included not only the American Indians but also Alaskan Eskimos and Hawaiians. Native American is both a social and legal entity and describes a diverse population.

By far the largest group within this population is the American Indian. Both American Indians and Eskimos trace their ancestry to the people already inhabiting the Americas when European explorers arrived. They number almost 2 million or 0.8% of the United States population (1990 U.S. Census). The American Indian population, living as tribes, was confined for a number of years to lands designated by law as reservations. These reservations have decreased in size over the years, forcing the people who lived there to move into non-Indian communities. Many tribes are currently attempting to reclaim their land through the courts. The Eskimo population historically wandered at will, following food supplies. In a major court decision, individual communities of Eskimos were awarded large tracts of their long-held lands in Alaska. Although traditional hunting and fishing continues, many communities are also establishing additional economic bases. A policy of the Bureau of Indian Affairs (BIA) to encourage assimilation was an important factor in motivating some young American Indians to move to urban areas, seeking both employment and the experience of living in an integrated environment. Native Hawaiians are descendants of the Polynesian people who were living in those islands when European explorers arrived. Regardless of cultural base, most people have strong feelings of loyalty to their personal ethnic history.

The *historical background* of American Indians is unique in that the BIA was established by the federal government in 1834 to oversee the affairs of more than 250 tribes. For many years there was no American Indian representation in the BIA, and far more effort went into negotiating treaties than into providing good health care, education, and other needed services. In 1955, after years of discontent on the part of American Indians who believed the BIA was not receptive to them or meeting their needs, the Indian Health Service was organized under the Department of Health, Education, and Welfare, now the Department of Health and Human Services (Fig. 33-2).

The goal of the Indian Health Service is to offer a comprehensive health services delivery system for American Indians and Alaska Natives. Because health maintenance of the American Indian population has continued to lag behind those in the general population, the agency has attempted to focus on preventive health care measures. The Indian Health Care Improvement Act, passed by Congress in 1976, has attempted to improve care by allocating funds to assist not only tribes living on reservations, but also American Indians living in urban communities. Providing adequate health care for American Indians continues to be a serious problem because of shortages of facilities, equipment, personnel, and funds.

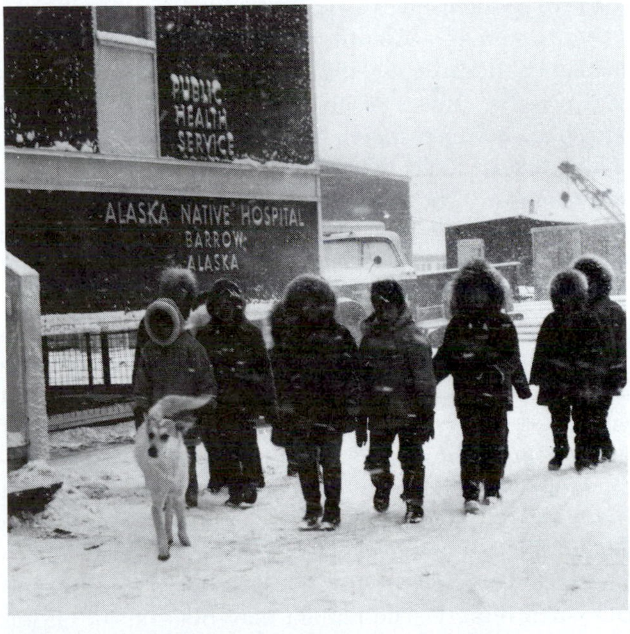

Figure 33-2. Health care for American Indian children is directed under the Indian Health Service, established in 1955.

Health Care and Incidence of Disease

There are differences between the general population and American Indians in both health care and incidence of disease. American Indians have a high incidence of many diseases that are either successfully treated or statistically under control in the general population. This disproportionate incidence is due in large part to living in overcrowded conditions, being economically disadvantaged, and having less access to health care. Although infant mortality figures for American Indians are slightly below the national rate, the rate of death for young infants is twice the national average. Much of this disparity has been attributed to poverty, which produces low birth weight and infections causing diarrhea (Spector, 1991). Preventive care such as early treatment of throat infections could reduce their incidence remarkably.

The United States Department of Health and Human Services reports that more American Indians suffer also from such illnesses and conditions as congenital anomalies (including cleft palate), alcoholism, flu, tuberculosis, impetigo (a skin infection), glaucoma (which can cause blindness), mental retardation, and sexually transmitted diseases. Because it is hard to gather accurate statistics due to the varied locations of these persons, the extent of alcoholism has only been estimated. Estimates suggest that alcoholism is the number one health problem among American Indians and Eskimos. Alcohol-related mortality rates are 23 times the national average in young adults of these ethnic groups. The domestic violence, suicide, and homicide rates are also above the national average, particularly among young persons. The incidence of certain of these conditions could be decreased with adaptations in living conditions and more funds for preventive health care.

Family

The family is important in American Indian culture and is generally broadly defined as consisting of a "community family." All children of the tribe may be conceived of as belonging to all members of the community, and the responsibility of childrearing may be shared. This practice derives from the era when widespread adult mortality resulted in the transferring of many parentless children to the care of another family. Most Indian children, having learned from the group what is acceptable and unacceptable behavior, need not be constantly reminded to behave.

It is often important to the Indian patient to have the family—sometimes a large group—gather at the bedside. The patient may believe it important to consult with the family on medical treatment before giving consent, and policy may have to be set aside to provide for this consultation.

Many tribes of American Indians are patriarchal, that

is, a single man or a group of men makes the decisions for the children and others in the tribe. Other tribes remain matriarchal, relying on a woman or women to make decisions. This distinction has important implications for nursing. To secure consent for treatment or general care, the health care team may have to involve very different persons than is the norm and often a group is needed. For example, if a child were being cared for, often a grandmother and even aunts might participate along with the birth mother in decisions concerning the child. The nurse's understanding of this custom leads to better relations with the family.

Communication

American Indians communicate using many tribal languages and dialects. Most also speak standard English although some idioms may be misunderstood. With non-Indians, the American Indian patient may be less verbal than with other American Indians.

We have spoken of the importance of body language. A quiet approach to the patient, combined with genuine interest and acceptance, is the best overture to communication. The nurse should be familiar with traditional forms of address for elders, women, men, youth, and children and should use them appropriately. An American Indian patient may be cautious in revealing information, thereby leading the nurse to the false conclusion that the patient is not interested in care. The truth is that Indians place much value on privacy; trust must be built slowly. To build trust, one must approach the patient in a quiet, thoughtful manner, respecting the person's sense of territoriality. Because the smile is a universal indication of caring and friendliness, it can be useful in bridging cultural gaps. Some members of this group view sustained eye contact as intrusive because old customs warned that such action could "control the spirit." You will soon note if your patient holds this belief, and in such a case you should use direct eye contact less frequently than you might otherwise. Emphasize positive body language with these patients. The family of an Indian patient may prove extremely helpful, offering you information to supplement the nursing history you gather from the patient.

Territoriality

Territoriality is an area to be highly respected when caring for a member of this group. Most American Indians are uncomfortable with touch and the close proximity of strangers. You should speak from approximately 3 feet distance until you have initiated communication. You should ask permission before touching the individual. Any manipulation or invasion of a body part may be considered by the patient to be a threat to territory. A procedure that requires disrobing, for example, should be undertaken only after complete preparation of the patient, including conscientious draping.

Diet

The American Indian diet has traditionally been composed of such natural foods as roots, grains, vegetables, and red meat and fish. Food also has a religious significance—for example—cornmeal may be spread around the bedside of the ill to aid recovery; it can be swept up, but should not be discarded (Backup, 1979). American Indians may eat only when hungry, and thus may not eat three meals a day at designated times. The nurse's expectations with regard to eating will have to be altered to individualize care. When the government attempted to introduce more protein into the American Indian diet by distributing dried milk and cheese, the program proved largely unsuccessful because not only did American Indians consider such unfamiliar food unappetizing, but many of their adults were found to have lactose intolerance (discussed more fully in Chapter 25), making them unable to digest milk easily.

Nurses need to know that Indians may attribute to certain foods not only medicinal properties but also religious significance. Because the specifics of these customs and beliefs vary from tribe to tribe, the nurse should openly consult with the particular Indian patient concerning foods that are either looked on favorably or restricted from the diet.

Spiritual Beliefs and Healing

Spiritual beliefs and healing beliefs are rooted in the culture base of the tribal nation. American Indians traditionally see themselves as part of nature; concomitantly, health is seen as a balance with nature and illness as an imbalance. Because evil thoughts and deeds are considered possible causes of illness, the ill person may feel punished. Because spirits, too, are perceived as causes of illness, the medicine man who appeases them is seen as a caregiver. The patient may not participate actively in scientific health care, viewing it as essentially unnecessary. Traditional American Indian treatments include exercise, dietary regimens, herbs, "sweating," symbolic *amulets*, and such rituals as prayers, chants, and dances.

The fact that few Indians live "by the clock" may interfere with the precise schedules usually associated with good nursing care. (This equation on the part of nurses is an expression of the dominant culture's preoccupation with efficiency.) Nurses need to understand that with the Indian culture, the concept of time may have a different, yet acceptable framework. The American Indian may believe that one sleeps when sleepy and eats when hungry. The patient may not consider it important to have appointments, medications, and meals at any particular time. Minimizing scheduled care and explaining clearly the rationale for procedures that must be done on time is the best approach.

Death and Bereavement

Death and bereavement are viewed by these persons as natural but sad life experiences. To the Indian, death is both a mystical experience and the natural end of life. The hereafter is not of overriding importance although it is consoling that the departed has been united with beloved ancestors. Some groups are demonstrative in grief; some are silent. Regardless of outward expression, the sense of loss is deeply felt throughout the community.

Burial practices vary widely from one tribe to another. The nurse should carefully inquire about what is customary. Because the body is considered a "whole" of nature, a body part or organ that has been removed may be requested for burial with the body. Some groups bury all the clothes of the deceased so that the spirit will have no reason to return. In view of this belief, all possessions should be carefully returned to the family. A few tribes still perform ritual wrapping of the body in ceremonial clothes, which may be done in the hospital. It is important to some Indians, and also a tribal custom, to be buried on the reservation of the tribe. Because *embalming* is usually forbidden and many states require embalming if the body is transported out of state, this custom may cause difficulties. The caring nurse will give special attention to these customs as well as to an appropriate bereavement period for Indian patients.

Asian Americans

The Asian American population is large and consists of many distinct groups that do not necessarily share the same cultural orientation. Within this ethnic group are Japanese, Chinese, Filipinos, Koreans, Southeast Asians, and South Pacific Islanders. In urban areas, many of the second and third generation families of these cultural groups continue to reside in communities made up largely of members of their own national background.

As *historical background*, the first Asian immigrants, mostly Chinese, received free passage to the United States in exchange for helping to build the railroads. Japanese immigration began with a trickle and soon swelled as the dream of a better life in America became, for some, a reality. By the time the transcontinental railroad was completed in 1869, thousands of Asians had become immigrant Americans. At about the same time, Filipinos were being recruited to work on Hawaiian plantations, at Alaskan canneries, and on California farmlands. These people received a pittance in pay, and many died of malnutrition and exposure to diseases for which they had no natural immunity.

Within the last 10 years many Laotians, Cambodians, and South Vietnamese have emigrated to the United States. Some of these immigrants have been referred to as the "boat people," for they escaped political oppression by traveling on small boats to politically freer countries near their own. Many of the lands to which the refugees fled have population saturation problems, leading many of the newer residents to seek asylum in the United States.

The problem of resettling and providing health care for the large number of political immigrants coming from Southeast Asia over the past several years has been a national concern. The current trend points to a continued increase in this population within the United States and Canada, a trend that will affect the delivery of nursing services.

Health Care and Incidence of Disease

Because Asian Americans are members of so many national groups, it will be necessary to speak in general terms about ethnic characteristics that one should consider in planning nursing care for these people. Many Asians have received inadequate health care. The language barrier and adherence to familiar native remedies causes many of them to forgo modern health care and pursue their traditional medical practice. The dominant concept in Asian medicine is energy. Because energizing the organs and senses is thought to prevent illness, sickness is typically perceived as a lack of energy.

Asian Americans appear to be prone to hypertension, tuberculosis, and diseases of the bone. The incidence of heart disease and cancer of the stomach has been lower than in the general population although the incidence of both has risen as more Asians have adopted westernized diets. Malnutrition has been reported in the elderly. Traditional health care may consist of the use of a combination of herbs, special foods, acupuncture, moxibustion, and conventional medicine. **Moxibustion** is the application of heated substances to the body. Acupuncture has been used for centuries among the Chinese as a method of instilling energy in designated portions of the body and as an analgesic agent. Its use by other Asians as an analgesic agent is relatively recent. Herbal broths are often administered. Among many traditional Chinese and other segments of the Asian American population, harmony with the five elements of nature—fire, earth, metal, water, and wood—is important, and these substances are often used in rituals of healing. Among all the ethnic groups, Asians have the lowest incidence of alcohol abuse.

Family

Asians consider the family to be an all-important unit. Even in adulthood, children feel a deep sense of obligation toward parents. Daughters remain at home until marriage. Moving away from the family geographically is sometimes discouraged and is generally a stressful occurrence.

It is typical in Asian families for the elderly to be treated with respect for having acquired great wisdom. The old and infirm are usually cared for within the family. Children are highly treasured; traditional families may value boys more than girls. In the traditional Japanese home, for example, males are sometimes served meals before females. Care of the sick is seen as a family and community responsibility.

Communication

Communication has at times been difficult, even within the cultural group because several dialects are used within the same Asian country or culture. For example, more than 40 dialects are spoken in the Philippines. This diversity poses problems in understanding one another and with providing interpreting aid. Asians are usually verbally polite to one another and to others with whom they communicate. They may be hesitant to ask questions for they may feel this reveals what might be interpreted as ignorance. The tone of the voice is important. Words should be softly spoken and not confrontational to be accepted. Having Asian clients paraphrase or repeat back what has been said is helpful to be sure they understand. Interpretation services are particularly useful when communicating with Asian clients.

In Asian cultures, the determination of whether or not to use eye contact is made on the basis of status or age. For example, younger persons often lower the eyes when meeting or communicating with an elder; students gaze downward when having a general conversation with a teacher. To lower the eyes and avoid eye contact signifies respect. It is considered acceptable for those of equal status or children to use eye contact when communicating.

Territoriality

Territoriality is an important part of Asian culture. A strong sense of social etiquette exists among Asians. It is considered rude, for example, for someone to drop in unexpectedly for a visit. If someone did drop in, however, Asians would consider it equally rude to confront the offender. Control of self and respect for others are high priorities in maintaining territoriality.

Asian American patients typically perceive physical and emotional privacy to have demarcated boundaries. The stereotype of communal baths to the contrary, Japanese patients tend to be extremely modest. Steps should be taken to provide maximum privacy. It is considered respectful and courteous to ask permission of an Asian patient to perform even routine care, for example, asking permission before opening the patient's bedside stand or closet. It is also important to solicit the patient's participation in decision-making.

Diet

The Asian diet has been considered to be more healthy than most western diets. Asian Americans tend to use a variety of seafood, pork, beef, and chicken in their diets, in combination with steamed vegetables. Raw vegetables are not used frequently. Rice and noodles are also included. Lactose intolerance is common among Asian Americans. Modifying the traditional diet may be a problem for those on sodium restriction for many dishes contain soy sauce, which is high in sodium content. Some Asians traditionally consider the ingestion of herbs and nutrition the most important aspect of maintaining harmony with nature. Foods are classified as *Yin* (cold) and *Yang* (hot) on the basis of each food's perceived nature, not its temperature. Because one must achieve a balance between the two for optimum health, a hot food, such as seasoned bean curd, might be served with a cold food, such as melon. (Some Asian national groups, such as Filipinos, do not subscribe to this concept.) Salads are not a typical Asian food. Entrails and organs are traditionally considered "blood-building."

Some foods are seen as having curative powers in certain illnesses. The powers of food are explained in detail to children. With Asian American patients, encouraging the family to bring in ethnic food, unless it is contraindicated, is helpful because food, which is viewed as "universal love," can be both physically and psychologically healing (Tien-Hyatt, 1987).

Spiritual Beliefs and Healing

Asians have deep spiritual beliefs that affect healing. Most of the people of Asia follow one of four predominant religions. We will briefly discuss them here since each is discussed in detail in Chapter 36.

Buddhism teaches that one's present life predetermines future lives. Buddhists believe that suffering is an inevitable part of existence, a view that may make the Buddhist patient reluctant to accept conscious relief from suffering. *Taoism* (from *Tao*, meaning "the path") is a Chinese religion based on the premise that the world is orderly and predictable, and passivity and simplicity are valued highly. *Confucianism* is a social belief system, centered around duty and loyalty to one's family and all other human beings. Confucianism sees the world as a place where human beings nurture one another. Finally, *Christianity*, primarily in the form of the Roman Catholic faith, is another religion of Asia.

Many individuals holding these various religious beliefs wear religious medals, amulets, or crucifixes. A rosary may be a special object for the Catholic Asian. Because healing powers are often attributed to these objects, they should not be treated carelessly or removed without the patient's permission. The thoughtful nurse always remembers to respect the beliefs of the patient.

Death and Bereavement

The concepts of death and bereavement are significant parts of the Asian culture. Death is viewed by most Asians as the process by which one is reunited with one's ancestors and thus as a transcendence to a better life. Weeping may be seen as weakness, particularly on the part of men, although grief is deeply felt. Once again, death practices vary from one group and even from one family to another; consult the family. Bells and incense may be used in the death ceremony, particularly by Chinese. In the Chinese culture, it is traditional for a male child to "guide" the parents' spirit into heaven at the time of death. Fast and lively music is often played at the funeral of some Asians to cheer the survivors. On special occasions during the first year after the death, a place may be set for the deceased at the table. Prayers are said for and to the departed.

African Americans

The term African American suggests the roots of this large group of Americans. It is the term most preferred because it identifies a cultural base that is important. Other terms are also used for this large group of the population. Many do not object to the all-inclusive title "black American" or even the simpler designation, "black."

African Americans constitute the largest minority group in the United States. According to the Bureau of the Census in 1991, blacks comprise approximately 12% of the population. Living predominantly in urban areas, black Americans, and especially black teenagers, continue to have a high unemployment rate despite advances in neighborhood and educational integration. The quality of nursing care for black patients may be limited by the fact that many nurses, despite their wishes to care for nonwhite patients, have had limited experience in providing such care. There is a growing need to graduate more black nurses who have the unique knowledge and sensitivity required to deliver quality health care to this minority group and share their knowledge with nonblack nurses.

The *historical background* of African Americans is documented in most school textbooks, which begin black history with stories of black slave trading. This is only partially complete. At least one black man sailed with Columbus, and many accompanied the European explorers who came to seek new land. Even before the African forced migration, some black people escaped African oppression and fled to Europe. Some escaped to North America and joined tribes and intermarried with the American Indians (Katz, 1987). Many blacks migrated to the West and became explorers, settlers, and cowboys (Durham and Jones, 1965).

The first black slaves arrived at the ports of New England in the early 1600s to be sold into bondage as commodities. Many whites did not regard blacks as full human beings with feelings like their own. The Quakers were among the first to raise a concerted outcry against inhumane treatment of blacks. The general outlines of subsequent black history in the United States are well known and hardly a source of pride for whites.

Black pride has blossomed over the past three decades, and past discriminatory practices are being redressed by equal opportunity laws and affirmative action programs in an effort to correct blacks' economic and educational disadvantages. Despite this, a great deal has yet to be achieved relative to fair social and employment practices.

Health Care and Incidence of Disease

There is national concern about the health care and incidence of disease among African Americans. The infant death rate of blacks is twice that of whites and comparable to that of American Indians. Even more startling, the maternal death rate of blacks is eight times that of whites. Diseases and conditions prevalent among blacks are sickle cell anemia, hypertension, obesity, heart disease, tuberculosis, and malnutrition. Although precise figures are not available, estimates of diabetes in blacks compared to whites range from 2:1 to as high as 5:1 (Roseman, 1984). Alcoholism and injection drug abuse are much more prevalent among blacks than among whites. Although there are few studies, alcoholism poses a serious problem in the black community (O'Brien and Chafetz, 1982). There are other alarming facts; African Americans have a higher level of domestic violence, and homicide is the leading cause of death among black males under the age of 18 (Fingerhut, Ingram, and Feldman, 1992).

Black patients may feel suspicious of the predominantly white health care system. Although there are more black physicians and nurses than ever before, the medical and nursing professions continue to be dominated by whites.

Health may be measured by black patients in terms of ability to work: to have to miss work means one is sick. Many blacks do not react to poor health until a crisis occurs, such as extreme pain, high fever, or bleeding. Otherwise, they tend to accept poor health as a fact of life. (This characteristic, like many of the others mentioned here, may be related more to low economic status and availability of health care than to racial background.)

Family

The family is an important factor in black culture. Black families have felt the impact of poverty and discrimination. Many African societies were matrilineal, tracing descent through the mother (Jacques, 1976). For this and complex other reasons, including greater employment discrimination against black men, many black families are headed by women. Children are often strongly encouraged to do well in school so that they can live better lives. The extended black family is a close unit. For those who remain within the family grouping, there is a strong sense of responsibility to one another (Fig. 33-3). Grandmothers often care for and at times raise their grandchildren to adulthood.

There are fewer black elders than there are whites in chronic care settings. One reason for this is that blacks have shorter life expectancy than whites. Another reason is that although elderly blacks appear to suffer more chronic illness than whites, nursing homes remain, for the most part, segregated facilities (Clavon, 1986). This situation is caused partly by the fact that many neighborhoods in urban areas remain segregated. Minority groups, including blacks, may not view the facility as a warm, welcoming, acceptable environment for long-term care. Another factor that results in fewer black elderly residents in nursing homes is the cultural tendency for family members to care in the home for those who are older and ill.

Communication

Because black patients and nonblack care providers both speak English, one might assume that communication would present few problems. However, communication is far more than mere words, and even words may cause lapses of communication. Many economically disadvantaged blacks speak *Black English*, a variation of English with unique inflections, sentence constructions, and vocabulary. For example, the sentence "She be sick," although incorrect in standard English, conforms to the grammatical rules of Black English. Much standard slang originates in Black English and spreads to the dominant culture.

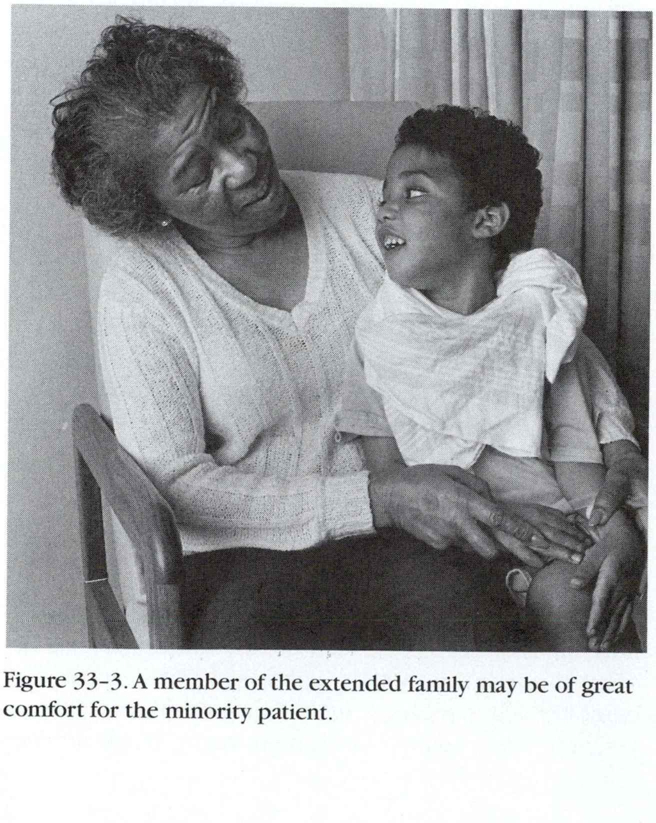

Figure 33-3. A member of the extended family may be of great comfort for the minority patient.

Mutual suspicion and awkwardness can attend communication between blacks and whites. If the nurse is straightforward, honest, and caring, most communication problems can be overcome.

Territoriality

Blacks, whose territoriality has often been brutally violated, tend to have mixed feelings about privacy. Until trust is built, a black patient may act aloof and suspicious of nonblacks. When trust has been established, however, the same patient may be open, verbal, and generous. Physical closeness and touching are common when trust has been established.

Diet

The traditional southern black diet consists of what is often called "soul food." The main meat of this diet is pork, which is cooked along with greens, okra, yams, lentils, and other vegetables. Grits, a porridge made from coarsely ground cornmeal, is served with most meals in the South, along with potatoes. Salt pork, bacon, and lard are used generously in food preparation and may contribute to the incidence of cardiovascular disease because these foods are high in saturated fats. Obesity can also occur from the long-term use of these products. The use of many pickled foods with high sodium content may be a problem for the many blacks who suffer from hypertension and cardiac problems. This diet is not restricted to southern blacks but is also used by others in the South. Because the diet is economical, its use is sometimes associated with persons who subsist at poverty levels, although this is not always so. Soul food is gaining in popularity although revisions are being made to make the diet more nutritious.

Although these traditional dietary patterns are still widely seen, many northern and urban black Americans are adopting different dietary patterns, which include less red meat and more fresh fruits and vegetables. Economically advantaged blacks appear to be following recommendations for a healthy diet.

Spiritual Beliefs and Healing

African Americans have established views concerning spiritual beliefs and healing. A large number of blacks live in the southern part of the United States and belong to conservative Christian groups, in which there is great emphasis on the Bible and its teachings. The church is a strong social as well as religious force. It is the primary support system among the black community, as church members visit and care for those who are sick or bereaved.

Many black persons may tend to have a fatalistic outlook regarding illness, that is, they may believe that whatever happens was meant to happen. Some equate illness with God's punishment. Certain African Americans may have a flexible time orientation, and thus may not see preventive health measures as expedient or meaningful.

A strong strain of black folk medicine remains in health and healing practices. Oils, herbs, and certain foods are thought to have medicinal powers, and preventive or curative powers may be attributed to certain objects. Spiritual health and physical health are seen as closely intertwined. Black medicine, which involves beliefs originating in Africa, is still used by a limited number of African Americans.

Death and Bereavement

The rituals surrounding death and bereavement help members of this group to cope with events. Death is no stranger to African Americans, whose life expectancy is 7 to 8 years less than that of the white population. Belief in the hereafter is strong and death is often referred to as "crossing over." The outlook that death is God's will and leads to a better life "on the other side" may be of great consolation to survivors.

When a death occurs, it is important for the family to come together. Those far away often have to sacrifice time and money, traveling long distances to fulfill this important obligation. The deceased person may have planned the clothing in which to be buried. Viewing the body and large funerals are common practices.

Bereavement may be expressed emotionally, even to the point of prostration. Such behavior may be upsetting to nonblacks who do not understand its significance for the family. Because viewing the body is important, the nurse should take special efforts to make this possible in the hospital and to prepare the body for viewing. All possessions should be returned to the family because they are valued as reminders of the deceased.

Hispanic Americans

The inclusive term Hispanic American is used to refer to people whose native language is Spanish or Portuguese and includes Puerto Ricans and immigrants from Mexico, Cuba, Central and South America, and Spain. *Chicano* refers to any person who is of Mexican descent and many, but not all, of these persons prefer this term. Some identify this term with the politically active segment of their group and choose not to use Chicano.

Easily distinguished by language and appearance, Hispanics have suffered from pervasive discrimination and disadvantage. The difficulty of integrating into the general population has caused many second and third generation Hispanics to remain in tightly knit communities known as *barrios*, primarily in the southwestern United States. Hispanics now comprise 9% of the general population (U.S. Census, 1991).

Spanish people have a unique place in the *historical background* of North America. By 1620, when the Pilgrims landed at Plymouth Rock, much of the Southwest had been explored, mapped, and colonized by the Spanish. Texas, California, Arizona, and New Mexico were under the Spanish flag long before the American Revolution. Thus, Hispanics were in a sense the first immigrants.

Many Mexican Americans have more recently entered the United States as farm workers. In the past, the relatively unguarded southern borders allowed easy illegal access to the United States and, therefore, illegal aliens from Mexico often lived and worked in the United States. In November, 1990, the United States Congress passed a general amnesty law that declared that those persons who had resided in the country for a year be granted permanent resident status. Many Hispanic immigrants entered the ranks of migrant workers, who move from one part of the country to another as crops need harvesting. Even more recently, Hispanic political refugees from several Central and South American countries have sought asylum in the United States. Many are seeking employment in the professions they practiced in their native countries.

Health Care and Incidence of Disease

Several factors influence the health care and incidence of disease among Hispanic people. Most Hispanics must contend with below-average family incomes and thus are particularly subject to diseases associated with the economically disadvantaged: obesity, hypertension, respiratory disease, and gastrointestinal disturbances. Diabetes is 2.8 times more frequent in Mexican American men than in white men and 1.5 times more frequent in Mexican American women than in white women (Stern, 1984). Language barriers can magnify economic barriers to high quality health care. Although high suicide rates usually accompany economic disadvantages, this is not the case with Hispanics, probably because of the religious belief that suicide is sinful.

Strongly Roman Catholic, most Hispanics tend to interpret health and illness as the "will of God." Many Hispanics regard *machismo* (maleness) and *hembrisma* (femaleness) as related to health. Belief in the **mal de ojo** (evil eye) is unique to Hispanic culture. **Brujas** are evil people able to cause illnesses, discomfort, and other problems. Hispanics who believe in such traditional interpretations of illness do not consider the established health care system beneficial for such conditions and thus use home remedies (**remedios**) and consult folk healers (**curanderos**), who derive their powers from God.

Amulets, charms, and other objects used by Hispanic patients should be considered cultural adjuncts to care. If they do not impede or contradict recognized health therapies, they may provide the Hispanic patient and the family a measure of psychological comfort not available from other sources.

Family

The family is the unit of support for the individual. Hispanic families tend to be patriarchal in that the father, regarded as strong and brave, is the decision-maker. Family honor is important and defended. The extended family concept is also apparent in that younger members provide for the care of older aunts, uncles, and grandparents. Hispanic children are a source of great pride and satisfaction and usually behave well so as not to dishonor the family. Religious holidays are times of family gatherings.

Communication

Communication is a problem for English-speaking nurses caring for Hispanics. Of the 104 languages spoken in Los Angeles County, most are of Hispanic origin. Many Hispanics, although they speak different dialects, can understand one another. Diaz-Duque (1982) writes that a secondary communication problem is that many Hispanics have a fear of the health care person that makes verbal communication even more difficult. Spanish and Portuguese are not difficult languages to learn, and it may be that the great influx of Spanish-speaking people will induce more nurses to acquire one of these languages. A small pocket dictionary may be helpful to the care provider in routine care. Using a translator is also a viable alternative for developing appropriate communication.

Territoriality

Although Hispanics are both open and effusive, there is a consideration for territoriality. Hispanic culture tends to be both expressive and inclusive. Hispanic patients usually welcome touch and may be offended if a handshake is withheld. Communication is expressive, and personal territory is generously shared in trusting relationships. Other patients and care providers who are more exclusively territorial may feel threatened by traditional Hispanic effusiveness.

Diet

The Hispanic family's diet often has cultural significance. Williams (1989) states that food has many meanings for these people, and decisions about which foods are to be prepared and when they are to be consumed are often based on cultural values (Fig. 33-4). Many foods are festive or holiday related. Nutritional deficiencies have been found among Hispanics, mainly lack of adequate calcium, vitamin C, and several of the B vitamins. These deficiencies have occurred primarily because Hispanics' low economic status has restricted their ability to choose a variety of more nutritious food items. For example, the diet of the Hispanic population tends to be dominated by beans, lentils, corn, and rice. Milk and milk products are often omitted. Meat may be limited in quantity. Garlic, once used by Hispanics to fight diphtheria, is now regarded as a general medicinal agent. Hispanics share with Asians an elaborate system relating "hot" foods and "cold" foods to the incidence and cure of disease. Much of the Hispanic diet is highly spiced.

Spiritual Beliefs and Healing

This culture has long-held beliefs about both religion and healing. Nearly all Hispanics are Roman Catholics. The Virgin Mary is the dominant religious figure, and prayers for health are offered up to her. Pictures of the Virgin are prominent in Hispanic homes. The patient may keep a crucifix at the bedside. The patient may find the sacraments for the sick comforting rituals, and prayers may be offered to the patient's patron saint.

Views of illness are different among different Hispanic groups. Some view ill health as punishment from God, whereas others attribute illness to "destiny." Hispanics may refuse hospital food, believing in the cura-

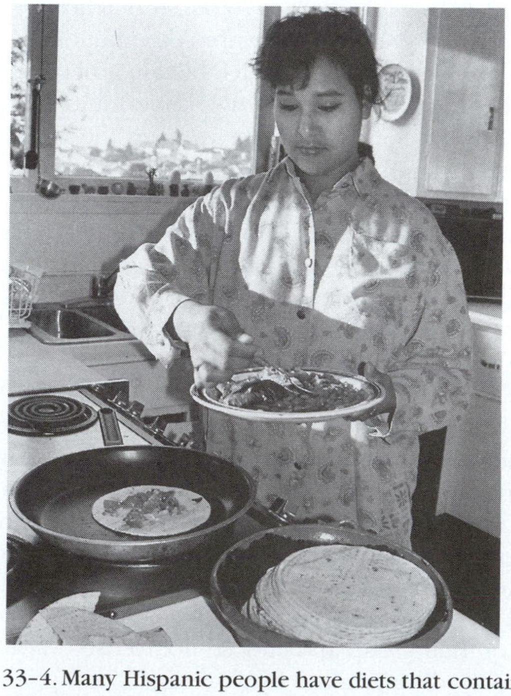

Figure 33-4. Many Hispanic people have diets that contain corn and bean products.

tive powers of "hot" or "cold" ethnic foods appropriate for the ailment to be treated. Folk healers are also often consulted. The Hispanic patient may appear somewhat resigned to the treatment regimen and may not participate in its intervention. Prayer is important for some; rituals to forestall "witchcraft" may be performed by others. The nurse should accept all of the patient's beliefs concerning healing unless they clearly interfere with recovery.

Death and Bereavement

Feelings about death and bereavement are deeply rooted. Death is often viewed by Hispanics as natural and as God's will. The body may be viewed privately by the family and close friends but is usually not viewed at the Mass. Death rituals may include such cultural traditions as fast and lively music, lighting of candles, and feasting. Grief is expressed openly, and weeping is widely accepted for both males and females. Body parts and organs are sometimes requested for burial because it is thought that the body cannot be disrupted if the spirit is to survive.

Other Subgroups of American Culture

Several other groups within our American culture have different needs. Some of these special groups are women, migrant people, the urban and rural poor, and the homeless. Many socially and economically disadvantaged Americans are also the victims of discrimination. Such people, members of all cultures, often suffer extreme hardship and stresses that lead to illness. This population's needs and problems must be addressed if this society is to equalize access to health care and promote health maintenance.

Women as a Subculture

Fifty years ago, most Americans would not have considered women a distinct cultural group. Many people still do not; yet women's political action and social support groups are an undeniable part of contemporary society. Attention on women's issues has crossed all social and ethnic lines and has persistently striven to give women equal representation in government and in the workplace. Many men have joined women in support of women's issues.

Several pieces of legislation in this country have been proposed to correct sexual inequities. One of these was the *Equal Rights Amendment* written in 1972. In 1978, Congress granted an extension for ratification by the states. In 1982, the amendment was defeated even though 62% of the population favored passage. The constitutional amendment would have banned all laws that give one sex rights denied to the other. Passage of the amendment would have had many implications. According to some economists, it would have substantially improved the economic situation of women. There is an attempt at present to revive this amendment for resubmission to the states.

Comparable Worth

The issue of comparable worth has been addressed in several states. **Comparable worth** means that those having comparable skill training or education and performing similar tasks or having similar responsibilities should receive equal compensation. It is clear that the persons who benefit the most under this concept are women and minorities. Because the majority of nurses are women and assume serious responsibility for the safety of others, the issue of comparable worth is a crucial one. However, to implement such a proposal is not without difficulties, although to many, the idea appears to have merit.

Nursing Research: *Implications for Practice*

Meleis, A. I. "Between Two Cultures: Identity, Roles and Health." *Health Care for Women International* 12, 4 (October-December 1991): 365–377.

The author has focused on the stresses experienced by women who are also immigrants. It is emphasized that immigrant women feel increased stress as they attempt to reconcile their relocation along with the many issues of also being a woman. With the increased population of immigrant women has come a renewed interest in balancing "values of their cultural heritage with those of the new host society."

Nurses should understand the increased stress imposed by circumstances on this population. The implication for the health care system and nurses is identifying high-risk immigrant women and developing ways to meet their needs that are congruent with their belief system.

Several states have passed comparable worth measures and retroactively compensated some workers under its decree.

Accomplishments of Women

The competencies and accomplishments of women are being increasingly recognized. More women are currently seeking and serving in political offices throughout the world than ever before. On a more local level, women are presently occupying more professional and management positions in the work force than before. A woman is now a Supreme Court justice and women are traveling into space. Women serve as chief executive officers of corporations and as mayors, governors, and senators. Women are also in the forefront of scientific and technological advance along with men.

Changing Roles of Women

Women's roles have changed dramatically over the past 10 years. One factor has been the increase in the number of women becoming single parents. The percentage of households headed by single women with children under the age of 18 has now reached approximately 90% of all single households. Almost one-half of all children in our country live in a single-parent household. Equally astounding is the fact that of the 10 million children living with a single woman, one-half reside in households living at poverty levels (U.S. Census, 1991).

Inflation and the rising cost of living have brought a large number of women into the workplace. They now constitute just over one-half of the labor force. Many single mothers are relatively unprepared for assuming full-time work outside the home to meet their financial needs. They must learn new skills and arrange for their children to be cared for in day-care centers during the day. Although some men are choosing to become single fathers, few women have a choice regarding single parenting. Considerable stress is produced for women trying to meet economic needs while caring for a young family alone. Wages remain consistently lower for women than for men. In addition, black women are paid even less, on the average, than white women.

Another group of women, who are highly educated and skilled, are entering the work force to secure job satisfaction and fulfillment. Occupations formerly limited to men are now more available to qualified women because of equal opportunity policies (Fig. 33-5). More women than ever before are delaying pregnancy or deciding to remain childless to meet the demands of a desired job or career. Women who work outside the home tend to have smaller families than those who do not work, and some people predict that in the future more women within the work force will choose to remain childless.

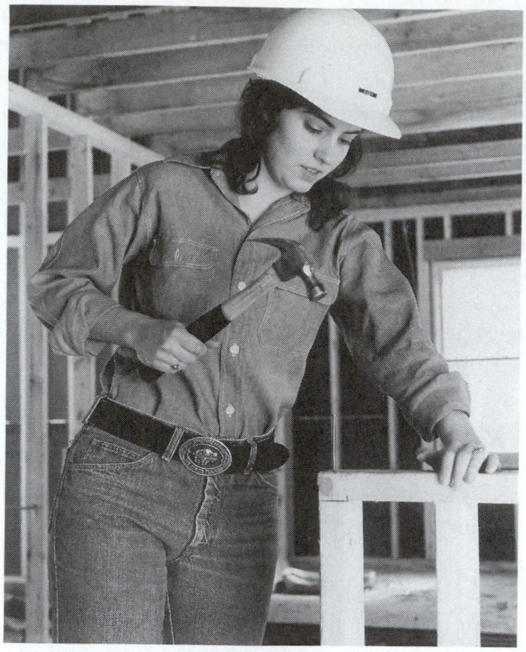

Figure 33-5. Women have entered many occupational fields that were formerly dominated by men.

Women's Health Care

More attention has been given recently to the special health care needs of women. Previously, the health concerns of women were thought to be the same as those of men. There was little awareness that women experienced a variety of unique health problems. Centers for research into women's health issues have escalated as more women have become invested in the importance of health care directed specifically to women.

As more women have become physicians (almost one-half of the students at large medical schools are women), women's health has gained increased interest. Because the anatomy and physiology of women differ from those of men, diseases and medical conditions also occur in different ratios among men and women. Statistically, women suffer more depression, lower back pain, and fractures than men. Several factors may affect these figures, however. First, women may report these medical conditions more often because women may be more apt than men to seek medical help. Second, women may have more skeletal problems because of decalcification of bone (osteoporosis, which is more common in older women because of estrogen deficiency) and general back strain because the protective muscle sheaths of their backs are not as strong as men's. Although heart disease is more prevalent in men, it is still the leading cause of death among women. Childbearing is becoming more a shared experience between mothers and fathers; however, women continue to have special needs during this time. Because of changing roles and their demands, women are experiencing new health problems. There are higher rates of physical illness in women as well as job-related stress that can further lead to physical illness.

Women have actively entered into issues of health for themselves. For example, the number of women surviving breast cancer has increased largely because of the breast self-examinations they performed. Women have become increasingly interested in exercise and diet programs that focus on maintaining health. At this time, there are more women than men in nursing but this is changing. Nurses have been instrumental in starting women's health clinics to address the preventive and maintenance health needs of women. Both male and female nurses have a vested interest in providing women with culturally relevant health care.

Table 33–2. Percentage of Adults and Children Living in Poverty—1989

All races	12.8%
White	10.0
Black	30.7
Hispanic	26.2
Children under 18 years of age	
All races	19.0
White	14.1
Black	43.2
Hispanic	35.5

Department of Commerce, Bureau of the Census, Washington, D.C.: 1992.

The Migrant Population

Migrants in North American society are not always regarded as a minority because they do not share a common cultural heritage. Thus, although they share many of the problems of other minority groups, they enjoy few of the benefits.

The mere fact of being migrant creates health care problems, such as unfamiliarity with the health resources of a community. Disease and unhealthy conditions may not be diagnosed promptly because of a lack of nearby facilities. Health records are frequently lacking. Because the lifestyle and cultural orientation of the migrant patient are different from those of the providers of health care, communication is likely to be poor.

Some migrant workers have not been legally admitted to this country and are fearful of retaliation if they consult a health care agency. These circumstances lead to poor health maintenance, fragmented treatment, and little or no follow-up care. Migrant health agencies are coming to the aid of migrant families in some areas, but the agencies' capacities are still far too limited to meet the need.

The Urban and Rural Poor

The numbers of those living in poverty increased in the United States from 1991 to 1992. Unemployment rates have climbed to 7.2% of the population. Fourteen percent live at or below the poverty level of $13,000 annually for a family of four in 1992, up from 12.8% in 1989. One of every four children under the age of 6 lives in poverty (U.S. Department of Economic Development and Bureau of the Census, 1992; Table 33-2).

It has clearly been documented that poor children have lowered self-esteem and because of poor nutrition and family problems, they are unable to learn as well as less deprived youngsters. For all ages, there are increased health problems because many diseases and conditions proliferate among the economically disadvantaged.

Many of the poor of our country belong to particular ethnic groups. Their poverty is caused by unemployment as well as the low pay in jobs held by minority persons. The number of poor younger women in our society is increasing because of marital disruption leading to the financial burden of caring for young children. There is concern both in individual states and nationally regarding the failure of working fathers to provide financially for their minor children. Laws concerning child support are being introduced into many legislatures.

Living quarters may make health care practices difficult, if not impossible, for the poor. Care of the homeless, particularly of those who move about from place to place, is another critical concern. Limited education may affect ability to understand illness and participate in care. Poor people may be reluctant to seek health care because they fear they will feel awkward or shabby, and transportation may be difficult. Another factor influencing lack of health care may be the feeling that "charity" health care is undesirable or an admission that one is poor. Nutrition may be inadequate because of limited income and lack of information about the purchase and use of correct foods.

Health problems, prevalent among the poor, include obesity (caused primarily by excessive consumption of high-fat, high-calorie cheap foods), malnutrition, diabetes, tuberculosis, depression, suicide, and homicide. Infant and maternal mortality rates among the poor are above the national average.

Poverty undermines dignity. Many of the poor must still laboriously justify their qualification for care and spend long hours waiting on clinic benches. They may receive sound medical treatment from community-based medical clinics but find their personal feelings and individuality ignored. This is, in all fairness, not always the case, and socially responsible health care providers are working toward changes to better serve the needs of disadvantaged patients. Each of us in nursing has a special mission provide sensitive care to those going through difficult economic times.

The Homeless Population

It is a sobering and unfortunate fact that of the 2.5 million homeless people in the United States, approximately one-third are families (Bassuk and Rosenberg, 1988). Although most of the homeless population reside in urban areas, some of the homeless are living in more rural neighborhoods.

Although the term homeless is interpreted as a lack of housing, the situation is much more complex (Lindsey, 1989). To be homeless means hopelessness and a dissociation from friends and family. This is particularly disruptive for the homeless parent with children. Health care providers have often stereotyped the homeless because formerly people with substance abuse or mental health problems were the homeless. Partly in response to attitudes of rejection, the homeless often fail to seek health care when needed. Nurses and other health professionals must become more knowledgeable concerning the homeless population to meet their special needs.

Hunter (1992) offers some suggestions regarding successfully interacting with the homeless. She reminds us that nonverbal messages are acutely interpreted by those who are embarrassed by having to ask for help. She poses questions and responses in a direct, understanding but nonthreatening manner. For example, rather than asking "What is your occupation?", it is kinder to simply ask, "Where do you get your money?" A major problem with care of the homeless is access to records. The homeless may move from one location to another so that medical recordkeeping is fragmented.

The homeless are particularly prone to many disorders. A portion may have substance abuse problems or be mentally ill. People who are without a home may suffer from an inhospitable environment, developing respiratory problems such as colds, flu, pneumonia, and drug-resistant tuberculosis. Inadequate sanitation and nutrition may lead to skin disruptions and gastrointestinal disturbances. Hypertension, seizure disorders, and diabetic crises are also more prevalent in this population. A major concern with the homeless is the incidence of foot problems caused by poorly fitting shoes, lack of foot care, and generally low health status. Nurses cannot realistically solve the multiple problems of the homeless population, but nurses can offer compassionate care and tap into community resources. With concerted effort toward providing quality care, nurses can play a vital role. Nurses can also support government programs designed to improve the plight of homeless people.

Assessment

Self-assessment

Assessing the needs of those patients from another ethnic group or culture requires special insight into your own attitudes as well as those of the patient. To assess effectively in these situations, nurses need to develop self-awareness and understanding and devote time and effort to understanding the ethnic group to which the patient belongs. Effort in these areas will enable you to develop an appropriately individualized plan of care.

To develop *self-awareness and understanding*, you must examine, with openness and honesty, your feelings toward the ethnic group to which your patient belongs. What past experiences have you had with people of this group? Were they positive or negative? How have these experiences affected your attitude? For example, suppose you were dissatisfied with the Italian auto me-

Nursing Issues and Trends: *Meeting the Health Needs of the Homeless*

Economic shifts have produced increasing numbers of homeless people (now estimated to be approaching 3 million). Once predominantly unemployed men with high rates of mental illness and alcoholism, the homeless now include many families, often single women with children. With homelessness comes increasing health problems. Both children and adults have more frequent respiratory and bladder infections as well as other illnesses than do people who are not homeless. A particular concern is that of foot care for homeless men. This may be due to ill-fitting shoes and exposure to a wet environment. Although it is hoped that the numbers of homeless will decrease over the next 10 years, we should become aware of the health issues unique to this special population so that that their needs can be addressed.

chanic who repaired your car; you felt he was uncaring and hostile. You admit you have already transferred some of your consequent hostility to the Italian patient in your care. You must then make a point of seeking out the individual characteristics that distinguish your patient from the auto mechanic, even though they share the same national origin. It may take reminders to yourself, until you know your patient better, that your patient has unique value and worth.

Understanding and gaining knowledge about the ethnic group to which the patient belongs provides data essential to patient care. The best way to gain understanding of the patient's ethnic group is to spend time reading and talking with other members of that group. Inaccuracies and myths you have long accepted may be dispelled. With a more open and accepting mind, you will be better able to develop an individualized nursing care plan and to relate it to the patient in a therapeutic manner. Keep in mind the effect of recency of immigration: for example, the customs and characteristics of a Chinese immigrant will be more traditional than those of a Chinese person born and reared in the United States who has adopted the manners, ways, and thinking of the white majority.

Interview

Interviewing patients from other cultures or ethnic groups should be carried out with genuine interest and sensitivity. This will help you understand what the ethnic group to which the patient belongs means to that individual. The ethnic group and dominant language of the patient is often apparent. The open-ended question can be the most effective way to gather data.

Health Care and Incidence of Disease

Basic questions such as "When have you last seen a doctor or been in the hospital?" can begin exploring the patient's health status. Questions to the patient or family regarding what they see as important in care identifies implementation that is congruent with that group's values. Noting what disorders have been experienced and the duration and treatment that helped are all important to the interview process.

Family

If the family is present at the time of the interview, you probably will get a sense of the degree of support and caring that exists among members. If the family is not present, you can ask, "Tell me about your family" or "Who is important to you?"

Many families not only appreciate being involved in care but like being included in the interview process. If the family is present to act as interpreters, the answers may include family attitudes as well as those of the patient.

Communication

Note the patient's or family's nonverbal communication such as body language. Does the patient look relaxed or anxious and fearful? What is the predominant language of the family and patient? Is another language spoken in the home? Will the patient need interpretive services, and if so, what language or dialect will be helpful? You can assess the family's willingness to help you communicate with the patient using simple words or symbols.

Territoriality

During the interview and later, during the physical examination, the patient's feelings concerning territoriality may become evident. Watch for the patient's response to your closeness and touch. At all times, you must respect the patient's "psychological safe space" or you will lose the patient's trust. Possessions may be considered personal and should never be taken for safekeeping or moved unless you are sure permission has been given. Questions asked without sensitivity can also intrude on territoriality.

Diet

The patient, family, and nutritionist can all give you assistance on finding food that is nutritious but also appropriate to the culture. Asking the patient about the family diet and what foods are most acceptable can help in planning menus while the patient is in the health care facility.

Spiritual Beliefs and Healing

During the interview, asking open-ended questions such as "Do you or your family have strong spiritual beliefs?" or "Tell me what you believe in." "How do these beliefs help you when you are ill?" "Has there been something in your life that seems to help healing that is different from the care that is usually given people?" Let the patient talk and listen attentively.

Death and Bereavement

Knowing about the culture's beliefs and practices regarding death and bereavement before the event is the most effective factor in providing support to the patient and the family. Sometimes, asking how you can help during this difficult time allows the person to share cultural death attitudes with you. Acceptance of practices unfamiliar to you can help resolve a death in a manner that is important to the group.

Physical Assessment

You will identify the patient's age and past history of physical disorders. The physical examination must be objective. You must not rely on your expectations of the physical characteristics of the culture but on your assessment skills. Skin color and other physical characteristics will be assessed in congruence with the person's ethnic heritage. For example, the presence of jaundice (a yellowing of the skin) may be more difficult to detect in the Asian than in the white person. The patient or family may be able to add to your data because they are more familiar with the person's usual appearance. The physical assessment will also give you data concerning the patient's nutritional and activity status.

Nursing Diagnosis

Many nursing diagnoses could be present in the patient from another culture. The plan of care should include those diagnoses that relate specifically to the problems related to ethnic or cultural diversity.

Impaired Verbal Communication

When using the diagnosis of Impaired Verbal Communication for the patient who is non-English speaking, you should add "related to foreign language barrier."

Anxiety

Another nursing diagnosis approved by the North American Nursing Diagnosis Association (NANDA) might be Anxiety related to unfamiliarity with environment. You would have to state specifically what knowledge the patient needs to decrease the level of anxiety. For example, perhaps the members of the health care team do not wear masks, gowns, and gloves when performing a procedure in the culture from which the person comes. Because of the ominous and strange appearance of a person wearing these in our health care setting, the patient may be anxious and need knowledge regarding the reasons behind this action.

Ineffective Individual Coping

Ineffective Individual Coping related to lack of culturally relevant support is appropriate for the person from another culture becoming a patient in the health care setting. The culturally diverse patient may become depressed and frightened because of the unfamiliar environment and the number of care providers who are not of the ethnic group and do not speak the same language as the patient. Separation from the family and more familiar surroundings may also contribute to difficulty in coping. Coping may become so ineffective that it interferes with care.

Social Isolation

Social Isolation related to difficulty interacting with others in the health care setting is an appropriate nursing diagnosis when the person cannot communicate with others. The patient feels isolated and some care providers may unintentionally decrease interaction with the patient because of the limitations of communication.

Noncompliance

Noncompliance as a nursing diagnosis for the culturally different patient only becomes appropriate if the etiology can be identified. The patient may be noncompliant because of anxiety. Another reason is that the care prescribed may not be culturally acceptable to the person. A common reason for noncompliance by the person is that because of a language barrier or unfamiliarity with the medical arena, the person may have a formidable knowledge deficit.

Knowledge Deficit

Knowledge Deficit is a category that is often directly related to unfamiliarity with a procedure, treatment, or areas of the plan of care. A language barrier can further complicate the teaching plan. Stating the etiology such as language, unfamiliarity, or no previous experience will help in planning and implementation.

Nursing Diagnoses Related to Care of the Patient From Another Culture

- Impaired Verbal Communication related to foreign language barrier
- Anxiety related to unfamiliarity with environment
- Ineffective Individual Coping related to lack of culturally relevant support
- Social Isolation related to difficulty interacting with others in the health care setting
- Noncompliance related to
  - anxiety concerning health care system
  - foreign language barrier
- Knowledge Deficit concerning unfamiliarity with medical procedure related to foreign language barrier

Planning and Implementation

The opportunity to plan culturally consistent care for the minority patient can be an enriching experience for the nurse. There are several culturally focused actions you can incorporate into the plan of care for this patient. The

Nursing Care Plan
Sample Nursing Care Plan Related to Ethnic Identity

Nursing Diagnosis

Impaired Verbal Communication related to foreign language barrier.

Supportive data:

Woman, age 47
Is Filipino
Arrived in the United States six months ago
Will be living with adult son
Speaks Tagalog as primary language. Speaks almost no English.

Desired Patient Outcomes

The patient will:

Relate basic needs to health care team within 2 days

Communicate feelings of acceptance and reduced frustration

Appear less anxious and fearful

Nursing Action	Rationale:
1. Explain communication problem to English-speaking son, Yen.	Involving English speaking family member may help in finding ways to communicate with non-English speaking patient.
2. Elicit help of staff nurse, Hulan, who speaks same language.	Asking help in communicating from staff nurse who speaks the same language as the patient is helpful in communicating medical and nursing terminology that may be unfamiliar to a family member.
3. Learn important words or phrases and post list on bedside table or over bed.	Learning key words and phrases spoken by the patient shows your interest in learning the patient's language and provides a limited degree of communication. Posting the list helps others communicate who do not speak the patient's language.
4. Know phone number and person to contact at community language resource (524-7300—Ming)	Seeking outside language resources facilitates more indepth communication.
5. Use gentle, nonintrusive touch.	If condoned by the ethnic group, touch can also provide a caring means of communication.

care plan can be individualized to accommodate to the patient's cultural or ethnic background and customs. Care can be planned and implemented around the areas discussed in this chapter (see the sample Nursing Care Plan Related to Ethnic Identity).

The desired outcomes in this setting include the following: the patient is able to communicate basic needs and is able to relate such feelings as acceptance, reduced frustration, and isolation (Carpenito, 1992); the patient can express coping concerns to the family or others, recognize strengths, and accept support to a level that leads to effective care; the patient's reasons for noncompliance are identified as well as ways of overcoming them; the patient is able to acknowledge a need for information and ways of providing that information are formulated.

Establishing Communication

To address these concerns, you must first establish communication. Imagine yourself as a patient in a large hospital where no one you see shares your ethnic background and you cannot understand the language. Communicating your needs is difficult to impossible, and you are unsure of what is expected of you. You long for a person who looks similar to you physically and with whom you can communicate. You may have to plan to involve someone from the family or a language resource agency to establish verbal communication with the patient to carry out health teaching.

Recognizing the Importance of the Family

Regardless of the culture, family is an important component to identity. What constitutes family composition, however, may be different from one culture to another. For example, the patient may consider family to mean not just the nuclear family but also extended family and friends. If the facility's policy is to allow only one or two family members at the bedside at any given time but the patient wants to have the entire family present, difficulties may arise. In such a case, restricting visitors may be detrimental to the patient. Sometimes, overcoming these obstacles requires reviewing the policies of the health care facility. Making exceptions to standard policy for the purpose of making care minimally disturbing to the minority group patient may have to have supervisory approval.

Conveying Respect for the Patient's Beliefs

Acknowledging the patient's values and beliefs may also require adaptation within the health care setting. If the burning of incense or the ingestion of herbs conflicts with policy, it may prove best for you to seek approval to waive this restriction for the purposes of patient comfort.

Knowing about the norms of territoriality is important so that you can build trust with the patient and the family. Intruding on what is spatially correct for that culture interferes with care.

Diet is another way of adapting to what is comfortable for the patient. You may want to consult with the dietary staff or ask the family for guidance. If the patient cannot eat because of the character of the illness, this fact may have to be explained also.

Respecting cultural feelings about death and bereavement is the final and most sensitive consideration you can offer the patient and those who survive. In general, health care facilities are becoming much more accepting of people society may view as different and more willing to amend and establish policies to prevent infringement of human rights, a fact that may help you in providing care for the patient who is culturally different.

Evaluation

Evaluation is a process of reviewing the desired outcomes established when you identified your nursing diagnoses. If a method of communication has been established so that the patient can make his or her needs known and appears less anxious and more comfortable in the care setting, then the evaluation of the plan is positive. Also, there is an unspoken trust that develops between the nurse and the culturally different patient and family that clearly affirms appreciation in the quality and sensitivity of care provided by the nurse.

Nursing Care Study
The Dietary Needs of a Hmong Woman

The Hmong were originally a rural tribal group living in the mountains of Laos. Many Hmong displaced by the war in Southeast Asia have come to the United States as refugees. Most adults have no formal education. Although the men may speak Lao and some English, the women often speak only the Hmong language.

Chi Vang was a 44-year-old Hmong woman who was hospitalized after the birth of her tenth child. This was the first birth for which she had ever received formal health care and her first hospitalization.

When Mrs. Vang's sponsor (a United States citizen helping with the refugee family's relocation) visited some hours after the birth, the nurses expressed serious concern that Mrs. Vang was not eating or drinking any fluids. They asked if the sponsor could help translate. The sponsor explained that she spoke no Hmong, but that she knew that the Hmong drink only hot water and that might be part of the problem. The Hmong believe that cold water will cause sickness. (This belief may be related to the effect of local water supplies in Laos.) She suggested that they try giving hot water to Mrs. Vang while she tried to contact Mrs. Vang's oldest son, Mao, who spoke English.

The nurse took hot water to Mrs. Vang and was pleased to note that Mrs. Vang immediately drank an entire cup. The nurse then put a notation on the care plan for hot water to be served to Mrs. Vang at frequent intervals.

(*continued*)

Nursing Care Study (continued)
The Dietary Needs of a Hmong Woman

Meanwhile, the sponsor had contacted Mao by telephone, and Mrs. Vang's food preferences were discussed. The nurse learned that the Hmong do not eat bread, potatoes, cereal, or raw vegetables and that rice is usually eaten at every meal. Fresh, not canned, fruits are eaten. Fish and poultry were the preferred protein foods. The nurse thanked Mao for his help and arranged to call him if the staff needed more information. The nurse then called the dietitian and explained Mrs. Vang's dietary preferences. A note was added to the care plan outlining Mrs. Vang's dietary preferences; included were directions to check Mrs. Vang's tray before serving the food.

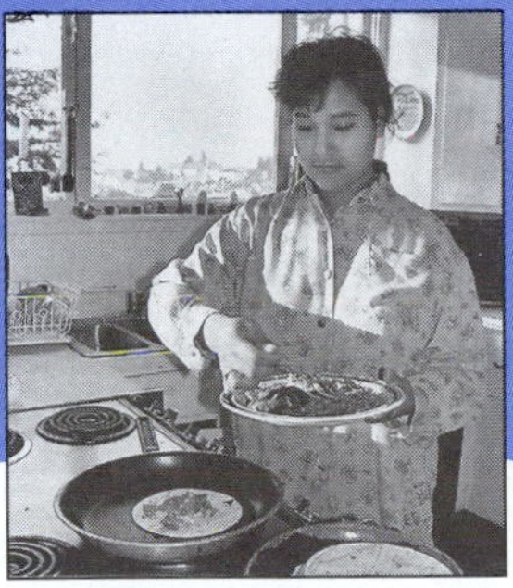

Key Points

- The specialty of transcultural nursing has sought to answer the nursing needs of many groups. Living in a diverse society has posed problems that also affect health care.
- Ethnocentrism, the belief that one's own group is superior to another, can lead to bias and prejudice, stereotyping, discrimination, and institutional racism.
- It is essential that nurses gain an understanding of the culturally different patients for whom they care and have an awareness of any personal prejudices that may interfere with care and an understanding of the ethnic group, its values, and its beliefs.
- Patients may vary in their approaches to health status, territoriality, diet, communication, health teaching, spiritual beliefs, and death.
- The American population is composed of many ethnic groups, including white Americans, American Indians and Eskimos, Asian Americans, African Americans, and Hispanic Americans.
- Against the historical background of each group, the nurse must look carefully at the person and family as they exist within their own cultural or ethnic environment, adapting care to the identity of the individual.
- The economically disadvantaged constitute another group of people with special health care needs and problems, although members of this group may not share much in the way of ethnic background. They are at risk for illness because of their impoverishment and stress.
- The migrant population, for whom health care is remote, and the urban and rural poor are special categories of persons needing care.
- Women have banded together as a group within American culture to seek equality in the home, the work setting, and government. The greater visibility of women nationally has led to improvements in health care, largely through the efforts of women themselves.
- Special assessment skills come into play as nurses care for persons who are culturally different.
- Nursing process is helpful when identifying problems that are specific to the patient from another culture. Several NANDA-approved nursing diagnoses such as Impaired Verbal Communication and Anxiety related to the unfamiliar health care setting are appropriate to consider when planning and implementing care.

Study Questions

1. Define the terms ethnocentrism, bias, prejudice, and stereotyping.
2. What measures could be taken, by the institution or by law, to end institutional racism?
3. List the characteristics in your own background that helped you gain knowledge of other ethnic groups.
4. What factors in the health care setting may interfere with care of the patient from a minority culture or ethnic group?
5. What provisions (if any) does your clinical facility make for assisting a patient who does not speak English?
6. In what ways might you include the families of ethnic minority patients in care?

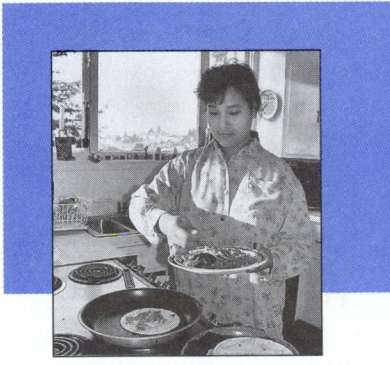

7. Compare bereavement rituals practiced by members of two cultural groups.
8. Briefly explain what you see as the issues in health care for the migrant population and the urban and rural poor.
9. What health issues are unique to women?

Critical Thinking Activities

1. Using the most recent census report for your community, identify the various ethnic groups represented and the percentage of the community belonging to each group. Research ways your community is meeting the health care needs of one minority group. How could health care delivery to this group be improved?
2. Visit a food market that serves a particular ethnic group. Compare the food items in the market to those found in a supermarket. Are any foods taken for medicinal purposes? Investigate the comparative costs and nutritional value of available foods.
3. Write a care plan in the areas of sociocultural needs for an elderly patient of an ethnic minority that is represented in your community. Identify the nursing actions that you could take to respond to the unique ethnic needs of the person.

References and Readings

Aber, C. S., and Hawkins, J. W. "Portrayal of Nurses in Advertisements in Medical and Nursing Journals." *Image* 24, 4 (Winter 1992): 289–293.

Afaf, I. M., Lipson, J. G., and Paul, S. M. "Ethnicity and Health Among Five Middle Eastern Immigrant Groups." *Nursing Research* 41, 2 (March/April 1992): 98–103.

Alexander, M. A., and Blank, J. J. "Factors Related to Obesity in Mexican-American Preschool Children." *Image* 20, 2 (Summer 1988): 79–82.

Anderson, J. M. "Immigrant Women Speak of Chronic Illness: The Social Construction of the Devalued Self." *Journal of Advanced Nursing* 16, 6 (June 1991): 710–717.

Andrews, M. M. "Cultural Perspectives on Nursing in the 21st Century." *Journal of Professional Nursing* 8, 1 (January-February 1992): 7–15.

Arnold, H. M. "I-Thou." *American Journal of Nursing* 70, 12 (December 1970): 2554.

Backup, R. W. "Implementing Quality Health Care for the American Indian Patient." *Washington State Journal of Nursing* (Special Supplement, 1979): 20–32.

Bassuk, E. L., and Rosenberg, L. "Why Does Family Homelessness Occur? A Case-control Study." *The American Journal of Public Health* 78 (June 1988): 783–788.

Bennett, S. L. "Comparable Worth: The Sex and Salary Debate." *Nursing and Health Care* 9, 5 (May 1988): 245–247.

Berne, A. S., Dato, C., Mason, D. J., and Rafferty, N. "A Nursing Model for Addressing the Health Needs of Homeless Families." *Image* 22, 1 (Spring 1990): 8–13.

Brown, L. P. "Collaborative Efforts of Law Enforcement and Health Care Professionals to Decrease Violence and Crime in the Black Community." *Journal of Black Nurses Association* 2, 1 (Fall 1988): 46–53.

Bullough, V. L. "Nightingale, Nursing and Harassment." *Image* 22, 1 (Spring 1990): 4–7.

Burns, B. M. "Reaching Educationally Disadvantaged Students." *American Journal of Nursing* 87, 10 (October 1987): 1359–1360.

Carpenito, L. J. *Nursing Diagnosis: Application to Clinical Practice.* 4th edition. Philadelphia: J. B. Lippincott, 1992.

Cerrato, P. L. "Suggest Diets with a Difference." *RN* 56, 2 (February 1993): 67–72.

Clavon, A. "The Black Elderly." *Journal of Gerontological Nursing* 12, 5 (May 1986): 6–11.

Coates, C. A. "Planting Seeds of Hope." *Nursing '92* 22, 8 (August 1992): 44–46.

Diaz-Duque, O. F. "Advice from an Interpreter." *American Journal of Nursing* 82, 11 (November 1982): 1380–1382.

Durham, P., and Jones, E. C. *The Negro Cowboys.* New York: Dodd, Mead, 1965.

Evans, M. *Homeless in America.* Washington, D.C.: Acropolis Books Ltd., 1988.

Felder, E. "Hypertension in Blacks: Implications for Health Care." *Association of Black Nursing Faculty in Higher Education Journal* 2, 1 (Winter 1991): 11–14.

Fingerhut, L. A., Ingram, D. D., and Feldman, J. J. "Firearm Homicide Among Black Teenage Males in Metropolitan Counties." *Journal of the American Medical Association* 267, 22 (June 10, 1992): 3054–3058.

Fong, C. M. "Ethnicity and Nursing Practice." *Topics in Clinical Nursing* 7, 3 (October 1985): 1–10.

———. "Nursing Needs Minorities." *Advancing Clinical Care* 6, 1 (January-February 1991): 19–21.

Francis, M. B. "Eight Homeless Mothers' Tales." *Image* 24, 2 (Summer 1992): 111–114.

Giger, J. N., Davidhizer, R. E., and Cherry, B. "Biological Variations in the Black Patient." 38, 2 (April-May 1991): 97–98.

Giger, J. N., and Davidhizer, R. E. *Transcultural Nursing: Assessment and Intervention.* St. Louis: C. V. Mosby, 1991.

Hamilton, C. L. "Nursing on the Navajo Reservation." *Imprint* 38, 2 (April-May 1991): 121, 174.

Harper, B. C. "Doing the Right Thing: Three Strategies for Increasing Minority Involvement." *Hospice* 1, 1 (Spring 1990): 14–15.

Horton, J. A. (Ed.). *The Women's Health Care Data Book.* Washington, D.C.: The Jacobs Institute of Women's Health, 1992.

Hunter, J. K. "Making a Difference for Homeless Patients." *RN* 55, 12 (December 1992): 48–53.

Jacques, G. "Cultural Health Traditions: A Black Perspective." In *Providing Safe Nursing Care for Ethnic People of Color.*

Edited by M. F. Branch and P. P. Paxton. pp. 115–124. New York: Appleton-Century-Crofts, 1976.

Katz, W. L. *The Black West.* 3rd edition. Seattle: Open Hand Publications, 1987.

Kus, R. J. "Nurses and Unpopular Patients." *American Journal of Nursing* 90, 6 (June 1990): 62–66.

Leininger, M. "Transcultural Nursing: Quo Vadis. (Where Goeth the Field)." *Journal of Transcultural Nursing* 1, 1 (January 1989): 33–45.

———. "Transcultural Specialists and Generalists: New Practitioners in Nursing." *Journal of Transcultural Nursing* 1, 1 (January 1989): 4–16.

———. "Transcultural Nursing: An Essential Knowledge and Practice Field for Today." *Canadian Nurse* 80, 11 (November 1984): 41–45.

Lindsey, A. M. "Health Care for the Homeless." *Nursing Outlook* 37, 2 (March-April 1989): 78–81.

Louie, K. B. "The Relation of Ethnicity and Ego Defensiveness of Female Registered Nurses to Their Attitudes Toward Ethnically Similar and Different Patients." Unpublished doctoral thesis, New York University, 1983.

Marchione, J., and Stearns, S. J. "Ethic Power Perspectives for Nursing." *Nursing and Health Care* 11, 6 (June 1990): 296–301.

Moccia, P., and Mason, D. "Poverty Trends: Implications for Nursing." *Nursing Outlook* 34, 1 (January-February 1986): 20–24.

Muecke, M. A. "Caring for Southeast Asian Refugee Patients in the USA." *American Journal of Public Health* 73 (April 1983): 431–438.

Mulligan, J. E. "Some Effects of the Women's Health Movement." *Topics in Clinical Nursing* 4 (January 1983): 1–12.

———. *New Our Bodies, Ourselves. The Boston Women's Health Book Collective.* New York: Simon and Schuster, 1984.

O'Brien, R. and Chafetz, M. *The Encyclopedia of Alcoholism.* New York: Green Spring Publishers, 1982.

Olds, S. B., London, M. L., and Ladeivig, P. W. *Maternal and Newborn Nursing.* Menlo Park, N.J.: Addison-Wesley, 1992.

Packett, S., Oswald, N., Bronson, S., and Kraushar, T. "A Problem Homeless Patients May Not Mention . . . Foot Ailments." *RN* 54, 11 (November 1991): 53–55.

Penckofer, S. and Holm, K. "What You Should Know About Women and Heart Disease." *Nursing 93.* 23, 6 (June 1993): 42–46.

Perry, F. "Black and White Issues." *Nursing Times* 88, 10 (March 4-10, 1992): 62–64.

Pizer, C. M., Collard A. F., James, S. M., and Bonaparte, B. H. "Nurses' Job Satisfaction: Are There Differences Between Foreign and U.S. Educated Nurses?" *Image* 24, 4 (Winter 1992): 301–306.

Pflug, C. C., Marsh, L., and Hofbauer, E. "Students Meet the Migrants." *American Journal of Nursing* 75 (July 1975): 1166–1167.

Rafferty, M. "Standing Up for America's Homeless." *American Journal of Nursing* 89, 12 (December 1989): 1614–1617.

———. "How Nurses are Helping the Homeless." *American Journal of Nursing* 89, 12 (December 1989): 1618–1619.

Rairdan, B., and Higgs, Z. R. "When your Patient is a Hmong Refugee." *American Journal of Nursing* 92, 3 (March 1992): 52–55.

Rhodes, S. "The Indian Health Program: The First 200 Years." *Imprint* 37, 3 (Summer 1990): 108–110.

Roseman, J. M. "Diabetes in Black Americans." In *Diabetes in America.* Washington, D.C.: National Institutes of Health, Department of Health and Human Services, 1984. (SN017–045–00102–1).

Scholz, J. "Cultural Expressions Affecting Patient Care." *Dimensions in Oncology Nursing* 4, 1 (Spring 1990): 16-26.

Smith, E. D. "The Role of Black Churches in Supporting Compliance with Antihypertension Regimens." *Public Health Nursing* 6, 4 (December 1989): 212–217.

Spector, R. E. *Cultural Diversity in Health and Illness.* Norwalk, Conn.: Appleton and Lange, 1991.

Stern, M. P. "Diabetes in Hispanic Americans." In *Diabetes in America.* Washington, D.C.: National Institutes of Health, Department of Health and Human Services, 1984. (SN017–045–00102–1).

Tannenbaum, I. "Women and HIV." *RN* 56, 5 (May 1993): 28–40.

Theiderman, S. B. "Workshops in Cross-cultural Health Care: The Challenge of Ethnographic Dynamite." *Journal of Clinical Education in Nursing* 18, 1 (January-February 1988): 25–27.

Tien-Hyatt, J. L. "Keying in on the Unique Care Needs of Asian Clients." *Nursing and Health Care* 8, 5 (May 1987): 269–271.

U.S. National Center for Health Statistics, Division of Vital Statistics, Washington, DC, 1992.

Tripp-Reimer, T., and Afifi, L. A. "Cross-cultural Perspectives on Patient Teaching." *Nursing Clinics of North America* 24, 3 (September 1989): 613–619.

Western Journal of Medicine (entire issue). Cross-cultural Medicine: A Decade Later. 157, 3 (September 1992).

Wetzel, R. C., and Rogers, M. C. "Gypsies and Acute Medical Intervention." *Pediatrics* 72, 5 (November 1983): 731–735.

Williams, S. *Nutrition and Diet Therapy.* 6th edition. St. Louis: C. V. Mosby, 1989.

Woods, N. F., and Shaver, J. F. "The Evolutionary Spiral of a Specialized Center for Women's Health Research." *Image* 24, 3 (Fall 1992): 223–228.

Wuest, J. "Joining Together: Students and Faculty Learn About Transcultural Nursing." *Journal of Nursing Education* 31, 2 (February 1992): 90–92.

Mental Health

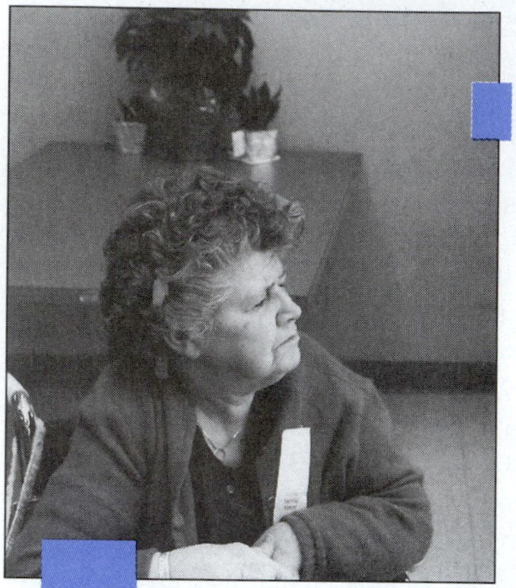

34

Objectives

After completing this chapter, you should be able to:

1. State and explain ten major mental health concepts.
2. Discuss threats to the patient's mental health.
3. Identify common behavior that is used for coping.
4. Outline data to be gathered for mental health assessment.
5. Define and describe alterations in emotional integrity.
6. Define and describe alterations in coping.
7. Define and describe alterations in meaningfulness.
8. Define and describe alterations in role performance.
9. Explain the steps in crisis intervention.
10. Discuss how therapeutic interaction can be used for assisting the person to maintain mental health.
11. Discuss the use of referral as a nursing intervention for mental health problems.

Study Terms

body image
compensation
conversion
coping
crisis
crisis intervention
defense mechanisms
depression
denial
displacement
fantasy
feedback
human dignity
identification
impaired adjustment
maturational crisis
mental health
mental illness
noncompliance
panic
primary role
projection
rationalization
reaction formation
regression
repression
restitution
role
role ambiguity
role conflict
role strain
secondary role
self-actualization
self-concept
self-esteem
social support
socialization
sublimation
substitution
suppression
tertiary role

Ellis, Nowlis: Nursing: A Human Needs Approach, 5th ed. © 1994 J.B. Lippincott Company

Outline

Mental health can be defined as a set of emotional and cognitive patterns conducive to effective functioning in one's own particular life situation. These patterns are positive for the individual in that they facilitate coping with life. Mental health encompasses thoughts, feelings, and responses to life and is closely related to physical health. Although many components of mental health have been identified, most can be seen as aspects of the human needs Maslow identified. When the needs for love, belonging, and self-esteem are met, positive patterns can develop.

The exact nature of positive patterns of thought and behavior varies from culture to culture. What is useful and constructive for functioning in one society might not be useful in another. For example, if submissiveness and deliberate submergence of one's personal views are a cultural norm, the person who deviates in the direction of personal assertiveness is likely to be considered abnormal; the result may be isolation from others and loss of self-esteem. In a culture that values aggressiveness, however, the individual who would be out of place in a submissive culture might be highly respected.

Mental health is also an individual matter. Whereas one person might derive satisfaction and a sense of belonging from dependence on someone else, dependence might arouse major inner conflicts in a person who views it as evidence of a personal deficiency.

The level of a person's mental health at any given time is usually ascertained by examining his or her ability to function in relationship to the self and the environment. The models used to describe health and illness in Chapters 5 and 6 also apply to mental health. **Mental**

illness is a state characterized by the inability to function in daily life due to psychological problems. This chapter focuses on the person who is basically healthy, but who may need assistance and support to function more effectively because of a life situation.

Basic Concepts in Mental Health

Let us consider some basic mental health concepts that are central to nursing in terms of human needs (Display 34-1).

The Whole Person

Mental health cannot be considered in isolation from physical health. *A human being is made up of interrelated components—physical, mental, emotional, and spiritual—and must be viewed as a whole person.* Problems that are basically emotional also affect physical health. Thus, it is never appropriate for a nurse to focus on one aspect of a person at the expense of another aspect. Because of the interrelationship between physical and mental health, actions aimed at relieving mental health problems may also help alleviate physical problems. The reverse is also true: when physical problems are under control, mental health is likely to improve. Thus mental health, like physical health, is a dynamic phenomenon, affected by events and always in flux.

Display 34–1
Major Mental Health Concepts

1. A human being is made up of interrelated components—physical, mental, emotional, and spiritual—and must be viewed as a whole person.
2. The concept of human dignity rests on faith in the individual's worth, regardless of race, sex, creed, culture, or behavior.
3. Feelings and sentiments are real and must be treated as such whether or not they appear to be based on fact.
4. Self-esteem is an important factor in coping with daily life.
5. Understanding oneself promotes an understanding of others.
6. Any mutilation or change in body structure or function will affect an individual's self-concept and relationships with others and must be understood in terms of the individual's feelings about the change.
7. Mental health requires that the individual have adequate means for communication with others and/or self-expression.
8. People respond and function both as individuals and as members of social groups.
9. All behavior has meaning and purpose for the individual.
10. Each individual has the basic capacity for growth.

Human Dignity

The concept of **human dignity** *rests on faith in the individual's worth, regardless of race, sex, creed, culture, or behavior* (Dunn, 1962). Recognition of the intrinsic worth of each individual is the basis of all supportive, helpful human relationships and is central to effective nursing. Belief in this principle underlies efforts that go unnoticed and supports work toward goals that are not realized. When acted on, the concept of *human dignity* promotes in others a belief in their own dignity and worth.

The Reality of Feelings

Feelings are subjective experiences of emotion, such as happiness, fear, or anxiety. Feelings are often verbally expressed, but they may also be indicated by *behavior.* It is generally much more difficult to identify others' feelings accurately when this must be done on the basis of behavior alone than when the person can express feelings verbally.

Feelings and sentiments are real and must be treated as such whether or not they appear to be based on fact. If we accept a person's feelings and sentiments without judging them to be right or wrong, we strengthen the interpersonal relationship and build mutual trust. It is usually easy to accept feelings—our own or others'—for which we can discern reasons; if we doubt the validity of the reasons, however, we may tend to label the feelings as inappropriate.

The Meaningfulness of All Behavior

All behavior has meaning and purpose for the individual. Behavior can solve problems, relieve anxiety, and help people cope with stress. Although you may not understand certain behavior or be able to discern its purpose, recognition that behavior has meaning to the individual can help you be more accepting even when your understanding is limited. Because behavior is not always understood by the individual who engages in it, your efforts to understand may guide the person to greater self-awareness. If you are attempting to help someone change his or her behavior, it may be essential to search for and understand the meaning and purpose of the behavior you hope to modify.

Self-concept

One's **self-concept** is one's total view of oneself—the psychological-spiritual-intellectual self as well as the physical self. *One's view of oneself directly affects one's ability to function.* If you see yourself as competent and resourceful, you will tend to behave in ways that reinforce this perception. Seeing yourself as incompetent, on the other hand, may make you reluctant to attempt tasks or even destine you to failure before you begin.

Your self-concept derives from many factors, among the most potent of which is **feedback**, or information about other people's impressions, responses, and opinions. When others respond to you in ways that indicate acceptance, you tend to see yourself as acceptable; if they reject you, you are likely to regard yourself as unacceptable.

Self-esteem, according to Maslow, is valuing oneself positively. We speak of those who attribute negative values to themselves as having low self-esteem. *Self-esteem is an important factor in coping with daily life,* and many aspects of life that affect self-esteem have pertinence for you as a nurse. Self-esteem is discussed more extensively in Chapter 35.

Another critical factor in self-esteem is the degree of *self-understanding* an individual possesses. Seeking self-knowledge tends to promote self-esteem in that it brings about recognition of one's positive features.

Self-understanding is particularly important for the nurse. *Understanding oneself promotes an understanding of others.* As a nurse you will be called on to understand others in many situations, and the basis for understanding others lies in understanding yourself. Self-understanding is not a static state but a dynamic process of striving to know yourself in relation to each new experience and each new person you encounter. Consider the applicability of all you learn about mental health to your own life and think about the ways such concepts can enhance your self-understanding. Then seek an understanding of how they apply to your relationships with family, friends, patients, and coworkers.

One's concept of one's physical self is called one's **body image**. In addition to feelings and attitudes about one's physical self, body image is based on sight, sound, touch, and proprioceptive input (stimuli from within the body). How one sees one's physical self is central to self-esteem.

Any mutilation or change in body structure or function will affect an individual's self-concept and relationship with others and must be understood in terms of the individual's feelings about the change. If a person undergoes a perceptible change in the body, such as the removal of a body part, he or she must be reoriented toward the body, must reappraise others' responses, and must adjust his or her self-concept. Body image changes may affect feelings about oneself as a sexual partner (see Chapter 37), as a worker, and as a family member. A minor change, such as a small appendectomy scar, may not cause difficulty. The loss of a leg, however, may create a major problem in adjustment. In assessing the seriousness of the difficulty and deciding whether or not the individual needs assistance in dealing with the change, the most significant factor is the meaning of the change for the individual (see Chapter 35).

The Need to Communicate

Mental health requires that the individual have adequate means for communication with others and self-expression. Some consider communication the most important single factor in mental health. Undeniably, anything that hampers communication with others—whether it is laryngitis, a language barrier, or a mental attitude—poses a threat to mental health. Inability to communicate significantly affects recovery from any illness.

Communication reflects one's belonging to the human community. Only communication can pierce an individual's isolation, allowing one person to feel close to another person. The nurse's responsibility is to help provide the patient with a means of communication. Doing so might require seeking the help of another person, such as the speech therapist, or using sign language, pictures, or gestures. For the patient in isolation, providing communication could mean setting aside time to talk together; for the deaf patient, you might provide a "magic slate" for writing messages. With patients whose mental attitudes block communication, the nurse must work skillfully and patiently to establish some form of communication.

Roles and Relationships

Social support is "the subjective feeling of belonging, of being accepted, loved, esteemed, valued, and needed for oneself, not for what one can do for others" (Moss, 1973). Every individual, according to Maslow, needs to feel loved and cared about. From infancy on, the feeling of being cared about is essential if the person is to thrive. The network of people who provide this support are the individual's social support system. Although the nurse cannot provide love and belonging in a patient's life, the nurse can certainly help meet this need through encouraging the support of family and friends and assisting the patient to reach out to others.

A **role** is a complex set of behaviors and expectations that form a particular position for the individual in society. A **primary role** is one that the individual possesses without choice, such as the role of woman or man, a person of a specific age, a son, or a daughter. Primary roles are always present throughout life. A **secondary role** is one that is ascribed to the individual and is expected to be a lifelong position, but it is one that can be altered, a role such as wife, friend, or member of a religious body. These secondary roles carry expectations for behavior and are a part of the way in which an individual participates in society. **Tertiary roles** are more transient and freely chosen than are primary and secondary roles. A person might be a sales clerk, a passenger on a cruise ship, or a member of a jury. The patient role or sick role is considered a tertiary role. As a nursing student you have chosen the tertiary role of nurse and you are learning expected behaviors of that role.

The behaviors appropriate to any role are learned through a process called **socialization**. Socialization into primary roles occurs mainly in the family; socialization into secondary and tertiary roles occurs in the wider society as well. Although individuals may choose to modify the way in which they behave in certain roles on the basis of decisions they make as adults, the basic role patterns learned in the family have strong effects on behavior.

People respond and function both as individuals within their roles and as members of social groups. It is important to see others as individuals whose responses grow out of their own experiences and to abandon expectations of behavior based on stereotyped views of "the good patient," racial and ethnic groups, or males and females. A nurse must not ignore the group to which an individual belongs. A person's family and ethnic group inevitably affect the way he or she responds and functions. Finding an appropriate middle ground between stereotyping and inattention to cultural backgrounds is a difficult task, as is distinguishing between behavior based on individual differences and behavior characteristic of the group to which the person belongs. However, a continuing effort to do so will help you deal more effectively with others. For example, some family groups respond to the illness of a member by gathering together and becoming intensely involved in the person's care. If the patient is placed in a unit where the number of visitors and length of visits are restricted, an understanding of this practice and its meaning to those involved may help you to work out some kind of modification of the rules. On the other hand, another patient from this same background may prefer that the family not be so intimately involved. Your responsibility is to ascertain what is important to the individual patient.

Many people derive a necessary sense of *belonging* from identification with a group. If nurses undermine this group identification in the care setting by "treating everyone alike," they are failing to recognize the importance of belonging for mental health. The nurse's attitude toward the group of which the patient is a member will also affect the patient's self-esteem because people typically interpret the value placed on their social group as the value placed on them as individuals.

Self-actualization and Capacity for Growth

According to Maslow, **self-actualization** is becoming what one is capable of becoming. Although self-actualization is often thought of as a remote end point, it is more helpful to see it as a process of growth. *Each individual has the basic capacity for growth.* As a person's immediate goals and needs are met, new ones arise to take their place. We are expecting growth when we ask individuals to adopt new ways of functioning, learn new skills, or deal with a variety of complex feelings and problems. If an individual does not appear to be striving for growth, the prevailing conditions need to be examined. Are the person's immediate needs going unmet? Is energy available for growth or is all the patient's available energy being devoted to maintenance? Are you providing a climate suitable for growth?

Threats to Mental Health Associated with Health Care

Becoming a patient requires a person to adopt a new role. The nature of this role may vary, depending on whether the setting is an outpatient clinic, the home, or an acute care hospital. People's responses to the patient role also depend on their families and cultural backgrounds, which teach them various interpretations of appropriate behavior for the sick person, and on their previous experiences with the patient role.

Individuals differ in their views of health and illness. A person with multiple handicaps who needs ongoing supervision by a health care team may consider himself healthy as long as he does not have an acute illness. His response to the patient role will be different from that of the person who perceives a sprained ankle as a serious threat to health and assumes a totally dependent role. When the patient's concept of health differs from that of the health care team members, conflict may result. This situation calls for the skillful use of interpersonal communication techniques to resolve the conflict. If altering the patient's perception is not possible or desirable, the health care providers may have to alter their expectations and approaches.

Changes in Physical Self and Functional Ability

Many individuals who are in contact with the health care system experience changes in the physical self, varying from the skin eruptions of acne to amputation of extremities. These changes require a readjustment in body image. Chapter 35 provides detailed information on the effects of physical changes.

Profound changes in function can be present even when there are no exterior signs of change. Changes in function may affect any organ system in the body. Some require modest revisions of lifestyle patterns, such as wearing corrective lenses when eyes function less well. Other changes affect the individual's entire self-image: "I can't fulfill my usual role in life. What will other people think of me? How will they treat me now?" The answers to these and other questions may require a change in the view of self. During a temporary illness, such changes may be minor and easily dealt with by the patient. A major illness, on the other hand, frequently requires profound changes, and patients may need assistance and support in dealing with their feelings. Your assessment of a patient's needs must consider the meaning that the change in function has for the individual.

Loss of Privacy

A second problem is the loss of privacy. The patient may be asked personal questions by a number of different people. Physical examinations may offend modesty. In the hospital, personal belongings are often carefully inspected, inventoried, and stored elsewhere for safekeeping. Elimination may have to take place while other people are present or separated only by a curtain. In brief, the hospital setting requires the patient to suppress a set of feelings and behaviors related to maintaining personal privacy and modesty.

Belief in human dignity and worth mandates protecting the privacy of the individual in every way possible. It requires that you be sensitive to the patient's feelings and recognize that they may differ from your own. With this principle as your guide, you will also provide a full measure of privacy to the individual who is not able to claim it independently: the comatose patient, the child, or the person without speech. Specifically, providing privacy means using blankets for draping, pulling curtains, and being discreet when you talk with the patient about personal matters.

Loss of Control

Adults in Western society are used to the sense of controlling their own lives. In the health care setting, tests may be ordered, forms filled out, and plans for care made by others; the person may have the sensation of being swept along on the tide. Giving consent does not necessarily mean that the patient thoroughly understands all that is happening.

Loss of control may also be a threat to the self-image and thus may create anxiety. This outcome can be prevented or alleviated by allowing patients to retain control over as much of their lives as possible. Whenever feasible, you can give the patient choices regarding care. For example, does he prefer a bath now or in an hour? In what order does she prefer the tasks of care? Too often such decisions are made arbitrarily by nursing personnel even when providing a choice is feasible. To help the patient feel more in control over the situation, you ought to introduce unfamiliar members of the health care team, describe their functions, and carefully explain all that is going to happen, including time schedules. You might also explain how beds and call lights work, where the bathroom is, and how the telephone operates.

Fear of loss of control over elimination is prevalent, especially in the elderly. Calm acceptance of such problems and shared planning to solve them can restore dignity and some control to the patient, even when physical control is lost. As for control over broader matters, review the Health Consumer Bill of Rights in Chapter 3 and consider how you can support the patient in the exercise of these rights.

Uncertainty About Expected Behavior

Patients also experience uncertainty regarding the behavior expected of them. "How is a patient supposed to act?" "Is it permissible to ask questions?" "Do I have to ask for pain relief, or can I expect it to be provided without asking?" You have faced such uncertainty yourself if you have ever sat in a doctor's examining room wondering what you should do next. "Am I expected to wait in the examining room until the doctor returns or should I get dressed and go to the desk?" Such uncertainty may be multiplied many times over when the entire environment is unfamiliar and one's previous contact with the health care system has been limited. Anxiety may be especially pronounced among individuals from cultural backgrounds other than those of the health care workers (Fig. 34-1).

You can assist the patient by describing the behavior you expect. The most routine admission to the hospital may be a completely new experience for the patient. "Am I expected to take all my clothes off under that gown?" "Can I leave my underwear on?" "Am I expected to go right to bed?" "Do I ring the buzzer or will you automatically come back?" Explanations of all such matters are necessary, as well as of any orders regarding activity, the policy on leaving the area, and the patient's

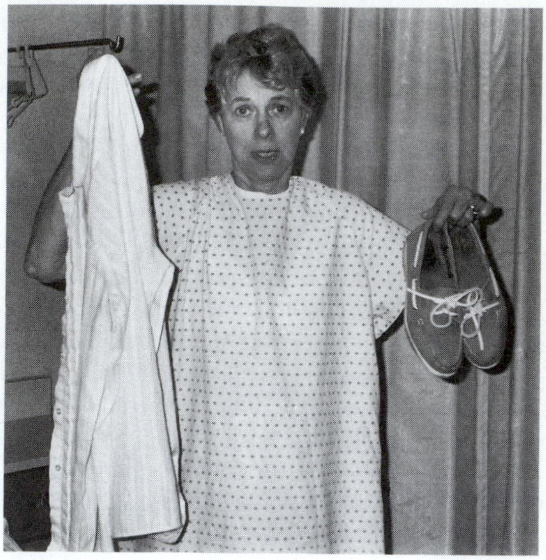

Figure 34-1. Uncertainty about the behavior expected in the health care setting creates stress.

responsibilities for his or her own care. Be sure to elicit the patient's questions and concerns as well.

Hospital admission is not the only time when expected behavior needs to be explained. Explanations are also needed when a new procedure or treatment is to be performed, when the patient is to go to another department for a test, and when changes occur in care. The need for clear statements of expected behavior continues throughout the patient's contact with the health care system.

Unfamiliar Routines

In the hospital the patient must adopt an entirely new pattern of living. The schedule may be drastically at odds with the patient's own. Despite attempts to individualize care, most institutions find that certain routines and schedules are necessary for smooth functioning. As a nurse, you might consider which of the patterns prescribed by the institution are really essential and whether it is possible to adapt them in any way to the needs and desires of the patient. Certain aspects of nursing routines are based on necessity, but others are unquestionably the result of long-standing traditions that have no rationale but have never been questioned.

Worry Over Expenses

A major problem facing the consumer of health care in the United States is its cost. Many individuals are without any health care insurance coverage. In addition, for most people, an extensive illness or hospitalization costs more than insurance pays, even when the person does have insurance. Health care costs have been rising much more rapidly than costs in most other sectors of the economy. Even those whose health care plans pay all the costs of illness may be subject to loss of income, expenses for child care, and the cost of homemaking services. The nurse is not usually in a position to alleviate a patient's financial concerns directly. However, the nurse can refer the patient to others with the ability and knowledge to do so, such as the social worker. Some hospitals employ individuals to help patients with their financial problems. Sometimes the patient can deal with such problems independently if he or she has access to the business office or insurance carrier. Developing a sound knowledge of available community resources can equip you to make appropriate referrals.

Uncertainty About Outcomes

Although some people enter the health care environment with relatively simple problems the favorable outcome of which is a virtual certainty, a great many patients carry a heavy burden of undisclosed fears. Sometimes such fears arise from realistic knowledge of the seriousness of the illness. A person who enters the hospital for treatment of kidney failure, for instance, may clearly recognize that the outcome cannot be predicted with certainty and that there is a possibility of prolonged treatment or death. Another patient may feel threatened by surgery the hospital staff regards as routine. For example, the person may fear never waking up from the anesthesia. Such fears are often exacerbated by physicians' caution about making absolute predictions. Full disclosure of the possible adverse effects of treatment may introduce or exaggerate fears. Uncertainty of this kind is threatening to most individuals. People are usually more successful at handling their anxieties when the nature of the problem is clearly stated.

Conflict With Developmental Tasks

In Unit 5 we discussed the development of individuals throughout the life span. At each age level different developmental tasks must be accomplished for satisfactory psychosocial development to continue. Illness and the need for health care may interfere in a variety of ways with the accomplishment of these tasks. For example, the adolescent is trying to establish an independent identity. If a major health problem forces dependence on others for basic needs, an adolescent may find it difficult to move toward self-understanding and independence. She might react by refusing the necessary dependency, thereby endangering her health status, or she may cease trying to master the developmental tasks appropriate for that age, thus endangering her development. Either of these behaviors is a problem.

Some health problems create conflict with developmental tasks at one age, but few problems at another age. For example, a young child expects to be dependent and accepts dependency without conflict. The young adult, however, is accustomed to being independent. A health problem creating dependency would create conflict for the young adult but would not be a concern for the young child. Long-term confinement to home because of illness would interfere with the development of the school-age child, whose developmental tasks require physical activity and interaction with peers. This restriction would not be as detrimental to the toddler, whose tasks still involve interacting with the family.

Threats to Relationships With Others

When health problems change one individual in a relationship, the relationship itself is changed. Although this may promote growth, many potential threats arise in these changes. The burden of maintaining the relationship may fall on the well person, and the ill person may have much greater needs for support. The health care system itself makes it harder for people to relate, compounding the problem of adjusting to these changes in roles and needs. Most health care settings have little privacy for personal sharing; the system may be strange and threatening; and the health problem itself may be poorly understood.

Physical separation alone is disruptive of interpersonal relationships. Most hospitals have recognized that a patient's support system is crucial to recovery and therefore allow liberal visiting hours. In the past, many intensive care units had rigid visitation rules, allowing perhaps one visitor for 5 minutes of every hour. This rigidity was convenient for nurses because it eliminated the need for assessment and decision-making in regard to the value of visitors for each individual, but it completely ignored the fact that patients benefit from feeling the love and support of family and friends.

Some patients must be separated from support systems because they have been transferred to major care centers away from home. This separation is especially likely in cases of major trauma, burns, spinal cord injury, and certain types of cancer. Patients who have been transferred because of one of these conditions are at particular risk for mental health problems due to separation from their support systems.

Communication is the basis of relationships. When communication is interrupted, it is difficult to sustain any kind of interpersonal relationship. Those who have their capacity for speech destroyed by a stroke lose more than words. Communication can also be interrupted by a hearing loss. Such a loss cuts the individual off from the thoughts and feelings of others and increases a sense of isolation. As a nurse, you will be responsible for developing some method of communication for the people for whom you care.

When one member of a family cannot continue in the tasks and responsibilities usually undertaken, all of the roles within the family must be realigned (Fig. 34-2). When family members have a background of flexibility or when the period of time involved is short, this realignment may not cause problems. However, on many occasions this realignment of roles creates high stress for the family, and many problems may ensue.

Threats to Self-actualization

When an individual is faced with illness, most energy must be devoted to maintenance and recovery. This leaves little energy available for personal growth. Even when energy is available, the health care setting tends to interfere with growth.

An environment in which there is nothing to do all day except watch television leads to boredom and despair. For those with long-term illnesses, this is a particular problem. In children, lack of stimulation results in irritability and bad temper. Adults often lose interest in their surroundings and may neglect care of themselves. Even when an individual is not able to engage in accustomed activities, it may be possible for the nurse to identify stimulating pastimes.

Even within the health care setting, individuals

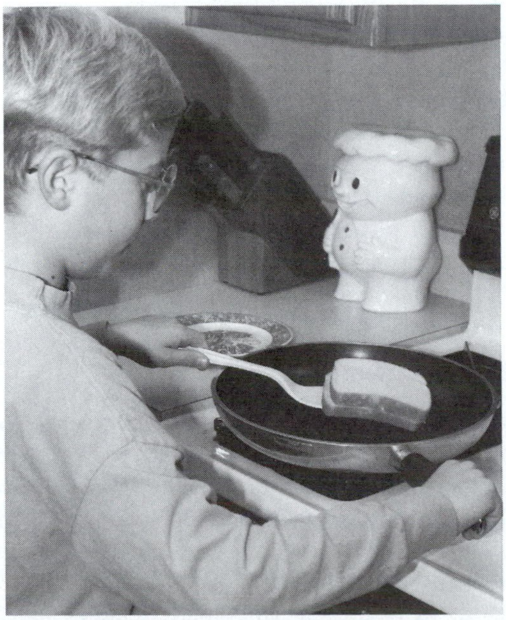

Figure 34-2. When one member of the family becomes ill, other family members often must learn to redefine their roles within the family.

grow through knowledge of their health status and understanding of their own care needs. Deprived of this information, they lose an opportunity for growth. Health teaching is discussed in Chapter 16.

Dependency in some aspects of self-care is essential in many illnesses. However, enforcing dependence when it is not essential creates regression and interferes with the individual's growth. In the past, dependency was commonly enforced in the mistaken belief that it would facilitate recovery. However, recovery is actually enhanced by the active participation of the patient; exercise and self-care are also conducive to feelings of self-esteem.

Coping Strategies

Coping is a process whereby the individual manages both internal and external stressors adequately and makes choices and decisions that are supportive of health and development. Effective coping requires that the individual master many different tasks. The person's self-concept must be maintained and satisfying relationships with others established. There is no one correct way to cope. Each person must cope on the basis of the individual circumstances of life and personal strengths and assets.

Lazarus and Folkman (1984) indicate that there are two basic types of coping behavior: problem focused and emotion focused. According to their work, problem-focused coping includes actions that would eliminate or decrease the strength of the stressor. Cognitive appraisal is the thought process used to evaluate the situation and determine the seriousness of the threat and the potential for alleviating the stressor. Through cognitive appraisal, the individual determines the source of the stressor, the possible choices of behavior, and whether help is available. Emotion-focused coping includes actions that alter the individual's personal feelings in response to the stressor (see Chapter 6). Emotion-focused coping includes both cognitive restructuring and defense mechanisms.

Problem-Solving

The most effective coping usually involves efforts to change or remedy the situation that creates problems. This problem-solving approach is the most positive and provides the longest-lasting remedy. Some individuals have many problem-solving skills and resources and bring these to the new health care situation. Others lack these skills or find their skills inadequate to meet new demands. The nurse may facilitate problem-solving through the use of therapeutic communication techniques. However, in many situations—particularly crises—the individual is not capable of problem-solving, even with assistance, and so other behaviors are manifest.

Cognitive Restructuring

When the situation cannot be changed, the individual is often able to cope effectively through cognitive restructuring. The person deliberately alters his or her own thinking about the situation to change feelings of distress. Identifying some problematic areas as not important, joking about or finding humor in the situation, and reframing the problems in less threatening terms are all cognitive strategies for coping. Although these strategies do not alter the situation, they do decrease feelings of stress and help individuals to use their energies in coping effectively with areas of life that are more amenable to problem-focused coping.

Defense Mechanism

Defense mechanisms are largely unconscious mental processes that relieve feelings of anxiety and tension. Although they do not solve the initial problems, defense mechanisms help to alleviate feelings of anxiety temporarily. Freud, who originated the concept of defense mechanisms, defined them narrowly as totally unconscious behaviors. Subsequently, various writers have expanded the list of defense mechanisms to include some that are not totally unconscious.

Most people begin to use defense mechanisms in childhood to handle anxieties. An individual will usually use only a few of the many mechanisms that have been identified. People typically continue to rely on those that have been successful for them in the past. For example, the person for whom repression was effective may use repression when faced with new stressors.

It is usually inappropriate to try to stop an individual from using defense mechanisms because the loss of defense mechanisms can arouse overwhelming anxiety. If defense mechanisms lead to dysfunction—that is, create more problems than they solve—they must be overcome for progress to be made. Professional counseling is often needed in such instances.

If consistent emotional support is available, a person will often abandon a defense mechanism independently when he or she is able to cope effectively without it. The defense mechanisms discussed are those most commonly encountered (Table 34-1).

Regression is a common response to illness. A person who regresses behaves in a way more appropriate to an earlier stage of development. An adult may become dependent, and a 3-year-old child may revert to drinking from a bottle. Although the person will need to reestablish age-appropriate behavior in the process of recovery, an episode of regression is not harmful to ongoing development.

Table 34–1. Common Defense Mechanisms

Defense Mechanism	Definition	Defense Mechanism	Definition
Regression	Exhibiting behavior characteristic of an earlier stage of development	Substitution	Consciously redirecting energy from a blocked goal to another endeavor
Rationalization	Offering intellectual justifications for behavior and/or feelings that are in reality based on unconscious thoughts and feelings	Projection	Attributing one's own feelings, ideas, or characteristics to another person
Repression	Unconsciously putting stress-provoking thoughts and/or feelings completely out of one's awareness to the extent that they cannot be voluntarily recalled	Displacement	Transferring feelings aroused by one person or situation onto another person or situation
Suppression	Consciously putting troubling thoughts and/or feeelings out of one's awareness on a temporary basis	Identification	Adopting attitudes and behaviors characteristic of an admired individual
Denial	Unconsciously refusing to acknowledge a painful truth or situation	Reaction formation	Adopting attitudes or behaviors diametrically opposed to those of a person or group with whom one is in conflict
Compensation	Emphasizing some personal trait to make up for perceived lacks in the self	Conversion	Developing a physical illness or disability to substitute for a painful emotional or mental conflict
Sublimation	Unconsciously redirecting energy from a blocked goal to another endeavor	Restitution	Relieving guilt by "making up" in some way for the actions that aroused the guilt
		Fantasy	Using one's imagination to create alternatives to reality

Rationalization means finding intellectual reasons to justify behavior and feelings that are in reality based on unconscious thoughts and feelings. For example, a person who works slowly and fails to finish a project on time may rationalize that it was done more thoroughly. Similarly, things that are desirable but unattainable may be characterized as unwanted or not valuable: a person who cannot afford a private room in the hospital may state that private rooms are undesirable because "you never get any attention there."

Repression is the process of putting stress-provoking thoughts or feelings completely out of one's awareness. Repression is not deliberate but unconscious, and the ideas repressed cannot be voluntarily recalled to awareness. If confronted with the repressed material, the person will truthfully declare that he or she has absolutely no recollection of it. An example is a student who was told that his clinical performance was unsatisfactory and later insisted that this was never said; the information was so threatening that the student repressed it.

Suppression is similar to repression in that the troubling material is withdrawn from conscious thought; the difference is that in suppression the withdrawal is a conscious or semiconscious act and the material can be recalled if needed. The person simply chooses to be impervious or not to remember. For example, a nurse with a serious personal problem might go to work, concentrate on performing well, and effectively exclude all thoughts of the personal problem until something recalls it to consciousness.

Denial is an unconscious mechanism whereby a person simply refuses to acknowledge a threatening reality. The event, situation, or feeling is treated as nonexistent. Denial is a common response to a severe shock or crisis. For example, the initial reaction to being informed of impending death is often to say, in effect, "No, there must be some mistake. It could not be true." Denial may be indicated by behavior as well as by words: a person who has been told that her illness is life threatening but continues to plan for the future, ignores directions for treatment, and acts happy and content may be denying the reality of the illness. Denial protects the person from an overwhelming reality.

Denial is often abandoned gradually; that is, the person may appear to acknowledge the reality of the situation in one instance and in another to behave as if it were not true. Denial is usually abandoned when it no longer protects the self from awareness of the situation. In some instances, however, denial may persist. If it interferes with recovery and rehabilitation, professional intervention may be necessary. Persistent denial may not be harmful, however, if there are no alternatives and the situation cannot be changed.

Compensation is emphasis on some trait or traits to make up for perceived lacks in the self. A member of a musical family who has little musical ability may strive for athletic proficiency. When the lack is real, compensation may be of value in redirecting the person's energies toward a sphere in which success is possible.

Unconscious redirection of energy from an unattainable goal to another endeavor is called **sublimation**. A person who wanted to have children but was unable to do so, for example, might sublimate by focusing all his energies on a job. This process would be unconscious, not deliberate.

Substitution is a consciously planned redirection of energies from a blocked goal to an accessible one. For example, a nurse who had planned to go to graduate school but was unable to do so because of family responsibilities might redirect energies into a course in coronary care nursing.

Projection is the attribution of one's own feelings, ideas, or characteristics to an other person. It is usually undesirable feelings and traits that are projected. For example, a man who is angry with others might perceive others as being angry with him.

Displacement is the transfer of feelings aroused by one person or situation to another person or situation. Displacement typically occurs when admitting the real object of such feelings would be too distressing. If a patient's anger is aroused by the perceived lack of support of close family members, expressing such anger toward them might further erode their support. The patient's anger may therefore be displaced onto the nursing personnel.

Admiration and affection for another person may prompt one to adopt attitudes and behaviors characteristic of that person. This is called **identification**. For example, a new graduate nurse who admires an experienced head nurse might begin to use similar expressions and gestures. Valuable behaviors might also be adopted in the process of identification. An important aspect of child development, identification originates unconsciously but sometimes affects conscious behavior. Conscious identification occurs when a person chooses to act like an admired role model.

Almost the exact opposite of identification, **reaction formation** is rejection in oneself of any characteristics one shares with a person or group one fears or despises and adoption of the diametrically opposed behavior and attitudes. Reaction formation also occurs when an individual is trying to establish independence or autonomy; in rejecting dependence, a teenager may also reject the person on whom he or she was formerly dependent, adopting behavior patterns highly antagonistic to those of the parent.

Conversion is the process by which a person experiencing painful emotions and mental conflict develops a physical illness or disability that then substitutes for the psychological problems. A psychological problem is thus converted into a physical one. A dramatic example is paralysis in a young army recruit ordered to participate in a military operation. Concern about his own survival, beliefs about duty and courage, and fear of what others will think of him may create an intolerable conflict, which the paralysis resolves by taking decision-making out of his hands. A person experiencing a conversion reaction is often amazingly calm and accepting of what most people would view as a major life crisis (such as paralysis) because, rather than representing crisis, conversion represents relief from crisis. Conversion is an unconscious mechanism.

Restitution is an effort to relieve guilt by means of behavior that makes up for the cause of the guilt. A woman who was angry at her husband just before he was injured in an accident may feel guilt over her anger; she may spend long hours at the hospital to compensate for her previous antagonistic feelings. Restitution is unconscious in origin.

Fantasy is the use of one's imagination to construct alternatives to reality. Children use fantasy a great deal, daydreaming about the present and the future and constructing elaborate scenes in which they star. Fantasies of the self as competent, resourceful, and capable can be productive for several reasons. First, the fantasy serves as a problem-solving forum in which alternative behaviors can be explored, allowing the individual to choose the best course of action. Second, fantasy can be self-fulfilling. Imagining oneself as a certain type of person makes one more likely to act in ways that will make the fantasy a reality. Seeing ourselves as strong and capable may result in our becoming exactly that. The converse is also true: fantasy that focuses on oneself as the victim of outside forces may have a negative effect on self-confidence and self-esteem.

Assessment

In assessing mental health status, you will need to gather information related to self-esteem as well as information about relationships to others. A wide variety of problems may be identified.

Validating Perceptions of Feelings/Emotions

The patient/client's feelings can usually be elicited by asking how the person feels. However, some people are not used to discussing feelings and may even lack a vocabulary to describe them. You might encourage the person to identify what the feeling is like, or when the feeling has been present in the past. Feelings regarding the self and relationships with others are important in assessing mental health. Display 34-2 lists words that might be used to describe feelings. When feelings are demonstrated through nonverbal behavior, you must validate with the patient the accuracy of your perception about feelings.

Understanding Thoughts/Cognition

Assessment also includes attention to the patient's thought processes and the content of thoughts. This is often referred to as *cognition.* In assessing cognition, you will want to determine whether the person is in contact with reality and has effective thinking abilities. This was discussed in Chapter 31.

Is there an ability to remember things from the past (long-term memory)? Can the patient remember things that have recently happened (short-term memory)? Does the patient understand time sequence and know the date and time? Does the patient know where he or she is and why? Is the patient able to understand what common items, such as a paper clip, are and what they would be used for? Does the patient understand cause and effect? Can he or she state possible problems that might be caused by certain behaviors? What are the patient's thoughts with regard to the illness itself and its cause? Are these realistic? What does the patient think are the major problems being faced? What does the patient believe are the barriers to effective functioning? What does the patient think will solve the current problem?

Identifying Significant Behaviors

Even more significant than statements of feelings are behaviors related to feelings. The nonverbal cues that indicate feelings are varied. As you consider each potential problem, consider the behavior that might indicate particular feelings. When possible you will want to observe interactions between the patient and others. Such observation may help you to understand whether the relationship is functioning well and is supportive to the patient/client. Of particular importance are whether the person is able to focus on problem-solving and whether behavior indicating high anxiety is present.

Developmental Tasks

You will need to review the developmental tasks you would expect to see the patient accomplishing and then look for evidence that the task is being performed. Sometimes you will identify patients who are functioning at a level different from the one their chronological age would indicate. A young adult may still be struggling with unfinished tasks of adolescence and be unable to move forward into the young adult framework until those tasks have been successfully accomplished.

Role Performance

Gordon (1991) identified the role–relationship pattern as one of the basic functional health patterns in her assessment schema. Roy (1984) identified the role pattern as one of the basic adaptive modes of the individual. In the writings of both of these nursing theorists, assessment to identify the roles in which the individual must function and the individual's ability to function in those roles is an important component.

To assess for role performance, you must first consider what roles the individual is currently performing. Consider primary, secondary, and tertiary roles and try to identify all those that are appropriate to this individual at this time. Then try to assess whether the person is expressing any difficulty in meeting the expectations of any of them. Consider whether any of these roles might be in conflict with any others or whether there might be a problem associated with clearly identifying the appropriate behaviors for this role. Is the person experiencing a new role, such as parent or caretaker, and does he or she feel uncomfortable with the demands of that new role?

Social Support System

You will need to identify the social support system the patient has available. Consider who the significant others are for the person. Significant others may be family members, friends, neighbors, or fellow members of a church or fraternal organization. You need to have a view of who will help to form a support system for the patient both in the facility and after discharge. In addition to knowing who the person's significant others are, meeting them when they come for a visit is helpful. Sometimes information should be directly sought from them (within the guidelines of confidentiality, of course), but in many instances what you need is simply to get a general view of the quality and strength of the relationships.

Situational Stressors

Health care problems create many situational stressors for the individual patient. Consider the threats to mental health discussed earlier and consider whether any of those threats are present for this patient. Consider whether there are physical or functional changes occurring. Is loss of privacy or loss of control a concern to this patient? Is the patient unfamiliar with the health care setting? Does the patient, therefore, have difficulties associated with the unfamiliar routines or uncertainty about expected behaviors?

Identifying when the patient has financial problems that might stand in the way of obtaining optimum care

Display 34–2
Words Used to Describe Feelings

Happy
brisk
buoyant
carefree
cheerful
comfortable
contented
ecstatic
elated
enthusiastic
excited
exhilarated
festive
glad
hilarious
jolly
joyous
jubilant
lighthearted
merry
optimistic
playful
pleased
satisfied
sparkling
spirited
thrilled
vivacious

Eager
aggressive
ardent
avid
desirous
earnest
enthusiastic
excited
impulsive
intent
keen
proud
zealous

Sad
blah
defeated
depressed
disappointed
discontented
discouraged
dismal
dreadful
dreary
dull
flat
gloomy
heavy-hearted
helpless
hopeless
ill at ease
in the dumps
low
melancholy
moody
mournful
out of sorts
powerless
quiet
somber
sorrowful
unhappy
useless
worthless

Hurt
aching
afflicted
crushed
despairing
distressed
heartbroken
injured
isolated
lonely
offended
pained
suffering
tortured

Angry
annoyed
awkward
belligerent
bitter
boiling
cross
enraged
frustrated
fuming
furious
grumpy
indignant
inflamed
infuriated
irate
irritated
offended
provoked
resentful
sullen
wrathful

Fearless
bold
brave
confident
courageous
daring
determined
encouraged
hardy
heroic
impulsive
independent
proud

Interested
absorbed
concerned
curious
engrossed
excited
fascinated
intrigued

Doubtful
distrustful
dubious
evasive
hesitant
indecisive
perplexed
pessimistic
questioning
skeptical
suspicious
unbelieving
uncertain
wavering

Affectionate
appealing
close
loving
passionate
seductive
sexy
tender
warm

Calm
complacent
peaceful
placid
reassured
relaxed
restful
secure
serene

Shame
appalled
ashamed
dismayed
doubtful
embarrassed
guilty
shameful

Afraid
alarmed
anxious
apprehensive
awed
fearful
fidgety
frightened
gutless
hesitant
horrified
hysterical
impatient
insecure
nervous
panicky
petrified
pressured
scared
shaky
shocked
terrified
threatened
worried

Miscellaneous
bored
cruel
distant
envious
humble
jealous
mixed-up
preoccupied
stubborn
sulky

and making referrals when appropriate are nursing responsibilities. However, people are sensitive in regard to their financial status and might interpret direct questions as prying or might mistake your interest for concern that the hospital bill will not be paid. On the face sheet of the chart, a section is usually marked indicating whether the patient has insurance coverage. This provides basic information. When discussing posthospital care you might comment, "Having to take so many medications is sometimes a strain on the budget. Is that a concern for you?" When suggesting a referral, you might first identify what the patient's cost will be and include that information in your discussion of the agency and whether a referral would be appropriate.

Nursing Diagnosis

When making a nursing diagnosis in relationship to a mental health problem, it is especially important not to determine a diagnosis based on only one sign or symptom. Remember that a nursing diagnosis involves a *cluster* of signs and symptoms. You will need to review carefully the descriptions of the various nursing diagnoses and the defining characteristics of them and compare these with the data you have gathered in regard to the patient. Look for the presence of critical defining characteristics; these are characteristics that must be present for this diagnosis to be made. They are essential parts of the definition of the diagnosis. When the appropriate nursing diagnosis has been made, you may then begin to plan nursing interventions designed to restore homeostasis.

The mental health-related nursing diagnoses we will discuss here fall into the general North American Nursing Diagnosis Association (NANDA) categories of emotional integrity, socialization, role performance, coping, and judgment. Mental health problems relating to self-concept are discussed in Chapter 35.

Alterations in emotional integrity include those feeling states that create distress in an individual. These diagnoses are appropriate when the feelings are a major source of discomfort or may be interfering with the person's ability to relate effectively to others.

The various alterations in coping indicate that the person or family is not able to manage stressors effectively. The person may make inappropriate decisions, fail to manage health care needs effectively, or be unable to maintain appropriate relationships with others. Alteration in role is the category that includes nursing diagnoses related to family processes and role performance.

Nursing Diagnoses Related to Mental Health

- Anxiety
- Fear
- High Risk for Violence
- Situational Depression
- Ineffective Individual Coping
- Impaired Adjustment
- Defensive Coping
- Ineffective Denial
- Potential for Growth in Family Coping
- Ineffective Family Coping
- Noncompliance
- Diversional Activity Deficit
- Altered Role Performance
- Altered Family Processes
- Parental Role Conflict
- Powerlessness
- Hopelessness
- Decisional Conflict
- Health-Seeking Behaviors

Anxiety

Anxiety is a subjective experience of apprehension initiated by a threat to oneself, whether physical, mental, emotional, or spiritual (Peplau, 1963). Because becoming a patient involves so many potential threats, you can expect most people to experience some degree of anxiety during their interaction with the health care system. Because of the interrelationship between physical and psychological well-being, the patient will feel anxiety whether the initial problem is physical or psychological. Helping the patient to reduce anxiety to a manageable level is an integral part of nursing practice.

The etiology of anxiety lies in an actual or perceived threat to the self. This threat may be to the self-concept or to the biologic self. The patient may also perceive a threat toward interpersonal relationships or socioeconomic status. Changes in the environment, such as hospitalization, may be perceived as a threat. In a **maturational crisis**, anxiety may center on fear of separation, if the patient is the young child, or it may be associated with sexual feelings in the adolescent.

To diagnose the presence of anxiety, your assessment should document physical, behavioral, and cognitive signs that indicate it. The client may also be able to describe emotions that indicate anxiety.

Physical signs of anxiety include increases in pulse and respiration rates, in blood pressure, and muscle tone. The patient may have difficulty sleeping or may report disturbances in normal sleep patterns. Some individuals may experience digestive disturbances, including nausea, vomiting, and diarrhea. Frequent urination, dry mouth, trembling, and diaphoresis (excessive sweating) may all accompany anxiety.

Behavioral signs include repetitive mannerisms, constant activity, and pacing. Nervous laughter, crying, angry outbursts, and criticism of others may occur. The person may exhibit irritability or impatience.

Cognitive responses include changes in perception and in learning ability. The person may be unresponsive to surroundings and unable to concentrate. He or she may have difficulty in remembering things and may tend to focus on the past rather than the future.

Emotional responses the patient might express include feelings of nervousness, tension, and loss of control. The patient may indicate that he or she feels apprehensive or afraid without being sure why. He may express that he is unable to relax and feels uptight. Some individuals may say that they are feeling anxious.

Table 34-2 provides an overview of anxiety. A condition of no anxiety at all is characterized by a calm, resting state. In this state the person is not alert or prepared for action. With the advent of mild anxiety, the pulse, respiration, and blood pressure rise slightly. Muscle tone and alertness increase and bring the person to a state of readiness. A person with mild anxiety focuses well, sees details, and is able to disregard extraneous material; learning is enhanced. This is the state that Hans Selye describes as "eustress." In this state the person develops problem-solving skills and learns new coping behaviors. These will be of value in future situations of anxiety and stress.

As anxiety increases, however, it becomes increasingly dysfunctional. With the advent of moderate anxiety, the person begins to suffer deficits in ability to function. Blood pressure rises and pulse and respiration are noticeably faster, demanding hard work of the organs. The increased level of muscle tension may lead to tension headache or low backache. Repetitive activities, such as pacing or jiggling keys, are often used to relieve some of the tension. The person feels nervous, tense, and somewhat upset. Focus narrows, which may cause the person to perceive only a portion of the situation. Learning slows.

Severe anxiety is characterized by extremely rapid, sometimes irregular, pulse. Blood pressure and respiration rate are both elevated. The person may feel extreme tension and be almost immobilized, or repetitive activity may increase in speed and intensity. The person feels that he or she is losing control and is upset. A severely anxious individual tends to focus on random details and is unable to perceive the whole situation. Learning is greatly diminished or absent altogether.

A **panic** state is one in which anxiety has risen so high that the individual is physically unable to maintain control. If immobilization has occurred, another person

Table 34–2. Characteristics of Anxiety

	No Anxiety (-)	Mild Anxiety (+)	Moderate Anxiety (++)	Severe Anxiety (+++)	Panic (++++)
Pulse	Resting rate	Slightly faster	Noticeably faster	Rapid, possibly irregular	Very rapid and irregular
Respiration	Resting rate	Slightly faster	Noticeably faster	Rapid and irregular	Very rapid, possible hyperventilation
Blood pressure	Resting level	Slightly elevated	Noticeably elevated	High	High; if profound, panic, may suddenly drop and cause fainting
Muscle tone and effect on activity	Flaccid, not ready to act; lethargic	Slight tension, ready to act; acts with purpose	Increased tension; may have headaches and other aches; may engage in repetitive mannerisms to release tension; may pace	Extreme tension—may be almost unable to move; no purposeful action; repetitive actions increased in speed and intensity	Extreme tension; either immobilization or eruption into erratic behavior; almost uncontrollable
Mood	Calm; may feel lethargic	Alert; feels ambitious and ready to act	Nervous, somewhat upset	Very upset, feels loss of control	Out of control, panicky
Effect on perception	Not alert, easily distracted	Alert, sees details well; extraneous material excluded from attention	Focuses more narrowly; may not perceive whole situation	Focuses on random detail; misses whole situation	Perception distorted
Effect on learning	Slow	Enhanced, optimal	Slow or limited	Greatly diminished or absent	No learning possible

may physically have to help the person to move from one place to another. If repetitive activity continues, it may become so extreme that another person has to control the behavior to keep it from becoming destructive. The panicked person's perception is not only narrowed, but seriously distorted. Learning is completely impossible. Intervention by another person is usually necessary to help relieve the panic state.

Fear

The threat in anxiety is diffuse and not identifiable; *fear* is a feeling similar to anxiety except that the source of distress is clearly identifiable. The physical signs of fear are similar to those of anxiety. The pulse and respiration rates increase and blood pressure rises. Fear has levels at which perception, behavior, and ability to learn all change just as they do with anxiety. Fear is usually adaptive because the person can identify the threat and take action to avoid or lessen it. But when a threat continues and is out of the person's control, the level of fear increases. Intervention by another person is usually needed.

Certain fears are a normal part of development. For example, fear of the dark is a common fear in childhood. With support during the time of fear, gradual recognition that harmful things are not present in the dark and increased feelings of control over the environment, a child's fear of the dark will disappear as the child matures. If the fear persists, additional intervention is usually appropriate.

Some fears are caused by stimuli that are not really a threat to the person. These types of fears are called *phobias.* A fear of cats is one such fear. These fears are considered pathologic, that is, destructive to health. Fears that persist after the threat has been removed are also pathologic. Such fears usually require intervention by a skilled professional. A staff nurse may be able to refer a patient to an appropriate resource for this problem.

High Risk for Violence

Individuals with a high risk for violent behavior require special attention from health care providers. A risk for violence may be the result of a physiologic abnormality such as a toxic response to a drug, damage to the brain, or hormonal imbalance. Violent behavior may also be related to psychosocial factors such as a catastrophic life event or rage directed at others. The person with a high risk for violence must be identified, both so that health care personnel can be safeguarded and so that the person can be assisted.

Early indicators of a high risk for violence are signs of hypervigilance by the person. Pupils may be dilated. The gaze may dart in all directions in an attempt to keep track of everything and everyone. Muscles are tensed even when the person is sitting quietly. Fists are sometimes clenched and the jaw may be tensed or clenched. Identifying these early indicators may help you to intervene before actual violent behavior has occurred.

More overt signs follow the subtle early signs. Agitation and increased motor activity begin. The alert person may make hostile comments and threaten violent action. The person with less awareness of surroundings may resist efforts to direct his or her behavior and try physically to prevent close contact or touch. Suspicion of others and the belief that others intend harm often accompany violent behavior. Pathologic fear of the environment may be present. The individual's anxiety level may be near the panic range.

A calm, quiet, nonthreatening environment is essential for the potentially violent person. The health care providers who contact the potentially violent person should be those who can demonstrate calm, nonthreatening behavior. The person should be separated from everyone except those who are working with the problem. This separation both reduces environmental stimuli and decreases the number of people at risk.

The first step is getting all nonessential people away from the potentially violent person. Personnel should stay out of reach of the patient and avoid being trapped between the person and an exit from the room. Removing objects that may be used for assault may be necessary. One designated person should talk to the patient in a slow, nonthreatening manner and encourage the person to talk about concerns and feelings. This may dissipate some of the tension. Sometimes this alone is enough to defuse the situation.

A "show-of-force" is bringing together a group of staff members who have been trained in techniques of managing a potentially violent person. This is done when the risk for violence is extremely high and the person does not show any indication of calming. This group of care providers should include enough persons with physical strength that they can clearly physically restrain the patient if necessary. Often their presence alone will diminish the potential for actual violent acts. The use of restraining devices may increase the risk of violent response; therefore, their use should be carefully thought out and other methods of control used first. When restraints are determined to be essential, they must be applied rapidly and with a nonpunitive attitude. Restraints are not punishment, but protection for others. Chemical restraints in the form of sedating drugs may be used in some situations.

Nurses and other health care workers may become victims of violence despite their best efforts. This most often happens in emergency situations when there are not adequate personnel or adequate time to assess an individual. It may also occur when deliberately violent criminal offenders are cared for in correctional facilities, emergency rooms, or walk-in clinics. Cognitively impaired individuals who suddenly lash out with fists or kicking may also injure others.

Health care personnel who become victims often need counseling assistance in addition to treatment for injuries. They may blame themselves for not preventing the violence. They may say "If I had been a better nurse, this would not have happened." In addition, colleagues may increase this guilt inadvertently by making suggestions such as "Why didn't you . . . ." We must understand that all violent behavior cannot be predicted or prevented. Health care workers need support and assistance in determining whether criminal charges should be filed in the case of criminal assault and in ensuring their own personal care. Facilities also have responsibilities in providing a safe working environment with the resources to handle potentially violent situations in those settings where they may occur.

Altered Role Performance

A variety of role problems may result in a diagnosis of Altered Role Performance. **Role strain** is the term used to describe a situation in which a person experiences difficulties while carrying out any role in life. **Role conflict** is one type of role strain in which the various roles a person must perform require conflicting or incompatible behaviors. For example, a woman may find that her role expectations for herself as a mother and her expectations for herself as a career woman are in conflict. Another type of role strain arises when the expectations about appropriate role behavior are not clear. This is called **role ambiguity**. Role conflict and role ambiguity may cause altered role performance.

Altered Role Performance is also diagnosed when an individual who is required to accept a role in life (*eg*, as a daughter) does not perform the appropriate behaviors or is unhappy with the expected behaviors. Altered Role Performance may also be diagnosed when an individual is having difficulty adapting successfully to a chosen role. Sometimes illness may cause changes in physical capacity to assume a role, thereby causing a problem.

The individual may express distress and unhappiness over the way the role is performed, with such comments as "I really would like to relate better to my mother, but I don't know how." Behaviors that indicate that the individual is not successful in the role may be observed. The individual may deny that the role is a part of his or her life.

Difficulties related to role performance may also result in the nursing diagnoses of Ineffective Coping as well as diagnoses of Altered Parenting and Altered Family Processes.

Altered Family Processes

The nursing diagnosis Altered Family Processes is used to describe a family that has functioned effectively in the past, but now is faced with a new and more challenging stressor. This nursing diagnosis is used when a family system does not adapt to a *crisis* or is unable to communicate effectively in the face of a new stressor. In addition, the family may not be able to meet the physical, emotional, or spiritual needs of all of its members. New coping skills may need to be developed. Sometimes the family does not seek help appropriately. Such factors as major illness of a family member that may include expensive or time-consuming treatments, trauma, or surgery may be contributing factors in this nursing diagnosis. The addition or loss of a family member through birth, death, adoption, or change in living arrangements may also contribute to alteration in family processes because these situations require the development of new modes of behavior.

Potential for Growth in Family Coping

This diagnosis describes a family that has effectively managed health problems, demonstrated adaptive changes in the past, and is exhibiting desire and readiness for the enhanced health and growth of the ill family member and of the family as a whole. The family members will indicate their recognition that this new situation requires new attitudes or behaviors, and they will be seeking information and assistance for their own growth. They will be choosing experiences and actions that will lead them toward health and wholeness.

Ineffective Family Coping

Ineffective Family Coping is the nursing diagnosis that describes a family with a pattern of destructive behavior when faced with stressors. The family demonstrates a failure to meet each other's needs; there may be abuse of and violence toward each other. Behavior problems in children and conflict between adults in the family may be present. The special needs of an ill family member or even the basic human needs of a member may be neglected.

The diagnosis of Ineffective Family Coping may be categorized as either compromised or disabling. In the compromised category, support is being offered, but it is ineffective, insufficient, or inappropriate. In the disabling category, significant persons in the family actu-

> ### ***Nursing Research:*** *Implications for Practice*
>
> Koller, P. A. "Family Needs and Coping Strategies During Illness Crisis." *AACN Clinical Issues in Critical Care Nursing* 2, 2 (May 1991): 338–345.
>
> Family needs and coping behaviors when faced with the stress of a family member's critical illness were studied. The top 10 needs identified by the families centered around the topics of assurance regarding care and condition, information about the situation, and being able to stay close to the individual. Hope was the most frequently used method of coping. The nursing interventions that families found helpful were provision of information, emotional support, competence of the nurse, and the manner of the nurse in relating to the family.

ally disable the ability of others to function as well as not functioning themselves.

Ineffective Individual Coping

A diagnosis of Ineffective Individual Coping indicates that the individual person is not managing stressors adequately and is making poor choices and decisions. The person may be taking actions that disturb interpersonal relationships with significant others. Characteristics that indicate this diagnosis include the presence of at least one of the following: verbalization of inability to cope, inappropriate use of defense mechanisms, and inability to meet the expectations related to one's roles in life. The usual communication pattern of the individual may also change. Additional manifestations of ineffective coping may be an inability to solve problems, inability to meet one's own basic needs, and an inability to ask for needed help. Frequent illnesses and accidents may also accompany ineffective coping. The person who is coping ineffectively may withdraw from social relationships and engage in destructive behavior toward the self or others.

Impaired Adjustment

The person with **impaired adjustment** is unwilling to modify lifestyle or behavior as necessary to manage a change in health status. The person may express the idea that he or she does not accept that the change in health status requires a change in behavior or may demonstrate the inability to make the needed changes in lifestyle. This person may be unwilling or unable to consider the future and may exhibit a prolonged period of shock or disbelief. Impaired adjustment is a response to a major change in health status such as loss of a limb, kidney failure, or cancer. It may also occur when support systems are inadequate or when they fail.

Noncompliance

When an individual decides not to follow the prescribed health care regimen in regard to activity, medications, or any other part of life, he or she is diagnosed as exhibiting **noncompliance**. Some nurses object to the term noncompliant because they believe it emphasizes a dependent role for the patient; being compliant is doing what one is told to do. These nurses prefer to use the term *nonadherence*. They believe that *adhering* to the health care regimen carries connotations of participating voluntarily after the patient decides that the regimen should be followed. Whichever term is used, the focus remains the same: the individual is not doing those things that would contribute to a healthier life. Here we will use the term noncompliance because that is the official NANDA diagnostic term.

Noncompliance has many different causes. Sometimes noncompliance results from a lack of correct knowledge of the nature of the regimen or its purpose. When understanding is gained, the individual then will choose to comply. However, the cause for noncompliance is usually more complex. You should investigate such factors as the time required, how the regimen fits into the individual's lifestyle, and the cost involved. Acceptance of the health problem and beliefs about health and self-determination are also important. You should also determine whether simply forgetting is a factor, whether the privacy needed for care is available, and whether the individual really wants to change. Some medications have adverse side effects that the person finds unacceptable. In trying to solve a noncompliance problem, you may have to consider ways in which the health care regimen can be adapted to fit the individual's lifestyle rather than how the lifestyle can be adapted to the health care regimen. Thorough assessment and accurate identification of the etiology in cases of noncompliance are essential to effective planning.

Decisional Conflict

The person experiencing decisional conflict is having difficulty determining the appropriate course of action in a situation that involves risk, loss, or conflict. There are real and difficult problems to be faced and the relative risks and merits must be weighed. The person exhibits symptoms of anxiety when discussing the decision and may be questioning personal values and beliefs as the decision is reviewed. This diagnosis is not appropriate when an individual is unable to make ordinary decisions of daily life. In this situation, the person is not coping effectively.

Diversional Activity Deficit

When an individual's life is changed by illness, often the person becomes unable to engage in usual pastimes. New long periods of free time may result in boredom. Not only is boredom uncomfortable for the individual, but it interferes with the positive outlook on life that is an asset to healing and recovery. This problem may result from external factors, such as a care setting with few opportunities for activity, or from internal factors, such as lack of motivation.

Depressed Mood

Depression is a mental state in which a person feels in low spirits, dejected, and even hopeless. Although depressed mood is not yet a NANDA-designated category, many nurses believe that depressed mood is a human response pattern for which nurses should be planning intervention. These nurses may make such a diagnosis using a variety of terminology in addition to depressed mood. Sometimes the term simple depression, situational depression, or reactive depression is used.

However, some nurses consider depression to be an indicator of the presence of another nursing diagnosis, such as Ineffective Coping. You will need to consult with your instructor and experienced nurses in your setting to determine whether depressed mood is being used as a nursing diagnosis.

Depressed mood used as a nursing diagnosis does not refer to the serious major depression that you will study as a psychiatric problem. Rather depressed mood is an expected response to loss and other sad life events. Most people feel this type of depression at times.

During a period of depressed mood a person is often internally sorting through feelings and information to cope successfully with the life event that precipitated the feelings. Such normal depression is not a problem but a functional life process. You can provide support for the depressed person, acknowledge the depression as an appropriate response, and assist with problem-solving as needed. The depression can be expected to recede as the person becomes able to respond to the situation effectively or as the situation changes. This common depression may create additional problems such as inability to cope effectively with daily living. In this situation, the nursing diagnosis Ineffective Coping related to depression is used.

Depression may also be pathologic, that is, related to abnormal functioning. Pathologic depression (or major depression) is much more extreme than would be expected in view of the prevailing circumstances or it occurs in the absence of any visible life problem. Pathologic depression renders the person unable to act effectively and self-esteem is low. Pathologic depression requires specialized professional help. The same cognitive, behavioral, and physical signs and symptoms characterize all depression (Table 34-3); the difference between simple depressed mood and major depression is in their severity and the length of time they persist. A depressed person is less able than usual to concentrate on the tasks at hand and exhibits a lack of interest in life. Learning is usually slowed. The entire thinking process may be slow, requiring more energy than is available.

A person who is depressed tends to move slowly and may sit for long periods of time doing nothing at all. Often, a person's sleep is disturbed. Although difficulty in getting to sleep is more common with simple depression, early morning awakening is more common with pathologic depression. With both conditions, the person may cry or sigh frequently, and appetite is typically poor. The posture of the depressed person is characterized by slumped shoulders and a tendency for the head to be bent. The person may appear to be carrying a great weight. The face seems to droop and the expression is typically sad (Fig. 34-3).

The physical changes in the body, also termed veg-

Table 34–3. Signs of Depression

Cognitive Signs	Behavioral Signs	Physical Signs
Decreased concentration	Slow movement	Slow pulse
Lack of interest	Inactivity	Slow respiration
Slowed learning	Sleep disturbance	Low blood pressure
	Early waking	Constipation
	Crying	Dry skin and hair
	Sighing	
	Slumped posture	
	Poor appetite	
	Bowed head	
	Sad expression	

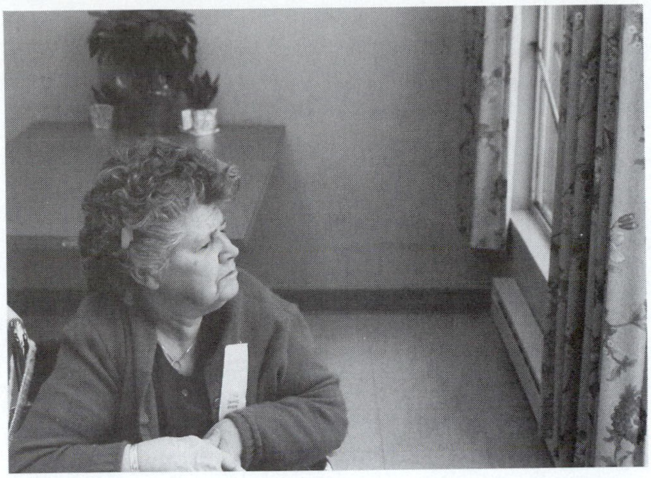

Figure 34-3. The person who is depressed exhibits characteristic physical signs.

etative signs, created by depression are most common when the depression has progressed beyond the simple situation and represents a major mental health problem that needs more advanced intervention. Body function may slow down, resulting in slow pulse, lowered blood pressure, and slowed respirations. Constipation is common. When depression persists for a long period of time, often the skin becomes dry and the hair lifeless.

Planning and Implementation

Desired outcomes for mental health-related problems are sometimes difficult to formulate. Remember that emotions and thoughts cannot be seen. Changes in emotions and feelings can be validated only through specific behaviors that can be objectively verified or through statements made by the patient of subjective feelings and thoughts.

For example, if a person is anxious, your outcomes should describe the behavior you would hope to see if the anxiety has been reduced. You could state the desired outcomes as "Decreased anxiety as evidenced by the following behaviors: 1) discusses problem in a calm voice, 2) does not pace the floor, 3) identifies possible actions that he can take to find child care." If the person is not coping effectively, you would use behavioral descriptions of appropriate coping. If a patient displays a particularly dysfunctional behavior, you might indicate that the absence of this behavior is a desired outcome.

In some instances, your outcome would indicate that the patient will speak of altered feelings or thoughts. You might indicate what statements the patient might make that would indicate decreased feelings of anxiety or improved coping.

Additionally you must make your desired outcomes realistic in light of the patient's situation. To do this, you might need to describe an outcome that does not represent complete resolution of the problem, but rather a lessening of it. If a patient is facing serious, major surgery, an absence of anxiety is not a realistic short-term outcome. The short-term outcome might be "*Decreased* anxiety as evidenced by the following behaviors: 1) expresses understanding of preoperative instructions, 2) sleeps during night before surgery." Thus the anxiety is still present, but the individual is able to understand the patient teaching and able to get needed rest.

If a patient is seriously depressed, an expected outcome related to absence of depression would reflect your lack of understanding of the seriousness of the situation for the patient. A better short-term outcome might be limited, such as "Discusses feelings of depression." You might also write a long-term outcome that would relate to behaviors that might be seen when the depression has been resolved.

To support the patient's mental health your primary tool will be yourself. Much of the art of nursing is in the use of the self as a therapeutic tool. In Chapter 13 we discussed the various approaches to communication skills. You will need to become skillful with the use of those communication techniques and be able to adapt them to the needs of the individual patient.

When planning for nursing interventions, you must always begin with establishing trust and a supportive climate. In determining what problems should take priority, you will want first to deal with any situation that threatens to overwhelm the individual. This is *crisis intervention.* The steps of the crisis intervention model presented here are also useful in other less acute situations. If anxiety is not high, you might start interaction by focusing on the second step in the crisis intervention model. Thus, this model is flexible and adaptable to many different situations.

In addition to crisis intervention, you will use communication techniques to help individuals with depression and coping problems. Providing skilled care assists to relieve anxiety and helps the person to use energies on problem-solving. Individuals can be helped to explore their role performance and to make effective decisions. You will refer patients and families to others when you determine that their problems need more long-term intervention or the skill of a specialty prepared care provider.

Establishing Trust and a Supportive Climate

To provide effective support to the patient and family, you must first establish a relationship in which the patient and family have trust in you. You create trust when your response can be relied on. You must endeavor to promise only what you can do, maintain confidentiality, and treat the patient's concerns as important. When you listen attentively to what the patient has to say, you convey an attitude that the patient is important. The patient will feel supported when you spend time listening and responding to concerns expressed. Remaining nonjudgmental about feelings will also provide needed support. Using the techniques of therapeutic interaction discussed in Chapter 13, you can help the person to resolve problems whenever possible.

Intervening in Anxiety/Crisis Situations

A **crisis** is "a situation which threatens to overwhelm the individual" (Aguilera, 1982). Specifically, it is a situation in which the coping patterns that proved successful in the past are no longer adequate. **Crisis intervention** is a specific set of nursing actions designed to assist the person toward more effective coping in the face of a crisis.

There are two types of crises. The first is the *maturational* or *developmental crisis*, which arises out of changes that occur in the context of the life span. You will recall from Chapter 17 that Erikson associates each stage in life with a characteristic developmental crisis. Developmental crises are thus relatively predictable in the life of the individual. For example, the adolescent can be expected to undergo a crisis involving the process of developing an identity as an independent individual. Conflicts and difficulties surrounding this process are not unexpected. By recognizing normal developmental crises, you will be better able to help an individual to resolve such a crisis successfully.

The other type of crisis is a *situational crisis*, which is one that involves specific occurrences in a person's life. The occurrence might be a single incident, such as an assault, or a particular stage in a relationship. In some cases, the precipitating incident itself may not appear overwhelming; the crisis occurs because the individual cannot cope with the sum total of accumulated stress.

In a crisis, a person becomes unable to function effectively in most areas of life. He or she might be unable to go to work or, once there, unable to do the job. Decision-making becomes almost impossible. Anxiety is typically very high, approaching the panic level.

Whatever the source of the crisis, some general guidelines for action are appropriate. The following general model will need to be adapted to the specific situation and the individual in question. Communication skills are the major tools for resolving a crisis. Therapeutic interaction is used.

Reducing Anxiety

The first step in anxiety reduction is to provide support (see the sample Nursing Care Plan Related to Reducing Anxiety). This includes staying with the person and not making demands. You should avoid anxious behavior and present a quiet, calming presence because anxious behavior on your part will increase the patient's anxiety. Speak slowly and calmly; use short, simple sentences and concise directions because the individual's ability to concentrate and to understand will be decreased. The use of gentle touch when it appears appropriate may convey empathy and concern and be a quieting influence. Decreasing the sensory stimulation may also help to lessen the anxiety.

Allow the person to walk, to talk, to cry, or to behave in whatever way will relieve tension. You may encourage the individual to engage in a physical activity, if that is possible, to dissipate tension and accumulated energy. If the person is hyperventilating, calmly coaching the individual in slow, deliberate breathing may help interrupt a pattern of escalating anxiety. When anxiety is brought down to a moderate level, the individual can respond meaningfully to therapeutic interaction (Display 34-3).

Encouraging Ventilating and Naming Feelings

Encourage the person to talk about feelings and to recognize the feeling being experienced as anxiety. An opportunity to express feelings and to be assured that someone else is concerned about those feelings may be all that is needed or possible. In any situation, ventilating feelings is always an important step for the individual. To help the person do this, you will need to use the skills of attentive listening and nondirective responses. Techniques such as reflecting and restating are often effective in encouraging people to express their feelings. When feelings are expressed, it is important to maintain an accepting attitude; remember that the validity of feelings is a central mental health concept.

Gaining Intellectual Understanding or Insight

Assist the individual to recognize the behaviors and other signs and symptoms that he or she is experiencing and help the individual to recognize the link between the feelings and the behaviors. You might describe the signs and symptoms you see and indicate that you believe that they reflect anxiety. Ask the patient to

Display 34–3
Steps in Anxiety/Crisis Intervention

1. Anxiety reduction
2. Ventilating and naming feelings
3. Gaining intellectual understanding or insight
4. Exploring ways of coping
5. Making decisions

Nursing Care Plan
Sample Nursing Care Plan Related to Reducing Anxiety

Nursing Diagnosis	Anxiety related to impending surgery **Supportive data:** Paces the floor constantly. Does not maintain eye contact when speaking; eyes dart around room. Pulse rate was 90 while resting. Patient informed of need for surgery by MD this AM.
Desired Patient Outcomes	**Anxiety decreased as evidenced by the following behaviors:** 1. Sits quietly. 2. Maintains eye contact. 3. Resting pulse is 80 or below. 4. Listens to explanations of pre- and postoperative care.

Nursing Action	**Rationale**
1. Encourage him to discuss feelings through nondirective techniques.	Verbalizing feelings assists an individual in effective coping with those feelings.
2. Move discussion to understanding of experience of anxiety.	Insight into a stresful situation itself will also help the person to cope more effectively.
3. Encourage patient to see self as a participant in successful outcomes through nondirective discussion.	Perceiving the self as competent and in control decreases anxiety.

think about those behaviors and validate your perception.

Insight into the stressful situation itself will also help the person to cope more effectively. To gain such insight, the patient must think through and explore the situation independently. For you to explain it is often of no value at all. Instead, the use of facilitating techniques can help the person to consider all aspects of the situation. At this point you may wish to use the exploratory responses, which help the person to consolidate information. If the patient is unwilling to work at this task, it is best simply to express concern and willingness to listen and plan to talk further when the patient is more ready to proceed.

Exploring Ways of Coping

When the patient has gained some insight into the predicament, it is appropriate to encourage him or her to recall successful methods of coping with stressful situations in the past. This approach encourages the person to see himself or herself as a capable person able to cope with stressful situations. It also helps the person to focus on specific actions rather than generalized concerns. Sometimes pointing out information in a nondirective manner is appropriate. For example, you might say, "Some people find that talking directly to the person they are angry with is helpful. Have you considered that approach?" Giving directions or direct suggestions ("You should . . ." or "You ought . . .") undermines the individual's autonomy.

Making Decisions

Remember that this person will have difficulty with effective decision-making and should not be required to make decisions at the onset of crisis if that can be avoided. Waiting for decision-making until the person is less anxious usually results in sounder decisions. However, in health care some decisions must be made even when the person is anxious. Acknowledge this fact and encourage the person to seek whatever advice and support is needed from his or her own social support system. When uncertainty is part of the etiology of a person's anxiety, making a specific decision will sometimes reduce the anxiety.

Again, the use of facilitating techniques is appropriate in encouraging someone to move toward a decision. When a decision has been made, it is helpful to summarize the process by which the person has arrived at it, reinforce the idea that he or she is capable and able to cope, and offer assistance if needed to implement the decision. Such assistance might include providing the name and telephone number of somebody to contact, obtaining appropriate booklets or pamphlets, or accompanying the person when he or she talks with someone else.

Responding to the Depressed Person

The person who is depressed is withdrawn and reluctant to talk. Therefore, pushing for interaction is often inappropriate and will be ineffective. The depressed person will tend to remain inactive, a state that increases the depression. The first avenue of intervention, therefore, is to increase activity (see sample Nursing Care Plan Related to Reducing Depression). Activity can provide evidence to the patient that he or she is still capable of functioning. Activity also tends to increase the production of neurohormones that contribute positively toward a more elevated mood. To increase physical activity, you might encourage the person to focus on the tasks required for daily living and the immediate present. Do not, however, ask the person to make decisions, because with depression decision-making is almost impossible. Simply state, "It is time for your shower. I know you do not feel like getting up, but this is important for your well-being." Then help the person to perform the task.

Nursing Care Plan

Sample Nursing Care Plan Related to Reducing Depression

Nursing Diagnosis

Ineffective Individual Coping related to depression associated with change in lifestyle needed for diabetes.

Supportive data:

Unwilling to discuss lifestyle changes.

Does not read any material provided regarding diabetes.

Sad expression on face.

Sits staring into space for long periods of time.

Does not voluntarily engage in any activity.

States, "I just can't seem to do anything. I feel so down."

Desired Patient Outcomes

Begins coping with diabetes, as evidenced by the following behaviors:

1. Reads literature.
2. Discusses changes in lifestyle.
3. Voluntarily practices injection technique and urine testing.
4. Performs self-care.

Nursing Action	Rationale
1. Give specific directions for self-care activities. Do not give choices regarding self-care.	Decision-making may be impossible for the depressed person. Inactivity tends to increase depression.
2. Set up specific times for practice and stay with patient, assisting with equipment if needed.	Repeated practice facilitates learning.
3. Express recognition that this is a major change and that feeling "down" is expected.	Feelings and sentiments are real. Acknowledging feelings as real supports self-esteem.
4. Stay with patient after activities and provide opportunity for discussion of feelings.	Verbalizing feelings assists an individual in effective coping with those feelings.

While acknowledging the depression as valid, you might also point out evidence that the person is coping effectively in some areas of life. This evidence reinforces self-esteem. You might say, "It is realistic to feel down; you have a really major change in your life. But you have started your physical therapy and that is the first step toward being independent again." Continuing evidence that you are willing to be future oriented and that you feel the person is worthwhile will help to reinforce feelings of self-worth. Activities that allow for positive accomplishment and thus support self-esteem are valuable.

When the depression lifts, you may be able to begin an approach directed at establishing more effective coping behavior. This would include helping the person gain intellectual understanding, explore ways of coping, and make decisions in regard to life.

If the depression fails to lift or if the depression appears to be deepening, referral to a mental health professional such as a psychiatric clinical nurse specialist for further assessment, planning for more active intervention, and possible referral to a psychiatrist becomes significant (see the information on referral below). Depression may become so great that the person contemplates suicide. If at any time a person indicates thoughts of suicide, this information should immediately be shared with others on the health care team and appropriate care should be initiated. Care of the seriously depressed or suicidal person is beyond the scope of this text and is part of studies in psychiatric nursing.

Responding to Anger and Hostility

Anger is a feeling of extreme displeasure with someone else, often stemming from the feeling of being "against" the person or a sense that the other is preventing the person from acting as he or she wishes. *Hostility* is viewing the other person as an opponent or enemy. Anger and hostility often go hand-in-hand. Neither of these states has been approved by NANDA as a nursing diagnosis. Rather, they are considered indicators of the presence of other nursing diagnoses.

Patients in health care settings may express anger toward their families, friends, and caregivers. Often anger is an appropriate response to events or circumstances. For example, a person who has been left lying on a stretcher in a hallway for 45 minutes while waiting for a test may be justified in feeling extreme displeasure toward the people responsible for the resulting discomfort and fatigue. If a file is misplaced, making it necessary for a test to be repeated, the patient's anger is appropriate—though it is inappropriate to direct such anger at the person who performs the repeated test if that person was not responsible for the original error.

When a patient expresses anger, your first response should be to examine the situation and determine whether the anger appears to be realistic. When it is, the health care team is responsible for trying to correct the situation (Fig. 34-4). If it proves impossible to do so, you should at least acknowledge to the patient that the anger is recognized and say that you will try to see that the situation is not repeated. This kind of response may prevent hostility and preserve a relationship in which the patient and the health care workers are "on the same team" rather than opponents.

When you cannot identify an objective provocation for a patient's anger, you might consider whether it is serving as a defense mechanism, such as projection or displacement. Anger that appears inappropriate is often a means of coping with anxiety. In this case, you would direct your interactions toward exploring the person's thoughts and feelings about what is happening to try to determine the nature of the underlying problem.

Supporting Effective Role Performance

Interventions to support effective role performance begin with clarifying with the individual the expected life roles. The patient must agree that the expected role is one he or she wants to perform. Then interventions are designed to assist the individual to learn behaviors appropriate to effective performance in that role (see sample Nursing Care Plan Related to Impaired Adjustment). Often the best action is referral for this purpose: to classes for learning parenting roles or to self-improvement classes to help individuals develop other roles. Individual counseling may be needed to help an individual develop new behaviors in relationship to others within the family or at the workplace. Sometimes roles are not performed effectively, not because the individual does not know what to do, but rather because feelings of low self-esteem make the person reluctant to try. In this case, your focus would be the problem with self-

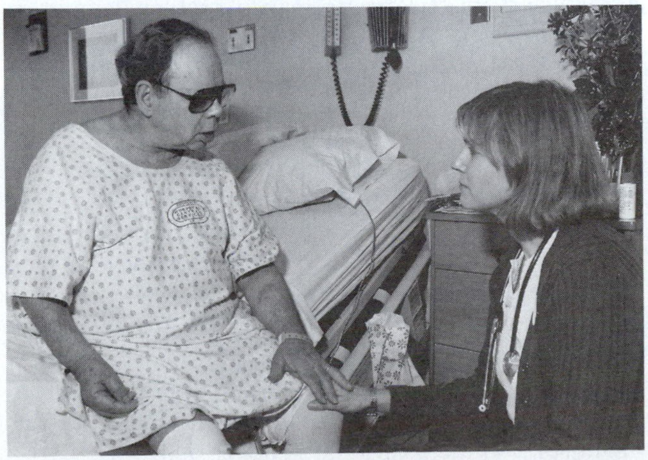

Figure 34-4. It is important to acknowledge when a patient's anger is justified.

Nursing Care Plan
Sample Nursing Care Plan Related to Impaired Adjustment

Nursing Diagnosis

Impaired Adjustment related to care for ileostomy and lack of support system.

Supportive data:

States: "I just don't know what to do—I can't handle all of this."

Refuses to practice self-care skills.

Says "I'll never be able to do it right anyway."

States she cannot think of anyone who could provide assistance or support.

Says, "I don't have any close friends and my family is hundreds of miles away."

Desired Patient Outcomes

1. Makes positive statements regarding own ability to manage self-care.
2. Practices self-care skills.
3. Identifies a source of personal support and initiates contact.

Nursing Action	Rationale
1. Encourage verbalization of feelings.	Verbalizing feelings assists an individual in effective coping with those feelings.
2. Assist her to review previous life problems and how she coped with them.	Perceiving the self as coping effectively in the past enhances self esteem.
3. Reinforce the value of previous coping skills in meeting this new situation.	Previously learned coping skills may often be adapted to new situations.
4. Help her to review the consequences of current behavior (*ie*, not learning self-care).	Identifying consequences may provide motivation for action.
5. Support realistic plans for learning self-care (such as one step at a time).	Realistic, attainable goals support feelings of competence. Unobtainable or remote goals may undermine feelings of competence.
6. Provide booklet on the local ostomy support group.	Written materials provide an ongoing resource for learning.

esteem and the role performance problem would be secondary.

Planning Appropriate Activities

Activities in which the patient can participate may be planned with the patient or may be planned for the patient by the nurse. Some activities are planned simply for their diversional nature. Other activities support mental health in a variety of ways. The person who has difficulties with communication that interfere with interpersonal relationships might be able to develop new skills of relating within the context an appropriate activity. An activity that promotes accomplishment of goals might support the individual's coping skills.

Consider the person's developmental level and lifestyle when planning for activities. You will need to consider a child's needs in terms of motor ability and development. In many settings there may be an activities director, a playroom coordinator, or an occupational therapist whose role is to assist with planning for appropriate therapeutic activities.

Projecting a Competent Manner

An important way to support the patient's mental health, often overlooked, is providing for his or her physical needs with a high degree of skill. When physical needs are met by a skillful caregiver, many anxieties are relieved and the person feels safe and able to relax. Energies can thus be directed toward the effort of coping with the illness and with recovery. When you experience uncertainties and doubts, they should be discussed with your instructor or an experienced nurse out of the

Nursing Issues and Trends: *Mental Health Care in the Community*

Community mental health centers were originally designed to provide assistance to individuals and families with a wide variety of threats to their mental health. This included those facing crises and specific problem situations in life as well as those who were diagnosed as mentally ill. Unfortunately, funding of these centers has severely limited their ability to serve the diverse needs of their communities. Nurses may have difficulty finding a referral organization that provides mental health support for those who do not have the ability to pay for services.

patient's hearing. When you are in the patient's presence, strive for a calm and confident attitude toward the tasks you are performing. This does not mean that you should be untruthful with your patients, but merely that your worries and uncertainties should not become problems for them.

Making Referrals to Other Professionals

Periodically you will conclude that the problem a patient is experiencing is beyond the scope of your own ability and understanding. In such a case, the appropriate step is referral to someone with the particular skills needed. For example, a mental health nursing clinician on the staff of the hospital may work directly with the patient or with the staff to develop appropriate nursing approaches to the patient. Alternatively, referral to a social worker or mental health therapist may be indicated. If a physician's order is needed for such a referral to be made, you will want to consult with the physician, presenting the data you have gathered and explaining your rationale for wishing to make such a referral. Remember that the best health care is a team effort with each individual contributing his or her special expertise for the patient's well-being (Fig. 34-5).

Evaluation

Evaluation of mental health must include careful attention to both the verbal and nonverbal cues to thoughts and feelings. You will want to be sensitive to the individual's responses to events and interactions. Behavior is also important in evaluating mental health status. As you observe the person, you will be comparing actual responses to the those you established as the desired outcomes. In evaluating emotional status, you will need to evaluate responses to individual interactions and adjust your communication to support the person.

Changes in behavior, thoughts, or feelings may not occur rapidly. You will need to develop skill in identifying small changes that may indicate progress. Do not become discouraged when positive responses are not forthcoming. Assisting people to resolve mental health problems often demands ongoing intervention and continuing support.

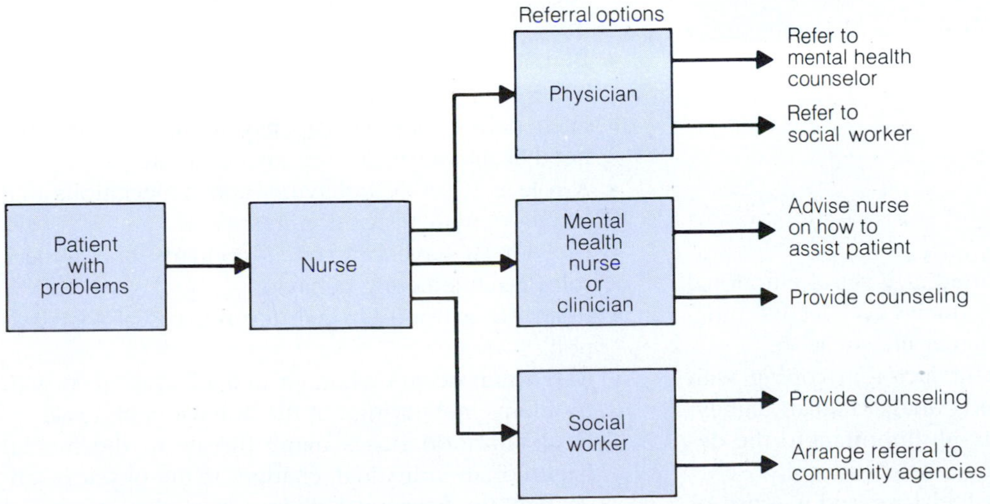

Figure 34-5. Referral is one avenue of intervention for patients with mental health problems.

Nursing Care Study
A Patient with Anxiety

Betty Westman was pacing the floor of her hospital room when Mary Cedino, the team leader, walked in. Ms. Cedino noted that Ms. Westman was breathing rapidly and had a tight, pinched expression on her face. Ms. Cedino knew that Ms. Westman had been told by her physician that she was to be discharged that afternoon. Ms. Cedino was also aware that Ms. Westman was a single parent with several preschool children at home. All these factors suggested to Ms. Cedino that Ms. Westman was anxious about going home. She validated this hypothesis by saying, "You look upset. Can you tell me how you're feeling?" Ms. Westman replied, "I just don't know what to do!"

"Could we sit down together and talk?" suggested Ms. Cedino. Ms. Westman nodded affirmatively. Ms. Cedino then pulled up a chair and said, "Please explain to me what is worrying you." After listening for a short while as Ms. Westman talked about how apprehensive she was about managing at home, Ms. Cedino decided to move from using general leads to trying to help Ms. Westman explore the situation and understand it more thoroughly. She encouraged Ms. Westman to discuss all the responsibilities at home that concerned her and to acknowledge that she was feeling anxious because she was worried about performing all the tasks of caring for her family.

Ms. Cedino then tried to help Ms. Westman think about previous occasions when she had been ill or away from home for a while and how she had managed then. Ms. Westman ventured that some jobs could be left undone and that once when she had been ill a neighbor had helped her with shopping. As the conversation progressed, Ms. Cedino encouraged Ms. Westman to identify actions she could take to make the home situation easier to manage. Ms. Westman decided that she would ask her neighbor to help with shopping again, hire a neighborhood teenager to take the children to the playground daily, and nap while the children were napping.

In conclusion, Ms. Cedino summarized the discussion and commented, "You have made some very constructive plans as we talked." Ms. Westman looked visibly more relaxed and replied, "Well, I've handled a lot of problems in my life and I guess I can handle this."

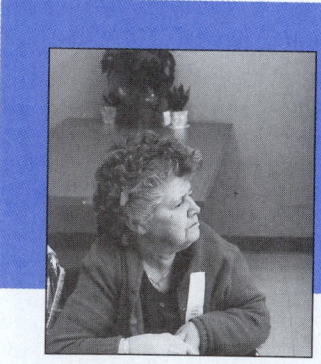

Key Points

- Mental health can be defined as a set of emotional and cognitive patterns conducive to effective functioning in one's own particular life situation.
- Self-esteem is an important factor in coping with daily life. Self-concept, body image, human dignity, and self-understanding are all important to the development and maintenance of self-esteem.
- Each individual needs to feel love and a sense of belonging.
- The ability to support an individual's mental health comes partially from a knowledge of individuality and partially from an understanding of group identification.
- Communication is an essential part of relating to others.
- Feelings are real and must be acknowledged as such even when there is no objective basis for them.
- Behavior has meaning and purpose for the individual; feelings are often revealed by behavior.
- Each person has the capacity for growth and the need to move toward self-actualization.
- A role is a set of behaviors and expectations that form a particular position in society.
- Individuals have primary, secondary, and tertiary roles, each affecting behavior.
- Roles are learned through the process of socialization.
- Role strain occurs when an individual is faced with problems in carrying out the behaviors of a role.
- Hospitalization poses many threats to the mental health of an individual: changes in the physical self, changes in functional ability, loss of privacy and control, uncertainty about expected behavior, unfa-

miliar routines, worry over expenses, uncertainty about outcomes, and conflict with developmental tasks may all threaten self-esteem.

- Hospitalization threatens self-actualization because of its nonstimulating atmosphere, its inadequate information for growth, and its enforced dependency.
- An individual's response to threats to mental health may include anxiety, fear, anger or hostility, potential for violence, situational reactive depression, ineffective individual or family coping, noncompliance, and impaired adjustment.
- When hospitalization causes role changes, the individual may experience altered role performance or altered family processes.
- Nursing process for mental health needs requires examination and validation of the individual's feelings, a willingness to provide support to the individual, and the setting of realistic short-term goals. In evaluation the plan of care, success may need to be measured in terms of relatively subtle changes in behavior and ability to cope.

Study Questions

1. Define mental health.
2. How does body image relate to self-esteem?
3. In what way does self-knowledge contribute to self-esteem?
4. What effect does a disruption of communication have on relationships with others?
5. What is an appropriate nursing response to an expression of a feeling?
6. What are the three types of roles one may possess?
7. List factors that tend to threaten the mental health of an individual who enters the health care system?
8. Name and describe at least four common defense mechanisms.
9. Discuss common responses to threats to mental health.
10. What factors should be considered when making an assessment related to mental health problems?
11. What is meant by using "the self" as a therapeutic agent?
12. What is a crisis?
13. Outline the steps in crisis intervention.
14. Describe appropriate nursing interventions for the depressed person.

Critical Thinking Activities

1. Write out goals for yourself aimed at increasing self-understanding. Establish a plan to meet these personal goals and try to achieve these goals during this term.
2. With a group of nursing students, participate in a discussion of mental health as it relates to you as a student and as a nurse.
3. Select a specific patient in the clinical area and identify a mental health concept that appears to be of primary importance in your relationship with this patient. List the reasons for your selection.
4. Recall the last time you were particularly anxious. Describe how you responded in terms of ability to focus on detail and to learn.
5. Identify defense mechanisms that you have used in the past and how they were or were not helpful to you.
6. Identify a mental health resource in your own community, learn about the resource including how referrals occur, the cost of the services, and the specific services offered. Report on it to your clinical group.

References and Readings

Aguilera, D., and Messick, J. *Crisis Intervention: Theory and Methodology.* 4th edition. St. Louis: C. V. Mosby, 1982.

Antai-Otong, D. "When Your Patient is Angry." *Nursing '88* 18, 2 (February 1988): 44–46.

Belaief, L. "Self-Esteem and Human Equality." *Nursing Digest* 6 (Fall 1978): 59–67.

Brownell, M. J. "The Concept of Crisis: Its Utility for Nursing." *Advances in Nursing Science* 6, 4 (July 1984): 10–21.

Bruss, C. R. "Nursing Diagnosis of Hopelessness." *Journal of Psychosocial Nursing and Mental Health Services* 26, 3 (March 1988): 28–32.

Carpenito, L. J. *Nursing Diagnosis: Application to Clinical Practice.* 4th edition. Philadelphia: J. B. Lippincott, 1992.

Carstairs, G. M. "Mental Health: What Is It?" *World Health* 26 (1973): 4–9.

Dobson, J. "Man and His Spirit: A Matter of Self-Esteem." Part 2. *Life and Health* 92 (February 1977): 28–29.

Dunn, H. L. *High-Level Wellness.* Arlington, Va.: R. W. Beatty, 1962.

Edel, M. K. "Noncompliance: An Appropriate Nursing Diagnosis." *Nursing Outlook* 33: 4 (July-August 1985): 183–185.

Geissler, E. M. "Crisis: What It Is and Is Not." *Advances in Nursing Science* 6, 4 (July 1984): 1–9.

Gordon, M. *Nursing Diagnosis: Process and Application.* 3rd edition. New York: McGraw-Hill, 1991.

Horsley, G. "Baggage from the Past." *American Journal of Nursing* 88, 1 (January 1988): 60–63.

Ignatavicius, D. D. "Meeting the Psychosocial Needs of Patients with Rheumatoid Arthritis." *Orthopedic Nursing* 6, 3 (May-June 1987): 16–21.

Issner, N. "The Family of the Hospitalized Child." *Nursing Clinics of North America* 7 (January 1972): 5–12.

Kane, C. F. "Family Social Support: Toward a Conceptual

Model." *Advances in Nursing Science* 10, 2 (January 1988): 18–25.

Kinkle, S. L. "Violence in the E.D.: How to Stop It Before It Starts." *American Journal of Nursing* 93, 7 (July 1993): 22–25.

Knowles, R. D. "Dealing with Feelings: Managing Anxiety." *American Journal of Nursing* 81 (January 1981): 110–112.

———. "Handling Anger: Responding vs. Reacting." *American Journal of Nursing* 81 (October 1981): 2196–2197.

Lazarus, R. S., and Folkman, S. *Stress, Appraisal and Coping.* New York: Springer, 1984.

Maynard, C. K. and Chitty, K. K. "Guidelines for Dealing with Anger." *Journal of Psychiatric Nursing* 17 (June 1979): 36–41.

McGee, R. F. "Hope: A Factor Influencing Crisis Resolution." *Advances in Nursing Science* 6, 4 (July 1984): 34–44.

McNett, S. C. "Social Support, Threat, Coping Responses and Effectiveness in the Functionally Disabled." *Nursing Research* 36, 2 (March-April 1987): 98–103.

Navis, E. S. "Controlling Violent Patients Before They Control You." *Nursing '87* 17, 9 (September 1987): 52–54.

Peplau, H. and Marshall, M. A. "A Working Definition of Anxiety." In *Some Clinical Approaches to Psychiatric Nursing,* edited by S. Burd, New York: Macmillan, 1963.

Powers, B. A. "Social Networks, Social Support, and Elderly Institutionalized People." *Advances in Nursing Science* 10, 2 (January 1988): 40–58.

Rosenbaum, M. "Depression: What to Do, What to Say." *Nursing '80* 10 (October 1980): 64–66.

Roy, Sr. C. *Introduction to Nursing: An Adaptation Model.* 2nd edition. Englewood Cliffs, N.J.: Prentice-Hall, 1984.

Schalling, D. "Anxiety, Pain, and Coping." *Issues in Mental Health Nursing* 7, 4 (1985): 437–460.

Seeger, P. A. "Self-Awareness and Nursing." *Journal of Psychiatric Nursing* 15 (August 1977): 24–25.

Sloboda, S. "Understanding Patient Behavior." *Nursing '77* 7 (September 1977): 74–77.

Smits, M. W., and Kee, C. C. "Correlates of Self-Care Among the Elderly: Self-Concept Affects Well-Being." *Journal of Gerontological Nursing* 18, 9 (September 1992): 13–17.

Snyder, J. C., and Wilson, M. F. "Elements of a Psychosocial Assessment." *American Journal of Nursing* 77 (February 1977): 235–239.

Volicer, B. J. "Patients' Perceptions of Stressful Events Associated with Hospitalization." *Nursing Research* 23 (1974): 235–238.

White, C. M. "The Nurse-Patient Encounter: Attitudes and Behavior in Action." *Journal of Gerontological Nursing* 3 (May-June 1977): 16–20.

Self-Concept

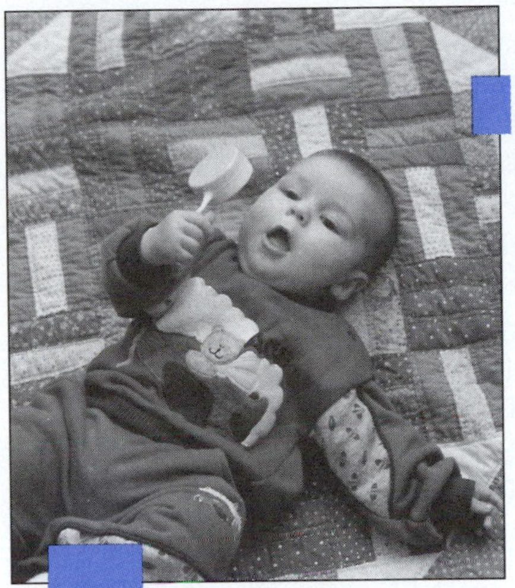

35

Objectives

After completing this chapter, you should be able to:

1. Define self-esteem and describe its development.
2. Identify situations in which self-esteem may be disturbed.
3. Define body image and describe its development.
4. Identify situations in which body image integrity may be disturbed.
5. Define personal identity and describe its development.
6. Identify situations in which personal identity may be disturbed.
7. Assess an individual patient with regard to self-concept including self-esteem, body image, and personal identity.
8. Define a disturbance in self-esteem.
9. Define disturbances of body image integrity.
10. List the five stages of response to disturbances of body image integrity.
11. Define a disturbance in personal identity.
12. Identify interventions to improve self-esteem.
13. List ways to prevent disturbances of body image integrity and to restore integrity if a disturbance occurs.
14. Explain interventions that may be used to support personal identity.
15. Define a disturbance in self-concept and identify situations in which this nursing diagnosis is appropriate.

Study Terms

acceptance
anger
body image
body image integrity
denial
depression
disbelief
kinesthetic feedback
perceptual feedback
verbal feedback
visual feedback
self-concept
self-esteem
shock
stimuli
therapeutic environment

Ellis, Nowlis: Nursing: A Human Needs Approach, 5th ed. © 1994 J.B. Lippincott Company

Outline

Self-concept was defined in Chapter 34 as one's total view of the self—the psychosocial-spiritual-intellectual self as well as the physical self. Self-concept is in a constant state of evolution as a person develops. In this chapter we discuss three areas of self-concept in which disturbances may occur. These are self-esteem, body image, and personal identity. We begin with understanding basic concepts, then look at situations that threaten the integrity of the individual's self-concept, and lastly examine how to use the nursing process in the area of self-concept.

Self-esteem

Self-esteem is the value an individual places on the self. Positive self-esteem is an essential foundation for meeting life's challenges with self-confidence and being willing to try alternatives and risk the possibility of failure. When you have high self-esteem, you see yourself as competent and capable; you see yourself as worth caring for and about.

The Development of Self-esteem

Self-esteem develops primarily from the perceptions you receive of the value others place on you. This begins, of course, in infancy and young childhood. Parents and other caretakers may give a child a sense of intrinsic worth and value through their recognition of the child's strengths, accomplishments, and attempts toward growth. This acceptance teaches the child to look for strengths in the self and to evaluate attempts at growth in a positive light. Additionally, self-esteem develops from your own evaluation of your competence and social acceptance. When you accomplish a task successfully or negotiate an interpersonal relationship successfully, your sense of self-esteem is enhanced.

Adolescence is another critical period in the development of self-esteem. With all the changes taking place and the attempts to adopt new behavior patterns, adolescents may easily evaluate themselves as inadequate and may have low self-esteem. Conversely, adolescents who receive family and societal support for emerging

Nursing Issues and Trends: Self-esteem For Adolescents

Self-esteem as a foundation for youth to engage in effective decision-making has received widespread attention in recent years. It is clear that those lacking self-esteem are less likely to complete their education and more likely to engage in behaviors that are personally detrimental. Schools and community agencies have instituted programs in which adolescents could accomplish tasks that contribute to their positive self-evaluation. But formal programs are not enough; self-esteem is complex and based on a lifetime of experiences and relationships. Adolescents need individual adults in their lives—adults who care and are willing to be involved as they struggle with their emerging identities. The best support for adolescent self-esteem may be support for family from its beginnings and support for parents as they strive to work effectively with their adolescent children.

independence and decision-making develop a positive sense of self.

In the adult as well as in the child and adolescent, self-esteem is enhanced by positive interactions and recognition of abilities and accomplishments. Self-esteem may be damaged by constant criticism and fault-finding. This may lead the individual to be excessively critical of the self and unable to accept any imperfections. Because perfection is unobtainable, an individual with unrealistic expectations of the self has persistently low self-esteem.

Situations That May Disturb Self-esteem

When individuals are faced with health challenges, threats to self-esteem abound. An individual's personal appearance may be affected by such factors as weight loss or weight gain, thinning of hair, changes in skin texture or coloration, and scarring. When this occurs, others may respond in ways that make the person feel less valued. The lack of energy or inability to accomplish tasks may make the person feel that he or she is not a contributing member of the family, the job situation, or community groups.

The older adult often has a decreasing ability to accomplish tasks because of fatigue and physical frailty. As the older adult's concrete contributions to the overall society lessen, the person may feel less worthwhile and self-esteem is damaged. This is often reinforced by a society that does not value the less concrete contributions of the older adult, contributions such as patience, wisdom, a sense of history, and a lifetime of effective problem-solving skills.

Caregivers may also affect a patient's self-esteem in the manner in which care is delivered. You may support self-esteem through positive approaches, avoiding criticism and supporting attempts at growth. When you offer frequent criticism and negative responses without recognizing the person's positive qualities, you may decrease the individual's self-esteem.

Nursing Research: Implications for Practice

Smits, M. W., and Kee, C. C. "Correlates of Self-Care Among the Independent Elderly." *Journal of Gerontological Nursing* 18, 9 (September 1992): 13–18.

The links between self-concept and self-care and between functional health status and self-care were investigated in a group of 48 independently living elders aged 65 and over. A strong, significant relationship was found between self-concept and self-care. No significant relationship was found between functional health status or demographic variables and self-care. These results suggest that the nurse may need to structure intervention to support self-concept as a basis for helping the person develop effective self-care behaviors.

Body Image

Body image was defined in Chapter 34 as a multidimensional view of one's body that considers its appearance, kinesthetic feedback, sensory feedback, and internal feelings. Appearance is the actual look of one's body seen directly and in a mirror. **Kinesthetic feedback** is the perceived location of one's body in relation to its surroundings and the relationship of body parts to one another determined through nervous system impulses received in the brain from the periphery. Sensory feedback is perception of the external environment through the five senses. Internal feelings include the full range of psychological responses to one's own body and appearance.

An individual who has an accurate and flexible body image that changes as the individual changes and who feels comfortable with his or her body is said to have **body image integrity**. Such integrity can be disturbed if the individual persists in viewing the body in a way that is no longer realistic.

Illness frequently causes changes in the body. Because these changes are usually undesirable and often happen suddenly, disturbances in body image integrity are common among ill people. As a nurse, you will need skill in 1) identifying situations in which body image integrity may be threatened, 2) assessing the patient's response to such a situation, and 3) intervening to prevent a disturbance or to help restore body image integrity if a disturbance occurs.

The Development of Body Image

One's body image changes throughout one's life as the body changes and as one's understanding of and feelings about the body change. Body image develops throughout life according to a pattern that roughly corresponds to the patterns of other aspects of development (review Unit 5 on the life span). The individual needs appropriate input at each stage of development to develop body image integrity.

Infancy

The infant is born without a body image. In the womb the infant and the environment are one, and the self is not perceived as a separate entity. The processes that lead to the development of the adult self-image begin at birth (Fig. 35-1).

The infant responds to the *internal* **stimuli** of pain and hunger and does not at first distinguish between them. Gradually the infant begins to identify those feelings of discomfort that are relieved by food and to distinguish them from other feelings. The same process occurs with regard to all other internal stimuli, and as a result the infant learns to trust his or her body and develops an understanding of its signals.

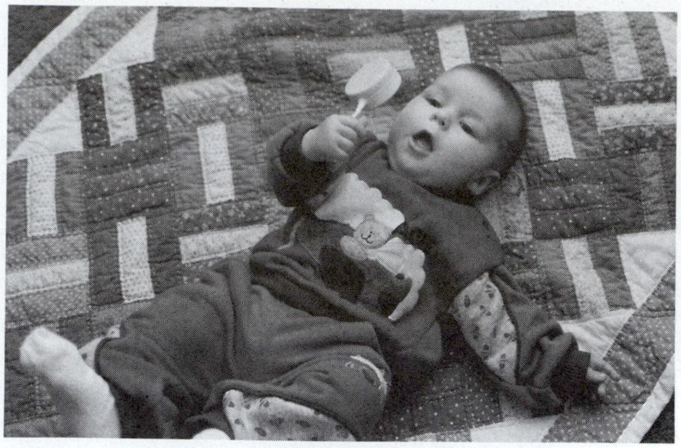

Figure 35-1. An infant must learn the limits of his or her own body.

External stimuli also help infants to identify their own bodies. Little babies sometimes cause themselves pain by biting their own toes, since they cannot distinguish the boundaries between the self and the nonself. The touch of those who care for the infant is central to the process of learning to differentiate self from nonself.

The Toddler

The toddler can distinguish self from nonself, has learned to trust feelings (one hopes), and begins to ascribe value to body parts. Some parts are seen as important, some as pretty, and some perhaps as unmentionable. These values are largely acquired from the people who are significant to the child and from the direct experience of pleasure or pain derived from body parts. The toddler typically perceives the limits of the body as more encompassing than does the adult. For example, feces, urine, fingernails, and hair are considered parts of the body, and their disappearance may be upsetting.

Early Childhood

Along with physical stature, the young child's body image is also changing. The child no longer feels like a baby and may ascribe this term to a younger sibling. Children of this age may see themselves as little adults, the boy pretending to act like his father and the girl imitating the activities of her mother. When there is no same sex role model in the household, the child often looks to others in the environment to identify appropriate ways to walk, talk, and behave.

Middle Childhood

By the time children reach school age, they have become highly aware of others' bodies and begun to make close comparisons between themselves and others. The child may be acutely aware of differences that are not even noted by the adult. Although the child has already begun to learn about the body's functioning at the beginning of this stage, real understanding is not achieved until age 9 or older. Before then, the child's ideas are often inaccurate and may be confused. Both boys and girls of this age group may seek out magazines and books that include pictures of the human body.

Adolescence

The adolescent undergoes many physical changes, both overt and internal, as discussed in Chapter 18. Plenty of physical activity and exercise can help teenagers become more comfortable with their changing bodies.

The changes associated with sexual development give rise to an intense awareness of and preoccupation with one's body. Adolescents often compare themselves with others, exhibit concern about whether or not they are normal, and develop exaggerated modesty. They may spend prolonged periods in front of the mirror and express profound dissatisfaction with their appearance. It is common for adolescents to feel dissatisfied with a particular facial feature—often the nose, which becomes more pronounced as adult features begin to emerge. Acne (pimples and other blemishes), which varies from mild and intermittent to severe and scarring, may cause particular distress. Adolescents with severe acne often withdraw from social contacts.

Adolescents are often confused by their sexual feelings and may control them poorly. There is considerable pressure, exerted through advertising, movies, music, and their peers, on American adolescents to act on their sexual feelings. Those who do not do so, for whatever reasons, may wonder whether they are normal in sexual feelings and function. Menstruation, seminal emissions, and erections at inopportune times can make the adolescent feel that his or her body has become unreliable and a cause for anxiety.

Young Adulthood

The body image of the young adult is deeply influenced by prevailing standards of beauty and value judgments about the body. Society judges appearance in various ways. Efforts to discern character on the basis of appearance have a dubious but long history; the belief that people with "beady" eyes are untrustworthy, for example, originated centuries ago. More recently, psychological studies of body types have been undertaken in an effort to legitimize such folk wisdom, but they have not succeeded in demonstrating a correlation between body and personal characteristics. Stereotyping is nevertheless common. (Health care workers who try not to respond to patients stereotypically sometimes forget that patients may respond to them, in turn, on the basis of stereotypes. Ideally all health care workers would be equally acceptable to a patient, but reassignments must be made if the patient's response to care is affected by his or her attitude to the provider of that care.)

In Western cultures, and especially in the United States, the young, beautiful body is idealized. For women, the standard is a very slim figure and conformity to a rather narrow definition of beauty. The spectrum of what is considered handsome in men is broader; for example, the older man with a slightly portly figure and graying hair may be seen as distinguished. However, height is often equated with leadership ability in men, and studies have shown that the short man may be handicapped in job advancement. (Those elected to the presidency of the United States have tended to be tall men.) These social stereotypes may influence the individual's view of the self. They may also prompt efforts to maintain physical fitness, control weight, and engage in other good health practices to maintain a body that is viewed positively.

Women seem to have clearer and more accurate images of their bodies than do men (Murray, 1972a). They are more acutely aware of physical changes, especially those that affect the face, than are men. Women also tend more to equate body with self; men tend to be less specific in their views of their own bodies and to relate self more to accomplishment and position in life. The women's movement and related phenomena may bring about a convergence of men's and women's attitudes toward their bodies. Pregnancy has a profound effect on a woman's body image. This subject is explored in texts on maternity nursing.

Middle Adulthood

Because of the physical changes occurring in the middle years (see Chapter 19), the body image may become more negative. The body may be perceived as less attractive, less able, and less valuable. The extent of these negative feelings is based on the individual's personality and how satisfactory life has been to this point. Many middle-aged adults see the changes as evidence of maturity and experience and are therefore comfortable with them. Today many middle-aged adults conscientiously work to "keep in shape," thereby avoiding the decreased function that comes from inactivity. Most middle-aged adults adjust gradually to the changes, with some feelings of regret for passing youth and some positive feelings about the values inherent in maturity.

Later Adulthood

The older adult is frequently faced with chronic illness as well as with diminished function and change in appearance. Sensory deficits (decreased hearing and visual acuity) are common in the older adult, and these may lessen the ability to participate in social functions and to enjoy such hobbies as music and reading. These changes are all distressing to the older adult and may lead to feelings of worthlessness and despair over lost abilities. On the other hand, the older adult may make realistic adaptations to decreased function and accept these changes along with the enhanced problem-solving and interpersonal skills that accompany experience, becoming a secure person, able to relate to others and positive in outlook.

Situations That Threaten Body Image Integrity

Some situations in life are particularly threatening to body image integrity. To determine how great the potential is for a problem in a specific situation, you will need to consider both the situation itself and the meaning of the situation to the individual involved.

Failure of Normal Development

Missing out on normal situations and interactions that would contribute to their development makes children prone to interrupted body image development during illness. The child may thus emerge from an illness having made no gains in psychological development. For example, an infant needs appropriate tactile input to learn to distinguish the body from the environment; touch is provided by cuddling, feeding, bathing, and playing with the infant. Insufficient touch retards development. Infants deprived of touch because of illness may still be exploring their own bodies when they should be ready to begin exploring the environment. The infant also needs to learn to identify feelings, such as hunger, that occur in the body. To do so, the infant must feel the discomfort, express it, be fed, and feel satisfaction. If fed according to a schedule without regard to the body's responses, the infant will not learn about them.

Such simple procedures as shaving a body part before surgery can upset a toddler, who considers hair part of the body and does not necessarily recognize it as expendable. The toddler may view an intravenous tube infused to the arm as part of the body and may need help understanding both its placement and its removal. The toddler needs from others an accepting attitude toward touching various body parts; it is important not to label some body parts good and others bad.

School-age children need contact with peers and reassurance that they are normal and acceptable. Lacking such support, they can be expected to suffer self-doubt and become withdrawn. Such children may exhibit behaviors usually associated with a child of a younger age. With an opportunity to engage in experiences that contribute to body image development, they will progress rapidly toward age-appropriate behaviors.

Changes in External Body Appearance

Disturbances in body image integrity can be caused by changes in external body appearance. The person who experiences formation of a scar, hair loss from chemotherapy, loss of a limb, or a colostomy (surgery to open the colon through the abdominal wall) will probably need some support and assistance to maintain body image integrity (Fig. 35-2).

To participate fully in life, one must accept such changes and incorporate them into one's self-image. Difficulty in doing so is a function of the individual's developmental level, previous life experiences, and previous body image. For example, a facial scar may be readily incorporated into the body image, and even worn as a badge of pride, by a young football star. The same scar on a teenage girl might elicit severe depression and cause her to withdraw from normal social life.

Certain changes in body structure are so great that they always cause some degree of problem with body image. Amputation of an extremity, a colostomy, or the removal of a breast can be expected to be a serious stressor to the individual. Those who appear to have no concerns or worries in regard to such a major change are often experiencing denial.

Changes in Body Function

Body image integrity can also be affected by changes in the body's functioning brought about by disease. Lung disease may limit physical activity, a stomach problem may necessitate dietary changes, or a medication may have side effects that include diminished alertness. The

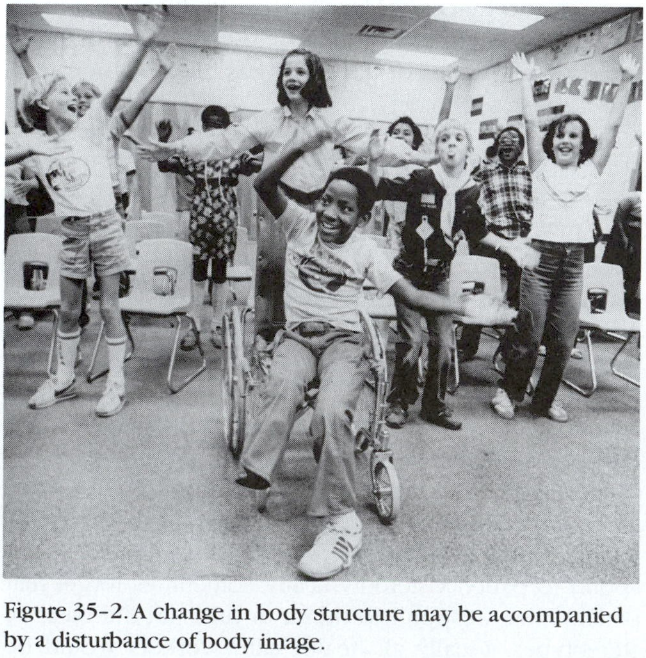

Figure 35-2. A change in body structure may be accompanied by a disturbance of body image.

body does not respond as it previously did and may be less acceptable. Some individuals deny such changes and jeopardize their health by failing to follow prescriptions for activity and diet. Others find the changes so overwhelming that they feel life is no longer meaningful.

Like certain structural changes in the body, certain illnesses cause changes so great that they universally require major life adjustments. Diabetes mellitus, with its demands for change in diet, medication, and lifestyle, is one illness that has a major impact on the life of any individual. Loss of reproductive ability is a concern to a large number of individuals. Loss of ability to function sexually is so great a threat to some that they will choose not to treat a life-threatening disease if the treatment is likely to result in such a disability. The person who is paralyzed by stroke or spinal cord injury suffers such a great change in functional ability that he or she may wonder whether it was worthwhile to have survived the injury.

Loss Associated With Body Changes

A change in the body evokes responses similar to those observed in a dying person who is coping with the total loss of self (see Chapter 41). The person who suffers a major physical change has lost the person he or she used to be and must come to accept and value the new person he or she has become. Although it is not uncommon for the dying person to remain in denial or die angry at the world, such an outcome would be unfortunate for the person with a body change for whom life goes on. The challenge is to find quality and joy in life despite the change.

Shock, Disbelief, and Denial

At first the patient may exhibit **shock**, **disbelief**, and **denial**. For a while, denial may actually be helpful; the patient whose energy is invested in coping with the physical problems of healing may not have adequate resources to cope simultaneously with psychological changes. But if denial persists for a long time and interferes with the patient's ability to participate in his or her own care, skilled psychological help may be needed.

Anger

As the reality of the change is acknowledged, the patient may express **anger**, more often at the world in general than at someone in particular. Such anger is characterized by a "Why me?" attitude. On occasion, anger may be directed at the most accessible targets, the nurse and the family. Although such anger is not really personal, the person at whom it is directed may have difficulty making this distinction, and families may need to talk to someone who understands what they are feeling. If you are the target of anger, you too may need someone with whom to discuss your feelings if you are to continue to function effectively with the patient. It is important that you not reject the patient at this time. Although the patient rejects others, he or she still needs their acceptance to move toward self-acceptance.

Bargaining

Bargaining is less common with body image disturbance than with other types of loss and impending loss. On occasion, a person might engage in bargaining for a period of time. A person with a new colostomy might say, for example, "If I am very careful about how I take care of myself, maybe the doctor will be able to operate and put everything back to normal." Although such bargaining may often be unrealistic, it should be accepted in light of the patient's feelings at the time.

Depression

Anger and bargaining may be followed by severe **depression** as the patient grieves for what was and might have been. Such a patient needs the constant concerned care and presence of others, even when he or she rejects them. Attempting to cheer up a depressed patient is inappropriate. Sitting with the patient in silence, with no expectation of response, may be especially helpful. Touch and other nonverbal forms of communication are particularly important.

Depression may be long lasting in the person with body image change and may be responsible for lack of progress in rehabilitation. The nurse can sometimes help by requiring the depressed person to participate in ordinary activities of daily living, to focus on small daily accomplishments, and not to look too long or too closely at the distant future. A matter-of-fact approach may help the individual to function in the face of depression; he or she should acknowledge the depression but refuse to dwell on it. Depression usually resolves as the person moves toward acceptance of the change (see Chapter 34 for information on supporting the person who is depressed). Skilled psychological counseling may be essential in making it possible for some individuals to make this adjustment.

Acceptance

Gradually the person develops **acceptance** of the new body image. Integrity is restored, and energy can be focused on rehabilitation or returning to the mainstream of life. Therapeutic interaction—to help the patient think about the entire experience, verbalize it, and give it meaning—is most effective at this time.

Health care workers sometimes make the mistake of expecting this entire process to be accomplished rapidly. Time is needed—time with others and time alone. Trying to hurry a person in the development of a new body image may only impede progress.

Personal Identity

Personal identity is the consciousness of oneself as a distinct and unique person. Identity is both consistent and dynamic. The consistent aspect includes a view of the kind of person one is and an attempt to remain consistent with one's values and beliefs. The dynamic aspect reflects the constant change and development that occurs in one's sense of identity.

Identity includes a sense of who one is as a man or woman. It requires an acceptance of that role in life and a view of how it is acted out. Identity also includes a sense of oneself as a sexual being and how that role is lived. Identity enlarges to encompass all the primary roles one plays. Secondary roles are also important in identity. For most individuals, tertiary roles are less central, but the entire identity of some individuals may be focused on a role as a worker or professional (see Chapter 34 for an explanation of roles).

The Development of Personal Identity

Adolescence is the time during which one's personal identity is first established. The adolescent identifies with the peer group and has an identity as a member of that group. This identity includes conforming to group behavior and group norms. In addition, the adolescent identifies with the family and community and looks for a sense of identity to the behavior and norms expected there. Integration of these various views of the personal self is necessary to establish a firm sense of oneself as an independent, unique individual.

As a person progresses into adulthood, additional roles and behaviors are incorporated into the personal identity, particularly in relationship to a job or career resulting in identity expressed as "I am a nurse," or "I am a sales representative." Some individuals may identify the self more closely with an occupation than others.

Primary roles of husband or stepmother, for example, emerge in adulthood and begin to form an important part of identity. Again, some individuals identify themselves more closely with one role than another. For example, the stepmother who has stepchildren living in the home and is the active parental figure in their lives may identify closely with the mothering role. Another individual may marry into a family with grown children. Although this individual is also a stepparent, this role may be insignificant in terms of identity. Whenever an individual adopts new roles in life, a change in personal identity occurs as these roles are incorporated.

Situations That May Disturb Personal Identity

During adolescence, conflict between the various expectations for behavior and a variety of values may make it difficult to establish a sense of personal identity. When illness intervenes during this developmental period, adolescents have increased difficulties in feeling confident of their independent selves. Cultural and social events may cause trouble with personal identity for both adolescents and adults. For the maintenance of personal identity, it is necessary to act on personal values and fulfill the behaviors one expects of oneself. When one's life situation changes and one does not meet one's own expectations for behavior, there may be interference with personal identity.

The loss of roles also causes changes in personal identity. This may happen in childhood, when the birth of a new child displaces an older child from the baby role. These roles ascribed by position in the family change when divorce and remarriage reconfigure the nature of the family. The death of parents causes the loss of the "child" role in a profound way, no matter what the age of the person. An individual who is laid off from a job or who retires must face the loss of the work role. If personal identity was rooted primarily in the occupational role, this change creates serious disruption.

Establishing personal identity may pose significant problems for gay and lesbian adolescents. There are many adverse societal responses to expressions of sexuality that differ from the majority. It is not uncommon for homosexual youth to be rejected by family and friends. Severe depression and even suicide may result.

Assessment

Assessment for all disturbances of mental health was discussed in Chapter 34. Many different factors must be considered in assessment related to self-concept. You will review the individual situation to identify whether aspects of the situation create high risk for problems. You will need to review the developmental level of the individual and the person's occupation and lifestyle. The person's strengths and weaknesses, the behavior the person exhibits, and the comments that reflect the person's perceptions about the self and the situation are also important aspects of your assessment.

Examine the Situation

Assessing the *situation* for its degree of risk to self-concept is the first step. What is the current situation for this individual patient at this time? You will need to closely examine what is happening to the patient and the nature of the illness. Consider the information regarding situations that place the individual at risk. Are any of these situations present for the patient?

Identify the Patient's Developmental Level

The individual's *developmental level* is crucial in all aspects of self-concept. What is the person's age? What are the developmental tasks of the individual at that age? What might be the primary needs and concerns based on that age? What is the evidence that the individual has met developmental tasks in the past? How are these developmental concerns related to the current situation? Is the patient, for example, a young adult just beginning to develop interdependent relationships with the opposite sex? If so, changes perceived as diminishing sexual attractiveness or sexual ability may be especially upsetting. In general, the removal of a uterus is likely to be less upsetting to a woman past childbearing age than to an 18-year-old who has never had a child, although, of course, the individual may differ from any usual expectation.

Explore the Patient's Roles in Life

Another area of concern is the person's *occupation or role*. A singer's throat is important to her, whereas a telephone lineman may consider his legs much more significant. The person whose occupation is sedentary will be less threatened by an illness that necessitates being sedentary than will someone whose previous job involved considerable physical activity. A businesswoman who considers it necessary to entertain frequently may be excessively upset by an ulcer that requires a special diet. Is the person a parent with responsibilities toward children? When a parent is unable to support children in school and community activities, there may be severe loss of self-esteem.

Identify Social Constraints and Supports

Cultural expectations may greatly affect a person's response to any illness. Because of Western society's definition of beauty in women, a woman who loses a great deal of weight might not be too upset. Conversely, Western society tends to equate large size in men with power. A man who associates large size with power might find weight loss to be of greater concern than weight gain.

As you assess the patient, consider his or her *strengths and weaknesses*. What assets will the person be able to bring to bear on the crisis? Some people have developed strength by confronting and successfully coping with previous crises. Others have the support of strong religious beliefs. Always try to meet the family or significant others in the patient's life and to assess their strengths. Some family members may be helpful; others will themselves need assistance in dealing with the crisis. Each individual has some strengths that can be used. A strong support system may enable an individual to cope with changes that could not be managed alone.

Some individuals do not have supportive families and friends. Some are undergoing other major crises in addition to body changes. Problems such as these will need to be considered when you plan for care of the patient.

Assess Individual Responses

When you have considered all of the significant background information, you will then use this to evaluate the responses you see in the patient. The individual's perception and feelings about the problem are primary factors in determining the seriousness of the problem. Statements of thoughts and feelings as well as behavioral responses are all important.

Always keep in mind that it is the person's own *subjective perception* of the situation that most profoundly affects his or her response. To determine how the individual sees the change and how he or she feels about it, an interview is essential. One colostomy patient may express fear that he will be unacceptable to others; another individual recovering from the same surgery may express relief that the colostomy will allow for social activity that was previously impossible because of chronic pain and diarrhea. The person may refuse to discuss the situation or, alternatively, become completely absorbed with it to the exclusion of all other topics.

Sometimes people look at very disfiguring surgery as the only alternative to death. Tierney (1975) found that in such situations the adjustment may move forward more rapidly than the extent of the change would lead one to expect. These individuals have made part of their adjustment before the surgery. The process can be likened to anticipatory grieving for a person who is dying (see Chapter 41).

You will want to encourage the patient to express feelings and thoughts about the situation. What does the patient see as the future consequences of the current illness? How does the patient feel about any changes in ability to function in accustomed roles? Does the patient believe that there are adverse responses from significant people?

If change or loss in body structure or function has occurred, identifying the particular stage the person is experiencing in the process of reestablishing body image integrity will help you to respond in the most helpful way.

Look for objective data. What are the patient's behavior patterns? Look for pacing the floor, chain smoking, and other signs of anxiety. What are the patient's facial expressions? Muscles may be tense and the lips tightly drawn if the person is upset and anxious. The entire face may droop if depression is severe. Does the person's reaction seem appropriate to the situation? For example, laughing and joking about the loss of a leg may indicate a serious problem. Such a loss is a major disability and requires considerable adaptation. Denial of the seriousness of the disability may be a barrier to rehabilitation. Are the behaviors congruent with feelings expressed? Sometimes an individual will state that there is no problem, and yet the behaviors indicate anxiety or distress.

Nursing Diagnosis

The North American Nursing Diagnosis Association (NANDA) has identified three major nursing diagnoses in the area of self-concept. They include Self-esteem Disturbance, Body Image Disturbance, and Personal Identity Disturbance.

Self-esteem Disturbance

The nursing diagnosis of Self-esteem Disturbance indicates that the person places a low value on the self and lacks confidence in his or her own ability to accomplish desired actions. Low self-esteem may be chronic or situational. Chronic Low Self-esteem is the diagnosis when this perception of the self has been in place for a prolonged time, usually many years. The individual responds to most of life's concerns with statements and behaviors that indicate a perception of the self as not capable, not worthwhile, and not likeable or loveable. Situational low self-esteem develops in the context of particular life events and therefore is not an ingrained part of the person's life responses.

Low self-esteem may result in self-destructive behaviors such as alcohol and drug abuse or, in adolescents, running away. The individual may withdraw from social contacts and be reluctant to meet new people. These patients may refuse to participate in their own care because they believe they can't do it right. The individual may make specific statements reflecting low self-worth, such as "I'm not important," "I really don't matter," "I can't do anything right," "Why would anyone care about me anyway."

Nursing Diagnoses Related to Self-Concept

- Situational Low Self-esteem related to inability to manage responsibilities of new infant
- Chronic Low Self-esteem related to family pattern of devaluing accomplishments
- Body Image Disturbance related to facial scars
- Personal Identity Disturbance related to adjustment problems of adolescence
- Self-concept Disturbance related to loss of employment

Body Image Disturbance

Body Image Disturbance is used as a nursing diagnosis when there are specific indications that the individual is experiencing a negative physical self-image. Such indications would include one or more of the following characteristics: a refusal to touch or look at a body part or to look in the mirror, an unwillingness to discuss the change in the body, a refusal to accept rehabilitation, and even denial of the change that has taken place.

Personal Identity Disturbance

A diagnosis of Personal Identity Disturbance indicates that the individual has difficulty in distinguishing between the self and others or feels unsure of his or her own identity. The person may express feelings of insecurity, for example, actually saying "I really don't know who I am anymore!" The person may also express confusion over just where he or she fits into the world. The person may have difficulty in making decisions and may vacillate back and forth, being unsure of what he or she really wants to do. At midlife a person may begin to question what accomplishments he or she has made in life and expresses confusion over identity.

Self-concept Disturbance

The three areas of self-concept mentioned above may be disturbed independently; the result would be those individual nursing diagnoses. However, there are situations when a more widespread or diffuse disturbance, involving self-esteem, body image, and personal identity together, exist. In other situations, self-concept is clearly disturbed, but data are insufficient to determine the specific problem. In working with these situations, many nurses use the nursing diagnosis of Self-concept Disturbance as a broader category, although it does not appear in the current NANDA list. The etiology of this broad nursing diagnosis may be multifaceted. Interventions also may be mixed, with interventions aimed at those behaviors and feelings that are the greatest problem to the individual.

Other Related Nursing Diagnoses

Other nursing diagnoses may be present that relate to the needs that are not met because the person's self-concept is disturbed.

Anxiety related to change in body image is common. The individual may show signs of acute anxiety, as discussed in Chapter 34. Such anxiety may result from feelings of being overwhelmed by the change and by the demands it places on the individual.

Dysfunctional Grieving related to change in body image may occur. The feelings associated with grieving are expected parts of the coping process and thus are not problems in themselves. Dysfunctional grieving occurs when a stage is prolonged and the person is not moving toward resolution of the grief. Grieving may also be considered dysfunctional when the person is not participating in personal care or rehabilitative efforts.

Self-care Deficits related to body change may be present. Major changes in structure or function often interfere with the person's ability to meet his or her own self-care needs. You may find it useful to specify the exact type of self-care deficit present in the individual.

Knowledge Deficit related to body change is a common diagnosis. The patient may obviously lack knowledge about the new skills needed for self-care. Less readily apparent is the person's need to know what is usual or normal. Many individuals are able to relax and give themselves permission to grieve and to adapt slowly if they know that such behavior is not unusual or indicative of weakness of character. Most people have never considered that grieving takes place when a change in a function, such as reproduction, occurs. An example was a man with a major back injury who was advised that he had to give up competitive sports and adopt a lifestyle in which activity was determined by what was or was not good for his back. He had considerable difficulty in adapting to this change and expressed displeasure with himself for having difficulty. He believed that he should have made the adjustment without any fuss. "After all, I am an intelligent man," he stated. After the concept of change in body function and body image and the idea of grieving over the loss of the self who was able to do "everything" were discussed with him, he was able to acknowledge his feelings and give himself permission to grieve.

Planning and Implementation

The desired outcome for a person with any kind of disturbance in self-concept is a modification of the individual's view of the self, increased ability to function, and emotional well-being. These general outcomes, however, are not measurable and so do not provide an adequate foundation for evaluation. You will need to consider what specific behaviors will indicate change in a particular individual.

For the person with low-self esteem, the desired outcome is that of a changed perception of the self and recognition of his or her own value. Most frequently this will be demonstrated by verbal expression of feelings about the self. An absence of statements that downgrade the self would also indicate progress. The desired outcomes you describe will need to be based on identifying changes in the signs and symptoms of low self-esteem that were exhibited by the individual.

Resolution of grieving and reinvestment in life represents a successful outcome of a body image disturbance. Because adjusting to changes in body image is a long-term process, you will usually find it helpful to write short-term outcomes and then review and revise them frequently. Some may be simple, such as "Discusses his new stoma in a matter-of-fact tone of voice" or "Looks at stoma and observes care being given." Other desired outcomes will be more complex, such as those related to the person's providing self-care.

The desired outcome of a disturbance in personal identity is that the individual resolves personal doubts and develops a clear sense of self as an independent person. Again this outcome describes inward feelings and perceptions.

A variety of nursing actions can be taken in regard to any disturbance in self-concept. Additionally, planning intervention requires that you give careful attention to the specific disturbance affecting the patient, that is, self-esteem, body image, or personal identity disturbance. As noted in the assessment section, it is vital for you to understand the patient's own subjective perception of a particular situation to formulate desired outcomes and nursing interventions that will be most effective.

Maintenance of a Therapeutic Environment

A **therapeutic environment** that helps the patient accept the current situation and supports the concept of self as a whole, competent person can be provided by promoting cleanliness, enhancing the patient's personal appearance, and performing other tasks that demonstrate respect. Providing privacy and preserving modesty are also important. Considerations of modesty are sometimes overlooked in the care of children, but they too respond to recognition of their personal modesty. All these measures reinforce the dignity and personal worth of the individual.

Establishment of Trust

The first step in helping another to improve self-concept is to develop a trusting relationship. This relationship will help the individual to feel safe with you and confide in you feelings that he or she may see as inappropriate or inadequate. Trust is established when you are genuine with the patient, expressing only feelings that are real and refraining from stereotyped comments and responses. You must be reliable, that is, when you state you will do something you carry through and do it. Maintaining confidentiality is another important part of trust. When you will share information, you say so and when information will not be shared you are direct about that.

Therapeutic Interaction

The nurse may be able to help the person understand what he or she is feeling through therapeutic interaction. The techniques of interpersonal communication (see Chapter 13) are valuable in this endeavor. One purpose of such interaction is to help the patient explore personal feelings. As the person explores feelings, insight is gained and this sets the stage for growth. Through therapeutic interaction you can assist the patient to make independent decisions about self-care, future plans, and methods of coping.

Identification of Strengths

Emphasizing unimpaired abilities and assets and putting no undue stress on any disabilities may help the person to see themselves in a broader light. Help the patient look for his or her own strengths by reviewing past life accomplishments and relating them to the current situation. When appropriate, remind the patient of previous occasions on which he or she has coped successfully with stress and of the family and friends available for support.

Teaching Family

The family and friends of a patient may deal more effectively with any problematic situation if they are adequately prepared before actually confronting it. It may thus be beneficial to describe the expected body changes or other concerns to the family in advance so they can maintain composure and provide support to the patient (Fig. 35-3). You may also counsel family and friends to help them understand the stages that the patient may experience when there is a body change. Sometimes they may benefit from explanation of the value of a therapeutic environment, trust in supportive others, and support of strengths.

Referral to Support Groups

A wide variety of voluntary organizations are oriented around specific health problems. Within these organiza-

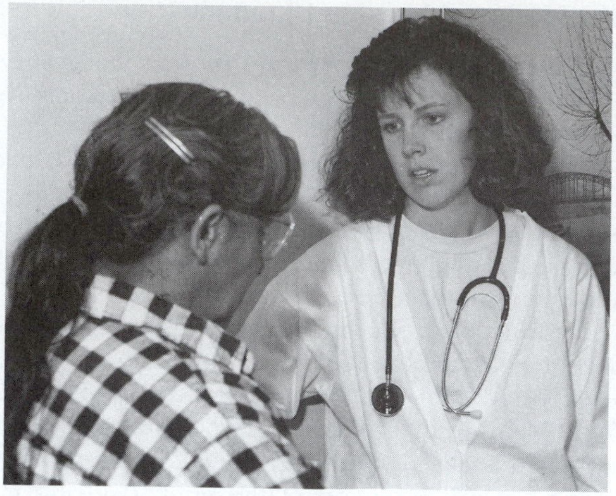

Figure 35-3. Preparing the family for situations they will encounter helps them be supportive to the patient.

tions are people who have confronted their problem with courage and dignity and who have much to offer others in terms of support. The support available from another person who has actually experienced the same or similar problem is different from the support that can be offered by a health professional, no matter how knowledgeable that professional is. For example, Reach For Recovery is an organization of women who have had mastectomies. When a representative visits a woman who has had a mastectomy, she can say, "I understand. I've been there too." In addition, for the person with the new surgery and still unresolved feelings, the visitor provides proof that life can go on and be rewarding and productive (see Appendix E for a list of voluntary organizations).

For any given group you will need to investigate the services offered, the costs involved in receiving services or becoming a member, and whether a physician's approval is necessary for the group to contact the patient. Most organizations that send visitors to the hospital require the physician's approval before they will come. Organizations that have general meetings at which members meet and share concerns and triumphs can usually be joined by anyone who wishes.

Enhancement of Self-esteem

In general, the individual with chronic low self-esteem may need the assistance of an ongoing counselor to resolve problems. You may act to enhance self-esteem in the current situation as discussed below, but referral to an ongoing support agency or staff member will be necessary to resolve the chronic problem.

Situational low self-esteem may be effectively resolved if identified early in the onset of the situation (see sample Nursing Care Plan Related to Low Self-

Nursing Care Plan

Sample Nursing Care Plan Related to Low Self-esteem

Nursing Diagnosis	Situational Low Self-esteem related to feeling unable to cope with care of new infant and toddler. **Supportive data:** Appears disheveled. Home looks unkempt. States, "I guess I just wasn't cut out to be a mother. I'm no good at it. I just can't keep up with things." Has 4-week-old infant who is eating every 3 to 4 hours around the clock. Two-year-old is also in diapers and is less independent than before baby was born.
Desired Patient Outcomes	States she does have strengths and lists two by 4/12. Sets realistic goals for self in relationship to child care by 4/12. Actively participates in at least one social activity by 4/30. Makes statements reflecting positive self-esteem by 5/12.

Nursing Action	Rationale
1. Assess support systems for their effect on her self-esteem and their ability to provide assistance.	Support persons may assist with tasks and lessen the demands placed on an individual.
2. Relate with supportive family members to increase support for her self-esteem.	Supportive family members may provide ongoing help when the health professional is not available.
3. Use facilitating techniques to help her discuss her expectations for self and explore whether these expectations are realistic or helpful.	Unrealistic expectations of the self cannot be attained and undermine self esteem.
4. Encourage her to set realistic goals.	Realistic goals that can be accomplished support self esteem.
5. Reinforce positive statements about self.	Reinforcement tends to cause behavior to continue.
6. Encourage her to plan some time for herself.	Personal time can be used to reduce stress and restore feelings of well-being.

esteem). After a trust relationship is established, you can encourage the person to share feelings. Remember that feelings are real, even when you do not believe they are based in fact. When the person expresses feelings of low self-worth, do not try to change these feelings by rational arguments, for feelings of self-worth are based, not on rational evaluations of the situation, but on individual perceptions arising out of the person's life experiences. You may respond that although the person sees himself or herself in that light, you do not share that perception. This presents an opportunity for the patient to test personal perceptions against those of others. When personal perceptions are not validated, then the individual is more likely to examine them.

In addition to encouraging the expression of the patient's feelings and stating your own perceptions, you will need to demonstrate through behavior that you value the person. You show this by making time for the person, treating concerns as important, and listening without judgment.

Another action that supports self-esteem is structuring experiences that will provide opportunities for the patient to respond in a successful manner. For example, you may give the patient responsibilities for aspects of

Nursing Care Plan

Sample Nursing Care Plan Related to Body Image Disturbance

Nursing Diagnosis	Body Image Disturbance related to feeling associated with total hysterectomy **Supporting data:** Had total hysterectomy 2 weeks ago. Physical recovery is progressing as expected. States has been having mood swings. Is exhibiting anger and depression. Says, "I don't know what is the matter with me. This isn't like me."
Desired Patient Outcomes	**For patient to verbalize understanding of grief:** States grief a normal, expected process after a major change. States grief may take a long time (year) to resolve and even then may occasionally return. **For patient to explore and express feelings over change:** Discusses feelings about hysterectomy and change in reproductive ability.

Nursing Action	Rationale
1. Explain concept of body image and change as related to grieving.	Intellectual understanding may provide a basis for developing coping strategies.
2. Use facilitating techniques to encourage her to discuss grieving and feelings about this change.	Verbalization of feelings assists an individual in coping with those feelings.

self-care. When the person is successful, you can point out the success thereby providing additional perceptional input as to self-worth. Whenever possible, try to recognize and point out instances that demonstrate that the individual is making appropriate decisions, striving for growth, or otherwise acting in positive and responsible ways. Through doing this, you are helping the individual to view the objective information and perhaps to develop a different perception of the self in that situation.

Support for Body Image Integrity

You can help the patient maintain body image integrity in many ways. Most interventions are valuable in preventing problems as well as in dealing with existing ones. Planning ahead for the maintenance of body image integrity may prevent the patient from experiencing severe difficulties (see sample Nursing Care Plan Related to Body Image Disturbance).

Anticipatory Interaction

When a body change is planned in advance, as is the case with surgeries, interactions in anticipation of the change can be planned. You might encourage the person to discuss feelings about the illness, about the change, and about coping. You would acknowledge feelings of anger, depression, and anxiety as normal or realistic. Such responses help the person to see himself or herself as an "OK" person. You would try to promote a positive self-concept by reinforcing feelings of being able to cope successfully and emphasizing the strengths the person brings to the situation. You may do this by helping the person to identify and then describe previous successful coping with difficult life situations. Thus, the adjustment to the change begins before the actual event.

Health Teaching Regarding Body Changes

Health teaching will focus on helping the individual understand the anatomy and physiology of any change that will occur. Explanations of changes in functioning should be at a level of sophistication appropriate to the patient. Such explanations should note possible changes in sensations and the effects that treatments and medications will have on functioning. Mistaken ideas often add greatly to the patient's fears and burdens.

Patient education will also be important after the change has occurred. There is a fine line between adequate preparation and frightening disclosures the patient is not ready for. The individual's response must be your guide in making the distinction. For example, a young woman refused to look at her colostomy for days after the surgery and would not consider learning to care for it herself. A nurse assessing the situation learned that the patient was envisioning a "horrible black mess" and explained that the colostomy is a rosy pink mucous membrane approximately 2 inches in diameter. The patient then looked at her colostomy, found it was not as bad as she had expected, and began learning self-care.

Keep in mind that learning information, although important, is not the main factor in an individual's change of attitude or belief. Therapeutic interaction described above will help the person to cope directly with feelings.

Providing Feedback

By avoiding an exclusive focus on one part of the body, you may help the patient retain a broad perspective on the self. If, on the other hand, everyone who contacts the patient is interested only in his or her bowel function, the patient, too, will focus on that alone. **Perceptual feedback** such as touching a scar or the stump of an amputated arm can provide valuable sensory input. Encouraging active movement of a changed part, such as an arm affected by a stroke, will provide for *kinesthetic feedback*. When active movement is not possible, passive movement (movement whose energy is provided by another person) is helpful. **Visual feedback** by means of mirrors allows the patient to face reality and not be overwhelmed by exaggerated imaginings. Feedback must be appropriate to the individual's level of development.

Verbal feedback on the movements being performed is valuable in establishing understanding of the body's new feelings. For example, while exercising a patient's leg, you may state, "Now I am bending your knee. Now I am straightening it out."

Facilitation of Insight and Understanding

The person experiencing a disturbance in personal identity needs opportunities to explore personal feelings and beliefs. Through talking with another, the individual is encouraged to explore, sort through, and make decisions relative to values. The person also needs opportunities to make decisions regarding the roles he or she chooses to assume. This is done through examining the various roles currently being experienced, determining whether or not those are desired roles, and then examining the behaviors within those roles that are consistent with the person's own values and beliefs. The objective is for the individual to say clearly, "This is who I am, what I believe, and how I will behave."

Evaluation

To effectively evaluate the person's responses in relationship to self-concept you will want to consider the particular nursing diagnosis and the desired outcomes you previously identified. You will observe for changes in feelings about the self or altered behavior in response to those feelings. Specific behaviors or statements of the individual that would demonstrate feelings are a necessary base for effective evaluation.

As is always the case, you will be comparing the desired outcomes with the actual results. In addition you will be identifying whether the patient is beginning to make some progress in relationship to the problem. Difficulties with such matters as self-esteem, body image, or personal identity rarely are resolved in a short time. Usually you will be looking for evidence that the patient has begun working on resolution of such problems.

Nursing Care Study
A Patient with a Disturbance of Body-Image

Eleanor Jacal, a student in a Fundamentals of Nursing course, is assigned Mrs. Katherine Meindl, age 48, who had a left mastectomy 3 days previously. In preparing to care for this patient, Eleanor notes the following:

1. A mastectomy involves removal of the entire breast.
2. A mastectomy is usually performed for a malignancy of the breast and there is likely to be considerable concern about the potential spread of malignancy.
3. Although mastectomy is extensive surgery, the patient usually is ambulating and performing self-care by the fourth postoperative day.
4. Movement of the arm on the operated side is usually ordered by the surgeon, and exercises are usually started in the postoperative period.

(continued)

Nursing Care Study (continued)
A Patient with a Disturbance of Body-Image

5. It is usual for the mastectomy patient to be upset about this change in body structure. She often feels a loss of femininity and concern over the response of significant family member, expecially her sexual partner. Depression is common.

In making her plans, Eleanor anticipates spending a great deal time with Mrs. Meindl, who will probably be sad and need support.

When Eleanor enters Mrs. Meindl's room the next morning, she is surprised to see a woman in a beautiful bed jacket, hair perfectly arranged and makeup expertly applied, although it is only 7:30 AM. Mrs. Meindl greets her with a smile and says, "I'm sure having a student will be fun. Of course, I'm not really a sick patient, so you won't have much to do." This is not at all the response Eleanor expected. She wonders if Mrs. Meindl is just an exceptionally well-adjusted woman.

When the surgeon arrives to change the dressings, Mrs. Meindl says, "You do what you must—I'm really not interested. Eleanor and I will just continue our chat." Mrs. Meindl looks the other way and ignores the surgeon's comments throughout the dressing change.

Later, when Eleanor is discussing with Mrs. Meindl her plans after leaving the hospital, the patient states that she expects to begin her old activities immediately. "You see, my daughter will be coming home from college for vacation. She doesn't know I've had surgery. I don't want her to know that she has only half a mother."

Ths staff nurse visits during the morning to say, "Mrs. Meindl, often women who have had a mastectomy wonder about the various kinds of breast prostheses available. There is an organization called Reach to Recovery made up of women who have had mastectomies. A member of that group would be glad to visit and would be able to discuss this with you."

"No!" Mrs. Meindl almost shouts. "I—I mean, no, thank you, I'm not interested," she continues, in a calmer tone of voice.

As Eleanor is preparing to report off to the team leader at noon, she reviews the assessment data she believes is significant.

1. Mrs. M. appeared cheerful and outgoing on first contact.
2. She refused to look at the surgical incision or to listen to the surgeon's discussion of the surgery.
3. Mrs. M.'s plans are to take up her former activities without a recuperative period. This is not realistic.
4. She has kept the operation a secret from a college-age daughter
5. She had called herself "half a mother."
6. Mrs. M. Appeared upset when a Reach to Recovery visitor was suggested.

Eleanor decides that Mrs. Meindl has a problem of body image integrity because she is not discussing or showing evidence of facing the physical change in any way and her emotional response to the problem appears to be interfering with her ability to be realistic about her care.

Because Eleanor will not be caring for Mrs. Meindl during the rest of her hospital stay, she decides to report her findings to the team leader. The team leader says, "I've been concerned about Mrs. Meindl. Her cheerfulness is too good to be true. After all, any surgery is serious and her attitude doesn't seem very realistic. I appreciate the specific information you've been able to give me. I do agree with your analysis of the problem. During our team conference this afternoon, we can bring this problem to the attention of the entire team and develop a plan for helping Mrs. Meindl.

The student nurse had researched background information, collected data on the patient, and analyzed the data, determining that a problem exists. In considering a plan of action, she recognizes her own limitations and reports her concerns to someone with the skill and opportunity to act. The process of assisting Mrs. Meindl with her problem has begun.

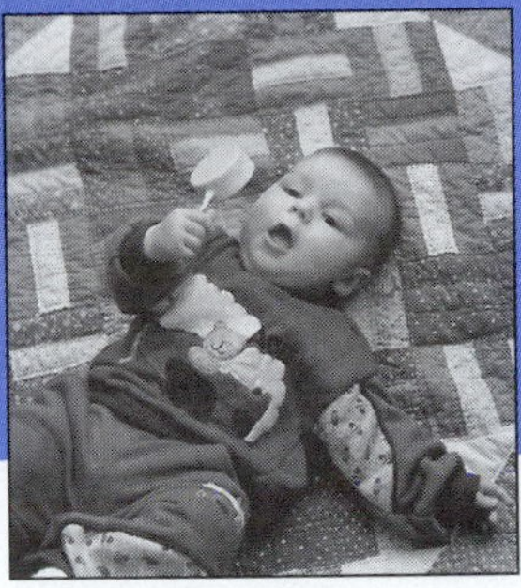

Key Points

- Body image is a multidimensional view of one's body that considers its appearance, kinesthetic feedback, sensory feedback, and internal feelings.
- Body image develops throughout the life span as the body grows and develops.
- The individual who experiences a change of body structure or function commonly moves through the same stages as the dying person from shock, disbelief, and denial through acceptance.
- Personal identity is the consciousness of oneself as a distinct and unique person, including one's sense of values, one's role as a man or woman and as a sexual being. It involves both identifying with some behaviors and norms and rejecting others.
- Identity continues to develop during life. Factors in development and in life situations may affect one's sense of personal identity.
- Assessment for self-concept includes gathering information related to the current situation and the individual's developmental level, consideration of cultural expectations, the person's roles in life, and the social support systems available. This background information is integrated with information about the individual's strengths and weaknesses, behavioral responses, and individual perceptions.
- Disturbance in self-esteem indicates that the person places a low value on the self and lacks confidence in his or her own ability to accomplish desired actions. This may be related to the specific situation or may be chronic.
- A disturbance in body image may be related to a failure of normal development, changes in external body appearance, or a change in body function. A disturbance in personal identity indicates that the individual has difficulty in distinguishing between the self and others or feels unsure of his or her own identity.
- A general nursing diagnosis of Self-concept Disturbance is used when the specific problem is still unclear or when several factors are intermingled. In addition, there are several nursing diagnoses that might be related to the self-concept problems such as Anxiety and Ineffective Individual Coping.
- Helping to improve any problem with self-concept begins with providing a therapeutic environment, establishing trust, using therapeutic interaction, emphasizing strengths, and mobilizing social support systems.
- To enhance self-esteem, the nurse can structure experiences that will provide positive evaluations of the self and point out abilities in self care and indications of effective problem-solving.
- Body image integrity may be supported by providing anticipatory interaction before the change occurs and providing perceptual and verbal feedback to help the person integrate the body change.
- A person must determine his or her own identity; one way to help do so is talking about it with a concerned listener. The listener can also help the person explore values and beliefs and identify those behaviors that are consistent with them.
- Successful resolution of disturbances in self-concept includes restructuring feelings and thoughts about the self. Appropriate outcome criteria define specific behaviors that indicate changes in feelings or thoughts and planning regarding the future.

Study Questions

1. What are the various components of self-concept?
2. Describe the development of self-concept.
3. Outline how you would assess an individual in relationship to self-concept.
4. Describe the nursing diagnoses related to self-concept.
5. List three types of situations that might cause a disturbance in body image?
6. What stage might a person be in if, after having a leg amputated, he laughs and states, "This isn't a problem. I'll be running with the best of them next year."
7. What nursing interventions might help an individual with a disturbance of body image?
8. What nursing interventions might help an individual with low self-esteem?
9. What nursing interventions might assist an individual with a disturbance in personal identity?
10. Describe desired outcomes for individuals with any disturbance in self-concept.

Critical Thinking Activities

1. List as many of your own physical characteristics as you can. Consider your appearance, sensations, and

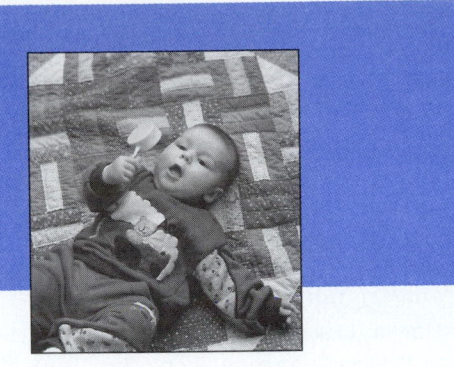

kinesthetic sense. Then identify those you believe to be your best features. Evaluate your own body image integrity.

2. Review the patients on a hospital unit, possibly during morning report. List those you consider prone to a disturbance in body image. Be prepared to discuss the reasons for your choice with your clinical group.
3. For a patient in the clinical area whom you have identified as suffering from a disturbance of body image, outline the appropriate nursing process. Include assessment, goal, plan for intervention, and evaluation.

References and Readings

Antonucci, T. C. "Physical Health and Self-esteem." *Family and Community Health* 6, 2 (August 1983): 1–10.

Blaesing, S., and Brockhaus, J. "The Development of Body Image in the Child." *Nursing Clinics of North America* 7 (December 1972): 597–607.

Bucy, N., Unruh, I., and McFadden, G. A. "Lead Your Maimed Patient Back to Independence." *RN* 40 (June 1977): 29–33.

Compton, C. Y. "War Injury: Identity Crisis for Young Men." *Nursing Clinics of North America* 8 (March 1973): 53–66.

Corbeil, M. "The Nursing Process for a Patient with a Body Image Disturbance." *Nursing Clinics of North America* 6 (March 1971): 155–163.

Craft, C. A. "Body Image and Obesity." *Nursing Clinics of North America* 7 (December 1972): 677.

Crouch, M. A., and Straub, V. "Enhancement of Self-esteem in Adults." *Family and Community Health* 6, 2 (August 1983): 65–78.

Dempsey, M. O. "The Development of Body Image in the Adolescent." *Nursing Clinics of North America* 7 (December 1972): 609–615.

Erikson, E. *Identity and the Life Cycle* (Reissue). New York: W. W. Norton, 1959 and 1980.

Fujita, M. "The Impact of Illness or Surgery on the Body Image of a Child." *Nursing Clinics of North America* 7 (December 1972): 641.

Gallagher, A. M. "Body Image Changes in the Patient with a Colostomy." *Nursing Clinics of North America* 7 (December 1972): 669–676.

Gilberts, R. "The Evaluation of Self-esteem." *Family and Community Health* 6, 2 (August 1983): 29–49.

Hill, S. "The Child with Ambiguous Genitalia." *American Journal of Nursing* 77 (May 1977): 810–814.

Honess, T., and Yardley, K. (Eds.). *The Self and Identity.* London: Routledge & Kegan/Paul, 1987.

Husted, G. L., Miller, M. C., and Wilczynski, E. M. "5 Ways To Build Your Self-Esteem" *Nursing '90* 20, 5 (May 1990): 152, 154.

Leonard, B. J. "Body Image Changes in Chronic Illness." *Nursing Clinics of North America* 7 (December 1972): 687–695.

Loxley, A. K. "The Emotional Toll of Crippling Deformity." *American Journal of Nursing* 72 (1972): 1839–1840.

McCloskey, J. C."How to Make the Most of Body Image Theory in Nursing Practice." *Nursing '76* 6 (May 1976): 68–72.

Miles, M. S. "Body Integrity Fears in the Toddler." *Nursing Clinics of North America* 4 (March 1969): 39–51.

Murray, R. L. "Body Image Development in Adulthood." *Nursing Clinics of North America* 7 (December 1972a): 651–660.

———. "Principles of Nursing Intervention for the Adult Patient with Body Image Changes." *Nursing Clinics of North America* 7 (December 1972b): 697–707.

Nev, C. "Coping with Newly Diagnosed Blindness." *American Journal of Nursing* 75 (1975): 2161–2163.

Norris, J., and Kunes-Connell, M. "Self-esteem Disturbance" *Nursing Clinics of North America* 20, 4 (December 1985): 745–761.

Riddle, I. "Nursing Intervention to Promote Body Image Integrity in Children." *Nursing Clinics of North America* 7 (December 1972): 651–661.

Robinson, K. M. "A Social Skills Training Program for Adult Caregivers." *Advances in Nursing Science* 10, 2 (January 1988): 40–58.

Smith, C. A."Body Image Changes after Myocardial Infarction." *Nursing Clinics of North America* 7 (December 1972): 663.

Smits, M. W., and Kee, C. C. "Correlates of Self-care among the Independent Elderly." *Journal of Gerontological Nursing* 18, 9 (September 1992): 13–18.

Stanwyck, D. J. "Self-esteem through the Life Span." *Family and Community Health* 6, 2 (August 1983): 11–27.

Taft, L. B. "Self-esteem in Later Life: A Nursing Perspective." *Advances in Nursing Science* 8, 1 (October 1985): 77–84.

Thorne, S. E., and Robinson, C. A. "Reciprocal Trust in Health Care Relationships." *Journal of Advanced Nursing* 13, (1988): 782–789.

Tierney, E. A. "Accepting Disfigurement When Death is the Alternative." *American Journal of Nursing* 75 (December 1975): 2149–2150.

Whitbourne, S. K. *The Me I Know: A Study of Adult Identity.* New York: Springer-Verlag, 1986.

Values and Beliefs

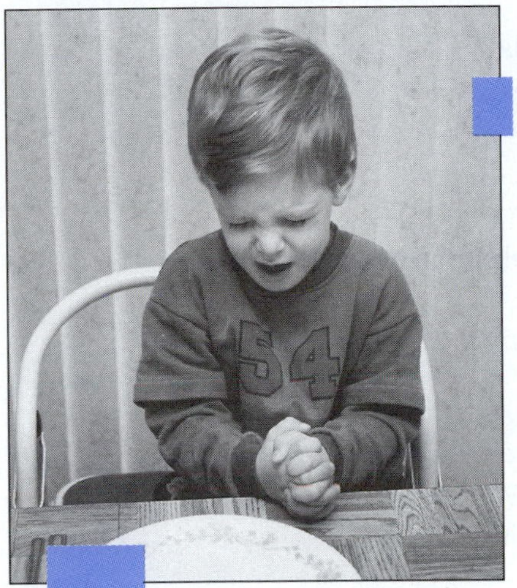

36

Objectives

After completing this chapter, you should be able to:

1. Identify common cultural values and discuss the ways in which they might affect health care.
2. Explain beliefs that might enhance health care and healing and those beliefs that might interfere with health care and healing.
3. Outline the major aspects of religious development.
4. Outline the major features that directly affect health care in the following religions: Roman Catholicism, Protestantism, Eastern Orthodoxy, Judaism, Islam, Hinduism, Buddhism, Animism.
5. Describe data to be gathered to identify spiritual distress, hopelessness, and powerlessness.
6. List the various resources that the nurse might use to assist in meeting the patient's needs relative to values and beliefs.
7. Discuss actions the nurse might take to help meet a patient's needs related to values and beliefs.

Study Terms

agnostic
Animism
Anointing of the Sick
atheist
belief
Buddhism
chaplain
Eastern Orthodoxy
elder
Hinduism
hopelessness
Islam
Judaism
laity
leisure ethic
Muslim
powerlessness
Protestantism
Roman Catholicism
rosary
values

Outline

Cultural Values Related to Health Care

Individuality Versus Community
Competition Versus Cooperation
Present Orientation Versus Future Orientation
Work Ethic Versus Leisure Ethic

Spiritual Beliefs and Health Care

Beliefs That Enhance Health and Healing
  Caring by God
  Life After Death
  Supernatural Healing
  Responsibility for Others
  Relief of Stress
  Effectiveness of Own Actions
  Respect for the Living Body
Beliefs That Interfere With Health Care
  Illness as Punishment
  Illness as Self-caused

Ellis, Nowlis: Nursing: A Human Needs Approach, 5th ed. © 1994 J.B. Lippincott Company

Recognition of the importance of that realm of life that deals with the inner spirit and humanity of the individual is central to an understanding of the total person. This inner life revolves around the beliefs and values of the individual. A **belief** is something that one places trust in and one accepts as true. **Values** are principles or standards of life that are highly prized. Beliefs and values may be based on an organized religious framework that focuses on beliefs about a supreme being and mankind's relationship to that being. Beliefs and values may also be based on a philosophical system unrelated to religion. For example, cultural values arising from a commitment to the free-enterprise system or a belief in the importance of hard work may be fundamental to the ways in which some people lead their lives. Whatever their source, beliefs and values are essential to effective human functioning.

Spiritual beliefs involve one's view of the meaning of life and one's place in the world. The spiritual aspect of life encompasses one's beliefs about who or what controls life and whether or not there is control. When one believes in God or a controlling force, then spiritual beliefs determine one's relationship with God or the controlling force. Spiritual beliefs are also a basis for one's beliefs about relationships with other people and one's responsibilities toward others.

Although most individuals learn values in their primary group or family, other values are assimilated from the culture or are embodied in religions that may not be explicitly taught in the family. Part of the search for identity in adolescence involves identifying those values that one will use to guide one's life. Identifying one's own values and finding meaning in life are essential to growth and development. For some people this search for values continues throughout life in the form of a careful examination of choices to be made.

Some people in scientific disciplines overlook or ignore the spiritual sphere of life in an effort to be objective. Nurses' efforts to care for the whole person, however, lead them to a recognition of the importance of values and beliefs and the spiritual dimension in life. The nurse's role is not to change the person, but to support the individual in achieving a sense of inner integrity.

Cultural Values Related to Health Care

Each individual holds personal values that affect his or her response to health care. These values frequently reflect the values of the society in which the person lives. Some individuals hold the values of a subgroup within society rather than those of the overall society. When the values an individual holds are different from the values of the caregivers, conflict may result. Health care professionals sometimes fail to understand that there is not a correct and an incorrect way of living but differing sets of values about ways of living. All sets of values have problems; all have strengths. The role of the health care provider is not to change an individual's values but to provide care that is congruent with those values.

The values discussed below are not necessarily held to the extreme or in isolation by any one individual. Often one individual holds competing values and the situation determines which one is acted on at a given time. Examining the opposite poles of a value will help you to better understand an individual who responds in a way different from what you would expect.

Individuality Versus Community

In Western society today, a strong value is placed on individuality and autonomy. Western culture encourages young people to move toward more independent modes of living and traditionally has frowned on the young person who continues to live in the family group into young adulthood. This has changed somewhat as economic problems have made it harder for individuals just beginning work life to financially manage independent life. Individuals are encouraged to make their own decisions and not to rely on others in decision-making. They are encouraged to make choices based on what is best for them as individuals.

Many people fail to perceive that the value on individuality is culturally rooted. In many cultures, such as in traditional Japan, the common group is valued more highly than the individual. This common group is usually the family. The individual is expected to live within the family group, sometimes even after marriage. Decisions are not made independently, but by the group as a whole, which especially relies on the older members of the family. Decisions are based not on what is best for the individual, but on what is best for the family group. The practice of viewing the group as more important than the individual may extend into schools and employment settings. *Community-based values* may conflict with the values of most health care providers in Western society.

Competition Versus Cooperation

Competitive behavior in which one person strives to be better than or attain more than another is highly regarded in most of Western society. *Competition* is often used to motivate people toward desirable goals. Prizes go to those who excel in competition and their achievements are celebrated. Not all people value competition, however. Competition may separate people and decrease the sharing of solutions to problems. Some individuals value *cooperation* and frown on evidence of competitive behavior. When confronted with people who do not value competition, you will want to devise motivational strategies that do not rely on a competitive spirit.

Present Orientation Versus Future Orientation

People who value a *future orientation* are motivated to put off current pleasure or comfort for the sake of future goals. Such people will tend to tolerate discomfort caused by treatment modalities or the side effects of drugs in the hope that the future will be different from the present. A strong future orientation may make an individual less committed to making changes for the sake of life in the present if you cannot offer a future (as in the case of the person with a terminal illness); hopelessness may occur.

The person who places high value on the present situation and is not motivated to worry about the future may not be willing to continue with health care medications and treatments that produce side effects or discomfort. This person may not wish to put off current pleasure for the promise of a future change. On the other hand, the present-oriented person may adapt well to a situation in which the future is uncertain. This person may find joy and pleasure in today's life regardless of what the future holds.

Work Ethic Versus Leisure Ethic

Historically the United States has been noted for a *work ethic*, a value system in which work is considered intrinsically valuable and an end in itself. From this value system arises the view that one should always do one's best in a job. A commonly used saying is "If it is worth doing at all, it is worth doing well." Pride in one's work and identification of oneself with an occupation accompany a work ethic. When asked to describe the self, a person operating within this framework will start by describing his or her occupation. For this individual, vacations may actually produce stress because the time spent is viewed as unproductive. A severe loss of self-esteem may accompany the loss of ability to work.

Other people see work as only a means to an end, that is, one works to be able to do something else. An individual who believes in a **leisure ethic** finds identity outside the workplace. Leisure time and the variety of experiences it permits are prized. This person may choose to work fewer hours or at a less demanding job to allow time to engage in leisure pursuits. A person subscribing to the leisure ethic would not choose to work if he or she could acquire sufficient income without working.

Individuals holding these two different value systems with regard to work often disagree about basic goals and directions. When a nurse with one orientation toward work cares for a patient with another orientation toward work, the nurse may have difficulty formulating patient-centered goals.

Spiritual Beliefs and Health Care

Folk cultures believe that spiritual forces are responsible for illness and for recovery or nonrecovery. In such cultures, the role of healer is combined with that of spiritual or religious adviser. Only in modern society have these two spheres of life been separated—a separation that involves losses and hazards for the ill person.

For many years the focus of medical research was on finding a single causative agent for each illness. This yielded important results in the field of infectious disease. However, this approach has proven inadequate to understanding the chronic illnesses that are now our major health problems. The modern study of illness focuses on multiple causes and individual susceptibility to the processes of illness. The better nurses understand the implications of this knowledge, the better able they will be to understand the importance of people's spiritual needs.

Beliefs That Enhance Health and Healing

Many people derive from their spiritual beliefs comfort and inner strength that help them to cope with illness. Religious beliefs sustain a person who is facing death. The force and value of personal faith should not be underestimated.

Spiritual belief is by no means limited to members of formal religions. Many people believe in the existence of God without necessarily subscribing to any particular faith's view of the nature of God. Others do not believe in God, but have a guiding philosophy of life. Many such people have highly developed personal beliefs about the meaning of life and ethical behavior.

Caring by God

A belief that God cares about an individual may support feelings of self-esteem. An individual may be able to tolerate separation from other people and even animosity from others because of this belief. An individual who believes in God's care will often state that he or she is not alone and has the help of God in facing problems.

Life After Death

A belief in a life after death may help patients and families who are facing terminal illness. They may be confident that the pain, distress, and disability of this life will end and that there will be well-being and closeness to loved ones in the hereafter. Those who believe in reincarnation may feel that their life here will be rewarded with an enhanced life to come.

Supernatural Healing

A belief in supernatural healing may help people to maintain hope and a positive outlook in the face of major illness. This belief can be a problem if it interferes with seeking or carrying out health care regimens. For many individuals, however, divine healing is sought while conventional medical care is being carried out. A large supportive group, such as a congregation, may be actively involved in prayer and support for the individual. Such prayer and support sustain the spirits and mental health of the person.

Responsibility for Others

Members of many religious groups feel a strong sense of responsibility for one another. Group members will often offer concrete assistance to the person who is ill, taking care of children at home, making frequent visits to the patient, and providing household help after discharge. Some groups, such as the Mormons, provide financial assistance as well because they do not believe in using government welfare systems. These social support systems sustain people through extraordinarily difficult times and often make it possible for individuals to return to independent living.

Relief of Stress

Many individuals with strong religious beliefs find relief from anxiety and stress in the practice of religious rituals and prayer and in the reading of Scripture. They are able to look beyond the immediate situation to what they see as eternal truths and values, and in this they find inner peace. This relief of stress, in turn, allows energy to be focused on problem-solving in relationship to health needs and on the tasks of healing.

Effectiveness of Own Actions

Some individuals believe that their own actions can be effective in changing their lives and their health status. This belief leads people to make changes in their lives and to learn how to care for themselves. A person with this basic belief will accept responsibility for diet, medications, and even complex care regimens in the expectation of preserving or attaining health. A parent with this belief will be open to learning effective parenting techniques to enhance the well-being of children. An older adult with this belief will enter enthusiastically into a rehabilitation program after hip replacement surgery. This belief provides the motivation for ongoing effort in difficult tasks.

Respect for the Living Body

Those who see the living human body as a unique, special entity that should be treated with care and concern are motivated to adopt good health care practices. They try to avoid those habits, such as smoking, known to be detrimental to the body. They are likely to adopt a lifestyle that includes regular exercise and attention to correct diet.

Beliefs That Interfere With Health Care

Some beliefs may prevent people from seeking health care or consenting to treatment. These beliefs may create conflict with health care providers who are asking patients to participate in their own care and recovery.

Illness as Punishment

The view of illness as punishment can be a barrier to effective health care. When those who adhere to such a belief are ill, their psychological status is likely to be at a low ebb; self-esteem is greatly diminished by guilt. Lowered self-esteem may in turn discourage the person from seeking health care or complying with the medical regimen. The individual may view the outcome of illness as dependent on the ability to identify and remedy wrongdoing. If this is not possible, the person may lose all motivation for health care. Guilt and low self-esteem may lead to depression, which interferes with healing.

This belief system presents a difficult dilemma for the health care worker. How can you interact with individuals to enhance their self-esteem and willingness to participate in care without interfering with their personal religious beliefs? One approach would be to help the person to think through his or her life and to focus on the positive roles he or she fills, such as wife or husband. Therapeutic techniques would be useful in such a situation. A member of the clergy might also be able to offer valuable guidance in such a situation.

Preschool and school-age children are likely to view illness as punishment, less because of religious teaching than because of the concrete interpretation of right and wrong typical of this age group. If you encounter this belief in a child, consult the child's parents to learn whether the belief has a religious component. You might say to the child, "From what I know about being sick, I don't believe it happens because you are bad," and then provide for the kind of open interaction that allows for discussion of the child's belief. You might also use a pragmatic approach such as encouraging a child to do all that is within his or her control to get better.

Illness as Self-caused

Some people believe that wellness is a person's natural state and that illness results from incorrect living and lack of religious faith. Christian Scientists, for example, do not seek health care from the conventional health care system. When illness strikes, they seek instead to strengthen their religious faith and purify their way of living. They may seek out a special religious healer to work with them in their efforts.

When those who believe they have caused their own illness do enter the conventional health care system, it is often with feelings of failure and a continuing reluctance to accept health care technology. Staff members often have difficulty accepting patients who do not willingly comply with treatment, but a supportive and accepting attitude on the part of the staff is essential to raise the self-esteem of these patients and to encourage them to engage in future interactions with health care providers.

Prohibition Against Blood or Blood Product Use

One of the most widely known restrictions on health care is the Jehovah's Witnesses' prohibition of the use of any blood or blood product as a part of care. This prohibition is based on their interpretation of the Bible. In the belief that violating this prohibition will result in God's punishment, Jehovah's Witnesses choose to die rather than accept a blood transfusion or the administration of blood products. When the patient is an adult, health care workers, even though they may be distressed by this position, must work diligently to be accepting of the patient's belief. When a child is involved, society—that is, the law—takes a different position. When a blood transfusion or blood product administration is considered essential to the survival of the child, a physician and hospital may take the case to the court. The court may then assume custody of the child for purposes of medical care and order the transfusion. The reasoning behind this approach is that the child's life should not be jeopardized when he or she is too young to make an independent commitment to a particular religious faith. In the case of an adolescent, however, the courts may be reluctant to intervene.

Trust in Miraculous Cures

As professionals trained in the sciences, nurses must be careful not to dismiss without thought the possibility that spontaneous remissions and cures can occur even

Nursing Issues and Trends: *Spiritual Beliefs and Health Care in Conflict*

What is the nurse's role when an individual's belief system comes into conflict with the health care system? When an individual refuses life-sustaining care based on religious convictions, should the nurse continue to be an advocate for that person's right to decide? Or should the nurse take the role of knowledgeable health care provider and try to help the individual to a new and different perception of meaning and value in life? When an actual situation arises, nurses may feel tremendous conflict and have difficulty determining what action to take. Who will serve as the support for the nurse and his or her individual values in that situation? The need for support for workers in health care increases as the potential for values conflict rises.

when objective evidence indicates a condition is irreversible. Although rare, there are, indeed, documented instances of spontaneous remission of many different types of illness. Belief in the possibility of such an occurrence is sustaining for many people.

At times, however, this belief prompts patients to abandon medical care. When health care workers become adversaries of a patient's belief system, trust may be destroyed. If, however, caregivers demonstrate respect for the patient and acceptance of the person's beliefs, it may be possible to encourage the patient to continue medical care while hoping for a miraculous cure.

Fate as Unchangeable

Some people strongly believe that life is predetermined and that changing one's fate or destiny in life is impossible. Although this belief may result in a calm acceptance of problems, it may also lead to a lack of attention to care and a reluctance to work at wellness. This belief may also lead to despair because it provides no avenue through which the individual can change what might happen. A sense of powerlessness may become a serious problem for this individual.

Religious Development

Religious development is difficult to characterize because it is so diverse. Much depends on what the individual is taught in childhood and on the importance of religion in the life of the family. Nevertheless, a general pattern can be discerned and correlated with the stages of cognitive and moral development.

Infants and Toddlers

Infants and toddlers are not yet able to think abstractly. Young toddlers can be taught to imitate adult actions, such as bowing the head and folding the hands in prayer. Toddlers are acutely responsive to the feeling associated with religious practices. If the family's attitude toward their religion is one of contentment and happiness, the toddler will usually exhibit a relaxed and happy attitude toward religious observance. If an attitude of fear and restriction surrounds religious practices, the toddler is likely to carry these feelings into later life.

Preschoolers

Preschoolers voluntarily imitate adult behavior when it is reinforced and thus may happily participate in religious rituals that are not too long or arduous. For example, a preschooler may enjoy saying a prayer before a meal or at bedtime, singing religious songs, or reciting short verses (Fig. 36-1).

The preschooler thinks concretely and does not conceptualize. God may be likened to a person the child knows, and religious thought typically centers on

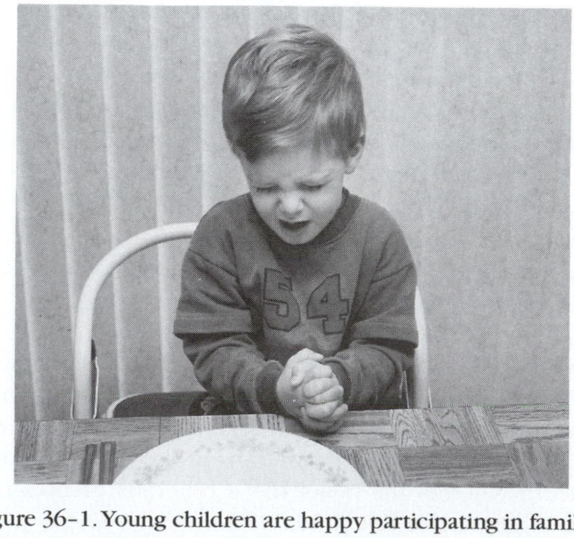

Figure 36-1. Young children are happy participating in family religious activities.

the self. Literal interpretation of the statement that prayers are answered, for example, may cause the preschooler to think that he or she can cause events by praying.

Preschoolers have developed a sense of right and wrong, heavily influenced by any religious teaching the family has offered. Firm beliefs about the consequences of wrongdoing are typical.

According to Murray and Zentner (1991), the preschooler is never spiritually neutral. This age child perceives the beliefs of the family and accepts them totally even when they are not explicitly stated. This wholehearted acceptance is an outgrowth of the preschooler's belief in the omnipotence of parents.

Caregivers should know what religious beliefs and observances are important to a hospitalized preschooler. If the child has religious rituals, such as a bedtime prayer, they should be continued in a hospital, because they provide security and continuity.

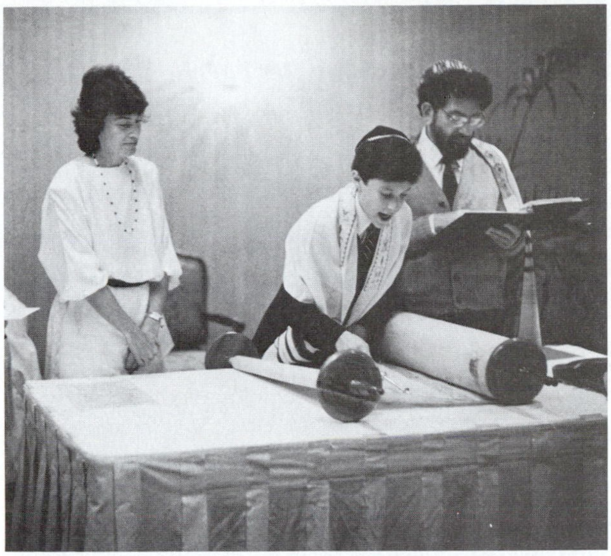

Figure 36-2. The adolescent may make a formal religious commitment in a ceremony such as this Bar Mitzvah.

School-Age Children

The school-age child is likely to have had formal religious instruction. Belief is still largely concrete in nature, but the child may be gradually moving toward an understanding of the abstractions associated with religious belief. The school-age child may hold conflicting beliefs simultaneously without questioning them or expressing concern. Caregivers ought not to challenge or point out inconsistencies in belief. Although inconsistencies may be of concern to an adult, the child will only become confused trying to sort them out. The family and religious teachers are the appropriate people to help the child do so as greater maturity is attained and religious instruction proceeds.

Certain religious rituals may be especially important to school-age children, who often believe in the magical value of ritual. Whenever possible, such rituals should be allowed the hospitalized child.

Adolescents

The adolescent is acquiring the ability to deal with intellectual abstractions and may be preoccupied with puzzling philosophical and moral questions. In general, adolescents are trying to figure out the world and their place in it. Typically, adolescents examine and challenge the beliefs with which they have been raised. Some adolescents are also able to make an independent decision to embrace a particular religious belief system. Many religions recognize this capacity in a formal way. In the Jewish faith, the ceremonies of Bar Mitzvah (for boys) and Bat Mitzvah (for girls) confer on adolescents the role of adult members of the congregation (Fig. 36-2). In some Protestant churches, *baptism* as an adult is performed during adolescence; in others, the capacity for independent decision-making is formally acknowledged by *confirmation*. Young people who make an emotional and intellectual commitment to a faith are likely to draw on their belief to answer the questions of identity and purpose that arise during adolescence. The opposite response is to deliberately reject the family religion, motivated by such factors as reaction formation, rebelliousness, the urge to be independent, and loss of belief. Thus the adolescent in a family with firm religious beliefs may refuse to attend church, declare that religion stifles independence, and profess atheism. Adolescents want to be treated as adults in religious matters. They want to make independent decisions and to be taken seriously when they express beliefs.

Adults

Spiritual life is not stagnant in adulthood. Throughout life, especially when confronting major crises, adults may reexamine their religious beliefs and practices. As caregivers, nurses must never make assumptions about a person's wishes with regard to religious needs. Membership in a particular religious group does not automatically mean that a patient will welcome a visit from clergy of that faith. Similarly, a hospitalized member of the clergy may not want to attend religious services in the hospital. Patients who have no formal religious affiliation may wish to talk to religious counselors. Do not make assumptions about another person's spiritual needs; instead, validate your perceptions through facilitating interaction.

The adult who has made decisions regarding spiri-

Nursing Research: *Implications for Practice*

Burbank, P. M. "An Exploratory Study: Assessing the Meaning in Life Among Older Adult Clients." *Journal of Gerontological Nursing* 18, 9 (September 1992): 19–28.

Meaning in life is a complex concept that many nursing theorists have linked with health and quality of life. The purpose of this study was to explore meaning in life among older people by identifying the factors perceived as meaningful and the degree of fulfillment experienced by older persons. The aspects of life that were identified as most meaningful included relationships, religion, service, and activities. For some individuals other aspects of life were most meaningful. Nurses need to assess clients in regard to what is meaningful to them and to plan interventions to support or improve areas meaningful to the older person.

tual needs with which he or she is comfortable and which provide support to the self will usually have a broad outlook on life and will have confidence in life's value and purpose.

Religions and Beliefs that Affect Health Care

Although individual members of the same faith differ in adherence to their faith's tenets, it is helpful for the nurse to have a general familiarity with specific religious beliefs as they relate to health care. An understanding of theology is not expected of the nurse. Most of the following discussion centers on the major religious groups in the United States, with which many Americans maintain at least nominal affiliation; we also briefly discuss other belief systems.

Roman Catholicism

Roman Catholicism is a religious body characterized by uniform beliefs and fairly formalized ways of dealing with health care problems. The specificity and uniformity of its guidelines facilitate appropriate action on the part of health care workers. Three Catholic *sacraments*—Baptism, Holy Communion, and Anointing of the Sick—are of special significance to the ill Roman Catholic.

Baptism

Baptism, which is considered essential, is usually performed on the young infant. If an unbaptized person wishes to be baptized, a priest will be willing to come to perform the rite. If the patient is in danger of dying, the priest will come immediately, for it is the Church's wish that no one die without baptism. If baptism is truly desired and it appears that the person will die before a priest arrives, any person may perform this rite. According to Roman Catholic doctrine, baptism has three essential components: 1) the sincere intent to baptize on the part of the person performing the rite; 2) sprinkling or pouring of any clear water over the head; and 3) recital of the words "I baptize you in the name of the Father, the Son, and the Holy Spirit" while the water is being sprinkled or poured. The baptism, is then recorded on the chart, and a priest is notified immediately. It is appropriate but not necessary for a Roman Catholic staff member to perform the rite. The Catholic church would accept the rite as valid no matter who had performed it.

Crises requiring such action occur most commonly in obstetrics, when a newborn child dies or a fetus is aborted. If the family is Catholic, the product of conception is baptized if there is any possibility that life is present. If it is known that the family is Catholic, baptism might be performed even if the parent cannot be consulted first (*eg*, the mother is under anesthesia and the father is not present). The fetus is buried by the family, and special arrangements must thus be made.

Holy Communion

The second sacrament of significance to the Roman Catholic patient is *Holy Communion* or the *Eucharist*. When Holy Communion is planned, the patient should be made presentable, the unit straightened, and a clean cleared table provided for the patient's use. The table may be covered with a linen hand towel if one is available. The patient is permitted to eat before taking communion, although some individuals may prefer not to. Privacy is necessary during the visit because the patient may wish to make a confession in conjunction with the sacrament. Communion is not commonly administered to the patient who is not allowed food because the communicant eats a bread wafer. An exception to the prohibition on food may be made in some circumstances. Communion may be administered by a priest or by a specially designated lay person who brings the prepared communion from the church. This lay person is termed a "eucharistic visitor."

Anointing of the Sick

The third important sacrament is the **Anointing of the Sick**, administered by a priest to a Catholic who is ill. The purpose of this sacrament is to provide a special blessing from God for the ill person. It is accompanied by prayers for healing and for spiritual well-being. If a dying patient is known to be Catholic, a priest is always called even if the patient is unable to authorize such a call. The Anointing of the Sick sacrament may be administered to an individual more than once, but it is usually performed only once in a particular episode of illness. In the past this sacrament was called Extreme Unction or Last Rites and was commonly administered only to those about to die. Many patients still be come frightened when this sacrament is suggested, viewing it as evidence of impending death. The nurse should be prepared for such a response, especially from the older patient. A note should be made in the patient's record after this rite has been administered.

Religious Objects

The Roman Catholic patient may use a **rosary**, which is a specially constructed chain of beads used as a guide to prayer, and may have various *religious medals* that commemorate particular saints. These items are important to the patient, providing reassurance and solace. Special care is needed to guard against their loss in the hospital.

Reproductive Issues

The Roman Catholic Church has a strong prohibition against any artificial means of contraception. Although contraceptive use among individual Roman Catholics is a matter of discussion, you should approach the subject with care and not make assumptions about the practices of the individual. The Catholic Church does accept contraception based on abstinence from intercourse during fertile periods. Much study is currently being carried out to try to make this method of contraception reliable. The Catholic Church is also strongly opposed to abortion for any reason other than to save the life of the mother.

Protestantism

Protestantism is a branch of Christianity that arose during the Reformation in reaction to perceived abuses by the Roman Catholic Church of that time. Protestant religious groups have the largest membership of any religious groups in the United States. It is difficult to be specific about Protestant religious beliefs because there are many denominations, each with its own beliefs and practices. Even within a single denomination, individual beliefs and practices differ; thus it is especially important to consult the individual patient about his or her wishes. Here we discuss some specific areas of concern.

Diet

Few Protestant denominations have dietary restrictions. The Seventh Day Adventists strongly advocate an ovolactovegetarian diet (see Chapter 25). The Church of Jesus Christ of Latter-day Saints, commonly called the Mormon Church, does not approve of drinking coffee, tea, chocolate, or cola beverages because they all contain stimulants. Many conservative Protestant groups disapprove of alcoholic beverages.

Baptism

Baptism is a sacrament in most Christian churches. Some Protestants believe in infant baptism and might wish to have a gravely ill infant or child baptized. Others, notably the Baptist churches, believe baptism should be deferred until the child reaches the age of responsible decision-making, usually considered to be about age 12 or 13. Thus infant baptism is not undertaken without explicit directions from the family. Protestant baptism is performed by ordained clergy. Some Protestant churches that do not have infant baptism do have a ceremony in which the infant is dedicated.

Communion

Communion, a sacrament in the majority of Protestant denominations, is conducted at a church with the congregation present. Communion may usually be provided by the pastor of the individual's church to a patient if the person desires it. Some churches only provide communion to their own members, whereas pastors of other churches will provide communion to another individual who desires it. Therefore, the particular policy of any church would need to be ascertained if you were seeking someone to provide communion for a patient who was not from the community or was not affiliated with a particular congregation.

Other Practices

Most Protestant groups do not routinely anoint the sick, but some may do so in special instances. Many Protestants take great comfort in reading the Bible. It is common practice to visit a sick member of the congregation in the hospital.

Reproductive Issues

Protestant churches vary greatly in their approach to reproductive issues. Most do not object to any method of contraception. Some groups, especially the more conservative and fundamentalist groups, however, are opposed to abortion for any reason other than to save the life of the mother. Other groups believe that abortion is an individual ethical decision and do not have a position against it.

The Church of Jesus Christ of Latter-day Saints discourages the use of artificial means of contraception although the prohibition is not as strong as it is within Roman Catholicism. They also are opposed to abortion for any reason other than to save the life of the mother.

Eastern Orthodoxy

There are several sects of **Eastern Orthodoxy**, a Christian religion based in Eastern Europe and the Middle East; each has a specific national origin, such as Russian Orthodox and Greek Orthodox. Because these churches are governed and function independently, the Eastern Orthodox patient will prefer a priest from his or her own church if a spiritual counselor is needed. If the community has no religious body of the individual's national background, the patient can be asked whether another Orthodox priest should be called. These churches do constitute a single faith, and in an emergency any Orthodox priest will serve the needs of an Orthodox patient.

The priest may perform confession and communion (or Holy Eucharist, as it is frequently called in the Orthodox Church) at the patient's bedside. There is also an ordinance for anointing of the sick, which is called Holy Unction. Preparation for these observances is the same for the Roman Catholic sacraments.

Judaism

There are several Jewish groups, which differ in the strictness of their adherence to the laws of **Judaism**, a religion based on the Torah and Talmud. The Orthodox Jew is the strictest and will usually wish to observe the laws concerning *kosher* food (see Chapter 25). Reform and Conservative Jews are less strict. The only Jewish ritual that might be performed in the hospital is circumcision of the male infant. Although usually performed after an infant is discharged, the ritual time for circumcision might occur if the infant is remaining in the hospital for some reason. Because a number of Jewish men, in addition to the *rabbi*, are present during the circumcision, special arrangements must be made. In areas where ritual circumcision is common, a routine has usually been established. If not, planning in consultation with the rabbi is appropriate. Such a plan must also be approved by the physician in charge of the infant's care.

The death of an Orthodox Jew presents a unique challenge: burial should take place within 24 hours of death and also before the Sabbath, which begins at sundown on Friday. If the death occurs early in the week, this is not difficult, but a death on Friday requires prompt action. Orthodox Jews usually do not permit autopsies to be performed. Jews do not object to contraception. There is no prohibition against abortion within Judaism.

Islam

Islam—the **Muslim** faith, based on the teachings of the prophet Mohammed—is the major religion in the Near East and North Africa. Islam emphasizes specific individual rituals and prayers, and the Islamic patient will wish to carry out these devotions in private. The only Islamic dietary restrictions are against alcoholic beverages and pork. There is a fasting period in the Muslim calendar, but the ill are exempt from this requirement.

Conservative Muslims believe in the strict separation of men and women in almost all areas of life. This applies to health care and in a Muslim country, a woman would be cared for by a woman and a man would be cared for by a man. This may become a problem in a Western health care facility that does not have personnel to support this practice. Women are also expected to wear clothing that covers the hair and the entire body and that does not reveal the shape of the body. Providing for the modesty of the Muslim woman is important. In traditional Muslim families, the man is the decision-maker and other family members are expected to abide by his decisions.

Many Muslims do not practice contraception, but there is no widespread prohibition against it. As in other family issues, using birth control or not is usually the husband's decision. Abortion is generally opposed but may be viewed as an individual decision by Muslims in this country. In Muslim fundamentalist societies the religious authorities would make this decision.

A large group of Muslims in the United States originated as an independent black religious movement known as the Nation of Islam. This group subsequently affiliated with the worldwide Islamic community and expanded its membership beyond the black community. Nevertheless, black pride, autonomy, and independence are still basic tenets of the faith, and the group remains somewhat separate.

Hinduism

Hinduism is an ancient religion that originated in India. The basic aim of life in Hinduism is to achieve Nirvana, a state of oneness with the universal life force called Brahmin. Individuals move toward Nirvana by leading lives of merit. After death the individual is reincarnated in another form. The nature of the new life form is based on the level of merit attained in previous lives. When sufficient merit is accumulated, Nirvana may be achieved. Prayer is an important aspect of achieving merit. Within the Hindu religion there are many gods that have power over individuals and what happens in their lives. Families may have an altar in the home and in India there are many shrines to different gods along the roads.

In addition, Hinduism has many sects that follow individual teachers. In the United States the Hare Krishna groups, who wear saffron-colored robes, shave their heads, and chant prayers, are a Hindu sect that follows the teacher Sri Raman Krishna. Within India many of these sects tend to be regional. The traditions of the individual are dependent on the particular sect to which he or she belongs. Some sects have traditional beliefs about balancing foods that are designated "hot" or "cold" as a way maintaining health.

Most Hindus are vegetarians and abstain from alcohol. They strictly prohibit killing of any animal life form, including insects, based on their belief in reincarnation. Most believe in cremation of the dead. They believe that fate, or karma, is unchangeable. This belief may lead them to avoid practicing birth control and may affect their approach to health care. Many individuals in the United States who are of a Hindu background may differ greatly in their adherence to Hindu traditions.

Buddhism

Buddhism is based on the teaching of the Lord Buddha. Buddha was a Hindu teacher who is believed to have achieved Nirvana. Buddhism has two major sects, and a wide variety of minor variations within these sects. Although Buddhism originated in India, most of the world's Buddhists are in Southeast Asia, China, and Japan. The number of Buddhists in the United States is growing. Many are of Asian background; others are young whites who have converted to Buddhism.

Many Buddhists follow the Hindu practice of vegetarianism. The belief that one's current actions affect one's later life and rebirth is also part of Buddhism. Buddhists generally attempt to be peaceful and cooperative in their daily living. This system of belief encourages calm acceptance of whatever life has to offer, and as a consequence, the Buddhist patient may not express needs or ask for care. The nurse must be especially alert to nonverbal indications of needs and problems.

Animism

Inhabitants of many of the more rural areas of Southeast Asia, such as the Hmong and Ming from Cambodia, who have emigrated to the United States are Animists. With few formal tenets and no written Scripture, **Animism** is considered a primitive religion. Animists believe that there are spirits in most of earth's objects. These spirits may be friendly or unfriendly, and it is possible to propitiate the spirits in ways that make them more friendly. There may be a complex system of taboos and required actions in an animist tribe. Animism has no clergy as such, although a wise person in the tribe may be sought out for advice regarding spiritual concerns.

Other Philosophical Systems

Some *fatalistic* philosophical systems view life as completely predetermined. "That's fate" and "What will be, will be" are common expressions that reflect this viewpoint. Adherents of such systems may not be willing to change their diets or lifestyles to improve their health in the belief that the future cannot be altered. Although concentrating on the present may enable you to assist such a person, you may not be able to change this attitude. Respect for philosophical beliefs is one of the rights of the patient.

An **agnostic** is a person who believes that human beings cannot know whether or not God exists. An **atheist** does not believe in the existence of God. A person who adheres to either of these beliefs bases ethical decisions on his or her philosophy of life. Such an individual will usually not wish to consult a member of the clergy, but may wish to share his or her feelings and thoughts with an interested, caring friend or health care provider.

Some individuals in contemporary society adhere to a wide variety of nontraditional belief systems. These belief systems may have an impact on the individual's response to health care. Some incorporate aspects of traditional religions, such as the reincarnation beliefs of Hinduism. Some focus on the inner strengths of the individual and the individual's ability to control and change life. You will be most successful in learning about a person's personal belief system if you remain nonjudgmental and encourage the person to explain those values and beliefs that are currently providing meaning and focus to his or her life.

Assessment

Nurses are often reluctant to ask about patients' spiritual needs or concerns, believing their questions may either be interpreted as prying or lead patients to erroneous assumptions about the seriousness of their illness. If you believe that it is a function of nursing to support the whole person, concern for the patient's spiritual needs will be a part of your nursing plan.

Many hospital admission forms provide a space in which to indicate religion. If the religious affiliation noted there would in some way affect health care, the affiliation should be considered when care is planned. The family can usually give you specific information about the patient's religious practices if the patient is unable to communicate (Fig. 36-3).

When you take a nursing history on the person's admission to the hospital, you might ask if religion is important to the patient or if the patient has a religious preference and wishes a religious adviser, pastor, or church notified of his or her illness. You might ask if the patient has any religious practices that he or she would like to continue while hospitalized. The responses will provide some information about the patient's spiritual concerns.

Observation of the patient's behavior provides additional information. Does the patient read the Bible or a prayer book? Does the person wear religious medals or insignia or use religious objects, such as a rosary? In conversation, does the patient discuss God or God's will? Does the patient talk about the meaning and purpose of his or her existence?

Reassessment of spiritual needs is appropriate when the patient must make a major decision or faces life-threatening problems. As you interact with the person about the problem, you would inquire whether there was anyone whom the patient would like to consult and indicate a member of the clergy or religious adviser as one of the possible options for support.

When a patient is facing difficult decisions regarding care, major changes in lifestyle, or impending death, you might encourage the person to think about his or her own basic values and beliefs. As the individual explores these, you may gain valuable understanding of the person and of what is of basic importance in that individual's life.

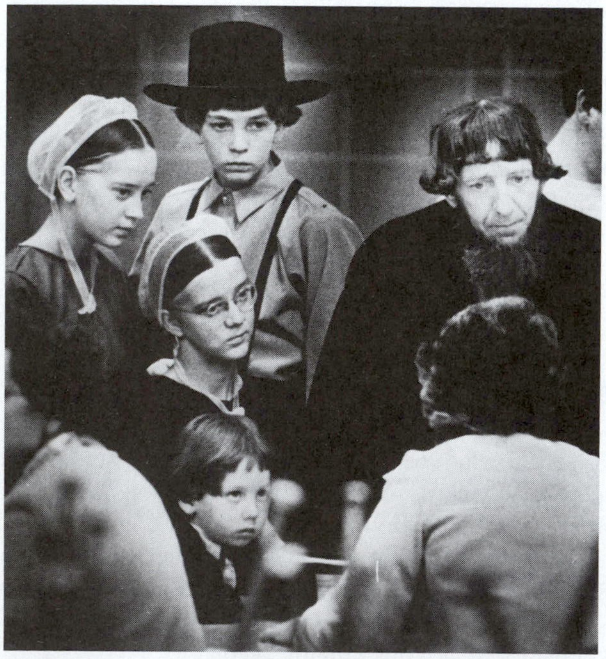

Figure 36-3. Sometimes individual members of a religion will permit medical treatment that is contrary to church teachings. These Amish parents allowed their children to receive polio vaccine, a practice forbidden by their religion (Wide World Photos).

Nursing Diagnosis

The nursing diagnoses that reflect values and beliefs are those relating to spiritual state and to the perception of the meaningfulness of life.

Meaningfulness is the perception that there is positive purpose and potential in life. The perception that life holds meaning is essential to meeting the need for growth and self-actualization. When a person perceives life as without meaning or ascribes to it meaning that is negative and does not hold potential for growth, the person will not be willing to engage in those activities that will promote health. Both a sense of powerlessness and a sense of hopelessness constitute alterations in meaningfulness.

Spiritual Distress

Spiritual distress is "the state in which the individual or group experiences or is at risk of experiencing a disturbance in the belief or value system which provides strength, hope, and meaning to life" (Carpenito, 1992, p. 802).

Spiritual distress may occur when an individual is unable to engage in valued spiritual practices because of the unavailability of clergy, physical inability to travel to a place of worship, or the seriousness of the illness. Sometimes a patient experiences embarrassment about

Nursing Diagnoses Related to Spiritual Needs

Spiritual Distress related to
- inability to practice religious rituals
- difficulty integrating feelings about illness with religious beliefs

Powerlessness related to
- erratic course of disease
- demands of the health care system

Hopelessness related to
- perception of expected course of illness as terminal
- belief that an active, productive life is impossible given the current disability

performing religious rituals around those who do not share the belief. The person may feel discouraged and express concerns about separation from religious practices. The person may feel a sense of loss or emptiness.

Spiritual distress may also occur when conflict exists between religious or spiritual beliefs and the health care regimen. The individual may express ambivalent feelings about both health care and religious beliefs. He or she may express anger that the conflict exists and be unable to make a decision about care.

Another situation that may precipitate spiritual distress is failure to make progress toward wellness. The person may be discouraged and question the credibility of his or her belief system. The individual may express resentment about suffering and become angry that prayer has not been answered.

Powerlessness

A feeling of a lack of control or power over one's own life is termed **powerlessness**. Although this feeling may be experienced in some degree by many ill persons, it represents a nursing diagnosis when the person is unable to respond constructively by seeking control over those aspects of life that can be controlled, but rather becomes apathetic and depressed and withdraws from the situation. The person may make comments such as "What's the use?" and "It really doesn't matter." The person may be unwilling to participate in decision-making. Even opinions may be withheld because the person perceives that these will not change the course of events. Some illness situations and some institutional policies create a setting conducive to the development of powerlessness.

Hopelessness

The nursing diagnosis of **Hopelessness** is "a sustained emotional state in which an individual sees no alternatives or personal choices available to solve problems or to achieve what is desired and cannot mobilize energy on own behalf to establish goals" (Carpenito, 1992, p. 489). The person who feels hopeless does not see any answers or solutions to problems, as opposed to the person who is powerless, who may see the solutions but perceives those solutions to be under the control of others.

The person who feels hopeless makes statements that indicate apathy and the perception that there are no solutions to problems, such as "I might as well give up, there is no way around this" or "What difference does it make, things will never be any better."

The person who feels hopeless may express emptiness and say that life has no purpose or meaning. The person's behavior may be passive, and there may be decreased verbalization and lack of initiative or lack of expressions of interest in anything. The person may lack the ability to think of any new ideas, to plan, or make decisions. Unwillingness to consider the future may occur because there is no belief that the future holds any promise for change or improvement.

Related Nursing Diagnoses

The nursing diagnoses in the area of personal identity grieving, and crisis may all have a dimension that is related to the values and beliefs that the patient holds. These problems may become more severe when the patient does not have a sustaining set of personal values and beliefs that serve as support during times of extreme stress. Values and beliefs may help the patient to find meaning in adverse events and a purpose and direction for life beyond the particular situation.

Planning and Implementation

When considering the outcome criteria for patients experiencing spiritual distress, hopelessness, and powerlessness, keep in mind the significance of a patient's values and beliefs in the overall ability of the patient to recover from illness. Desired outcomes should include not only a reduction in distress but also an overall increase in the patient's ability to adapt and to cope with the present illness because personal spiritual needs have been met satisfactorily.

Criteria for evaluation will be based on the specific nursing diagnosis identified. If the spiritual distress is related to inability to carry out religious practices, the desired outcome might be that the person carry out religious practices. In addition, criteria should be established relating to the person's subjective feelings in regard to spiritual state. For example, the goal might be for the person to state that he or she feels at peace or is satisfied with the present spiritual state. For the person whose spiritual distress was related to a conflict in values or to feelings of guilt, resolution would be identified by statements indicating that the conflict was resolved or that feelings of guilt and anxiety were lessened. When patients express feelings of hopelessness or powerlessness, outcome criteria will most often focus on the feelings expressed by the patient.

Planning will need to include setting aside the necessary time to identify the patient's spiritual needs through thoughtful questioning and attentive listening. A wide variety of options are available to help the person with spiritual needs. These might include referral to others as well as independent actions that you, as a nurse, might take.

Nursing Care Plan
Sample Nursing Care Plan Related to Spiritual Needs

Nursing Diagnosis	Spiritual distress related to feelings of guilt and remorse. **Supportive data:** States feels guilty over not participating in religious activities. States, "God probably doesn't care about me any more. I haven't been a good person." Patient is Roman Cathlolic.
Desired Patient Outcomes	States he feels better about his relationship with God. Expresses hope that God cares about him. Makes positive statements regarding the future.

Nursing Action	Rationale
1. Contact priest for immediate visit.	A Roman Catholic priest is able to help the Roman Catholic patient deal with the feelings of guilt and remorse.
2. In talking with patient encourage him to identify positive aspects of his past life (i.e., role as good worker, caring son to older parents).	Identifying positive roles in life supports self esteem.
3. Arrange for patient to attend church service when he wishes.	Church services provide a resource for individuals to meet spiritual needs.

Referral

When planning to meet spiritual needs for the patient and family, remember that you are not the only resource. In some situations, you can effectively intervene. In others, a spiritual adviser such as a member of the clergy, will be more effective in assisting the person.

Members of the Clergy

Many large hospitals have as a member of the health care team a **chaplain**, whose task is to identify and, if possible, meet patients' spiritual and religious needs. The modern chaplain has usually had special education in dealing with the spiritual needs of those who are ill. Familiar with a wide variety of religious beliefs, the chaplain is prepared to contact other members of the clergy when patients have specific needs. Furthermore, the chaplain's understanding of health care makes him or her a valuable participant on the health care team. Some large hospitals may have more than one chaplain, representing several religions.

Chaplains' methods of operation vary, depending largely on the philosophy of the hospital. Often the chaplain visits each newly admitted patient. Although an ordained member of the clergy of a particular faith, the chaplain does not restrict his or her attention to members of the same faith. During the initial visit, the chaplain greets the patient and explains the role of the chaplain. A patient who has religious needs will often indicate them to the chaplain at this time.

The chaplain is also available for referrals by the nurse or consultations with the staff about problems related to patients' religious needs. The chaplain may spend time with the patient simply visiting, reading Scripture, or ministering in a variety of ways. A skilled chaplain assesses the patient's needs and relates in the way that is most helpful to the patient. In some settings the chaplain also helps the staff cope with the stresses of caring for patients who are critically ill.

When there is no hospital chaplain, members of the clergy in the community usually undertake to fulfill the chaplain's role. Because they are often unfamiliar with hospital routine, these persons may need special assistance from the nurse in planning what they will do. If the patient wishes to see a member of the clergy, the patient, the family, or the nurse (with the patient's permission) may call one. If the patient is affiliated with a specific congregation, its clergy should be called. If the patient is far from a personal congregation or does not belong to one, you may ask a few questions to ascertain the patient's general beliefs and then suggest several churches with similar beliefs whose clergy have expressed willingness to serve the needs of the sick.

Not all those with strong religious affiliations wish a member of the clergy to visit. For example, Jewish clergy are basically teachers of their congregations and have few special religious powers exceeding those of other Jews. Thus a Jewish patient may wish to see his or her own rabbi, but be uninterested in seeing any other rabbi.

Occasionally, a member of the clergy may lack skill in dealing with the sick and may upset rather than support the patient. In such a case, the nurse must tactfully explain to the clergy member that the patient is upset and suggest that he or she limit or abandon visits.

Lay Visitors

Those who are not professional clergy in a religious body are called the **laity**. A lay visitor is a member of a religious body who seeks to minister to the spiritual needs of the individual. Some religious groups, including the Latter-day Saints (Mormons) and Christian Scientists, do not have professional clergy. Instead, these denominations appoint lay people to minister to the sick, and their religious function should be recognized by the health care worker. In Christian Science, this role is undertaken by the *reader*. Among the Latter-day Saints (Mormons), this person might be an **elder**.

Well-intentioned but misguided members of some religious groups sometimes wish to visit many patients without regard for individual patients' wishes. Patients who would deny strangers entry into their homes often feel unable to control access to their hospital bedsides. Thus it is the nurse's responsibility to protect the patient's privacy.

Spiritual Teachers

Many individuals seek answers to spiritual questions of meaning and purpose in their lives through individual spiritual teachers. These individuals may not be part of any larger spiritual or religious belief group. Through the teaching and life pattern that the spiritual teacher presents, the individual may find inner peace, stability, and a sense of meaning and purpose.

Nontraditional spiritual teachers can pose sensitive problems, because some persons purporting to be spiritual teachers are, in fact, engaged in defrauding the public for personal gain. Your role is not to question the patient's spiritual beliefs, but if fraudulent practices come to your attention, you will want to consult with someone else as to how to proceed to assist the patient in the situation.

Quiet Rooms

Many hospitals have a chapel or quiet meditation room for use by patients, families, and staff. This quiet room is usually nondenominational, so that a wide variety of people will feel comfortable using it, although this may not be the case if the hospital is sponsored by or affiliated with a specific religious group. Such a room can be of value to those who need a few moments of quiet thought, as well as those who wish to worship. It may be the only place where privacy and refuge from the hectic pace of the hospital are available to a family that has just lost a loved one. Wise use of this peaceful environment will be supportive to many people. Staff members, too, may need a few moments' refuge to gather strength for difficult situations (Fig. 36-4).

Attendance at Worship Services

Worship services are held in some large hospitals and nursing homes. These services may be nondenominational, or separate services may be held for different religious groups. If such services are held, the nurse should offer information about them to the patient and the family. The nurse is also responsible for planning the patient's care so that attendance is possible. A desire to attend religious services should be treated as a special need when priorities for care are determined.

Individual Nursing Responses

Sometimes a patient requests that a nurse read *Scripture* to him or her. Most people would not consider doing so as constituting participation in a religious observance, but the individual nurse must decide how to respond in light of the specific situation. It is the nurse's responsibility to seek someone to meet this need if he or she feels uncomfortable meeting it personally. Often a vol-

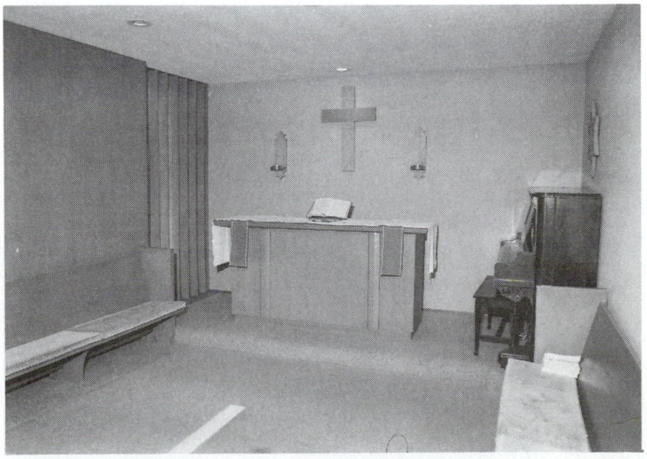

Figure 36-4. Quiet rooms provide privacy and refuge for hospital patients and their families.

unteer will read Scripture, or the patient's congregation will locate a member willing to do so.

If the patient has religious symbols or medals, their loss can be seriously upsetting. Every effort should be made to keep track of these items and to ensure that they are not inadvertently lost. Occasionally, a patient will request permission to take a religious object to the operating room. Although this is not common practice, arrangements can usually be made with the surgeon, operating room staff, and recovery room staff. This alone may make a significant difference in the patient's ability to tolerate severe stress.

Patients may ask you to pray for or with them. If your religious beliefs coincide, you might join the patient in prayer. If your beliefs differ greatly, you might simply offer to stay while the patient prays. If you also find this difficult, you can seek another staff member who would be more comfortable in this role. If the patient asks you to pray on his or her behalf and you do not feel that it is appropriate for you to do so, you might say that you will continue to keep the patient in your thoughts and offer to contact a member of the clergy or other person who could meet this need.

If a patient feels guilt with regard either to illness or to some other aspect of life, a member of the clergy is often best able to assist in its resolution. Some religions have prescribed means of absolving guilt; in others the process is less formal. All major religions address issues of guilt and conscience and attempt to assist the individual in confronting them. The serious anxiety that guilt can arouse can be a barrier to healing. Thus resolution of guilt, which is a religious problem, contributes to recovery from physical illness.

Occasionally religious beliefs cause patients to behave in ways that create problems for the nurse. If a patient attempts to convert the nurse to the patient's own religious beliefs, the nurse faces the difficult task of maintaining simultaneously a helpful nurse–patient relationship and personal religious or philosophical integrity. Acknowledging the importance of the patient's beliefs and redirecting the conversation to focus on the patient's health status needs is an effective way to deal with this problem.

When a member of the clergy or another person with a religious vocation, such as a nun, becomes a patient, health care workers may have unrealistic expectations of their behavior. Such an individual is sometimes expected to continue to act in a supportive way toward others and to be exemplary in behavior and free from anxiety. This expectation is far from realistic. Members of the clergy are people, with varying degrees of ability to tolerate and deal with the stresses of illness. Natural feelings of anxiety will be present, and the support and aid of others will be needed. Reducing staff expectations of exceptional behavior and carefully assessing the individual will ensure realistic care.

Your implementation will take several different forms. You might spend time with the person in therapeutic interaction, helping the person to identify concerns and come to personal conclusions. You might facilitate attendance at religious services or time for personal religious devotions. Alternatively, you might refer the patient to another person who is more closely identified with the spiritual sphere of life, such as a member of the clergy. In a wide variety of ways, your actions will help the person to move toward spiritual wholeness.

Evaluation

When evaluating the patient's resolution of problems related to values and beliefs, you will be identifying whether the specific desired outcomes have been met. Is the person now able to perform spiritual practices? Does the person express a lessened level of spiritual distress? Does the person feel at greater peace?

When evaluating those who feel hopeless or powerless, it will be important to examine the individual's behavior. Those who feel less powerless may be taking increased control in their own lives. This may include making decisions relative to health care and to daily living. The person who feels less hopeless may begin referring to the future, may be willing to make plans, and may be thinking positively about possible outcomes.

Nursing Care Study
A Patient Manifesting Spiritual Needs

Ms. Jennifer Nakima, a student nurse on the medical unit, was assigned to care for Mr. Stephen MacDougal. In the course of her assessment, she noted that Mr. MacDougal kept a well-worn Bible at his bedside. His admitting information sheet gave his religious preference as Protestant. She also noted that when she entered his room he would often put his Bible away and fold his hands expectantly.

MS. NAKIMA: "Mr. MacDougal, I notice that you read your Bible a lot. It seems to be an important part of your life."

MR. MACDOUGAL: "Yes, it is. I was raised as a Christian and have been one all my life. Other people may be wishywashy, but not me! I was an elder in my church for many years, but lately I've been sick too much to be able to take any responsibility."

MS. NAKIMA: "Are you used to attending church on Sundays?"

MR. MACDOUGAL: "Never miss! Except now, of course."

MS. NAKIMA: "Did you know that there is a nondenominational church service here in the hospital every Sunday?"

MR. MACDOUGAL: "No–who goes?"

MS. NAKIMA: "Well, it's for patients mainly, but visitors and staff are welcome to attend, too. Ministers from different churches conduct the service."

MR. MACDOUGAL: "When do they have it?"

MS. NAKIMA: "It's at 1:30 in the afternoon because most people are done with treatments and things and the staff can help them get there. Would you like to go? I could arrange it."

MR. MACDOUGAL: "Well . . . do you have to get dressed up to go?"

MS. NAKIMA: "A robe and slippers are what most people wear."

MR. MACDOUGAL: "I'd like to go, then, if it isn't too much trouble."

MS. NAKIMA: "I'll make the arrangements with the team leader who will be here Sunday and mark it on your care plan. Maybe you could remind the person who is taking care of you on Sunday, too. That would make a double check."

MR. MACDOUGAL: "Sure, I won't forget, that's for sure."

In this instance, the nursing student assessed the patient's spiritual needs and identified an appropriate way to meet them. Her actions were carefully planned and made use of the unit's communication system to facilitate implementation. The patient was included at all points in the process; Ms. Nakima validated her assessment with him, he participated in making the plan, and he had a role in carrying out the plan.

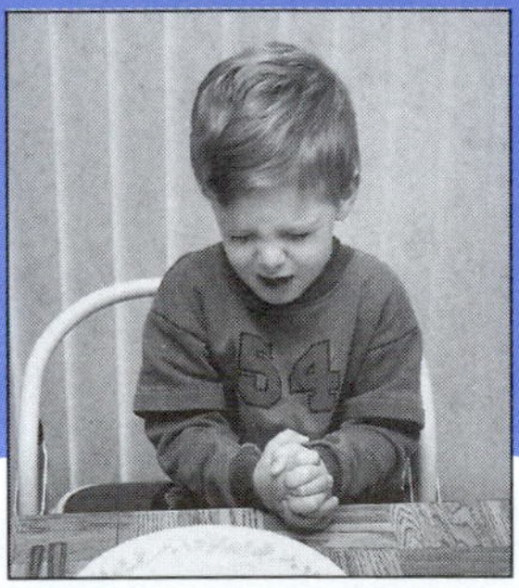

Key Points

- The spiritual aspect of life concerns the beliefs and values of the individual. Whether based on an organized framework of religion or on a general philosophical system, these beliefs and values are essential to effective human functioning.
- Cultural values relate to health care in that an illness or disability is handled more or less effectively based on those values. Some people value individuality and emphasize individual autonomy, whereas others value the community and actions taken for the common good. Western society values individuality over community, and competition is valued by many as a motivation for excellence. Others feel that competition interferes with cooperation.
- People who value a present orientation may not be motivated by concern about the future but may adapt well when facing an uncertain future, as when faced with a serious illness. Those who are oriented to the future may tolerate present difficulties for the promise of a better future but may be adversely affected by a situation that does not offer future promise.
- Cultural values also come into play when people who value the work ethic highly identify with their occupation and suffer loss of self-esteem if working

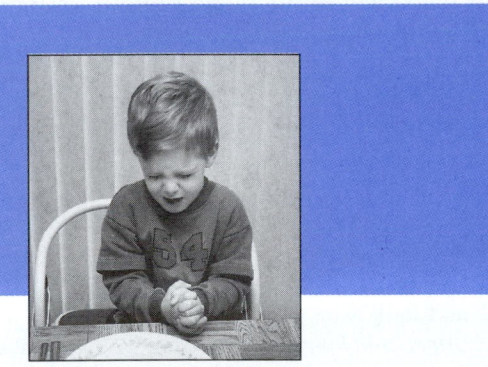

is no longer possible. Those who value a leisure ethic may be comfortable working fewer hours or at a less demanding job for the sake of being able to engage in desired leisure pursuits.

- Spiritual beliefs that enhance health care and healing include belief that God cares about the individual, belief in life after death, and belief in supernatural healing. Belief in the effectiveness of one's own action in changing life can provide motivation to care for oneself. Respect for the living body as unique and special may stimulate the adoption of sound health practices and avoidance of things harmful to the body.
- Some spiritual beliefs interfere with health care. Those who see illness as punishment may have lowered self-esteem and may be discouraged from attempts to change what is happening. Those who believe illness is self-caused may see themselves as failures and be reluctant to accept health care technology.
- Nurses must be aware of particular beliefs that preclude some kinds of treatment. For instance, the Jehovah's Witnesses prohibit the use of blood or blood products. Other beliefs that can interfere with health care include trust in miraculous cures to the exclusion of health care and the belief that fate is unchangeable.
- Religious development progresses throughout the life span, including adulthood.
- Roman Catholicism, Protestantism, Eastern Orthodoxy, Judaism, Islam, Hinduism, and Buddhism are the major religious groups in the United States. Basic knowledge about these religions and other philosophical systems, such as agnosticism or atheism, will increase your understanding of those who do not share your belief system and help you in planning their care.
- Assessment of the patient's needs related to values and beliefs includes gathering data about religious beliefs and background as well as exploring the individual's basic values and beliefs.
- Nursing diagnoses related to an individual's values and beliefs include Spiritual Distress, Powerlessness, and Hopelessness.
- In planning to meet spiritual needs, you may use the services of the clergy, lay visitors, the facilities available, and your own actions. Criteria for evaluation are based on the specific etiology of spiritual distress.
- Recognizing and meeting spiritual needs, or making referrals to those who can meet them, is an aspect of caring for the whole patient and may significantly enhance the patient's ability to deal successfully with illness.

Study Questions

1. How might valuing the community over the individual affect a person's decision-making?
2. How might a competitive value affect motivation?
3. What effect might a work ethic have on a person's response to a disabling illness?
4. List four beliefs that may enhance health and healing, and explain how they might help.
5. List four beliefs that may interfere with health and healing, and explain how they might interfere.
6. Outline what might be used to assess for spiritual needs.
7. How might the clergy be used to assist in meeting a patient's spiritual needs?
8. What actions might the nurse take independently to meet a patient's needs relative to values and beliefs?
9. What resources may be available to help meet a patient's needs relative to values and beliefs?

Critical Thinking Activities

1. Choose a religious group to contact for information about its response to illness and special help for those who are ill. Summarize this information and present it for class discussion. (Each group member should choose a different religious group.)
2. Interview a nurse to determine what he or she sees as the most significant actions nurses can undertake with regard to spiritual needs. Compare and contrast this with what is presented in the text. Synthesize your own view of the nurse's role in relationship to meeting spiritual needs.

References and Readings

Belgum, D. (Ed.). *Religion and Medicine: Essays on Meaning, Value, and Health.* Ames, Iowa: Iowa State University Press, 1967.

Berkowitz, P., and Berkowitz, N. "The Jewish Patient in the Hospital." *American Journal of Nursing* 67 (November 1967): 2335.

Betz, C. L. "Faith Development in Children." *Pediatric Nursing* 7 (July 1981): 22–23.

Bowers, C. C. "Spiritual Dimensions of the Rehabilitation Journey." *Rehabilitation Nursing* 12, 2 (March-April 1987): 90–91.

Brooke, V. "The Spiritual Well-Being of the Elderly." *Geriatric Nursing* 8, 4 (July-August 1987): 194–195.

Burkhardt, M. A. and Nagai-Jacobson, M. G. "Dealing with

Spiritual Concerns of Clients in the Community." *Journal of Community Health Nursing* 2, 4 (April 1985): 191–198.

Carpenito, L. J. *Nursing Diagnosis: Applications to Clinical Practice.* 4th edition. Philadelphia: J. B. Lippincott, 1992.

Damsteegt, D. "Pastoral Roles in Pre-Surgical Visits." *American Journal of Nursing* 75 (August 1975): 1336–1337.

Dickinson, Sister C. "The Search for Spiritual Meaning." *American Journal of Nursing* 75 (October 1975): 1789–1793.

Dillenberger, J., and Welch, C. *Protestant Christianity.* New York: Charles Scribner and Sons, 1955.

Donley, R. "Spiritual Dimensions of Health Care: Nursing's Mission." *Nursing and Health Care* 12, 4 (April 1991): 178–183.

Hammer, M. L. "Spiritual Needs: A Forgotten Dimension." *Journal of Gerontological Nursing* 16, 12 (December 1990): 3–4.

Highfield, M. F. "Spiritual Needs of Patients: Are They Recognized?" *Cancer Nursing* 6 (March 1983): 187–189.

Hover, M. "If a Patient Asks You to Pray with Him." *RN* 49, 4 (April 1986): 17–18.

Karvis, P. S. "Building a Foundation for Spiritual Care." *Journal of Christian Nursing* 8, 3 (Summer 1991): 10–13.

MacInnis, K. "Prayer." *American Journal of Nursing* 87, 9 (September 1987): 1256.

Morris, K. L. and Foerster, J. D. "Team Work: Nurse and Chaplain." *American Journal of Nursing* 72 (December 1972): 2197–2199.

Murray, R., and Zentner, J. *Nursing Assessment and Health Promotion Strategies Through the Life Span.* 5th editing. Englewood Cliffs, N.J.: Prentice-Hall, 1991.

Naiman, H. L. "Nursing in Jewish Law." *American Journal of Nursing* 70 (September 1970): 2378–2379.

"Patients' Religious Beliefs—Nurses' Responsibility." *Regan Reports on Nursing Law* 14 (April 1974): 2.

Pederson, W. D. "The Broadening Role of the Hospital Chaplain." *Hospitals* 42 (September 1968): 58.

Peterson, E. A. "The Physical, the Spiritual: Can You Meet All Your Patient's Needs?" *Journal of Gerontological Nursing* 11, 10 (October 1985): 23–37.

Peterson, E. A., and Nelson, K. "How to Meet Your Client's Spiritual Needs." *Journal of Psychosocial Nursing and Mental Health Services* 25, 5 (May 1987): 35–40.

Piepgras, B. "The Other Dimension: Spiritual Help." *American Journal of Nursing* 68 (December 1968): 2610–2613.

Pumphrey, J. B. "Recognizing Your Patient's Spiritual Needs." *Nursing '77* 12 (December 1977): 64–69.

Raciappa, J. D. "A Total Ministry." *American Journal of Nursing* 73 (April 1973): 645.

Rew, L. "Exercises for Spiritual Growth." *Journal of Holistic Nursing* 4, 1 (Spring 1986): 20–22.

Saudia, T. L., Kinney, M. R., and Brown, K. C. "Health Locus of Control and Helpfulness of Prayer." *Heart Lung* 20, 1 (January 1991): 60–65.

Shaffer, J. L. "Spiritual Distress and Critical Illness." *Critical Care Nursing* 11, 1 (January 1991): 42–43, 45.

Voelkel, M. A. "Four Keys to Inner Wholeness." *Journal of Christian Nursing* 3, 4 (Fall 1986): 16–19.

Wald, F. S. and Bailey, S. S. "Nurturing the Spiritual Component in Care for the Terminally Ill." *Caring* 9, 11 (November 1990): 64–68.

Ware, T. *The Orthodox Church.* Baltimore: Penguin Books, 1972.

Westberg, G. E. *Nurse, Pastor and Patient.* Rock Island, Ill.: Augustana Press, 1955.

Human Sexuality

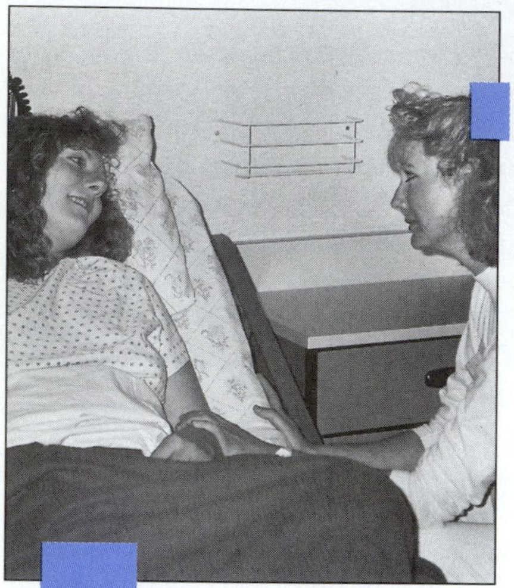

37

Objectives

After completing this chapter, you should be able to:

1. Differentiate among sexual behavior, sexuality, and sensuality.
2. Name and describe in general terms the four stages of the sexual response.
3. Define androgyny and two views regarding sexual identity.
4. List five factors that affect sexuality and their relationship to nursing practice.
5. Discuss the impact of sexually transmitted diseases on sexual behavior.
6. Explain how common problems may affect sexuality, libido, and sexual behavior.
7. Explain how assessment regarding sexuality may be conducted with sensitivity.
8. Identify the major nursing diagnoses that relate to sexuality.
9. Describe how the nurse can intervene for problems of sexuality.
10. Outline the process of evaluation in regard to problems of a sexual nature.

Study Terms

androgens
androgyny
asexual
bisexuality
conjoint therapy
dyspareunia
inhibitory ejaculation
paraorgasm
premature ejaculation
sensuality
seropositive
vaginismus

Outline

Ellis, Nowlis: Nursing: A Human Needs Approach, 5th ed. © 1994 J.B. Lippincott Company

Common Problems Affecting Sexuality

Chronic Illness and Disability
Drug Effects
Sexually Transmitted Diseases
Sexual Problems of Men
Sexual Problems of Women
Cardiac Disease
Sexuality and the Surgical Experience

Assessment

Interview
Physical Assessment

Nursing Diagnosis

Sexual Dysfunction
Altered Sexual Patterns
Impaired Verbal Communication
Altered Family Processes
Situational Low Self-esteem
Anxiety
Knowledge Deficit

Planning and Implementation

Effective Listening
Building Trust
Therapeutic Communication
Acceptance of Body Changes
Referral to Sexual Counselors

Evaluation

Sexuality is an integral aspect of every person. All human beings have a need for some means of sexual expression. The components of sexuality are awareness of one's body as a source of pleasure, perception of oneself as feminine or masculine, and a sense of how one can comfortably express those feelings.

Sexual behavior is the expression of sexuality through communication, intimate touch, and use of the sexual organs. To state that sexuality is an important part of every person does not mean that every person must be sexually active.

Sensuality is often confused with being sexual. **Sensuality** is pleasure perceived through the senses and may or may not be sexual in nature. For example, watching the beautiful concentric circles formed on the surface of a pond by a falling leaf is a sensual experience, but not a sexual one. Gazing at a Henry Moore sculpture with its smooth, rounded facets may be a sensual experience to some and suggest sexuality to others.

Increasing recognition that sexuality is a fundamental component of the human character has led to a new awareness of individual and group needs for sexual expression. Certain groups of people—the elderly, the handicapped, and those who are disadvantaged by other circumstances—have gained recognition of their special needs, including sexual needs, thereby securing greater control over their lives. Individual sexual needs also have been reexamined and, as a result, sexual attitudes are changing. A new openness about sexuality is allowing people to explore their sexual feelings honestly. Such matters as abortion, family planning, and alternative sexual lifestyles, until recently considered unmentionable in polite society, are now discussed frankly and openly. Most nursing programs include sexuality as a basic need in their curricula.

The Reproductive System

The reproductive systems of the male and female have remarkable symmetry. They arise from the same embryonic tissue and have many commonalities as well as differences. Stimulation of hormones can cause masculinizing of the female; stimulation of female hormones will cause feminizing of the male.

The Female Reproductive System

The external female sexual organs are termed the *vulva*. There are several external structures that make up the vulva (Fig. 37-1). Skin covering fatty tissue over the symphysis pubis is called the mons veneris. Loose skin forms exterior folds on either side of the perineum called the *labia majora*. Within these folds are another set of folds covered by mucous membrane called the *labia minora*. Another part of the vulva is the clitoris, a tiny organ posterior to the mons within the labia minora, which is sensitive and important to sexual arousal. Just posterior to the clitoris is the urinary meatus, and just posterior to that is the entrance to the vagina. On each side of the vaginal orifice are Bartholin's glands, which secrete a lubricating fluid.

A thin fold of tissue called the hymen borders the opening of the *vagina*. The hymen usually separates at the time of first intercourse, causing some mild discomfort. The vagina itself is a tubelike structure that lies anterior to the rectum and posterior to the urinary urethra and bladder. It is lined with folds of mucous membrane.

At the upper end of the vagina is the *cervix*, a round, doughnut-shaped structure that forms the lower portion of the uterus. The cervix has two openings: the external os opening into the vagina and higher, the internal os opening into the uterus.

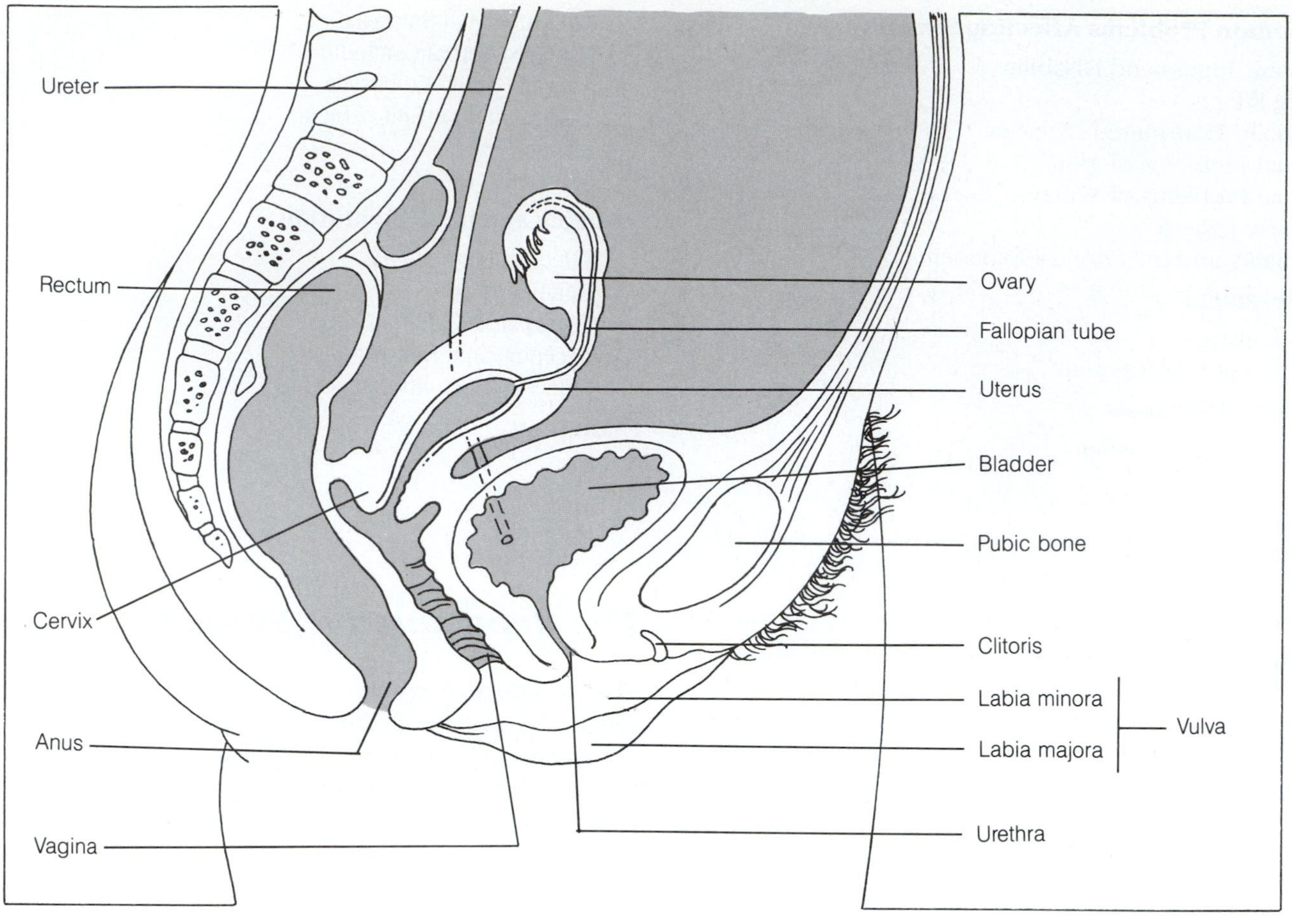

Figure 37-1. The female sexual organs.

Extending upward from the cervical opening is the remainder of the *uterus*, which is a pear-shaped organ, the rounded upper part of which is referred to as the fundus. The uterus is composed of an epithelial lining called the endometrium, a thick center layer of smooth muscle called the myometrium, and an outer covering of serous membrane called the perimetrium.

Attached to the upper outer angles of the uterus are the *Fallopian tubes*, which are made up of the same three layers as the uterus. These tubes serve as ducts for the ovaries; the upper end of each tube wraps up and over an ovary but is not attached. Small fringelike projections collect the egg (ovum) deposited by the ovary.

The ovaries themselves are the actual organs of reproduction for the female. Each is approximately the shape and size of an almond. The ovaries both produce the ova and secrete female hormones. The manner in which the ovum is formed, fertilized, and develops into the fetus and the actual process of birth are covered in studies of maternal—child nursing.

The Male Reproductive System

The external male sexual organ, which is also the organ of urinary elimination, is the *penis* (Fig. 37-2). The tip of the penis is called the glans and is covered by a loose folded skin referred to as the foreskin. This foreskin is surgically removed if circumcision is performed. A ridge called the corona separates the glans from the penis body. Both the glans and the corona provide sensitive areas for arousal. The penis contains three long internal chambers as well as the urinary urethra.

The *scrotum*, a pouch made of skin that contains the *testes*, is suspended below the penis. The testes are the actual reproductive organs of the male; they produce male sperm cells and also manufacture the sex hormone, testosterone, which is an **androgen** (male hormones).

The sperm produced by the testes enter the *epididymis*, a tube estimated to be 20 feet in length, which is tightly coiled on and about the testes. The sperm mature in this tube and then enter another tubelike structure, the vas deferens.

The *vas deferens*, which contains the sperm, follows a

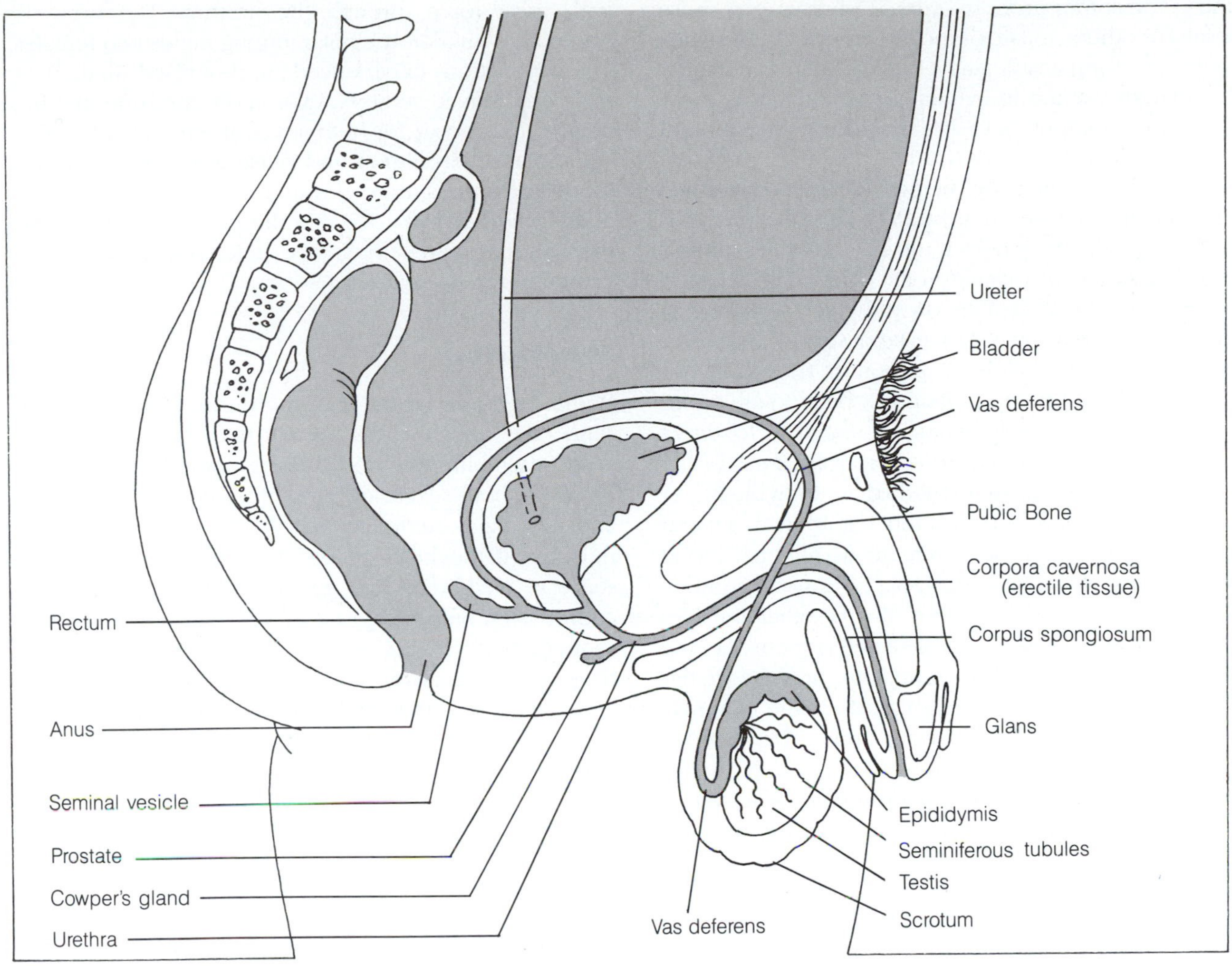

Figure 37-2. The male sexual organs.

circuitous route over the pubic bone and through the prostate gland. Here the sperm mix with fluid from two small saclike structures called the seminal vesicles as well as with fluid from the prostate gland. The sperm then exit from the vas deferens through the ejaculatory duct. This mixture of sperm and fluid, called semen, is then propelled or ejaculated through the urethra at the time of intercourse.

Gender Differences in the Body

There are both hormonal and anatomic differences between the sexes. Briefly, the female's breasts are more enlarged than the male's, although both female and male breasts can be used for *erotic* stimulation. Males, in general, have greater bone density, more muscle mass, coarser skin, wider distribution of hair over the body, broader shoulders, narrower hips, and lower voices than do females. Of course, these characteristics can overlap so an individual male may not differ from an individual female in all these areas.

Sexual Response

Two researchers, William Masters and Virginia Johnson (1966), have made considerable contribution to the research on sexuality. Through the use of scientific observation and data gathering, they described more clearly than anyone before them the physiology of human sexual response. Their research demonstrated that the sexual responses in men and women are more similar than had been formerly thought. Their work defined four stages of sexual response: excitement, plateau, orgasm, and resolution.

Excitement

Arousal can take place in response to many stimuli. Some persons are sexually aroused by certain smells. Among these odors are perfumes, fragrant flowers, incense, some fabrics such as leather, and the smell of the body. Other people are sexually aroused by specific sounds. For some, erotic words or phrases can cause arousal; for others, music or individual instruments such as bells or string music may be sexually stimulating. Sights that arouse are individual. Erotic literature, movies, and photographs have been sold for their arousal capabilities. Which materials are erotic and which are pornographic is currently being debated. Unclothed bodies, in our culture, may be very sexually provocative, although this may not be the case in other cultures in which persons are usually naked or lightly clad. A great deal has been written on the role of fantasy in arousal. The person may fantasize a sexual encounter with someone who has been important in the past or someone with whom the person has been totally uninvolved. Arousal can also occur in response to direct touch of the genitals, touch to other erotic areas of the body (which differ from individual to individual), or thoughts. Both men and women experience general vasocongestion in the pelvic organs as regional blood flow increases, as well as myotonia, or muscle contraction, primarily of the pelvis but also of other muscles throughout the body as a part of sexual response. In the male, during the period of *excitement*, or *arousal*, the penis becomes erect when the tissues of the channels called the corpus cavernosum and the corpus spongiosum suddenly become engorged with blood. The physical response to sexual arousal in the female is that vasocongestion causes fluid to move through the semipermeable membranes to the vaginal wall, lubricating the tissues. Engorgement of the clitoris similar to that of the male penis occurs. The nipples also become erect. Rates of respiration, pulse, and blood pressure increase for both sexes. There are other changes, such as swelling of the scrotum of the male and of the labia of the female. Visual accommodation narrows considerably.

Plateau

The *plateau* stage involves further intensity of vasocongestion. In the male, the testes enlarge, the penis becomes more firm, and the Cowper's glands emit a small amount of lubrication. The female's breasts temporarily enlarge, and the color and size of the labia change. At the end of the plateau stage, tension is sufficient to allow orgasm.

Orgasm

Masters and Johnson described the stage of *orgasm* for the male as having two components. The first occurs when the vas deferens, seminal vesicles, and prostate contract, forcing the semen into a bulblike structure at the base of the urethra.

Second, rhythmic contractions propel the ejaculate with great force through the urethra. The orgasmic stages are remarkably similar among males and females. The contractions experienced are described similarly by male and female subjects; even more amazing, the first contractions occur for both sexes at intervals of exactly 0.8 second. Respiration and pulse are more rapid and blood pressure is more elevated than at any other time. Many other changes occur in the pelvic tissues of both men and women during this stage, but these are not central to the present discussion.

Resolution

Within seconds after orgasm, during the *resolution* stage, the body begins to return to the preorgasmic state, resembling the body's more natural physical condition. In both sexes, swelling of tissues subsides, color and vital signs return to near normal ranges, and the muscles of the body relax. Most individuals report a sense of well-being and general relaxation after intercourse. Men enter a *refractory stage* during which subsequent performance is not possible. Women do not have this refractory stage and are able to become aroused again with sufficient erotic stimulation. That females are capable of being multiorgasmic is a widely known fact.

Masturbation

Masturbation is self-stimulation for the purpose of sexual pleasure, possibly terminating in sexual *climax*. Once thought harmful, masturbation is now accepted as a natural component of psychosexual development and a useful outlet for sexual tension for some individuals. Nevertheless, cultural taboos still surround masturbation, and it remains an emotionally charged subject. It may happen that you observe patients masturbating. Small children and psychologically disturbed patients for whom cultural values are not for the moment important may masturbate. Developmentally impaired and brain-damaged people sometimes masturbate openly. Only if such behavior becomes excessive and, in adults, is preferred to normal relationships does it pose a problem. When the patient improves and reestablishes a sexual relationship, masturbation usually diminishes.

When masturbation is performed visibly, the family and the staff may become upset, viewing such behavior as indelicate. Understanding the person's age and emotional and intellectual state may explain this behavior. For example, a 19-year-old young man has considerable brain damage due to a motorcycle accident. As his state of awareness improves, he begins to engage in masturbation. His mother, embarrassed and upset, asks the nurse to do something to stop him. When the nurse explains that such behavior is not unusual in brain-injured patients and could be a sign that the patient is becoming more aware of himself and progressing toward fuller consciousness, his mother can become more accepting.

What if the nurse happens in on an adult patient in the act of masturbating or engaging in other sexual activity? Leaving the patient in privacy is an appropriate response. Such behavior should be regarded as satisfying an immediate need, and no response should be made that might cause the patient to feel guilty or ashamed. The same principles apply in the case of the elderly man or woman who engages in masturbation. Sexual interest continues late in life, and some elderly people have no appropriate way to express this other than masturbation. Because the elderly who are institutionalized may suffer sensory deprivation, sexual self-stimulation can be therapeutic. Although encounters with masturbating patients will probably occur infrequently, the nurse should be prepared to deal with the situation knowledgeably and in an understanding manner.

It is important for nurses to know that some male patients may experience an involuntary erection during care. Such nursing tasks as cleansing the areas of elimination and the genitals can make both the nurse and the patient uncomfortable. It is not uncommon for a male patient to experience an erection of the penis during such care. This reflex should not be construed as a sexual overture. The erection mechanism is both voluntary, arising from the cerebral cortex, and involuntary, originating in the lumbar portion of the spinal cord. Even very young infants have erections, and adult men may experience them during the REM sleep stage. Adult men sometimes awaken with an erection due to a distended bladder. An erection during care is usually simply a reaction to the stimulus of touch and not an expression of erotic feelings. If the patient shows signs of embarrassment or makes an apology, the nurse may want to put the patient at ease by maintaining a professional manner and perhaps mentioning that such an occurrence is not uncommon and is due to a reflex that is not under his control.

Sexual Identity

Anatomic sexual identity is usually obvious at birth although with some congenital abnormalities genitalia are ambiguous. However, whether an individual's psychological sexual identity (*ie*, feelings, beliefs, and attitudes about his or her gender that lead to behavior deemed male or female) is present at birth is a controversial question. Recent research is focusing on identifiable differences in brain structure and brain hormonal distribution in those who identify with a particular sexual identity. Some people believe that physical characteristics are the determinants of later sexual behavior. Others believe that regardless of the imprinting at birth of sexual assignment, early social interaction largely determines gender identification and behavior. In support of the latter view, a number of studies report that parents and society behave differently toward boys than they do toward girls. These differences cause gender-specific behavior. For example, a little girl may be told that playful wrestling is not ladylike, yet a brother enjoying the same activity will receive parental encouragement. Brothers are told to take care of their sisters.

Behavior Related to Sexual Identity

Behavior related to sexual identity can be a reflection of the culture. Within a particular culture, the expectations for male or female behavior may be rigid. Different cultures, however, have different expectations. For example, consider the passivity of the Japanese woman, who in silence serves tea to only the male members of the family. This behavior is different from that of the German woman who enthusiastically serves dinner to the entire family of males and females. In many of these countries, sexual mores are vastly changing, particularly in large cities. For example, Japanese women are highly visible in universities, seeking positions in business and medicine. Changes in the German economy have opened up opportunities for women to compete with men for high positions in the workplace.

Despite this, prescribed norms for male and female behavior persist. People seem to feel more comfortable when they clearly know the sexual roles of those around them. These roles are largely defined by observable behavior. Gradually, however, as the limitations on acceptable sexual behavior have lessened, people have striven for more individuality regardless of their sexual orientation.

Appearance and attire are often sexually oriented. Clothing for females is often made of softer fabrics, such as silks, whereas male clothing has been dominated by the use of gabardine and woolens. Some designers are presenting clothing in materials and styles not exclusive to one sexual orientation. Although both sexes are currently sharing preferences for many of the same colors, colors for infants follow the ageless adage of blue for boys and pink for girls. Trousers and pants are worn by both sexes, but the styles, as with hair, are usually not the same.

You need to realize that the need for sexual behavior or to be sexually active is not as fundamental as the needs for oxygen and circulation, which are necessary for survival. Although most individuals do have a need to express their sexuality and sensuality by engaging in acts of intimacy, this need is by no means universal.

Sexual energy can be redirected on a short- or long-term basis. Many people, such as members of Catholic religious orders, those intensely involved in careers, or those lacking an appropriate sexual partner, may choose to be sexually inactive or only intermittently active. Yet these persons retain their sexual nature and enjoy the sensual experiences of life. Still others, usually those who have set a high priority on maintaining consistently active sexual behavior, become frustrated and distressed when their sexual pattern is disrupted. Human beings can express their sexual activity in a variety of ways.

Language and conversation can be sexually oriented. Women are sometimes stigmatized for telling "off-color" stories, whereas men may encourage one another to the point of a joke-telling competition. Many phrases and words are used almost exclusively by one sex or the other. For example, men rarely use the word "cute" when describing another man.

Role responsibility means that each of the sexes, because of expectations, undertakes certain tasks or responsibilities. The fact that the wife traditionally took responsibility for managing the home gave rise to the word housewife. Men have more traditionally overseen yard work and car maintenance. Today, however, with more women working full time, many couples divide household and yard responsibilities. Financial responsibilities are another arena in which change is occurring. For the first time, statistics show that a significant number of women in the United States make more money annually than their partners. Women are assuming managerial tasks, a divergence from the traditional pattern.

Dowling (1990), in a book called *The Cinderella Complex*, writes that because the role of women has been influenced by early conditioning, many women seek out partners who will take care of them and, in so doing, fail to fully develop their own potential. Attitudes about appropriate male and female behavior may also account for the view that men should initiate sexual encounters and women should be more passive. This particular aspect of gender-specific behavior is changing, however, as interviews with men reveal that many men find sexual initiation by their partner exciting. Kohlberg (1966) demonstrated that once a gender role is established, youngsters are motivated to behave as expected in that role. For example, a man or woman may ask, "How are boys or girls expected to act in our society and how can I be like that?" Gender identification and behavior are complicated matters and may be influenced by a combination of congenital, developmental, and societal factors.

Some of the more sensuous areas of behavior were once felt to be predominantly female. These include touch, giving service, and nurturing. Nowlis (1983) found that a woman, usually the adult daughter, functioned as the primary relationship person to an elderly individual three times as often as a man. Although the nurturing and service role has been culturally assigned in the past to women, men in increasing numbers are becoming involved in traditionally female occupations and professions such as education and nursing. The fact that more men are entering schools of nursing points out that sensitivity crosses all sexual lines. It may be helpful if you think about yourself as a sexual person and what behaviors are most comfortable for you. What situations cause you discomfort, both in society and in the patient care situation? Nurses can become more authentic with others if they are willing to examine their own sexual behavior and recognize its meaning.

Androgyny

It has long been recognized that both male and female characteristics exist in varying degrees with in each of us. The term for this phenomenon is **androgyny** from the Greek *andreios*, meaning male, and *gune*, meaning woman. To be androgynous is to be a fully masculine or feminine person and yet enjoy those components of the personality that are usually identified with the opposite sex. One example is the woman who enjoys the intense competition of running track; another is the man who creates delicate flower arrangements. A more interesting aspect of androgyny is revealed by the research of Bem (1974), who concluded that people who were more androgynous than others have the "flexibility to exhibit either masculine or feminine behaviors, depending on what the situation calls for . . . and thus, are better able to function effectively in a wider range of situations."

Sexual Orientation

Sexual orientation refers to the gender to which one is sexually attached. *Heterosexuality*, sexual response to members of the opposite sex, is the sexual orientation of most people in our society. Years ago, people engaging in sexual intercourse were married; today more and more heterosexual couples are having intercourse before or without marriage. Premarital intercourse has brought about reactions varying from disapproval to qualified acceptance to indifference. It is unclear if the increased acceptance of young people living together (cohabiting) before marriage has contributed to the rise premarital intercourse. The sexual practices of heterosexual persons are also far more varied than was once acknowledged. Current data reveal that heterosexual people spend a longer time during intercourse and use a greater variety of positions and techniques than those who are homosexual or bisexual.

Two other sexual lifestyles are also present in society: *homosexuality* (gay), that is, sexual orientation toward members of the same sex, and **bisexuality**, sexual attraction to members of both sexes. It is unclear whether more people are homosexual and bisexual now than in previous generations or whether greater public acceptance has simply made sexual lifestyles more apparent. Recent studies estimate that from 5% to 10% of the male population is homosexual. Statistics on women are more difficult to determine because of the hesitancy of some women to reveal their sexual orientation. Bisexuality is easily kept covert or hidden, and therefore the statistics that have been gathered are considered inaccurate. Until recently, both homosexuality and bisexuality were considered deviant behavior. In the last few years, homosexuals, most of whom prefer to be called *gays* (either sex) or *lesbians* (women), have formed groups for mutual support and to protest practices that discriminate against them. One important step in regard to gay rights was the affirmation by the American Psychiatric Association (APA) in 1973 of the position that homosexuality in and of itself does not constitute mental illness. This opinion remains valid today.

Sexual stereotyping, unwise in any situation, is particularly futile when one tries to guess another person's sexual orientation. The notion that a particular behavior pattern in men or women denotes that they are gay is simply false. Studies of gay people reveal no overwhelming preponderance of particular traits. These findings underline the wisdom of accepting people as they are, without preconceptions.

Although some individuals in society find it difficult to accept the homosexual person as an equal, with similar attitudes and feelings, society as a whole has become much more accepting of homosexuality. Many gay persons are revealing their sexual orientation and openly entering the political arena. Others are speaking out for gay rights, seeking recognition as contributing citizens to our society.

Despite this openness, the homosexual patient is sometimes psychologically ostracized by the nursing staff. This happens more often when the patient has a partner of the same sex, and affection is openly displayed between the two. Some nurses are uncomfortable with this behavior, so a degree of relief is sometimes evident when the patient is discharged.

Nurses and Sexual Awareness

If we consider nurses sociologically, we can better understand the sources of the attitudes nurses sometimes exhibit toward people whose sexual lives differ from the majority. The roots of nursing were in religion; many schools of nursing were originally church based. Also, nurses are largely drawn from the middle class; few are very wealthy or very poor. The characteristic values of the middle class have tended to be conservative, particularly in the realm of sexuality. Social changes are usually initiated at the fringes of society and make their way into the mainstream gradually. Nurses, as representatives of the mainstream, may accept social change somewhat reluctantly.

Nurses come from all sectors of society and reflect the same variety of sexual preferences that exists in society at large. Just as a certain percentage of the general population is homosexual or bisexual, so some members of the health care team, including nurses, may be. It is impossible, of course, to suppress one's emotional and sexual lives entirely when practicing nursing.

It has been said that many nurses appear **asexual** or sexless and prefer to regard patients in the same light. Perhaps some nurses exaggerate their professional demeanor as an emotional defense to facilitate performing intimate tasks for patients. Nurses' attitudes unavoidably influence their interactions with patients and with peers. You must understand that nurses should never impose their sexual views on their patients. Although remaining objective and nonjudgmental is not always easy, nurses should regard patients as people with problems who need care, regardless of their sexual orientation or lifestyle. Similarly, nurses should evaluate one another in terms only of nursing proficiency, not of sexual orientation. As a part of society, nurses are becoming increasingly aware of differences in sexual orientation and the impact of these differences on health care.

It is incumbent on nurses to recognize that individuals have the right to fulfill their sexual needs however they desire, as long as others are not coerced or harmed in any way. It is important, furthermore, to respond objectively and professionally to gay patients and others whose lifestyles are differ from the majority.

Inappropriate Sexual Behavior

Sexuality can sometimes be used in a harmful way to intimidate others. Although these behaviors are sexual, they may primarily be acts of power seeking or anger and have both social and legal consequences.

Sexual Harassment

Sexual harassment issues have been addressed by the federal Equal Employment Opportunity Commission (EEOC). Although the majority of victims of sexual harassment are women, men may also be subjected to sexual harassment. Any of the following may be considered forms of sexual harassment:

1. Unwelcome sexual advances
2. Requests for sexual favors
3. Unnecessary touch
4. Offensive sexual graffiti
5. Offensive, disparaging remarks about one's gender

6. Physical aggression such as pinching, patting, or grabbing
7. Sexual innuendos made at inappropriate times
8. Written communications with sexual overtones
9. Verbal sexually abusive remarks disguised as humor
10. Obscene gestures

Female and male nurses, in particular, are vulnerable to such behavior, partially because their job entails care that is often sensitive and intimate in nature. Harassment may come not only from patients but from peers and those in supervisory positions. One would like to believe that such situations are rare, but recent court cases reveal that they occur frequently. It must be pointed out that "the line between subtle seductive behavior and harassment is a fine one." When harassment comes from patients, "there is considerable room for interpretation—and confusion—on the part of both patients and nurses" (Heinrich, 1987).

There are initial things you can do to stop such actions before consulting your supervisor on the nursing staff. Pretending such an incident did not occur is usually not helpful because it allows the same behavior to be repeated. It is usually more effective to confront the situation, saying calmly that you care about the patient professionally but that personal advances are inappropriate and may even interfere with care. If you express your concern for the patient as a person and do not respond to such an incident with rejection, a working relationship and a friendly professional atmosphere can usually be reinstated. Setting limits allows the patient and the nurse to feel more comfortable.

You must closely examine your own dress and behavior to ensure whether, even unconsciously, you are not sending messages that could be construed as sexually provocative. In general, women express sexuality more visually than do men; men express sexuality more verbally. For example, a female nurse in a short, form-fitting uniform may convey a highly sexual image to the patient. A male nurse may exhibit his sexuality by making a lighthearted but sexually suggestive remark to a patient. Neither is behaving professionally. Patients, who are typically bored and unable to pursue their usual forms of sexual release, are especially vulnerable to both visual and verbal nuances. Any frank sexual remark or overture to a patient by any nurse or the same behavior to a nurse by any patient, regardless of the sex of either, is extremely inappropriate and unprofessional.

Sexual Coercion and Domestic Violence

There are private relationships in which one partner uses sexuality as a coercive device. Two situations could be coercive. The first involves one person demanding favors from a partner who is unable to resist the advances. This person may have low self-esteem resulting in powerlessness to decline to participate or be in a position in which one has to agree to sexual participation to preserve the relationship for social, retaliative, or economic reasons. Often, the reason for a married person is attributed to maintaining an intact home for children. Although physical violence may not have occurred, this situation is currently called the battered woman (or man) syndrome.

The second situation is one in which one of the partners uses sexual attraction or performance to gain power over the other. For example, a woman (not a prostitute) may willingly participate in sexual performance to gain approval or a feeling of being needed. The coercion may be to gain material things in life such as expensive clothing or an automobile. Each of these situations uses sexuality in an inappropriate manner because they use sexuality to manipulate another person.

In the extreme, coercive sexual behavior can lead to sexual assault. Domestic violence is often of a sexual nature and may include physical harm. The couple may be married or unmarried. There is growing concern about the increasing domestic violence throughout the world. Studies have shown that domestic violence increases during periods of economic strain. Personal pressures experienced by individuals may also lead to this kind of activity.

As a member of a helping profession, you should never participate in such a relationship nor should you ignore clear evidence that a patient is a perpetrator or victim of violence. If you are personally involved in a destructive relationship in which there is a threat or an actual event of violence or you identify cues from a patient, action is appropriate. If you are in the situation, it is clear that changes must be made. If the person is a patient, it is best to not confront such a sensitive issue yourself. Persons on the staff or in the community have special education concerning these issues and your input and referral to someone knowledgeable is a service to the patient.

Sexual Assault

Sexual assault can occur within or without an established relationship. It can involve a person unknown by the victim or not recognized as an appropriate sexual partner such as a relative, neighbor, or coworker.

Sexual assault, the imposition of any sexual behavior on an unwilling person, includes acts ranging in severity from simple exposure to rape. It is important to understand that these acts of sexual assault are more hostile and violent than sexual in motivation. Statistics on the incidence of sexual assault are difficult to gather; the majority of cases are not reported because the victim feels fear, guilt, or humiliation. Recent attention has been focused on date rape, in which one partner is assaulted by another within the confines of an arranged social event that was not intended to include sexual activity.

As a nurse, you may be consulted by a patient or a friend seeking counseling or support for a victim. Sexual assault violates the dignity and bodily integrity of the victim and can be highly damaging emotionally. Subsequent sexual problems may arise between the victim and the usual sexual partner. The person may develop socially incapacitating fears. For these and other reasons, the victim should be strongly encouraged to seek professional help. A physical examination should be performed to rule out the presence of sexually transmitted disease (STD) and pregnancy; psychological help is highly desirable to offset emotional trauma. Nurses can provide support and caring for victims of sexual assault.

Large urban areas have sexual assault clinics or rape relief agencies whose purpose is to aid victims medically, psychologically, socially, and legally. Privacy is respected. You should encourage the victim or the family to make use of such community resources, which can do a great deal to minimize the trauma of sexual assault.

Factors Affecting Sexuality

A number of factors affect sexuality; some are internal, and some external. *Libido* (the desire for sexual activity) can be affected as well as sexual performance. We shall not attempt to discuss such factors as childhood influences or choice of partners, not because they are unimportant, but because they are complex and lie outside the intent of this text. For nurses, some of the more important factors that affect sexuality are age, relationships, the environment, and current health status.

Age

In the past, the span of years available for sexual performance and procreation was much shorter than it is today. Over the past 100 years, puberty has occurred much earlier in the life span and longevity has approximately doubled. This lengthening of life expectancy is due in large part to the increased emphasis on personal hygiene and the decreased incidence of contagious disease, as well as to the strides in modern technology that have produced better diets and generally healthier lives. Because sexual performance is possible from the time of puberty into the later years, many have suggested that these changes make it unrealistic to attempt to confine sexual expression to the married years or to make sexual performance acceptable only within marriage. Whether society will continue to strongly expect sexual behavior to be confined to marriage is open to question. Difficult problems are bound to arise when the sexual norms and moral standards of society do not provide an outlet for those with an age-related physical potential for sexuality.

Even with the wide use of birth control pills and other birth control methods, statistics show that one in every three pregnancies among young people is unplanned and involves a single mother. Some researchers place this figure even higher. The recent massive increase in pregnancy and STDs among teenagers is a matter of deep concern to health care professionals, public policymakers, parents, and teenagers alike. In addition to the problems unplanned pregnancy can cause young people themselves, there are the developmental health problems of the infants, the incidence of which tends to be high among infants of teenage parents. As a nursing student or practicing nurse, you may be consulted by teenagers or their parents with regard to sexual matters. You should listen with empathy to their problems and serve as a resource person, providing referral to a professional counselor or agency.

Young adulthood and the middle years may also be characterized by a variety of sexual crises. Many couples experience sexual incompatibility or differing desires with regard to frequency of intercourse, although divorcing couples cite money and children more often than sexual problems as causes of estrangement.

Although separation and divorce can occur during the life span of any adult, they are statistically more frequent in young adulthood and the middle years. Once a separation or divorce has occurred, many sexual issues arise. "When deprived of regular sexual relations, persons respond with a variety of stress reactions and symptoms. Life style changes become an immediate reality. Personal values are challenged. Dating becomes a new challenge or threat depending upon the reaction of the individual" (Turner, 1980). The pursuit of sexual gratification is usually a hidden agenda in these new relationships.

Sexual activity between people past childbearing age was once thought to be not nice and not necessary, but such attitudes no longer prevail. Both partners may continue to enjoy sexual activity into their eighties and beyond. Thus, it is unjustifiable to assume that an elderly patient is no longer interested and has no active sexual life. Some elderly couples have, for health-related or psychological reasons, mutually decided to conclude their sexual activity. In other cases, such a decision is made unilaterally, causing friction between the partners. Physiologically, the aging process causes structural and hormonal changes in the sexual organs that may bring about some decline in libido and frequency of performance.

In the woman, *estrogen* production decreases as the

ovaries become less active, causing changes in the sexual organs. The vaginal walls become thinner and less elastic than during the productive years. At this time *menopause* is occurring. The woman may also notice less lubrication at time of intercourse; commercial lubricants can be used. Physicians may choose to prescribe replacement estrogen for their patients. This decision does carry some risk, such as carcinoma of the uterus, so patients taking estrogen, except for those who have undergone hysterectomy (removal of the uterus), should be under close surveillance.

In the man, testosterone production decreases, increasing the time needed to achieve erection and extending the refractory stage. The volume of semen also decreases, and the testicles become somewhat smaller in size. Unlike the woman, the man may have some difficulty in maintaining the frequency of intercourse of the earlier years, but he may enjoy it more because of increased control over *ejaculation.*

Masters and Johnson (1966) revealed an interesting fact about both men and women; those older persons who were previously sexually active on a regular basis and had their sexual relationship interrupted were able to resume sexual relations with another partner fairly easily, whereas those who had never been sexually active or were not recently active found performing sexually to be much more difficult.

Because women are likely to live longer than men, the problem of losing the sexual partner in later years is of particular concern to this group. Older women outnumber available men, so that it is more difficult to replace the lost partner. Because older women are often more reluctant to pursue a partner than older widowed men, women are even more sexually isolated. Sexual outlets for these women are fairly limited although some enjoy masturbation. Others find that this activity causes anxiety, guilt, and shame, so that abstinence is the most acceptable chosen path. This seems to indicate that the unavailability of a sexual partner on a regular basis, leading to abstinence, may be a strong factor in giving the impression that older persons are not interested in sexual matters. Those who are older need to know that sexual activity in the later years is acceptable, enjoyable, and natural, and nurses need to dispel any preconceptions to the contrary.

Relationships

Relationships are a primary factor when considering the area of sexuality. Certainly, a good and supportive relationship is eloquently expressed when partners join together in a mutually satisfying sexual experience. The sexual act is both gratifying to the individual as well as a giving, caring response to the other person. A sexually gratifying partnership has a greater chance of survival than does one with sexual problems.

Studies have shown that both men and women can remain sexually active through advanced age. However, some individuals who are young or older, choose not to be sexually active for a variety of reasons. These persons can continue to feel sexually secure in their relationship to others and relate in a sexual manner without being sexually active. Regardless of the decision concerning sexual activity, relationship remains an essential part of sexuality.

Environment

The major changes that illness causes in the patterns of daily living are exaggerated by the unfamiliar environment of the hospital. Not only is sexual activity postponed but work, hobbies, and family and community responsibilities are also interrupted. For the sexually active patient, long-term interruption of sexual activity can be a stressor that intensifies the illness (Fig. 37-3). Many people in health care view the hospital or chronic care setting as an inappropriate place for sexual interaction. Some acute and chronic care settings do allow conjugal visitation between sexual partners. Rooms can also be shared by partners. This arrangement is mutually agreeable to all involved, including staff, and privacy is provided.

Another option is to provide home passes for hospitalized patients. The patient remains registered on the census record of the hospital but visits home for a predetermined period of time. Passes are frequently issued for a variety of reasons. This alternative is particularly valuable for patients undergoing intermittent treatment or lengthy rehabilitation. For the patient unable to go out on pass, lack of a comfortable, stress-free environ-

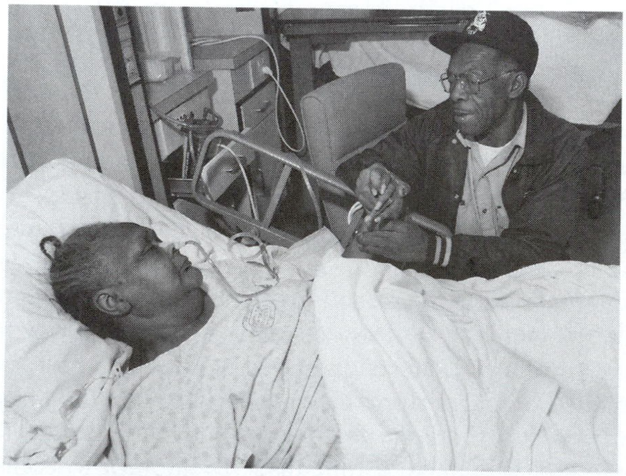

Figure 37-3. The hospital environment may cause a temporary disruption in sexual activity.

ment for purposes of intimacy continues to be an unanswered problem in most institutions.

It has been suggested that residents in long-term care facilities have access to a special room for *conjugal* visits with the sexual partner. Several prisons in this country have had this arrangement for some time, and it seems no less important for those who are medically confined over a long period of time. It is unfortunate when nurses view the patient role as one without sexual needs.

Current Health Status

Interest in sexual matters and sexual performance are enhanced by a state of physical and psychological well-being. When illness intrudes, both general and specific sexual problems can arise.

Among the most common components of illness are fatigue and general malaise or listlessness, neither of which is conducive to sexual activity. The body's resources are all engaged in combating the illness; the patient's mind is focused on regaining health and possibly also on missing work and the burden the illness represents for the family. Illness is also typically accompanied by some degree of mental depression, which is known to reduce libido.

Common Problems Affecting Sexuality

Nurses should be familiar with common medical problems that are sexual in nature. Both men and women may experience low libido. The need for sexual activity varies greatly from one individual to another and may become a problem when it is perceived as such by the individual. There are also distinct medical sexual problems that are experienced by both men and women.

Chronic Illness and Disability

Certain chronic illnesses can affect sexuality. Diabetic men, for example, experience more sterility and impotence than the general population, and women whose diabetes is poorly controlled tend to give birth to larger-than-normal infants.

Sexual performance provokes anxiety in some epileptics, who equate sexual excitement with the advent of a seizure. However, there is no evidence to substantiate the notion that seizures are brought on by sexual activity. Living as normally as possible is desirable for the epileptic individual.

Many patients suffer from chronic illnesses such as emphysema and arthritis. These individuals need not necessarily forgo sexual pleasure; with variations in frequency and technique, they can continue to be sexually active. Having an understanding partner is of great benefit in these situations.

Many people are *disabled* by chronic conditions and diseases of the muscular, skeletal, cardiovascular, and nervous systems that render them disabled. Of necessity, their lives consist of numerous adaptations and adjustments to function as normally as possible. Health care personnel have traditionally focused primarily on helping handicapped patients ambulate, dress and feed themselves, and perform basic hygiene. Only recently have those caring for the disabled begun to consider their sexual needs. It must be remembered that the patient's sexual needs usually involve another person equally and fully. With therapy and walking devices, some patients may learn to walk again. But this could be only a hollow triumph in the wake of a broken marriage or the loss of a meaningful relationship.

There are certain preconditions for the development of a friendship that leads to a caring sexual relationship. The disabled face some unique problems establishing such a relationship—problems with body image, conveying sexuality, finding a partner, and sexual performance.

Body image is one's concept of one's physical self. Achievement of a body image that is both favorable and realistic is one of the central tasks of development, particularly in adolescence. Such a body image in turn contributes to a strong self-concept. For the disabled, as for everyone else, body image is deeply influenced by the reactions of others. Furthermore, a sense of control over one's body is central to one's self-concept (Bogle and Shaul, 1979). People disabled since birth or early childhood may be less prone to body image disturbance than those disabled in adulthood. Coming to terms with disability in a realistic and accepting way frees a person to reach out for friendship that can grow into a sexual relationship.

Visible disability can be a barrier to *conveying sexuality* in such a way that it attracts another person into an intimate relationship. Inability to stand may hinder the initial sexual phase. To make eye contact with someone in a wheelchair or bed, the nondisabled person must sit. If the upper limbs are affected, embracing is left to the nondisabled partner. The disabled can, however, learn to use expressive body language.

Appliances such as braces convey a feeling of being cold, hard, and angular, characteristics that do not convey sexuality. More often, sexuality is thought of in terms of warmth, softness, and roundness. Appliances and body distortion, such as limb atrophy, can be frightening to people unaccustomed to physical disabilities.

Finding a partner may also be a problem for some

Nursing Research: *Implications for Practice*

Hahn, K. "Sexuality and COPD." *Rehabilitation Nursing* 14, 4 (July-August 1989): 191–195.

Hahn formed a pulmonary support group of 18 persons and their partners, focusing on exploring sexual matters. The content was presented through the use of diagrams, video tapes, and handouts showing possible adaptations during sexual intercourse. The participants were then divided into two groups for discussion—persons with breathing problems and partners of those persons. The questions asked of the groups were "What has changed about your sex life since breathing problems entered it?" and "What has helped you and your partner most in dealing with those changes?"

When the two groups merged for a final and lengthy discussion, it was clear that "good communication (between partners) facilitates healthy, satisfying adjustment in sexual relations." "Health professionals needed to present information to patients with less reluctance and more knowledge."

This study emphasizes the important role of the nurse as a facilitator so that adequate communication can occur between partners when sexual adaptations are necessary. It also places on the nurse the role of teacher. To teach effectively, the nurse must attain the confidence and comfort needed to assess and talk more openly with patients concerning sexual matters.

who are disabled. Transforming a friendship into an intimate sexual relationship is a delicate process. The process usually begins with subtle probing to find out whether the desire for a relationship is mutual. There may follow a covert testing period, which can provoke anxiety. If the relationship does not become sexual, the disappointed partner often suffers feelings of rejection and unworthiness. In addition to these universal problems, the disabled have the added disadvantage that many nondisabled people consider them incapable of sexual arousal or performance.

Adaptations may have to be made regarding *sexual performance*. A disabled person with a willing, accepting partner can find sexual variations that will prove mutually satisfying. Although each case is entirely individual, recent studies are optimistic about sexual activity for the handicapped. New sexual techniques must often be learned and adaptations made, but the joy of relating sexually need not end. Such adjustments may be as simple as trying a new position or as delicate as accommodating to the presence of a catheter or stoma. Some disabled people have succeeded in enhancing the *erogenous* potential of parts of the body other than the genitals, even to the point of experiencing orgasmic equivalents in such areas as the abdomen, buttocks, and ears. This experience is called a **paraorgasm**.

Drug Effects

Few, if any, drugs are without side effects. Such side effects are at best distressing to the patient and at worst dangerous. Physicians often choose to prescribe a certain drug, regardless of its side effects, because it is the best agent for a specific condition. Drugs commonly cause skin rashes, blood disorders, nausea, respiratory depression, and a host of other reactions and can cause changes and problems in every system of the body. Drugs can also affect libido or sexual performance. Other types of drugs may also change sexual response.

More than 200 *prescription drugs* can cause some degree of change in libido or sexual performance. Steroids are widely used as anti-inflammatory agents. These drugs often bring on a sense of well-being that enhances sexual performance. Steroids also tend to be antiandrogens, which may reduce libido. These opposite effects can cause different responses in different individuals.

Antihypertensive drugs are known for reducing potency in men and it is suggested that women also experience lowered sexual response. Anticholinergics, which are used in reducing the incidence of peptic ulcer, in the treatment of urinary and gastrointestinal distress, and for glaucoma symptoms, do not alter libido but can have an effect on performance. Other classes of drugs that decrease sexual adequacy are *antidepressants*, *antihistamines*, *sedatives*, and *anorexics* (these reduce appetite, but some are amphetamine related).

Prescription drugs are used in other ways that affect sexuality. Several hormones we have discussed, such as testosterone and other androgens, are often used to retard malignant or abnormal cell growth. When used for this purpose, a hormone predominant in the opposite sex may be prescribed in rather large dosage. Some masculinizing effect on the female and feminizing effect on the male undergoing such therapy is almost unavoidable, and a supportive, empathic attitude on the part of the nurse is essential.

Although many of the potential side effects of drugs are mentioned to the patient so that he or she will be sure to inform the physician if they occur, there is disagreement about whether information on potential sexual alterations should be provided in all cases. The issue is whether such information might be suggestive enough to trigger problems not otherwise caused by the medication. On the other hand, patients taking some of these drugs have been known to become upset over decreased libido and difficulty in sexual performance, not realizing that such changes are drug induced.

The drug information circulated by pharmaceutical companies citing sexual difficulties due to certain drugs usually focuses on the male response—lack of sexual desire, failure to attain or maintain an erection, and ejaculation of semen too early or not at all. Such deficiencies in men appear to be more readily measurable than are deficiencies of response in women, but lack of sexual desire and inability to attain climax may occur in the woman to an equally distressing degree.

A trusted nurse is often the one person to whom the patient confides sexual problems. Patients may express great relief when you explain that it is possible that such problems may be drug related. When the physician is consulted, the drug may or may not be discontinued, depending on its importance in the treatment of the underlying condition. If the drug is not withdrawn, the patient and the partner may need continuing support and counsel with regard to the resultant sexual problem.

You may help patients by keeping in mind the drugs each is taking and by monitoring side effects. One strong argument for ongoing assessment is that problems of a sexual nature are thus detected before they cause the patient undue emotional distress and anxiety.

Since early times, people have sought out compounds or foods that could heighten sexual desire and improve performance. These substances are called *aphrodisiacs*. A true aphrodisiac has not been found, but we do know that testosterone, one of the group of hormones called androgens (normally found in both sexes but more substantially in the male), can sometimes increase sexual performance in the male. A synthetic preparation of another androgen to increase the libido of women has been tried with mixed success. Side effects occur with both drugs.

Many who use *illicit drugs*, also called *recreational drugs*, do so in the hope of improving their sexual performance. Data are still inconclusive as to the degree of change occurring with any one drug. One reason for this is that "drugs in small dosages and used infrequently may produce one effect; in large dosages and used habitually they may produce an opposite reaction" (Siemens and Brandzel, 1982). "Poppers," or inhaled amyl nitrite from ampules, are used by males to enhance orgasm. Amyl nitrite is a vasodilator that increases blood flow to the pelvic organs. Marijuana increases blood testosterone levels for those who are light users. Many of these persons report increased sexual capability, but this may happen because the drug brings about a state of relaxation that removes sexual inhibitions. Male chronic heavy users of marijuana have decreased levels of testosterone, a condition that can cause decreased sexual activity. Whether this decrease is caused by lowered libido or decreased ability to perform is not clear at this time.

Cocaine and the *amphetamines* are stimulants that increase circulation to the genitals and raise blood pressure. Both have been credited by some with increasing sexual performance, but again, the causes may be their tendency to relax those using them and to give these persons a false sense of well-being.

Opiates constitute perhaps the most dramatic group of drugs that negatively alter normal sexual activity. The "rush" obtained by the user has been described as erotic, so some addicts actually substitute this experience for their usual sexual activity. Both men and women under the influence of opiates cannot achieve the physiologic stages of excitement and orgasm.

Nicotine, a vasoconstrictor, usually taken in through smoking tobacco, may delay erection and ejaculation so that sexual performance for the male is delayed and libido for the female is decreased. *Alcohol* is considered to be the most abused drug in our country today, with over 7 million people (7% of the population) having a drinking problem (Siemens and Brandzel, 1982). Alcohol, a depressant, commonly causes impotence in males. Although women appear to have fewer physiologic problems with alcohol, their drinking is often closely tied to feelings of sexual inadequacy. A large number of identified alcoholics have long-term sexual dysfunction. Unfortunately, altered sexual performance is only one consequence of excessive alcohol intake. Many other life-threatening effects make this social habit one with serious consequences.

Sexually Transmitted Diseases

Various STDs have been treated by the health care system for many years. Many of these diseases have existed throughout history. There are more than 100 STDs, ranging from viral to bacterial disorders. Some common ones that affect both males and females are genital ulcers, the chlamydial infections, syphilis, and gonorrhea. Other sexually transmitted infections include bloodborne diseases such as human immunodeficiency virus (HIV) and hepatitis B virus.

The STDs are detected through a complete history

that includes an interview, physical examination, and laboratory examination. Because STDs are increasing in number, the media and educators have given them considerable attention in an attempt to decrease their incidence.

Infection with HIV is currently of extreme concern to most of the inhabitants of the world as well as to health care professionals. Although this disease can be transmitted in a variety of ways such as through injection drug abuse, contaminated needle stick injuries, contaminated blood transfusions, and from the mother to the unborn child, sexual transmission continues to be a major concern.

The first documented case of acquired immunodeficiency syndrome (AIDS) was described in 1979. Since that time, the number of persons infected with HIV has grown so relentlessly that it is estimated that 2 million persons or more have been infected in the United States alone. Accurate worldwide statistics are not available although there is a continuing effort to monitor the extent of this epidemic. Persons who have been exposed to the HIV virus and have developed antibodies are by definition infected, although they may not manifest symptoms of AIDS.

Researchers are presently unsure how many persons exposed to the virus and infected will eventually develop this fatal disease. In June 1992, a new definition of AIDS was proposed by the Centers for Disease Control and Prevention (CDC). Under this definition, any person whose T cell lymphocyte count tested at 200 or below could be designated as having AIDS. The use of this definition will drastically increase the number of individuals diagnosed as having AIDS. Although many important facts about this disease are unknown at this time, we do know about some characteristics of the virus and how it is transmitted.

Originally AIDS occurred in the gay population in North America. The practice of having many sexual partners, which was common in the gay population in the late 1970s and early 1980s contributed to the spread of the virus within this group. Homosexual transmission may also be high because of the practice of anal intercourse and the potential for injury to the rectal tissue. The virus in the semen is then able to enter the bloodstream more easily.

The incidence of AIDS is now increasing among heterosexual individuals. It is more likely that a man will transfer the virus to a female partner than vice versa, because the vaginal wall is full of blood vessels and can be injured during intercourse. In addition, semen carries a larger total quantity of virus than does vaginal fluid. However, cases have been reported in which the woman has transmitted the virus to the man.

Data have indicated that approximately 90% of babies born to mothers positive for the HIV antibody will receive maternal HIV antibodies and of these, approximately one-half are infected with the virus and will develop the disease. In 1992, the CDC announced that research had revealed that the virus is present in breast milk so that infected pregnant women are discouraged from breast-feeding their infants. The naturally immature immune system of infants may intensify the effects of the virus on the body, giving these children a short life expectancy.

To have contracted the HIV virus and become antibody positive (**seropositive**) can be devastating to the individual. At present, various proposals for testing individuals are being considered. Many see mandatory testing as a practice that could place an infected person at risk of job loss, in jeopardy for loss of insurance coverage, and at risk of social alienation.

The fear of contracting the virus has caused intense interest in methods to prevent spread of the disease. Protective precautions intended for avoiding transmission of the virus are effective also in preventing the spread of other STDs. The AIDS epidemic has drastically changed sexual practices among many people. Perhaps no other issue than risk of acquiring the AIDS infection has so completely affected thinking about sexuality.

By far the safest sexual practice is to abstain, or not participate in sexual intercourse. To many persons, this is not an acceptable option. The next safest practice is to engage in sexual activity only within an established monogamous relationship with an uninfected partner. Sexual activity that does not include intercourse or exchange of body fluids is believed to be safe.

If an established monogamous relationship does not exist, sexual activity should be entered into with only one partner, who has practiced low-risk behavior. Low-risk behavior means abstaining from sexual intercourse with infected persons, with those who have used injection drugs, with those with a history of multiple sexual partners (especially prostitutes), or with those who have had multiple blood transfusions before testing procedures were available.

Those who do not establish a monogamous relationship are more at risk. The greater the number of sexual partners, the greater the risk, particularly when the sexual history is unknown. The most hazardous sexual practice is to engage in sexual intercourse with multiple partners, unprotected by a latex condom and a spermicidal product such as nonoxynol-9. (This product has been proven very effective in destroying sexually transmitted microorganisms.)

The CDC recommends that men wear latex condoms whenever intercourse occurs regardless of high or low risk. There is also an approved female condom. A further recommendation is to use nonoxynol-9 with a condom if there is any uncertainty regarding the partner's sexual history. Anal sex is thought to be more hazardous than vaginal sex because of the greater incidence of trauma, among other factors.

Nurses and those who care about them have felt a wave of fear related to the care of HIV seropositive and AIDS patients. Because the disease is fatal, this fear is understandable. However, public awareness and better education concerning AIDS have done a great deal to dispel unreasonable fear. Nurses can protect themselves. The current guidelines recommended by the CDC and legally mandated by the Occupational Safety and Health Administration were discussed in Chapter 21. These practices provide protection for health care workers from HIV as well as any disease transmitted by blood or body fluids. At a time when attention is being focused on the sexual transmission of diseases through the interchange of body fluids, nurses must be knowledgeable about safe sexual practices to fulfill their teaching responsibilities.

Sexual Problems of Men

By far the most common sexual problem for men is *impotence*, the inability to produce or maintain a penile *erection*. Although it is commonly believed that impotence is usually psychological rather than physical in origin, disorders of the endocrine system, such as too little testosterone or overactive thyroids should not be overlooked. Impotence can also be caused by motor nerve disruption, as in cases of spinal cord injury and by circulatory problems such as atherosclerosis. A variety of medical and surgical treatments are available for impotence.

Studies have found that occasional impotence is present in most of all sexually active males among the general population and is considered normal. Masters and Johnson (1966) reported that among the men they studied experiencing impotence, the most, by far, had what they termed "secondary impotence," which they defined as erectile problems occurring during sexual encounters at least 25% of the time. Secondary impotence deserves to be treated. Because society places great value on male potency, impotence has profound psychological impact. This impact also makes study and treatment a complicated matter.

The second most common problem is **premature ejaculation**, usually defined as ejaculation of semen within 30 to 60 seconds of *intromission*, or penetration of the vagina. Premature ejaculation is a problem because it interferes with the satisfaction of one or both partners and may be caused by anxiety or other psychological mechanisms as well as by physical problems.

Less common is **inhibitory ejaculation**, which can take the form of either delayed ejaculation or inability to ejaculate. This problem may interfere with the mutual satisfaction of the partners and is often psychological in origin.

Sexual Problems of Women

Frigidity is a term that is no longer widely used by health care personnel because of its broad definition encompassing a variety of problems from low desire to dissatisfaction with sexual relations. Much of the newer terminology focuses on orgasmic ability.

Masters and Johnson (1966) use the term *primary orgasmic dysfunction* to identify the woman who has never experienced an orgasm by any means—masturbation, foreplay, or intercourse. *Secondary orgasmic dysfunction* refers to a woman who has experienced at least one orgasm by whatever means but no longer does. A *nonorgasmic* woman may have a strong libido and yet not be able to achieve an orgasm.

The response of women with secondary orgasmic dysfunction and those who are nonorgasmic is similar. Both may have sexual desire and both may find great pleasure in intimacy. Nonorgasmic women differ in that some have never had an orgasm, whereas others can achieve orgasm only with difficulty. Some women who do not achieve orgasm through intercourse alone can do so with other forms of sexual play and may prefer such alternatives to intercourse. Accurate data are difficult to obtain, but several studies report that from 10% to 20% of women either have never experienced an orgasm or have done so only intermittently. A woman may also feel satisfied without attaining an orgasm. Being nonorgasmic becomes a problem, in large part, only if the woman or her partner perceives it as one.

Vaginismus, meaning severe and painful spasm of the vaginal orifice brought on by attempts at intercourse, is a less common sexual problem and usually psychological in origin. Painful intercourse, or **dyspareunia**, is often due to inadequate lubrication of the vagina, which in older women may be a consequence of estrogen deficiency. Occasionally, dyspareunia is caused by structural defects.

The causes of sexual dysfunction in women are complex. Each individual has to be evaluated separately for appropriate solutions to be reached. Most dysfunctions have underlying causes, including traumatic sexual experiences as a child or as an adult, repressive attitudes imposed early in life, fear, depression, and unsatisfactory interactions. The increasing documentation of sexual abuse today suggests that such abuse may be a more important cause of female sexual dysfunction than it had traditionally been thought to be.

Cardiac Disease

Men are statistically more at risk than women for heart attacks. Because a heart attack can happen during the excitement and energy expenditure of intercourse, many of these patients experience sexual anxiety after surviving the event. First, they wonder, "Can I ever perform sexually again?" and then, "If I do, will I have another heart attack?" If this anxiety reaches high levels, psychological impotence can occur.

Nurses who practice in coronary care units are specially educated to give health instruction to postcardiac patients. A teaching program should include information on sexual activity and its effect on the heart. The physician determines what instructions are appropriate for a given patient, but it is rare that medical status dictates that sexual activity be entirely eliminated. Depending on their cardiac status, some people resume sexual relations almost immediately, whereas others must delay doing so. If there is risk for a patient, the partner can be encouraged and instructed to assume the more active role in intercourse. Audiovisual materials are available to teach the patient and the partner sexual adaptations if necessary.

Sexuality and the Surgical Experience

Some surgical procedures that involve the genitourinary system have an undeniable effect on sexuality. Moreover, any surgical procedure that alters body image can alter the patient's feelings about his or her sexuality.

The male patient who undergoes a bilateral *orchiectomy* (removal of both testicles) may have alterations in sexual performance due to psychological factors or a decrease in *androgens*. He may or may not receive hormonal supplements, depending on the characteristics of his illness.

The woman who undergoes *surgical menopause* (removal of the uterus, fallopian tubes, and ovaries) may experience a decline but not a total loss of libido, depending on her particular hormonal system. Again, hormonal supplements may or may not be administered. Whenever libido is lost partly or completely, sexual counseling is appropriate to minimize feelings of failure, guilt, or inadequacy.

Other sexually related conditions requiring surgery, although they have no direct physiologic effect on libido or performance, have real psychological implications that can bring about sexual problems even in medically sophisticated patients. The impact of such psychological factors must never be minimized. For example, a man who chooses to have a *vasectomy*, an interruption of the tubes that deliver sperm for purposes of contraception, may encounter unexpected problems with sexual performance following the procedure. In fact, this consequence is so common that physicians now recommend a brief counseling session before the procedure is performed.

Women sometimes experience decreased libido after a *hysterectomy*, or removal of the uterus, which does not physiologically affect sexual interest. Particularly in a society that equates the breasts with womanliness, the woman who must undergo a *mastectomy*, or removal of a breast, may experience sexual trauma. She may feel that she is no longer the woman she once was and is therefore diminished sexually. The emotional support of her sexual partner is essential.

The patient, male or female, who has had a *colostomy* needs very special attention from the health care team with regard to sexuality (Fig. 37-4). A colostomy, which is performed for many medical conditions, is the surgical interruption of the intestines, a portion of which is brought through the lower abdominal wall to form a new opening for the excretion of feces. The intestinal opening or *stoma* appears moist, deep pink in color, and varies in size from individual to individual.

In all cases of amputation, scarring, and incisions that violate the body's integrity, there are potential problems of body image and consequently, sexuality. Each surgical patient warrants a realistic assessment for potential sexual problems.

Assessment

Information regarding sexuality is obtained in a variety of indirect and direct ways. Assessment for sexual problems may be more difficult for you than assessment for other human needs because you generally need to rely more on subtle and subjective data. In addition, you find yourself more uncomfortable with the topic. As in

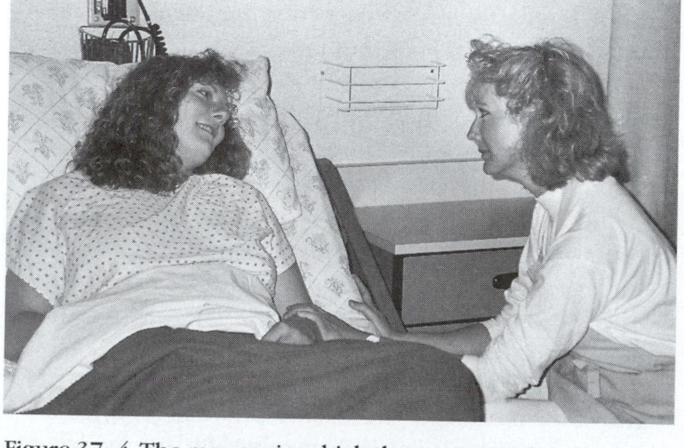

Figure 37-4. The manner in which the care provider responds to the colostomy affects the patient's self-concept.

other areas, self-assessment and self-understanding are crucial.

Interview

Because sexuality is a delicate and emotion-laden subject, sexual information from patients is rarely solicited by means of direct and detailed questions. Counselors in sexuality interview patients in a detailed fashion, but this is usually not a task of the staff nurse. Many patients would consider the nurse's asking direct sexual questions an invasion of privacy.

However, the nurse's assessment is important. The question, "How has this (health problem) affected you as a man (or as a woman)?" is often a nonintrusive way to open the door to concerns about sexuality. With medical or surgical conditions involving the reproductive or sexual organs and potential alterations in self concept (see Chapter 35), the nurse can assess more directly with a leading remark such as "Some patients who have this surgery are concerned about how their sexual life might be affected. Have you and your physician talked about this? Is there anything I can help clarify for you?"

Your interview may also provide cues regarding the patient's general state of health, presence of a sexual partner, and sexual awareness. Areas to consider as the nurse interacts with the patient include:

1. Does the patient have a significant intimate relationship?
2. Is that person caring and supportive?
3. Is the present condition one that might affect sexuality?
4. Is the patient taking any medications that might affect sexuality?
5. What is the patient's drug and alcohol use pattern, past and present?

The repetitive telling of sexual jokes and nonverbal behaviors may be signs of feelings of sexual frustration. Some patients may openly express such feelings, whereas others are more private about these matters. Sexual frustration is commonly related to separation from, loss of, or lack of a partner.

Physical Assessment

A portion of the physical assessment will be provided by the medical record. The medical diagnosis may be one that involves or influences sexual concerns. Maturational sexual development will be apparent when the patient's physical assessment is performed. The physical assessment will also reveal any obvious disruption of organs related to the sexual response. For example, the man who has undergone a bilateral orchiectomy will not have testicles. The woman who has had a hysterectomy may perceive a change in sexual feelings and response.

Nursing Diagnosis

The North American Nursing Diagnosis Association (NANDA) has approved two nursing diagnoses in the sexual area—Sexual Dysfunction and Altered Sexuality Patterns. Other possible diagnoses are Impaired Verbal Communication, Altered Family Processes, Situational Low Self-esteem, Anxiety, and Knowledge Deficit.

Sexual Dysfunction

The diagnosis of Sexual Dysfunction is defined as "the state in which an individual experiences or is at risk of experiencing a change in sexual function that is viewed as unrewarding or inadequate" (Carpenito, 1992). This definition includes physical inability to perform, feelings about not fulfilling a sexual role, not feeling desirable, value conflict, and many other issues. The statement is an excellent foundation on which to base assessment of other nursing diagnoses. Nursing diagnoses in such categories as coping, knowledge deficit, and anxiety may be appropriate.

Altered Sexual Patterns

A nursing diagnosis identified as Altered Sexual Patterns is often associated with a specific cause such as stress, illness, surgery, perinatal factors, and others. This diagnosis is appropriate for the person who is experiencing frustration at separation from a sexual partner. Specify-

Nursing Diagnoses Related to Sexuality

Sexual Dysfunction related to
- decreased communication with partner secondary to lack of privacy
- feelings of sexual undesirability secondary to recent surgery

Altered Sexuality Pattern related to
- death of partner
- physical disability
- extreme fatigue

Anxiety related to intrusive nature of procedures involving the body

Knowledge Deficit regarding alternative sexual techniques for possible use after discharge ing the defining characteristics would further clarify the problem. For example, a person with a serious, chronic illness may have a defining characteristic of a change in physical appearance that is a barrier to adequate sexual function.

Impaired Verbal Communication

Intimacy is a form of communication and the sexual act an expression of communication. But for sexuality to be truly fulfilling, there must be verbal and nonverbal communication between partners. Sometimes inadequate communication may occur because the person's illness has caused that person to feel distanced, or emotionally apart, from the other. A nursing diagnosis centered around Impaired Verbal Communication with a partner can be a valid identification of a problem. In the health care facility, decreased communication may be related to a lack of privacy. Patients may become upset about the restraints imposed, and some are unable to verbalize their frustration.

Altered Family Processes

The nursing diagnosis Altered Family Processes is also an appropriate nursing diagnosis regarding sexuality when illness or separation has intruded on the intimacy of a relationship. The individual may experience depression related to the inability to fulfill the sexual role. The patient and sexual partner may experience serious disruption in their patterns of relating based on changes in sexual function.

Situational Low Self-esteem

When people feel less than well, they often have low self-esteem, which intrudes into their sexual feelings as well. Situational Low Self-esteem is a nursing diagnosis that may be applicable to those with alterations in sexual performance. Often, such feelings are transient, disappearing as soon as the person feels well again or recovers from a surgical procedure. With the more chronically ill, seeing oneself as not desirable can escalate to become a major problem and an important nursing diagnosis.

Anxiety

The diagnosis of Anxiety may be appropriate within the area of sexuality. The many health care procedures involving the body and inquiries of a personal nature can cause sexually oriented anxiety. Both men and women may feel apprehension and anxiety based on vague sexual feelings that the body is being invaded and privacy lost. The etiology may be such things as the intrusive nature of procedures that are sexual in nature. Lack of privacy within the health care facility may also cause sexual anxiety.

Knowledge Deficit

The nursing diagnosis Knowledge Deficit is often related to the need to have certain information about sexual matters. Subjects range in scope from family planning to sexual techniques. For patients who have had surgical procedures that alter the usual sexual response or act and those suffering cardiac or other disability, the nursing diagnosis should be written with a statement regarding the specific knowledge needed by the patient or the patient and the partner. This sometimes involves information about alternative means of sexual expression.

Planning and Implementation

Desired outcomes in the area of sexuality must be individualized to the person's view of self and of life. There is no right answer. Each individual must determine what he or she believes is an appropriate expression of sexuality consistent with personal values. The individual must determine what a satisfactory outcome would be in the specific situation.

Certain desired outcomes are important with any sexual problem. One is for the patient (and sometimes the partner) to recognize the problem and be willing to explore and become more comfortable with ways to resolve the problem. In some situations, an outcome may be for the patient (and partner) to enter into a counseling setting to both explore options and gain information regarding any needed changes in sexual matters.

At one time, little was written for the health professional regarding sexual dysfunction. The current plenitude of articles on the subject in the health literature is welcome because sexual dissatisfaction has played a prominent role in the dissolution of many marriages and caused unhappiness for many single people as well. Patients are increasingly likely to discuss sexual problems with nurses or physicians in an effort to seek help. Your interventions may include acceptance of body changes, effective listening, therapeutic communication, and appropriate referral (see the sample Nursing Care Plan Related to Sexuality).

Effective Listening

As a nurse your role will not usually be to correct a sexuality problem, but rather to help the person in coping with whatever changes or concerns are present. Listening can be, in itself, a form of intervention for sexual problems. Attentive listening can provide patients with the opportunity to hear themselves articulate concerns that may have been hidden or suppressed (Fig. 37-5).

Nursing Care Plan
Sample Nursing Care Plan Related to Sexuality

Nursing Diagnosis

Altered Sexuality Pattern related to death of partner.

Supportive data:

Man, age 51.

Wife died 2 years ago.

Verbalizes presence of libido.

States that becoming sexually active again "would not be fair to his wife."

Active in political group composed of both men and women.

Attracted to woman friend in group.

Desired Patient Outcomes

Long term:

Resume satisfactory sexual relationship.

Short term:

Attends sessions with grief counselor.

Makes statements indicating acceptance of self as an attractive person who is capable of finding a new relationship.

States that pursuing a new relationship does not imply lack of love for his deceased wife.

Nursing Action	Rationale
1. Spend time with the patient to explore the feelings he is expressing.	Spending unhurried time with the patient conveys caring and allows him to share feelings of grief that affect sexuality.
2. Show interest in his group involvement and in his new friend within the group.	Showing interest in patient's new group and new friend encourages continuing participation and conveys a sense of acceptance.
3. Explore the possibility of referral to a bereavement counselor who could be useful in helping him resolve the grief/sexuality conflict.	Seeking a bereavement resource and giving this information to the patient may result in patient's receiving needed support.
4. Be available to the patient for further interaction regarding the problem.	Being available to the patient will provide open communication during which the patient can feel free to express feelings of anxiety and grief about loss.

Building Trust

Some patients may be reluctant to discuss sexual topics. If this is the case, the best way to help may be to build a trusting relationship with the patient and signal your availability to explore any problems the patient may have. Other patients, or their sexual partners, may talk to you about sexual problems without prompting. A man may be more comfortable talking to a male nurse; women might also prefer to speak with a nurse of their own sex, although this is not always the case. In the obstetric setting, issues of sexuality are important. Discussions regarding sexuality and contraception are a routine part of care.

Therapeutic Communication

Sometimes the nurse's role is to facilitate communication about sexual matters between the patient, the patient's sexual partner, and perhaps the physician. At other times it may be to offer information, emotional support, and health teaching, particularly if sexual adap-

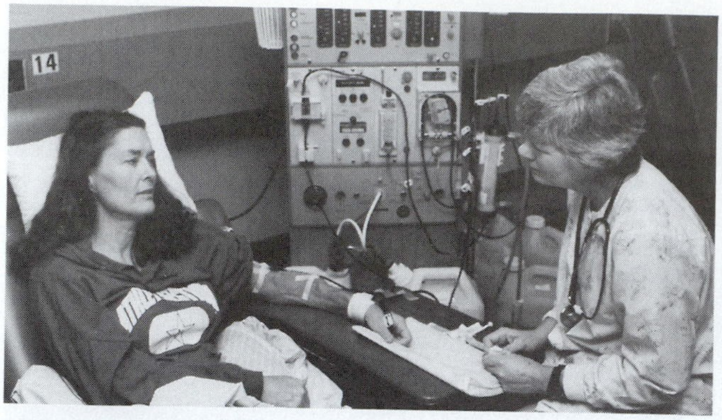

Figure 37-5. Sexual concerns are shared by patient and nurse.

tations are necessary. The nurse can often talk honestly and openly with both partners, together or separately, to help reinstate the patient's feelings of sexuality. For a discussion of communication, see Chapter 13.

We have noted the decrease in libido caused by illness, fatigue, and hospitalization. It is not uncommon for this circumstance to be followed by its opposite. For example, a recovering heart patient under orders for bed rest, who feels refreshed and no longer extremely anxious, may begin to joke or talk about sexual matters. The nurse should realize that this behavior may indicate accumulated sexual tension or worries and problems the patient wants to address. This situation calls for an effective response.

First, you should acknowledge the patient's behavior by saying something like "You certainly have quite a repertoire of jokes" or "You must be improving to be showing so much interest in sex." You might go on to say that it is not unusual for patients who are beginning to feel like their old selves again to experience renewed interest in sexual matters. This opening can lead to discussion if the patient wishes to talk.

Communication with the physician may also be important. If your assessment reveals a problem that may be related to a drug used in care, you will want to discuss this with the physician. It may be possible for the physician to alter the drug or the dosage to modify side effects. If the drug cannot be altered, then the physician might spend time with the patient explaining the reasons for the drug and discussing the problem being experienced.

Acceptance of Body Changes

Your responsibility for helping the colostomy patient maintain sexual integrity begins when you perform the first dressing change (see sample Nursing Care Plan Related to Sexuality). If your face reflects acceptance, without a flicker of aversion, you have taken a significant step toward acceptance on the part of the patient. The displacement of the intestine is no minor matter for the patient psychologically, and the patient's emotional status should be treated as a priority. After discharge from the hospital, unexpected excretions, the wearing of ostomy appliances, and possible odor may affect sexual desire on the part of both partners. Ideally, such problems are of short duration. A light dressing or attractive underclothing to cover the stoma can minimize any feelings of repugnance. Pamphlets on daily living after colostomies, including information on sexual activity, are available from several organizations.

Referral to Sexual Counselors

Individuals with the onset of major disability and certain types of illnesses as well as those who express serious sexual concerns should be referred to appropriate sexual counselors or agencies. Most facilities require that the patient's physician agree to a referral for sexual counseling. You should know how to refer couples or individuals looking for a competent sexuality therapist. Most large hospitals and university medical centers now have sexual dysfunction clinics, and many private clinics treat sexual dysfunction and other mental health problems. In all probability, smaller communities now also have such resources. A telephone call to the nearest university, large hospital, or medical society will usually elicit the names of one or more practitioners or groups trained in treatment of sexual dysfunction.

It is important to warn patients to avoid or carefully check the authenticity of a sexual dysfunction clinic that publicly advertises. Regulations establishing guidelines for sexual therapists have not yet been implemented, and disreputable persons use questionable techniques. Sound counseling, however, has enabled large numbers of people to find new satisfaction in their sexual lives.

The guidance of a counselor in sexuality can often help troubled couples reaffirm their relationship and achieve mutual sexual satisfaction. Sexuality counselors use many techniques. **Conjoint therapy** is the treatment of a couple by a male and a female therapist, one or both of whom are physicians. Often the nonphysician is a nurse with special training. Each sees the patient of the same sex alone, after which the four interact to resolve problems.

Individual psychotherapy is also available to address the particular needs of one individual. The intent of psychotherapy is to explore past or present issues that are having a damaging effect on sexuality. Psychotherapy sometimes raises concerns that are not strictly sexual and should be undertaken only with a reputable professional. Nurses who choose to specialize in the treatment of sexual dysfunction can now receive special education in this area and have proved to be a valuable addition to this type of practice.

Nursing Care Plan
Sample Nursing Care Plan Related to Sexuality

Nursing Diagnosis

Sexual Dysfunction related to feelings about colostomy.

Supportive data:

Verbalizes concern about no longer being sexually attractive.

Diverts eyes when colostomy dressing is changed.

Does not initiate conversation with husband.

Appears quiet and depressed.

Desired Patient Outcomes

Long term:

Able to resume satisfactory sexual relations.

Short term:

States more positive view of self as a sexual partner.

Able to look at colostomy stoma during dressing changes.

Takes increased interest in appearance.

Communicates more freely with husband.

Becomes more outgoing and cheerful by discharge.

Nursing Action	Rationale
1. Spend 15 minutes to 1 hour per day shift with patient so concerns can be explored.	Establishing regular times for communication as part of the plan of care allows the patient to express concerns regarding surgery.
2. After giving reassurance, ask if patient would like to see incision site.	By offering reassurance, the nurse shows understanding of the difficulty in accepting a change in body image. Allowing the patient to decide whether or not to see the surgical site provides the patient with a sense of control.
3. Affirm patient's attractiveness and encourage resumption of use of makeup, etc.	Affirming that the patient remains attractive supports self-esteem. The use of makeup and appealing clothing gives the patient control in maintaining an acceptable appearance.
4. Allow privacy and time with husband for communication.	Privacy and time spent with the husband can promote communication and uninterrupted sharing of concerns.
5. Be available for further interaction and need for counseling referral.	Adaptation to major body changes often requires time and professional support.

Biofeedback is another form of treatment often used with men experiencing impotence and with anorgasmic women. The biofeedback process allows the person to focus on thoughts he or she considers erotic in an environment that is nonthreatening and to get in touch with his or her body and how a response is possible. Later, these techniques are transferred to an interpersonal encounter.

With newly paralyzed or incapacitated patients, the first step after separate interviews with the partners is usually to create a climate in which each can share with the other fears about their sexual status. The male patient might be thinking, "Am I really still a man at all?" "Will my partner leave me if I can no longer satisfy her sexually?" or even "Is it fair to her for us to remain together?" His partner may be thinking, "Can he ever be the man to me he once was?" or "I feel it's wrong for me to have sexual longings when he cannot participate in sexual performance," or even "There is no way I can leave him now without unbearable guilt" or "I'm locked into a relationship no longer sexually alive." The airing of these guilt-provoking thoughts allows the couple to begin to come to grips with the problem they share. Constructive therapy can then begin. The problem may be less severe if it is the woman who is disabled because she may still be capable of enjoying and participating in receptive sexual activity. When the man is handicapped, the wife may be encouraged to assume a more active role and to take the superior position during intercourse. Social stereotypes sometimes make it difficult for the man to be sexually receptive and the woman active without feelings of humiliation on both parts. Sexual counselors often use instructive films when recommending changing sexual roles. The long-term guidance of a trained counselor can often lead couples to reaffirmation of their relationship and mutual sexual satisfaction.

Evaluation

If the nurse has a long-term relationship with a patient, it may be possible to evaluate the progress of a sexual concern. More often, progress in resolving sexual problems is seen and evaluated by the patient, perhaps the partner, and the counselor within the therapy setting.

Evaluation of sexuality may only be possible with some patients after discharge from the health care setting or at a time when health has been regained or a stabilization stage has occurred.

Nursing Care Study
A Patient in Need of Sexual Counseling

Ed Jefferson, a 27-year-old quadriplegic (a person with paralysis of all four extremities), is in a rehabilitation unit. He has an attractive wife, who visits regularly, and a young daughter. During the 7 weeks since his injury, he has been highly motivated in his sessions with the physical therapist and has talked about regaining all function. A minimal degree of shoulder movement has returned, but the physician has told Mr. Jefferson that he will probably never regain the use of his legs.

Ms. Stevens, a registered nurse, has been caring for Mr. Jefferson. She perceives a potential problem in the physician's statement and the patient's subsequent depression. Ms. Stevens knows that although many quadriplegics can maintain a penile erection, Mr. Jefferson's sexual function may be compromised.

Ms. Stevens notices that Mr. Jefferson is becoming increasingly quiet. He develops a headache or nausea just before the therapist's visits and pleads not to have therapy. He no longer initiates conversation, simply answering direct questions and making his immediate needs known. He watches less television than he once did and spends long periods of time awake but with his eyes closed. Just before his wife's daily visit, he complains about all sorts of minor matters. He appears edgy and apprehensive at these times; his wife also appears unusually quiet and at times uncomfortable. They talk together primarily about their child.

The possibility that the patient's sexual function may be compromised appears to be affecting the psychological status of both husband and wife and the relationship between them. Ms. Stevens decides that nursing intervention is needed. She recognizes that she cannot provide sexual counseling but knows that a sexual counselor is available in the community.

While bathing Mr. Jefferson one day, Ms. Stevens says, "You know, many people who are paralyzed worry a great deal about whether or not they'll be able to function sexually. It's certainly normal to have this concern, and if you have had some feelings about this, would you like to talk to someone educated in this area who can guide both you and your wife toward some solutions?" In the process of validating her conjecture, she has formulated an appropriate plan to refer the couple to someone equipped to offer counseling.

A look of relief comes over Mr. Jefferson's face as he admits that sexual functioning has been one of his primary concerns. After consulting with the physician, the nurse makes a referral to a therapist in sexual counseling. Ms. Stevens feels satisfaction as she realizes that her goal has been reached: Mr. Jefferson and his wife will receive help. Evaluation of her nursing action is positive.

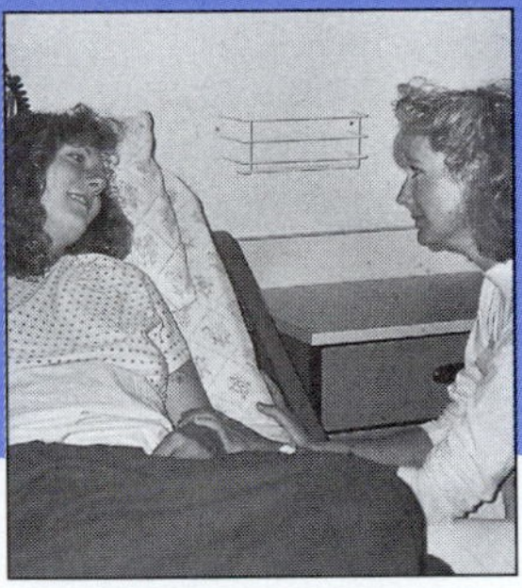

Key Points

- Sexuality is a universal human need involving the awareness of one's feelings of masculinity or femininity; sexual behavior is one expression of sexuality.
- There are basically four stages of sexual response: excitement, plateau, orgasm, and resolution.
- The determination of sexual identity in the individual is not fully understood, but research indicates that there are genetic, societal, and family influences.
- In Western society the three main categories of sexual orientation are heterosexuality, homosexuality, and bisexuality.
- Nurses have a personal and professional responsibility to be sensitive, aware and accepting of differences in sexual orientation.
- Sexually transmitted diseases and AIDS in particular are of great concern to health care professionals. Nurses need to be knowledgeable about both the ways in which they are transmitted and the methods of prevention so that they can provide sensitive care and up-to-date health teaching.
- Factors affecting sexuality include drugs, age, current health status, disability, and the constraints of the environment. Medical conditions and surgery may affect sexual functioning.
- A stable, caring relationship can enhance sexual sharing while a destructive relationship can be coercive. A growing concern in our society is the increase in sexual assault.
- Nurses can use the nursing process to help patients with sexual dysfunction. A thorough assessment of sexual problems based on data about health status as well as cues from the patient or partner may identify appropriate nursing diagnoses. Planning and implementation may involve listening and, with the physician's approval, referral to a sexuality therapist.
- The disabled may have special problems related to sexuality. Some of these concern body image, difficulty in conveying sexuality, finding an appropriate partner, and actual sexual performance. Emotional support, creativity in sexual matters, and a positive outlook can promote satisfactory sexual adjustment for most persons.
- Knowledge concerning human sexuality can provide nurses with both insight into their own feelings and the ability to offer support to the patients in their care.

Study Questions

1. What is the difference between the terms sexuality and sensuality?
2. Describe two differences between the sexual responses of females and males.
3. What is meant by the term "androgyny," and how does this concept fit in with modern society?
4. Based on your understanding of sexually transmitted diseases, what information might you give a patient regarding safer sex practices?
5. Describe the usual patterns of sexual development for different ages of life: the toddler, adolescent, young adult, middle adult, and older adult.
6. How might sexuality be affected for the young man who has recently had a leg amputated?
7. What might be the sexual concerns of a woman who has just had a hysterectomy?
8. If a male patient said to you, "I don't think my wife will ever find me sexually appealing again because of my colostomy," how might you respond?
9. In what ways do you see society and the health care system not meeting the sexuality needs of the disabled?
10. What resources could you use to explore the availability of sexual counseling in your community?
11. Describe three situations regarding sexuality that may occur in the practice of nursing.

Critical Thinking Activities

1. Visit a sexual dysfunction clinic in your area and interview a counselor. Analyze the educational preparation needed. Identify the age and lifestyles of the clients being served. Write a brief paper on your visit and share it with a small group of fellow students.
2. Obtain from your school or public library the most recent HIV/AIDS Quarterly Epidemiology Report from the Centers for Disease Control. Compare the reported cases in your state compare with national statistics. Include age, race, and exposure category.

3. If an adolescent patient has shared with you the fact that she is not practicing safe sex, what information and attitudes could you present that might guide her to change her sexual behavior?

References and Readings

Barnard, M. U., Clancy, B. J., and Krantz, K. E. *Human Sexuality for Health Professionals.* Philadelphia: W. B. Saunders, 1978.

Bem, S. L. "The Measurement of Psychological Androgyny." *Journal of Counseling and Clinical Psychology* (August 1974): 155–162.

Berger, R. "Realities of Gay and Lesbian Aging." *Social Work* 29, 1 (January 1984): 57–62.

Blanchard, M. G. "Sex Education for Spinal Cord Injury Patients and Their Nurses." *Supervisor Nurse* 7 (February 1976): 20–28.

Carpenito, L. J. *Nursing Diagnosis: Application to Clinical Practice.* 4th edition. Philadelphia: J. B. Lippincott, 1992.

DiIorion, C., Parsons, M., Lehr S., Adame, D., and Carlone, J. "Measurement of Safe Sex Behavior in Adolescents and Young Adults." *Nursing Research* 41, 4 (July/August 1992): 203–208.

Dolan, M. B. "An Eternal Flame...The Elderly and Sex." *Nursing '85* 85, 1 (January 1985): 104.

Donohoe, G. "Sensitivity Can Break the Rules: Female Sexual Problems and Treatment Approaches." *Professional Nurse* 7, 5 (February 1992): 304–308.

Dowling, C. *The Cinderella Complex: Women's Hidden Fear of Independence.* New York: Summit Books, 1990.

Fogel, C.I., and Lauver, D. *Sexual Health Promotion.* Philadelphia: W. B. Saunders, 1990.

Freda, M., and Rubinsky, H. "Sexual Function in the Stroke Survivor." *Physical Medicine and Rehabilitation Clinics of North America* 2, 3 (August 1991): 643–658.

Gilliss, C., and Rankin, S. "Social and Sexual Activity after Cardiac Surgery." *Progress in Cardiovascular Nursing* 3, 3 (March 1988): 93–97.

Glass, J. C., and Dalton, J. "Sexuality in Older Adults: A Continuing Education Concern." *Journal of Continuing Education in Nursing* 19, 2 (March-April 1988): 61–64.

Hahn, K. "Sexuality and COPD." *Rehabilitation Nursing* 14, 4 (April 1989): 191–195.

Heinrich, K. T. "Effective Responses to Sexual Harassment." *Nursing Outlook* 35, 2 (March-April 1987): 70–72.

Katzin, L. "Chronic Illness and Sexuality." *American Journal of Nursing* 90, 1 (January 1990): 54–59.

Kinsey, A. C., Pomeroy, W. B., and Martin, C. E. *Sexual Behavior in the Human Male.* Philadelphia: W. B. Saunders, 1948.

Kinsey, A. C., Pomeroy, W. B., Martin, C. E., and Gebhard, P. *Sexual Behavior in the Human Female.* Philadelphia: W. B. Saunders, 1953.

Kohlberg, L. "A Cognitive-Developmental Analysis of Children's Sex-Role Concepts and Attitudes." In *The Development of Sex Differences*, edited by E. E. Maccoby. Stanford, Cal.: Stanford University Press, 1966.

Larson, J., McNaughton, M. W., Kennedy, J. W., and Mansfield, L. W. "Heart Rate and Blood Pressure: Responses of Coronary Artery Disease Patients During Sexual Activity and a 2-Flight Stair Climbing Test." *Heart Lung* 9, 6 (June 1980): 1025–1030.

LeMone, P. "Human Sexuality in Adults with Insulin-Dependent Diabetes Mellitus." *Image* 25, 2 (Summer 1993): 101–105.

Lewis, H. R., and Lewis, M. E. "What You and Your Patients Need to Know about Safer Sex." *RN* 50, 9 (September 1987): 53–58.

Martin, F. "When the Solution is Prosthesis." *RN* 53, 3 (March 1990): 32–35.

McCracken, A. "Sexual Practice by Elders: The Forgotten Aspect of Functional Health." *Journal of Gerontological Nursing* 14, 10 (October 1988): 13–18.

Masters, W., and Johnson, V. *Human Sexual Response.* Boston: Little, Brown, 1966.

Nowlis, E. A. "A Study to Determine How Care Providers for the Elderly Perceive and Use Information Resources." Unpublished dissertation, Seattle University, 1983.

Perkins, J. L., Bennett, D. N., and Dorman, R. "Why Men Choose Nursing." *Nursing and Health Care* 14, 1 (January 1993): 34–38.

Renshaw, D. C. "Sex, Intimacy, and the Older Women." *Women and Health* 8, 4 (August 1983): 43–54.

Reznichek, C., and Reznichek, R. "The Problem Most Men Won't Talk About." *RN* 53, 3 (March 1990): 28–32.

Rieve, J. F. "Sexuality and the Adult with Acquired Physical Disability." *Nursing Clinics of North America* 24, 1 (March 1989): 265–276.

Shell, J. A. "Sexuality for Patients with Gynecologic Cancer." *Clinical Issues in Perinatal Women's Health Nursing* 1, 4 (April 1990): 479–494.

Shipes, E. "Sexual Function Following Ostomy Surgery." *Nursing Clinics of North America* 22, 2 (June 1987): 303–310.

Siemens, S., and Brandzel, R. C. *Sexuality: Nursing Assessment and Intervention.* Philadelphia: J. B. Lippincott, 1982.

Stein, A. P. "The Chlamydia Epidemic: Teenagers at Risk." *Medical Aspects of Human Sexuality* 2, 25 (February 1991): 26–34.

Steinke, E. E. "Older Adults' Knowledge and Attitudes about Sexuality and Aging." *Image* 20, 2 (Summer 1988): 93–95.

Stevens, P. E., and Hall, J. M. "Stigma, Health Beliefs and Experiences with Health Care in Lesbian Women." *Image* 20, 2 (Summer 1988): 69–73.

Tietze, M. "Human Sexuality—Female Nurses' Responses to Their Male Dialysis Patients." *American Association of Nephrology Nurses and Technicians Journal* 10 (June 1983): 19–22.

Woods, N. F. *Human Sexuality in Health and Illness.* 3rd edition. St. Louis: C. V. Mosby, 1987.

Special Needs

VIII

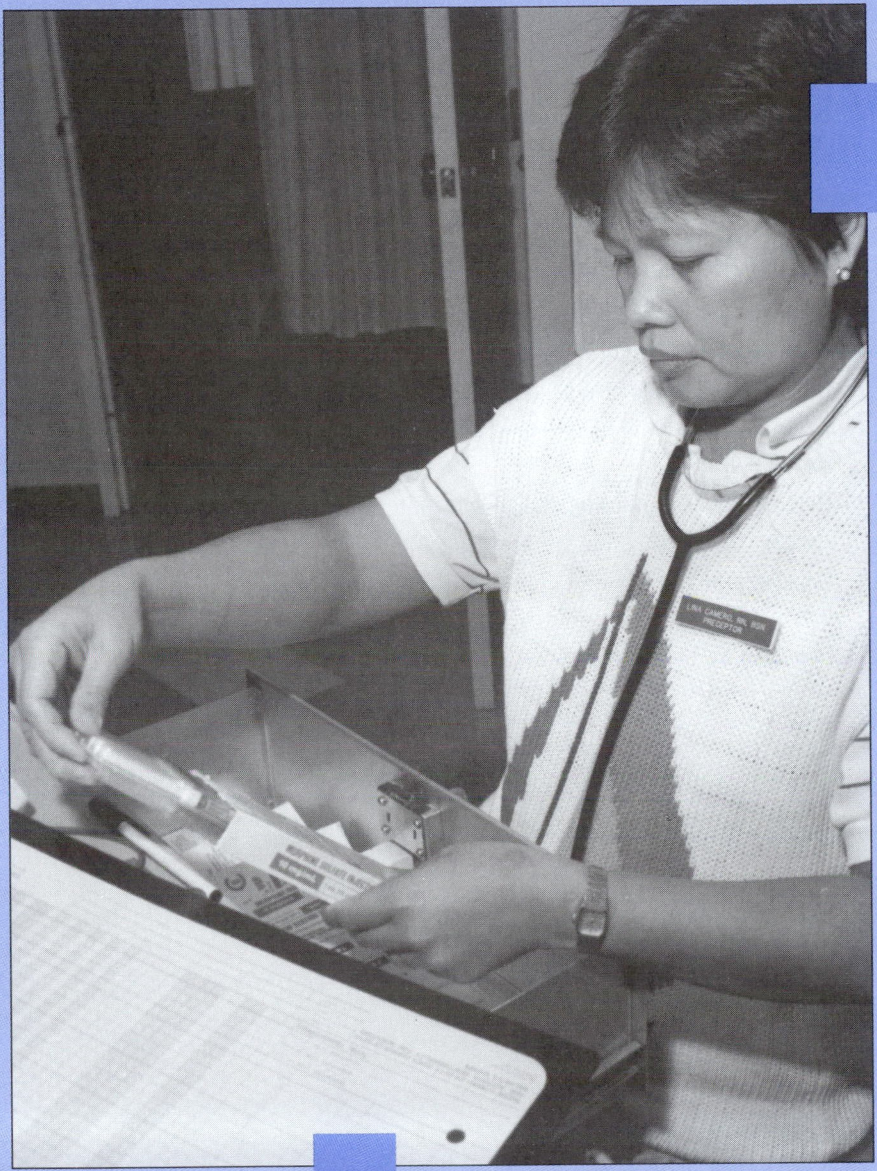

Diagnostic Testing

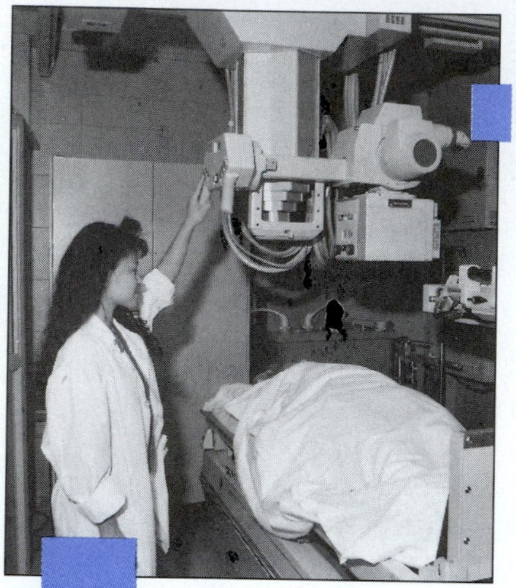

38

Objectives

After completing this chapter, you should be able to:

1. List resources that can be used for information about diagnostic tests.
2. Describe six types of diagnostic tests.
3. Explain when consent for a procedure is necessary.
4. Describe the procedure used for scheduling tests.
5. Explain appropriate assessment of the patient who is to have a diagnostic test performed.
6. Discuss common nursing diagnoses related to diagnostic tests.
7. Explain the nurse's role in preparing a patient for a diagnostic test.
8. Describe the nurse's role in health teaching the patient regarding diagnostic tests and procedures.
9. Describe nursing care needed after diagnostic tests.

Study Terms

allergy
aspiration
biopsy
CAT or CT scan
contrast studies
ECG or EKG
EEG
EMG
endoscopy
fiberoptic scope
guaiac
MRI
markers
NPO
occult blood
PET scan
radiopaque contrast material
rigid scope
trocar

Outline

Types of Diagnostic Tests

Diagnostic Imaging
Measurement and Recording of Electrical Impulses
Special Visual Examinations (Endoscopy)
Tests Involving Aspirations and Biopsies
Miscellaneous Tests of Specific Body Function
Tests Initiated by Nurses

The Nurse's Role in Tests and Procedures

Resources for Information
Scheduling Diagnostic Tests
Consent for Procedures

Assessment

Interview
Physical Data

Nursing Diagnosis

Knowledge Deficit
Anxiety
Pain
Ineffective Airway Clearance
Potential Complications

Planning and Implementation

Ellis, Nowlis: Nursing: A Human Needs Approach, 5th ed. © 1994 J.B. Lippincott Company

Nurses are directly involved in the areas of patient care that pertain to diagnostic testing. Various diagnostic tests are used to aid in the determination of the patient's diagnosis or identify problems. "As health care becomes more and more technical, the multitude of diagnostic procedures and laboratory tests continues to grow" (Corbett, 1992, p. 9). Student nurses and nurses in practice must keep current about the many new and technically complex diagnostic tests being done today. A firm knowledge base provides safety for the patient undergoing a diagnostic test. With some exceptions, diagnostic tests are carried out either by the physician or by the nurse with an order from the physician. Some diagnostic tests can be performed at the discretion of the nurse.

Types of Diagnostic Tests

Numerous diagnostic tests are now available, making it impossible for the nurse to have full knowledge of every procedure without consulting a resource. We discuss categories of the more common tests. Lists in this chapter will be helpful in learning about the various tests, the organ studied in each test, and the purpose of the test. We have also outlined guidelines for preparation, the method used in the testing examination, and any special nursing concerns. For additional tests specific to a particular organ or system, consult a diagnostic testing reference book.

Diagnostic Imaging

Radiography produces a film that shows images of the outlines of various structures whose different densities allow varying amounts of radiation to penetrate through to the film. Most x-rays are simple images of body parts, for example, x-rays of the chest and extremities to identify fractures. The desired view or patient position is usually designated by the physician.

Some organs do not appear on routine x-rays because they are not sufficiently dense to block any radiation. In these cases, **contrast studies** are performed: a **radiopaque contrast material** (sometimes called a dye) is introduced into the organ so that a clear outline of it can be seen on the x-ray. The functioning of an organ can sometimes be studied by taking a series of x-rays as the contrast material moves through the organ. Intravenous contrast materials are potent and can cause severe allergic reactions (Table 38-1).

Other diagnostic imaging tests can be performed. Each can be done with or without using a contrast medium. One of the most common diagnostic procedures is the **CAT** or **CT scan** (computed axial tomography). The scanner rotates 180° around the patient's body, recording multiple x-ray images that are converted into a three-dimensional film. The test is noninvasive and without risks unless a contrast medium is used. If contrast materials are used, the patient should always be observed for signs of any complications, particularly those involving the cardiovascular or respiratory systems. The patient is placed on a padded traylike device

> **Nursing Issues and Trends:** *Health Care Costs and Diagnostic Testing*
>
> Health care costs are a major concern for all Americans. One hindrance to control is the cost of multiple diagnostic tests. Third-party payers (health insurance companies) claim that this increase in tests is one cause for the increases being charged for health care insurance coverage. The use of many diagnostic tests is often defended as essential to protect against possible legal claims of malpractice. (This is frequently referred to as practicing "defensive medicine.") This issue continues to be a dilemma for physicians, nurses, and consumers as the country attempts to create a national health care plan that will best serve the needs of all.

Table 38–1. Diagnostic Imaging Methods

	Organ Studied	Preparation	Method	Special Nursing Concerns
Angiogram	Blood vessels. Usually used to examine a system of veins and arteries within an organ.	Usually NPO. Sometimes surgical preparation of site.	Catheter is threaded into artery (often the femoral), and contrast medium is injected under pressure into the organ's vascular system.	Allergic reaction to contrast medium. Bleeding from puncture site. Thrombus formation.
Arteriogram	Arteries (but often used as a synonym for angiogram)	Same as for angiogram.	Same as for angiogram.	Same as for angiogram.
Barium enema (lower bowel)	Large intestine	Measures to cleanse bowel completely begun evening before and completed morning of test.	Barium is given as enema. Large plug is inserted in rectum to prevent loss of barium.	Barium causes severe constipation or even obstruction, if not removed by means of enemas or laxatives.
Bronchogram	Bronchi	NPO. Routine preop. General anesthesia usual. Dentures out.	Contrast medium is inserted through bronchoscope, then suctioned out.	Same as for bronchoscopy. Also irritation from contrast medium causes increased secretions. Retained contrast medium may cause pneumonia.
Cholangiogram	Bile ducts	NPO. Preparation for surgery. Usually done during gall bladder surgery.	Contrast medium is injected into bile ducts themselves.	None usual.
Cholecystogram (Gallbladder series)	Gallbladder	NPO. Fat-free meal evening before. Oral contrast pills evening before as directed.	Material excreted in bile is given in pill form. X-rays are taken to determine whether gallbladder contains the material. Then a fatty liquid is given, and further x-rays are taken to observe function of gallbladder. Constrast medium IV may be given just before test.	Pills often cause nausea and vomiting. Vomiting of pills makes test invalid. Burning on urination as contrast medium is excreted.
Computed tomography (CT scan)	Any area of body	NPO if contrast media used.	Computer controls exposure of multiple x-rays providing clear view of soft tissue.	A noninvasive test
Cystogram	Bladder	None usual.	Patient is catheterized and contrast medium inserted through catheter.	Encourage fluids to prevent infection.
Intravenous pyelogram (IVP)	Kidney, ureters, and bladder	NPO. Measures to cleanse bowel completely evening before test.	Contrast medium is injected intravenously and excreted by kidneys. A series of x-rays is made of entire urinary tract.	Contrast medium can cause urinary irritation, Encourage fluids.
Magnetic resonance imaging (MRI or MI)	Any area of body	Patient cannot wear metal. Report presence of metallic implants (Such as pacemakers, meta joints). Report patient very obese.	Patient is placed in large machine, which may evoke uncomfortable feelings. Test is noninvasive.	None

that moves slowly through a large tube containing the scanner. When preparing patients, they should be told that a clicking noise may be heard and that they are required to lie still during the test. Remaining motionless for a lengthy period of time can be stressful for the patient. If the person is claustrophobic, the test may produce some anxiety. Some laboratories have used music and placed colorful stickers with messages on the inner core of the tube to relax patients. The CT scan can visualize any part of the body.

A similar diagnostic test is done by a **PET scan** (positron emission tomography). The patient is injected with a small dose of radioactive material that emits positrons (electrons having a positive charge), which are detected by the scanner. The film produced is in color and considered more accurate and detailed than is the CT scan. It reflects function not simply structure.

A third diagnostic test that is increasing in use is the **MRI** (magnetic resonance imaging). This is a noninvasive test that uses radio waves and a large magnet. The patient is enclosed in a specially designed room that prevents interference with the magnetic environment that has been created. As with the CT scan, the patient having an MRI reclines on a padded surface that is passed through a tube containing the magnet. When the radio waves are introduced, a variety of sounds occur, which can be disturbing to the patient. Music or ear plugs help the situation. The images are produced when the radio waves are activated within the magnetic field. These images are then converted to film. Very obese persons or those with implanted metal objects such as pacemakers are not appropriate for MRI at this time.

In tests using radioactive materials, small amounts of specific radioactive substances are injected or ingested into the body and a scanning device that registers the presence of radioactive particles is used to determine their distribution. Some substances are simply circulated in the bloodstream to allow circulatory pathways and changes or interruptions in those pathways to be seen. In other tests, differential rates at which the specific radioactive substance is absorbed by different tissues allow rates of activity, types of tissue, and ability to function to be determined. The amounts of radiation are so small that they pose no hazard to personnel or patient. However, caution must be used in recommending such a test for a pregnant woman.

Measurement and Recording of Electrical Impulses

When functioning, some organs of the body generate electrical impulses that can be measured and evaluated (Table 38-2). Illness and some diseases can either decrease or alter these impulses. Because these changes in electrical potential can be significant in arriving at a medical diagnosis and treatment, devices are available that identify the various patterns.

A common test done is the electrocardiogram (**ECG** or **EKG**), which measures the electrical impulses from the heart. During rest, the heart muscle is polarized or charged. A signal from the sinoatrial node causes contraction or depolarization of the muscle. The cardiographic strip shows this process of intermittent polarization and depolarization. Some physicians routinely perform an ECG on all patients before surgery or on patients older than age 40. If a patient has heart disease or is seriously ill, a continual cardiac monitor may be used, which shows a continual tracing on a oscilloscope.

Another example of this type of test is the electroencephalogram (**EEG**), which measures the electrical impulses emitted from the cortex of the brain. Electrodes are affixed to the scalp with fine needles (sometimes called pins) or glue and a recording is made. Another example and similar to the EEG is the electromyogram (**EMG**). With this test, electrodes are placed on muscle groups so that alterations in electrical conduction to muscles can be detected.

Special Visual Examinations (Endoscopy)

Endoscopy is the direct visualization of hollow organs that open to the body's exterior surface (Table 38-3). A sedative is usually given before the procedure to make the patient more comfortable. Endoscopy is done by inserting a scope or tube containing a light and of a diameter appropriate for the test being performed. Scopes are of two basic types: rigid and fiberoptic. The **rigid scope** is a metal or plastic tube and the passageway into the organ must be straightened to allow entry of the inflexible tube. The light illuminates the inside of the organ, which is visually inspected. It is also possible to insert a special instrument to obtain a specimen of tissue. This procedure is called a *biopsy* (see next section).

The **fiberoptic scope** is a flexible tube containing a bundle of fibers that reflect light. These fibers are so perfectly aligned that the image at the bottom of the tube is clearly seen at the top. Fiberoptic scopes can conform to the shape of the passage or organ and can thus be inserted into areas of the body not accessible to metal scopes. These scopes cause less discomfort than do rigid scopes and also have attached instruments to take tissue samples.

Tests Involving Aspirations and Biopsies

Aspiration is the removal of fluid from the body through a needle for purposes of inspection and testing. We have defined a **biopsy** as the removal of tissue for the same purpose (Table 38-4). Because of the size of

Table 38–2. Methods of Measuring and Recording Electrical Impulses

	Organ Studied	Preparation	Method	Special Nursing Concerns
Electrocardiogram (EKG or ECG)	Heart	None usual	Electrodes are secured to the chest wall with electrode past and tape or suction cups. Other electrodes are attached to the extremities. The machine then records the electrical activity of the heart.	None
Electroencephalogram (EEG)	Brain	None usual	Electrodes are attached to the scalp with small needles or paste. The patient is at rest in a darkened room, and may be asked to deep breathe (hyperventilation) or watch a flashing light (photic stimulation) at certain times.	None
Electromyogram (EMG)	Muscles	None usual	Electrodes are attached to the muscles to be tested with small needles or paste, and the electrical impulses are recorded.	None
Myelogram	Spinal canal	NPO. Sedative given. Usually not general anesthesia.	Lumbar puncture is done, some spinal fluid is removed, and contrast medium is injected into canal. Patient is positioned on tilt table, which is tilted to allow contrast medium to flow to desired level.	Same as for lumbar puncture (see Table 38–4). Allergic reactions to dye. Check for specific type of dye used for special needs.
Pneumoencephalogram	Ventricles of brain	NPO. Sedative given. Full: 100 cc of air, general anesthesia. Limited: 10–15 cc air, local anesthesia.	Lumbar puncture is done, some spinal fluid is removed, and air is inserted. Air rises to ventricles when patient is placed in upright position.	Headache until air is absorbed. Pain medications are given. Quiet and darkened room and flat bed rest are usually helpful.
Retrograde pyelogram	Kidney	NPO. Laxatives to clear bowel.	Cystoscopy is performed. Ureteral catheters are inserted, films are taken of catheters, and contrast medium is then injected into renal pelvis for films.	Same as for cystoscopy.
Upper GI	Esophagus, stomach, duodenum	NPO after midnight.	Barium is swallowed. Films are taken as material fills upper gastrointestinal system.	Same as for barium enema.
Ventriculogram	Ventricles of brain	Complete surgical preparation as for neurosurgery.	Burr holes are drilled in skull, and cannula is inserted to inject contrast medium into ventricles.	Complete postop care for a neuro patient (see a medical-surgical textbook).

Table 38–3. Types of Special Visual Examinations (Endoscopy)

	Organ Studied	Preparation	Special Nursing Concerns
Bronchoscopy	Bronchi and (with fiberoptic scope) lung segments	NPO and sedatives. If general anesthesia, routine preop. If local, special explanation of procedure. Dentures out.	If performed with local anesthesia, do not give fluids or food until gag rellex returns. Complications to watch for include bleeding due to tissue trauma, laryngospasm, and respiratory distress. Also, in any procedure that uses a local anesthetic, watch for allergic reaction.
Colonoscopy	Entire large bowel (with fiberoptic scope)	Measures to cleanse bowel completely begun evening before and completed morning of test.	Bleeding due to trauma.
Cystoscopy	Bladder	Same as for bronchoscopy.	Urinary tract irritation from scope. Possible infection. Encourage fluids.
Esophagoscopy	Esophagus	Same as for bronchoscopy.	If performed with local anesthesia, do not give fluids or food until gag reflex returns.
Gastroscopy	Stomach (with fiberoptic scope)	Same as for bronhcoscopy.	Same as for esophagoscopy.
Laryngoscopy	Larynx	If general anesthesia, routine preop. If local, special explanation of procedure.	If performed with local anesthesia, do not give fluids or food until gag reflex returns. Complications to watch for include bleeding due to tissue trauma and laryngospasm.
Proctoscopy	Rectum	Measures to cleanse bowel completely begun evening before and completed morning of test.	Bleeding due to trauma.
Sigmoidoscopy	Sigmoid colon and rectum.	Same as for proctoscopy.	Same as for proctoscopy.

the needle (a very large bore needle is called a **trocar**), a local anesthetic is administered before the needle is inserted. If the patient is especially anxious, a low dosage of sedation may be given before the procedure is begun. Aspirations and biopsies can be done at the same time as other types of tests are performed. These procedures may also be performed independently. Regardless, aspirations and biopsies are performed by a physician following the careful sterile technique appropriate to minor surgical procedures. If you are assisting, you must also observe strict sterile technique. Care and transport of any specimens may also be your responsibility.

Miscellaneous Tests of Specific Body Functions

Many tests have been devised to examine the functioning of body processes (Table 38-5). The urinary and endocrine systems alone have numerous procedures that may be used to arrive at the medical diagnosis or monitor the patient's progress. New research has developed procedures that can detect what are called markers. **Markers** are substances that are in a person's tissues or body fluids that may predict the possibility of developing abnormal cell growth or disease. Procedures may involve obtaining samples of blood, body fluids, or tissues. It is hoped that cancer in certain organs will be detected and treated much earlier through the use of marker procedures. For purposes of this text, we have listed only a few of the more common tests performed in the hospital today.

Tests Initiated by Nurses

There are many simple, noninvasive tests that you may perform without a physician's order. Most agencies have a policy that you can consult regarding this. Although an explanation to the patient for your actions is appropriate, these noninvasive tests performed at your discretion should not cause the patient discomfort or anxiety.

For example, a commonly performed test in this category is the hematest performed on urine, feces, or other body fluids. It is done to test for the presence of **occult** (hidden) **blood**. The blood present is undetectable by simple observation. When a chemical agent is placed in contact with a small specimen of the patient's body substance, a color change occurs when blood is

Table 38–4. Types of Tests Involving Aspirations and Biopsies

	Purpose	Method	Special Nursing Concerns
Abdominal paracentesis	To remove fluid that has accumulated in the peritoneal cavity	With the patient in a sitting position, the needle is inserted through the abdominal wall. A three-way stopcock, syringe, and tubing may be attached to the needle to allow aspiration of the fluid.	The patient should void first. Shock may occur during the procedure (see a medical-surgical text). The wound must be dressed afterward. Be alert to the amount of fluid removed.
Bone marrow biopsy	To obtain a sample of bone marrow tissue to examine its production of blood components	The patient is lying down. The sternum or the iliac crest is commonly punctured.	The procedure may be upsetting to the patient. Some pain is felt when the bone is entered, and the aspiration of tissue may be painful. The sound of bone penetration may be upsetting. Afterwards pressure is applied for 5 minutes to prevent bleeding.
Lumbar puncture	To puncture the spinal subarachnoid space to remove a sample of fluid for study or to inject dye for a contrast x-ray	The patient lies on side in a flexed (bowed) position to allow access to the lower spine. During the procedure, a measurement of spinal fluid pressure is made.	Afterwards the patient is kept flat for a time. The prone position is preferred to allow "welling" of the puncture site, preventing further loss of fluid. Fluids are encouraged to facilitate replacement of spinal fluid. Headache occurs infrequently as a complication.
Thoracentesis	To puncture the pleural space to remove fluid or allow for the insertion of chest tubes	With the patient usually sitting up and leaning over a table, the puncture is made in the lower posterior chest to remove fluid and in the upper anterior chest to remove air.	Possible respiratory distress and pain during aspiration.

Table 38–5. Miscellaneous Tests of Specific Body Functions

	Purpose	Preparation	Method
Basal metabolism rate (BMR)	To test the rate at which the body uses oxygen at complete rest (not sleep) to measure metabolic rate	NPO. Test performed first thing in the morning. No activity allowed preceding test.	The nose is clamped; the patient breathes through a mouthpiece so the oxygen consumption can be measured.
Gastric analysis	To measure and analyze the stomach's production of gastric juices	NPO.	A nasogastric tube is inserted in the stomach. All gastric contents are aspirated and saved over a period of time. Samples are taken at specified time intervals according to laboratory procedure.
Glucose tolerance test (GTT)	To measure the ability of the body to metabolize a glucose "load"	NPO.	A fasting urine sample is obtained, and a blood sample is drawn for a fasting blood sugar test. Then a solution containing a known amount of glucose is drunk by the patient. At intervals specified by the laboratory, urine samples are taken and blood samples are drawn (usually by the laboratory technician).
Indirect gastric analysis (tubeless gastric analysis "Diagnex Blue," "Azurea")	To measure the production of gastric acid by determining the rate at which the dye material is absorbed and excreted	NPO	Dye material is given as directed by the manufacturer. Urine is saved for 24 h and sent to the labortory for analysis. Urine will continue to be blue for several days after the test.

present. You may hear the term, **guaiac** used to refer to the hematest. This is an older term when the chemical guaiac was used to perform the test. Although other chemicals are now also used, the term remains to describe the procedure. A positive result signifying the presence of blood in the substance may help with the diagnosis or can be one indicator of the medical status of patients.

The Nurse's Role in Tests and Procedures

Whether performing diagnostic procedures independently or assisting with special tests and procedures performed by the physician or other members of the health care team, the nurse has specific responsibilities in regard to diagnostic tests. These responsibilities include being informed, understanding when consent is needed, and planning for scheduling.

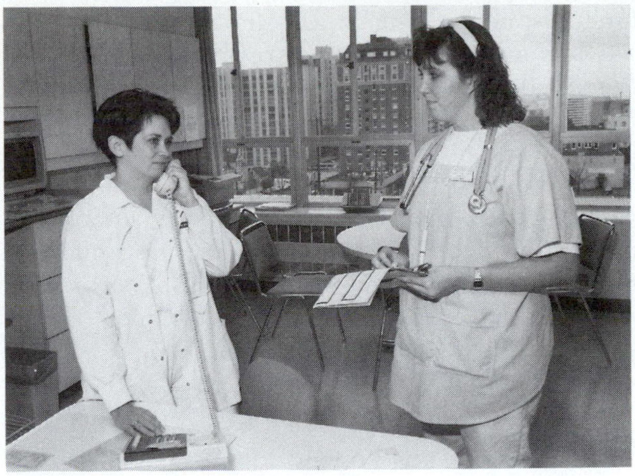

Figure 38-1. The nurse is calling another department for additional information about a diagnostic test.

Resources for Information

The nurse needs adequate knowledge about all diagnostic tests to teach the patient, to prepare the patient when needed, and to perform or assist with the test when appropriate. To learn about the variety of tests performed in other departments of the agency, a number of resources are available. Basic nursing texts may describe the more common tests. Nursing laboratory test reference books provide comprehensive information. Many nursing units have laboratory manuals that outline the various tests and preparation that needs to be done by the nursing staff. If necessary information cannot be found, the department where the test is to be performed can be contacted (Fig. 38-1). New procedures are constantly being done so more than one resource may have to be used. The nursing instructor who is supervising students may encourage them to accompany patients to tests or to arrange to observe as many as possible because this provides first-hand knowledge of the various procedures.

Important information to be gathered includes exactly what test or procedure is to be performed, the purpose of the test, how long it will take, and whether it is invasive or noninvasive. An invasive test is one during which a body cavity is entered by a catheter, needle, or radiation that may alter body function. A noninvasive procedure is done without insertion of a device into a body cavity or without radiation and will not affect the body's functioning. Invasive tests place the patient at a higher risk of complications than do noninvasive procedures.

It is important to know who is responsible for carrying out any preparations before the test. This includes what type of equipment will be needed and the proper positioning of the patient for the test. To gain patient cooperation, it is important to know to what extent the patient will be asked to participate in the procedure. For example, some organ biopsies require that patients have the ability to hold the breath for a few seconds while the needle is inserted through the anesthetized skin. If this knowledge is known and shared with the patient beforehand, the patient will feel much more prepared and less anxious at the time of the procedure.

A resource can also outline any risks that may accompany a procedure. Special care may be necessary after a test with appropriate parameters to be used for monitoring the patient.

Scheduling Diagnostic Tests

Either the nurse or unit secretary may schedule tests that are to occur in another department. A test that is to be performed by the physician may be planned for a time according to his or her schedule. The patient's plan of care may have to be revised to accommodate the time of the test. Patients should know when tests are to be performed so that they can anticipate any physical preparation necessary and can prepare psychologically.

Consent for Procedures

In most facilities, consent for x-rays and other noninvasive, uncomplicated procedures is covered by the general consent form signed by the patient on admission. However, specific informed signed consent is required for any procedure that is invasive or complex.

Similar to obtaining consent for a surgical procedure, the patient signing consent for a diagnostic procedure must not be a minor as defined by the law of the state and must sign before any premedication is administered. The patient has the legal right to know any risks that may accompany the procedure. Although it is not the nurse's primary responsibility to obtain consent for testing procedures, sending the patient to another department for a test without appropriate authorization may lead to delay and increase patient discomfort. Remind the physician involved as soon as it becomes apparent that a consent has not been obtained. Consent was discussed in some detail in Chapter 3.

Assessment

Part of the nursing responsibility is adequate assessment before the diagnostic test. You will need to both interview the patient and check the record and medical order before you begin your assessment (Fig. 38-2).

Interview

During an interview, the patient and the family, if this is appropriate, appreciate your interest and willingness to clarify any questions they have regarding a planned diagnostic test. Assessment of knowledge level and feelings are both important.

You should assess the patient's knowledge level regarding the test to be performed. This should include determining whether or not the patient has had the testing procedure before and knows what is entailed. The patient also should know the time the test is scheduled.

You will need to determine the patient's feelings about the test. Does the patient view the test as a positive step that may lead to an understanding of what is wrong? Is the patient distraught or anxious about the preparatory restrictions or procedures before the test or about the possibility of the test's revealing serious health concerns?

Physical Data

Assessing the patient's current medical status in relationship to the planned procedure is also important. General assessment of the patient's ability to tolerate the test may be a question. This may involve assessment of respiratory and mobility status. It may also include collecting data relative to other systems than that being tested. If, for example, your patient with severe neurologic agitation is scheduled for rigorous respiratory tests in the morning, you should notify the physician of the patient's present condition, which might result in the physician's treating the agitation or having the tests delayed until the patient can be more cooperative and understanding of the importance of the scheduled procedure.

An important assessment regarding safety is to ascertain if the patient has a known **allergy** (abnormal body hypersensitivity to a specific substance) that might be relevant to testing substances being used. Many diagnostic contrast materials are iodine based. People who are allergic to seafood, which contains iodine, may react adversely to these substances, occasionally to a life-threatening degree. Any indication of an allergy should be documented in writing on the patient's record and promptly reported to the physician and the testing department before the test. A decision can then be made as to whether or not to use a specific contrast medium or whether to use another type that does not contain iodine.

Nursing Diagnosis

Most of the nursing diagnoses for patients undergoing diagnostic tests or procedures are associated with the potential for complications resulting from the tests. Some diagnoses involve psychosocial concerns such as anxiety or knowledge deficit.

#1 BARIUM ENEMA/COLON

Category I:
1. Liquid diet 3 days if possible.
2. Day before exam take 2 oz castor oil or "Go lightly."
3. Encourage fluids until midnight.
4. Morning of exam—enemas until clear.

If for gross bleeding follow Category II.

Category II:
1. 2 oz castor oil 4 PM day before (or "Go lightly" can be substituted).
2. Encourage fluids until midnight.
3. Light liquid dinner.
4. NPO after midnight.
5. Morning of exam—enemas until clear.
6. 2 oz. Milk of Magnesia should be taken after exam.

For obstruction or partial obstruction, conditions 1 and 2 may be eliminated.

Figure 38-2. Directions for preparing patient for diagnostic tests.

Knowledge Deficit

Many patients are uninformed about the test they are to undergo, the purpose of the test, and any necessary preparations. The nursing diagnosis Knowledge Deficit is important for the nurse to consider. Patients who have knowledge about the diagnostic test can participate more fully and be more knowledgeable about any risks and complications arising from the test. The informed patient will also be able to receive the results of the test in an intelligent manner so that any decisions can be made regarding further study or treatment needed. The nurse has a collaborative role in providing basic information relative to diagnostic testing.

Anxiety

Each diagnostic test provides different information and must be interpreted in association with the patient's symptoms or along with other tests to reach accurate conclusions. A diagnostic test may be only one piece of the process for reaching a diagnosis. Patients may not understand this and develop unrealistic anxiety about individual tests. Patients may also become confused and anxious concerning the risks in having diagnostic tests performed. They do not understand the concept of a risk–benefit ratio. This means that there are risks with having a variety of tests, but the benefits of the information gained may outweigh potential risks. The physician should clearly point out risks *and* benefits to patients who are scheduled for any test that includes risks. The nurse is often in a position to support the physician's decision to perform the test.

Most patients have some degree of anxiety about having a diagnostic test performed. Even a simple, uncomplicated x-ray can produce a mild degree of anxiety. Removing all or part of the clothing for any type of test can make the patient feel vulnerable and unprotected. Tests that require confinement to a small area such as the enclosure of a CT scan can produce anxiety. Any test that may entail physical pain produces anxiety. Anxiety can be particularly high if the results of a diagnostic test can signal the presence of a disease process that will mean a significant change in health status or lifestyle for the patient.

Pain

This nursing diagnosis requires a statement regarding a defining characteristic. The patient may have head pain following the performance of a lumbar puncture. It is possible for the patient to have flank pain after a kidney biopsy. The location, type, and intensity of pain may be very different in each of these situations so that identifying statements add to the specificity of the nursing diagnosis and suggest appropriate interventions.

Ineffective Airway Clearance

The nursing diagnosis High Risk for Ineffective Airway Clearance is appropriate if the patient has had a bronchoscopy because the bronchoscope can cause irritation of the respiratory passages, resulting in edema and increased secretions. This is an at-risk problem because most patients do not have difficulty breathing or expectorating secretions after the test.

Potential Complications

Specific complications may occur after certain diagnostic tests. When an oral contrast medium is given to x-ray the bowel, that material may cause severe constipation or even a bowel obstruction if it is not eliminated. The possibility of bleeding is always a concern for the patient having certain invasive diagnostic tests. It is more of a concern with tests that involve vascular organs. For example, if a bone marrow aspiration or a liver biopsy has been performed, there is a greater risk for internal bleeding than a test involving a less vascular area. Tests such as an x-ray or MRI do not carry this risk because they are noninvasive. Knowing about tests and how they are performed allows the nurse to determine the specific potential complications.

Planning and Implementation

When any diagnostic test is ordered for a patient, desired patient outcomes must be established. A practical outcome is that the test will be properly scheduled, the patient or family notified, and the test carried out safely and successfully with the least amount of discomfort. Another desired outcome is that the test will be without complications, both during the test and in the period afterward. By setting criteria for evaluation at this time, evaluating the patient's response to the procedure can be more effective.

Planning for a Diagnostic Test

The equipment to be used, the appropriate physical environment, and the time needed for the procedure must all be accounted for in a plan. If the patient is going to another department such as x-ray, the department personnel will take responsibility for the equipment and the environment. The nurse will also need to plan what information the patient needs and what adjustments in the daily schedule or routine are essential. For example, if medication times are missed, should medications be given early or held until the procedure is over? The physician or diagnostic department may need to be consulted about some aspects of the plan. For example, if a medication needed at a precise time is due when the test is scheduled, arrangements can be made with the department to give the order appropriately so that the medication schedule can be maintained properly.

Physical Preparation

The best way to physically prepare the patient for the test is to be knowledgeable regarding the scheduled procedure. Preparations vary greatly; a simple x-ray or brain scan does not require special preparation, yet other tests do. Many tests require that the patient must be **NPO** (nothing by mouth) for a period of time before the procedure. For some tests, this means that the patient cannot have any nourishment or water whatsoever. In other instances, the physician will allow sips of water for taking oral medications only. This is particularly true when the medications are ones that should not be omitted or for which the medication schedule should not be interrupted. You should clarify this with the physician for a specific patient. If a patient is dehydrated, especially a young child or an older person, not taking fluids for a length of time could be hazardous. If these people have been ordered NPO and a test is delayed, notify the physician so that a decision can be made regarding fluid status. A few tests require that fluids be encouraged before the test. This is done to dilute a contrast medium that is to be used, enhancing visualization.

Some tests require that nursing procedures be done in preparation. For example, an x-ray of the lower gastrointestinal tract may necessitate a cleansing enema to remove feces so the outline of the tract can be more easily visualized. Other tests require that catheterization or gastric intubation be done beforehand. If premedication is needed before the procedure, the physician will write an order appropriate to the patient's mental status, age, and anticipated discomfort that may be caused by the diagnostic test.

Health Teaching

With knowledge and sound rationale for the test that is to be performed, the nurse is in the unique position to listen to the patient and actively teach regarding the test. There may also be questions that can be answered, allaying anxiety. Before proceeding with the preparation of the patient, you should obtain information about tests.

You will also want to consider the age of the patient. Explanations to a child should be given in language that is direct, honest, understood by the child, and yet, not frightening. The person in midlife who is experiencing hospitalization for the first time may be unfamiliar with medical terminology, yet feel hesitant about asking for clarification. The elderly may view tests as invasive and an indication that something is clearly wrong with their body. In each instance, adjusting your health teaching to the individual person's life stage and needs is crucial. The nurse's responsibilities do not end with the completion of the diagnostic test. Health teaching may be related directly to the test, such as informing the patient to be aware of any signs or symptoms that should be acted on and the reasons prompt reporting is important. This includes signs such as bleeding, nausea, weakness, or discomfort.

Health teaching may continue as a nursing function after the completion of the test. The results may require alterations in daily living based on the results of the test. For example, if an EEG revealed a seizure disorder, information about seizures, seizure precautions, and living a full but regular lifestyle will be in order.

Anxiety Intervention

The nurse can be useful in relieving anxiety by sharing information about the test and its preparation and recognizing and accepting any psychological distress the patient may have. Responsibilities include being knowledgeable concerning diagnostic tests as well as preparing the patient for the test and providing comfort and continued monitoring after the procedure has been concluded. In addition the techniques for anxiety intervention discussed in Chapter 34 can be used to assist the patient.

Performing a Diagnostic Test

On some occasions the nurse has the responsibility of making the decision to perform a diagnostic test. These tests more commonly involve performing the hematest on fluids to detect the presence of blood or testing the urine for specific gravity or for the presence of glucose. Performing a finger stick or blood glucose test during which the finger is penetrated with a small lance or needle is considered invasive and requires a physician's order. Consult a procedure manual or Module 20, Performing Common Laboratory Tests, of *Basic Nursing Skills* for descriptions of these procedures.

If a procedure is to be performed by the physician on the nursing unit, you may be asked to assist. Even though the physician has talked with the patient and obtained consent if this is necessary, it is your responsibility to visit the patient to carry out your own assessment and answer any questions.

Most of the equipment needed for routine tests is standard within the facility but may need to be ordered.

Nursing Research: Implications for Practice

Wakefield, B., Wakefield, D. S., Booth, B. M. "Evaluating Validity of Blood Glucose Monitoring Strip Interpretation by Experienced Users." *Applied Nursing Research* 5, 1 (February 1992): 13–19.

This study examined the accuracy of patients and registered nurses in interpreting blood glucose monitoring strips (BGMS). An important part of the study is that patients often bisect or cut lengthwise the test strip as a cost-saving measure. Thirty-two patients read an intact strip and one that had been cut. Three registered nurses read 32 strips that were intact and 32 strips that had been cut. The readings of each group were compared with the readings from a reflectance meter.

The results revealed a difference in visual interpretation, with each group underestimating the glucose values. Patients or their spouses underestimated readings by as much as 20% on both intact and cut strips. All three nurses also visually read BGMSs below the reflectance meter readings on all strips, but particulary on the cut strips.

This study has important implications for nurses because insulin administration is often determined by glucose values. Nurses should not only monitor their own proficiency in glucose monitoring but health teach patients and their families more efficiently so that patients learn to only use intact strips and know how to read them accurately

Allow time to gather all the equipment so that the test can be carried out smoothly without interruptions. If there is some question about an item or the size of a piece of the equipment, clarify this with the physician so that you will have everything that might be needed.

Drape the patient to provide privacy and offer psychological reassurance both before and during the procedure. Standing by, holding the patient's hand, or placing your hand lightly on the shoulder are all indications that you care about the patient's welfare and that the patient is safe (Fig. 38-3). Unfamiliar procedures can be intimidating even though explanations have been given. It is also your responsibility to carefully observe the status of the patient during the test while the physician focuses on performing the procedure. It may also be appropriate to take vital signs during the procedure to ensure that the patient's status is free of complications to vital functions.

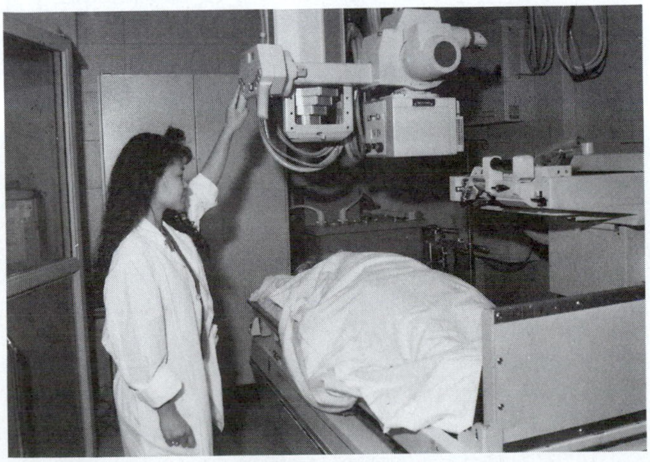

Figure 38-3. A patient in the radiology department.

Positions vary with the procedure performed so that, again, your knowledge of the particular procedure is crucial. You may want to use pillows to support various parts of the body for comfort. If the patient is a child, it may or may not be appropriate for a parent to be present or help hold the child. This will have to be an individual decision.

A specimen of fluid or tissue in a fluid medium may be obtained during a diagnostic procedure. These specimen containers should be carefully labeled and handled. The Centers for Disease Control and Prevention have recommended that all specimens be treated as if the person has a blood-borne infection. Therefore, all specimen containers are placed in leakproof plastic bags to protect others. Specimens should be sent promptly to the laboratory before time can cause alterations in the specimen.

Caring for the Patient After a Diagnostic Test

The primary consideration for care of the patient after the procedure is always safety. Some tests carry more risk for adverse aftereffects than do others. After a biopsy of a highly vascular organ such as the liver, for example, the risk for bleeding may be a concern.

Side effects from other procedures may be uncomfortable but not dangerous. After a lumbar puncture, the patient is ordered to remain in bed with the head flat or only slightly elevated for a period of time. This is done to allow time for the cerebrospinal fluid volume to equalize so that the patient does not experience head pain. After some noninvasive procedures such as x-rays, there are no side effects for which caution should be taken.

If there are significant risks stemming from any procedure or if the patient's pretest status was precarious, you should make frequent observations as well as take frequent vital signs. Each facility has guidelines that you can follow for care after a specific diagnostic procedure.

Documentation

Although the person carrying out the procedure will record it, the nurse will also document that the test has been done and any assessment related to the procedure. This is also true when the nurse assists the physician. Data are entered on the progress notes and include the name of the procedure, the time, date, and physician's name.

If the patient was transported to another department for a test, this should also be documented on the record before the patient and the record leave the unit. When the patient returns, you should document any observations and ongoing assessments that you perform.

If you are performing a single test such as the hematest, you can record this as an observation on the progress notes. If you are performing tests at specific intervals, such as testing urine for glucose, a parameter sheet may be used listing the date, time, and the results (see Module 6, Documentation) for information about recording continuous data.

Evaluation

Evaluation of the technical success of the procedure is the responsibility of the person carrying it out, but the nurse will evaluate the response of the patient to the entire procedure. The patient's status will be compared with baseline status and the criteria established during the planning phase. The nurse may need to continue to monitor important parameters such as pulse and blood pressure for a period of time after the procedure to determine the patient's response.

Nursing Care Study
The Patient Scheduled for a Diagnostic Test

As Pamela Nelson left the unit for home late at night, she noticed the light was still on in Mr. Atwood's room so she stopped in to briefly visit with him. She had cared for Mr. Atwood for several evenings but had not this evening because she had been busy caring for postop patients.

Mr. Atwood was nervously playing cards and did not seem as relaxed as he usually appeared. "I noticed that you are going to have an x-ray of the gallbladder in the morning so maybe you should get some sleep," Pamela remarked. At this, Mr. Atwood replied, "You know, that's why I can't get to sleep. The last time I had that test, I had a reaction or something. I felt short of breath and before I knew it, everyone got excited and they gave me shots and started some oxygen. I was really scared and I hope that doesn't happen this time. Of course, that was in another hospital."

"Did you tell your doctor about what happened?" asked Pamela. "No, I didn't want him to think that I didn't trust him to do a good job," said Mr. Atwood. "Believe me, Mr. Atwood, it sounds like you had a reaction and I can understand your being frightened. It may have been due to the dye that was used. I think your doctor should know about this so I'm glad I stopped by and you mentioned it to me. I will call him and let him know what happened. He might choose to use another type of dye for the test." "Golly, I didn't know it could be serious and happen again."

Pamela stayed to call the physician and record her concern on the patient's record. Later than she had intended, Pamela left the hospital with a feeling of satisfaction that her patient would now be safe.

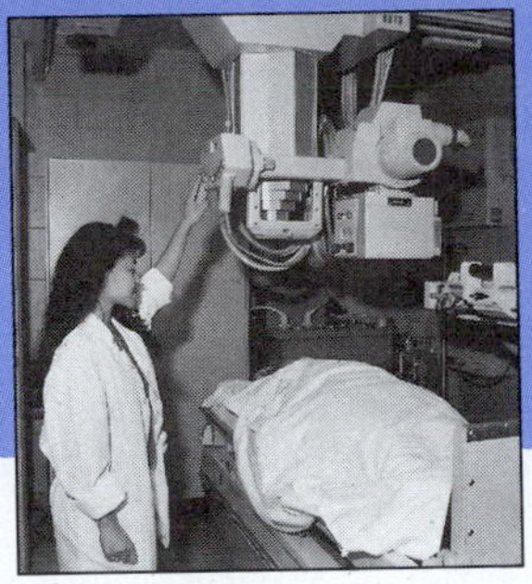

Key Points

- Nurses have specific responsibilities in regard to assisting with diagnostic tests and procedures, including being knowledgeable about the test ordered, assessing the patient's anxiety level and knowledge about the test, and providing for the patient's safety.
- Some of the types of diagnostic tests available include tests using radioactive material; tests that measure and record electrical impulses; tests involving endoscopy, aspirations, and biopsies; and tests to measure specific body functions.
- The policy for scheduling tests and the responsibility for obtaining consent should be clarified for a specific procedure.
- The nursing process is a helpful framework for carrying out the nurse's involvement with diagnostic tests.
- The patient should be assessed for readiness, medical status, the presence of allergies, and age-related factors.
- Planning for diagnostic tests includes providing knowledge to the patient regarding the test, clarifying information for the patient when questions arise, allotting time for preparatory nursing procedures, and carrying out the physician's orders on fluid intake and medications. The nurse must also consider the time necessary for a test so the daily plan of care can be adjusted if necessary.
- Implementation involves providing privacy for the patient, conducting ongoing assessment for tests that involve any risk to the patient, positioning the patient properly, reassuring the patient, ensuring patient comfort, assisting the physician, caring for specimens correctly, teaching the patient about complications from the test or implications for changes in lifestyle mandated by the test results, and observing and monitoring the patient to ensure safety after the diagnostic test is completed.
- The nurse documents that the diagnostic procedure was performed and its preparatory procedures carried out. An evaluation of the patient's response to the procedure is also carried out.

Study Questions

1. If you learned that your patient was scheduled for a diagnostic test about which you had little knowledge, where would you go for information?
2. Why is questioning the patient about the presence of any allergy so important when carrying out assessment?
3. Name and discuss two of the imaging diagnostic tests.
4. Why are tests using magnetic resonance imaging (MRI) more accurate than regular x-rays?
5. Compare the preparation needed for an x-ray of the lower gastrointestinal tract with that needed for an EEG.
6. What is your role as a nurse when assisting a physician with performing diagnostic tests?
7. What specific instructions should you give the patient before aspiration biopsy?
8. Give one example of how the plan of care might be revised so that a diagnostic test can be scheduled.
9. What information should you document after a physician has completed a diagnostic procedure on your patient?
10. Name two areas for health teaching the patient after a diagnostic test has been performed?

Critical Thinking Activities

1. Select a diagnostic test performed commonly on the unit where you care for patients. Compare the preparation for this diagnostic test on a young child with that needed by an older adult. Consider language and specific areas of information that would be included with each patient and patient's family.
2. Compare the preparation needed for an x-ray of the lower gastrointestinal tract and that needed for an EEG. Explain what anatomical information is being sought in each and relate this to the type of preparation that is appropriate.
3. Write a teaching plan for the patient with "Knowledge Deficit regarding scheduled liver biopsy."
4. List five diagnostic tests in order of the degree of risk to the patient. For each test, identify the specific benefit that would occur for the patient.

Relevant Sections in Modules for Basic Nursing Skills

References and Readings

Baer, D. M., and Belsey, R. E. "New Requirements from the JCAHO." *RN* 54, 6 (June 1991): 19–22.

Carr, P. "When Overcompliance Means Trouble." *Nursing* 90, 3 (March 1990): 65–66.

Corbett, J. V. *Laboratory Tests and Diagnostic Procedures with Nursing Diagnoses.* 3rd edition. Norwalk, Conn.: Appleton-Lange, 1992.

Gawlikowski, J. "White Cells at War." *American Journal of Nursing* 92, 3 (March 1992): 44–51.

Griffith, H. W. *Instructions for Patients: Medical Tests and Diagnostic Procedures.* Philadelphia: Lea and Febiger, 1989.

Henry, P. F. "Abnormal Laboratory Test Results: Going the Extra Mile." *Nurse Practitioner Forum* 2, 1 (March 1991): 5–7.

Horowitz, L. "Runaway Medical Testing." *Health* 20, 10 (October 1988): 46–47.

Kee, J. L. *Laboratory and Diagnostic Tests with Nursing Implications.* 3rd edition. Norwalk, Conn.: Appleton and Lange, 1991.

Kee, J. L., and Hayes, E. R. "Assessment of Patient Laboratory Data in the Acutely Ill." *Nursing Clinics of North America* 25, 4 (December 1990): 751–759.

Kestel, F. "Using Blood Glucose Meters: What You and Your Patient Need to Know." *Nursing '93.* 23, 3 (March 1993): 34–41.

Kobos, P. B. "On Noncompliance." *American Journal of Nursing* 89, 11 (November 1989): 1594.

Korniewicz, D. M. et al. "Integrity of Vinyl and Latex Procedure Gloves." *Nursing Research.* 38, 3 (May/June 1989): 144–146.

Nicholson, C. and Coleman, C. A. and Mack, M. "Are You Ready for Video Thoracoscopy?" *American Journal of Nursing.* 93, 3 (March 1993): 54–57.

Treseler, K. M. *Clinical Laboratory and Diagnostic Tests: Significance and Nursing Implications.* 2nd edition. Los Altos, Calif.: Appleton-Lange, 1988.

Pharmacotherapeutics

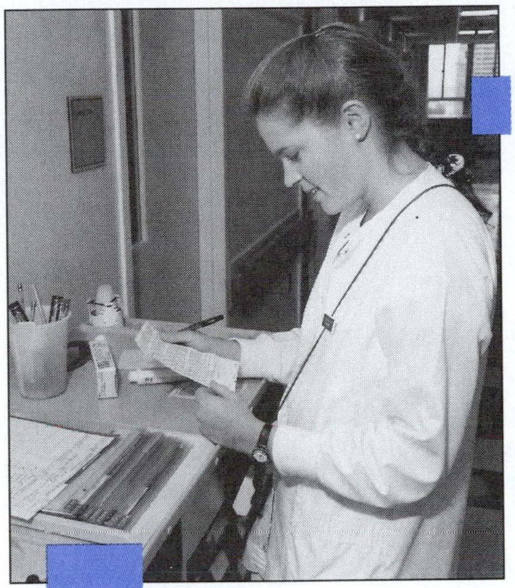

39

Objectives

After completing this chapter, you should be able to:

1. List the organizations in the United States and Canada that have drug regulatory function.
2. Explain the relationships of drug classification, generic name, and trade name.
3. Name and briefly describe the five categories of controlled substances.
4. Discuss the resources the nurse can use for information about medications.
5. Discuss what is meant by the benefit–risk ratio in regard to prescribing drugs.
6. Describe the needed assessment in regard to medications.
7. Discuss common nursing diagnoses in relationship to medications.
8. Describe methods used by the nurse for transcribing and checking medication orders.
9. Discuss factors to be considered in decision-making regarding the administration of PRN medications.
10. Describe the procedure for administering medications, emphasizing actions for safety.
11. Explain what action should be taken if a medication error occurs.
12. Discuss the information about their medications that the nurse should teach to patients.

Study Terms

allergy
contraindication
dosage
efficacy
five rights
pharmacotherapeutics
quality assurance form
side effects
sliding scale
standing orders

Outline

Organizations for Regulating Drugs
Classifications of Drugs
Names for Drugs
Schedules for Controlled Substances
The Nurse's Role in Pharmacotherapeutics
Resources for Information
The Benefit–Risk Ratio
Assessment
Interview
Physical Assessment

Ellis, Nowlis: Nursing: A Human Needs Approach, 5th ed. © 1994 J.B. Lippincott Company

Nursing Diagnosis

- Knowledge Deficit
- Noncompliance
- Ineffective Management of the Therapeutic Regimen
- Altered Comfort
- Altered Nutrition
- Diarrhea
- Constipation
- Sleep Pattern Disturbance
- Impaired Skin Integrity
- Other Nursing Diagnoses

Planning and Implementation

- Verifying the Drug Order
- Obtaining Drug Information
- Transcribing the Drug Order
- Obtaining the Drug
- Administering Drugs
- Using PRN Drugs Effectively
- Documentation
- Health Teaching
- Medication Errors

Evaluation

An important responsibility of the nurse is supporting the medical treatment plan through the administration of drugs. The treatment of the patient through the use of drugs is called **pharmacotherapeutics**. Pharmacotherapeutics may be used to cure disease, to arrest disease, or to control symptoms. The overall goal is to restore the person to an optimum state of health.

The administration of drugs is a serious endeavor for the nurse because of the potentially serious effects they may have on the person. Any substance that causes changes in the body may cause adverse as well as positive responses. Drugs themselves may create disorders that were not present originally. Although the physician is responsible for diagnosing disease and prescribing drugs, others in the health care team have critical responsibilities in ensuring that drugs are given correctly, monitored carefully, and evaluated purposefully.

Organizations for Regulating Drugs

Both the United States and Canada have governmental agencies that regulate drugs. In the United States, drug standards have been set by the federal government. Since 1952, the Federal Food, Drug, and Cosmetic Act has been given extensive power to regulate all substances promoted as having therapeutic properties to protect the consumer. Under this act, the United States Pharmacopeia (USP) and the National Formulary (NF) have been designated official standards. Since 1970, the Controlled Substances Act has mandated monitoring and action to suppress the illicit use of harmful drugs, including narcotics.

In Canada, similar agencies exist. The Canadian Food and Drug Act requires that all drugs manufactured and marketed in Canada must comply with standards set forth by the Canadian Pharmacopeia and Formulary. Since 1961, narcotic possession in Canada is controlled by the Canadian Narcotic Control Act.

In both countries, drugs cannot be marketed until the manufacturer submits research data regarding the safety and effectiveness of the drug. Some drugs are approved for experimental use, some for prescription use, and others for over-the-counter (OTC) use. The United States and Canada differ in regard to some drugs that have been approved by one agency and not the other. The greatest majority of drugs are approved in both countries although their brand names may differ.

Classifications of Drugs

Drugs are classified, named, and regulated in various ways in regard to their potential to cause harm. These systems may be confusing to nurses and those concerned with ordering and administering drugs to patients. Drugs are organized into groups based on their actions and sometimes on their chemical structure. These groups are called drug classifications. For example, the drugs in a group that is used for controlling high blood pressure are classified as antihypertensives; the drugs used for decreasing water retention within the body are classified as diuretics. Drugs used for treating depression are called antidepressants. Within the classification of antidepressants is a subgroup called tricyclic antidepressants. These drugs all share a similar chemical structure.

Using information about classifications helps simplify the learning of various drugs by nurses. Most textbooks and drug reference texts use the classification system for presenting their content. By learning about a major classification and its uses, it is possible to have information that can then be generalized to all of the drugs within that group. Although each one will have specific differences, the similarities assist you in your learning.

Nursing Issues and Trends: Orphan Drugs

An important current issue for nurses regarding drugs is that of "orphan drugs." Orphan drugs are a small number of drugs that are very costly to develop and produce and are used to treat rare disorders or diseases. The questions center around the exorbitant cost of developing these drugs that benefit so few people. Questions also being asked about orphan drugs are who is to pay the high price of researching and developing these drugs and what part, if any, should the government play. There is also the issue of providing these drugs to those people who are afflicted with these rare diseases and cannot pay their cost. Nurses should be cognizant of the advent of these unusual drugs and become involved in decisions about orphan drugs because they directly affect comprehensive health care for everyone.

Names for Drugs

One drug can have four different names. By far the most descriptive is the drug's *chemical name.* This is a name that identifies the chemical composition of the compound. One of the most familiar chemical names for a drug is acetylsalicylic acid. The *generic name* is the official name approved by the regulatory agency. The generic name for acetylsalicylic acid is aspirin. The drug manufacturer then gives the drug its third or *brand* name. The brand name is intended to be simple to remember and easy for health care providers to remember to facilitate marketing. Pharmaceutical companies often name their products in such a way that the drug's action is implicit in the name or that the name is similar to others in its classification.

Unfortunately, some drugs have similar names although they are completely different in function or dosage. It is not only confusing but may lead to errors when the generic or brand names of two drugs are similar. The nurse should be careful of drug names when preparing to administer drugs.

Schedules for Controlled Substances

Drugs that have potential for addiction or abuse are more closely regulated and controlled than are other drugs. Prescribers are carefully identified and the drug supplies are monitored, counted, and controlled at all points in their manufacture and distribution. Drugs that are regulated in this way are called *controlled substances.*

These drugs are ranked in five schedules or classes. *Schedule I* drugs have the highest potential for addiction and abuse and are not available for regular therapeutic use. Some are used for research purposes. Heroin, marijuana, and LSD are examples.

Schedule II contains the major narcotics such as morphine, meperidine, hydromorphone, and codeine. Schedule II drugs must be individually prescribed and must contain a warning label; the prescription cannot be automatically refilled.

Many of the *schedule III* drugs contain schedule II drugs but in lesser quantities combined with nonnarcotic drugs. Common schedule III drugs include acetaminophen with codeine and aspirin with codeine. In addition, there are other schedule III drugs such as paregoric. These drugs must be ordered by prescription and are limited to one month's use. The prescription, if not used, expires in 6 months. A warning label is required. The prescription may be renewed five times.

Drugs that cause relaxation or induce sleep are in *schedule IV.* These drugs have a limited supply of one month and a warning label is required. They may be refilled only five times. Examples of schedule IV drugs are diazepam (Valium) and phenobarbital. Finally, *schedule V* drugs are those considered to have less abusive potential but still must be ordered by prescription. These drugs often contain small amounts of narcotics or other scheduled drugs. Included in this schedule are some anticough preparations and medications for treatment of diarrhea and allergic reactions.

The Nurse's Role in Pharmacotherapeutics

The administration of drugs to patients is a nursing task accompanied by a high degree of responsibility. The nurse must know about the drug itself, its actions, and its potential adverse effects. A knowledge of the safe dosage of the drug is also essential. In addition the nurse needs to understand why the particular drug is being used for the individual patient to evaluate the effectiveness of the medication. The nurse uses this information to double check the medication order. An informed nurse and a knowledgeable pharmacist work as a team with the physician to ensure that errors in medications do not occur.

Patients also need information regarding their drugs to participate effectively in their own health care. They must know what to look for in their own responses, what to report, and how to avoid adverse effects. Patients often take drugs brought to them by the nurse without question. It is essential that nurses be able to teach patients regarding their medications.

Resources for Information

The number of drugs available, both new and variations of those that have been used for a long time, is startling. Keeping current with so many drugs is not only difficult for the beginning nursing student but for practicing staff nurses. Because principles of safety must be maintained, the nurse must continually update information regarding drugs and their actions. A variety of resources can be used to learn the classifications, names, actions, and **side effects** (effects of a drug other than those for which it is given) of medications. Also important are the interactions of different drugs given to the same patient. Pharmacology textbooks give lengthy and detailed information about drugs, their chemical composition, and their action. Drug reference books are easier and faster to use but are limited in their information concerning a classification. They are particularly useful regarding dosages and side effects. Nursing journals contain monthly drug updates on newer drugs that become available.

If the nurse is unable to find sufficient information or lacks information on a new drug, the pharmacist is an invaluable source of information and will research specific questions for the nurse on request. Talking with the pharmacist is particularly helpful when an experimental drug has been prescribed. You are legally responsible for having knowledge of the drugs you are administering.

The Benefit-Risk Ratio

When the nurse gathers information about drugs, there may seem to be conflicting facts. For example, there may be a statement that caution should be used or even that the drug should not be used if the patient has a particular disease or condition. The risk may be accepted because of potential benefits to the patient or the drug may be withheld if the physician thinks the risk is not warranted. The relationship of the benefits and risks is called the *benefit–risk ratio.*

With the numerous drugs in use and the assortment of reactions that occur, these warnings are becoming more frequent. The warnings should not be ignored and if you are concerned, the physician ordering the drugs should be consulted to clarify the order. However, remember that these warnings are general and the individual benefits to the patient must be considered.

You must be aware of any interactions with other drugs the patient is receiving or contraindications to the drug's use. A **contraindication** is an indication of a situation in which administration of a drug carries a higher than normal risk of adverse responses. If the medication ordered is contraindicated for any reason, it is the nurse's responsibility to bring this circumstance to the attention of the physician. If the physician is aware of the conflict, the nurse should request an explanation of the rationale for giving the medication. If, after hearing the rationale, the nurse is still reluctant to give any medication, the nursing supervisor may be contacted for advice and direction. It is the privilege and responsibility of the nurse not to administer a medication he or she firmly believes will be harmful to the patient.

Another type of adverse reaction that may occur is the idiosyncratic reaction. This means that the particular individual has a specific individualized reaction to a drug. Idiosyncratic reactions to drugs are identified through careful assessment.

Assessment

When administering drugs that have been ordered for the patient, following the nursing process will be helpful in giving the drug safely. Reviewing the process will enable you to identify your responsibilities in administration.

Interview

Patients should be asked during the interview what medications they are currently taking and for what purpose. The patient may have daily medications from home and these should be stored and monitored according to the policy of the facility. Information should also be gathered as to how long the drug has been taken and in what dosage. All drug information should be carefully documented as part of the patient's record.

A history of drugs that have been taken in the past is crucial. The patient can often remember if there has been a problem with allergic or untoward reactions to a particular drug or a classification of drugs. The patient can have either an allergic reaction to a drug or an unpleasant side effect such as nausea and vomiting. Any reaction can become more severe with subsequent exposure to a drug that has not been tolerated in the past. If a medication is ordered that has produced reactions in the past, the physician should be consulted.

Patients may report that they cannot take penicillin, not realizing that many other drugs would produce similar reactions because they are related to the penicillin group. Attention to possible allergies to medications can prevent unfortunate and sometimes tragic mistakes. However, some adverse effects that the patient reports as an **allergy** (hypersensitivity to a specific substance) may not be a true allergy that threatens life, but rather have been a known effect of the drug that was dosage related. For example, constipation is a common adverse effect of narcotics but is not an allergy.

Drugs are perceived in many different ways by individuals. Many people view drugs as unnecessary and even harmful, whereas others often have taken various drugs for years and sec them as the "quick fix" for medical problems. Your assessment interview must include the patient's perception of taking drugs and expectations of how useful they will be.

The nurse can also assess willingness and ability to take the ordered drugs. A patient may refuse an order for a drug and has the right to do so. For example, a patient may perceive a sleeping pill ordered to be given each night as unnecessary. At other times, the patient may be noncompliant because of confusion or agitation.

The patient's prior knowledge of drugs is an important part of complete assessment. For example, if a patient was ordered to have a thyroid hormone replacement drug, you would want to find out what the patient knew about the drug, its use, and its side effects.

Information may be needed about when and how to take the drug. Drugs may be ordered to be given at specific times and over a limited course of time. Other drugs such as replacement drugs may be needed indefinitely throughout the patient's lifetime. Medications must sometimes be taken with food to avoid nausea, whereas other medications are taken when the stomach is empty so that absorption is more complete. Certain medications have interactions with food that are important for planning menus. When assessing for knowledge deficit in regard to drugs, you must have complete information to determine what knowledge would be needed by the patient to effectively use the drug in treatment.

The patient may be unaware of the desired effects of the drugs. A patient who does not understand the expected effect of a medication is unable to evaluate personal response to the drug. Does the person know when the desired effect should become apparent? Will the effect need to be determined by laboratory or diagnostic tests? If so, does the patient understand how these will be used and when they must be done?

You will need to determine whether the patient understands the possible adverse effects of the drug and how to manage them. If the adverse responses cannot be avoided, such as hair loss with some cancer treatments, then does the person have information about the problem and how to manage it? A patient must have the knowledge necessary to recognize potentially serious side effects early to be able to report them. What would be the earliest indicators of adverse response? Are there measures the patient can take to prevent adverse reactions and does the patient understand these?

Physical Assessment

The nurse should obtain information from the record concerning the patient's diagnosis and physical examination. This information will often give clues to the reason certain medications are ordered. In some cases you will need to measure vital signs immediately before administering a medication to determine whether the medication should be administered. These data will also provide a baseline for monitoring and evaluating drug effects.

The physical ability to take a medication can be assessed. The ability to swallow is especially relevant for safety. Many drugs are available in liquid form so that if the nurse assesses swallowing difficulties (dysphagia), the physician can order the same drug in liquid form. If a feeding tube is in place, medications must be either liquid in form or must be dissolved to be administered orally.

Other physical difficulties can create problems. If the patient has difficulties in coordination or is paralyzed, assistance will have to be provided. An individual may be unable to sit up to swallow making it impossible to take oral medications.

When injections are ordered, part of your assessment must include whether the person has adequate tissue for appropriate absorption of the medication. An emaciated patient may not be a good candidate for routinely receiving intramuscular injections. If intravenous medications are ordered, you will need to check what type of intravenous access is present. Is there an ongoing intravenous fluid line, a heparin lock, or is no access present?

Specific assessment needs to be conducted in regard to the need for PRN medications that have been ordered. Some PRN medications are ordered to alleviate symptoms that may be present. Other PRN medications are given based on specific laboratory test results or parameters such as blood pressure. To use PRN medications effectively, you must know what drugs have been ordered, what their purposes are, and then thoroughly assess the patient.

Nursing Diagnosis

Many of the common nursing diagnoses related to drug therapy have to do with knowledge deficit or the adverse side effects caused by drugs. All are equally important.

Knowledge Deficit

The diagnosis Knowledge Deficit regarding a specific drug is common. It may be that the patient has incorrect knowledge concerning a drug, or the patient may be totally unfamiliar with a drug that has been ordered. One of the difficulties for the hospitalized patient is the volume of important information regarding a drug. The patient needs information to be a knowledgeable partner in care. You will want to identify the knowledge that is most essential and focus your attention there initially.

Noncompliance

Noncompliance refers to the situation in which a patient decides not to take a drug. Noncompliance has many causes and should be investigated carefully. Is the drug causing unpleasant side effects that have not been disclosed? Sometimes drugs are expensive and a low-income person may decide to forgo medication because it is a lower priority than basic needs. Does the person clearly understand the purpose of the drug and its potential for improved health? What are the beliefs about medications? Some individuals have unrealistic fears about drug dependence when using any medication on a long-term basis.

Nursing Diagnoses Related to Pharmacotherapeutics

Knowledge Deficit: Lack of information related to antihypertensive medication

Noncompliance related to unpleasant side effects of prescribed drug

Ineffective Management of the Therapeutic Regimen: Fails to remember to take prescribed medication

Altered Comfort: Nausea related to antineoplastic medication

Altered nutrition: Less Than Body Requirements related to nausea and vomiting secondary to medications

Diarrhea related to side effects of medication

Constipation related to iron supplements and decreased intestinal motility

Sleep Pattern Disturbance: Insomnia related to effects of bronchodilators

Impaired Skin Integrity:Fine body rash related to medication side effects

Ineffective Management of the Therapeutic Regimen

The individual who forgets to take drugs, who takes them incorrectly, or does not follow directions in regard to dietary restrictions or other self-care activities related to prescribed drugs may be experiencing this diagnosis. Often nurses assume that all ineffective management is related to a knowledge deficit. This is not the case. Carrying out a therapeutic regimen is affected by many different life factors. The better you know the patient the more accurately you can identify the etiology of ineffective management.

Altered Comfort

The most common disruption of comfort caused by drugs is nausea and vomiting. The nurse could write this nursing diagnosis as Altered Comfort related to medication effects, as evidenced by nausea and vomiting. Many of the antineoplastic drugs used in the treatment of cancer cause these side effects. Other drugs are often given before administration or during the administration of these agents to decrease the discomfort.

Altered Nutrition

When drugs cause loss of appetite (anorexia) so that the patient cannot consume a nutritious diet for a lengthy period of time, the nursing diagnosis Altered Nutrition: Less Than Body Requirements related to anorexia is present. A person may also have altered nutrition related to persistent nausea or vomiting secondary to medications. Because adequate nutrition is so essential to the restoration and maintenance of health, this can become a serious problem.

Diarrhea

Some medications can also cause abdominal cramping and diarrhea. Antibiotics are prominent in this group. However, many other drugs also create this problem. In some instances, the drug must be continued and therefore treatment of the diarrhea is needed. The nurse must be alert for the possibility of additional problems that occur secondary to diarrhea, such as fluid and electrolyte imbalance and impaired skin integrity.

Constipation

Many common drugs such as narcotic analgesics and iron preparations can cause constipation. This is particularly true for the elderly person who also has decreased intestinal motility. The nursing diagnosis Constipation related to medication effects is used. The pregnant woman may become constipated from a combination of medication and the pressure of the growing fetus on the intestines. The individual may note that bowel movements are spaced further apart and the stool is hard and dry. When other problems are prominent for the patient, constipation may sometimes be ignored until it becomes a serious problem for the individual.

Sleep Pattern Disturbance

The nursing diagnosis Sleep Pattern Disturbance is appropriate when the patient's sleep is disturbed because of the ordered drugs. Some drugs act as stimulants, thus interfering with sleep. Some of the bronchodilators cause feelings of agitation, which results in insomnia. The patient often describes this as "feeling jittery."

The diuretics, medications that increase urinary excretion of fluid, also can interfere with sleep because the patient has to urinate several times during the sleeping hours. It is better to give these drugs during the waking hours so that sleep can occur more normally and not be disturbed, but this is not always possible.

Impaired Skin Integrity

One of the most common allergic responses to drugs is a skin rash. The presence of rash and itching can cause the person to scratch the skin so that its integrity is impaired. Impaired Skin Integrity: Fine rash related to medication effects becomes appropriate when this is the situation. Other medications, either topical or systemic, may be ordered to alleviate the rash and itching. Itching may also contribute to sleep disturbance and create severe discomfort.

Other Nursing Diagnoses

Other nursing diagnoses are related to side effects of drugs. Drugs such as the antihypertensives can cause changes in libido, leading to a diagnosis of Sexual Dysfunction. Occasionally, a drug causes or increases confusion, prompting a diagnosis of Altered Thought Processes. When an individual is confused, a nursing diagnosis of High Risk for Injury may be appropriate. Each individual should be carefully assessed in relationship to these common problems created by drugs.

Planning and Implementation

The desired patient outcomes for drug administration are important. The patient should receive the maximum **efficacy** (therapeutic results) from a drug with the fewest side effects. Another outcome is that the patient is knowledgeable about a drug and willingly complies with its administration.

Verifying the Drug Order

With some exceptions, drugs in the hospital setting are ordered by the physician and administered by the nurse. Some drugs are routine standing orders for every patient of a specific physician, or some drugs can be given at the discretion of the nurse, relying on accurate assessment of the patient.

The nurse has several specific responsibilities relating to the drug therapy ordered by the physician. These include checking the original order for the drug. You should carefully check the name of the drug, the dosage, and the administration schedule. If there are abbreviations you do not understand, check them out with the physician. Whether the nurse is to administer the medication or the patient is to self-administer, the accuracy of the order is the responsibility of the nurse.

Because some patients are admitted with their own medications from home, the policy in your agency will have to be consulted regarding how this situation should be handled. The policy may allow the patient to keep these drugs at the bedside for self-administration if the physician so designates, or they may be stored under the nurse's supervision until the patient is discharged. Whatever the policy, you will need to verify the physician's order regarding the medications to be taken by the patient.

Obtaining Drug Information

After determining the drug to be given, you will need to obtain information about the drug (Fig. 39-1). As you become more experienced, you may find that you are familiar with the common drugs used where you practice. However, new drugs are constantly being approved and no nurse can expect to have all information about all drugs memorized. The resources for obtaining information were discussed previously.

You will need to know the route and intended action of the drug, its usual purpose, and effects and side effects. Also, your recognition that any medication delivered intravenously carries additional safety risks is criti-

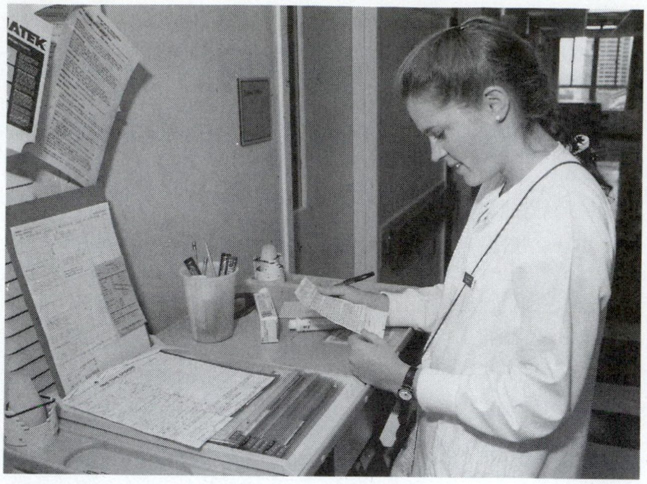

Figure 39-1. The nurse sets up medications at the cart and reviews drug information for unfamiliar medications.

cal. The fact that intravenous drugs are infused directly into the circulatory system, have instant absorption, and cannot be retrieved makes safety a special concern in their administration.

When looking at information in regard to a specific drug for a specific patient, you will be determining that the drug is not contraindicated for this patient. When you have specific information, you are able to identify desired effects and potential side effects.

Another responsibility of the nurse is to know the correct **dosage** of a medication and have knowledge of basic mathematic equivalencies (Table 39-1). Errors in dosage can occur because of incorrect transcription of orders from one place to another, poor penmanship, or simple human fallibility. The nurse who knows the correct dosage and checks the order is often able to catch such errors and contact the physician to correct them.

Knowing dosages is particularly important for nurses working with children. Children's dosages are so much smaller than adults' that even slight errors can cause serious problems. We have presented a table of equivalencies for your use in working with dosages.

Transcribing the Drug Order

After a physician writes a drug order, the nurse has many further duties with regard to it. The nurse may transcribe the order from the patient record to the card index (Kardex), other medication administration record (MAR; Fig. 39-2), or a computer. In other settings, the task of transcribing is assigned to the unit secretary and subsequently checked for accuracy by a registered nurse. In either case, the ultimate responsibility for checking the correctness of the transcription belongs to the nurse.

In addition to transcribing the specific information in the physician's order, the nurse is responsible for identifying appropriate administration parameters such as times of administration. The order may written for

Table 39–1. Equivalencies for Common Units of Measurement

Metric Doses and Apothecaries' Equivalents

Liquid

Metric	Approximate apothecaries' equivalents
1,000 ml	1 quart
500 ml	1 pint
250 ml	8 fluidounces
30 ml	1 fluidounce
15 ml	4 fluidrams
5 ml	1 fluidram
1 ml	15 minims
0.06 ml	1 minim

Solid

Metric	Approximate apothecaries' equivalents
30 g	1 ounce
15 g	4 drams
4 g	60 grains (1 dram)
1 g	15 grains
0.5 g	7½ grains
60 mg	1 grain
30 mg	½ grain
15 mg	¼ grain
10 mg	1/6 grain
8 mg	1/8 grain
1 mg	1/60 grain
0.6 mg	1/100 grain
0.4 mg	1/150 grain
0.3 mg	1/200 grain
0.2 mg	1/300 grain
0.1 mg	1/600 grain

Approximate Household Measures

1 teaspoonful	1 fl dr	4–5 ml
1 tablespoonful	½ fl oz	15 or 16 ml
1 jigger	1½ fl oz	45 ml
1 cup	8 fl oz	240 ml

Prescription Abbreviations

gr	grain or grains
gtt*	drops
ʒ	dram
℥	ounce
$\overline{aa}$	equal parts
$\overline{ss}$	one half
cc†	cubic centimeter
g	gram
mg	milligram
mcg	microgram
ml	milliliter
mEq	milliequivalent
♏	minim

*Gutta(e)

†Although technically not exactly equivalent, ml and cc are often used interchangeably.

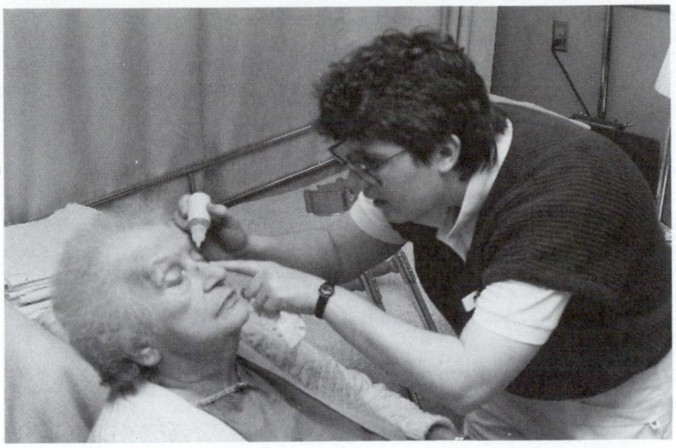

Figure 39-2. The nurse is administering eye medication to a patient.

"four times a day." The nurse determines whether this should be four times around the clock (every 6 hours) or four times during the waking time (every 4 hours), based on knowledge of the drug and its effects. If a question arises, the pharmacist is consulted.

If the order has previously been transcribed, a routine for checking the accuracy of the transcribed record may have been established. In some facilities, this step is eliminated and the order is written directly on the record from which the medication is given. The medication order must be transmitted to the pharmacy in some way. A carbon of the order may be used for this purpose or a computerized ordering system may be in place. The pharmacist is then able to check the physician's order also.

Obtaining the Drug

You will have to locate the drug and check to determine if it is the exact drug ordered. The medication may have already been delivered by the pharmacy to the unit or if it is a new order, you may have to obtain the drug from the pharmacy. Careful checking of drug names and dosages is essential for safety.

Administering Drugs

Once you have ascertained that you have the correct information, you may begin the procedure of administering the medication. Whatever its structure, the system of drug administration is designed to provide the **five rights**: the right medication in the right dosage, by the right route, at the right time to the right patient. You will need to learn the exact system or procedure of any facility in which you are employed. Whatever the system, the nurse's responsibility is to use it correctly so that the chances of error are minimized (Fig. 39-3).

For a detailed discussion of the procedure for administering medications, see Modules 49 through 54 in *Basic Nursing Skills.*

Using PRN Drugs Effectively

If the drug is one that is ordered PRN, planning involves personal assessment and may include consultation with the patient. Your observations are essential. When a patient is in pain, the nurse should not quickly administer a medication prescribed for pain without considering other options that may be used for relief of pain along with the drug or as an alternative. PRN is derived from *pro re nata,* which means *for the situation needed.* Based on assessment, the nurse can make the decision whether or not to administer an ordered medication. The medications most often written as PRN are drugs to control pain, laxatives, antacids, and antipyretics to control fever.

The PRN physician's order carries with it an added responsibility for accurate assessment and appropriate

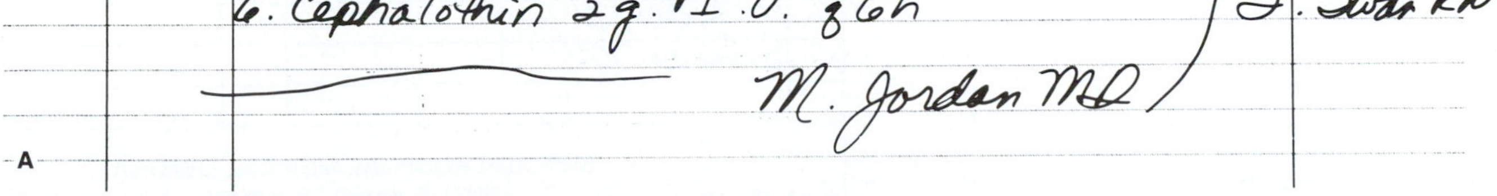

DATE	TIME	PHYSICIAN'S ORDERS	NOTED BY
5/20/94	0900	1. Bowel care per standing orders, PRN	
		2. Maalox 2 tsp. q2h prn	5/20/94
		3. Prednisone 5mg. t.i.d.	
		4. Metaproterenol inhaler 2 puffs q4h	0930
		5. O_2 per nasal prongs @ 2 L.	
		6. Cephalothin 2g. I.V. q6h	S. Swan RN
		M. Jordan MD	

A

Figure 39-3. **A**: An example of a physician's orders for medications. **B**: Recording the ordered medications on a medication administration record.

DIAGNOSIS: Pneumonia, Asthma

ALLERGIES: Mold

A = Rt. Dors/Glut
B = Lt. Dors/Glut
C = Rt. Deltoid
D = Lt. Deltoid
E = Rt. Thigh
F = Lt. Thigh
G = Rt. Vent/Glut
H = Lt. Vent/Glut

Page ___ of ___

MEDICATION AND STRENGTH: ROUTE & DIRECTIONS	SHIFT	Date:	Date:	Date:
5/20/94 Prednisone 5 mg. t.i.d. 09-13-17 S.S.	24/07			
	07/15	09 AR 13 AR		
	15/24			
5/20/94 Metaproterenol Inhaler 2 puffs q4h 01-05-09-13-17-21 SS.	24/07			
	07/15	09 AR 13 AR		
	15/24			
5/20/94 Cephalothin 2g. I.V. q6h 03-09-15-21 SS	24/07			
	07/15	09 AR 15 AR		
	15/24			
	24/07			
	07/15			
	15/24			
	24/07			
	07/15			
	15/24			
	24/07			
	07/15			
	15/24			
	24/07			
	07/15			
	15/24			
5/20/94 Maalox 2 tsp. q 2h PRN S.S.	24/07			
	07/15	09 AR 1300 AR 11 AR 1500 AR		
	15/24			
5/20/94 Bowel care per standing orders. PRN S.S.	24/07			
	07/15	09 M.O.M. AR 30 ml.		
	15/24			

INITIAL	NAME:	INITIAL	NAME:	INITIAL	NAME:
AR	A. Rider RN				
SS	S. Swan RN				

SWEDISH HOSPITAL MEDICAL CENTER
SEATTLE, WASHINGTON 98104

P-346 Rev. 1/91
STOCK NO. 5630

B

Figure 39-3. (continued)

follow through to provide effective resolution to the patient's concerns. PRN orders provide the nurse with additional autonomy in caring for patients' increased decision-making ability.

Sometimes the PRN order is specifically written for a situation which provides guidelines for administration. For example, "Tylenol 2 tabs. for temperatures over 101°." At other times, the nurse's planning is an important piece of decision-making. You may receive an order for analgesics stating that you can give an analgesic of a variable dosage for the patient's pain. This means that based on the assessment of the level of the patient's pain, you may legally administer the dosage within the dosages specified in the order. This is called a **sliding scale** medication order.

Some facilities have standing orders for certain medications. A **standing order** means it is ongoing and is sometimes written as an order on the patient's record. Some surgeons provide a stamped list of standing orders for their postoperative patients. Standing orders can also take other forms; a nurses' bowel care standing order may be the administration of selected laxatives as well as options for the administration of enema procedures.

Documentation

All drug administration must legally be documented by the nurse as soon after administration as possible. After administration of the medication, a record is made of the medication, dosage, time, and route (oral, IM, IV). This legal record must be signed by the person administering the medication. The importance of accurate recording cannot be overemphasized. Failure to record might result in a patient's receiving an ordered medication twice, with potentially serious effects.

Omission of a medication must also be recorded, along with the reasons for omission. Medication documentation policies vary from one facility to another so that you will want to have sound knowledge of the policy of your institution. If a medication has been refused by the patient or not given for some other reason, this also should be documented on the patient's record. Patients have the right to refuse a medication. Documentation should indicate that the medication was refused and the reason. Your will also note your action concerning assessing the patient's declining the drug as well as notification of the physician.

Health Teaching

The nurse plays an important role in teaching the patient about drugs that are ordered. The public media is constantly involved in not only educational programming that adds to the patient's knowledge but also in advertising, which can communicate inaccuracies or encourage false hopes in pharmacotherapeutics.

Therefore, the nurse can present unbiased and scientific information to the patient. Some health teaching may simply involve methods for continuing the medications after discharge. Many hospitals require a registered nurse to review, both orally and in writing, the patient's medications with the person or the family before discharge. During the health teaching session, the nurse can also answer any questions the patient may have about drugs being given. Health teaching also provides the nurse with additional time for assessment of possible future problems that may be encountered. There may be a problem with access to a pharmacist or payment for drugs that are needed for treatment. The nurse can supply this important information. This should be done in such a way that the patient does not become alarmed and yet is knowledgeable about side effects that can occur and can report concerns promptly.

Medication Errors

Because of the complexity of modern medication regimens, errors do occur. A distinction is made between *errors of commission*, such as giving a wrong medication or an incorrect dosage, and *errors of omission*, such as failing to administer medication.

However a medication error occurs, your immediate concern must be the well-being of the patient. The patient's status must be assessed in light of the nature of the error. If an overdosage was administered, are there signs of adverse reactions? If a medication was omitted, are there possible adverse consequences for the patient? When the patient's immediate status has been assessed, the nurse must plan the course of action. Sometimes immediate measures should be taken. When, for example, a medication to relieve muscle spasm was to have been given at 8:00 AM and the nurse discovers at 10:00 AM that it was omitted, the nurse might elect to give the medication immediately because the patient needs relief. Other errors may require other types of action. It may be sufficient to make a notation on the nursing care plan or card index to alert other nurses to watch for particular problems.

The plan of action must always include notification of the physician. The nurse should be prepared to give the physician a complete assessment of the patient's condition and a summary of any action taken and to consult with the physician on further action. If the problem is not serious, notification may be postponed until the physician's next visit. Otherwise, notification should be made immediately. If the physician is not available, the nursing supervisor and another physician may be called.

Another part of the nurse's plan will be to fill out a

Nursing Research: Implications for Practice

Walters, J. A. "Nurses' Perceptions of Reportable Medication Errors and Factors That Contribute to Their Occurrence." *Applied Nursing Research* 5, 2 (May 1992): 86–88.

Using a questionnaire to gather data, the researcher surveyed 238 registered nurses to identify: 1) the nurse's estimate of the number of medication errors made and reported over a 12-month period, 2) perceptions of major causes of medication errors, and 3) the practice of reporting medication errors.

Forty-nine percent of the respondents averaged 1.5 medication errors over a 12 month period, whereas 51% reported making no errors. According to the data, the major causes of errors that should have been reported according to hospital policy were:

Received late from pharmacy	43.3%
RN being too busy	39.1%
RN forgetfulness/oversight	35.3%
Unclear medication record	35.3%
System problems	21.8%
RN disorganization	12.6%

Only 13% responded that they would report all of the categories listed above. However, 97% would report the error if it involved a life-threatening situation; 95% would report the error if it interfered with treatment.

This study suggests that hospital administration and nurses be more aware of the occurrence of medication errors and revise policies and procedures, on both the management and practice levels, to decrease their occurrence, prioritize their importance to safe care, and increase accurate reporting.

special incident form for the hospital or facility. Some hospitals call these forms **quality assurance forms**. The primary purpose of such forms is to gather data on problems so that steps can be taken to eliminate them. They also serve as a legal record for the facility.

Evaluation

To evaluate the effectiveness of medications you administer, you must know the expected reaction to the drug and establish criteria for ascertaining its effectiveness. For example, to evaluate codeine's effectiveness for a patient, you need to know that codeine is given to reduce pain. Knowing how long a medication takes to become effective also helps you establish specific evaluation criteria, such as "pain relief obtained within 30 minutes."

Side effects and allergies to drugs are common complications of drug therapy. Familiarity with the problems that can result from a given medication will enable the nurse to recognize their presence in a patient during the evaluation process. The earlier a problem is recognized, the sooner appropriate action may be taken to combat it. It is always the responsibility of the nurse to discontinue any drug that has dangerous or serious adverse effects until the physician can be notified and consulted. The physician may wish to lower the dosage, discontinue the medication altogether, or even order other medications to counteract a given reaction.

Nursing Care Study
The Patient Who is Noncompliant Regarding an Ordered Drug

Julie Powers entered Mr. Owens room to greet him as a new admission to her unit and to begin the assessment interview. Mr. Owens was age 40 and being admitted for a hernia repair. When she asked about drugs taken in the past, the patient appeared somewhat anxious and said, "About a year ago, the doctor put me on some blood pressure pills but I quit taking them." Julie asked Mr. Owens to say more about why he discontinued the drug. "Well, those pills really bothered me; I really didn't feel like a man and had trouble with relations—you know, with my wife."

During the physical examination, Julie discovered that Mr. Owens' blood pressure was 164/88. When Mr. Owens asked how high his blood pressure reading was, Julie told him and asked that he tell the physician about not taking his medication. After Dr. Stewart's visit to the patient later in the afternoon, Julie checked to be sure Mr. Owens had reported his discontinuing the antihypertensive medication.

Dr. Stewart had been informed by the patient and Mr. Owens had clearly stated his reasons regarding the drug's side effects. Dr. Stewart told Julie that he had told the patient the serious risks of high blood pressure but appreciated the patient's concern. He assured Mr. Owens that another less aggressive drug would be tried for one month along with other methods for lowering his blood pressure, such as salt restrictions and relaxation techniques. Mr. Owens said he had not realized that serious physical events could happen and he was willing to try the new drug being offered.

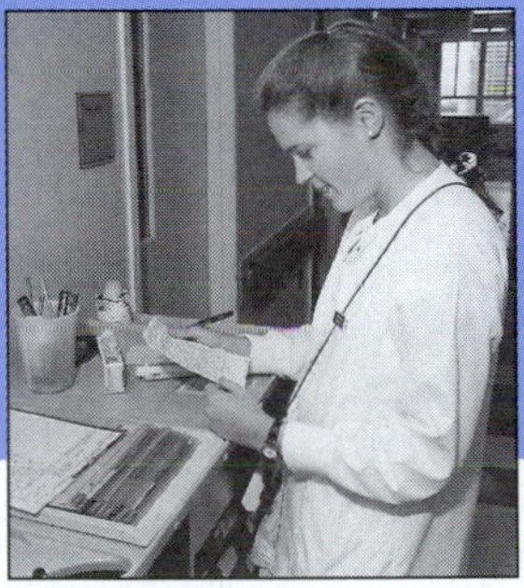

Key Points

- Administering medication safely and conscientiously demands that the nurse be knowledgeable, responsible, and accountable.
- Assessment for drug therapy includes interviewing the patient to determine medical status, the presence of allergies, and age.
- Nurses must have a knowledge of organizations and agencies that regulate available drugs in the United States and Canada, as well as basic knowledge of drugs and dosages.
- Each drug administered should be given according to safe protocol and individualized to the patient's need.
- Proper documentation of drug administration is an important legal concern.
- Knowledge of drug side effects makes it possible for the nurse to recognize undesirable effects early so that corrective action can be taken.
- When a medication error occurs, the nurse needs to know the steps to take to protect the patient and to meet legal responsibilities. Corrective action may involve completing an incident report, sometimes referred to as a quality assurance form.

Study Questions

1. What is the primary purpose of organizations like the United States and Canadian Pharmacopeia and Formulary?
2. What resources could you use in the hospital setting for obtaining information about drugs.
3. Name one specific drug that illustrates the concept of the benefit–risk ratio.
4. What is a nurse responsible for knowing in regard to a medication to be administered?
5. What are the "five rights" and how do they apply to drug administration?
6. Why is Knowledge Deficit an important nursing diagnosis related to drug therapy?
7. Explain terms "standing order" and "sliding scale."
8. What are four common side effects of drugs?
9. What is the appropriate action for a nurse if the dos-

age of a medication is larger than is that recommended by the manufacturer?

Critical Thinking Activities

1. Visit a retail pharmacy and notice how drugs are displayed for the consumer. Write a brief paper identifying which classifications of over-the-counter drugs that appear to be most frequently purchased based on number of brands and amount of shelf space. Compare the cost of different brands of one common medication and whether or not the information printed on the containers is easy for the average consumer to comprehend. Share your observations with that of other students.
2. Lead a small group discussion in which each student presents information on a commonly used drug, giving its classification, action, side effects, and interactions with other drugs.
3. Review the procedure in your facility for administering medications to patients. Analyze how the patient is protected from errors by the procedure.
4. Identify an adult patient in the clinical area who is being discharged with three or more prescriptions. Write a health teaching plan regarding these medications.

Relevant Sections in Modules for Basic Nursing Skills

References and Readings

Azzarello, J. "Reviewing your Patient's Medication Regimen: A Systematic Approach." *Home Healthcare Nurse* 7, 6 (November-December 1989): 24–26.

Baer, D. M., and Belsey, R. E.. "New Requirements from the JCAHO." *RN* 54, 6 (June 1991): 19–22.

Carey, N., Jones, S. L., and O'Toole, A. W. "Do You Feel Powerless When a Patient Refuses Medication?" *Journal of Psychosocial Nursing* 28, 10 (October 1990): 19–25, 40–41.

Carr, P. "When Overcompliance Means Trouble." *Nursing* 90, 3 (March 1990): 65–66.

Cohen, M. R. "Do We Still Need the Apothecary System?" *Nursing '93.* 23, 2 (February 1993): 57–58.

Conn, V. S. "Older Adults: Factors that Predict the Use of Over-the-Counter Medication." *Journal of Advanced Nursing.* 16, 11 (November 1991): 90–96.

DiStasio, S. A. "Zofran Makes Chemo Bearable." *RN.* 56, 5 (May 1993): 56–57.

Drass, J. "What You Need to Know About Insulin Injections." *Nursing '92* 22, 11 (November 1992): 40–45.

Hayes, J. D. "How to Ask Drug Companies for Help." *American Journal of Nursing.* 93, 1 (January 1993): 38–41.

Kobos, P. B. "On Noncompliance." *American Journal of Nursing* 89, 11 (November 1989): 1594.

Koska, M. T. "Drug Errors: Dangerous, Costly and Avoidable." *Hospitals* 63, 11 (June 5, 1989): 24.

Kudzma, E. C. "Drug Response: All Bodies Are Not Created Equal." *American Journal of Nursing.* 92, 12 (December 1992: 48–50.

Leadbeater, M. "Increasing Knowledge . . . Self-administration of Drugs." *Nursing Times* 87, 30 (July 1991): 32–35.

Messner, R. L., and Gardner, S. S. "Start with the Medicine Cabinet." *RN* 56, 1 (January 1993): 50–53.

McGovern, K. "10 Golden Rules for Administering Drugs Safely." *Nursing '92* 22, 3 (March 1992): 49–56.

Morelli, J. "Pediatric Poisoning: The 10 Most Toxic Prescription Drugs." *American Journal of Nursing* 93, 7 (July 1993): 26–29.

Nursing '92. "Documenting Telephone Orders." Charting Tips. 22, 8 (August 1992): 21.

Nursing '93. Patient Teaching Aid. "Tips for Taking O.T.C. Analgesics." 23, 3 (March 1993): 70–75.

Nursing '93. Poll Report: "What You Said About the Apothecary System." 23, 7 (July 1993): 56–58.

O'Donnell, J. "Adverse Drug Reactions." *Nursing '92* 22, 8 (August 1992): 34–39.

Rodman, M. J. "Cough, Cold and Allergy Preparations." *RN* 56, 2 (February 1993): 38–41.

Smith, M., and Buckwalter, K. C. "Medication Management, Antidepressant Drugs, and the Elderly: An Overview." *Psychosocial Nursing* 30, 10 (October 1992): 30–36.

Stewart-Fahs, P. S. and Kinney, M. R. "The Abdomen, Thigh and Arm as Sites for Subcutaneous Sodium Heparin Injections." *Nursing Research.* 40, 4 (July/August 1991): 204–207.

Walsh, M. and Johnson, M. "Update on Antimicrobial Agents." *Nursing Clinics of North America.* 26, 2 (February 1991): 341–359.

Williams, B. "Medication Education." *Nursing Times* 87, 29 (July 1991): 50–52.

The Experience of Surgery

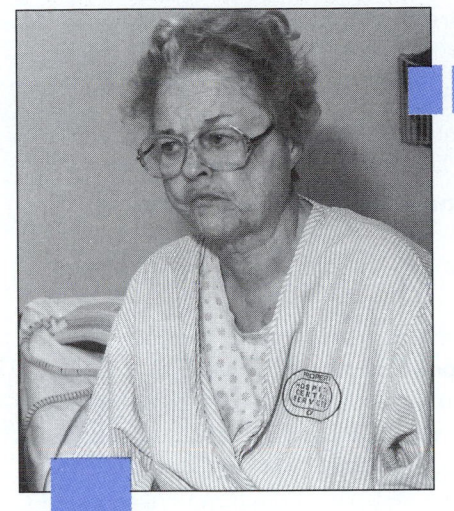

40

Objectives

After completing this chapter, you should be able to:

1. Discuss changes in the health care system that have affected surgical care.
2. Outline the concerns of the person experiencing surgery.
3. Outline the nurse's responsibilities in the preoperative period.
4. Differentiate between local, regional, and general anesthesia and the risks of each.
5. List common risks of surgery.
6. Discuss the roles of the personnel in the operating room.
7. Describe complete assessment of the postoperative patient.
8. Identify the common nursing diagnoses and potential complications that may occur in the postoperative period.
9. Explain nursing actions used to prevent and treat postoperative nursing diagnoses and potential complications.
10. Describe criteria that may be used for evaluating care in the postoperative patient.

Study Terms

adipose
general anesthesia
local anesthesia
regional anesthesia
atelectasis
circulating nurse
craniotomy
day surgery
debridement
dehiscence
evisceration
fixation
hiccoughing
intraoperative period
laparotomy
laser
nurse anesthetist
paralytic ileus
perioperative period
postanesthesia recovery room (PARR)
postoperative period
preoperative period
pulmonary embolus
recovery room (RR)
reduction
risk–benefit
scrub nurse
singultus
surgicenter

Outline

Surgery affects thousands of individuals every day. In the past, surgery was always accompanied by long hospital stays and the prospect of additional time during which activities were restricted. Although there are still many major surgical procedures performed on very ill or debilitated individuals where this pattern is essential, that is not always the case in today's health care system.

Many of today's surgical procedures present a much different picture. More surgeries are performed for outpatients than are performed on those who have overnight hospital stays. This is often referred to as **day surgery** or *outpatient surgery.* The surgery may be performed in a specialty surgery clinic, sometimes referred to as a **surgicenter**, or in a hospital setting. Many procedures are completed with small incisions and little disruption of surrounding tissue. The person is admitted, has the surgery, stays in the setting until stable, and then is discharged for recovery at home. Healing is rapid and return to function equally fast. Day surgery creates a new set of concerns about discharge planning and home care.

At the same time that some individuals are avoiding hospital stays altogether, a few selected patients are having ever more complex surgeries with long recovery periods. These include vascular reconstruction, microscopic surgery of the brain, organ transplants, and limb reattachments. In addition, surgeries are performed on individuals whose general health state may greatly increase their risk of adverse responses and who therefore require advanced technologic monitoring and skilled care. These complex situations have presented enormous challenges to all members of the health care team in terms of adequately preparing patients and their families for the surgical experience and setting the stage for them to effectively care for themselves postoperatively.

To become an expert nurse for the patient during the **perioperative period** (that time before [**preoperative period**], during [**intraoperative period**], and immediately after [**postoperative period**] the surgery), you will need theory relative to disease processes, specific surgical procedures, and specialized nursing techniques. In addition, you must develop the technical skill to move rapidly in a fast-paced environment. However, you may participate effectively as a beginning nursing student in caring for patients experiencing surgery through mastering basic principles. That is the purpose of this chapter.

The Person Experiencing Surgery

The person experiencing surgery has a variety of goals and expectations and faces many challenges. One major challenge is the anxiety created by the surgery itself and the by the disruption of job and family life. Another major challenge is the physical stress of the surgery and the demand placed on the body by the needs for healing.

Patient Goals and Expectations

What are the goals and expectations of the patient who is admitted for a surgical procedure? When a surgery is planned in advance (termed an *elective* surgery) the patient has an opportunity to consider the possible outcomes and make plans. For an *emergency* surgery (one that must be done within 24 hours), the patient may be shocked and not know what to expect as an outcome.

However, all patients expect that their care providers will be knowledgeable and skilled. They hope for the best possible surgical outcome with return to overall health. Sometimes this expectation may be unrealistic. Helping people to cope with a surgery that may result

Nursing Issues and Trends: *Too Much Surgery?*

Surgery is costly both in terms of dollars and in terms of individual patient pain and recovery. In recent years many questions have been raised about whether some surgery is performed when less invasive treatment would be as successful. In an effort to control costs, many health insurers now require that a second opinion be obtained for any elective surgery. Women's groups have challenged the number of hysterectomies performed, suggesting that many are unnecessary. The federal government's Agency for Health Care Policy has supported development of general criteria for decisions about surgery in some specific illnesses. Many physician's are concerned about decision-making by any outside agency that becomes binding on an individual. What are reasonable constraints to prevent unnecessary surgery and what are unwarranted intrusions into individual medical practice?

in a life-threatening diagnosis, permanent disability, or a change in body structure and function is a major challenge for nurses. You will need to focus on maximizing health as much as possible for the individual. Part of your initial nursing assessment should include ascertaining the patient's goals and expectations regarding the surgery so you can work effectively with patients toward their achievement or appropriate modification.

Anxiety Related to Anticipation of Surgery

When an individual first learns that surgery will be needed, the reaction is most commonly anxiety. Most individuals are at least marginally aware of the risks that surgery poses. People usually know that anesthesia is needed, pain may occur, and the body will be subjected to cutting. In fact, you may hear people speak fearfully of going under the knife. A specific surgery that is seen as particularly hazardous, such as brain surgery, may increase anxiety. Enumerating specific risks for the purposes of informed consent may add to anxiety in some individuals.

Anxiety is further exacerbated by worries over missing time from work and possibly losing income (Fig. 40-1). For some individuals this may be a major family problem. Family life and relationships may be disrupted by one person being ill and unable to fulfill usual responsibilities. When a parent in a family is recovering, child care may be a problem. When a previously active individual must be more dependent, the role change may be uncomfortable. In single-parent families, surgery for the parent is even more disruptive. There may be no other person to share responsibilities or assume physically demanding tasks. Elderly persons facing surgery may live alone and have multiple chronic illnesses that complicate their ability to manage self-care after surgery. Any one of these factors will create anxiety. Many individuals face several of these concerns.

Preparing for the Physical Challenge of Surgery

The person who is to undergo a surgical procedure will have the best recovery if preoperative health is optimum. Although the ideal situation would be one in which the individual has always maintained health, this is not always the case. When surgery can be planned in advance, the nurse may be in a position to support the individual in improving overall health status in preparation for surgery. One of the actions that would be most helpful would be not smoking to allow the lungs to be in good health before the anesthetic agent is administered. Regular exercise such as brisk walking daily will help to strengthen the cardiovascular system and improve muscle tone and circulation. Attention to sound diet will ensure that the body is in the best condition for healing and that the gastrointestinal system is functioning well.

For the very ill individual or the person for whom

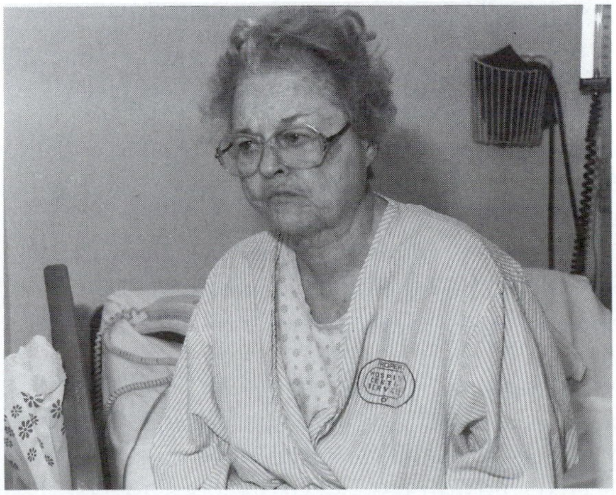

Figure 40-1. Most patients experience preoperative anxiety.

surgery is not planned in advance, these preparations are not possible. Careful interviewing and assessment to determine the physical problems that exist will assist in planning actions that will support the individual whose health is not optimum. When these concerns are identified preoperatively, planning for postoperative care can be directed toward effective support for the individual.

Common Surgical Risk Factors

Because much of care in the perioperative period is focused on prevention of complications, you need to understand the health risks that surgery poses to the person. There are realistic risks to any surgery; however, some surgeries do have more risks than others. The surgeon will discuss risks and benefits (the risk–benefit ratio) specific to the individual surgery with the patient or family, but you should be aware of some of the major risks that apply to all surgical patients.

In addition to these general hazards, each surgical procedure has its own particular risks related to the specific anatomy that is disrupted, the physiology that may be altered, and the complexity of the surgical procedure.

Bleeding

Cutting into tissue always creates some bleeding. This is minimal in some surgeries, but in others where extensive tissue dissection is needed, bleeding may be significant. Although this is a problem for anyone, those who already are anemic, have problems with clotting, or have cardiovascular illness are at an even higher risk should bleeding be extensive.

Infection

Whenever skin or mucous membranes are opened, the body loses one of its major defenses against invading organisms. Postoperative infection is always a potential hazard. It becomes a greater hazard when an area, such as the bowel, with its high population of microorganisms is within the surgical site.

Pain

Pain is another common accompaniment to surgery. Different individuals respond differently to the same surgical procedure, but pain is expected for all. One of the roles of the nurse is to plan with the patient for a realistic method of pain management. This was discussed in detail in Chapter 32.

Obesity

Obesity is an additional risk because the obese person requires more anesthetic agent, more tissue needs to be dissected, and **adipose** (fat) tissue does not heal as well as muscle and skin. The obese person may also find that breathing is more restricted, making the lungs more susceptible to postoperative complications. The overweight individual may be asked to lose weight to decrease these problems in the postoperative period when the surgery has been planned far in advance.

Coexisting Illness

Coexisting illnesses, especially those affecting the heart and lungs, are considered serious risk factors for surgery. The chronic illness may make recovery and healing progress more slowly and the surgery may exacerbate the chronic illness. When individuals are currently taking medications for their chronic illnesses, these medications may interact adversely with anesthetic agents, adding to the potential for negative results from surgery.

Complications of Anesthetics

An additional risk is the effect on the body of *anesthetic agents* that remove all sensation. There is no perfect anesthetic agent. Each has its benefits and each its adverse effects. Anesthetic agents are administered in several different ways.

General Anesthetics. **General anesthesia,** given as an inhaled gas or intravenously, has its effect on brain tissue and creates an unconscious state. There is always a chance of an adverse central nervous system or cardiovascular response to general anesthetic drugs. Individuals may have allergies or simply increased susceptibility to their effects and side effects. These adverse responses can include impairment of breathing, blood pressure, heart rate, and temperature regulation. Most anesthetic agents place a load on the liver to detoxify them for excretion.

The heart must cope with changing blood volume created by bleeding, with vasodilatation created by the profound relaxation, and with the lack of muscle activity to promote venous return. The kidneys often must respond to the increased load of intravenous fluids. The surgery invokes the stress response with its attendant problems, including fluid retention, decreased inflammatory and immune response, and changes in metabolism. When the anesthetic agent is inhaled, it causes some irritation to lung tissue, increasing the production of mucus and susceptibility to pneumonia if these secretions are retained. For the young, otherwise healthy person, these risks may not pose a serious hazard, but for the elderly or those with currently existing illness, this added stress may threaten life.

Local Anesthetics. When the anesthetic agent is injected into a specific nerve pathway, a local or regional area is anesthetized. **Local anesthesia** refers to anesthesia in the area of injection only. These same local anesthetic agents may also be injected into the spinal canal as *spinal anesthetics,* creating anesthesia in the lower part of the body. Although it is an uncommon complication, these agents can anesthetize nerves in unintended areas, such as those controlling respirations.

Autonomic responses to spinal anesthetics may create severe hypotension.

A local anesthetic agent may also be infused into the area outside the dura along the spinal cord. This provides *epidural anesthesia* as the anesthetic agent is absorbed across the dura and acts on the spinal cord. Epidural anesthesia may be given as a bolus dose but may also be maintained by continuous infusion of an anesthetic agent.

Regional Anesthetics. **Regional anesthesia** refers to anesthesia in an entire section of the body such as an entire arm. With these types of anesthesia, there is the risk of damage to nerves injected. Motor reflexes and responses may be impaired. Allergic and adverse responses to locally injected anesthetics also occur.

Concerns Related to Age

Surgical concerns also vary based on the age of the patient. Surgery has increased risks for infants because their adaptive mechanisms are immature, and they may react adversely to many anesthetics and other medications. Fluid balance is much more critical because even apparently small amounts of intravenous fluid may cause fluid excess. Technical aspects of surgery must be adapted to the small size of the child or infant.

Separation from parents or caregivers creates high stress in infants and young children. Teaching and planning are directed toward parents, who are encouraged to stay with the child as much of the time as is possible. Teaching for young children must be designed for their cognitive and emotional level and focus on those aspects that are of immediate concern to them.

The elderly are also at high risk for complications from surgery. Their healing processes are often slower. They may have a wide variety of chronic illnesses that compromise their ability to tolerate anesthesia and the stress of surgery. In addition, the elderly may have fewer social supports and thus need more planning for care after discharge.

Preoperative Care

Successful recovery from surgery begins with the first contacts the patient has with the health care system. Effective preoperative care has clearly been demonstrated to reduce the risk of postoperative complications.

The first opportunity to begin preoperative care is when the physician determines that surgery will be needed to correct a health problem. As the surgeon begins the explanation of the surgery, he or she is establishing a relationship that has the potential to allay anxiety, mobilize the patient's personal resources, and set the stage for what is to follow. In the surgeon's office, a nurse may be involved in preoperative planning and teaching. Nurses in the day surgery or hospital setting will be involved in the entire perioperative process including preoperative care, intraoperative care, and postoperative care. The discussion here focuses on the nurse in this setting.

Preoperative Assessment

When a patient is admitted for surgery, the first nursing responsibility focuses on assessment. Your preoperative assessment will include a review of the record to learn what surgery is being planned to ensure that you have basic information about it. Complete information on care will be found in a medical-surgical text; however, a basic definition and explanation may be found in a medical dictionary.

Verifying the date and time of the procedure and the name of the surgeon is also a nursing responsibility. A specific surgical time may be indicated or the surgery may be designated as a "to follow" or "TF" surgery. This means that the surgery will be done immediately after the previous one scheduled, but that the exact time the prior surgery will be finished is uncertain. The operating room personnel usually notify the unit when it is clear when the "to follow" surgery will occur. Nurses are responsible for coordinating care so that the patient is ready when it is time for the procedure.

The patient's chart contains preoperative physician's orders for the specific procedures that must be completed and medications that must be administered preoperatively for the individual. Additionally, the individual surgeon may have general preferences that affect preoperative preparation. Many surgical units have a reference file indicating routine preparation that is expected by individual surgeons for all of their patients having a given surgery.

For some patients preoperative preparation may be elaborate and require an overnight stay in the hospital. However, for many surgeries, these procedures are explained to patients in the surgeon's office or during a preoperative appointment with a nurse at the hospital and then the patient completes them at home before being admitted for surgery.

The patient's record should also contain a medical history and physical examination report (H & P). If this is not on the record, you might need to check as to whether it was dictated and has not yet been typed for inclusion in the chart. The presence of the history and physical is a legal safeguard indicating the patient was examined and evaluated for possible factors that might complicate the surgery. In emergency situations, it may not be possible to do a complete medical history and physical examination, but the physician will ask some pertinent questions and will do a rapid physical examination.

Laboratory tests may be an essential part of preoperative preparation for some procedures or for patients with particular health problems. The patient may have necessary laboratory tests performed in the week before surgery or at the time of admission; the reports of these tests should be obtained and included in the record. If needed tests have not been done, the nurse arranges to have them completed before the scheduled surgery.

The nurse then performs a preoperative nursing assessment of the patient. Some essential aspects of this assessment are the indicators of anxiety level, knowledge level in regard to the surgical procedure and postoperative care, history of previous surgeries and blood transfusions, the presence of allergies, smoking habits, and alcohol and drug intake. Information about the patient's support system and plan for postdischarge care will be needed to plan discharge teaching.

The preoperative physical assessment is usually the same as any admission assessment with particular emphasis on assessing lungs and vital signs. You should also check that the patient is wearing a correct and accurate identification band. This will be important for maintaining safety.

Preoperative Planning and Implementation

When the assessment is completed, you will be able to identify the nursing problems that are present. Intervention for specific nursing diagnoses are discussed throughout the text. Here we will focus on general areas that are needed for almost all preoperative patients.

Verifying Informed Consent for Surgery

Informed consent has been discussed previously. Remember that the surgeon is responsible for informing the patient of the purpose of the surgery, the potential risks, and the potential benefits. However, it is common for patients to be uncertain about exactly what they have been told, to not understand terminology used, or to forget information. Nurses augment the surgeon's teaching and reinforce important information.

In some facilities the nurse obtains a patient's signature on a surgical permission form. This does not make the nurse responsible for providing the information about the surgery itself. This remains the responsibility of the surgeon. The nurse's responsibility in this situation is to ask whether the person was given information, have the patient sign the form, and witness that the named person signed the permission. This must be done before any preoperative sedation is administered in order for the person to be legally responsible. If the nurse determines that the patient does not seem to be informed, the nurse is responsible for notifying the surgeon so that the patient can be appropriately informed before signing the permission form.

Anxiety Intervention

A major nursing focus in the preoperative period is the reduction of anxiety to a manageable level and the support of the person who continues to be anxious. A total absence of anxiety is an unrealistic nursing goal; a more appropriate goal may be that anxiety be reduced to a level at which the person is able to cope more effectively. The anxiety intervention techniques discussed in Chapter 34 will be effective in helping the patient experiencing preoperative anxiety. Providing information may relieve anxiety if a cause of the anxiety is fear of the unknown. However, in some instances, increased information about potential risks and specifics of the surgery may increase anxiety. You will need to carefully weigh the potential impact of information to determine what is appropriate for you to give. Details are often not needed for informed participation and may contribute to increased anxiety.

Nursing Research: *Implications for Practice*

Cupples, S. A. "Effects of Timing and Reinforcement of Preoperative Education on Knowledge and Recovery of Patients Having Coronary Artery Bypass Graft Surgery." *Heart and Lung* 20, 6 (November 1991): 654–660.

Because studies of patients having major life-threatening surgeries indicated that this situation undermined the effectiveness of preoperative teaching, these researchers disigned an experiment to test different approaches to preoperative teaching. One group received routine preoperative teaching after admission. The other group received both preoperative teaching before admission and again after admission. The group receiving teaching both before and after admission had significantly higher preoperative knowledge levels, more positive mood states, and more favorable physiologic recoveries. Recognizing this difference will guide nurses as they plan for preoperative teaching for patients facing life-threatening surgeries.

Preoperative Teaching

Teaching the patient assumes primary importance in the preoperative stage (Fig. 40-2). The informed patient is better able to participate in the recovery process and therefore experiences fewer complications. The most important components of preoperative teaching are the experiences the patient will have and the ways in which he or she can best enhance recovery. The following are standard parts of preoperative teaching; additional information will be necessary related to the specific surgical procedure. In many large centers, preoperative teaching is being planned for groups of patients. These classes may be provided on a routine schedule and patients attend a convenient class sometime before their surgery.

The overall progression of care from transport to the operating room, to the postanesthesia recovery room (PARR), and then return to the unit should be explained. Knowing that this is the standard procedure alleviates worry that PARR care indicates special problems. For children, familiarization with the clothing (especially the head coverings and masks) worn by personnel in the operating room is of primary importance.

Deep breathing has many benefits in the postoperative period and is often difficult because of pain. Doing ten deep breaths in a row will fully expand all alveoli, mobilize secretions, and improve oxygenation. Practicing preoperatively helps the patient to deep breathe more effectively. When respiratory problems are anticipated, an *incentive spirometer* (IS) that gives visual feedback on the volume of air inhaled may be used to encourage deep breathing. The patient will be asked to deep breathe frequently in the postoperative period.

Coughing is necessary when secretions are accumulating in the lungs; they must be mobilized and expectorated to prevent the secretions from becoming a medium for microorganisms to grow. However, severe coughing may collapse alveoli (**atelectasis**) and be painful. Coughing is more effective and creates fewer problems when the person has been taught this procedure (see Module 41, Respiratory Care Procedures, for information on how to teach deep breathing and coughing).

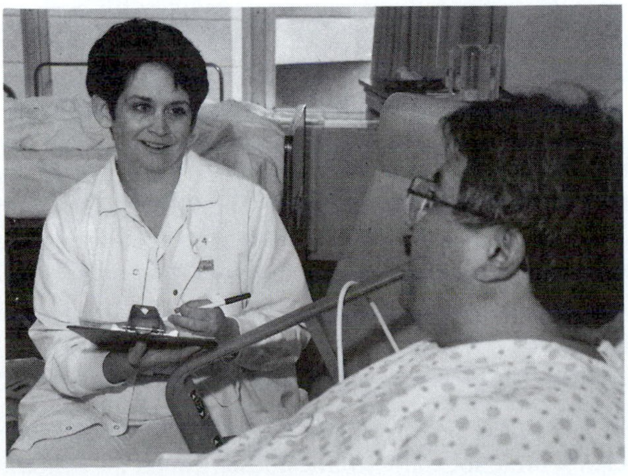

Figure 40-2. Preoperative teaching improves surgical outcomes.

A surgical site located in the abdomen or chest will make deep breathing and coughing painful. The sharp movements caused by these maneuvers create pulling on the incision. "Splinting" by holding flat hands or a pillow firmly over the incision will decrease movement in the incisional area and lessen pain. Teaching this procedure in advance helps the patient to be prepared to participate more effectively in postoperative care.

Leg exercises increase circulation to the lower extremities and promote venous return. During the surgery and while the patient is inactive postoperatively, blood tends to pool in the large veins of the legs. Therefore, postoperatively the calf muscles, gluteal muscles, and quadriceps muscles are exercised to promote venous return. These exercises are called calf pumping, gluteal setting, and quadriceps setting, respectively. Each group of muscles is contracted and held for approximately 6 to 8 seconds and then released. This provides a mechanical pumping effect on the large veins running through the muscle area. These isometric exercises can be done even when active exercise is not possible.

Pain management plans are important to the patient. The patient should understand that pain will interfere with the ability to move and participate in care. Some patients must be taught that the narcotics used for surgical pain management do not pose addiction problems and therefore should not be avoided for this reason. The importance of maintaining pain control and not letting pain mount should be taught. If a patient-controlled analgesia (PCA) pump is to be used, the administration process must be taught.

Teaching of techniques for moving adapted to the particular surgery will make it easier for the patient during the immediate postoperative period. Using side rails for support and using extremities to provide momentum can lessen the stress on a surgical site during movement and therefore lessen pain.

If any postoperative equipment, such as suction devices, intravenous lines, and catheters, is expected, the patient will need to be taught about these devices to prevent anxiety. If some item of equipment is used in only some but not all similar surgeries, you may indicate that this may be used and that its use does not indicate a complication.

Immediate Preoperative Preparation

When the patient is ready to go to surgery, the nurse is responsible for ensuring that all critical aspects of care have been completed. Most hospitals or care centers have a checklist that outlines the essential items that must be completed.

The nurse ensures that all records are complete.

This includes the consent for surgery, the history and physical examination, and the laboratory test results. Specific information from the preoperative nursing assessment such as the skin assessment, the patient's mental and emotional condition, and allergies may be recorded on the list.

Vital signs are measured and recorded as a baseline. The patient is asked to void to begin surgery with an empty bladder. Nails are checked to be sure nail polish has been removed so that nail beds can be checked for circulation during surgery.

Bobby pins, hair combs, jewelry, false teeth, glasses, hearing aids, and any other items are removed. Items of value are either given to the family or placed in an official safe storage location (often the business office). These items may harbor bacteria, fall out into areas where they injure the patient, or become lost if not removed. If the patient wants to keep an item, such as a hearing aid, in place until actually in the operating room, the nurse must arrange for this with operating room personnel.

Preoperative skin preparation is completed if ordered by the physician. This may include a bath or shower with antibacterial soap to lessen the potential for infection. Shaving or using a depilatory (chemical hair remover) is needed in some surgeries. This may be done in the holding area immediately before the surgery itself.

Any preoperative medication is given and recorded. When the preoperative medication includes sedatives and narcotics, special attention must be given to patient safety. Side rails are raised and the patient is instructed to not get up without help. When the patient leaves the unit, two individuals commonly check the patient's identity.

Intraoperative Care

As a beginning nursing student, you may be offered an opportunity to observe a patient having a surgical procedure. You will want to be familiar with the roles of the various people in the operating room to more accurately identify their specific role in the procedure you are watching. In addition you will want to understand the anesthetic agents and medications administered to the patient and the surgical procedure itself. Observing this entire process may assist you in providing more knowledgeable and sensitive care to patients both preoperatively and postoperatively.

The Nursing Role in the Intraoperative Period

The *nursing role* in the intraoperative period includes managing the environment, assessing for patient needs, planning for the support of the patient, and maintaining safety during the surgical procedure itself. Before the patient arrives, the operating room nurse ensures that the room is appropriately set up for the type of surgery to be performed, the appropriate supportive personnel are available, and that all essential supplies and equipment are available.

When the patient arrives at the operating room, the nurse ensures that the patient is correctly identified, quickly reviews the assessment of the preoperative nurse, and reviews the chart for pertinent information. The nurse personally assesses those indicators that might have changed during transport. Additional assessment at this time is most often needed for the critically ill patient. If problems have arisen, the operating room nurse is responsible for ensuring that they are managed or referred to the physician for management.

The nurse directs the positioning of the patient for maximum safety as well as appropriate access to the site for the surgeon. The initial preparation of the surgical site may be done by the nurse at this time. This preparation is designed to decrease the potential for infection in the postoperative period.

During the surgery, one role for the nurse is termed the **circulating nurse** because it includes moving about the room to obtain needed supplies and serving as the communication link between the operating room and the rest of the unit. The circulating nurse administers medications and intravenous fluids or provides for their administration by the person giving the anesthesia. A second role during the surgery is the **scrub nurse**. This nurse has "scrubbed in," that is, done the surgical scrub and is wearing sterile garments. This role includes managing the instruments and supplies, handing them to the surgeon, and providing assistance within the sterile field (Fig. 40-3).

As part of the safety checks in the operating room, the circulating nurse counts instruments and gauze sponges as the surgery progresses. This ensures that none are inadvertently left in a wound. When tissue is removed, the nurse assumes responsibility for correctly labeling it and directing its transport to the laboratory for examination. In some surgeries, a section of tissue is sent to the laboratory to be quick frozen and then examined while the surgery is in progress to allow the surgeon to determine the extent of surgery necessary. The circulating nurse conveys this report to the surgeon. After the surgery, the operating room nurse ensures the safe transport of the patient to the recovery area.

Roles of Other Personnel in the Operating Room

The person who administers anesthesia is either a physician with a specialty in anesthesia, called an *anesthesiologist*, or a nurse with advanced specialty education and certification, called a **nurse anesthetist**. The anes-

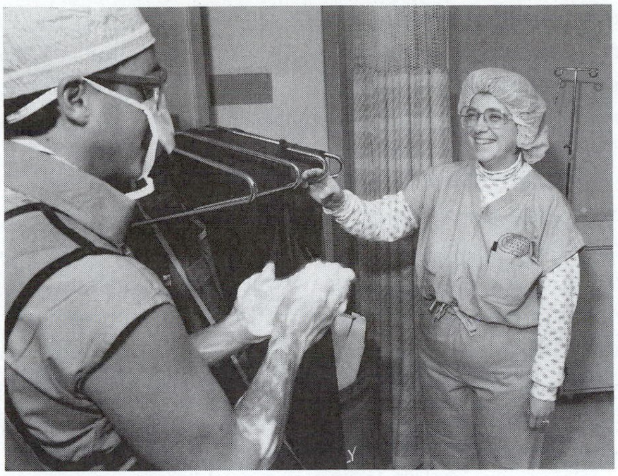

Figure 40-3. The registered nurse has an important role in the operating room.

thesiologist or anesthetist does a preoperative assessment of the patient and discusses the anesthesia. They generally rely on the written report of medical history and complete physical examination done by the surgeon and limit their examination to those specific areas that they have determined are of concern. If the patient is hospitalized, this may be done the night before surgery. If the patient is admitted just before the surgery, this may be done in the admitting area or in a holding area just before the patient enters the operating room.

The anesthesiologist or nurse anesthetist is responsible for continuous assessment of the patient during the surgical procedure. This includes monitoring vital signs, color of skin, mucous membranes, and nail beds, and maintaining intravenous infusions. In many surgeries the patient is connected to a cardiac monitor and additional monitoring equipment may be used as appropriate for the specific surgery and the patient's condition. In addition, the person administering the anesthesia gives medications to control heart rate, blood pressure, muscle relaxation, urinary output, and other essential functions throughout the surgical procedure. After the surgical procedure, the anesthesiologist or anesthetist accompanies the patient to the recovery area and ensures that the patient's condition is stable. In a real sense the anesthesiologist or nurse anesthetist is responsible for the whole person during surgery.

The *surgeon* performs the actual surgery. During the surgical procedure, the surgeon is in charge of the operating room. Legally the role of the surgeon has been likened to the role of the captain of a ship. Although other professionals are responsible for their actions, the surgeon is responsible for knowing exactly what is being done by each person and directing the entire process.

The *first assistant* to the surgeon assists with tying sutures, holding retractors that help expose the operative field, and working within the operative field itself. In most cases the first assistant is another surgeon or a physician in a surgical specialty training program who is called a *resident.* Traditionally, this has been required because the first assistant might need to complete the surgery if the surgeon becomes incapacitated. In some states, nurses can serve as first assistants for certain surgical procedures. Another surgeon is available within the hospital if someone were needed to complete the surgery. In these instances the nurse is commonly an employee of the surgeon and works with that individual only. This nurse may also have a role in both preoperative and postoperative management of the patient.

A *surgical technician* is usually an employee of the hospital but may also be employed by an individual surgeon. In some facilities this role may be referred to as the *scrub technician* because the individual has done a surgical scrub and is clothed in sterile garb. This person sets up the tables of instruments, assists the surgeon during the procedure by handing instruments and supplies to the surgeon, and discards used materials. Increasingly hospitals are using surgical technicians in place of scrub nurses.

Understanding the Surgical Procedure

An understanding of some simple prefixes and suffixes will help you to better understand the exact nature of the surgical procedure. These are usually attached to Latin anatomic terms making it possible to understand what is being done. An *otomy* is opening an area. Therefore, **craniotomy** is opening the cranium or skull. A **laparotomy** is opening the abdomen. An *ectomy* is removal of a part. Therefore, an appendectomy is removal of the appendix and a colectomy is removal of the colon. An *ostomy* is the creation of a new opening between two areas. Therefore, a *colostomy* is the creation of new opening between the surface of the abdomen and the colon. A *gastrojejunostomy* is an opening between the stomach and the jejunum. Any surgery that repairs or reconstructs an area is termed a *plasty.* Therefore, a *pyloroplasty* is the reconstruction of the pyloric valve, and a *rhinoplasty* is the reconstruction of the nose. **Lasers** (devices that produce light of specific frequencies focused into narrow bands) are used for precise dissection and also for coagulating blood vessels to close them. A **fixation** refers to securing parts in correct anatomic alignment. This is most commonly used in relationship to bone fractures (see Appendix D for other terms of importance).

Postoperative Care

Immediate postoperative care takes place in the **postanesthesia recovery room (PARR)**, which is part of the surgical suite and is provided with emergency equipment and supplies. Sometimes the PARR is referred to as the recovery room (RR). Patients receive continuous monitoring by nurses with expert abilities in assessment for and management of postoperative complications. Vital signs are taken as frequently as every 5 minutes. The anesthesiologist continues to be available for immediate intervention in any emergency. The PARR nurse commonly uses a flow sheet with a scoring system to help evaluate the patient's progress and readiness to be moved to a less closely monitored setting (Fig. 40-4). When the patient's condition is stable, he or she is transported to a postoperative unit.

Receiving a Patient on a Postoperative Unit

The postoperative patient unit routinely contains equipment to take vital signs, an emesis basin, tissues, an intravenous stand, and suction equipment. The bed is placed in a high position and made with linen arranged to facilitate transfer of the patient from the stretcher. Often the nurse in the PARR will telephone a report on a patient before the patient is transferred. This ensures that the unit can be prepared for any of the patient's special needs and personnel are available to receive the patient.

When the patient is received on the unit, the receiving nurse does an immediate assessment. Although the patient was assessed before leaving the PARR, the process of transportation may cause the patient's condition to change. When the nurse has determined that the patient is stable, a schedule for ongoing assessment and care to prevent complications is established. Display 40-1 lists the immediate observations to be made when the patient arrives on the unit. Display 40-2 lists significant information that can be obtained from the postoperative chart.

One major focus of immediate postoperative care is preventing complications when possible and identifying them at the earliest possible time when you cannot prevent them. A second major focus is managing the nursing diagnoses common in the postoperative period. Both potential complications and nursing diagnoses for which the patient is at high risk should be considered when assessing and planning for nursing care.

Assessment and Planning for Postoperative Care

General assessment to identify the progress and problems in the postoperative patient is outlined below. The specific potential complications (collaborative problems) and nursing diagnoses for which the patient is at high risk are shown in the two displays accompanying this discussion. More information on each of the specific nursing diagnoses can be found in the chapter focused on that particular human need and in Module 47, Postoperative Care. Standard interventions used to prevent problems are outlined below for your use in planning.

Alterations in Circulation

Because of the seriousness of the circulatory complications, high priority is given to assessing pulse and blood pressure, looking for signs of bleeding, and identifying indications of changes in peripheral circulation such as changes in skin, nail beds, and mucous membrane color that could indicate hemorrhage and shock. Identifying the estimated blood loss (EBL) during surgery from the surgical record, provides a baseline for evaluation of these parameters. The dressings are checked for blood and the bed under the patient is checked to be sure that blood is not seeping unnoticed under the patient.

Sudden movements of the patient in the immediate postoperative period should be avoided because they may precipitate adverse circulatory responses such as a drop in blood pressure. Intravenous fluids must be monitored to maintain appropriate fluid balance to support blood volume and blood pressure.

The lower extremities are examined for indications of thrombophlebitis such as heat, redness, pain, and swelling over the calves and thighs. Isometric exercises and early ambulation help to maintain venous circulation, and adequate fluids prevent increased blood viscosity that can predispose to spontaneous venous clotting.

Alterations in Oxygenation

Respiratory complications are always a major concern. While the patient is still unconscious, assessing for airway patency is a critical focus. To identify oxygenation effectiveness, you will assess respiratory rate, depth of respirations, chest excursion, respiratory effort, breath sounds, and color of mucous membranes and nail beds.

Hypoventilation is common in the postoperative period because of sedation and pain. Narcotics also predispose to hypoventilation. Assisting the patient to deep breathe effectively and cough up secretions will help to prevent ineffective airway clearance and the complication of hypostatic pneumonia. Often pain management and splinting of incisions are critical to effective deep breathing. These measures decrease the discomfort created by moving the area of the surgical wound. Early activity also promotes movement of respiratory secretions and stimulates deeper respirations. Prolonged coughing, however, may cause the collapse of alveoli and predispose to more widespread atelectasis.

Alterations in Comfort

Pain management is one of the single most important factors in postoperative care. Effective pain management allows the person to move more, to deep breathe

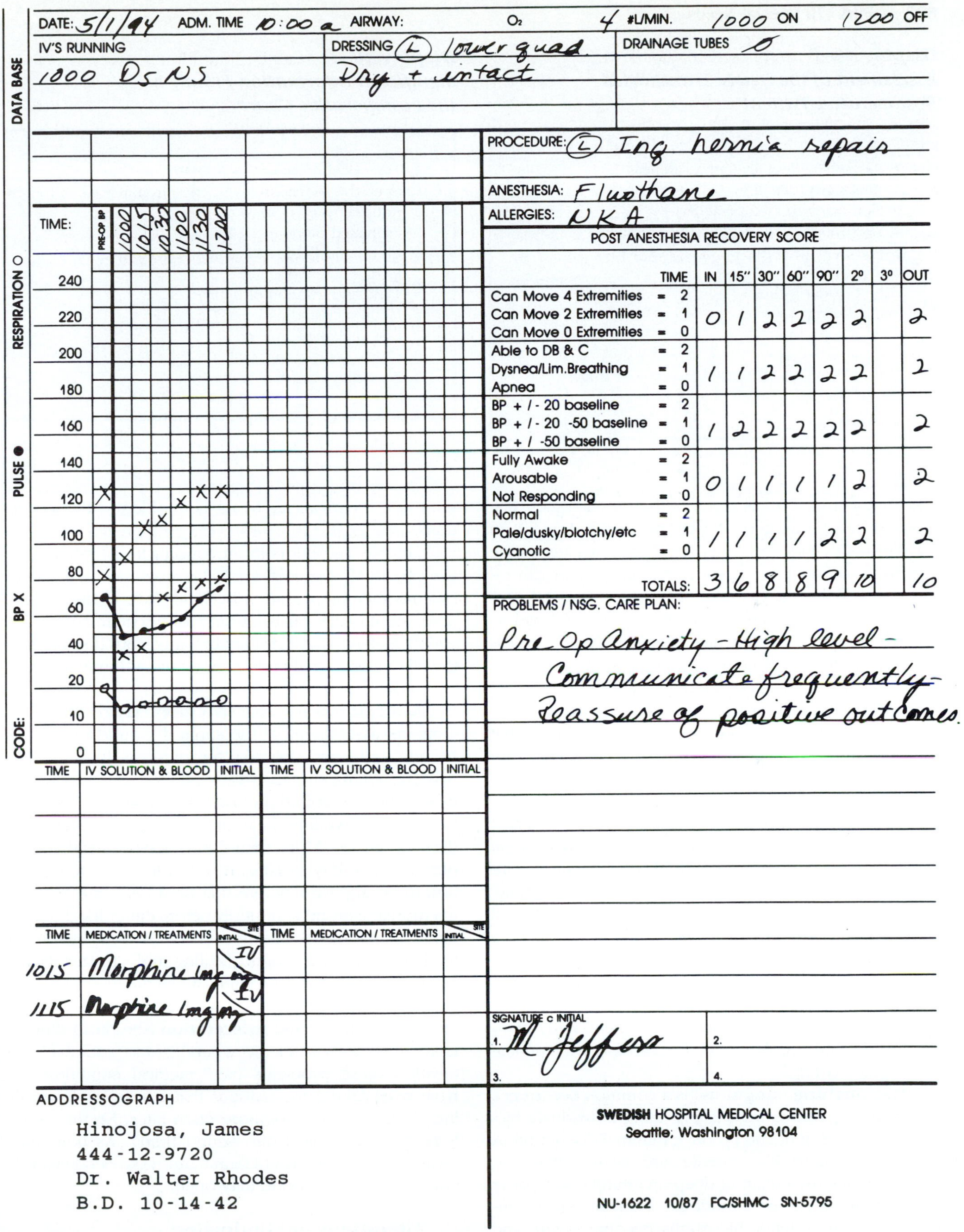

DATA BASE

DATE: 5/1/94 ADM. TIME 10:00 a AIRWAY: O2 4 #L/MIN. 1000 ON 1200 OFF

IV'S RUNNING: 1000 D5 NS

DRESSING: (L) lower quad. Dry + intact

DRAINAGE TUBES: 0

PROCEDURE: (L) Ing. hernia repair

ANESTHESIA: Fluothane

ALLERGIES: NKA

TIME: PRE-OP BP, 1000, 1015, 1030, 1100, 1130, 1200

CODE: BP X PULSE ● RESPIRATION ○

240, 220, 200, 180, 160, 140, 120, 100, 80, 60, 40, 20, 10, 0

POST ANESTHESIA RECOVERY SCORE

TIME	IN	15"	30"	60"	90"	2°	3°	OUT
Can Move 4 Extremities = 2 Can Move 2 Extremities = 1 Can Move 0 Extremities = 0	0	1	2	2	2	2		2
Able to DB & C = 2 Dysnea/Lim.Breathing = 1 Apnea = 0	1	1	2	2	2	2		2
BP + / - 20 baseline = 2 BP + / - 20 -50 baseline = 1 BP + / -50 baseline = 0	1	2	2	2	2	2		2
Fully Awake = 2 Arousable = 1 Not Responding = 0	0	1	1	1	1	2		2
Normal = 2 Pale/dusky/blotchy/etc = 1 Cyanotic = 0	1	1	1	1	2	2		2
TOTALS:	3	6	8	8	9	10		10

PROBLEMS / NSG. CARE PLAN:

Pre Op Anxiety – High level –
Communicate frequently –
Reassure of positive outcomes.

TIME	IV SOLUTION & BLOOD	INITIAL	TIME	IV SOLUTION & BLOOD	INITIAL

TIME	MEDICATION / TREATMENTS	INITIAL	SITE	TIME	MEDICATION / TREATMENTS	INITIAL	SITE
1015	Morphine 1mg	mj	IV				
1115	Morphine 1mg	mj	IV				

SIGNATURE c INITIAL
1. M Jefferson 2.
3. 4.

ADDRESSOGRAPH

Hinojosa, James
444-12-9720
Dr. Walter Rhodes
B.D. 10-14-42

SWEDISH HOSPITAL MEDICAL CENTER
Seattle, Washington 98104

NU-1622 10/87 FC/SHMC SN-5795

Figure 40–4. A PARR flow sheet includes a scoring system to determine the patient's readiness for transfer to the regular unit.

Display 40–1
Assessment of the Newly Transported Postoperative Patient

1. Responsiveness/level of awareness
2. Vital signs
3. Skin color and temperature
4. Surgical site and condition of dressings
5. Presence and function of any devices
   a. IV
   b. bladder catheter
   c. drainage tubes
   d. other
6. Comfort level
7. Positioning in relationship to type of surgery and airway

Display 40–2
Significant Information From the Postoperative Chart

1. Type of surgical procedure performed and postoperative diagnosis
2. Anesthetic agent used
3. Estimated blood loss (EBL)
4. Blood and fluid replacement in surgery and PARR
5. Type and location of drains
6. Medications administered in PARR
7. Last vital signs in PARR
8. Urinary output in PARR
9. Physician's orders

and cough, and relieves much of the psychological distress created by surgery. According to the Acute Pain Management Guideline Panel (1992) " . . . an aggressive approach to pain assessment and management can reduce such pain, increase patient comfort and satisfaction, and in some cases contribute to improved patient outcomes and shorter hospital stays." Although excess narcotic administration may have adverse consequences, this is an uncommon problem. The patient's subjective statements regarding comfort are most important, but you should also be alert to nonverbal cues that indicate pain. Remember that prevention of severe pain is more effective than treatment after it has occurred (see Chapter 32).

Nausea and vomiting in the postoperative period are primarily problems of comfort. They rarely become severe enough to compromise fluid balance because intravenous fluids are usually being provided at the time. For the short postoperative time in which nausea and vomiting occur, they usually do not pose a threat to overall nutritional status. The underlying cause of nausea and vomiting is often the central nervous system effects of medications. Therefore, antiemetic medications are often the best choice of treatment. Early identification of the problem and intervention are essential to adequate control.

Hiccoughing (singultus) is a common occurrence in the postoperative period. For most individuals hiccoughs are transient and produce minimal discomfort. A variety of nonintrusive remedies are usually attempted early. Holding the breath or deep breathing into a paper bag to increase carbon dioxide level is sometimes helpful. For some patients, hiccoughs become severe and prolonged. When this occurs, rest is disturbed and comfort is disrupted. When the nonintrusive measures do not work, the physician treats the problem with medications.

Thirst is another comfort concern in the postoperative period. Most patients are NPO for a period of time and mucous membranes often become dry and uncomfortable. Mouth care can alleviate this discomfort until the patient is able to have oral fluids. Intravenous fluids during the NPO period will prevent any fluid volume deficit.

Alterations in Skin Integrity/Hygiene

Ongoing assessment of the surgical wound reveals its healing status and potential for infection. In an appropriately healing surgical wound, the edges are approximated and the wound is closed. The wound is observed for redness, swelling, heat, and drainage that might indicate infection. Most wound infections occur the third postoperative day or later. It is rare for a wound infection to be apparent before that because contaminating microorganisms must multiply before either local or systemic symptoms of infection occur. Review Chapter 6 for information on wound healing and Chapter 22 for assessment related to infection. When the wound fails to heal, the patient is at risk for **dehiscence** (separating of the wound edges) and **evisceration** (the protruding of internal organs out of the wound.) Most patients who develop these problems have medical conditions or have been taking medications that interfere with healing. Again, this occurs more often after the third day. Initially sutures hold the wound firmly. As time progresses, if healing has not begun, this hold becomes less effective and the wound may open.

Alterations in Elimination

The abdomen is observed for distention and auscultated for bowel sounds. The return of bowel sounds indicates

Nursing Diagnoses Related to the Postoperative Patient

Circulation

Altered Tissue Perfusion: Peripheral venous stasis related to immobility

Fluid Volume Deficit related to inadequate fluid intake

Fluid Volume Excess related to rapid infusion of IV fluids

Oxygenation

Ineffective Breathing Pattern: Hypoventilation related to pain and immobility

Ineffective Airway Clearance: Retained secretions related to painful coughing or decreased cough reflex secondary to narcotics

Comfort

Pain related to incision/surgical procedure

Altered Comfort: Nausea and vomiting related to anesthetic agents, pain medications

Altered Comfort: Abdominal discomfort related to retained gas

Altered Comfort: Hiccough (singultus) related to phrenic nerve stimulation secondary to dilation of the stomach or irritation of the diaphragm

Altered Comfort: Thirst related to NPO status

Skin Integrity/Hygiene

Impaired Skin Integrity related to surgical wound

Elimination

Constipation related to inadequate fluids and bulk, effects of anesthesia and analgesics on the bowel, or decreased activity

Urinary Retention related to recumbent position or effects of anesthesia and analgesics on the bladder

Activity and Rest

Impaired Physical Mobility related to surgery

Psychosocial

Ineffective Individual Coping related to medical diagnosis, physical status, hospitalization

Anxiety related to pain and discomfort or possible outcomes of surgery

Situational Depression related to illness, surgery, change in body image, or effect of medications

Potential Complications for the Postoperative Patient

Circulation

Potential complication: hypovolemic shock

Potential complication: thrombophlebitis

Oxygenation

Potential complication: pulmonary embolus

Potential complication: atelectasis

Potential complication: hypostatic pneumonia

Skin Integrity/Hygiene

Potential complication: dehiscence

Potential complication: evisceration

Potential complication: wound infection

Elimination

Potential complication: paralytic ileus

Potential complication: urinary tract infection

that the gastrointestinal tract is returning to function. In general, no oral intake is encouraged until bowel sounds have returned. Patients may identify that they feel uncomfortable from the presence of gas. Activity is the best remedy for distention from gas because it stimulates peristalsis. When this alone is not successful, the physician may order return flow enemas or medication to stimulate peristalsis.

Close observation of voiding patterns and output are important in the postoperative patient. If the patient does not void, the abdomen is checked to determine whether the bladder is distended. If the bladder becomes overdistended, catheterization may be needed until normal bladder function returns. If a bladder catheter has been left in place, the patient must be observed closely for the possibility of infection.

Alterations in Activity

The patient's ability to move about in the bed and to get up and return to usual activity patterns is important. There may be impaired physical mobility after surgery. Early return to usual activity promotes more rapid healing and generally enhances health and well-being. Patients may be reluctant to move for fear that this will be increase pain or cause the incision to open. In these cases you will want to teach the patient how important activity is in the recovery process.

Alterations in Psychosocial Status

After surgery psychosocial concerns continue. Therapeutic interaction and observation of nonverbal behavior will help you to identify the feelings and concerns of the patient. If there has been an adverse diagnosis as a result of the surgery, the patient may react with denial, despair, anger, or any variety of emotions. The patient may need to adapt to new health maintenance activities and health care practices. You may identify changes in coping ability, anxiety, and depressed mood. Nurses are in a unique position to use the self in a therapeutic manner in supporting successful adaptation.

Evaluating Outcomes for the Surgical Patient

Patient outcomes for the person experiencing surgery include specific desired outcomes of the surgery itself and outcomes related to prevention of complications and effective management of the nursing diagnoses that occur. Individualized outcomes will help structure the evaluation related to the specific patient and should consider the patient's goals and expectations as well as those of the health care team.

Standardized desired outcomes have been developed for surgical patients. These standardized outcomes are often used to evaluate the entire hospital service as well as the care of a specific patient. For example, a desired outcome in any surgery is "No postoperative infection, as evidenced by temperature within normal range, white blood cell count within norms, wound clear and showing evidence of healing without swelling, inflammation, or purulent drainage." In addition to evaluating this for the individual patient, the entire surgical population could be examined to determine infection rates and the effectiveness of infection control measures in the facility.

Care pathways pose a series of nursing actions and desired outcomes with specific timelines for a particular type of surgery. Care pathways are being used to manage the care of individuals more effectively and thus decrease the overall cost of care. Figure 40-5 provides an example of the education and discharge planning components of a care pathway for a person with a total hip replacement surgery. The outcomes are designated

	Day of Surgery	Post-op Day 1	Post-op Day 2	Post-op Day 3	Post-op Day 4	Post-op Day 5	Post-op Day 6
EDUCATION (patient and/or caregiver)	Patient performs: [coughing & deep breathing exercises independently]						
Education: Total Hip Replacement	[Calf pumping exercises independently]	Total Hip Precautions	→	→	→	→	[Patient/caregiver verbalizes and/or demonstrates understanding of total hip replacement precautions, lifestyle changes, safety precautions, and home exercise program.]
		exercise program	→	→	→	→	
Education: Post-operative	Patient/Caregiver indicates understanding of: [diet progression, activity progression, types of equipment and purpose, medication regimen, expected length of stay]		transfers (bed to stand, stand to sit)	→	→	→	
			ambulation with assistive device	→	stair ambulation	→	
				activities of daily living	→	→	
DISCHARGE PLANNING			Re-evaluate DC plan and plan for transportation arrangements at discharge;	→	→	[DC plan finalized: Home caregiver identified; arrangements for assistance at home completed; transportation to home arranged]	
			Pt. Services consult prn	→	VNS referral initiated prn	→	[DC to home with caregiver and/or VNS]
					Initiate transfer to SNF if LOS expected to be > 7 days	→	[DC to SNF]

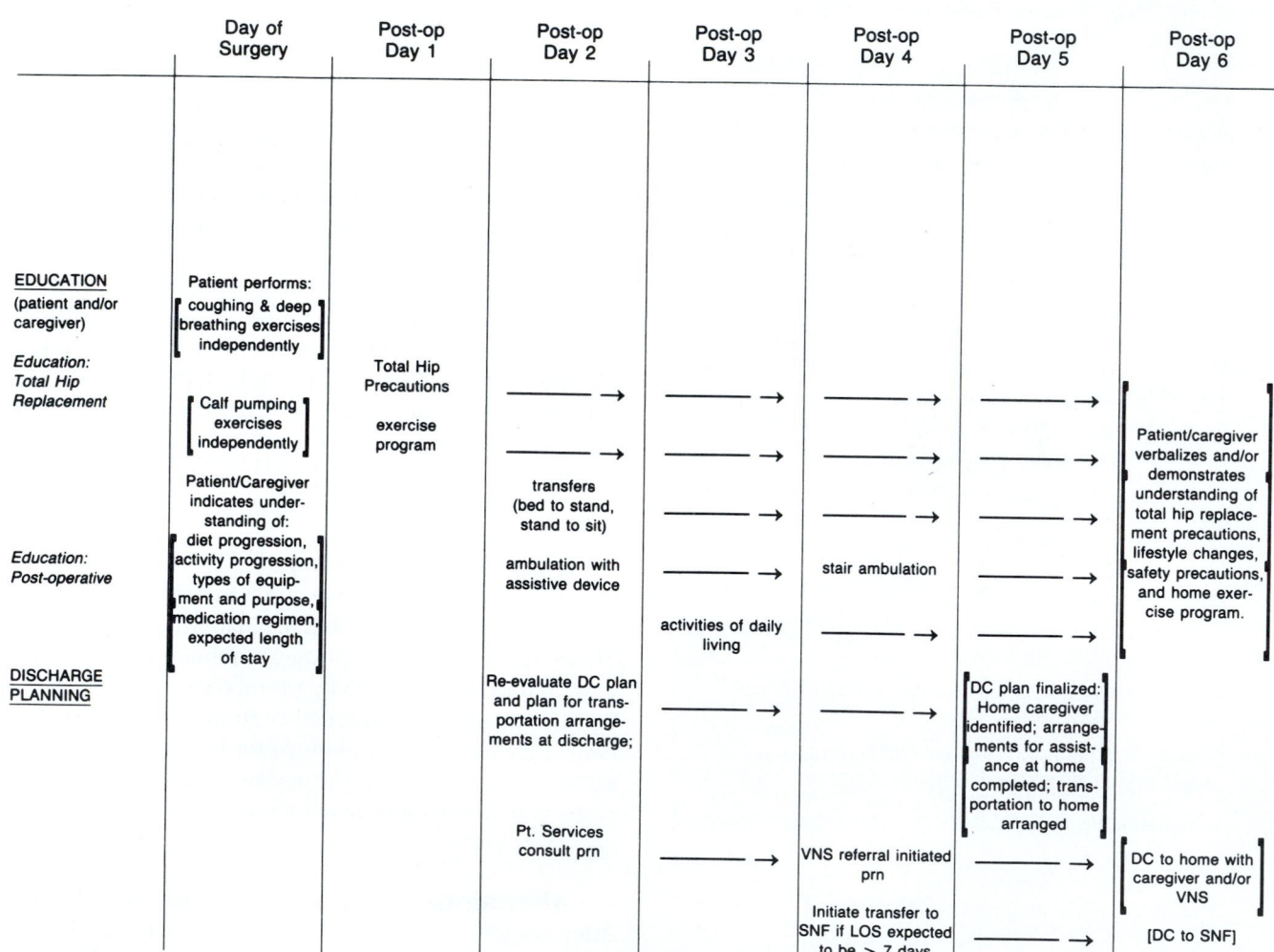

Figure 40-5. Two aspects of a care pathway for a surgical patient (Swedish Hospital Medical Center).

by brackets. Arrows indicate the continuation of the actions previously instituted. Note that planning for discharge to a skilled nursing facility (SNF) is begun on day 4 if the length of stay is expected to be greater than 7 days. This prevents the length of stay in the acute care facility from being extended because a suitable long-term care setting has not been procured. The desired outcomes can only be reached if appropriate care was begun in the preoperative period.

Nursing Care Study
Preoperative Care in a Day Surgery

The day surgery unit bustled with activity as patients were being admitted and prepared for surgery. Admitting had just called and said that Edith Anderson had arrived and would be at the unit in approximately 10 minutes. Mary Hinojosa, the nursing student assigned to Mrs. Anderson's care, began reviewing her notes. The surgery itself, a breast biopsy with possible lumpectomy was a fairly simple procedure. The patient would be expected to recover rapidly and would return home that day. The future treatment and emotional implications were much more complex. If the breast lump were cancerous, then major decisions would be required regarding treatment plans. Mrs. Anderson would be anxious about much more than today's procedure! Mary began to review what she knew about anxiety intervention.

Mary greeted Mr. and Mrs. Anderson as they arrived on the unit. Mrs. Anderson explained that her husband was going to stay with her the entire time. Both had worried looks on their faces. Their posture was rigid. They moved rapidly and jerkily. Mary recognized that she needed to consider both individuals as she talked with them and completed Mrs. Anderson's admitting assessment.

First Mary gave clear directions as to each step of the admitting process. She guided them through the admission interview carefully, making sure they understood all of the questions. She completed her physical assessment with quiet competence and then sat down beside them. They had been well informed about the surgical procedure. Mary explained the general plan for care and taught deep breathing and coughing. She emphasized the importance of early mobilization and activity. Pain management was a major concern and she explained how Mrs. Anderson could be active in helping to manage pain effectively. She encouraged them to express their concerns and ask questions.

They were worried about the possible diagnosis of cancer. Their daughter was expecting a new baby and they had planned to be a support to her. Now they saw themselves as caught in a whirlpool that threatened to drag them down, unable to help themselves, much less anyone else. Mary encouraged them to review their own coping abilities and to identify other crises they had managed in the past. She asked what supports they had in the larger family and community. As they talked, their faces visibly relaxed. When it was time for Mrs. Anderson to go to the operating room, Mary walked with them. Walking to the OR emphasized that Mrs. Anderson really was a well, capable person and that surgery was a temporary problem. As they walked, Mr. Anderson said, "Well, nothing can make this OK, but you really helped, Mary. I wasn't sure we were going to make it through this morning without falling apart. Now it seems like we'll make it. Thanks!"

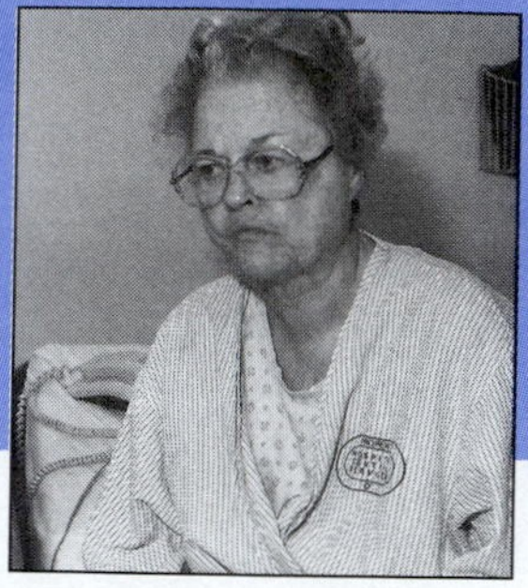

Key Points

- Modern surgery is often accomplished during a short hospitalization or on an outpatient basis, and even patients with longer hospitalizations are now encouraged to resume moderate physical activity and self-care soon after surgery.
- Within the health care setting, nurses must be aware of the goals and expectations of the patient as well as those of the health care team.
- Nurses must be aware of the specific problems that the patient's physical condition or age may create when surgery is part of the medical treatment.
- Nurses are responsible for careful assessment before surgery, including interviewing the patient, reviewing records, and performing a physical assessment.
- Anxiety intervention and preoperative teaching are major aspects of preoperative nursing care.
- Patients need information that will help them to participate in their own recovery following surgery, including how to move, exercises that can be done safely, deep breathing and coughing techniques, pain management, and postoperative routines and equipment.
- Immediately before surgery the nurse is responsible for completing the activities listed on the preoperative checklist in the facility, which ensures that all last minute details have been completed and the patient's safety is maintained.
- To care for surgical patients, the nurse needs an understanding of the common risk factors for any surgery, the types of anesthesia, and the surgical procedure itself.
- The primary nursing role in the intraoperative period is managing the environment, assessing for patient needs, planning for support of the patient, and maintaining safety.
- The circulating nurse's duties in the operating room include moving about the room to obtain supplies, serving as the communication link, administering medications, and maintaining safety checks.
- Other personnel in the operating room include the surgeon, the anesthesiologist or anesthetist, the first assistant, and the scrub technician. Nurses sometimes serve in the role of scrub nurse and, in some settings, as first assistant to the surgeon.
- Postoperative nursing care is directed at assessing for and preventing potential complications and managing common nursing diagnoses associated with surgery.
- Complete physical assessment and a careful interview are essential in identifying the many different patient problems that may occur postoperatively.
- Careful nursing care can prevent many complications of surgery. When complications do occur, they must be identified at the earliest possible time so that appropriate treatment can be instituted.
- Evaluation of outcomes for the individual surgical patient is essential. General outcomes may be written that apply to many patients and used a basis for both individual and overall evaluation. Outcomes specific to the individual are also important and should consider the patient's goals and expectations that have been identified.

Study Questions

1. Describe four changes in the health care system that have affected surgical care.
2. Discuss the essential preoperative assessment.
3. What are the primary risk factors of each type of anesthesia?
4. What are the effects of anxiety in the postoperative patient
5. Describe the role of the nurse in the operating room.
6. How might you prevent postoperative complications?
7. What assessment data would reveal postoperative problems related to elimination?
8. What nursing actions could prevent postoperative complications?
9. How might a care pathway be used for evaluating care of a postoperative patient?

Critical Thinking Activities

1. Review the surgical schedule at the hospital where you have clinical practice. List all of the different items of information that are available on this form. Identify how this information would be used in planning nursing care.

2. Choose a specific surgical procedure. Research information about the exact procedure and the related nursing care. Report on this surgery to a group of fellow students.
3. Obtain a copy of the preoperative check list used in the facility where you have clinical practice and review the actions that must be taken before a patient is sent to surgery. Compare this to the information given in the text. Determine the rationale for any differences.
4. Arrange with your instructor to observe a surgical procedure. Identify the various nursing roles you see and how the nurses meet patient needs in that setting.
5. Arrange with your instructor to observe in a PARR. In particular, observe the assessment done and the criteria used to determine when a patient is ready to be discharged from that unit. Compare your skill level to the skill level of the nurses in that setting. Identify areas for personal growth.

Relevant Sections in Modules for Basic Nursing Skills

Volume II Module
- Respiratory Care Procedures 41
- Surgical Asepsis: Scrubbing, Gowning, and Gloving 45
- Preoperative Care 46
- Postoperative Care 47

References and Readings

Acute Pain Management in Adults, USDHHS, Public Health Service, AHCP&R, Pub. No. 92–0018. Rockville, MD, 1992.

Bailes, B. K. "Perioperative Nursing Research, Part 4, Intraoperative Phase." *AORN Journal* 49, 5 (May 1989): 1397–1399.

Edel, E. M. "Perioperative Documentation: Incorporating Nursing Diagnosis into the Intraoperative Period." *AORN Journal* 50, 3 (September 1989): 596–600.

Gallagher, M., and Kahn, C. "Lasers: Scalpels of Light." *RN* 53, 5 (May 1990): 46–52.

Kneedler, J. A. "Perioperative Nursing Research, Part 2, Intraoperative Chemical and Physical Hazards to Personnel." *AORN Journal* 49, 3 (March 1989): 829–836.

Kneedler, J. A. "Perioperative Nursing Research, Part 3, Potential Intraoperative Biological Hazard to Personnel." *AORN Journal* 49, 4 (April 1989): 1066–1067.

Litwack, K., Saleh, D., and Schultz, P. "Postoperative Pulmonary Complications." *Critical Care Nursing Clinics of North America* 3, 1 (March 1991): 77–82.

Noah, V. "Preoperative Teaching Is the Key to PCA Success." *RN* 53, 5 (May 1990): 60–63.

Noriega, L. and Mudd, D. L. "Perioperative Nursing Research, Part 7, Postoperative Care" *AORN Journal* 50, 2 (August 1989): 370–381.

Richards, M. L. "Perioperative Nursing Research, Part 6, Postoperative Phase." *AORN Journal* 50, 1 (July 1989): 120–122.

Rothrock, J. C. "Perioperative Nursing Research, Part 1, Preoperative Psychoeducational Interventions." *AORN Journal* 49, 2 (February 1989): 597.

Silo, H. M. "Perioperative Nursing Research, Part 5, Intraoperative Recommended Practices." *AORN Journal* 49, 6 (June 1989): 1627–1636.

Wild, L., and Coyne, C. "The Basics and Beyond: Epidural Analgesia." *American Journal of Nursing* 92, 4 (April 1992): 26–34.

Coping with Loss

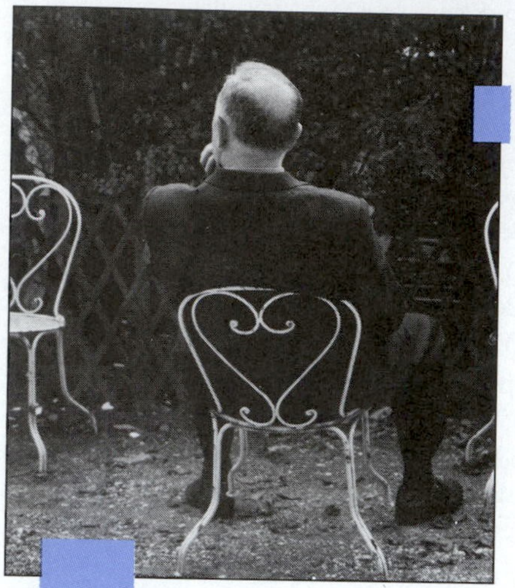

41

Objectives

After completing this chapter, you should be able to:

1. Give an example of how each of the six stages of dying might affect nursing care.
2. Explain how the concept of trajectory affects care of the dying patient and the family.
3. Identify common physical and psychological problems of the dying patient.
4. Explain the special needs of children who are dying.
5. Discuss the implications for nurses of the issue of death with dignity.
6. Explain assessment needed for the dying person.
7. Discuss the nursing diagnoses that are commonly present in the dying person.
8. Identify nursing actions that provide support to the dying person.
9. Briefly discuss the impact of the hospice philosophy on care related to death and dying.
10. Compare Worden's tasks of mourning with Engel's stages of grief.
11. Compare normal and abnormal grief.
12. Describe assessment needed for the grieving person.
13. Discuss nursing diagnoses seen in the grieving person.
14. Explain how nurses can help persons with the grieving process.

Study Terms

acceptance
advance directive
anticipatory grief
bargaining
burnout
code
death care
denial
disengagement
euthanasia
grief
hospice care
integrative therapy
interdisciplinary team
life review
mourning
natural death acts
resignation
resolution
restitution
symbolic language
trajectory

Ellis, Nowlis: Nursing: A Human Needs Approach, 5th ed. © 1994 J.B. Lippincott Company

Outline

Life is a series of losses. We lose the shelter of childhood, financial support from parents, the freedom of being single, youth. At some time during our lives, many of us lose our jobs, homes, pets, friends, and even a loved one. With illness, we may lose independence and the expected functioning of part of our body.

Death is the ultimate and loneliest experience of loss all human beings face. Human beings are the only species aware of their own mortality, and this knowledge may bring not only feelings of loneliness and helplessness but also outright fear of annihilation. However, even these feelings can be accompanied by growth—a growth in perceptiveness leading to a feeling of relative contentment and acceptance. It is to these ends that nurses must direct their actions. Nurses are often in closest contact with dying patients and their families, offering sensitive care during this most difficult time. Asked why they have chosen nursing as a profession, most nursing students quickly and understandably reply that they wish to help people get well. Today's society is recovery oriented. Medicine is designed to cure or at least to prolong life. Nurses must realize that the inability to cure does not mean that we do not care.

New technology has greatly extended the capacity to prolong life, compelling people in general, and those in health care, to look more closely at end-of-life issues. A thoughtful controversy continues regarding questions never before raised.

Society and Death

In primitive societies, death was accepted as the natural conclusion to life. Death occurred daily in villages, to animals and human beings alike, usually within full view of members of the community. Observance of the loss was in direct proportion to the value of the deceased to the community; a young hunter or prestigious leader elicited an outpouring of grief not paralleled by grief for the elderly or even children. Except for those wounded on hunting expeditions or in accidents and worthy of salvage, dying people who could no longer feed themselves were rarely helped to eat; instead they were allowed to die.

In contemporary society, death is no longer so visible, except on television and in films. Although it is not unusual to read—from the comfort of the living room—about the death of thousands in a natural disaster, many people live their entire lives without viewing a dead person. Thus, death is often depersonalized in our culture. That is, death is perceived as something abstract that happens only to others, and even thinking about it can be consciously avoided.

The language used today is evidence of a death-denying culture. Such phrases as "passing on" and "no longer with us" reflect an attempt to protect ourselves emotionally from the reality of death. Commercial sympathy cards avoid the use of the word death, and many funeral homes have a "slumber room" where the dead person looks lifelike.

"Institutionalized and given over to professional caretakers, death is kept apart from the rest of us." In 1900, two-thirds of deaths were those of persons less than 50 years old, and most people died at home (DeSpelder and Strickland, 1989). Today, on the other hand, most deaths are those of older persons, and in urban areas almost 90% die in an institutional setting. These figures indicate the importance of the role nurses play in relating to the dying and those who are significant in their lives (Fig. 41–1).

Who is Dying?

In reality, we are all moving through our lives toward death. The capacity of modern technology to prolong life far beyond the natural course of disease makes the classification of dying persons less clear. A troubling situation nurses and families frequently face is preparing psychologically for the impending loss of the patient and then watching the person live on indefinitely, sometimes in pain and hopelessness, with the help of life-sustaining devices.

Equally disturbing are situations in which patients who might be expected to respond to lifesaving medical measures die when such measures are either not available or not used because of a decision by the patient, family, or physician. And there are those with life-threatening conditions whom the nurse does not perceive as

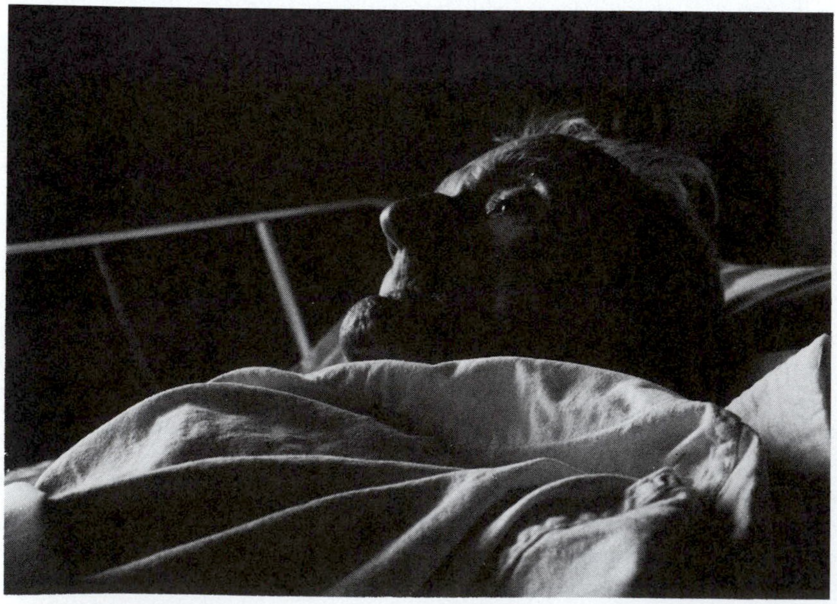

Figure 41–1. Death can be the ultimate and loneliest experience all human beings face.

dying but who are experiencing the same feelings and reactions as those close to death. In this situation, the nurse must interact with seriously ill patients by sharing both fears and cares and, at the same time, accepting the uncertainty of the prognosis. This is a difficult task.

Stages of Dying

In the late 1960s, Kubler-Ross (1969) identified five stages of dying, which are helpful as guidelines when one is caring for the terminally ill. The stages are denial, anger, bargaining, depression, and acceptance. There is sometimes a sixth stage, disengagement. Not only the patient but also the family and care providers experience these stages, although not necessarily simultaneously. For example, at the same time the patient is sharing feelings about dying with the nurse in an open and realistic way, the family may be talking about taking the patient on a trip as soon as she gets well. We discuss the process of trajectories later in this chapter.

Nurses—as observers, sharers, helpers, and supporters in the dying experience—must understand that not all patients pass sequentially through the various stages or experience every stage. It is common for a dying person to revert from apparent acceptance back into a state of depression. Bargaining may punctuate the dying process, only to be replaced by depression or anger. The family and members of the health care team may in a sense accompany the patient through the stages of dying, sharing many of the patient's feelings.

Because each of these stages is a mechanism for coping, premature intervention is unwise. Only if the patient's outlook is interfering with necessary aspects of care and treatment, or if it is disrupting the family, should intervention take place. Any direct intervention should be undertaken by a skilled person who can point out an alternative outlook and behavior. The patient should have the right to die in his or her own way. The uniqueness of the individual patient, in dying as well as in living, is an absolute principle in nursing care.

Denial

During the stage of **denial**, the individual is consciously or unconsciously denying that something of serious consequence is occurring. This is the "No, not me!" stage. Denial usually lasts a relatively short time because events make the truth apparent so that denial is no longer possible. The stage of denial may "buy time" during which the patient can come to terms with the reality of the situation (Callanan and Kelley, 1992).

During this stage the patient may seek other professional opinions, request the repetition of certain tests, or flatly state that there has been a mistake and the test results are someone else's. Within certain limits, denial should not be contradicted but allowed to subside slowly as the patient gradually adjusts to the upsetting news.

Anger

No other stage is as difficult for nurses to deal with as *anger.* This is the "Why me?" stage. It seems blatantly unfair to the patient that he or she has been chosen to die while those around remain healthy. The feeling of anger becomes almost intolerable at times, and the nurse may be the receiver of these negative feelings. The family is sometimes protected from those feelings because the family's love makes such outpourings unacceptable to the patient. The physician may or may not escape anger. The physician may be viewed as the one person who may be able to help and whom the patient does not dare to alienate. At other times, the physician is the target of anger.

The patient's anger is often focused on the nurse, taking the form of excessive demands or complaints about care. The nurse may become uncomfortable, feeling angry in return and regretting that the person will not recover so an appropriate response can be made. Making use of effective communication skills, you can tell the patient with firmness and kindness that you understand that he or she is seriously ill and angry about the consequent restrictions and that you would like to provide the best possible care. However, some limitations must be set so both your goals and the patient's can be accomplished. Such a confrontation is not disconcerting to the patient, and at times a patient will express relief at being treated as a person who can still elicit feelings in others. Clearing the air, in such instances, is therapeutic.

Bargaining

The third stage, **bargaining**, may be short or intermittent. The patient may be bargaining for a reprieve or postponement—even a cure. During this stage, there may be a resurgence in actively seeking out a new therapy or diet or making a change in one's belief system. The patient may say, "If only I were a better person . . . ." A special event may be set as a goal for survival, such as "If I can only live until my son's graduation."

Depression

When bargaining fails to delay the course of the illness or bring about a cure, impending death becomes a reality that can no longer be avoided psychologically. The sense of losing one's life, family, and total earthly environment is understandably accompanied by feelings of deep depression and profound sadness. To do your own grief work but remain close to the patient is an important nursing achievement. Crying during this stage denotes awareness, and it is therefore inappropriate for the nurse and family to admonish the patient not to cry. The stage of *depression* may be lengthy and may persist in some patients. One hopes, however, that the patient will pass through this stage to acceptance.

Acceptance

Acceptance should not be confused with **resignation** (passive submission to a situation). The period of **acceptance** can be a time of contentment, final sharing with close friends and family, and conclusion of unfinished business. It is hoped by all that the pain is controlled and that the struggle, which can be exhausting, is almost over. The patient's circle of interest narrows, and attention is given only to events and people close to the person. The family may need additional support during this period because they may not have reached comparable acceptance of the loss.

Disengagement

The period of acceptance, the final stage described by Kubler-Ross, is sometimes followed by a sixth stage that could be called **disengagement**. This stage often occurs shortly before death. The dying person may become quiet, even withdrawn, but not necessarily sad. The terminal person wants to see only intimates or no one at all, is apathetic, and appears aware that the end is near. A dying teenager said to his father, "Take the radio home, Dad; I won't be needing it anymore," and died within a few hours. The dying person has, in fact, passed beyond the stage of acceptance.

These stages clearly affect the way the patient, family, and nursing staff see the course of the illness. The process of developing an idea of the course of the disease is called forming a trajectory.

Trajectories Related to Death

Trajectory means path. Each person has a trajectory reflecting a view of the path that the remainder of life will take. Most healthy individuals see their trajectories as ascending toward their most productive years, plateauing, and then entering a period of gentle decline, only to end in a peaceful death at home with loved ones gathered about.

When someone is dying, trajectories often are influenced by the stages of dying. A terminally ill person in the disbelief, anger, or bargaining stage may have a different trajectory from someone in a period of depression or acceptance of impending death. These variations also hold true for family and nurses, who experience similar stages as they relate to the person with a terminal illness.

Persons who are facing the closure of their lives incorporate into their trajectories, consciously or unconsciously, a vision of how much time remains. For a while, this trajectory may undergo frequent modification as intervention delays death or alarming new symptoms indicate the close of life. This process is useful to the individual, who needs to estimate time available to complete unfinished business or to grieve the loss of self.

Family members and friends close to the person also have trajectories. Each senses, in his or her own way, the course of the illness suffered by the loved one and how much time may remain for relating. Again, the formation of a trajectory allows significant persons to allocate time well and share thoughts that might have remained unsaid.

The staff, too, forms trajectories regarding the patients for whom they provide care. Even though nurses have access to the plan of care, individual caregivers may possess either realistic or unrealistic trajectories, depending on their psychological investment in giving care and the degree of hope for survival.

When the patient, family, and nurse have different trajectories, problems can develop in communication patterns and interpersonal relationships (Fig. 41-2). For example, let us suppose some type of medical intervention that was tried before with only limited success is to be tried again. The patient, who is in the stage of acceptance and sees only peace in dying, may not be able to change the trajectory. The family members, still in stages of anger and bargaining, may view the treatment as providing possible salvation from death and quickly change their trajectories. The nurses, who had some reservations about the treatment before, may have a variety of trajectories different from both the patient's and the family's. Despair may lead one nurse to develop a short trajectory ending in death; denial may lead another to generate an extended trajectory culminating in recovery.

The Dying Child

Children die of many causes: congenital defects, injury, suicide, cancer, and other diseases of the major systems of the body. It is painful to contemplate children dying, and it takes a special nursing team to provide the support the child and the family need. Although it is beyond the scope of this chapter to deal in depth with a child's death, some observations are appropriate.

A child's concept of death depends on the age of the child as well as the influence of the family, culture, religion, and past experiences. However, even very young children perceive that there is something seri-

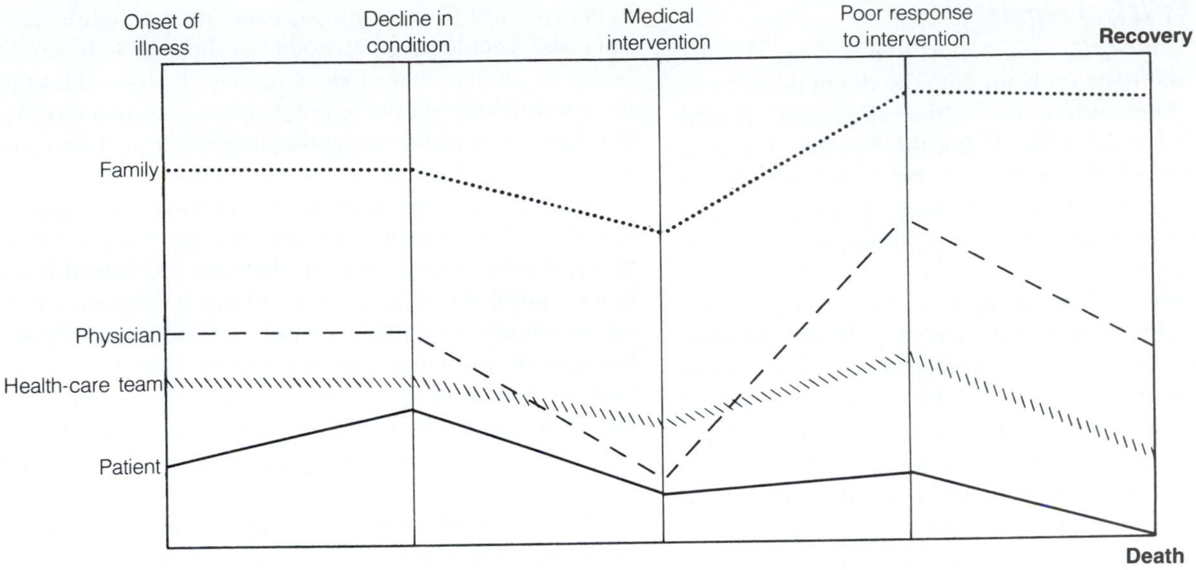

Figure 41-2. Different trajectories relative to the dying experience can lead to problems in care.

ously wrong because of the way they feel physically or the behavior of those significant to them. Young children quickly receive messages from those about them and respond to them. If the parents are fearful and upset, the child also feels fearful and upset. Older children often discuss their fears more with peers than with adults, perhaps to avoid intensifying the anxiety of the adults about them. Another reason children often share upsetting feelings with peers may be because the peer group is important; children relate closely to those of their own age group. Sharing should be encouraged not only between the child and family members but also between the child and peers. Family members should be made to feel welcome within the health care setting, for they may form the primary support system for the child (Fig. 41-3).

It is important to remember that siblings are also important members of the family. Kubler-Ross (1983) states that these children may react with increasing negativity to the terminally ill child when parents react to the illness with "excessive pampering" of the ill child. Parents often have to spend considerable time away from the home visiting the hospitalized child. The well children of the family can feel disruption and rejection unless an effort is made to provide continuity in the home. Giving parents permission to be away from the hospital to sustain lines of communication with the other children in the family is a part of care that has beneficial consequences later.

At age 8 or 9, the child begins to understand the finality of death. A dying child of this age or older may exhibit anger, regression, withdrawal, anxiety, and sadness. Children who have learned to associate being hurt or punished with being bad may harbor feelings of guilt; this response is particularly characteristic of young children. Letting the child talk about these feelings with a trusted staff member is helpful. It must be emphasized to the child that being sick is *not* a punishment for bad behavior and that family and friends recognize that the child is good. As with adults, realistic hope should never be taken away.

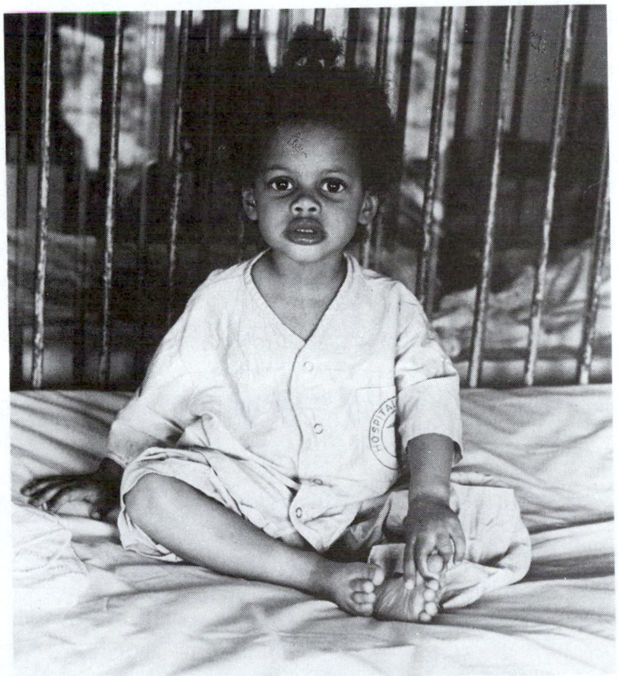

Figure 41-3. Children often face death with openness and honesty.

Death With Dignity

For nurses, the issues surrounding the dying person can be difficult. The abiding wish is that all patients should recover and not die. Confronting the fact that a patient has an illness for which little can be done medically is frustrating and painful for the nurse. A question those who provide care must answer is "What is dignity for the dying?"

Some believe that dignity is to be left alone with private thoughts. Others maintain that dignity involves self-determination, that is, letting the person decide what he or she wishes to do in the remaining time and who should be included in that final relationship. Many feel strongly that dignity includes being physically clean and pain free. It is helpful to get to know the patient and family well so that what they perceive as dignity becomes clearer. Thinking about yourself and what dignity means to you in a personal sense may give you empathy toward the patient. There is no single definition of dignity, but whatever definition you embrace must include respect as well as many of the above factors.

Euthanasia

No current ethical issue except abortion is of more immediate concern to nurses than **euthanasia**, which means good death. It is essential to recognize that there are two kinds of euthanasia: *active* (*positive*), which is the use of toxic substances or other methods to end life, and *passive* (*negative*), which is the withdrawal of or decision not to use extraordinary means to prolong life.

Active euthanasia is legally murder. Public sentiment, as well as that of the medical community, appears to be growing in support of negative euthanasia, which is, in fact, practiced and made possible by the use of advance directives, which we will discuss. Local medical societies and many religious denominations have spoken out against the dehumanization brought about by the use of extraordinary means when no reasonable hope for recovery is possible.

Another difficult task is differentiating between ordinary and extraordinary means to prolong life. Figure 41-4 shows a continuum of methods used to assist patients who are ill. You should examine this figure carefully and decide at what point on the line you would begin to define measures as extraordinary. Although most individuals would agree that being connected to a ventilator is extraordinary, other aspects of treatment are less clear-cut. Ten nurses would probably define extraordinary measures as beginning at six to seven different places on the continuum. Bioethicists usually define extraordinary as any measure that one ordinary human being cannot do for another. From this standpoint, intravenous fluids, although common, remain extraordinary because an ordinary person cannot provide this service to another. Not all people are comfortable with this definition of extraordinary. Often a court is asked to decide what will be considered extraordinary in an individual situation.

Kaplan (1987) raised the sensitive question of positive euthanasia when he explored the possibility of providing life-ending drugs to rational and suffering terminally ill patients. The necessary mechanism for this, Dr. Kaplan envisions, is the legalization of euthanasia so that the dignity of patients will be maintained and the dilemma faced by nurses and physicians ended. Others believe that the answer to suffering is to provide appropriate pain management and this would eliminate the need for positive euthanasia. This question is being addressed in the United States courts today.

Until such time as a consensus is legally mandated, nurses will remain in the arena of conflicting beliefs. Individual nurses must be true to themselves. No nurse should participate in any decision or practice he or she considers ethically unacceptable.

Resuscitation

When aggressive resuscitation methods are needed to save the life of a patient, a **code** was historically used in hospitals to summon a team to begin resuscitation. This was designed to prevent anxiety among patients and visitors. Today the code is used to facilitate rapid communication. "Code 99 in room 220" may indicate cardiopulmonary arrest in room 220. A code may be announced over the public address system or the advanced life support team may be summoned by

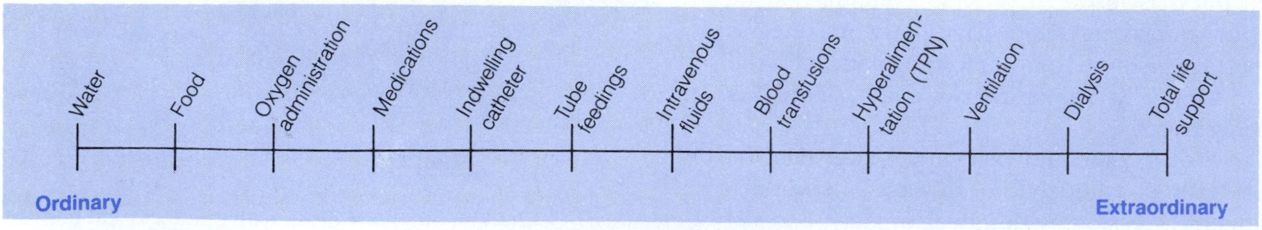

Figure 41-4. Continuum of ordinary/extraordinary means to support life.

pagers. Calling a code is usually a nursing function because the nurse most often discovers the patient in distress. The advanced life support term hurries to the area and begins whatever measures are needed to attempt resuscitation. This includes the use of cardiopulmonary resuscitation (CPR), drugs, and mechanical ventilation.

For many patients who have sudden, sometimes unexpected cardiac or respiratory arrest, attempts to resuscitate the patient are certainly appropriate. But whether a terminally ill patient who does not wish to have such intervention should be resuscitated is a controversial issue. The selected references at the conclusion of this chapter are but a few of a growing number on the topic.

Recent changes are making it easier for nurses to handle such sensitive situations. When a person is obviously at risk of not surviving, physicians in many hospitals are attempting to determine with the patient or family before an emergency arises, what resuscitative procedures should be undertaken. Although such questions should be posed to the patient first and the family second, it is only honest to say that in the past, the patient has not always been included in the decision-making. The inclusion of patients in this important decision is now mandated by law through the Patient Self-determination Act. This law requires that when individuals are admitted to a health care agency, they be given an opportunity to state their wishes in regard to resuscitative procedures.

A number of studies have been done that question the resuscitation procedure. Data indicate that if attempts at resuscitation have been made for 30 minutes or longer and there has been no response, people do not survive. Lung disease also appears to be an indicator for nonsurvival. Although age in and of itself does not appear to be a survivor factor, the frail elderly have proven to have a poor resuscitation outcome (Donius, 1992-1993). Studies question the appropriateness of some codes, wondering if pursuing this option is a kindness for families when a successful outcome is unrealistic.

State Natural Death Acts

A factor that has been important in the trend toward assigning decision-making to the person concerned has been the enactment of **natural death acts** in most states. These laws use language similar to that of living wills, which were not legally binding. Although the titles and wording vary from state to state, their purpose is to allow a person to declare his or her wishes before—or, in some states, during—the terminal illness. The declaration is called an **advance directive** for health care and is legal if signed in the presence of two witnesses, neither of whom can be a relative or gain financially from the person's death (Figs. 41-5 and 41-6). Call your legislative offices to receive a copy of the law if your state has advance directives (see Chapter 3 and Chapter 36).

The confrontation with the sensitive issues surrounding death gives those in nursing continuing concern. You should carefully examine your own feelings regarding the prolongation of life and be respectful of the views of others.

Care at the Time of Death

However long expected and emotionally prepared for, the actual death of the patient may be difficult to accept by the family and care providers. Whether the moment of death is sad but memorable or painful and distressing is, to some degree, influenced by your nursing care. Some people close to the dying patient feel a deep need to be present at the moment of death. Their presence allows for a decisive, final letting go and for the beginning of a new phase of grief that will eventually be resolved. The nursing staff should make every effort to honor these wishes. Families frequently say that they have been comforted by a nurse who talked with them about the death and stayed with them during the final moments. Because most people today have not wit-

Nursing Issues and Trends: *Implementing the Patient Self-Determination Act*

The Patient Self-Determination Act became a federal law in December, 1991. The law assures patients and residents of facilities who participate in Medicare or Medicaid the right to be informed of their option to refuse treatment through enacting a legal advance directive. Other parts of the law address staff education, policies, and records and prohibit discrimination on the basis of individual decision-making regarding end-of-life issues. Making sure that this law is conscientiously implemented within each facility is a vital part of providing complete and sensitive care to the patients we serve.

Directive to Physicians

Directive made this ________ day of ______________________________ (month, year).

I ____, being of sound mind, willfully and voluntarily make known my desire that my life shall not be artificially prolonged under the circumstances set forth below, and do hereby declare:

1. If at any time I should have an incurable injury, disease, or illness certified to be a terminal condition by two physicians, and where the application of life-sustaining procedures would serve only to artificially prolong the moment of my death and where my physician determines that my death is imminent whether or not life-sustaining procedures are utilized, I direct that such procedures be withheld or withdrawn, and that I be permitted to die naturally.
2. In the absence of my ability to give directions regarding the use of such life-sustaining procedures, it is my intention that this directive shall be honored by my family and physician(s) as the final expression of my legal right to refuse medical or surgical treatment and accept the consequences from such refusal.
3. If I have been diagnosed as pregnant and that diagnosis is known to my physician, this directive shall have no force or effect during the course of my pregnancy.
4. I have been diagnosed and notified at least 14 days ago as having a terminal condition by

   ________________________________, M.D., whose address is ______________________________

   ____ and whose telephone number is __________________

   I understand that if I have not filled in the physician's name and address, it shall be presumed that I did not have a terminal condition when I made out this directive.
5. This directive shall have no force or effect five years from the date filled in above.
6. I understand the full import of this directive and I am emotionally and mentally competent to make this directive.

Signed ____

City, County and State of Residence ____

____

The declarant has been personally known to me and I believe him or her to be of sound mind.

Witness ____

Witness ____

This Directive complies in form with the "Natural Death Act" California Health and Safety Code, Section 7188, Assembly Bill 3060 (Keene).

Figure 41-5. Natural Death Directive in use in California.

nessed a death and thus feel some fear, the nurse may explain what it might be like: that death usually comes quietly and that the patient is often unresponsive and pain free but probably able to hear. Everyone should be aware that the dying person's hearing may be intact and that they should speak with respect and say only what would be appropriate for the person to hear.

The children of the family should also be allowed, if the family wishes, to share the natural end of life. Their presence should depend, of course, on their prior preparation as well as their relationship to the dying person.

Allowing the family to view the body in the care setting is becoming more widespread as a way of helping families through the grieving process. After caring for the body, the nurse may want to join the family and others in visiting or sitting with the body. Confrontation with the body is a healthy part of the grieving process. It sharpens the reality of death. Some families, however, prefer to view the body later in a church, a funeral home, or not at all. Nurses should respect the rights and wishes of all those involved.

The health care team grieves together with the family and others who were close to the patient. Crying denotes awareness of the loss. Nurses and physicians often weep with the family.

Guidelines for Signers

The DIRECTIVE allows you to instruct your doctor not to use artificial methods to extend the natural process of dying.

Before signing the DIRECTIVE, you may ask advice from anyone you wish, but you do not have to see a lawyer or have the DIRECTIVE certified by a notary public.

If you sign the DIRECTIVE, talk it over with your doctor and ask that it be made part of your medical record.

The DIRECTIVE must be WITNESSED by two adults who (1) are not related to you by blood or marriage, (2) are not mentioned in your will, and (3) would have no claim on your estate.

The DIRECTIVE may NOT be witnessed by your doctor or by anyone working for your doctor. If you are in a HOSPITAL at the time you sign the DIRECTIVE, none of its employees may be a witness. If you are in a SKILLED NURSING FACILITY, one of your two witnesses MUST be a "patient advocate" or "ombudsman" designated by the State Department of Aging.

Figure 41-6. Instructions accompanying the Natural Death Directive.

Death care, the cleansing and preparation of the body after death, may be simple or detailed, depending on the hospital. Sometimes it is referred to by the Latin term *postmortem*, meaning after death. It is best to check the procedure of the facility where you practice. After the patient is pronounced dead by the physician, usual practice is that all equipment is disconnected, clean dressings are applied, teeth and eyeglasses are sent with the body, and valuables are signed for and given to the nearest relative. It is a nursing responsibility to see that the body leaves the unit properly and with dignity. For a description of the tasks and procedures involved in caring for the body, consult Module 33, Postmortem Care.

Assessment Related to the Dying Patient

The most beneficial care one can give the terminally ill is that which is planned to meet the needs of the patient directly and expediently. The concerns of the terminally ill are many. For purposes of assessment, we shall consider the three major categories—physical, psychological, and social—with the understanding that they overlap and have an impact on one another and that each is as important as the others. Not all patients have problems in all three areas, but assessments must be made in each to ensure total care of the patient. The dying person's psychological needs are often less well understood than physical and social needs. One reason may be that the nurse often feels uncomfortable dealing with what may be psychologically disturbing to the patient. The dying person wants to be treated as a contributing person and to be involved in decisions regarding the community, family and most of all, self, as long as possible.

Assessment of the terminally ill person must be done unobtrusively and with sensitivity. It is essential that the family be included. Once a relationship based on trust and honest communication has been established, these special patients will share their concerns with the nurse.

Throughout the text, we have discussed techniques for assessment and each of these methods is used for the terminally ill patient. You must place special emphasis on any assessment of any symptoms that cause the patient discomfort or distress or interfere with daily living. These data will help you write accurate nursing diagnoses that will be incorporated into the plan of care. There is also assessment of high risk situations. For example, activity intolerance may result in the patient's experiencing more fatigue and spending more time in bed than is desired. Many of the unique problems of the dying require coordinated implementation with other members of the health care team.

Interview

The interview can be helpful in assessing the patient's problems. After discussing the physical, psychological, and social problems you assess, an open-ended question usually elicits the specific concerns of the person. A question such as "What bothers you the most?" can reveal an area that should be a priority part of the assessment process. The patient may answer, "That I can't walk as far as I'd like," or "That I had to give up my job" or "My friends seem to be uncomfortable when they visit me."

Interviewing the family or those closest to the patient is also helpful. Listening carefully to their concerns signifies you care about them during this painful time. Beginning the interview by saying, "This must be a very hard time for you; tell me what is the most difficult current problem as you see it," can be a good beginning in showing your interest and developing trust. Often, the nurse can help solve a problem identified in the interview. It may be contacting a community resource or talking with the physician regarding pain management. The interview fulfills a vital purpose for care of the patient with life-threatening disease.

Physical Assessment

The physical changes that may accompany serious illness can understandably be alarming to the patient and the family. The systems of the body are not functioning as they should.

Weakness and Fatigue

The ill person may feel moderate to extreme physical weakness and fatigue related to the disease process itself or the treatment, such as radiation or chemotherapy. The patient may feel anxious or depressed because the weakness or fatigue interferes with daily life. The use of assistive devices such as canes, walkers, or wheelchairs may become necessary. Participation in social or diversional activities, once enjoyed, may no longer be possible because of the symptoms.

Weight Loss

Deterioration evidenced by extreme weight loss signals that a decline in health is occurring. The patient's body image is also changing in response to weight loss, and accommodation to these changes is difficult. Your assessment may be done by observing the patient's behavior. Some patients refuse to look in mirrors or are reluctant to have visitors. Other patients strive to compensate for physical deterioration with mental competence. Accompanying weight loss may be generalized weakness and inability to perform many daily functions.

Discomfort

Although no attempt is made to assign priorities to physical problems, pain must be a top priority for assessment and treatment. Pain influences and interrupts all aspects of a relationship. As a dying woman put it, "Pain consumes you." Chronic pain is different from other pain in that it has no beginning and no end.

Pain has different meanings for different individuals. It may mean that the disease is progressing, that things are getting worse. That death is imminent is an understandable interpretation, and occasionally a welcome one if the illness has been long and painful. But pain is ordinarily unwelcome to the dying, destroying hope and draining the individual of energy that could be used to relate to family and friends.

Just as one's previous experiences with death affect one's dying, past experiences with pain affect response to pain. For example, a patient who has experienced only infrequent moderate pain, which has been satisfactorily controlled, is unlikely to be fearful that pain will get out of control. On the other hand, the patient who has had severe, uncontrolled pain fears it and lacks trust that it can be controlled.

It is important that the patient help you accurately assess the degree of pain so that appropriate nursing actions can be taken. Using a rating scale, such as described in Chapter 32, provides participation in assessment by the patient. Other indications that the patient is having pain include nonverbal communication and changes in vital signs. Frequent interaction with the patient is important because pain levels can change rapidly. Continuous assessment of this area by the nurse is essential.

Skin Changes and Edema

In the later stages of disease, many patients experience skin changes or edema. If the liver or pancreas is involved, your assessment may reveal that the skin has taken on a yellowish tinge and the patient is said to be jaundiced. This color change appears first in the sclera (white portion) of the eyes and then becomes more generalized. Assess for *itching* or *jaundiced skin*, which can be particularly distressing for the patient.

Edema, the presence of fluid in the interstitial tissues, may be detected first in the upper buttocks and later in the lower extremities, particularly the ankles. You may also see swelling around the eyes (periorbital edema). If edema progresses or becomes severe, swelling of the ankles occurs, which becomes more prominent when the lower extremities are in the dependent position. Patients sometimes remark that they feel the rings on their fingers are tight.

Respiratory Function

Dyspnea is a common problem for persons with a terminal disease. Shortness of breath can be caused by physical limitations but is always exacerbated by apprehension and emotional distress. Dyspnea itself is subjective, so simply understanding what causes it physically does not tell you how the patient perceives its severity. When you are assessing for problems in breathing, have the patient rate the difficulty on a scale of 0 to 5, 0 representing no difficulty. (A similar scale can be used to rate pain.)

Objective data are also important. These include rate, depth, rhythm, chest sounds, and respiratory effort. These are discussed in detail in Chapter 28.

Bowel Function

Abdominal distention, which may be a final symptom of terminal disease, is particularly distressing for the patient because it causes bloating and can interfere with breathing and eating. Distention may be caused by gas, large amounts of feces due to intestinal immobility, free-floating fluid in the abdominal cavity (ascites), or tumor mass.

Ask the patient about how well pain is being managed and factors that may be interfering with sleep. All the drugs used to control chronic terminal pain cause some degree of constipation. If the dosage is high, the constipation may be profound and impaction is not uncommon (see Chapter 26). The inability to drink adequate fluids or eat a diet containing fiber also adds to the incidence of constipation for the seriously ill.

Assessment for constipation requires that you find out what elimination pattern is normal for the patient and how the patient perceives the problem. This information, along with documentation of the number and types of stools produced, will identify whether or not a problem exists.

Cognitive Status

Cognitive impairment, most often demonstrated by confusion, occurs in approximately 85% of terminally ill patients (Martin, 1990). The confusion in the terminally ill usually occurs rapidly and can change throughout a 24-hour period. The person may have disturbances in attention, orientation, and sleep pattern or become agitated, combative, or lethargic. Confusion can be caused by the underlying disease process that may alter electrolytes. Laboratory reports should also be a part of assessment because they may reveal electrolyte imbalances that can be reversed. During assessment, you can use a mental status examination similar to the one presented in Chapter 31.

Other Assessment Data

First, assessment must be made related to the effects of the feelings the patient is experiencing. The person may experience interruption of sleep, which may be related to physical factors such as pain or psychological factors such as anxiety. Often, the patient will become withdrawn or not participate in daily care, even losing interest in maintaining basic hygiene. Careful assessment of past interests can help you plan activities with the patient that will help that person to continue to feel productive.

Assess other psychological concerns. Fear of dependency and powerlessness are common concerns of persons who are seriously ill. Explore the importance of spirituality and what part faith has had in the person's life. Identifying the persons who are important to the patient is necessary because these people may be supportive as illness continues. A pet may be an important part of the patient's life and separation from the animal can be stressful.

Assess communication patterns without being intrusive. The patient may tell you that there is a lack of communication with the family. The patient's behavior may also tell you there are communication problems. The patient may talk with you only about aspects of care instead of feelings or may be more withdrawn when some individuals are visiting. Careful listening techniques are essential to assessment of this area.

The family may ask for your assessment of the patient's interest in being a part of planning death rituals, such as a funeral or a memorial service. One woman, a mountain climber, planned a memorial service consisting solely of beautiful music accompanied by slides of the patient, smiling, at the summit of a mountain. Her family and friends found this personal remembrance extremely moving. This is a highly individual and personal decision that is to be made by the patient and the family.

Although each of us has social needs, some people require more social integration than others. A person who is gregarious by nature may as a patient retain more interest in social activities and relationships than a more solitary person, who may be content to limit the social portion of life. However, most patients who discover they have a disease from which they will not recover experience some degree of social isolation. A primary reason for this isolation is that some healthy people feel uncomfortable and threatened by contact with people they know are dying. The feeling that "it could be me" is disturbing and people may feel uncertain about what to say or how to act. This behavior is unfortunate because it occurs precisely when the patient most needs closeness to family and friends.

Again, assessment centers around the level of social interaction before the illness and if the patient perceives a problem. Some patients find comfort in not having to respond to a large number of visitors and recognize their need to be solitary and rest. Others miss the social activity formerly enjoyed. Assessment includes that you observe who visits the patient and how receptive the patient is to the visitor. The patient may share feelings with you about the level of social activity.

Nursing Diagnosis Related to the Dying Patient

Because care of the dying is a highly emotional process, a nurse may overlook the importance of establishing nursing diagnoses on which to base care. Most of the nursing diagnoses for those with terminal illness are similar to those diagnoses for other ill patients. It is important to remember, however, that the etiologies for the diagnoses may be related specifically to the disease process or treatment.

Nursing diagnoses related to terminal illness may be specific or general. Specific diagnoses are appropriate as guides for physical or psychological care of the person, whereas more general nursing diagnoses may be

Nursing Diagnoses Related to the Dying Patient

Activity Intolerance: Weakness related to muscle wasting

Altered Nutrition: Less Than Body Requirements related to anorexia

Pain related to metastasis to the spine

Ineffective Breathing Pattern

Constipation related to pain medications

Self-care Deficit: Partial or Total

Altered Role Performance

Powerlessness

Situational Low Self-esteem

Hopelessness

Personal Identity Disturbance

Decisional Conflict

Altered Sexuality Patterns

Ineffective Individual Coping

Spiritual Distress

needed for social problems. Many of the nursing diagnoses for the terminally ill are psychosocial. To make these diagnoses accurately, the nurse must validate the patient's feelings through open communication. Psychosocial diagnoses may be less concrete than diagnoses of physical conditions. With any nursing diagnosis, it is important for the nurse to identify desired patient outcomes. Throughout the illness, the outcome may be one of maximizing the quality of life through providing comfort, leading to a peaceful death.

Activity Intolerance

If the patient is weak and fatigued, which leads to decreased mobility, the nursing diagnosis Activity Intolerance is appropriate. Identifying whether the activity intolerance is related to progression of the disease or a side effect of treatment will help the nurse determine the duration of the problem and suggest methods for increasing mobility.

Altered Nutrition: Less Than Body Requirements

Anorexia is a common concern for the seriously ill patient. Inability to eat a regular diet leads to weight loss and resultant muscle wasting. If the patient is in the hospital, alternative feeding methods may be ordered; this is an ethical dilemma that should be considered by the patient and the family.

Altered Nutrition: Less Than Body Requirements related to anorexia may also be secondary to effects of chemotherapy treatments. This nursing diagnosis, along with others, should be written to give special guidance to nursing actions.

Pain

The pain that these patients experience may be difficult to manage so that knowing the type and origin of the pain is helpful to the nurse. Pain related to metastasis to the spine implies a deep, dull, bone pain that is intensified with movement. If the nursing diagnosis relating to pain specifies that the pain is originating from the stretching of soft organs such as the pancreas, the implementation will be different.

Other Physical Nursing Diagnoses

A variety of other physical nursing diagnoses are appropriate for persons with terminal illness. Ineffective Breathing Pattern is a nursing diagnosis when the patient's respirations become labored or compromised. If the person experiences bladder retention or incontinence or bowel problems such as diarrhea or constipation, the nursing diagnosis is specific such as Diarrhea or Incontinence related to the factor causing the problem. A common nursing diagnosis is Self-care Deficit when the person can no longer partially or completely give self-care. High risk states should also be included. High Risk for Injury: Falls may be a realistic nursing diagnosis when the patient is unsteady or confused.

Altered Role Performance

Another nursing diagnosis may be that of Altered Role Performance. As serious illness encroaches on lifestyle and role responsibility, disturbances in work, family, and social relationships may arise. The nursing diagnosis should identify specific areas in which difficulties are present. Distress surrounding the person's having to relinquish control in some areas of life is a prominent problem.

Most people find dependence—relying on some one else to meet most of their needs—depressing. You can assess dependency by identifying realistically how many of the patient's tasks have been assigned to others. Physical assistance can have dependency meaning for the patient. If the person is no longer independent in feeding or dressing, it can have genuine impact on feelings of dependency. If the family is making major decisions without consulting the patient, this also can be psychologically disturbing to the ill person. You should also carefully listen to the patient as an important part of your assessment. After trust has been established, many persons will tell you how they feel about what they view is intrusion on their remaining independent. Not only becoming dependent but *fears* about becoming dependent are important issues included in assessment.

Powerlessness

Closely related to independence is *control.* Beginning in the toddler years, an individual values control. The zest of life is tied to the ability to choose, within reasonable limits, one's relationships, occupation, ways of spending leisure, and pattern and style of daily living. With any disability, some control is sacrificed. Adjustments have to be made.

For those who are terminally ill, giving up some control over life is more difficult because of the permanency and extent of the adjustments. First, recognition of the loss of control over parts of the body and function is particularly painful; it is even viewed by some as bodily betrayal. Most dying persons reluctantly adjust over time. However, many still have to confront the dehumanizing loss of control over simple but important things such as daily schedule, choice of clothing, and activities throughout the day.

Low Self-esteem

Self-esteem Disturbance is another commonly seen nursing diagnosis. Problems in self-esteem or difficulty accepting oneself as ill, particularly seriously ill with death as a possibility, may be related to health perception.

In conjunction with the need for independence, terminally ill patients also have a need to feel productive and should be encouraged to continue their jobs as long as possible. One dying woman continued to fold letters, soliciting funds for a charitable organization until shortly before she died. An elderly man reported to the occupational therapy department in his wheelchair each morning to work on a doll house for his granddaughter; 3 days after gluing the chimney, he peacefully died. Nurses should appreciate the need for *productivity* because it is universal and a vital part of self-esteem.

Hopelessness

Of all human needs, perhaps none is more important than *hope.* Patients hope that their illnesses will be brief or their surgery successful. Disabled people hope for maintenance of function and mobility. Nurses share these hopes with their patients. Realistic hope may be for pain to be relieved and for meaningful interactions with family. Again, through observing the patient's behavior and attentive listening, your assessment of the degree of hope the patient and the family has maintained can be identified.

Personal Identity Disturbance

Every dying patient grieves loss of self. As part of the grieving process, most feel a need to review their lives. The family, too, may feel a need to reflect on the past with the patient. They may look at photographs together. This process is referred to as **life review** and appears to be a way of "letting go," giving meaning to life and death and making certain one will be remembered. Assessment of this stage can be made by showing interest in the patient as a person. Through building trust and knowing the patient over a length of time, you can more easily assess this important process.

Decisional Conflict

Although Decisional Conflict is not approved by the North American Nursing Diagnosis Association (NANDA), Carpenito (1992) discusses the extreme stress imposed on patients, families, and nurses when end-of-life decisions have to be made. Health–illness perceptions and the perceived trajectory of the patient will affect the plan of care and interpersonal relationships with family members. Denial can bring about noncompliance with the care plan. The patient's vision of the illness is an important area to explore when writing diagnoses for the terminally ill.

Altered Sexuality Patterns

Separate from the diagnoses of physical sexual problems related to the medical condition, nursing diagnoses are also written to identify problems associated with the person's changing feelings toward sexual adequacy. These nursing diagnoses may be Sexual Dysfunction or Altered Sexuality Patterns. Nursing diagnoses concerning sexuality may be related to those concerning self-esteem.

Ineffective Individual Coping

The nursing diagnosis Ineffective Individual Coping should be used with caution. Many persons cope amazingly well under these stressful circumstances, making the diagnosis inappropriate. Given the extreme stress accompanying serious illness, nursing diagnoses related to ability to cope are sometimes appropriate for both the patient and those significant to the patient.

Spiritual Distress

Serious life-threatening illness can often change a person's values and belief system. Individuals may strengthen their belief system to be sustained throughout the troubled times of the illness. Occasionally despair will cause people to change or abandon long-held belief systems that were formerly important to them. Although values and beliefs must be respected by care providers, those that clearly interfere with comfort or appropriate treatment can be identified as diagnoses of Spiritual Distress.

Planning and Implementation Related to the Dying Patient

Planning must always include identifying the desired outcomes of care. Common desired outcomes include that the person will be pain free and that other symptoms will be controlled. Further desired outcomes might include that the individual will express feelings and concerns and have the opportunity to relate to significant others. Outcome criteria are important when evaluating the current plan of care and considering revision that will more clearly meet the needs of the patient. The physical and emotional status of terminally ill patients continually changes so that frequently reviewing the outcomes will result in more effective ongoing care by the entire health care team.

In planning care for the dying person, you must recognize that although problems will fall into the three areas of physical, psychological, and social concerns, the specific problems will be different with each patient for whom you care. Individualizing the plan of care and being flexible enough to review continuously and change it are essential in maximizing the quality of life of your patient.

Managing Weight Loss

Many terminal individuals have extreme loss of appetite, often because of the effects of radiation or chemotherapy. You can help the patient with *weight loss* and *lack of energy* by performing several nursing actions. It is important that you offer reassurance so that these patients know that they remain valuable and important individuals despite any changes in physical appearance. To increase weight, diet supplements can be used to provide extra calories. For the anorectic patient, obtaining special preferred food items or having the family bring favorite dishes to the facility may improve intake. Spacing ambulation activities may lead to strength building, and the use of assistive devices can enhance activity for nutritionally weakened patients.

Managing Pain and Discomfort

Establishing techniques for managing the *pain* of the terminally ill is an essential component of planning care. Although it is generally recognized that terminally ill persons rely on large dosages of pain medications, dependence is not a concern. These people do not show the aberrant behavior of the chemically addicted person. Many terminally ill persons who are taking what would ordinarily be near-lethal levels of narcotics remain mentally intact and able to relate to those about them. Knowing this, nurses should become comfortable about providing liberal amounts of pain medication to make the remaining time more comfortable for terminally ill patients.

If *itching* is present, special drugs can be administered along with soothing baths. If *edema* becomes generalized in the later stages of illness, the nurse must remember that the tissues cannot readily absorb medications by injection. The patient with edema may prefer long-sleeved garments for the sake of appearance. The lower extremities should not be in the dependent position but be kept elevated on a stool to reduce edema when the patient is sitting.

Supporting Breathing

Breathing problems are difficult for the patient. Poor oxygenation can cause restlessness, anxiety, and fear. Placing the person in a high position, administering oxygen, and staying with the patient and giving reassurance all help relieve symptoms of dyspnea. A calm and supportive manner on the part of the nurse or family caregiver is essential. Some dying patients develop increased respiratory secretions, which produces in the final hours of life what has been called a "death rattle." This process may be more disturbing to the family than to the patient who is often unresponsive. Oxygen is sometimes given but usually has little effect because respiratory exchange may be compromised. However, this measure may comfort the family.

Suctioning can increase secretions because of irritation and should be used sparingly. During the patient's final hours, the physician may order a drug that dries secretions. This drug may cause the pulse to increase and the face to become mildly flushed, but these effects are not a concern in the dying person.

Maintaining Mobility

Maintaining the patient at the highest level of mobility is important. A higher degree of mobility can be attained if the patient's activity is performed at the time of highest energy. This is usually in the morning. Sometimes the person can be more active by using assistive devices such as a cane or walker. Mobility aids appetite, breathing, and elimination so that this area should be an important part of care (see Chapter 23).

Maintaining Bowel Elimination

If *distention* is a problem, regardless of the cause, conservative nursing actions are often helpful. These include positioning the patient high in the bed and encouraging ambulation. If the cause is gas, a nasogastric tube may be ordered to provide some relief. The use of suppositories may bring about defecation and expulsion of gas. If the cause of the distention is fluid in the abdominal cavity, you may be assisting the physician in performing a paracentesis (introducing a large needle into the abdomen to withdraw the fluid) to make the patient more comfortable. Paracentesis is at best only a temporary measure because the fluid usually reaccumulates; it also depletes the patient of needed protein, which is a major constituent of the fluid. The benefits of paracentesis are the reduction of fluid, which improves both appearance and breathing.

Pain-relieving medications as well as decrease in physical activity and poor diet may lead to *constipation*. Such nursing actions as increasing fluid intake and fiber in the diet and promoting ambulation and exercise are all helpful. Suppositories and enemas can be used to relieve the constipated patient. Laxatives are often prescribed as a preventive measure along with the medications used for pain. If, for medical reasons, the patient cannot pursue these actions, constipation can become a serious problem. The patient feels both psychologically and physically unwell because regular elimination is a component of most people's concept of wellness.

Intestinal obstruction may occur in cases of abdominal or pelvic tumor, which causes inability to eat or drink without pain or cramping. If the obstruction occurs early in the illness, surgical intervention is sometimes undertaken. The physician bypasses the obstruction or, if possible, removes the tumor mass that is occluding the passage. If the patient's physical condition contraindicates surgical intervention, a nasogastric tube is sometimes used to relieve the gas and distention caused by the obstruction. If the obstruction occurs late in the disease process, near death, a treatment being used with increasing frequency is to give the patient diphenoxylate hydrochloride (Lomotil), a drug that stops motility of the bowel. The patient becomes more comfortable and can take small amounts of fluids so that the insertion of a nasogastric tube may be avoided.

Maintaining Cognitive Function

Although *cognitive impairment* may have a physiologic cause, the patient's disorientation or confusion may affect the quality of life, interaction with the family, and compliance with care. In situations such as electrolyte imbalance, drug toxicity, or poor pain management, consulting the physician is appropriate so that changes can be made in the plan of care to diminish the cognitive problem. Drug dosages may have to be reduced or different drugs prescribed. Medications that decrease anxiety or drugs that promote sleep may be appropriate.

Other nursing actions are also helpful. Frequent contact with a supportive family is consoling to the patient and may decrease confusion. Nurses who care for the confused terminally ill are most effective if they are calm and caring and have the ability to individualize the plan of care.

Supporting Autonomy

You should try to maximize *independence* and *control* for dying patients by encouraging them to make decisions about care and to participate in their own care. For example, the patient should decide how far he or she is able to walk within the facility or whether or not to visit a local library in the community. Too often the family, in an effort to protect the patient from stress, excludes him or her from family decisions. Such behavior is a disservice to the patient because it underscores the dependent role.

Nursing actions can also affect the fear of *loss of control*. Nurses can be of the greatest help to persons toward the end of life by offering the patient control in all areas of life where this is still possible, thus minimizing loss of control. Because nurses are such ardent care providers, they sometimes find it difficult not to take unwarranted and excessive control. The smallest matter is of consequence and should be thoughtfully examined and explored with the person before he or she relinquishes control. For more on the control issue, see Chapter 34.

Overcoming Barriers to Communication

What should the patient be told? Interviews with dying people reveal that most know they are dying. However, some persons do not want to be told that they have a terminal condition and some families do not want the patient to be told. Deciding whether or not to tell the patient the extent of the illness and the prognosis is primarily the responsibility of the physician, and ideally, should involve the family. Even though it is the patient's right to know of his or her condition, the kindest and most reasonable approach on the part of the physician is to reveal whatever the patient wants and is willing to know, which varies from patient to patient. Nurses often find themselves in the uncomfortable position of not knowing exactly what the patient and family have been told. It is appropriate to ask the attending physician what information has been shared with the patient and the family. Experience in interacting with dying people will enable you to discern how much the patient knows or is willing to know about the diagnosis.

A great deal of communication takes place between the patient and the family, and the nurse can be helpful in assessing problems with the essential connection. Losing a loved one is a heart-wrenching experience for the family and can be nearly unbearable in cases of extended terminal illness when the goodbyes seem never ending. If the family is unable to be in touch with the dying person, the consequence can be true isolation. Long after the patient accepts and wants to talk about dying, the family may deny the fact of approaching death. Family members may talk endlessly about the patient's coming home. Or they may keep all conversation superficial, saying nothing that is meaningful to the patient. Visits become shorter.

Nurses and other health care providers are sometimes uncomfortable talking with the dying. One social worker wrote, "I know he wanted to talk to me . . . the patient knew and I knew, but as he saw my desperate attempts to escape, he took pity on me and kept to himself what he wanted to share with another human being. And so he died and did not bother me" (Kubler-Ross and Warshaw, 1978). Nurses often express the fear that, if the patient asks a direct question, they won't know what to say. Such direct questions are fairly infrequent.

Using Therapeutic Interaction

Although each case is unique, certain guidelines for communication can be offered. Probably the most valuable action the nurse can do is to plan sufficient time to sit with the patient and listen undisturbed. It is all too common for nurses to enter the patient's room only to perform a task and then leave immediately after completing it, fearful that the patient will confront them about the illness. Keep in mind that, even with very critically ill patients, you do not know whether or when they will die. Thus it is risky, for your own peace of mind as well as the patient's, to make rigid predictions. It is far better, if the occasion arises, to let the patient know you understand that he or she is seriously ill. Nurses are often so concerned about giving information that they fail to simply listen to the patient, which is the essence of therapeutic communication with the dying. Patients really do not expect their caregivers to have the answers to their philosophical questions, but they do appreciate someone who will explore the profound "whys" with them. With the support of the nurse, many families are able to maintain contact with their loved one, finding out for themselves that patients do not talk about dying at great length but only want to communicate their feelings on occasion to those who mean the most to them. Referral to a counselor or agency that provides visits and communication may be appropriate.

Using Symbolic Language and Integrative Therapy

The use of **symbolic language**, which focuses on hopes and fears, has been used extensively in interacting with dying children and adults suffering life-threatening illness and their families. Symbolic language, in the form of poetry, stories, or drawings, can reflect thoughts that may not be consciously apparent. The person or family as well as the care provider can learn a great deal by reviewing the words or images. Invaluable insight can be gained that may dispel fears, decrease anger, and help patients to "let go" while at the same time, affirming the joy of life. Many seriously ill persons and their families who have difficulty verbalizing troublesome thoughts may be able to consciously or unconsciously express them through drawing (Fig. 41-7).

Petzold (1982) used a similar technique with patients of all ages, which he called **integrative therapy**. Patients are encouraged to write poetry and prose, expressing angry feelings or any others kinds of feelings. All work is viewed in a nonjudgmental way. Writing one's feelings in words, sometimes by attributing them to characters in a story format, is therapeutic. Having patients work with clay to sculpt meaningful forms is another technique this researcher has used in his work with the dying.

Emphasizing Strengths

Emphasizing *strengths* rather than weaknesses is an important part of caring for the terminally ill. Too often nurses focus on the patient's weaknesses because they are the source of the patient's problems. However understandable, such an emphasis can be detrimental to the spirits of the dying patient. Every person retains many strengths until the final hours of life, and emphasizing those strengths is essential. If, for example, the patient expresses sadness and discouragement about no longer being able to drive a car, you can remind the patient that short walks and outings can still be enjoyable. It is important not to deny or dismiss a patient's statements in an effort to emphasize the positive. One patient, too weak to write letters to close friends, was able to use a tape recorder to send caring messages; it was the nurse who suggested doing so and procured the recorder and tapes. When designing a plan of care plan for a terminally ill patient, the nurse should attempt to incorporate the many strengths of the person (Fig. 41-8).

Maintaining Hope

Maintaining hope and a sense of self for the terminally ill person is an important part of the plan of care. Hope for long-term survival many not be realistic, but this

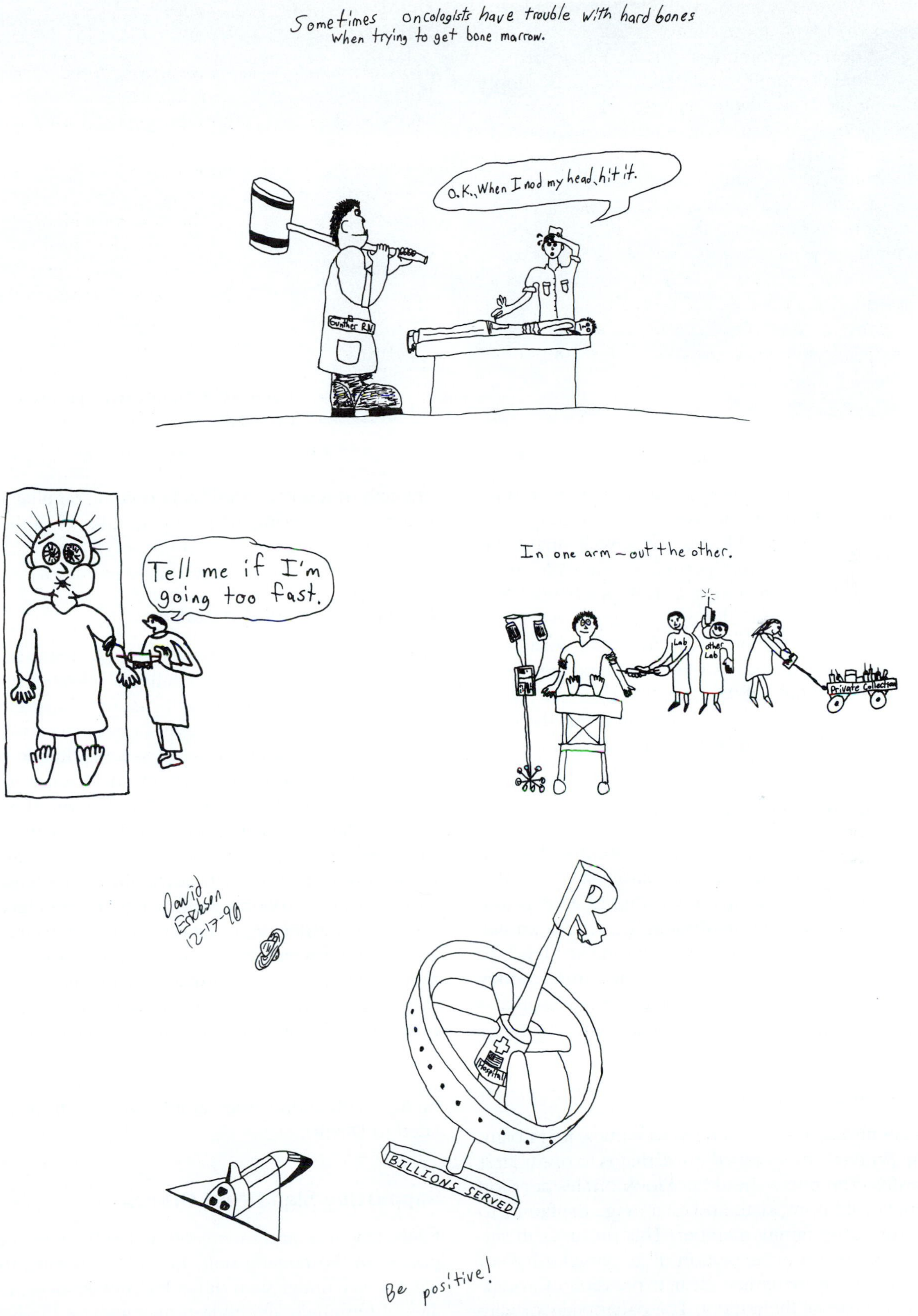
Sometimes oncologists have trouble with hard bones when trying to get bone marrow.
O.K., When I nod my head, hit it.
Gunther RN
Tell me if I'm going too fast.
In one arm – out the other.
Lab
other Lab
Private Collection
R
Hospital
BILLIONS SERVED
Be positive!

Figure 41-7. Self-expression through art. Here a boy with cancer used art to express feelings.

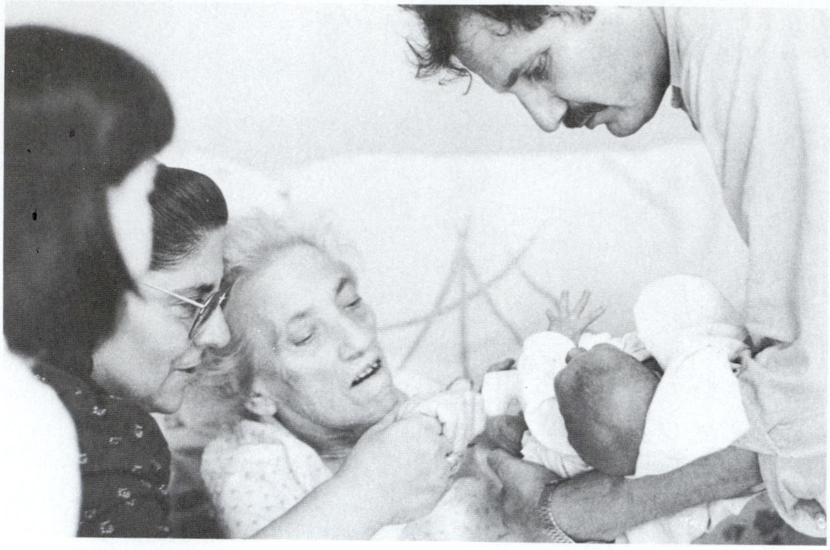

Figure 41-8. There can be joy, even in the last days of life.

does not mean that hope is impossible. There are other things for which to hope, such as a brief return home, a talk with a long-estranged loved one, a walk unaided to the dayroom, or a pain-free period of time with friends and family. Hope is contagious, as is hopelessness. If, as a care provider, you lose all hope, so might the patient and the family. Nurses are in the fortunate position of being able to turn hope into action. Hope can be as sustaining as nursing skill and creativity permit. The ultimate hope in nursing the terminally ill is that the quality of the patient's life can be maintained.

Facilitating Life Review

Because the nurse is likely to be an objective listener, the patient may find the nurse a particularly valuable participant in *life review*. The reviewing process is also valuable for the nurse by increasing the nurse's knowledge of the patient. The process of life review tends to have the beneficial effect of eliciting **anticipatory grief**, grieving before the actual death. We will discuss this in more detail later in the chapter.

Planning Death Rituals

Many patients express a real need to participate in planning the *funeral or memorial ritual* that is to occur after their deaths. The nurse should not look on this decision as morbid or inappropriate and encourage the family to include the dying family member. This process can signify the completion or resolution of grieving for loss of self. Making such plans is a clear expression of acceptance on the part of the patient. The patient may or may not feel this need, but many do have a genuine need to make their wishes known regarding death rituals. You can only assess this need by becoming familiar with the patient and allowing the patient to talk about these matters.

Decreasing Social Isolation

Nursing actions can also be taken to decrease social isolation. In the hospital, dying patients are often placed far from the nursing station in an unconscious attempt to minimize contact. Studies have shown that nurses spend less time in the rooms of dying patients than in those of patients who will recover (Glaser and Strauss, 1965).

The degree of isolation a dying patient experiences depends largely on the person's social lifestyle before the illness. If the patient has always been outgoing and enjoyed strong support from family and friends, such support usually continues. For a patient who has been a quiet, private person, isolation can be profound. Occasionally the reverse is true; a popular, outgoing patient may frighten off social contacts, whereas an introspective person may know better how to cope with loneliness and isolation. The nurse may become close to the patient when others find closeness too painful, and the nurse's caring can alleviate the patient's feelings of being totally alone (see sample Nursing Care Plan Related to Death).

Supporting Significant Others

Peers, teachers, and friends of the family may need support from the nursing staff. Because it is hard to know what to say under such difficult circumstances, the families of terminally ill children may also be inadvertently isolated.

Children, including teenagers, who have the sup-

Nursing Care Plan

Sample Nursing Care Plan Related to Death

Nursing Diagnosis

Social Isolation related to lack of visitors to the hospital.

Supportive data:

17-year-old boy.

Diagnosis: Leukemia for which interventions are no longer successful.

Appears withdrawn and depressed.

States, "I wish more of my friends would come and visit me."

States, "I must look terrible."

Only one young male friend and one young female friend have visited since admission one week ago.

Desired Patient Outcomes

Short term:

For visits by peer group to increase to one time each day or to tolerance level of patient.

For patient and visitors to state that visits are mutually enjoyable.

Long term:

For patient to convey that he feels more comfortable with appearance.

Nursing Action	Rationale
1. Talk with patient and get more data concerning friends and names of those he would like to see.	Involving the patient in determining those who are important to him and that he would like to see provides personal control.
2. Explore feelings regarding his perceptions of how illness is causing isolation.	Communicating feelings helps the individual to cope more effectively.
3. Assure patient that appearance, although altered, is good and socially pleasant.	Reassuring the patient that he is socially acceptable in appearance enhances self concept.
4. Ask permission to talk with family and friends who visit concerning his desire for more social contact.	Asking permission to share patient's concerns with family and friends maintains the patient's dignity and confidentiality.
5. If #4 is positive, a) greet friends and convey patient's desire to extend visits, including others and b) talk with family about other friends who might like to visit patient.	a) Communication with the nurse may decrease anxiety of visitors and foster greater contact with the patient. b) because the family is usually psychologically closest to the patient, family members may provide the most accurate information regarding who among the patient's friends may be appropriate to visit.
6. Share resource books regarding illness with family and friends.	Books provide an additional source of information.
7. Explain to patient how seriously ill persons can become isolated from friends and importance of remaining in contact.	Explaining that social isolation is a common concern for the seriously ill may reassure the patient who is feeling lonely.
8. Communicate with others on the health care team.	Documentation provides a record for the health care team so that useful interventions can continue as part of the patient's plan of care.

port of a loving family and a sensitive, caring health care team approach death with amazing openness, honesty, and acceptance. Nothing is so sad, yet so inspiring.

Again, one concern is the feelings of the siblings of the terminally ill child. Research reveals that these youngsters often feel guilty about the death. Sometimes it is a feeling best reflected in the thought "Why my brother instead of me, as I have always been the one who got into trouble?" Parents may be too involved in the process of grieving over one child to talk with their other children honestly to remove guilt. Consulting a counselor may help prevent future difficulties over these issues if they can be explored during the illness instead of after the death.

Hospice Care

Hospice care programs offer alternative types of care and care settings for dying individuals that allow individuals and their families to direct their energies toward maintaining quality of life for the dying person rather than seeking unrealistic cures. Aroskar (1985) states, "Individual freedom of choice has several identifying characteristics that indicate how to implement respect for persons who seek an alternative to care from the traditional acute care hospital setting where cure is generally the guiding philosophy." Both the dying and the grieving processes are central to the *hospice* concept.

The Hospice Philosophy

Hospices embody a unique alternative philosophy for care of the dying. The philosophy encompasses 1) self-determination by the patient, 2) inclusion of the family and those significant to the dying, 3) an interdisciplinary approach, 4) pain and symptom control, and 5) bereavement services.

Self-determination. The hospice philosophy holds that the person who is leaving life—letting go—knows best what remains important and is the person best able to make decisions concerning management of the illness. On the basis of this principle, the essential decisions governing quality of life for the person in the time remaining are left to the patient. For example, the patient decides where he or she wishes to be and whom he or she wants near. This philosophy is difficult for the traditional health care team, which often sees that care is provided rather than allowing the patient to identify what care is most needed and actively assist in planning care.

Inclusion of Family and Significant Persons. Death involves not only the patient but the family, friends, and community. When you plan care that includes other important persons, you will see that each finds strength in the others and thus prepares more completely for the final loss. The family is encouraged to join in giving as much physical and emotional care as possible. At the same time, the hospice care team provides comfort to these persons.

Interdisciplinary Team. The hospice approach recognizes that it takes an **interdisciplinary team** to meet the needs of the dying sufficiently. The central hospice team, whether inpatient or outpatient, is usually composed of a primary hospice nurse, a social worker, a medical doctor, and a member of the clergy. Professionals such as nutritionists, physical therapists, occupational therapists, and others are added to the team to enhance the strengths of the patient as well as the quality of care. An essential element is a devoted group of volunteers, who perform many tasks in the home and with other members of the family. These persons also give an enormous amount of time and comfort to the patient.

Pain and Symptom Control. The hospice concept stresses the management of pain and symptoms. Because distressing pain and symptoms interfere with relating to others and with the enjoyment of life, the team, together with the patient, devotes much energy to managing pain and any symptoms that arise.

Bereavement Services. The intimacy of the patient, family, and hospice team make bereavement services a natural extension of the care that has been provided. All grieve in their own special ways, including the hospice team. The end of life is not the end of care. Contact and caring continue until those who remain find some degree of resolution and the strength to build new lives.

The Nursing Role in Hospice

Hospice care provides the nurse opportunities for a broadly expanded role. It requires special education, often given by hospice organizations. The methods of assessing patients' needs and assigning priorities to care are different from those of traditional nursing. Emphasizing the quality of life, rather than cure, requires some adaptations of standard nursing practice. For example, rather than carefully describing chest sounds, the hospice nurse focuses on what the patient sees as a problem and how it is affecting his or her life.

Hospice care allows the nurse to develop and apply new skills in bereavement counseling and understanding of family dynamics. The nurse also grows through the experience of loss, learning the wider meaning of care, growing close to families, and developing the inner strength to terminate that relationship when it is no longer needed and to move to new experiences.

Types of Hospice Programs

From the start, funding problems have been the most discouraging part of hospice development. Third-party payers (insurance companies) did not provide payment for hospice patients. In 1982 the government, through its Medicare program, recognized hospices and initiated a funding system for hospice care for those past age 65. This action was the first public recognition of hospices as a viable option to traditional care, whether in the hospital or at home. Since that time, many insurance carriers have begun supporting hospice services.

Many different hospice models have been developed. Some offer home care as well as inpatient care. Some are part of a hospital's services. Some hospices have special clinics where outpatients, their families, and the staff can share concerns. Day care services are being developed that provide a full day of physical, occupational, recreational, and medical management. These day care centers also offer nutritional advice, individual counseling, and other services. Some hospices with inpatient units offer respite care, which is short-term inpatient care designed to provide special attention to a patient's specific needs or a rest for family members who have been caring for the patient at home.

The National Hospice Organization

In several regions and states hospices have formed organizations to share developmental problems and successes. In an effort to coordinate the development of hospices in the United States, the National Hospice Organization (NHO) was established in 1978. According to the NHO bylaws, the organization has four main purposes:

1. To promote the principles and concept of hospice care for the terminally ill and their families.
2. To act as a clearinghouse for the dissemination of information and ideas to groups and individuals dedicated to the hospice concept.
3. To develop and promote educational projects for professionals and the public, focusing on the concepts of hospice care.
4. To oversee legislation relevant to hospice development.

Inherent in the general goals of the organization is a commitment to establishing and promoting standards for quality care. Hospice programs continue to seek adequate funding for existing programs and expansion of the movement.

Evaluation Related to the Dying Patient

The problems and nursing diagnoses change frequently in the plan of care for the dying patient. This occurs because the patient's condition may fluctuate and some needs are resolved while new ones emerge. You should review outcome criteria for problems frequently so that accurate evaluation can be made and the plan of care revised to daily meet the patient's needs.

Unique to the care of the dying, an important outcome criteria can be the attainment of peace and contentment. This is often obvious as the family lovingly comforts the patient and each other at the end of the person's life.

Support for Professional Care Providers

It is also important to give physical and emotional support to professionals who care for the terminally ill. Now that care of the terminally ill has become a specialty within the practice of nursing, the **burnout** syndrome has been identified. Burnout occurs because nurses are sensitive people who feel the loss of their patients deeply. This is as it should be. However, the experience of repeated losses can give rise to such signs of stress as fatigue, irritability, and insomnia. Some nurses have reported disruption of personal relationships.

In some facilities, nurses caring for dying patients regularly meet with a therapist as a group to explore their feelings. On a more informal basis, staff nurses provide mutual support by recognizing one another's feelings and encouraging each other to share losses. Research is continuing on burnout among nurses who are repeatedly subject to high stress, including loss, in their work. Ways are being sought to minimize this syndrome among nurses and other professionals.

The majority of nurses do not care exclusively for terminally ill patients. But even the loss of one patient can bring on feelings of despair and regret that more could not have been done. These feelings are natural but should be kept in perspective. Nurses should remember that they have made a difference by allowing the person and family to be more comfortable with one another in a supportive environment.

To be able to continue effectively in a stress-related profession such as nursing, you have to allow time for self-renewal. Taking time to engage in pursuits you enjoy and to talk with a peer or close friend (taking care to maintain confidentiality) is essential. As you share your feelings, you will develop a greater understanding of yourself and your personal philosophy about death.

For care providers who are family members or close friends of the person or child who is terminally ill, there are a variety of support groups. These care providers experience much of the same pain as do nurses. In addition, they may have a long history of personal involvement, so that questions like "Why is this happening to our family?" or "What more can I do to make things better?" are both natural and painful inquiries. Groups that include others going through the same process of losing someone have proven to be supportive and helpful. Sometimes these groups are led by nurses, often from hospices, who are skilled and knowledgeable regarding problems of loss. To refer a family member or friend, call your local cancer agency or a hospice group.

Grief and Mourning

Grief is a feeling of despair that begins at the moment when a person perceives a loss. It has been described by some as mental suffering and distress. This feeling is not always associated with death. **Mourning** is the normal psychological process that follows a loss and accompanies the feeling of grief. Mourning involves a series of tasks as one tries to resolve feelings of grief. The terms grieving and mourning are sometimes used interchangeably.

Life is, among other things, a series of losses: loss of a prize in school, loss of a desired position in one's working life, loss of a relationship due to divorce, and so on. Again, how one has coped with previous losses largely determines how one copes with the loss of a beloved person.

Benoliel (1985) states, "Loss is important because it signifies the departure or removal of someone or something that gave meaning to an individual or group. Both individuals and groups vary in their capacities to adapt in growth-producing ways to the losses associated with terminal illness." Martocchio (1985) lists two major purposes of grieving: first, it allows "facing the pain and recognizing what is happening is a normal part of life" and second, "grieving allows participating in the full range of feelings."

In the health care setting, grief is not confined to those who are dying and their families. Grief can be an appropriate response to other losses. The elderly stroke patient with a flaccid and useless arm is bereaved. The woman who loses a breast to cancer grieves. Hospitalized children separated from their parents grieve. The person losing sight grieves.

Some grieve over loss of health or independence almost as acutely as if it were loss of self (death). To grieve is a natural response to the loss of body parts and to illness-related changes in self-image and roles. Nurses should allow patients to feel sad and support them as they experience some of the tasks and stages described by Engel and Worden. To limit these only to the death experience indicates a lack of understanding grief.

The resolution of other losses often involves finding strengths to replace what has been lost. The young amputee may find new challenge in becoming a competent skier with the use of special devices. The physically limited person who has grieved well may seek new horizons through writing or painting. Losses can provide an opportunity for change that is both creative and rewarding.

Stages of Grief

The stages of grief are not very different from the stages of dying because in dying one grieves for oneself. This is a time to touch and be close to the survivor. The nurse should convey understanding that this is a difficult and sad time. Reassurances that tomorrow will be better ring hollow and are not helpful. Allowing survivors to share their feelings of rejection and depression and move through these feelings is of real value.

Engel (1964) described grief in terms of four stages: shock and disbelief, developing awareness, restitution, and resolution.

Shock and disbelief can accompany expected death as well as sudden death. Nurses are sometimes surprised when a family that has long expected a loved one to die expresses disbelief at the time of the death, but disbelief is a normal stage of grief. Sometimes people have to disbelieve before they can believe. This stage may recur days later, when a family member may say, "I still can't believe this actually happened." Quiet support is needed during this period (Fig. 41-9).

The unconscious mind, functioning protectively, allows painful reality to enter consciousness gradually. This mechanism of **developing awareness** explains why some people do not cry until some time after a death. As awareness becomes more complete, the survivors often feel fear, abandonment, or deep depression. Such depression is a painful but normal reaction and should not be considered abnormal.

Restitution is recognition of the death. Formal observance of the death may take the form of a funeral or memorial service, or a simple gathering of friends and family to share memories of the deceased. Some form of restitution is important to complete the grieving process. Death counselors report that families that abstain from any type of gathering, thereby denying themselves and others an opportunity to focus on the loss, do not come to resolution as soon or as smoothly as families that grieve more openly.

Resolution is sometimes referred to as replacement. This term is by no means intended to suggest that the loved one can be replaced, but rather that the survivors need to find replacements, different from what has been lost, in their lives. For example, a large number of widowed people return to school, some remarry, and others make career changes. Parkes (1973) calls one stage of resolution that may occur "the search," during which the survivor "seeks out" the deceased. There may be repetitive dreams of the deceased or the survivor

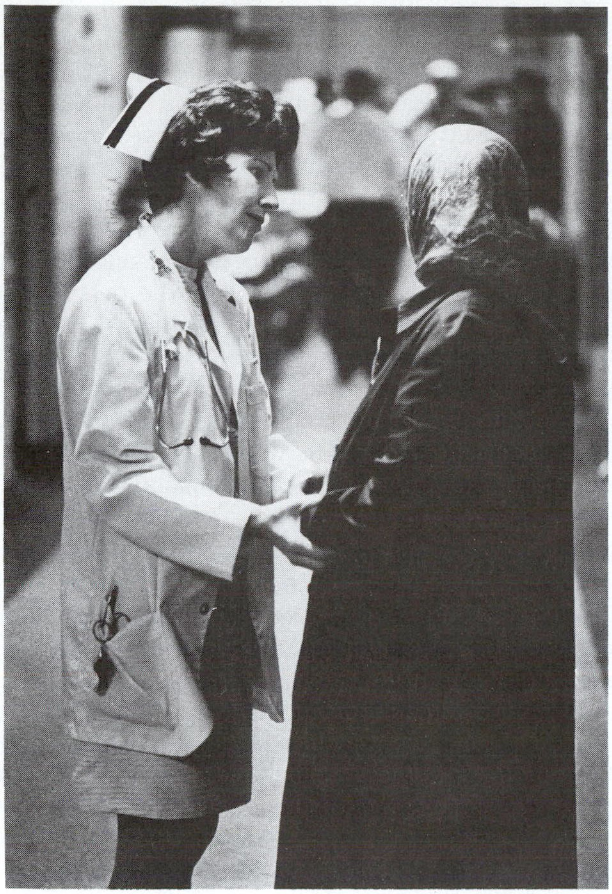

Figure 41–9. Family members need nursing support at the time of death.

may suddenly see someone who resembles the dead person and fleetingly but piercingly hopes that he or she is still alive. Callanan and Kelley (1992) also describe this process as being normal for some people. The nurse may have to reassure the survivor that this is a normal experience.

As a part of resolution, the survivor may make a frantic attempt to regain control of life by means of hasty decisions, such as selling a beloved home, and may turn to the nurse for advice. The nurse can be most helpful by trying to refocus the survivor's thoughts on the everyday changes that must occur rather than major ones that might be regretted later. Major decisions should be delayed. Realistic and constructive adaptive changes in the lives of the survivors should be supported, but it is not up to the nurse to suggest such changes.

Tasks of Mourning

Worden (1982) stated that mourning is necessary and that there are certain "tasks of mourning" that must be completed to regain equilibrium. These tasks of mourning go hand in hand with the feelings associated with grief.

Task I is to *accept the reality of the loss.* Denial may be an important temporary task as the person finds acceptance of the loss difficult. Even though the survivor may have a strong belief system and look forward to being united with the deceased in a life after death, the realization that this person is not ever again going to share life in the present is an important and difficult one. The survivor may feel anger at the loss incurred, but this anger can mean that there is beginning realization of the true reality of death.

Task II is to *experience the pain of grief.* Feeling the pain of the loss, although distressing, is normal and natural. The pain reflects recognition of what has ended and affirmation of the importance of that which has been. The care providers should be comforting and sharing but should not attempt to take away the sadness of this stage (which is not possible). Accepting the pain of bereavement can assist one in moving on to a new stage, that of adjustment.

Nursing Research: *Implications for Practice*

Aber, C. S. "Spousal Death, a Threat to Women's Health: Paid Work as a Resistance Resource." *Image* 24, 2 (Summer 1992): 95–99.

In an effort to determine if the paid work role had an impact on successful resolution of the death of the spouse, 157 bereaved widows, ages 55 to 75 were studied. The paid work role had previously been described as a role that increased self-esteem and well-being; was a source of income, personal identity, satisfaction; and gave life meaning. Instruments were designed to measure work history and work attitude. An analysis was also conducted of other variables, such as age and education. The study summary indicates that "paid work provides benefits to health during bereavement. By encouraging the paid work role for women, health care professionals may be directing women toward health-promoting and health-sustaining behaviors".

Task III is to *adjust to an environment in which the deceased is missing.* The intensity of this task depends on the relationship the survivor had with the person who died. Once the survivor clearly recognizes that the environment is not the same without the missing person, the task also becomes clear—to make adjustments in life to regain some level of comfort. This task moves the person away from preoccupation with the former life and relationship and on to a different, more viable orientation.

Finally, task IV is to *withdraw energy and reinvest it in another relationship.* Fulfilling this task does not necessarily involve direct replacement, but it is a refocusing of energy so that life takes on new meaning. Widows and widowers are often reluctant to remarry, perhaps because of fear of dishonoring the dead or fear of subsequent loss (Fig. 41-10). Worden quotes the Harvard Bereavement Study, which showed a 25% remarriage rate among those widowed, as compared to a 75% remarriage rate among those divorced. The care provider should remember that the choice is an individual matter and should support whatever the survivor chooses.

Normal and Dysfunctional Grief

To promote normal grieving or identify grieving factors that are abnormal, you should know what generally is considered normal and dysfunctional grief. Hofling and Leininger (1967) compared the person experiencing normal grief to the captain of a ship that has lost its anchor in a heavy sea. The person must put aside other things for a time and attempt to right the floundering ship. A substitute anchor is found and the sea also calms.

It is not unusual for much of the grieving process to occur even before the patient is biologically dead. The end of the relationship, because of coma or disengagement, may begin the grief mechanism. During the period of bereavement, the nurse may note the survivor becoming temporarily more dependent. In addition, the grieving person may develop symptoms or mannerisms of the deceased. Disturbances of the digestive tract, insomnia, heavy sighing, pacing, and unresponsiveness to others are other signs that may be seen. The person may want to talk about the deceased and spend a great deal of time discussing the attributes of the person who died. There may be an unrealistic view of the deceased as almost perfect or saintly. All these are normal reactions to grief. This may continue for months and then the individual gradually refocuses attention on reality. The grieving individual begins to return to usual functioning. Such phrases as "the way he would have wanted me to be" and "carrying on for her" are common.

When should grieving be over? The estimates of those who have studied the subject of death and dying vary widely. Some say that by the end of one year, sufficient grieving should have been accomplished. Others say that the length of time varies and the loss has been grieved for when the mourner has moved through the tasks and arrived at a level of comfort and productivity. It may be said that grieving has taken place satisfactorily when the survivor can remember the deceased comfortably, recalling both the pleasures and the disappointments of the relationship. However, as with most human processes, grief is not necessarily a linear process. Individuals may seem to have moved forward and then reexperience severe feelings of grief. This is particularly apt to happen on significant anniversary dates such birthdays and holidays or on dates when a significant event would have happened, such as a graduation. This does not mean that the person is not successfully resolving grief, but rather that some new loss (such as the loss of a hoped for graduation celebration) has just been acknowledged.

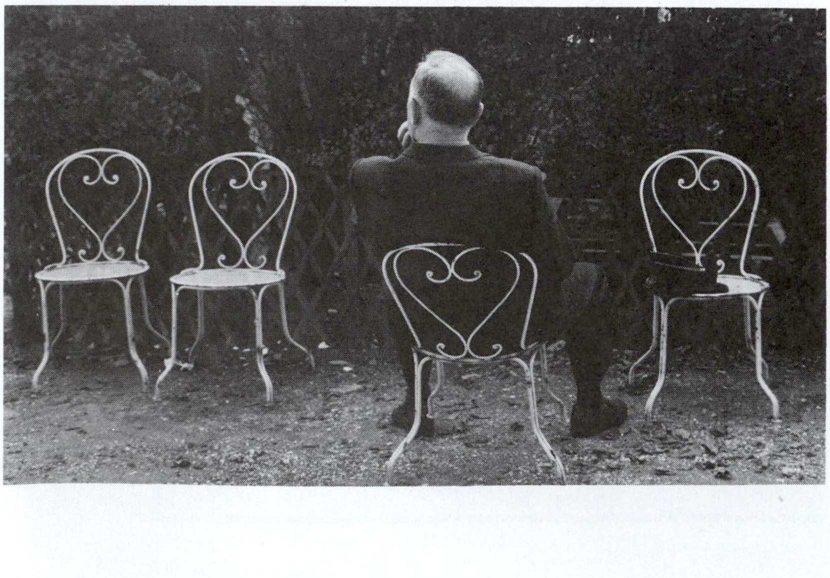

Figure 41-10. Replacement is often difficult for the elderly.

You will need to recognize incomplete or abnormal coping to provide help or possibly to refer the person to a grief counselor. Extreme exaggerations of the normal grief process, such as dependence to the point of nonfunctioning, persistent symptoms or mannerisms of the deceased, and constant dreams or even hallucinations of the deceased, constitute unsuccessful coping and may indicate a need for help. If the person is making self-destructive choices or failing to cope with daily living, then the grieving can be termed dysfunctional. Dysfunctional or abnormal grieving will be discussed as a nursing diagnosis.

Factors Affecting Grief

Several factors influence both the process and the resolution of grief. These factors have to do with past grief experiences, the investment in the person who has been lost, and sociocultural orientation.

Those who have had losses and resolved their grief in the past still experience pain with the new loss, but they may grieve in a different way from those for whom feelings of deep loss are new. In dealing with experiences, individuals tend to revert back to those coping behaviors that were successful in the past, and the grief experience is no exception. Older persons who have had recurrent grief often manage their grief well.

The extent of the survivor's investment in the individual who is being grieved for has an impact on the intensity of the grief. The grief response may be more intense, for example, for the young wife with children who had projected much of her life around having a family with a husband provider than for the young, financially independent wife who has a career of her own. This is not to suggest that each does not feel the pain of the loss, but rather that the pain is different.

The social and cultural background of the survivor often determine the style of grieving appropriate for that person. It is certainly not accurate to say that all Mediterranean persons grieve openly and vocally or that Northern Europeans grieve stoically. However, cultural patterns relating to grief have been observed. Social patterns predispose some persons to become immersed in neighborhood and community grieving, and others to remain isolated. For more discussion of social and cultural variables, see Chapter 33.

Finally, among other factors, the kind of death directly affects the bereavement process. There may be little or no time to prepare when the death is sudden. The absence of a time for anticipatory grief means that the first psychological "blows" caused by the sudden loss may have to be telescoped into a few brief minutes. The denial period may be elongated and resolution understandably delayed.

Assessment Related to Grieving

When there has been a loss or a perceived future loss, the person may experience normal grieving, anticipatory grieving, or abnormal grieving. Many areas should be considered when assessing the process of grieving, including an unobtrusive interview and assessment of any observable physical or emotional unresolved problems.

Interview

An informal interview is usually the most appropriate during the painful time of bereavement. You will often gather data by establishing a relationship that will allow a comfortable sharing environment. The interview should be focused on the survivor, identifying the physical and mental status of the survivor and determining ways that the nurse can help facilitate the normal grieving process. Each situation is different but the following guidelines may be useful during the interview or talking with others who are close to the bereaved person.

Previous losses experienced by the family or the person and coping mechanisms that were used. If there have been repeated losses within the family such as the loss of other family members or the loss of a job, the patient and family probably have developed a variety of coping skills. If the loss is a new family experience, not only are current coping skills used but new ones may have to be learned.

Cultural and religious background. Always assess the patient and the family's cultural and spiritual background. The terminally ill person may be associated with a different faith than the family's but hold past cultural connections. A variety of death beliefs associated with culture are discussed in Chapter 33.

Life span of family members; presence of elders or children. The experience of a family member's death from either an elder or child's view is unique. It is no less painful for an older parent to lose an adult child than if there is no age difference. Children who have been included throughout the person's dying process and allowed to grieve with the family have the opportunity for therapeutic resolution. You should assess the ages of the family members and the intergenerational relationships.

Relationship of the grieving person and other members of the family to the deceased. The grieving process is directly influenced by the type and quality of relationship to the deceased. This can be negative for the person who holds old grudges and on the death, feels guilty. Children can feel abandoned by the parent who is no longer present. A positive relationship can foster growth. Many survivors go forward with new purpose because the relationship was one in which support and love continue to endure.

Behavior that is withdrawn, disinterest in others in the environment, and change in dress or grooming. Assessment also includes behavior that may be considered normal for the immediate period of grieving after a death. If appropriate and confidential, you may want to talk with other trusted family members relative to your concerns.

Evidence of the appearance of physical problems. You will also assess the presence of any physical problems, particularly if these problems were not present before the illness and death of the terminally ill person. These signs may include excessive anorexia, nausea and vomiting, constipation or diarrhea, sleeplessness, fatigue, or weight loss.

Feelings being expressed such as anger, guilt, depression, fear, lack of self-worth, or suicidal thoughts. Survivors can feel overwhelmed so that their behavior or thoughts express negative and sometimes self-destructive tendencies. Your assessing and identifying such situations can help the person enter a counseling setting and resolve conflicts.

Physical Assessment

Physical concerns often evolve from the interview. The survivor may appear tired and listless. It may be apparent that the person has lost considerable weight and reports not feeling well. The extent and duration of the person's physical concerns is of importance because a degree of physical distress will occur with the normal grieving process. Because grieving is a normal and necessary process, caution must be used in writing accurate nursing diagnoses.

Nursing Diagnosis Related to Grieving

Two approved NANDA nursing diagnoses related to the grieving process are Anticipatory Grieving and Dysfunctional Grieving. Within each of these categories, you must additionally specify the etiology that is causing the individual to grieve. The overall category of grieving is used by some nurses as a nursing diagnosis when normal grieving is occurring.

Nursing diagnoses related to grieving have broad and appropriate application. A definition of grief written by Carpenito (1992) states, "A state in which an individual or family experiences an actual or a perceived loss (person, object, function, status, relationship)." From this definition, it is valid to use a nursing diagnosis at other times than a death event.

Nursing Diagnoses Related to Grieving

Grieving

Anticipatory Grieving

Dysfunctional Grieving

Alteration in Nutrition: Less Than Body Requirements related to recent loss of partner

Sleep Pattern Disturbance

Ineffective Individual Coping

Spiritual Distress

Grieving

Although grieving is a general category, not a specific nursing diagnosis approved by NANDA, many nurses believe that this human response pattern needs to be identified and appropriate nursing support planned for the individual. Increasingly nurses are suggesting that nursing diagnoses should not all pertain to abnormal or problem situations. The person who is experiencing a normal grief reaction would be assigned the general nursing diagnosis of Grieving, and appropriate nursing actions would be planned. Grieving itself is a genuine need for resolution and not an abnormality (see the sample Nursing Care Plan Related to Grief).

Anticipatory Grieving

The diagnosis Anticipatory Grieving describes a person needing "grief work" before an actual loss. The terminally ill patient goes through the grieving process because he or she is losing self. Others experience grief because they perceive the loss of someone who is important to them. Anticipatory grieving is truly grieving. It allows individuals to begin to come to terms with the anticipated loss before it occurs. In some instances, individuals have done so much anticipatory grieving that their period of mourning after the actual loss is shortened.

Dysfunctional Grieving

The diagnosis of Dysfunctional Grieving indicates that the grieving process is interfering with daily living and effective functioning. Problems arise when grief is prolonged or causes physical or emotional disruptions in

Nursing Care Plan

Sample Nursing Care Plan Related to Grief

Nursing Diagnosis	High Risk for Dysfunctional Grieving related to recent loss and no family members close by. **Supportive data:** Male survivor, 57 years old. Wife died 2 days ago. Has son living in city, daughter en route for memorial services from another state. States, "I think I'm losing my mind. I can't concentrate on anything, get done all I'm supposed to do."
Desired Patient Outcomes	**Short term:** To enter decision-making only to tolerance and comfort level. **Long term:** Successful resolution of grief to allow resumption of preloss mental functioning. States feels more like self, more confident. States feels more positive about being able to cope on a daily basis.

Nursing Action	Rationale
1. Assure patient that his feelings are normal grief reactions and that he is not "crazy."	Patient will feel relief when nurse, as a professional, assures person that grief reactions are "normal" and that sanity is being maintained.
2. Explore with patient, in a quiet environment, what decisions and tasks he feels are important for him to do and what might be delegated.	Allowing patient to determine tasks that are needed to be done but delegating maintains a level of control. Delegation conserves energy needed by the patient to move through the grief period.
3. With son, make list of tasks son can do and have patient approve.	Eliciting input from the patient's son validates accuracy of list of tasks so that priorities can be set.
4. Consult with daughter on arrival concerning patient's wishes.	Consulting daughter, on her arrival, helps her feel included and helpful in the family process of grieving.
5. Continue to tell patient you recognize his great loss and will support him and his family in any way possible.	Continued support of the grieving person facilitates successful resolution of grief.

life. The individual experiencing dysfunctional grieving may be creating problems rather than solving them, may be immobilized, or may be suffering severe somatic symptoms. The individual may personally identify that grief is dysfunctional because of the level of discomfort being experienced. There may be difficulties in concentration, labile affect, developmental regression, and alterations in sleep and dream patterns. You may identify that grief is dysfunctional by observing the person's responses and by careful interviewing in relationship to feelings and daily functioning.

Other Nursing Diagnoses

Diagnoses often present the disturbance as the problem and anticipatory or actual grief as the cause of the problem. For example, Altered Nutrition: Less Than Body Requirements related to recent loss of partner is one diagnosis. Another may be Spiritual Distress: Questions long-held belief system related to anticipated death of wife.

Planning and Implementation Related to Grieving

Desired outcomes for the person experiencing grief are certainly that in the long-term the grief will be successfully resolved and that the person will reinvest in life. However, short-term outcomes should also be identified and include the individual's coping with the demands of daily living. Additionally, the individual needs to be engaged in the process of grieving. Short-term outcomes might revolve around each of the tasks of grieving outlined previously.

Outcome criteria on which you can measure evaluation of actions also have to be considered in relationship to the individual. Outcomes include the willingness to express feelings and describe the meaning of the anticipated or real loss to the individual. Another outcome is the willingness to explore changes that will occur because of the loss. Finally, an important outcome may be the willingness to seek counseling to assist the person through the time of crisis.

Nursing encompasses all dimensions of human emotions. The joys of birth, growth, and recovery are parts of nursing that nurses are privileged to share. But the limitations of illness and the despair people experience in grieving are also integral parts of nursing that the nurse must accept. The nurse must also accept his or her own humanness and not hold back feelings of grief on losing a patient in whom nursing skills, hopes, and emotions were so heavily invested. In grieving along with the survivors, the nurse gives them perspective, strength, and comfort. With each loss, the nurse is enriched and becomes a better care provider.

Listening

The grieving individual benefits from the presence of a concerned listener who will listen to thoughts and feelings without judging them. Accepting the reality of the loss (Worden's task I) often requires that the individual talk about the event many times. Intervention demands careful listening to both the patient and the family so that you can determine whether or not there might be a problem with the grieving process. Often, you will find yourself as the support person when death is pending or has occurred.

Therapeutic Interaction

The techniques of therapeutic interaction are well suited to providing support to the individual who is grieving. Those not familiar with the work of grieving often discourage a person from discussing feelings in the mistaken belief that this makes them worse. Experiencing the pain of grief (Worden's task II) requires that the individual explore personal feelings. An opportunity for reviewing relationships, expressing sadness, anger, or guilt will assist the person to accomplish this task. Grief is painful, but talking about the pain does help the individual come to terms with it. This is not a one-time need, but will emerge again and again as new feelings arise and threaten to overwhelm.

Adjusting to an environment in which the deceased is missing (Worden's task III) requires that the individual explore potential actions, solve problems in difficult situations, and plan for life changes. These are tasks that many individuals accomplish more effectively when they are supported through therapeutic communication. You can help with encouraging effective problem-solving and guiding a person to avoid making drastic decisions while severely grief stricken.

Withdrawing energy and reinvesting it in another relationship (Worden's task IV) may not happen for a long time. When the individual does begin to consider this kind of change, a first step is often to discuss it in a relationship of trust. Survivors often feel disloyal or as if they are betraying the memory of the deceased when they prepare to move on with life. Acceptance of these decisions from others helps to reinforce that this is an appropriate life choice.

Supporting Physical Well-being

There are a variety of things you can do for survivors to preserve their physical well-being. Arranging for adequate nutrition, rest, and sleep is important because grieving requires both physiologic and psychological energy far above levels needed for daily life. Sometimes individuals will need help with contacting support persons in their family or community. You can encourage the individual to accept offered help such as the meal prepared by a friend or assistance with transportation.

Referral

You may refer a grieving person to a variety of resources for assistance. Sometimes the resources are to meet practical needs such as the social service worker who might help with finding emergency child care. The resource might be from the person's own social support network such as a trusted clergy member who could provide ongoing support. A support group of other individuals who have faced a similar loss may be useful. For example, Compassionate Friends, an organization for those who have lost children, provides ongoing support.

If you decide the dying patient or family needs special counseling, you can make a referral to someone educated in end-of-life issues. Some nurses have expertise in the practice of bereavement counseling. Others are also skilled in this area. Most communities have such services available through hospice programs, home health care agencies, churches, and clinics.

Evaluation Related to Grieving

It is difficult to evaluate many of the long-term outcomes but you can often evaluate more short-term criteria. Reviewing the outcomes, you will be aware of expressions of grief and the person's perception of the changes that will occur because of the loss. You will also be knowledgeable regarding whether a referral is needed and the willingness of the survivor to seek additional help.

Nursing Care Study
Managing Death Through a Team Effort

Tom Simmons was only 36, too young to die, thought Peg Johnson, RN, as she reviewed the physician's orders and prepared to write the nursing care plan for tomorrow's team conference. Tom was a new admission. She read over the nursing interview and began.

Physically, pain was the priority problem and the reason for admission. Tom's pain medication was not providing adequate pain relief. Tom was irritable and demanding with his wife, Sue, who was close to tears most of the time.

Socially, Tom has been at home, dealing not only with the pain, which kept him from sleeping, but also with boredom. He had been an engineer in a busy computer design firm and had lots of friends, but calls and visits from these friends over the last 7 months had diminished to the point of nonexistence.

Tom's mother visited daily, however, trying to cheer him up and talking about how the entire family would go up to the island next summer. "Doesn't she know I'm not going to have another summer!" Tom would yell after his mother left. Sue would rush from the room in tears.

Psychologically, Tom's boredom was increasing, along with his concern over his two sons, aged 8 and 11. Tom usually saw the boys only on Sundays, since his mother had taken them to stay with her until "Tom feels better." Although Sue did not like this arrangement, she agreed rather than make an issue of it. The school principal reported acting-out behavior problems on the part of the older boy, which had not existed before his father's illness. The younger boy was acting withdrawn.

The following morning, Mark Vatalie, a social worker, took a chair from the lounge and joined the others: Dr. Phil Bennett; Peg Johnson; Joan Seward, RN; Ken Tratner, the hospital chaplain; and Dick Brown, the hospital pharmacist. Peg presented her care plan assessment data; the discussion began. Over an hour later, the plan was complete and the team was anxious to start.

Peg would be the primary care nurse, relating directly to Tom's changing needs. Joan would provide backup and play a special advocacy role with Sue. Mark would consult with the teachers at school. Ken would introduce himself to the family, be available for any religious needs they might have, and consult with a family pastor if indicated. Dr. Bennett, after consultation with Dick on the best pain management, would coordinate the team and evaluate progress.

The next month brought hard work but considerable satisfaction. Much of the intervention went more smoothly than the team had anticipated. After trying various combinations of agents, the team found a pain medication that almost totally controlled Tom's pain. With his pain under control, Tom became much more communicative and able to express deep feelings of guilt over leaving Sue with the boys. Ventilating these feelings with Peg released much of his anger, and visits with Sue took on a new ease and meaning for them both.

Joan and Sue began to spend coffee breaks together, and Sue soon released her pent-up anger toward her mother-in-law. Joan and Sue decided it was time for the boys to be at home and to begin visiting their father, who would not be with them much longer. Tom's mother was a capable and well-meaning woman who wanted to help but could not accept the death she knew was approaching. Joan asked Tom's mother to join them for a coffee break and suggested that if she had some free time while at the hospital, the unit was badly in need of volunteer help to shop and write letters for other patients. Sue then said she was feeling alone

(continued)

Nursing Care Study (continued)
Managing Death Through a Team Effort

with Tom in the hospital and that if the boys could come home and Tom's mother could help with dinner two nights a week, she would appreciate it. Tom's mother turned to Sue with tears in her eyes. "Oh, it's so good to have you ask me to do something. It's so hard to lose a son, you know." She gently put her arms around Tom's mother and said how good it felt.

Mark met twice a week with the boys' teachers and also spent considerable time with the boys, both separately and together. He drove them to soccer on Saturdays, after which they had a good talk over hamburgers and went to the hospital to see Tom. Mark and the teachers decided not to discuss the changes in their behavior with the boys but simply to be available and supportive. Apparently as a result of the changes in Tom and Sue and their new relationship with Mark, the boys' behavior in school began to improve; though behavior changes were still apparent, they seemed to Mark a natural response to the home crisis.

Tom left the hospital 4 weeks after his admission. Home care nursing services were provided. Peg thought a great deal about Tom and Sue, and the team often asked her what she had heard. Two weeks after Tom's discharge, Sue called Peg to invite her to a small gathering to celebrate Tom's thirty-seventh birthday. Sue had invited a few friends and wives from the office, "And they're coming!" she said excitedly. It was a quiet, good time. Peg loved the evening, so different from the first day on the unit.

Tom died peacefully 6 weeks later at home, with his family and Peg nearby.

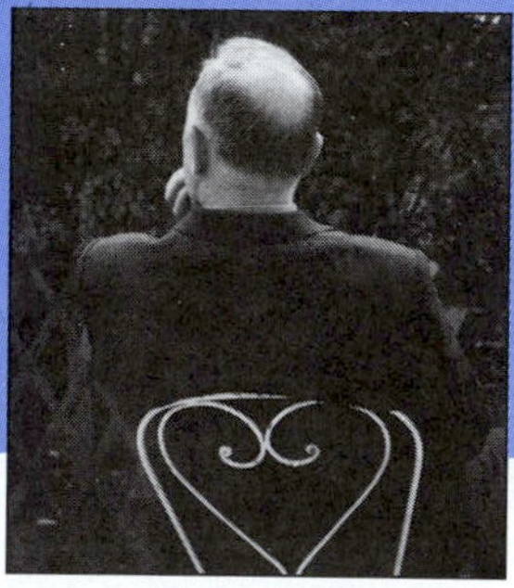

Key Points

- Persons facing the end of life, as well as their families and care providers, experience several stages: denial, anger, bargaining, depression, acceptance, and disengagement.
- Dying persons and those significant to them form a trajectory or perception of the course of the illness and its outcome. When the patient, family, staff, and nurses all have different trajectories, problems can develop in communication patterns and interpersonal relationships.
- Nursing process for the care of the dying addresses both the comfort needs of the patient and the psychological and spiritual needs. Nursing interventions are directed toward both the patient and the family and must be modified with the changing status of the patient. Ongoing evaluation is critical in the care of the dying to make timely changes in care.
- Nursing care of the dying child includes caring for the parents and siblings as well.
- The ability to communicate with dying children and their families can be greatly enhanced through the use of symbolic language. Troublesome thoughts and fears can be identified through a child's drawings.
- Nurses and families of the terminally ill must recognize the physical and emotional toll of caring for the patient. Taking time for enjoyable pursuits and sharing with others are helpful ways of dealing with this stress.
- The ethical issues resulting from the availability of modern medical technology have led to the development of advance directives for health care. When a patient signs an advance directive, it allows the physician to discontinue aggressive care when death is imminent and quality of life has decreased.
- Grief begins when an individual perceives that a loss is to occur. According to Worden (1982), grieving successfully involves the completion of the following tasks: accepting the reality of the loss, experiencing the pain of grief, adjusting to an environment in which the deceased is missing, and withdrawing energy and reinvesting it in another relationship.
- Factors affecting grief include past loss experiences,

the degree of investment in the deceased, and the social and cultural background.

- Abnormal grief responses often require intervention by specially educated persons.
- Hospice care is a new area in the care of the dying that encompasses self-determination for the dying person, inclusion of the family, an interdisciplinary approach, pain and symptom control, and bereavement service.

Study Questions

1. Give an example of the behavior a patient would exhibit during each of the six stages of the dying experience.
2. What is meant by the term "trajectory?"
3. Name the six stages of the dying process.
4. List three physical symptoms, other than pain, that are distressing to terminally ill person.
5. List three psychosocial problems that are commonly experienced by terminally ill persons.
6. Using knowledge of effective communication, discuss responses that are most facilitating when you are communicating with the terminally ill.
7. How do small children perceive that they are seriously ill?
8. List three needs each of the dying child, the parents, and the siblings.
9. What is "symbolic language" and how is it used in death/grief therapy?
10. What can care providers do to manage the burnout that can occur among people caring for dying patients?
11. What are natural death laws and why were they enacted?
12. When does grieving begin?
13. List Engel's four stages of grieving.
14. What are some of the characteristics of abnormal grief?
15. What is meant by hospice care?

Critical Thinking Activities

1. Read a book about death and dying after checking your selection with your instructor. In a small group, give a verbal report on your reading. Include the reason for the author's writing the book, the intended readers, and whether or not you agree with the manner in which the topic is presented.
2. Write a care plan for a seriously ill patient with the nursing diagnosis of "Powerlessness." Identify nursing actions that will help the person feel more in control.
3. Using references, write a five- to eight-page paper on one of the following topics. If another topic seems more appropriate or compelling, check with your instructor.
   a. Communicating with the dying patient.
   b. Supporting the family of the dying patient.
   c. Hope in relation to dying.
   d. Dying with dignity.
   e. I have just been told I have a fatal disease.
   f. My personal views about death (or what dying means to me).
4. Talk with a person in your community whose job or profession involves confrontations with death. Ask that person to share with you the education or training involved in preparation for the position and how he or she views the services provided to patients or families. Compare the information you have received with that of another student who interviewed a person in a different death-related profession.
5. Locate in your area two agencies or persons who provide bereavement counseling. Compare methods of referral, costs, methods of counseling, and types of clients served. Discuss these community resources in your clinical group.

Relevant Sections in Modules for Basic Nursing Skills

Volume 1 Module
Postmortem Care 33

References and Readings

Anthony, M. L. "No Code: Helping the Family Understand What It Means." *Nursing '93* 23, 2 (February 1993): 42–47.

Archer, D. N., and Clark, A. C. "Sorrow Has Many Faces." *Nursing '88* 18, 5 (May 1988): 43–45.

Aroskar, M. A. "Access to Hospice." *Nursing Clinics of North America* 20, 2 (June 1985): 299–309.

Badjek, L. A. "What You Need to Know About Advanced Directives." *Nursing '92* 22, 6 (June 1992): 58–59.

Bailey, M. M. and Arbour, R. "Getting Through Your First Code." *Nursing '93* 23, 6 (June 1993): 60–61.

Benoliel, J. Q. "Loss and Terminal Illness." *Nursing Clinics of North America* 20, 2 (June 1985): 439–448.

Blackburn, C., and Copley, R. "One Precious Moment." *Nursing '89* 19, 9 (September 1989): 52–54.

Britt, J. "What To Do When Your Patient Codes." *Nursing '90* 20, (January 1990): 42–43.

Callanan, M., and Kelley, P. *Final Gifts.* New York: Poseidon Press, 1992.

Carpenito, L. J. *Nursing Diagnosis: Application to Clinical Practice.* 4th edition. Philadelphia: J. B. Lippincott, 1992.

Cate, S. "Death by Choice." *American Journal of Nursing* 91, 7 (July 1991): 32–34.

Constantino, R. E. "Comparison of Two Group Interventions for the Bereaved." *Image* 20, 2 (Summer 1988): 83–87.

Descheneaux, K. "How Do I Ask?" *Nursing '89* 19, 1 (January 1989): 70–75.

DeSpelder, L. A., and Strickland, A. L. *The Last Dance: Encountering Death and Dying.* Palo Alto, Calif.: Mayfield Publishing Company, 1989.

Donius, M. "CPR Has Poor Outcome for Frail Elderly." *Oregon Geriatric Education Center* 4, 1 (Winter 1992-1993).

Engel, G. L. "Grief and Grieving." *American Journal of Nursing* 64 (September 1964): 93–98.

Gifford, B. J., and Cleary, B. B. "Supporting the Bereaved." *American Journal of Nursing* 90, 2 (February 1990): 48–55.

Glaser, B., and Strauss, A. L. *Awareness of Dying.* Chicago: Aldine Press, 1965.

Grassman, D. "Turning Personal Grief into Personal Growth." *Nursing '92* 22, 4 (April 1992): 43–47.

Hamilton, C. L., and Neubauer, B. J. "Hospice Nursing: Serving Ambivalent Clients." *Nursing and Health Care* 10, 6 (June 1989): 321–322.

Heiney, S. P. "Helping Children Through Painful Procedures." *American Journal of Nursing* 91, 11 (November 1991): 20–24.

Hofling, C. K., and Leininger, M. M. *Basic Psychiatric Concepts in Nursing.* 2nd edition. Philadelphia: J. B. Lippincott, 1967.

Jones, P. S., and Martinson, I. M. "The Experience of Bereavement in Caregivers of Family Members with Alzheimer's Disease." *Image* 24, 3 (Fall 1992): 172–176.

Kaplan, H. "It's Time We Helped Patients Die." *RN* 50, 11 (November 1987): 44–51.

Kowalski, S. "Assisted Suicide: Where Do Nurses Draw the Line?" *Nursing and Health Care* 14, 2 (February 1993): 70–76.

Kubler-Ross, E. *On Children and Death.* New York: Macmillan, 1983.

———. *On Death and Dying.* New York: Macmillan, 1969.

Kubler-Ross, E., and Warshaw, M. *To Live Until We Say Goodbye.* Englewood Cliffs, N.J.: Prentice-Hall, 1978.

Lillis, P. P., and Prophit, P. "Keeping Hope Alive." *Nursing '91* 21, 12 (December 1991): 65–66.

Linquist, D. "Frankie Was Never Satisfied Until She Made a New Connection with Life." *Nursing '92* 22, 7 (July 1992): 60–62.

Mahaney, B. "Working with Kids Who Have Cancer." *Nursing '90* 20, 8 (August 1990): 44–49.

Maher, M. E., and Strong, S. "Organ Donation: A Nursing Perspective." *Journal of Neuroscience Nursing* 21, 6 (December 1989): 357–361.

Maltz, A. "When the Patient Doesn't Want to be Resuscitated." *RN* 54, 2 (February 1991): 65–67.

Martin E. W. "Confusion in the Terminally Ill: Recognition and Management." *The American Journal of Hospice and Palliative Care* 7, 3 (May-June 1990): 20–24.

Martocchio, B. C. "Grief and Bereavement." *Nursing Clinics of North America* 20, 2 (June 1985): 333–341.

McKerracher, B. "How to Lend Support in a Crisis." *Nursing '90* 20, 11 (November 1990): 62–64.

Meyer, C. "'End of Life' Care: Patients' Choices, Nurses' Challenges." *American Journal of Nursing* 93, 2 (February 1993): 40–45.

Norris, G. "How to Manage Tissue Donation." *American Journal of Nursing* 89, 10 (October 1989): 1300–1301.

Parkes, C. M. *Bereavement: Studies of Grief in Adult Life.* New York: International Universities Press, 1973.

Petzold, H. G. "Gestalt Therapy with the Dying Patient: Integrative Work Using Clay, Poetry Therapy and Creative Media." *Death Education* 6, 3 (Fall 1982): 249–264.

Pfost, K. S., Stevens, M. J., and Wessels, A. B. "Relationship of Purpose in Life to Grief Experiences in Response to the Death of a Significant Other." *Death Studies* 13, 4 (April 1989): 371–378.

Post, H. "Letting the Family in During a Code." *Nursing '89* 19, 3 (March 1989): 43–46.

Quill, T., Cassel, C. R., and Meier, D. E. "Care of the Hopelessly Ill." *New England Journal of Medicine* 327, 19 (November 5, 1992): 1421–1427.

Snyder, R., and Westerfield, J. "Should Nurses Pronounce Death?" *Nursing '90* 20, 6 (June 1990): 41.

Strother, A. "Drawing the Line Between Life and Death." *American Journal of Nursing* 91, 4 (April 1991): 24–25.

Ufema, J. K. "Meeting the Challenge of a Dying Patient." *Nursing '91* 21, 2 (February 1991): 42–46.

———. "Helping Loved Ones Say Goodbye." *Nursing '91* 21, 10 (October 1991): 42–43.

Waltman, R. "When a Spouse Dies." *Nursing '92* 22, 7 (July 1992): 48–51.

Weber, G. "Tips on Implementing the Patient Self-determination Act." *Nursing and Health Care* 14, 2 (February 1993): 86–91.

Worden, J. W. *Grief Counseling and Grief Therapy.* New York: Springer, 1982.

Coping with Chronic Illness

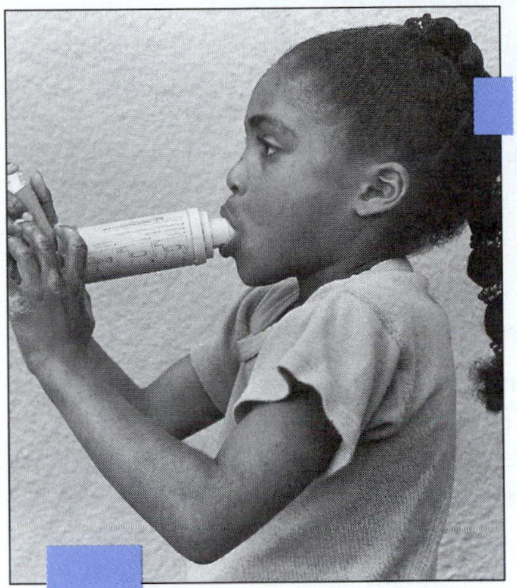

42

Objectives

After you have completed this chapter, you should be able to:

1. Define chronic illness.
2. Discuss the incidence and severity of chronic illness.
3. List four possible courses chronic illness may take.
4. Discuss factors that may influence the course of chronic illness.
5. Explain the special needs of the chronically ill person.
6. Describe the different ways in which the family and the client may deal with chronic illness.
7. Identify common nursing diagnoses related to chronic illness.
8. Discuss how nursing actions may be modified for the chronically ill person.
9. Explain differences between home nursing care and institutional nursing care.
10. Discuss the special needs of a caregiver in the home.
11. Outline and explain the factors that contribute to quality of life in a residential long-term care facility.

Study Terms

adherence
caregiver role strain
chronic illness
compliance
crises
deterioration
disease course
exacerbation
legitimizing
normalizing
quality of life
remission
respite care
social isolation

Outline

Ellis, Nowlis: Nursing: A Human Needs Approach, 5th ed. © 1994 J.B. Lippincott Company

- Avoidance and Management of Crises
- Control of Symptoms
- Adherence to Prescribed Care
- Management of Finances
- Time Management
- Legitimizing Versus Normalizing
- Education

The Family and Chronic Illness

- Negative Experiences Related to Chronic Illness
- Positive Experiences Related to Chronic Illness

Assessment

- Physical Assessment
- Interview

Nursing Diagnosis

- Altered Health Maintenance
- Dysfunctional Grieving
- Chronic Low Self-esteem
- Altered Role Performance
- Body Image Disturbance
- Noncompliance
- Ineffective Management of Therapeutic Regimen
- Powerlessness
- Social Isolation
- Impaired Home Maintenance Management
- Altered Parenting
- Altered Family Processes
- Ineffective Family Coping
- Caregiver Role Strain

Planning and Implementation

- Adjustment of Health Care Routines
- Health Teaching
- Nondirective Communication
- Assistance With Decision-making
- Support for Personal Resources
- Use of Community Resources

Evaluation

Home Health Care

- The Nurse's Role in Home Care
- Assessment in the Home Environment
- Planning and Implementation in the Home
- Caregivers in the Home

Residential Long-term Care

- Resident Versus Patient or Client
- Quality of Life

Chronic illness was defined by the 1956 Commission on Chronic Illness as "all impairments or deviations from normal which have one or more of the following characteristics: are permanent, leave residual disability, are caused by non-reversible pathological alteration, require special training of the patient for rehabilitation, may be expected to require a long period of supervision, observation, or care" (Mayo, 1956). This definition still identifies the hundreds of different conditions that can be considered chronic illnesses.

Some of the conditions that can be considered chronic are minor annoyances in the lives of individuals rather than major health problems. The seriousness of the problem may depend on the attitude of the person as well as the severity of the illness. For example, mild hay fever is uncomfortable and annoying, but it is not life threatening. However, it is a permanent condition and must be treated if the patient is to be comfortable and receive adequate rest. If the person with hay fever perceives it as a major problem, stays home from work and school, and expects others to assume all responsibilities, then the disease can become a major problem. On the other hand, an individual with severe arthritis may stay active, maintain all responsibilities, and view the arthritis as just one of life's difficulties. This person may not consider the arthritis to be a major problem in life.

Understanding Chronic Illness

The Incidence of Chronic Illness

Chronic conditions are present in individuals at every age level, but they occur more frequently as people grow older. These conditions vary in severity from nonspecific, dry, itching skin to heart rhythm disorders; many individuals have more than one chronic condition. Table 42-1 identifies the incidence of chronic conditions in differing age groups. Because the number of elderly persons in our society is increasing, chronic illness is a growing health problem.

Chronic illness does not always cause limitations in activity. In fact, the majority of those with chronic illness carry on lives that they do not perceive to be limited (Table 41-2). Limitations in activity caused by chronic conditions are much more prevalent in the older population (Table 42-3), a fact that has major implications for nurses as they plan for care of individuals with chronic conditions.

Table 42–1. Incidence of Selected Chronic Conditions* by Age

Age (years)	Cases of Chronic Conditions
Under 18	515.7
18–44	1283.8
45–64	2934.7
65–69	3362.8
70 and over	3977.6

*56 of the most common chronic conditions were included in the survey question that produced these figures. Reported in cases per 1000 population. Some individuals have two or more chronic conditions. Data from National Center for Health Statistics, *Vital and Health Statistics: Current Estimates from the National Health Interview Survey, 1990*. Series 10, No. 181, Table 57, p. 82, Hyattsville, Md.: USDHHS, Public Health Service, Centers for Disease Control, December, 1991.

The Course of Chronic Illness

Each chronic illness has a course, which may be affected by many factors. By the **disease course** we mean the ongoing subjective and objective evidence of the illness, which is indicative of the progression of the disease process within the body. Usually a person is not aware of the course of a disease unless there are manifestations such as signs or symptoms. Depending on the illness and the person, courses may vary greatly. Some illnesses start on one course and change to another. Some chronic illnesses follow a relatively certain course.

The course of *remission* and *exacerbation* is one of fluctuation. When the illness is in **remission**, symptoms are partially or completely absent. When there is an **exacerbation**, symptoms intensify. Either frequent or infrequent remissions and exacerbations may be associated with chronic illness. With some conditions, the fluctuations themselves undergo changes: for example, the exacerbations become generally less or more intense and the periods of remission longer or shorter. Two conditions that typically follow a course of remission and exacerbation are multiple sclerosis, a degenerative nervous system disease, and arthritis.

A course of **deterioration** is one in which restoration does not occur. The progression of the disease is downward as it becomes more severe and creates more problems. Severe cases of diabetes and renal disease often take a gradual downward course. Remission and exacerbation may combine with a deteriorating course. Each exacerbation leaves a more serious condition as further tissue destruction takes place. Some forms of multiple sclerosis combine remissions and exacerbations with a course of deterioration.

Some chronic illnesses have an *uncertain future*. Some individuals experience steady deterioration, yet others experience remissions and exacerbations. Often the reasons for these differences are not clearly understood. Many of the rheumatic disorders such as rheumatoid arthritis and lupus erythematosus fit this pattern.

Some diseases that have gradual deterioration result in a *terminal outcome*. This happens with chronic obstructive pulmonary disease (COPD) that gradually moves the person toward death. However, not all conditions causing deterioration lead to death. The person with severe rheumatoid arthritis may become more and more disabled, but life is not threatened by the condition. Diseases that have remission and exacerbation may also have a terminal outcome when a particular exacerbation is extremely severe. For example, a person with chronic high blood pressure may have an exacerbation of extremely high blood pressure that results in death through rupture of a small vessel in the brain.

Table 42–2. Self-assessed Health Status

Age (years)	Excellent	Very	Good	Fair	Poor
	(Percent of persons in each category)				
Under 5*	53.2	28.1	15.8	2.6	0.3
5–17*	52.3	28.0	17.4	2.0	0.3
18–24	44.6	31.1	20.3	3.5	0.6
25–44	41.6	31.2	21.0	4.9	1.3
45–64	29.2	27.1	27.7	10.9	5.1
65 and older	17.1	22.9	32.3	18.7	8.9

*Health Status determined by parent in child too young to respond.
Data from National Center for Health Statistics, *Vital and Health Statistics: Current Estimates from the National Health Interview Survey, 1990*. Series 10, No. 181, Table 70, p. 112, Hyattsville, Md.: USDHHS, Public Health Service, Centers for Disease Control, December, 1991.

Table 42–3. Persons with Activity Limited by Their Chronic Illness

Age (years)	% With No Limitation	% With Activity Limitation
Under 18	95.1	4.9
18–44	91.2	8.8
45–64	78.2	21.8
65–69	64.1	35.9
70 and over	61.7	38.3

Data from National Center for Health Statistics, *Vital and Health Statistics: Current Estimates from the National Health Interview Survey, 1990.* Series 10, No. 181, Table 67, p. 106, Hyattsville, Md.: USDHHS, Public Health Service, Centers for Disease Control, December, 1991.

Factors that Influence the Course of Chronic Illness

Various factors influence the course of chronic illness for any individual. These include the presence of other illness, other life stressors, compliance, attitudes, social support, and the availability of treatment.

Presence of Additional Illness

The presence of an additional illness may change the course of a chronic illness, causing a less favorable outcome. For example, if a person with severe diabetes also develops COPD, the risk of respiratory infections is increased. The decreased ability of the body to subdue infections because of the diabetes may alter the course of this person's COPD to one of terminal outcome.

The individual with a neuromuscular disorder that makes movement and locomotion difficult may experience a severe deterioration in ability during a time immobilized by a fracture. Sometimes this deterioration may be impossible to reverse. The elderly person with marginal function may fall, break a hip, and subsequently never be able to live independently.

Presence of Other Stressors

The number of other stressors in life can also alter a disease's course. Chapter 6 discusses the hazards of accumulating stressors. The chronic illness itself is a major stressor and minimizing or adding other stressors will affect its course. Many individuals with chronic illness identify that when stress becomes high their illness worsens. Conversely, decreasing stress may cause a reduction in the symptoms of a chronic illness. An example is the person with a chronic back injury. During times of low stress, this individual may remain pain free through exercise, appropriate rest, and careful body mechanics. When severe stress occurs, these measures alone may no longer be sufficient to preserve pain-free function and anti-inflammatory medications may also be needed.

Degree of Compliance

The degree of *compliance*—that is, to what extent the ill person follows a prescribed regimen of treatment—can affect the course of a disease. Where a treatment has been proven effective, the acceptance of such treatment may offer an individual the chance to change the course of the illness to one with a more favorable outcome. The diabetic who carefully manages insulin and diet to maintain a normal blood sugar level has fewer complications than the one who does not maintain control. The person with hypertension who takes medications and keeps blood pressure under control will have a lower risk for adverse consequences, such as stroke.

Attitudes

The chronically ill person's view of the disease and general outlook on life have strong potential for actually changing the course of the illness to some degree. Although holistic health does not preclude illness, a positive mind set can affect one's health. Health, itself, can be a state of mind (see Chapter 5 for a full discussion of this topic). Cousins (1979) explored this concept from a personal viewpoint, focusing on the power of humor to change the course of illness. His management of his own chronic illness was characterized by taking personal control and developing a positive mental state.

Various writers have explored the concept of "attitudinal healing," by which they mean altering one's perception of what is happening. One study (Ellis, 1990) found that perception of health status in individuals with rheumatoid arthritis was more closely related to their perception of personal control in their lives than to their physical disabilities.

Availability of Treatment

The treatment modalities available or appropriate to the illness are a strong factor in determining its course. New treatments for chronic illness are being investigated and developed constantly through medical research. One rather extraordinary example is the dramatic strides being made through organ transplant programs. A limited number of chronically ill individuals have had the organs from deceased persons transplanted to replace their own diseased organs. Although transplant is usually a last resort, organ transplants may create a "turnaround" in the course of an illness.

Much less dramatic, but equally important, are those who have seen their lives changed through the federal support for orphan drugs. These are drugs that will benefit only a few individuals with a rare illness and therefore would not be profitable for companies to research and produce without subsidy. Since the federal government has strengthened support for programs of research and development, increasing numbers of drugs are being made available.

Trajectories of Chronic Illness

In Chapter 41, we discussed trajectories—the way the person perceives the path or course of the illness. The person who is chronically ill has a *trajectory* or perception of the direction of that course. Other people who have relationships with the chronically ill person also have trajectories. As terminally ill persons grieve for loss of self, chronically ill persons mourn loss of body function. Trajectories may be influenced by the factors that affect the course: the presence of other conditions, the appearance of symptoms, the effectiveness of treatment, the burden of other stressors, and the manner in which the person and those who have relationships with that person feel about the illness.

At times, the chronically ill person may optimistically believe that the illness is beginning to remit or improve. The sign of a new symptom or the awareness that someone who is close is in despair about the situation may deflect the trajectory to one of hopelessness. In forming trajectories, it is important to include hope. Beland (1981) states that "hope is real and involves becoming involved in a process" (p. 175). Trajectories based on hope are to be encouraged when one is dealing with chronic illness. This is no less true for the family and significant others than for the person who is chronically ill.

The trajectories of the family and the ill person may be the same sometimes and at variance at other times. For example, if a new symptom appears, the chronically ill person may suddenly see a more foreboding trajectory. The family members who are not as directly involved with the symptoms and who have dealt repeatedly with such crises may not change trajectory, leading the ill person to view them as unsympathetic.

Nurses who care for the chronically ill form trajectories, just as they do for terminally ill patients. These may agree or disagree with the trajectories of the chronically ill person and the family. Disparity in trajectories of the course of a chronic illness is just one of the issues that can be a problem for patients, families, and nurses.

Factors that Influence Adaptation to Chronic Illness

The ability to make the many adaptations needed for chronic illness is affected by a variety of factors in life. Larkin (1987) pointed out some of the most significant. She included the care received, the technology available, social support, developmental level, communication abilities, and economic resources.

Care Received

The care received by a client is an important factor in adaptation to chronic illness. The physicians and nurses who help this person may assist toward independence and self-care or may foster dependence on others as a mode of action. The physician may provide current therapy and monitoring that minimizes symptoms and complications. Nurses may provide education, monitoring, and other aspects of care to give continuing support. If quality care is lacking, the individual may be unable to manage the illness, leading to increased symptomatology, increased complications, and lessened independence.

Technology Available

Technology is important in today's health care world. Technologic innovations are able to help many chronically ill persons to lead more normal lives. Insulin pumps for diabetics and continuous ambulatory peritoneal dialysis for some individuals with kidney failure are just two examples of the ways in which technology may support greater wellness in the chronically ill person. Robotic devices are being developed to assist those with spinal cord damage. The continued improvements in technology and the appropriate use of current devices are important in assisting the chronically ill to adapt.

Social Support

Family relationships provide the undergirding social support that enables individuals to use their energies for adaptation. When families work well, they provide the chronically ill person with enhanced self-esteem and assist with effective problem-solving. When families can work together and agree on goals and priorities, they are more likely to be effective than when they disagree.

Families are not the only source of social support. Friends, neighbors, fellow church members, and coworkers may all be a significant part of the individual's social support network. These people may provide contact with the world, encouragement, friendship, and a sense of self-worth for the individual as well as providing more concrete assistance in the form of transportation, assistance with some tasks, or daily monitoring telephone calls.

The support (or lack thereof) and attitudes of those around the chronically ill person can alter the course of illness. Many of the cues a person gets from others have emotional effects that then affect a physical state of illness or well-being. Social support enables a person with chronic illness to adjust the burdens of life when necessary. Caring concern from others may support personal feelings of worth and enhance self-esteem. Conversely, being seen as incapable may undermine personal resources and create feelings of powerlessness and hopelessness.

Developmental Level

Developmental level is a significant factor in the ways in which the patient and significant others respond to chronic illness. Our society expects children to be untouched by chronic illness or death and may unintentionally isolate the child and family faced with either of these circumstances. Special fears are associated with chronic illness in children. Will physical growth patterns be interfered with? Will the child's intellectual potential be fully realized?

The child may feel disadvantaged because of interference with the normal activities of childhood. These feelings may elicit different responses from different children. Some children may become overly demanding of attention, often to the detriment of siblings. Others find their limitations an opportunity for growth and development of special talents and skills (Figs. 42-1 and 42-2). The family also may respond to the chronically ill child in different ways. Parents may feel unrealistic guilt for the presence of the illness and become too involved in the demands of the child. Parents can find their own lives restricted because of problems such as the difficulty of finding baby sitters for their chronically ill child. Other parents encourage their chronically ill child to pursue interests the child might not have experienced had he or she not been confined or limited by illness.

Although the response of the chronically ill young or middle adult are more mature than those of the child, they may be similar in basic content. Chronic illness can excuse the person from ordinary responsibilities and create demands that family and friends be oversolicitous. On the other hand, many chronically ill persons relate deeply to others because they have a special appreciation for life.

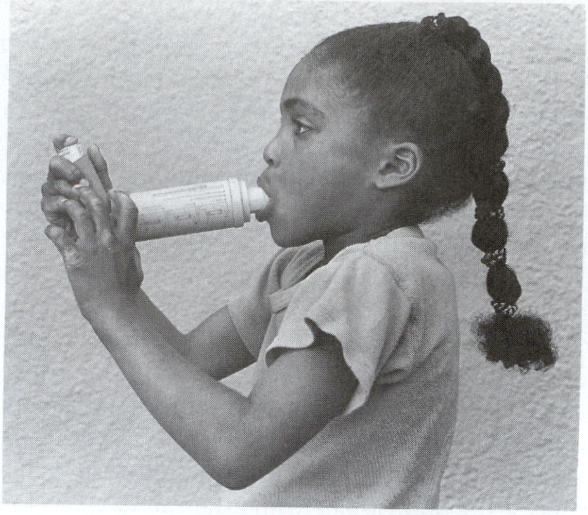

Figure 42-1. This child does not perceive life with a disability as limited.

Unfortunately, chronicity has come to be viewed as almost normal as the life span has stretched into the 80s and beyond (see Chapter 20). Actually, adjusting to chronic illness in the later years is difficult, particularly because older persons are also experiencing other losses, such as the death of significant persons. Adult children may view the onset of chronic illness in the parent as threatening to them as well. They may be forced to assume more of the care of the older person, which can result in intergenerational disruption. Fortunately, even with the burden of chronic illness, many older persons call on strong coping behaviors from earlier years and react with persistent emotional strength and good humor.

Communication With Others

Much of the adaptation to chronic illness relies on communication with others. Communication may assist the individual with self-esteem, provide a window to a wider world, and support the feelings that others care. Communication from caregivers, friends, and family members helps the individual to be a positive participant in the world.

Economic Resources

The cost of care for a chronic illness may be high. Medicines, medical devices, special foods, alterations in the home environment, and bills for medical services and

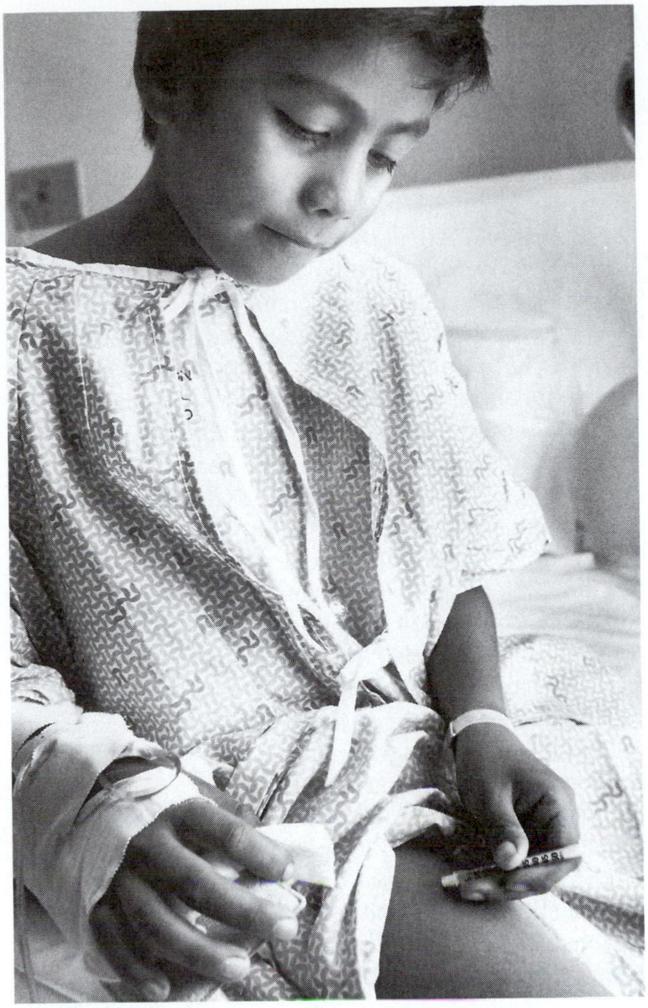

Figure 42-2. Even children must learn complex techniques of health care.

ongoing care are costly. Those who have the economic resources for the health care required will have an easier time with adaptation. A current concern is the lack of available economic support for many aspects of chronic illness.

In countries with some form of national health coverage, such as Canada, health care costs may be adequately covered. However, when people must rely on private health insurance, as in the United States, many problems arise. Most health insurance plans are structured so that there is good coverage for accidents, emergencies, and hospital care, but little coverage for continuing care of a chronic illness. Some individuals with chronic illnesses are unable to obtain health insurance at all because most policies exclude coverage for preexisting conditions. Still others are uninsured because they are unable to work and are not able to afford insurance. This then leaves the individual without financial resources for acute illness or exacerbation.

Special Needs Created by Chronic Illness

Strauss (1984) and others have written extensively about the special needs of those who have chronic illnesses. Although not all authors have identified the same set of needs, most speak to the particular difficulties the chronically ill have in meeting their basic needs for a normal life as well as the special needs imposed by their illnesses.

Strauss and colleagues identified avoiding and managing crises, controlling symptoms, adhering to prescribed care, managing finances, managing time, legitimizing versus normalizing, and education as the seven major needs of the chronically ill person.

Avoidance and Management of Crises

Most chronic illnesses are characterized by acute **crises**, times when active disease seriously interferes with daily living. These crises usually require medical care and often require hospitalization. They may also cause deterioration in the patient's overall health status, leaving the person more disabled than before the crisis. Therefore, a large part of the management of chronic illness is aimed at the basic goal of avoiding these crisis situations.

Adherence to prescribed details of care is often important in avoiding crises. Controlling the contributing factors such as stress is also important. However, care alone is not always enough. Crises may occur because of a change in the disease itself. The person and the family members need to learn what to do to try to avoid these crises. It is also important that they be able to recognize the development of crises early to obtain health care before the situation becomes overwhelming. When crisis occurs, the entire organization of life may have to be changed. Some family members may have to assume different roles. The ill person can no longer meet obligations to family, friends, and employer. If crises occur frequently, the whole of life may be disrupted.

Control of Symptoms

Symptoms may be controlled by medications or treatments or by lifestyle changes. A problem with gas from a colostomy, which is socially embarrassing, may be managed by careful attention to diet. Unavoidable symptoms may be managed so that they are not disruptive to the person's lifestyle. For example, incontinence may be managed by the use of waterproof, disposable undergarments.

Coping with constant symptoms requires many resources, financial as well as personal. Part of coping is managing the physical symptoms themselves, but perhaps an even greater part is managing the feelings associated with having symptoms as part of one's life. The difficulty of the latter task is greatly affected by the degree of visibility of the symptoms.

Adherence to Prescribed Care

Adherence—or **compliance**—is a subject of concern to most health professionals who work with the chronically ill and refers to carrying out all treatments conscientiously, taking medications as ordered, and modifying life activities as directed. Although many health professionals act as though nonadherence resulted only from *lack of knowledge*, that is only one of many possible reasons for nonadherence. Simple forgetting may cause noncompliance on the part of someone with the best of knowledge and intentions. Sometimes exercises are omitted because an individual is busy and is unwilling to take the time for them. Some therapies recommended are expensive, and the person may not have the financial resources for them. Health care practices that are visible to others may be omitted out of embarrassment or feelings of modesty. Sometimes a person omits prescribed care because of a wish to feel normal, not different. We will discuss some of these special concerns individually.

The Health Belief Model explains the likelihood of an individual taking action to either prevent illness or promote health. This model, originally proposed by Becker and others (1977) and further adapted by Pender (1984), identifies factors that influence compliance. An important aspect of this model is the identification of compliance as a complex issue in which many different factors affect behavior. Individual perceptions about the importance of health, the significance of personal control, the threat of disease, personal susceptibility, the benefits of the actions, and the value of early detection are all significant. These perceptions are modified by age, gender, ethnicity, education, and interpersonal and situational variables. The model also identifies that barriers to taking action exist as well as cues that support taking appropriate health actions. As nurses work with individuals to support compliance, their assessment must include these many factors. Some of these factors may also be altered to increase the likelihood of the person taking appropriate health action.

Management of Finances

As discussed previously, anyone with a chronic illness is faced with ongoing costs for medical supervision, medications, treatments, and equipment. For some people such costs may amount to thousands of dollars a year. In addition to the costs of health care, there may be hidden costs. Transportation to medical appointments creates additional expense. Household assistance may have to be procured because of inability to carry out all tasks. Wages may be lost because of absences. Food costs may be higher because of special dietary needs. These are just a few of the ways that life becomes more costly for those with chronic illness.

The individual and family must learn to set priorities for spending and seek out resources within the community. A disproportionate share of the family's resources may go for support of the family member with a chronic illness. Although others may agree that this is essential, they may at times resent that their share is limited.

For some, the financial demands are not a matter of reordering priorities, but a matter of life and death. They simply do not have the money to pay for the care needed. Elderly people on limited Social Security incomes may find themselves faced with a monthly income of $500 and bills of $250 for rent and $200 for medical treatment. The choice may be between food and medicine. Social service programs providing care for those with long-term chronic illnesses are limited and tend to be fragmented.

Often no solution is apparent for the chronically ill who are attempting to manage part of life independently. If they are unable to work at all and are therefore eligible for financial assistance, they receive help with medical care. If they have some means of personal support, they are usually not eligible for financial assistance for medical care. Assistance for kidney dialysis treatment is one exception. Through a federal law often called "Medicare-Kidney," dialysis is paid for everyone who needs it, regardless of financial status, through the Medicare program.

Time Management

Many of the treatments, exercises, and care procedures prescribed for the person with chronic illness are time consuming. Particularly if they need to be carried out at specific times of the day, the rest of life must be organized around the time demands of the illness. Even when some flexibility in time is possible, the individual may be reluctant to be flexible for fear that excessive flexibility may lead to exacerbation of symptoms or even a crisis. The time demands affect not only the person with the chronic illness, but also the entire family. This is especially true when the ill person is a child. Not only may daily life be changed, but taking vacations and attending special events may become impossible because of the time demands of caring for the person with a chronic illness.

Legitimizing Versus Normalizing

Strauss (1984) identified two opposing needs of the person with chronic illness—the need to legitimize and the need to normalize—that are often in conflict within the person. **Legitimizing** is establishing the illness and disability as real and acceptable to others. **Normalizing** is establishing that one is a normal individual able to live a normal life despite the illness.

Legitimizing often requires that the person share symptoms with others, explain the illness, and set limits to activity. In doing this, the individual is focusing on the illness and the ways in which it creates differences from others. Doing this is necessary to gain social approval for not willingly participating in all aspects of life. For example, the man with a low back injury that is invisible to others must explain it carefully to find acceptance when he allows his pregnant wife to carry the groceries. Legitimizing seems to encourage the display of symptoms and may result in secondary rewards for remaining in the sick role. However, legitimizing may be necessary for a person to continue to manage symptoms and prevent crises. If a person has COPD, it may be essential to legitimize this condition in the minds of coworkers to establish a nonsmoking work environment successfully.

In normalizing, the person tries to create the impression of being a completely normal person without disability. This process tends to support a full and positive lifestyle. It encourages independent action and not being dependent on others. However, it may lead to actions that are not compatible with optimal control of symptoms and prevention of crises. For example, on a camping trip with friends, a diabetic teenager overwhelmingly concerned with normalizing may eat what everyone else is eating and neglect to take insulin.

It is easy for the objective observer to say that what is needed is an appropriate balance between these two needs. But for the person with the chronic illness, the exact nature of the proper balance may be difficult to determine. It often takes trial and error and help from others to finally arrive at a workable balance. This balance may change from time to time. A person may need to normalize in a work setting and legitimize with family members, or legitimize when symptoms are exacerbating and renormalize when symptoms have receded. Individuals may make conscious choices regarding the effect of legitimizing on the quality of life. Certain people may choose a course that is likely to lead to earlier death because of a strong belief that the current quality of life obtained through normalizing is more important than the additional length of life that might be obtained through legitimizing.

Education

The child with a chronic illness has special educational needs. Fatigue and symptoms may make daily participation in class a problem. Exacerbations may interfere with school, causing poor performance or failure. Disabilities may make attendance in a conventional classroom difficult. The child may have special physical needs that create concerns for the teacher. Some children with chronic illness have learning difficulties related to brain function. In the past, these children were often denied adequate educational opportunities and therefore were handicapped in additional ways as adults.

There have always been some special schools for children with multiple handicaps. These were associated with a university or were expensive private facilities. Although they provide a fine education, they are accessible to only a small number of children.

In recent years, society has recognized that education is a right of all children no matter what their illnesses or disabilities. This has resulted in laws that require schools to make accommodations for students with disabilities and adapt education to special needs. Special classes are available for those with vision and hearing problems. Support is provided for teachers who have children with disabilities in the mainstream classroom. Children often need a strong advocate to ensure the provision of adequate educational opportunities.

The Family and Chronic Illness

Because of its ongoing nature, often of lifetime duration, and the need for adaptations to meet the demands of daily living, chronic illness creates both negative and positive experiences for the family, nuclear and extended. Experiences vary greatly, depending on the person, illness, and lifestyle, but we can look at some important experiences that commonly occur when one member of the family has a chronic illness.

Negative Experiences Related to Chronic Illness

Perhaps most visible are the negative experiences such as the financial drain and demands on personal resources. The illness usually affects the financial resources of the family. The need for intermittent health care, medications, and possibly assistive devices may impose an extreme burden on some people. Families may have to reevaluate spending practices, setting aside some pleasures to pay for items necessary for the afflicted person to maintain function. The many financial demands were discussed in terms of the individual person's needs.

Either consciously or unconsciously, the ill person can become manipulative. Manipulation is the use of indirect behavior to control other people against their will. The chronically ill may want or even demand unreasonable consideration. Sometimes relationships or activities may be changed. The patient's admonishment that something would be done "if you really cared about my health" is an obvious example of manipulative behavior, in which instilling guilt is being used to control a family member's behavior. The family's activities may change to accommodate to rather than adjust to the health status of the ill person.

Illness may require that persons in the family assume roles with new or different responsibilities. Sometimes changes are unwelcome and accepted reluctantly. To take on more of the household tasks, teenagers may have to give up some of their social life, which is important at their developmental level. Responsibilities for the yard and gardening, once a joy to the ill person, may have to be assumed by a member of the family who finds them arduous and unpleasant. Roles may reverse, with children taking care of parents. Such a reversal may be tolerable for a short period of time, but the ongoing responsibility often turns it into a more negative experience.

With the chronic illness of one member may come lifestyle changes for the entire family. A once outgoing and community-involved family may become isolated as collective attention is focused on the ill member. Adaptations may have to be made that remove other family members from friends and activities that were important in their lives. For example, the family may have to move to a structurally different type of housing adapted for the handicapped.

The family is faced with an ominous negative feeling that the future is uncertain. People like a sense of stability in their lives, and living with a chronically ill person undermines that feeling. Unexplained friction and frequent irritability may result, making daily living difficult.

Positive Experiences Related to Chronic Illness

In the face of numerous potentially negative experiences, many families of those with chronic illness respond with growth and maturity. They find joy in what life presents and report that many positive experiences are related to living with chronic illness in the family.

The state of being chronically ill can provide new opportunities for creativity. The chronically ill person may find new projects or activities that the entire family can enjoy. Music and art may substitute for the hiking once shared. Although other members may choose to continue hiking trips, and they should be encouraged to do so, learning to experience music and art through the one who is no longer able to hike benefits the family. In other ways, compensatory activities and interests may be developed. Some of these compensatory activities may lead to new life choices for occupation or education.

The presence of chronic illness and its threat to the health of a family member may result in an affirmation of the family by each person. Members of the family may reexamine the reasons why each is important to the other. New individual strengths evolve, and family values are strengthened. Friendships developed with others who have similar problems may be particularly deep and lasting because they are based on sharing of problems and inner feelings.

The presence of chronic illness can bring about a reassessment of values. What is really important in life? Who is important? Illness may force the family to define the quality of living. Many people have stated that only through the ongoing crisis of a chronic illness was true satisfaction in living reached, both for the ill person and for the family.

Family members may find that the illness of one member requires that other members learn new skills. These might be in relationship to caregiving but may also be in relationship to daily living. A person who has never driven may learn to drive and gain independence and increased self-esteem through this new ability. The learning of new skills required because of the illness can affect many other areas of life on a permanent basis. Family members may see this as a positive benefit to themselves.

The illness of any family member may highlight the value of wellness for other members of the family. They may recognize that wellness is not to be taken for granted and may change their health practices in the direction of improved health. They may have regular checkups, use seat belts, or adopt other such health-sustaining practices. They may state that they better appreciate being well and are more aware than they used to be of the daily advantages that good health provides.

Assessment

The assessment of the person with chronic illness should focus on the manner in which that person is dealing with the illness and its disabilities. Rather than identifying deficits as singular problems, it is more appropriate to assess the adaptations to the deficits and the strengths of the individual.

Physical Assessment

Physical assessment should include all need areas discussed in the text. Special attention should be given to those areas that are affected by the disease state. You will want to learn what ongoing symptoms are present and how the person is currently managing these. Those problems for which the person has not found solutions should be clearly identified.

Interview

Communication techniques are used to make your psychosocial assessment of the individual with chronic illness. The patient's feelings about the illness and how it is affecting life are as important as physical status. You will need to learn how the person is coping with the chronic illness and the many stressors it brings.

Of particular relevance in your assessment are indications of grieving. Many potential losses are associated with chronic illness: the loss of the invulnerable self, the loss of ability, the loss of occupation, the loss of relationships. As the individual confronts these losses, grieving occurs. Successful resolution of this grief supports effective adaptation.

The interrelationship between patient and the family and the family's response to the illness and to the patient are especially meaningful in chronic illness. In addition to interviewing the patient, it is helpful to interview family members. The patient may be present when the family is interviewed, but people may be more open in discussing their feelings if the interview is private.

Nursing Diagnoses Related to Chronic Illness

Altered Family Processes related to the chronic illness of a family member (specify illness and which family member)

Altered Health Maintenance related to lack of interest in or knowledge regarding routine health care

Altered Parenting related to child with (specify chronic illness)

Altered Role Performance related to (specify disability)

Body Image Disturbance related to (specify chronic illness)

Caregiver Role Strain related to (specify personal problems with care giving)

Ineffective Management of Therapeutic Regimen related to difficulty in time planning

Impaired Home Maintenance Management related to symptoms of chronic illness (specify symptoms)

Ineffective Family Coping (compromised or disabling) related to chronic illness of a family member (specify chronic illness and which family member)

Noncompliance related to belief systems about own ability to control symptoms or prevent crises

Powerlessness related to uncertain course of chronic illness (specify illness)

Social Isolation related to symptoms associated with chronic illness (specify symptoms and illness)

Nursing Diagnosis

The chronically ill person may have any of the nursing diagnoses that have already been identified in relation to the specific psychological and physiologic needs of the person. However, the nurse needs to be particularly alert to the possibility of some problems related to the special needs of the chronically ill. Some of the diagnoses identified by the North American Nursing Diagnosis Association (NANDA) are especially pertinent to the chronically ill; a brief discussion of these follows.

Altered Health Maintenance

A diagnosis of Altered Health Maintenance relates to managing those areas of life that are not part of the disease state and includes all health promotion activities. For example, a chronic illness that increases fatigue may interfere with proper exercise, which is essential for health maintenance. The long-term consequences of lack of exercise affect many aspects of health. Or a child with a chronic illness may not have had appropriate immunizations. Health maintenance needs to be recognized as important to the individual regardless of the status of the chronic illness.

Dysfunctional Grieving

Some individuals continue to grieve in ways that interfere with their coping with chronic illness. The person may express distress over the loss and have difficulty in meeting basic needs and performing self-care activities. Recognition that grieving is normal and supporting normal grief resolution will assist in preventing dysfunctional grieving.

Chronic Low Self-esteem

Chronic Low Self-esteem is the diagnosis used to describe the person who has negative feelings and thoughts about the self on an ongoing basis. Because the illness is chronic, negative feelings about the self may also persist. Negative thoughts and feelings might be identified by the statements the person makes about self-esteem or by behaviors that indicate denial of reality. The patient may express hostility toward those who are healthy and may be unable to make decisions.

Altered Role Performance

The diagnosis of Altered Role Performance reflects a perception of the self as unable to function in appropriate roles in life. Of particular importance in this diagnosis is the recognition by care providers that the perception of the client is the key factor. Factors such as dependency or the attitudes of others and loss of physical abilities to carry out previous life tasks might underlie this perception of self. For example, if a woman with a chronic illness states that she is unable to function effectively as a mother because she cannot engage in active play with her children, this diagnosis would be appropriate. Perhaps you believe that the central element of effective mothering has nothing to do active play. This might help you to formulate strategies for nursing intervention but would not negate the presence of the nursing diagnosis.

Body Image Disturbance

Because chronic illness creates visible physical changes in many instances and changes in function in others, body image disturbance is common. One patient with body changes created by the corticosteroids used in her treatment kept a picture of herself from before the treatment. She showed this to all visitors and care providers, saying "This is what I really look like!" She was disturbed by her current appearance and found it difficult to accept. Body image disturbance is discussed in Chapter 34.

Noncompliance

Noncompliance is an informed decision not to follow a prescribed health care regimen. Noncompliance and its many causes were discussed in the previous section. Noncompliance is an appropriate nursing diagnosis when the individual is not carrying out the prescribed plan of care. Identifying the etiology of noncompliance is essential to planning intervention (see sample Nursing Care Plan Related to Compliance With Prescribed Medication).

Ineffective Management of Therapeutic Regimen

The individual with a diagnosis of Ineffective Management of the Therapeutic Regimen demonstrates a pattern of choices in daily living that are not effective in meeting the goals of treatment. The person may be aware that choices turn out poorly and seek help or may indicate that he or she is having difficulty in managing the treatment plan. In other instances, health care providers become aware that personal health management is ineffective when complications or adverse effects occur. Further assessment then reveals that the person is not managing the therapeutic regimen effectively.

Powerlessness

A chronic illness may progress in a manner that leaves the patient feeling totally without power to change any aspect of life. The person who feels powerless will not make decisions, expressing the belief that results would not be changed by any decisions made. Powerlessness is reflected in statements such as "It doesn't make any difference what I think" or "I don't care; do anything you want to." Health care providers may inadvertently reinforce feelings of powerlessness by communicating an attitude that only professionals are really able to understand and plan for care. More often the literature is reporting on programs in which even complex care is put in the hands of patients. These programs demonstrate that patients do not need to be powerless (see Chapter 36 for further discussion of powerlessness).

Social Isolation

People become socially isolated by their chronic illnesses for a variety of different reasons. Social interaction requires energy and time, and some individuals just do not have enough of either to relate to others. Transportation may be difficult; lack of money may restrict leisure pursuits. Some chronic illnesses are visible, and embarrassment or fear about the reactions of others may lead to social isolation. Those suffering from **social isolation** may indicate that they have few friends. When asked about support persons, they may not be able to think of anyone they could ask for assistance in any way.

Impaired Home Maintenance Management

The individual may independently identify difficulties with home maintenance and seek help in resolving them. Those who do not seek help and keep saying that they will be able to manage independently may be trying to normalize. The key factor in deciding whether the diagnosis is appropriate is whether health or safety is threatened by the inability to manage the home. Comfort is another consideration, but it must be defined by the individual involved. For example, a person with severe arthritis may have a house in which you would not be comfortable because it does not meet your standards

Nursing Care Plan

Sample Nursing Care Plan Related to Compliance with Prescribed Medication

Nursing Diagnosis	Noncompliance with self-administration of diuretic related to distress over effects of medication. **Supportive data:** Has gained 4 lb since last visit. Ankles "puffy." States does not take diuretic because "I can't leave the house when I have to go to the bathroom so often.
Desired Patient Outcomes	**Short term:** Takes diuretic as ordered. **Long term:** Shows no signs of fluid retention (no edema, no weight gain, no fluid in lungs). Expresses feelings of satisfaction over control of health problems.

Nursing Action	**Rationale**
1. Review reason diuretic is needed—to decrease load on heart.	Understanding of rationale for medications may increase compliance.
2. Discuss her pattern of response to diuretics.	Individuals may respond uniquely to medications. Understanding these individual responses provides a basis for individualized planning.
3. Discuss at what time in her schedule having to urinate would be least disruptive.	When the health care regimen does not disrupt daily living, adherence is more likely.
4. Encourage her to select a time for taking diuretic based on her schedule for the day.	Adherence is supported by personal control over actions.
5. Inform her that occasional omission (not more than once per week) for important occasions is acceptable.	An overall pattern of compliance is more effective in maintaining health than is an erratic schedule.

of neatness and cleanliness. However, if the person expresses satisfaction with the home and the home is clean enough to be healthy and neat enough not to pose safety hazards, a diagnosis of Impaired Home Maintenance Management is not appropriate.

Altered Parenting

Parenting a child who has a chronic illness is extremely difficult. Even the ordinary tasks of feeding and bathing can be surrounded in complications when the child has a serious health problem. Coping with the problems of discipline and setting limits are even more difficult for parents. How do you discipline a child who has breathing difficulties whenever she feels stress? How do you provide opportunities to explore the environment to a child with motor deficits? How do you provide growing independence to a child with blindness? These are just a few of the problems facing parents of chronically ill children. A child should not be raised without limits and discipline, and normal developmental needs should be met. Learning to manage parenting with a special child often requires outside help and support.

Altered Family Processes

The special time requirements, the needs for special care, and the lessened ability of the ill person to perform some tasks often lead to changes in family processes. This is true no matter which family member has the chronic illness. Family members may have less time, energy, and ability to relate to one another. The result may be a lack of communication, changes in roles with resulting discomfort, and feelings of fear, anxiety, or anger. Quarrels may develop within the family. Family members may express feelings of guilt or anger to health care personnel. Interaction between family members may be limited. If these patterns continue, they will be destructive to the family unit and to the individuals within that family unit. This diagnosis applies to families in which members were previously able to relate to one an other and work together to resolve problems.

Ineffective Family Coping

When the family engages in destructive behaviors, family *coping* may be compromised. Problems usually relate to the fact that personal resources are inadequate to manage the stressors involved. Tension arises within the family. A diagnosis of Ineffective Family Coping relates to a family that was not functioning well before a family member was diagnosed as having a chronic illness and then is further disrupted by chronic illness. NANDA has suggested that this diagnosis can be modified to indicate whether the family is compromised or completely disabled by the situation.

Caregiver Role Strain

Caregiver Role Strain is a nursing diagnosis that refers to the caregiver's felt difficulty in performing the caregiver role. The individual may report that he or she does not have the resources to provide care or may report that caregiving interferes with personal life. The caregiver may perceive conflict either internal or with the family around issues related to caregiving. Feelings of stress and loss related to the changes that caregiving has caused are common. **Caregiver role strain** may occur when the caregiver does not have the physical resources for the task because of age or personal health problems. The caregiver may not be developmentally able to provide care for another. Poor relationships between the care recipient and the care provider contribute to role strain. When role strain is not already present, but factors exist that contribute to caregiver role strain, the diagnosis of High Risk for Caregiver Role Strain is used.

Planning and Implementation

Strauss (1984) points out that the individual with chronic illness often receives fragmented care in the current health system; most care is directed to a specific health problem, and no one looks at the overall relationship of the health problem to quality of life. The definition of nursing developed by Carnevali (1993) outlines the domain of nursing as the "interface between health status and daily living." This definition of nursing suggests that the nurse is the health care worker who should accept responsibility for working with a chronically ill person in such a way as to enhance the quality of life.

The nursing diagnoses listed in this chapter did not relate to management of specific symptoms or organ dysfunctions but to the problems an individual might develop in the totality of life. In planning intervention for these nursing diagnoses, you need to look at the person's total lifestyle as well as the health care status.

Adjustment of Health Care Routines

In some instances nursing intervention will be aimed at adjusting the health care routines to make life more acceptable. The nurse can be a liaison with the physician and others on the health care team to help interpret the patient's needs in regard to life in general. Adjustments can range from rescheduling appointments to modifying dietary prescriptions.

Health Teaching

For those working with the chronically ill, a large part of nursing care will always be health teaching. However,

Nursing Issues and Trends: *Empowering Individuals With Chronic Illness*

Chronic illnesses are responsible for the majority of the disability and death in all of society. Medical care does not have cures for those with chronic illness. Actions by health care professionals do not create the most long-lasting improvement or change in well-being. Chronic illnesses must be managed by the individual with support from professionals. We need to refocus our attention to strategies that empower individuals to evaluate all recommendations in light of their own experiences, to take charge of their own lives and health, and to seek optimum wellness.

you must be prepared for patients who know more than you about their own condition. Patients are the experts on their own feelings and responses. In addition to being experts in regard to their own feelings, they may also be experts on the disease process itself. Many have lived with their conditions for many years and have experienced forms of therapy that are only history to today's health care workers. They may know from personal experience just what the side effects of drugs are and how certain treatments affect them. Approaching such patients as if they know nothing is demeaning to their integrity. However, blindly assuming that an individual has all the necessary knowledge is also a disservice. The key is to assess thoroughly before beginning any health teaching (see Chapter 16).

Nondirective Communication

Often the chronically ill person or a family member is in need of a nonjudgmental person with whom to explore concerns and express feelings. Most people do not see nurses as authoritative or threatening, and thus they often will talk freely with a nurse. The nurse may have a long-term relationship with the person through a home health agency or an outpatient setting. Setting the stage and providing time for interpersonal communication is not always easy. Reimbursement for nursing care from insurance companies and other funding sources tends to be focused on tasks the nurse does, and the "talking" nurse may not be valued as much as the "doing" nurse. Having a supportive and knowledgeable listener helps to relieve anxiety and tension. Just knowing that someone else cares about the burdens being experienced may be enough to help the person with adjustments that are necessary (see Chapter 13).

Assistance with Decision-making

The nurse may be sought out for advice in decision-making. Giving advice is a grave responsibility and should not be accepted unless you have the background and experience to understand the total situation. In many instances, giving advice is inappropriate because the decision should be based on the values and beliefs of the patient. In such a situation, you would use communication skills to assist the person to solve problems and make a personal decision. This process was discussed in Chapter 13.

However, giving advice in regard to care is an important part of providing support to those with chronic illness in the family. A nurse can be helpful by answering factual questions about appropriate treatment, side effects of drugs, dietary needs, and so forth. When patients ask questions such as "What foods can I substitute for . . . ?" "How do I get a child to swallow that medicine?" "Should I go to see the physician?" and "Is this considered an emergency?", they need accurate, clear, and direct responses.

Support for Personal Resources

Miller (1992) sees overcoming powerlessness as a central factor in coping with chronic illnesses. She identified power resources that may be maximized by effective nursing care. These resources include physical strength, social support, psychological stamina, positive self-concept, knowledge and insight, energy, motivation, and a belief system that supports hope. Some of these have been discussed specifically above. A patient can preserve energy by planning for rest and by carefully identifying which activities have priority. A belief system that affords hope and positive self-regard supports coping.

Use of Community Resources

A wide variety of government, private, social, and personal resources are available, but many individuals lack understanding of what they are, how they relate, and how to use them. There are groups that discuss problems such as parenting a chronically ill child, groups that provide social activities in a safe environment, and groups that provide motivation and support for those with specific conditions (Fig. 42-3). Chapter 15 and Appendix E list some national voluntary organizations that may have local chapters in your area. You should explore the health care resources in your own community to inform patients whose needs they could meet (see sample Nursing Care Plan Related to a Family Coping With Chronic Illness).

Two major resources for caring for those with chronic illnesses that cause continuing symptoms and disability are home care and residential long-term care facilities or nursing homes.

Evaluation

One of the adjustments that those who work with the chronically ill must make is in the type of desired outcome established. Health care workers as a whole tend to be oriented toward achieving wellness. Wellness in the sense of absence of disease or absence of signs and symptoms is not a possibility for many with chronic illnesses. Wellness must be defined by the person involved in terms of quality of life and desired lifestyle (Fig. 42-4).

Long-term comprehensive outcomes are needed in the care of the chronically ill person. The entire health care team, the patient, and the family should work together to develop these outcomes. Such outcomes help to direct activities of health care workers and patients alike. For example, a comprehensive outcome for an

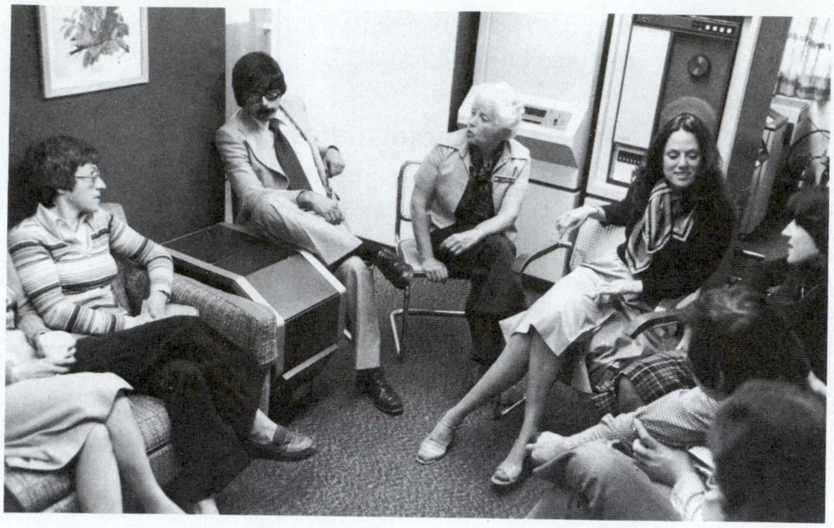

Figure 42-3. A support group may be an appropriate community resource to assist the patient.

adult with a stroke might be "Return to complete self-care in the home environment."

In addition, short-term outcomes are needed to provide more concrete guidance and feedback on performance. One aspect of self-care with which the nursing staff might be working is transferring. A short-term outcome might be "Transfers self from bed to wheelchair without assistance." Sometimes even smaller increments must be identified as desired outcomes. Each part of the transfer may be listed as a desired outcome. Achievement of these small goals reinforces that progress is being made.

When evaluating the desired outcomes you have established in regard to nursing diagnoses for the chronically ill person, a critical aspect is evaluation by the patient. This is the person who must live with and manage the chronic illness. Therefore, that person's evaluation will guide you as you determine whether additional planning or intervention is needed. From your perception, you may believe that the person has made adequate progress, but for the individual involved it may not be enough. Conversely, you may think that much more should be accomplished at the current time, yet the patient is content with the progress made. Sensitivity to these differences will make you a more effective partner in health care with the person who has a chronic illness.

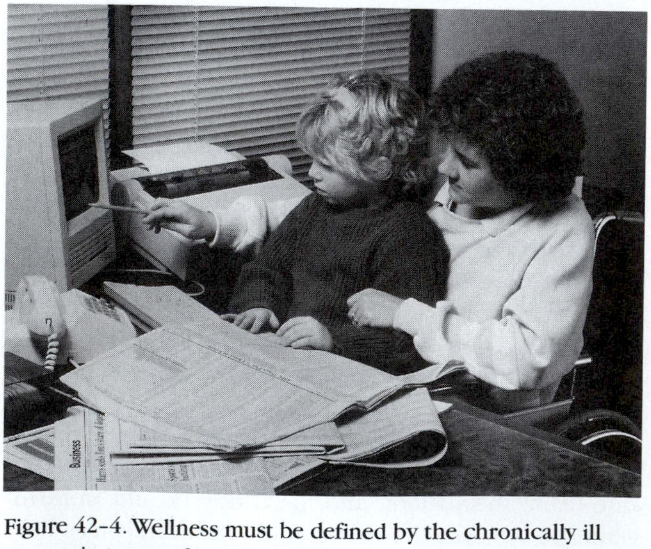

Figure 42-4. Wellness must be defined by the chronically ill person in terms of quality of life.

Home Health Care

Care of individuals with illness or disability in the home is not a new phenomenon. Families have been providing health care in the home as far back as we have records. Since early in this century, professionals have provided some care in the home through private duty nursing or periodic nursing visits. What is new about home health care is the extent to which sophisticated treatments are being performed in the home and the amount of professional involvement in teaching individuals to provide their own quality health care. One reason for this change is that hospital stays are shorter, with the result that patients are being discharged with many health care needs unmet. Another factor is the recognition that support in home care may make the difference between an individual's being able to remain independent in the community and needing some type of residential care. The underlying purpose in all home health care is to provide quality health care in the least restrictive setting while maintaining maximum independence for clients and their families.

To do this, home health care agencies typically provide a wide variety of services, ranging from home

Nursing Care Plan
Sample Nursing Care Plan Related to a Family Coping with Chronic Illness

Nursing Diagnosis

Altered Family Processes related to care of wife with multiple sclerosis.

Supporting data:

Patient now requires assistance for all activities of daily living.

Teenage daughter fixes all meals and cleans house.

Husband provides all direct care and works evenings, so daughter is home when he is at work.

Daughter stated, "I know I should be more understanding, but sometimes I just get tired of being responsible."

Desired Patient Outcomes

Family discusses feelings about caring for patient.

Family develops realistic plans for time off for both husband and daughter.

Patient care remains of high quality as defined by the patient.

Nursing Action	Rationale
1. Arrange specific times to talk with husband and daughter to encourage expression of feelings.	Verbalizing feelings assists individuals in effective coping with those feelings.
2. Inform family of family support group at Multiple Sclerosis Society headquarters.	Support groups may provide an avenue for more effective individual coping.
3. Contact the Visiting Nurse Service regarding regular assistance for time off.	Respite for caregivers helps to prevent caregiver "burnout."
4. Talk with patient regarding her expectations from family.	Identifying expectations clearly will form a basis for planning.
5. Encourage family to discuss problems and feelings openly and to plan for time off for husband and daughter.	Open family communication is an effective avenue for resolution of problems and concerns.

health aides, who will assist with personal care and simple household tasks, to registered nurses and therapists, who provide skilled care. With the use of home health care services, many individuals are able to stay in their own homes or in the homes of family members and avoid residential care. No matter how fine the quality of care in a long-term residential facility, most individuals prefer the independence and autonomy provided by an independent living situation.

The Nurse's Role in Home Care

The nurse who goes to the home of a client is in one sense a guest in another's home. This distinguishes the relationship from what it is in a care facility, where the client is the person who enters the health care environment. At home, the client is on familiar territory and will feel more comfortable and less anxious than in the facility. However, the reverse may be true for the nurse.

The nurse also has far less control over the environment as far as care is concerned and also over how care is managed between visits. The nurse may suggest that living arrangements be altered, identify other community resources that may provide assistance, and develop plans for ongoing care. However, the decision to follow through on those suggestions is controlled by the client and family. Until the nurse recognizes this and accepts it as a positive factor, frustration may occur.

Some home health care nurses begin a home care relationship by outlining the services they can provide and telling the ways in which they believe nursing would assist the client and family. The client is then asked to consider whether this meets what he or she perceives as care needs. When a decision is made by the client, a contract may be written to outline the responsibilities of each party in the care relationship.

Most reimbursement programs for home care provide registered nurse care for three distinct areas: skilled monitoring of signs and symptoms to detect complications, deterioration, or problems that require intervention; skilled technical care, such as intravenous medications; and health teaching for both the client and the family to ensure that they possess the knowledge and skills needed for home care. Home health care nurses recognize that support for psychosocial needs may also be important for maintaining the client's independence. However, reimbursement is difficult to obtain for these needs.

Another emerging role for the nurse in home care is that of case manager. When many individuals and organizations are involved in care, the process operates more effectively if one person coordinates services. Because the nurse has the skills for assessment, the opportunity for assessment in the home visit, understands the health care system, and has the skills to work with others in the system, the nurse has been the logical choice for this role in many agencies.

Assessment in the Home Environment

Assessment in the home requires more attention to the environment than does standard assessment in the institutional setting. In the institution you may be able to take for granted the lighting, heating, and adequate plumbing. This is not true in the home environment, where the major obstacles to self-care may lie in parts of the environment that the client sees as unchangeable. The creative nurse may perceive ways in which the environment may be adapted to better support independence and self-care.

Physical assessment must be made without some of the tools taken for granted in the institution. Lighting may be less than ideal for observation. Quiet, to be able listen to breath sounds, may be impossible to achieve. These are challenges to the nurse responsible for physical assessment in the home.

Psychosocial assessment may take on added depth and be more comfortable in the home. Rather than relying on verbal reports, the nurse is able to observe interactions, see responses to stressors in daily living, and observe coping strategies in action. The entire realm of social and cultural life for the patient and family may also be observed. You may see the religious beliefs displayed, the health beliefs acted on, and the values unveiled.

Planning and Implementation in the Home

Creative planning is often required when adapting care procedures to the home environment. Equipment is available through rental or purchase, but not all types of equipment will be economically feasible for a client. The nurse may need to understand insurance and Medicare and Medicaid reimbursement rules. When equipment is needed on an ongoing basis, it is more reasonable to obtain it for home use than when its need is for only a single treatment or short time. Thus, the nurse may help a client to obtain a commode for elimination, but for another client there will not be a handy intravenous pole to hold an irrigation container. The nurse will have to devise an alternative within the home setting.

Supplies such as sterile dressings may be expensive. To some individuals receiving home care who are changing their own dressings over leg ulcers, clean technique, rather than sterile, is taught. When the client uses careful clean technique, his or her own immune system may be able to resist the small number of familiar organisms that are introduced. The patient's home is different from the institutional setting, where concern for the wide number of different organisms and the presence of drug-resistant organisms makes sterile technique essential.

Techniques may need adaptation for patients with a variety of physical disabilities. Those with vision difficulties may need special adaptive devices to learn to use an insulin syringe. An individual with one arm paralyzed from a stroke will need to manage tasks in a new way. Although the initial teaching of individuals with these kinds of problems occurs in the hospital, often hospital teaching can only be introductory because of the patient's early discharge.

Health teaching encompasses not only the simple aspects of daily living, but also instruction in highly technical skills. Infants who still need ventilator support are being sent home in some areas of the country. Individuals with cancer who have surgically implanted central intravenous lines requiring care are now commonly cared for at home. Some individuals are now being taught to administer intravenous drug therapy and nutritional solutions at home. Therefore, home health care nurses must have a wide variety of technical skills.

Caregivers in the Home

Most of the care for individuals disabled by chronic illness is provided by family members in the home. They are the ones who are present 24 hours a day and 7 days a week. More attention is currently being addressed to needs of the *caregivers* in these situations. Their task is

Nursing Research: *Implications for Practice*

Gaynor, S. E. "The Long Haul: The Effects of Home Care On Caregivers." *Image* 22, 4 (Winter 1990): 208–212.

Women with the experience of caring for a spouse with a long-term physical or cognitive disability were studied. Younger women found the caregiving more burdensome than did older women. In addition, those with longer caregiving experience had more personal physical health problems. In assessing families where an individual provides care on a ongoing basis, the physical and emotional health of the caregiver must be addressed. The author suggests that nursing interventions be addressed to prevent a decline in the caregiver's health.

often arduous, draining both physical and emotional resources.

Nurses in home care provide family caregivers with emotional support as well as education. One important role the nurse assumes is assisting caregivers in preventing *burnout* and assessing them for the possibility of burnout. Burnout may result in poor care for the patient or premature institutionalization of a person who has many care needs. Institutionalization is both expensive and emotionally distressing for all people involved.

To prevent burnout, caregivers need time for themselves and opportunities to maintain their own lives independent of the caregiving situation. Sometimes they need a professional to reassure them that this rest is indeed appropriate and that they are not being selfish in wanting some personal life. This may be particularly true when spouses are caring for one another. The healthier spouse may feel guilt for enjoying life when the disabled spouse is unable to do so. This attitude may be held by the ill person also, and guilt may be invoked by statements such as "If you really cared about me . . . ." The nurse may assist in resolving the interpersonal stresses and supporting the caregiver in leading a more balanced life.

Respite care is temporary care that allows a caregiver to have time away from the ill person while someone else takes the responsibility for care. Respite care may last for hours, days, or even for a brief vacation trip. Caregivers for respite care may come to the home or, in the case of longer periods of time, respite care may involve short-term admission to an institutional setting. Respite care is especially valuable to the parent of a disabled child who may be facing long years of caregiving and the person caring for an individual with cognitive impairment such as Alzheimer's disease.

Adult day care may be used during weekdays to provide both the ill older person and the caregiver with an alternative. In a group day care setting, the person with chronic illness may have opportunities to socialize, may be involved in positive experiences such as exercise classes, reality orientation, or validation therapy, and will receive supervision for medications and meals. The caregiver is assured that the person is being well cared for while the caregiver works, tends the home, shops, or is otherwise occupied. Day care may be offered from 1 to 5 days a week. Some adult day care facilities even provide clients with transportation to and from the center.

Disabled children may be enrolled in special developmental preschool programs at an early age. These programs provide skilled assistance to the child in learning age-appropriate developmental tasks. In addition, they provide guidance to parents in how to continue to support the child in development at home. The parents benefit also from the having respite from care demands. Respite child care is also available in many communities. These programs provide skilled professionals to care for children with special needs to allow the parents to have a day, an evening, or even a weekend without the care responsibility.

To assess for caregiver burnout, the nurse will look for the presence of warning signs. Sleep disturbances and loss of concentration may occur. The caregiver may suffer from anxiety or depression and may have a low energy level. Loss of appetite and subsequent loss of weight may indicate burnout. Abuse of drugs or alcohol may occur. The caregiver may report increasing difficulties in managing in the form of being irritated or angry over little things, feeling that no matter what is done it is not enough, and no longer feeling pride in providing care. The caregiver may feel very much alone or may say that relationships are breaking down.

When indications of possible burnout occur, the nursing diagnosis of Altered Family Processes is appropriate, and nursing interventions are planned that will assist the caregiver. Planning together for a means for the caregiver to receive some relief from the burdens of care will be necessary. The nurse may know what community resources are available, the caregiver will know what family and financial resources might be used, and the caregiver must make the psychological adjustment to seeking care alternatives.

Residential Long-term Care

It has been estimated that one of four elderly persons will be a resident in a nursing home for some period of time (Fulmer, 1987). This rate is expected to increase as the population of elders increases as individuals live to an older age. The majority of those entering long-term residential care facilities are 80 years of age or older. They enter because of multiple chronic illnesses and disabilities, which result in their being unable to manage activities of daily living even with support. The most common reasons for nursing home care are dependence in three or more functional areas (such as bathing, toileting, eating, and so forth) and cognitive impairment that can no longer be managed in the home environment. Some enter for limited periods of time for rehabilitation and convalescence after discharge from an acute care hospital.

Resident Versus Patient or Client

The term client has the connotation of one who freely contracts for professional services, usually on an episodic basis. Although the person who enters a long-term care facility may be client to the physician or the therapist, who are seen at intervals, the majority of caregivers are not chosen by the individual, and the institution with which the agreement for care is made is often detached from day-to-day living. For those who rely on some form of government financial assistance for care, even this distant contractual relationship may be missing. The facility may be designated through contracts between a government agency and the facility.

The term patient connotes one who is ill and receives health care. The person in a long-term care facility may be ill, but often perceives himself or herself as having disabilities and being in a stable, well state in relationship to the individual's own standards. The term patient may also connote that this person should be dependent and follow directions for care.

More and more often, long-term care facilities are using the term *resident* rather than either patient or client. Resident implies that this institution, whatever its size, structure, governance, or method of payment, is now the home of the person. The standards for a good home are far different from standards for something we call a health care institution. The difference is a focus on total **quality of life**, that is, the extent to which life provides the attributes valued by the individual, rather than just quality of care.

Quality of Life

Quality health care is one aspect of the quality of life, but by no means the most significant aspect. To maintain care of high quality in an intensive care unit, some aspects of personal living are placed "on hold." For a 5-day stay in an acute care hospital, whether roommates like one another may not be important. This is not true in long-term care facilities. For most residents, the facility is now home. Whatever life the individual now has will remain within that context despite visits elsewhere for brief periods of time. Therefore, the quality of the relationship with the roommate becomes important.

The National Coalition for Nursing Home Reform asked more than 400 nursing home residents to identify the factors that provided quality of life. They identified seven areas:

1. Quality interactions with competent staff
2. Respect for privacy and individual dignity
3. Having choices and options
4. Maximizing independence in activities of daily living
5. Having a variety of social and recreational activities
6. Maintaining accustomed roles
7. Clean, safe physical environment (Institute of Medicine, 1986)

Those who care for individuals in nursing homes need to look carefully at the routines, policies, and procedures to ensure that they support these indicators of quality of life.

Nursing Care Study
A Patient With a Chronic Illness

Johnny Jefferson, age 8, was admitted last evening for his asthma. He was given intravenous medication and oxygen. His mother stayed in the hospital all night long. Mrs. Jefferson is sitting by Johnny's bed, gazing into space, while Johnny lies sleeping. Steve MacKenzie, RN, enters to check on Johnny. After he has done his assessment and determined that Johnny does not need any attention, he turns to Mrs. Jefferson. "You look awfully tense. How about coming down to the family room and having a cup of tea? Johnny is sleeping now and you need to have a break."

Mrs. Jefferson replies, "Do you think it will be all right to leave him?"

"I'll make sure he is checked on frequently and we'll call you right back if he needs you," Steve states.

In the family room, Steve sits down with Mrs. Jefferson and opens the conversation by saying, "This must have been an upsetting night for you. How are you feeling now?"

Almost as if a dam is breaking, Mrs. Jefferson begins to talk about her fears that one day Johnny may not respond and will die in one of his asthmatic episodes. Steve encourages her to explore her feelings and to describe how Johnny's care is managed at home. He perceives that there is a problem with Powerlessness related to the sudden, unexpected onset of asthmatic episodes. Mrs. Jefferson communicates that she feels life is totally out of control.

After Mrs. Jefferson has returned to Johnny's room, Steve places a call to the clinical nursing specialist for respiratory care. He explains the problem he has identified in Mrs. Jefferson and asks the nursing specialist to come for a conference to assist in planning intervention. He says that he perceives that the family may have multiple problems with coping and that he hopes to initiate a plan that may follow the family back to the community and assist them in daily living with a child with severe asthma.

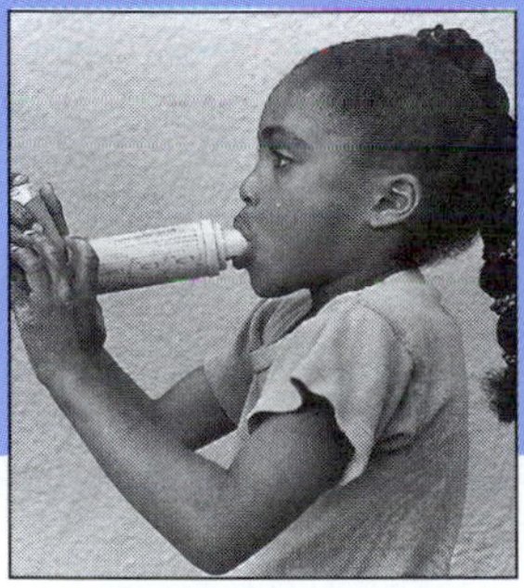

Key Points

- Chronic illness can be defined as an illness that is permanent, leaves nonreversible residual disability, is caused by pathology, or requires special rehabilitation.
- Some chronic illnesses necessitate considerable life adjustment and can follow an erratic course.
- The incidence of chronic illness increases with age.
- Each chronic illness has a course; a person's perception of that course is the trajectory.
- Remission may be followed by exacerbation, or the individual's health may steadily deteriorate.
- Factors influencing the course of chronic illness include the presence of a concurrent illness and the addition of other stressors in life.
- Data strongly support the theory that the outlooks of the person who is ill and of those around that person play an important part in determining the severity and course of the illness.
- Persons with a chronic illness have special needs, including the need for management of an acute crisis, the need to control symptoms, financial needs, the need to reconcile the drive to legitimize and the drive to normalize, and in some cases the need for special education.
- Financial drain and manipulative behavior on the part of the ill person can create difficulties for the family of the chronically ill.
- Some of the positive experiences that chronic illness can give rise to are enjoying compensatory activities, forming stronger bonds with others, reassessing values, and learning new skills.
- Nursing Assessment for chronic illness should include both physical and psychosocial data.
- Nursing diagnoses for chronic illness may include Altered Family Processes, Altered Health Maintenance, Altered Parenting, Chronic Low Self-esteem, Ineffective Family Coping, Noncompliance, Powerlessness, and Social Isolation.

- Planning and implementation for chronic illness are often ongoing and complex. Possible nursing interventions include adjusting health care routines, health teaching, interpersonal communication, giving advice, and identifying resources.
- In the home health care setting, the nurse must adapt to a new role and adapt both assessment and implementation to the requirements of the home environment.
- An important function of the home health care nurse is support of the caregivers in the home to prevent burnout.
- Residential long-term care requires an emphasis on the quality of the resident's life. Seven factors identified as being important are quality interactions with competent staff, respect for privacy and individual dignity, having choices and options, maximizing independence in activities of daily living, having a variety of social and recreational activities, maintaining accustomed roles, and having a clean, safe physical environment.
- Evaluation within the entire context of care of the chronically ill person must focus on the achievement of small goals and the maintenance of maximum independence.

Study Questions

1. Define chronic illness.
2. What are the differences between the response to chronic illness of the young child and that of the adult?
3. What percentage of children have a chronic illness?
4. What is meant by the course of a chronic illness?
5. Explain four possible courses for a chronic illness.
6. How does the degree of compliance affect the course of a chronic illness?
7. How does the support of families and others affect the course of a chronic illness?
8. List seven special needs created by the presence of a chronic illness.
9. What factors may influence compliance with the prescribed care regime?
10. List negative experiences related to chronic illness.
11. List positive experiences related to chronic illness.
12. What special points of psychosocial assessment are relevant to chronic illness?
13. How are family processes altered by chronic illness?
14. What special problems of parenting occur when the child has a chronic illness?
15. Describe situations in which it is appropriate for a nurse to give advice to a chronically ill patient or the patient's family.
16. What are indications of burnout in a home caregiver?
17. List factors important to quality of life in a residential long-term care facility.

Critical Thinking Activities

1. Identify a community resource that could be used by a person with a chronic illness. Learn how a referral can be made, what services are provided, and what services cost. Report on this to a small class group.
2. Take a survey in one of your classes. Find out each person's general age range, whether the person has any kind of chronic illness, and, if so, whether the illness causes any disability. Compare the percentages with the ones cited in the chapter.
3. On a hospital unit, go through the admitting medical diagnoses of all of the patients and count the total number of patients and the number with chronic illnesses. Determine the percentage of patients who have been admitted for chronic illness.
4. In your library, locate and read the autobiography of a person with a chronic illness.

References and Readings

Becker, M. H., Haefner, D. P., and Kasl, S. V. "Selected psychosocial models and correlates of individual health related behaviors." *Med Care* 5 (January 1977): 27–46.

Beland, I. *Clinical Nursing: Pathophysiological and Psychosocial Approaches.* New York: Macmillan, 1981.

Brannon, M. "A Hands-on Rehab Technique That Really Works." *RN* 52, 11 (November 1989): 65–69.

Burckhardt, C. S. "Coping Strategies of the Chronically Ill." *Nursing Clinics of North America* 22, 3 (September 1987): 543–550.

Carnevali, D. *Diagnostic Reasoning and Treatment Decision-Making.* Philadelphia: J. B. Lippincott, 1993.

Carnevali, D., and Patrick, M. *Nursing Management for the Elderly.* 2nd edition. Philadelphia: J. B. Lippincott, 1986.

Clubb, R. C. "Chronic Sorrow: Adaptation Patterns of Parents with Chronically Ill Children." *Pediatric Nursing* 17, 5 (September-October 1991): 461–466.

Cooper, M. C. "Chronic Illness and Nursing's Ethical Challenge." *Holistic Nursing Practice* 5, 1 (October 1990): 10–16.

Corbin, J. M., and Strauss, A. L. "Collaboration: Couples Working Together to Manage Chronic Illness." *Image* 16, 4 (Fall 1984): 109–115.

Cousins, N. *Anatomy of an Illness.* New York: Bantam Books, 1979.

Dambroski, B. "Knock, Knock." *American Journal of Nursing* 87, 2 (February 1987): 205.

Eggland, E. T. "Home Health Care." *Nursing '87* 17, 10 (October 1987): 75–81.

Ellis, J. R. *Health Status, Health Behavior, Multidimensional Health Locus of Control and Factors in the Development of Personal Control in Individuals with Rheumatoid Arthritis.* The University of Texas at Austin. Dissertation 1990. UMI #9031563.

Friedman, J. "Guiding Patients through the Labyrinth of Home Health Care Services." *Nursing and Health Care* 7, 6 (June 1986): 305–306.

Fulmer, T. "Lessons from a Nursing Home." *American Journal of Nursing* 87, 3 (March 1987): 332.

Gaynor, S. E. "The Long Haul: The Effects of Home Care on Caregivers." *Image* 22, 4 (Winter 1990): 208–212.

Given, B., and Given, C. W. "Creating a Climate for Compliance." *Cancer Nursing* 7, 2 (April-May 1984): 139–148.

Gull, H. J. "The Chronically Ill Patient's Adaptation to Hospitalization." *Nursing Clinics of North America* 22, 3 (September 1987): 593–602.

Hilton, B. A. "Perceptions of Uncertainty: Its Relevance to Life-threatening and Chronic Illness." *Critical Care Nursing* 12, 2 (February 1992): 70–73.

Institute of Medicine. *Improving Quality of Care in Nursing Homes.* Washington, D.C.: National Academy Press, 1986.

Johnson, J. "The Effects of a Patient Education Course on Persons with Chronic Illness." *Cancer Nursing* 5, 4 (April 1982): 117–123.

Lambert, C. E., and Lambert, V. A. "Psychosocial Impacts Created by Chronic Illness." *Nursing Clinics of North America* 22, 3 (September 1987): 527–534.

Larkin, J. "Factors Influencing One's Ability to Adapt to Chronic Illness." *Nursing Clinics of North America* 22, 3 (September 1987): 535–542.

Lewis, K. "Grief in Chronic Illness and Disability." *Journal of Rehabilitation* 49, 3 (July-September 1983): 8–11.

Mayo, L. "Problem and Challenge." In *Guides to Action on Chronic Illness,* pp. 9–13. New York: National Health Council, 1956.

McNamara, R. M. "Working in a Long-term Care Facility." *Nursing '86* 16, 12 (December 1986): 53.

Miller, J. F. *Coping with Chronic Illness.* 2nd edition. Philadelphia: F. A. Davis, 1992.

Mitchell, P. H. "Crisis Management for Families Living with Chronic Illness." *Washington State Journal of Nursing* 54, 2 (Summer-Autumn 1983): 2–8.

Nick, S. "Long-term Care: Choices for Geriatric Residents." *Journal of Gerontological Nursing* 18, 7 (July 1992): 11–18.

Pender, N. J. *Health Promotion in Nursing Practice* 2nd ed. East Norwalk, CT: Appleton-Lange, 1987.

Pereira, Sr. B. "Loss and Grief in Chronic Illness." *Rehabilitation Nursing* 9, 2 (March-April 1984): 20–22.

Piano, L. A. "Adult Day Care: A New Ambulatory Care Alternative." *Nursing '86* 16, 8 (August 1986): 60–62.

Pollack, S. E. "Human Responses to Chronic Illness: Physiologic and Psychosocial Adaptation." *Nursing Research* 35, 2 (March-April 1986): 90–99.

Pruitt, R. H., Keller, L. S., and Hale, S. L. "Mastering Distractions That Mar Home Visits." *Nursing and Health Care* 8, 6 (June 1987): 345–347.

Rancour, P. "Guided Imagery: Healing When Curing Is Out of the Question." *Perspectives in Psychiatric Care* 27, 4 (April 1991): 30–33.

Rinke, L. T. "Replacing a Failing Old Pattern with a New Paradigm: Home Care." *Nursing and Health Care* 8, 6 (June 1987): 331–333.

Robertson, J. F., and Cummings, C. C. "What Makes Long-term Care Nursing Attractive?" *American Journal of Nursing* 91, 11 (November 1991): 41–46.

Rosenberg, G. "The Known and Unknown About the Chronically Ill." *Social Work in Health Care* 15, 3 (March 1991): 1–7.

Sargis, N. M., Jennrich, J. A., and Murray, K. M. "Housing Conditions and Health: A Crucial Link." *Nursing and Health Care* 8, 6 (June 1987): 335–338.

Selcher, D. M. "Helping Your Patients Dress for Success." *RN* 54, 8 (August 1991): 43–45.

Soeken, K. L., and Carson, V. J. "Responding to the Spiritual Needs of the Chronically Ill." *Nursing Clinics of North America* 22, 3 (September 1987): 603–612.

Strauss, A. L. *Chronic Illness and the Quality of Life.* St. Louis: C. V. Mosby, 1984.

Strumpf, N. "A New Age for Elderly Care." *Nursing and Health Care* 8, 8 (June 1986): 444–449.

Swayze, S. "Helping Them Cope: Developing Self-help Groups for Clients with Chronic Illness." *Journal of Psychosocial Nursing and Mental Health Services* 29, 5 (May 1991): 35–39.

Taira, F. "Teaching Independently Living Older Adults About Managing Their Medications." *Rehabilitation Nursing* 16, 6 (November-December 1991): 322–326.

Thompson, L. E. "When Caring Is the Only Cure." *Nursing '87* 17, 1 (January 1987): 58–59.

Thorne, S. E. "Constructive Noncompliance in Chronic Illness." *Holistic Nursing Practice* 5, 1 (October 1990): 62–69.

Vital and Health Statistics: Current Estimates from the National Health Interview Survey, 1990. Series 10, No. 181. Hyattsville, MD: U.S. Department of Health and Human Services, Public Health Service, Centers for Disease Control, December, 1991.

Warner-Beland, J. A. (Ed.). *Grief Responses to Long-term Illness and Disability.* Reston, Va.: Reston Publishing, 1980.

Glossary

abduction The act of drawing away from the median line or center of the body. (23*)

absorption The process by which nutrients are moved from the interior of the digestive tract into the blood stream. (25)

acceptance Affirmation of a belief in a situation or state. (35, 41)

accommodation 1) A term used by Piaget to describe the needed adjustment in thinking to reconcile old and new information. 2) The second stage in the life of a group when individuals adjust their own behavior to work more effectively with others. 3) Pupillary; changes in pupil size and lens thickness to adjust retinal focus of objects at different distances. (14, 17)

accountability The state of being responsible or answerable for one's actions. (1)

accreditation Approval by a recognized body of a program or facility that meets certain standards.

acid–base balance The balance of the acidity and alkalinity of the body fluids for optimum homeostasis. (30)

acid mantle A descriptive term used to describe the protective properties of the slightly acid surface of the skin. (21)

acidity The property of giving off hydrogen ions or being acidic, measured as less than 7.0 on the pH scale. (30)

acidosis A disturbance of the acid–base balance resulting in the accumulation of acids in the body; a serum pH of less than 7.35. (30)

active assistive exercise Movement that one accomplishes by oneself, with the assistance of another. (23)

active exercise Voluntary movement of a body part resulting from muscular contraction and relaxation.(23)

active immunity Resistance to a specific microorganism resulting from the body's production of a specific antibody. (6)

active participation Personal involvement in a task. (16)

active transport An energy-consuming process for moving substances across a cell wall against the concentration gradient. (30)

activities of daily living (ADLs) Those tasks necessary to meeting personal basic needs. (9)

acupuncture A technique for relieving pain or providing regional anesthesia by inserting needles into specific points in the body. (7, 32)

acute care Health care for a condition that requires treatment of a fairly intensive nature for a limited time span. (2)

acute illness Illness that is usually of rapid onset, requires short-term treatment, and resolves itself with no apparent residual. (7)

*Numbers in parentheses indicate chapter(s) in which term is discussed.

adaptation The processes by which the body attempts to maintain and restore homeostasis. (6)

adaptive forces Any forces, internal or external, that tend to maintain or restore homeostasis. (4)

adaptive response A response by a person that tends to restore homeostasis.

addiction Dependence on a substance for daily functioning such that illness results from withdrawal of the substance. (32)

adduction The act of drawing toward the median line or center of the body. (23)

adherence Following the prescribed regime for selfcare of a health problem. (42)

adipose Referring to fat or fatty tissue. (40)

administrative law Rules and regulations developed by a governmental agency to carry out their legislated responsibilities. (3)

adolescent A person in the age group from 12 to 18. (18)

adrenals A pair of small endocrine glands, one of which is located on the top of each kidney. Each adrenal is composed of a center called the medulla and an exterior layer called the cortex. Each portion functions as a separate endocrine gland. (6)

advance directive for health care A legal document in which an individual makes known his or her wishes in regard to health care and especially in regard to the use of extraordinary measures at the end of life. (3) (41)

adventitious sounds Abnormal sounds, as in the lungs. (28)

advocate An individual who speaks or acts on the behalf of another. (1, 15, 28)

aerobic bacteria Designating bacteria that live only in the presence of free oxygen. (21)

aesthetic needs In Maslow's hierarchy, the highest level needs, relating to beauty and artistic endeavor. (5)

affective learning Designating the type of learning that relates to attitudes and values. (16)

affirm To recognize and declare the value and positive aspects of another person. (13)

ageism A derogatory attitude toward those of advanced years. (20)

aggregate A number of people who have no common goal but are found in one place and considered collectively. (14)

aggression Expressing a viewpoint or insisting on an action in a manner that infringes on the rights of others. (13)

agnostic An individual who neither accepts nor rejects the existence of God or a higher being. (36)

agonist/antagonist effect The ability of some drugs to act similarly to narcotics in some respects but to antagonize other narcotic actions. (32)

agreeing-disagreeing Giving a personal viewpoint on a statement made by another person—a blocking response when used in regard to feelings. (13)

AIDS (Acquired Immune Deficiency Syndrome) A disease caused by the HIV virus that attacks the immune system and eventually other susceptible body cells. (21)

aids to decision-making Facilitating responses that assist another person to plan a course of action. (13)

airborne Designating a route of transmission whereby pathogens are transmitted via dust particles in the air. (21)

air embolus A bubble of air moving through the circulatory system. (25)

alarm reaction The first stage of Selye's General Adaptation Syndrome (GAS). (6)

albuminuria The abnormal presence of protein in the urine. (27)

alcoholism Chronic dependence on excessive amounts of alcohol. (33)

aldosterone An adrenocorticosteroid hormone that causes salt and water to be reabsorbed and potassium to be excreted by the kidney tubules. (6)

alignment The position of body parts in relationship to one another. (23)

alkalinity The property of being basic, measured as greater than 7.0 on the pH scale. (30)

alkalosis A disturbance of the acid–base balance resulting in an accumulation of bases in the body; a serum pH greater than 7.45. (30)

allergy An abnormal body hypersensitivity to a specific antigen that is ordinarily harmless. (38, 39)

allocation of resources An ethical decision determining who in society will benefit from health care funds, donor organs, and other aspects of health care. (3)

alopecia Loss of hair; baldness. (20)

alveoli Small pouches of thin, single-layered membrane in the lungs where the exchange of gases occurs. (28)

Alzheimer's disease A disease afflicting primarily elderly persons, characterized by mental deterioration and changes in brain tissue that can be identified on autopsy. (19, 20)

ambulation Walking. (23)

amino acids A compound composed of both the amino group and the carboxylic group, found as an essential component of the protein molecule of foods. (25)

amulet An object worn as a charm against evil or injury. (33)

anabolism The process of building up tissue. (25)

anaerobic Designating pathogens that grow best in an oxygen-free atmosphere.

anal stage Freud's psychosexual stage of the 2- to 3-year-old, when the anal and urethral areas provide sensual satisfaction. (18)

analgesia Absence of pain sensation. (31)

androgens Male hormones. (37)

androgyny Having both male and female characteristics. (37)

anesthesia Loss of all sensation. (31)

anger A subjective feeling of extreme displeasure toward a person or situation. (35)

Animism A primitive religious system without formalized beliefs in which spirits are believed to reside in objects in nature. (36)

anion An ion with a negative charge. (30)

ankylosed Designating a joint in which the bones are fused to make it immovable. (23)

Anointing the Sick A sacrament or ceremony of several Christian groups in which prayers are said and oil touched to the ill person. (36)

anorexia Lack of appetite or interest in food. (25)

anorgasmic Designating a woman who is unable to achieve an orgasm. (37)

antropometric measurements Measurements of various body parts to identify problems. Height, weight, and skin fold thickness are measured to assess nutritional status. (25)

antibiotics Drugs that are effective in inhibiting the growth of or destroying bacteria. (21)

antibody A protein of specific structure that is produced by the body and interacts with a specific antigen to destroy or inactivate it. (6)

anticholinergics A classification of drugs that block acetylcholine receptors and therefore reduce the transmission of impulse in the parasympathetic nervous system. (27)

anticipatory grief Feelings of grief that occur when it is perceived that a loss may be imminent. (41)

antidiuretic hormone (ADH) A hormone secreted by the posterior pituitary that causes the kidneys to reabsorb water independently of solids. (27)

antiemetic A substance that prevents and controls nausea and vomiting. (25)

antifungal Designating agents that inhibit the growth of or destroy fungi. (21)

antigen Any substance that can cause the body to form an antibody. (6)

antihistamines A group of drugs that depress the action of histamine in the body, resulting in decreased secretions and decreased swelling of mucous membranes. (6)

antihypertensive Tending to counteract high blood pressure. (29)

antimicrobial Capable of suppressing the growth of microorganisms. (21)

anuria Total absence of formation of urine by the kidneys; urinary suppression. (27)

anxiety A subjective experience of apprehension initiated by a threat to oneself, whether physical, mental, emotional, or spiritual. (7)

apex of heart The lower, more pointed end of the heart. (29)

aphasia Inability to use language caused by brain dysfunction. (31)

aphrodisiacs Agents thought to enhance sexual performance. (37)

apical pulse The heart rate as counted by listening to the heart over its apex. (29)

apnea Absence of respiration. (28)

appetite A subjective desire for or interest in food. (25)

approving–disapproving Giving a value judgment on a statement made by another person—a blocking response when used in relationship to feelings. (13)

arousal The state of being sexually excited. (37)

arteriosclerosis Thickening and hardening of the inner and middle wall of vessels, narrowing the opening through which blood flows. (20)

arthritis Inflammation of the joints. (23)
artificial insemination Introducing semen into the female without sexual contact. (3)
artificial tears A neutral, sterile solution used to lubricate the eyes. (22)
ascending fibers Those nerves in the spinal cord that transmit impulses up to the brain. (32)
ascites The accumulation of excess fluid in the peritoneal cavity. (29)
asepsis Absence of all disease-producing microorganisms. (21)
aseptic conscience In the practice of nursing, feeling an obligation to be the strictest and most rigid judge of whether or not aseptic technique has been broken. (21)
asexual Lacking sexual awareness. (37)
Asians A large, diverse group consisting of Japanese, Chinese, Filipinos, Koreans, and Southeast Asians. (33)
aspiration 1.) The inhalation of a foreign substance into the respiratory passages. 2.) Withdrawal of fluid from the body through a needle or catheter. (38)
assault A threat to do bodily harm. (3)
assertion Expressing a viewpoint or performing an action in a manner that clearly establishes one's own autonomy without infringing on the rights of others. (13)
assessment The first step of the nursing process, which includes collecting data and making a nursing diagnosis. (8)
assimilation Piaget's term for the process by which information is absorbed. (17)
assisted living centers Living facilities for the elderly that offer minimal levels of services, yet provide supervision of care needs. (20)
associate degree program A college-level education of approximately 2 years in length for which an associate degree is awarded. (1)
associate nurse A nurse who assumes the responsibility for a patient's care when the primary nurse is absent. (1)
astereognosis The inability to identify small objects by touch, without looking. (31)
asynchrony Growth that is disproportionate, although normal for early childhood. (18)
ataxia Difficulty with gait or walking. (23)
atelectasis The collapse of portions of the lung due to lack of air in the alveoli; often the consequence of secretions blocking the airways and absorption of air distal to the plug. (28, 40)
atheist An individual who believes that there is no God or higher being. (36)
atherosclerosis A condition in which plaques of a cholesterol-based material are deposited in the interior of the arteries. (20)
atony Lack of muscle tone. (23)
atrophy The condition of becoming smaller in bulk or size, such as through the wasting or deterioration of a body part. (23)
attentive listening Focusing one's thoughts on the person who is speaking to clearly understand what is being said, and exhibiting behavior that encourages the other person to express thoughts and ideas. (13)
attitude An internal feeling or mental position toward a person or idea. (13)
audiovisual aids Objects or methods to provide visual and auditory information for learning. (16)
audit A method of evaluating by checking what care was provided and comparing it to a previously established standard for care. (8)
auditory Pertaining to hearing. (31)
auditory input Input received through the ears; sounds. (31)
authoritarian leadeship Autocratic. (14)
authority The power to accomplish an action. (1)
autocratic leadership A style of leadership in which decision-making and authority are located in the leader. (14)
autogenic training A set of exercises designed to help one focus on physical sensations, shut out psychosocial stressors, and induce the relaxation response. (6)
autoimmunity A state in which antibodies are produced. (7)
autonomic nervous system The involuntary part of the nervous system that sends and receives impulses from the heart muscle, smooth muscles, blood vessels, and hollow organs, as well as controlling the secretions of glands. (4)
autonomic responses Involuntary body responses controlled by the autonomic nervous system. (32)
autonomy Erikson's term for the toddler's goal of becoming important to self and developing assertiveness. (18)
autonomy vs. shame and doubt state The second of Erikson's stages of psychosocial development seen in the toddler. (18)
autotransfusion The transfusion of one's own blood, that was donated previously. (29)

baccalaureate program A college-level education approximately 4 years in length, for which a bachelor's degree is awarded. (1)
bacteria One-celled microorganisms, the most numerous of all pathogens. (21)
bacteriuria The presence of bacteria in the urine. (27)
balanced solution An intravenous electrolyte solution that provides water, calories, and electrolytes in concentrations commonly found in the body. (30)
Baptism A sacrament of Christian churches in which water is used and prayers are said to receive the individual into the Christian faith. (36)
bargaining Negotiating for a change in circumstances in return for changes in behavior or feelings. (41)
baroreceptor Sensory nerve that responds to pressure. (28)
barrier 1) A boundary or limit. 2) A technique for limiting the spread of microorganisms. (21)
barrio A Spanish-speaking community within a larger community. (33)
base A substance that releases the OH^- radical in solution; an alkaline substance. (30)
base (of heart) The wider, superiorly located end of the heart. (29)
base of support A foundation that supports the body weight. (23)
Basic Four A simplified framework for planning meals to include all essential nutrients in adequate amounts. The four groups are bread, meat, milk, and fruits and vegetables. (25)

basic life skills The abilities needed to manage one's time, finances, and interpersonal relationships. (13)

basic needs The essential physiologic requirements for survival. (5, 9,10)

battery Touching or harming a person without consent. (3)

behavior modification An approach to changing conduct by using manipulation of the environment, especially by manipulating the consequence of the conduct. (6, 16, 32)

belief Placing trust or confidence in something. (35)

belittling A blocking response in which a person's feelings or problems are categorized as not major or less than those of others. (13)

belongingness A need to feel a part of a social group, described by Maslow as part of the hierarchy of needs. (5)

benign pain Pain that does not represent a life threatening problem. (32)

bereavement Grief or mourning. (41)

bias Adverse judgments or opinions without knowledge or facts; prejudice. (33)

bilingual Having the ability to communicate in two languages. (33)

bioethics A field of study dealing with questions of right and wrong that relate to human life. (3)

biofeedback A mechanical means of providing information on specific body processes. (6, 7)

biopsy The removal of tissue for examination or testing. (38)

biorhythms Regularly recurring patterns of biologic functioning within the individual, some annually, some monthly, some on a daily basis, and others on a less than 24-hour pattern. (24)

Biots' respirations Similar to Cheyne-Stokes respirations except that the respirations between the periods of apnea appear normal (see Cheyne-Stokes respirations). (28)

bisexual Having sexual feelings toward members of both sexes. (37)

Black English A variation of English having certain words, phrases, and sentence structure that are special to some African-Americans. (33)

blanching Pallor of the skin in a limited area created by a decrease in circulation. Often a result of the application of pressure that occludes blood vessels. (22)

blocking behavior Actions that tend to interfere with or halt communication. (13)

blocking responses Responses that tend to inhibit another person from sharing thoughts and feelings. (13)

blood-borne pathogens Pathogens that are present in blood and certain other internal body fluids. (21)

blood gases The gas components of the blood, primarily oxygen and carbon dioxide. (28)

blood pressure The pressure exerted by the blood against the walls of the blood vessels. (29)

body image A multidimensional view of one's body that takes into account its appearance, kinesthetic feedback, sensory feedback, and internal feelings. (19, 34, 35)

body image integrity A situation in which an individual has an accurate perception of his or her physical self and has adapted successfully to that reality. (35)

body mechanics The analysis of the action of forces on the body parts during activity. (23)

bolus 1) A concentrated solution of medication or tube feeding given over a short period of time. 2) A rounded mass of food passing through the gastrointestinal system. (25, 26)

bonding The forming of a strong emotional attachment such as between an infant and parent. (18)

bradycardia An abnormally slow heart rate, usually below 60 beats/min in the adult. (29)

bradypnea Slow respirations, usually below 16/min in the adult. (28)

bridging A method of supporting the body parts on pillows so that areas where pressure usually occurs are bridged between the pillows. (22)

Brompton's mixture An oral solution of heroin, cocaine, an antiemetic, and other needed drugs in an alcohol-based syrup used in England for terminal pain. Modified Brompton's is a mixture similar to Brompton's, but with morphine or methadone substituted for the heroin. (32)

brujas Persons viewed by some Hispanics as capable of causing illness or discomfort. (33)

Buddhism A religion based on the teachings of Siddhartha Guatama Buddha, who lived in India about 500 BC. (36)

buffer A substance that can combine with either a strong acid or a strong base and bring it closer to a neutral pH of 7.0. (30)

burnout Symptoms of emotional, social, and physical exhaustion due to the stress of the role of the care provider. (2, 41)

calculi Stones. (21)

callus A soft tissue formed between the ends of broken bone as part of the healing process. (6)

calorie counting A method of planning a reducing diet by keeping a record of the calories contained in food and planning menus that stay within a specific calorie range. (25)

carbohydrate A compound of carbon, hydrogen, and water used by the body for energy. (25)

carbohydrate counting A method of planning a reducing diet in which only the grams of carbohydrate are monitored and limited. (25)

carcinogenic Cancer-causing. (7)

cardinal signs of inflammation Five indicators of the presence of inflammation: Redness, heat, swelling, pain, and loss of function. (6)

cardiopulmonary resuscitation (CPR) A combination of rescue breathing and external cardiac massage. (29)

cardiovascular conditioning Activities designed to make the cardiovascular system function more effectively. (29)

caregiver Any individual who provides ongoing personal, physical, and psychological support to a patient/client. (42)

caries The decay of bone or teeth. (22)

carrier An infected person without signs or symptoms who is capable of transmitting a disease to another person. (21)

care management A mechanism for monitoring and directing health care for an individual patient to accomplish desired outcomes with the greatest efficiency of time, energy, and resources. (1)

casts Small dish-shaped, hardened mucus particles formed in the renal tubules and discarded in the urine. (27)

CAT scanner Computed axial tomogram scanner, a noninvasive instrument for discerning abnormalities of the brain and other body tissues. (38)

catabolism The process of breaking down tissue. (25)

cataract A condition in which the lens of the eye becomes opaque. (20)

catheterization The process of inserting a catheter, most commonly into the bladder. (27)

cation A positively charged ion. (30)

Caucasian Ethnic group consisting of persons who are not people of color. (33)

cell-mediated immunity A delayed immune response dependent upon the action of the T-lymphocytes and directed against cancer cells, viruses, and foreign tissue. (6)

center of gravity A point in an object or person at which gravitational pull functions as if the entire weight of the object or person were at that single point. (23)

centering A part of Piaget's preoperational stage in which the person is unable to see a complete situation and sees only those aspects pertaining to the moment. (17)

central nervous system The division of the nervous system pertaining to central neurologic control—the brain and spinal cord. (31) (32)

central venous pressure The pressure of the blood in the vena cava and right atrium, normally 5 to 10 cm of water. (29)

cephalocaudal development Relating to the neuromuscular motor development from the head downward to the feet, evident from birth to age 2. (18)

certification A process of obtaining a credential attesting to ability in a specialized field. (1, 2)

challenging A blocking response in which a person's statements of concerns or feelings are questioned. (13)

chaplain A member of the clergy who has a specific relationship with or is employed by the health care facility to assist in meeting the spiritual needs of the patients, families, and staff. (36)

chemical theory of sleep The theory that sleep is brought on by increased carbon dioxide levels in the blood. (24)

chemoreceptor Sensory nerve that responds to specific substances. (28)

chemotaxis Movement of a white blood cell toward a microorganism or foreign substance because of chemical responses. (6)

chemotherapeutic agents 1) The treatment of disease through the use of drugs with a chemical base. 2) A classification of drugs used to combat neoplastic disease. (39)

Cheyne-Stokes respirations Respirations that gradually taper off to the point of cessation and then, after a period of apnea, gradually return to become deep and rapid. (28)

Chicano A Mexican American. (33)

cholesterol An animal sterol which, when elevated, may place persons at risk for heart disease. (25)

choosing In the NANDA taxonomy, a human response pattern of selecting alternatives. (10)

chordotomy A surgical procedure that severs afferent pain nerves. (32)

Christianity A worldwide religion that follows the teachings of Jesus Christ. (36)

chromosomes The portion of the nucleus of body cells that determines inborn characteristics. (17)

chronic illness According to the 1956 Commission on Chronic Illness, an illness that has one or more of the following characteristics: a) is permanent, b) leaves residual disability, c) is caused by nonreversible pathologic alteration, and/or d)may be expected to require a long period of supervision, observation, or care. (7, 41)

chronic obstructive pulmonary disease (COPD) A group of respiratory diseases involving obstruction to airflow and therefore difficulty in breathing. (28)

chyme A gruel-like semiliquid that is composed of secretions of the digestive system and food that has been acted on by gastric enzymes. (26)

circadian rhythm The approximately 24-hour cyclic pattern of rest and activity in human beings. (24)

circulating nurse The nurse who manages the care of the patient undergoing surgery and coordinates the function of the operating room. (40)

circulatory overload A condition in which the volume of fluid circulating in the body is more than the heart can pump adequately. This condition can develop if a large volume of fluid is infused over a short period of time or if heart disease is present. (29)

circumduction A circular movement of the eye or a body part. (23)

citrated blood Blood that is prevented from coagulating by the presence of citrate-phosphate-dextrose or acid-citrate-dextrose. (29)

clergy Individuals who have fulfilled the requirements to become full-time, paid workers for their religious groups. (36)

clichés Routine social phrases or responses that tend to block communication. (13)

climacteric A time in middle age characterized by a decrease in the production of sex hormones resulting in menopause in women. (19)

climax Sexual orgasm. (19)

clotting factor One of several compounds necessary for the clotting process to occur. (39)

clubbed fingers A sign of chronic low oxygenation in which the angle at the base of the fingernail changes and the end of the finger assumes the appearance of a club. (22)

cocaine A crystalline powder with psychoactive properties, originally derived from coca leaves.

codes A hospital system for summoning a specially educated team to resuscitate a person who has had a cardiac or respiratory arrest. (41)

cognition Rational thinking processes or knowledge. (31)

cognitive learning The type of learning that relates to knowledge. (16)

cohesion A mutual attraction that holds a group together. (14)

colitis Inflammation of the colon. (26)

collaborative problem A patient/client problem that requires the cooperative intervention of nurses and physicians. (10)

colleague A fellow member of the health professions. (2)

colloid A large-molecule substance that cannot pass through a semipermeable membrane. (30)

colloidal osmotic pressure (COP) The osmotic pressure created by the presence of colloids on one side of a semipermeable membrane, causing water to move through the membrane to the colloids. (30)

colonization The growth of organisms on the surface of a tissue; does not always indicate infection of the tissue. (21)

colostomy A surgically created opening of the colon onto the abdominal wall. (26)

colonoscopy The direct visualization of the walls of the colon through a specialized endoscope called a colonoscopy. (26)

coma A level of awareness in which a person no longer responds to external stimuli except, in some cases, painful stimuli. (31)

combining power The number of positive or negative ions in a molecule of a substance. (30)

common law The broad area of common knowledge, customary procedure, and judicial decisions on which a current legal decision may be based. (3)

communicating In the NANDA taxonomy, a human response pattern of sending messages. (10)

communication The process by which one person makes thoughts, feelings, and concerns known to another. (13)

community The general group in which one functions. (33)

comparable worth A concept that monetary compensation should be equal for jobs requiring similar amounts of skill and energy expenditure. (33)

compensation Emphasis on a trait or traits to make up for perceived deficiencies of the self. (34)

competition Striving to be better than or superior to others. (36)

complementary functioning Acting in a way that serves to complete the function of another. (1)

complementary role A function or position that serves to complete the function of another. (1)

complete blood count (CBC) A measurement that establishes the values of a variety of components of the blood, usually including red blood count, white blood count, hemoglobin, and hematocrit. (29)

complication An unexpected negative sign or symptom of an illness or injury. (7)

concrete operational stage Piaget's cognitive stage of the 7- to 11-year-old, during which a person can understand the physical environment in relation to technology. (17)

concurrent review An evaluation process that takes place during the patient's stay, usually done by auditing (examining) records. (8)

conduction The transfer of nerve impulses by neurons. (4)

confidentiality The protection of the patient's privacy through careful use of both written and oral communication. (3)

Confucianism A religious group that follows the teachings of the Chinese philosopher Confucius.

congenital defect Present at birth but not inherited.(17)

conjoint therapy The treatment of a couple by a male and female therapist. (37)

conjugal A sexual relationship between two married partners. (37)

consciousness The state of being awake, alert, and able to communicate. (31)

consensus A decision reached by general agreement of all group members. (14)

consent A decision to accept an offered plan of care. (3)

considering consequences A facilitating response in which a person is helped to look realistically at the potential result of a particular course of action. (13)

constant fever A fever in which the temperature remains elevated at a uniform level. (4)

content The topics discussed, decisions made, and actions taken by a group. (14)

continuing care communities (CCC) Living facilities for the elderly that offer a variety of options ranging from retirement apartments to long term care. (20)

continuing education (CE) Learning programs undertaken after graduation from a basic program to maintain or expand competence. (1)

continuing education unit (CEU) A measure of credit for continuing education programs in which one unit represents one hour of instruction. (1)

continuous quality improvement (CQI) An organizational process directed at examining every facet of the organization and its functioning with the purpose of improving outcomes through improving structure or process. (12)

contraception Prevention of impregnation. (37)

contracture A shortening of a muscle that causes distortion or deformity of a joint. (23)

contraindications Indications that a certain plan of treatment is inadvisable. (2, 39)

contrast material A radiopaque substance that will be visible on an x-ray. Injected or instilled into an organ or system to allow visualization of soft tissue. Often referred to as "dye." (38)

contrast studies Radiologic tests which use contrast materials or dyes. (38)

convection Heat transfer caused by the movement of air carrying heat away from the body surface and its replacement by cooler air. (4)

conventional level Kohlberg's level of moral development that incorporates the need to please or be accepted by others. (17)

conversion The development of a physical illness or disability as a substitute for a psychological problem. (34)

cooperation Working with others for a common goal. (14)

coordination 1) The ability to voluntarily move the extremities and body parts in a balanced and effective manner. 2) Facilitation of the functioning of the health care team to provide better care. (15)

coping Dealing effectively with stress and problems. (6, 34)

coping mechanisms Any action that assists an individual in tolerating a stressor and relieving unpleasant feelings. (6)

cornea The central, clear convex surface of the eye over the pupil and iris. (31)

cortex Thin outer layer of the brain. (31)

cortisols The corticosteroid class of drugs. (6)

cost containment Actions taken to decrease the rate at which health care costs rise. (2)

cough reflex The involuntary reflex that prevents foreign bodies from lodging in the respiratory tract. (28)

course of the illness The way in which signs and symptoms may appear, remiss, and disappear during an illness. (7)

crackles A sound similar to hair strands being rubbed together heard upon auscultation of the lungs and indicating moisture in small airways. (28)
craniotomy A surgical procedure that involves opening the skull (cranium). (40)
credential Written evidence of one's qualifications issued by a recognized institution or regulatory body. (2)
Credé's maneuver Manually exerting pressure on the bladder to force out urine. (27)
crisis A situation in which previous methods of coping are no longer useful and problems threaten to overwhelm the individual. (34, 42)
crisis intervention A process for assisting the individual faced with a crisis in coping effectively with the situation. (34)
criteria Specific standards on which an evaluative judgment may be based. (11)
critical pathway A sequence of standardized short-term patient outcomes that will lead toward an overall long-term outcome and that can be used to manage care. (12)
critical thinking A thinking process characterized by a determined attempt to be logical, to seek relationships, to be open to new ideas, and to examine information in light of both its source and other knowledge. (8)
cryoprecipitate A frozen preparation of clotting factor used in the treatment of hemophilia. (29)
curanderos Folk healers of the Hispanic culture who derive their powers from God. (33)
cutaneous (superficial) pain Discomfort occurring in surface tissue. (32)
cyanosis A bluish discoloration of the skin due to oxygen deficiency. (28, 29)
cystic fibrosis An inherited disorder which causes the glands of the body to produce a thick type of mucus which can obstruct ducts. (28)
cystoscope A fiberoptic lighted scope which is inserted through the urethra so that the inside bladder wall can be visualized. (27)

dangling Sitting on the side of the bed with the feet and lower legs hanging off the edge. (23)
data base Information gathered about a patient and used to establish a plan of care. (15)
data collection Gathering information—a part of the first step in the nursing process. (9)
Davenport nomogram A graph used for plotting blood chemistry values to determine acid–base status. (30)
day surgery A surgical unit in which patients are admitted, have surgery, and are discharged in the same day. Also the surgery performed in a day surgery unit. (40)
dead air space The portion of the airway in which gas exchange does not take place. (28)
death care The cleansing and preparation of the body after death. (41)
debridement The removal of dead tissue from a wound. (22)
decerebration Deep coma progressing to total or partial interruption of the connection of the spinal cord tracts to the brain. (31)
deciduous teeth Temporary teeth. (18, 22)
decorticate Deterioration of the internal capsule of the brain stem, resulting in a posture showing adduction of the upper extremities on the chest with flexion of the elbows, wrists, and fingers. The lower extremities are also adducted. (31)
decubitus ulcer An open sore or lesion developed from lying in one position for a prolonged period of time. (22)
defending A blocking response in which one person opposes another by rebutting critical statements made. (13)
defense mechanisms Largely unconscious behaviors that relieve feelings of anxiety and tension. (6, 34)
defining characteristics Those signs and symptoms that indicate that a particular nursing diagnosis is present. (10)
dehiscence The splitting open of a wound, usually of the abdomen. (40)
dehydration A shortage of body fluids caused by an undue loss of body water. (30)
delusion Faulty thinking pattern inconsistent with reality. (31)
demanding an explanation A blocking response in which a reason for feeling and behavior is strongly requested. (13)
democratic Pertaining to the form of rule in which decisions are made by all group members. (14)
denial An unconscious refusal to recognize a happening or circumstance. (35, 41)
deontologic approach A method of ethical decision-making in which duty is considered to be of primary importance. (3)
dependency The inability to function satisfactorily without the aid of another. (7)
dependent functioning Working under the direction of another individual. (1)
deposition A legal testimony given in written form. (3)
depression A state of being in low spirits, feeling dejected, and often lacking hope. (7, 34, 35)
dermis The inner, thicker layer of the skin. (22)
desired outcomes Those specific measurable, objective events or states that are the sought for result of planned actions, also called goals. (8, 11)
despair Erikson's term for the unsuccessful outcome of the later years in which the older adult feels useless and loses hope. (19)
desquamation The process of shedding or peeling of the top layers of the skin. (22)
detoxify Commonly used to describe a process by which persons who use alcohol or drugs excessively are treated by removal of toxic agents. (27)
developing awareness Gradually recognizing reality and making changes related to that recognition. (41)
development A pattern of positive changes in the human being which are functional and organizational in nature. (17)
developmental crisis A crisis arising out of the changes that occur within the life cycle. (17)
developmental self-care requisites In Orem's theory, those things needed by any person of a given age to continue successful development. (9)
diagnosis-related group (DRG) A category of illnesses that

have been determined to require approximately the same level of and length of care. Used to determine payment in a prospective reimbursement system. (2)

diagnostic process (10) The process of moving from a broad set of assessment data to specific statements of diagnosis.

diagnostic test A procedure designed to provide information that will aid in the identification of a disease process. (38)

dialysis A procedure for replacing kidney function. (27)

diaphragm 1) A muscular membranous partition that separates the abdominal and thoracic cavities and functions in respiration. 2) On a stethoscope, the flat, drumlike head that is used most often for listening to blood pressure and to lung and bowel sounds. (28)

diaphoresis Perspiration. (22)

diarrhea Pathologically excessive evacuation of watery feces. (26)

diastolic Pertaining to the period when the heart muscle is relaxed between contractions. (29)

diastolic blood pressure The pressure exerted by the blood against the walls of the blood vessels between contractions when the heart muscle is relaxed. (29)

diet order The physician's prescription for diet, including *content:* the kinds of foods to be eaten; *form:* whether the daily intake is to be in three meals, six meals, three meals plus snacks, or any other pattern; and *texture:* whether the food is pureed, chopped, or regular. (25)

Dietary Goals Recommendations for diet for Americans published by the United States Department of Agriculture in 1979. (25)

Dietary Guidelines Recommendations for diet for Americans published by the United States Department of Agriculture in 1976. (25)

dietary history A complete record of the eating patterns, likes, and dislikes of an individual. (25)

differential blood count A report on the white blood count including the percentages of each type of white blood cell present. (29)

diffusion The movement of particles from their area of greater concentration to their area of lesser concentration. (30)

diploma program A basic education of approximately 3 years in length, associated with a hospital, for which a diploma is awarded. (1)

direct care audit Evaluation of care through checking the actual care given. (2)

disabled Handicapped; having a physical or mental abnormality that interferes with optimal function. (7)

disbelief A subjective state in which an individual does not believe that an event has taken place. Often a response to an overwhelming distressing event. (35)

discharge planner An individual with the responsibility for planning for care of the patient after discharge from the facility. (15)

discrimination Taking actions directed by bias, prejudice, or stereotyping. (33)

disease course See course of illness.

disengagement A natural withdrawal from the environment. (41)

displacement Focusing feelings related to one person or situation on another person or situation. (34)

dissolution stage The final stage in the life of a group, during which the group is ended. (14)

distress A level of stress within the body great enough to disturb homeostasis. (6)

diuretic A drug that increases the production of urine. (27)

diverse Varied or different. (33)

diverticulum An abnormal pouchlike formation extending outward from the wall of an organ, commonly found in the colon. (26)

documentation Recording information of significance demonstrating the health status of an individual and the health care provided. (15)

dorsal column stimulator (DCS) A battery-powered electrical device with an electrode surgically placed at the spinal nerves that produces electrical stimulation, thus interfering with pain impulses; used for intractable chronic pain. (32)

dorsiflexion The act of bending or moving a part in a backward direction. (23)

dosage A specified quantity of a therapeutic agent, prescribed to be taken at one time or at stated intervals. (39)

doubt Erikson's term for the unsuccessful outcome of early development in which the toddler becomes uncertain and distrusts others. (18)

douche A stream of water applied to a part or a cavity of the body for cleaning or medicinal purposes, most frequently the vagina. (37)

DRG *See* diagnosis-related group. (7)

droplet The moisture of a sneeze or cough which provides a means of transmission of pathogens. (21)

drug abuse The use of drugs for purposes and in a manner other than those for which they were intended. (32)

drug dependence A response to long-term administration of a drug, in which physiologic changes have occurred within the body such that adverse symptoms, called withdrawal symptoms, will occur if the drug is no longer administered. (32)

dwarfism Arrested physical growth usually related to hormonal deficiencies. (17)

dyspareunia Painful intercourse. (37)

dysphagia Difficulty in swallowing. (25)

dysphasia Difficulty in using language. (31)

dyspnea Difficulty or pain when breathing. (28)

dysuria Difficulty or pain on urination. (27)

Eastern Orthodoxy A Christian religion based in Eastern European and Mideastern countries. (36)

ecchymosis A bruise. (22)

ECG An electrocardiogram. This test records the electrical activity of the heart. Also referred to as an EKG. (38)

edema An excessive accumulation of serous fluid in the tissues. (22)

efficacy The potential for an action, treatment, or drug having the desired effect. (39)

ego As defined by Freud, the conscious self. (17)

egocentricism A part of Piaget's preoperational stage in which the self is seen as the central focus. (17)

ejaculation discharging of seminal fluid.

EKG Also referred to as an ECG An electrocardiogram. Records the electrical activity of the heart. (38)

elder A member of the laity within certain religious groups who has special duties and responsibilities. (36, 40)

elder abuse Imposed physical or emotional injury by others to those of advanced age. (20)

electroencephalogram (EEG) A recording or tracing of the electrical output of the cortex of the brain. (38)

electroencephalograph The device or machine that produces the electroencephalogram. (38)

electrolyte A charged particle capable of conducting an electrical impulse. Specific electrolytes are essential to body function. (30)

electromyogram (EMG) A recording of the electrical activity created by muscle function. (38)

elemental formula (enteral feeding) A formula composed of simple food substances that can be absorbed directly without the need for digestion. Vivonex is a popular brand. (25)

emancipated minor An underage person who is financially independent and does not live in the parent's home. (3)

embalming Introducing certain substances into the circulatory system of a corpse for purposes of preserving the body. (41)

embolus An object moving in the blood stream; for example, a moving blood clot. (29)

emesis Vomiting. (25)

emotional Pertaining to feelings. (34)

empathy The ability to participate in the feelings of another. (13)

emphysema A chronic respiratory disease in which the walls between alveoli are broken down and there are large spaces within the lungs. (28)

enacted law Laws passed by a legislative body. (3)

encouraging comparisons A facilitating response in which the person is asked to compare current experience with other experiences. (13)

endocrine system The body system composed of the ductless glands that secrete hormones which regulate body processes. (4)

endoscopy A procedure for visualizing the interior of hollow organs through the insertion of a tubular instrument that contains a light source. (26, 38)

enema A procedure whereby a fluid is instilled into the colon through the rectum, usually for the purpose of cleansing. (26)

enteral feeding Any food substance fed by a tube directly into the gastrointestinal tract. (25)

entry into practice The issue of what basic educational credentials should be required of a nurse beginning practice. (1)

enuresis Involuntary urination during the nighttime hours. (24, 27)

environment All of the physical, biologic, and social surroundings. (16)

epidural analgesia The administration of narcotics into the epidural space for purposes of pain relief. (32)

epilepsy A condition characterized by seizures.

equianalgesic A dosage of one analgesic drug that provides comparable pain relief to a given dosage of another analgesic drug. (32)

equilibration Piaget's term for the process of making thought consistent. (4, 17)

erection The enlargement and hardening of the penis as it fills with blood. (37)

erogenous zones Areas of the body that can be sexually aroused. (37)

erotic Arousing sexual feelings. (37)

eschar A dry scab over a wound. (22)

esophagogastroduodenoscopy (EGD) The direct visualization of the esophagus, stomach, and duodenum through a specialized endoscope called a gastroscope. (26)

esophagostomy A surgically made opening into the esophagus from the skin surface, usually beside the trachea above the clavicle. (25)

esteem needs In Maslow's hierarchy, the middle level of nonphysiologic needs related to feelings of self-worth. (5)

estrogens Female hormones, produced mainly by the ovaries, that are responsible for the menses and secondary sex characteristics. (37)

ethicist One who studies or is knowledgeable about ethics. (3)

ethics The study of the moral choices to be made by an individual. (3)

ethnocentrism A belief that one's ethnic group and pattern of behavior are superior to others. (33)

etiology The source or cause of a problem. (10)

eudaimonistic definition A definition of health that centers around the concept of self-actualization.

eupnea Normal breathing. (28)

eustress A level of stress in the body that tends to make it more able to protect itself. (6)

euthanasia 1) *Active:* the use of toxic substances or other methods to end life. 2) *Passive:* the withdrawal of or the decision not to use extraordinary means to prolong life. (41)

evaluation 1) The process of examining or judging to decide the value of something. 2) Examining the result and ascertaining the success of the nursing intervention—the fourth step in the nursing process. (8, 12)

evaporation Heat loss or cooling of the skin by the dissipation into the air of perspiration or moisture. (4)

eversion The act of turning in an outward direction. (23)

evisceration The protrusion of an internal organ (viscera) through a dehisced wound to the surface of the body. (40)

exacerbate To become worse or enter an acute phase. (42)

exacerbation An acute phase of a chronic illness. (42)

exchange menu A diet plan in which foods are organized into categories within which the foods are approximately equivalent nutritionally and therefore interchangeable. (25)

exchanging In the NANDA taxonomy, a human response pattern of mutual giving and receiving. (10)

excitement The first stage of the sexual response as described by Masters and Johnson, during which arousal takes place. (37)

exhaustion (stage of . . .) The third stage of Selye's General Adaptation Syndrome in which the body's resources are depleted by response to stressors and death results. (6)

expectorant Drugs that promote coughing up and secretion of respiratory fluids. (28)

expiratory reserve The volume of air that can be expired with maximum effort after a normal expiration. (28)

exploratory responses A variety of facilitating responses that help a person to understand the current situation. (13)

expressive responses Behavior that gives overt evidence of pain, such as crying, moaning, grimacing, swearing, and screaming. (32)

expressive role The collection of behaviors that serve to assist others to express feelings. (13)

extension The act of straightening or extending a limb. (23)

external cardiac massage A process of applying rhythmic pressure to the chest to compress the heart and circulate the blood. (29)

external influences on learning Those factors outside the person that decrease or increase learning. (16)

external respiration The exchange that takes place when room air reaches the alveoli. (28)

extracellular fluid The fluid found in the circulating blood and lymph and interstitial spaces. (30)

extrapersonal factors Those factors having an effect but residing outside of the person. (4)

facilitating behavior Actions that tend to encourage and enhance communication. (13)

facilitating responses Verbal replies that tend to encourage another individual to communicate. (13)

false imprisonment Holding people, either physically or through threats, against their will. (3)

false reassurance A blocking response in which general statements that "all will be well" are made. (13)

fantasy Make believe or imagination. (34)

fat A compound composed of glycerol and fatty acids and used for energy in the body. It may be either plant or animal in origin. (25)

fear A feeling of distress due to an objective danger or threat. (7)

fecal incontinence Involuntary passing of stool. (26)

feces Waste excreted from the bowels. (26)

feedback 1) Information provided to the source of a process about the process itself. 2) Information provided to an individual regarding progress. (14, 16, 34)

feedback theory of sleep A theory that sleep takes place when, after a period of neuronal activity during which electrical impulses are relayed throughout the system, fatigue sets in. (24)

feeling In the NANDA taxonomy, a human response pattern of subjective awareness of information. (10)

fetus The unborn child. (18)

fever Abnormally high body temperature. (21)

fiber A complex carbohydrate formed by plants that is not digestible in the human gastrointestinal system. (25)

fiberoptic endoscope A flexible tubular instrument that contains fibers that transmit light and images, used for performing endoscopy. (38)

fibrin A protein formed from fibrinogen by the action of thrombin, creating a fibrous network for clotting and for wound healing. (6)

fibrinous exudate Fluid containing fibrin that is secreted into an area of inflammation. (6)

field dependent A learning style in which a person learns more effectively if the entire picture is presented first and then component parts are presented. (16)

field independent A learning style in which a person learns more effectively if individual components are presented in an ordered fashion and then the entire picture is presented. (16)

filtration A process of using pressure to pass a liquid or a gas through a substance to remove certain particles. (30)

filtration pressure The pressure created by the blood pressure that causes fluid to move out of the capillary into the interstitial space. (30)

first intention healing Healing of a wound to the point at which edges are approximated and there is no evidence of inflammation. (6)

five rights A safety checklist used to ensure that drugs are administered correctly: 1) The right drug is given 2) in the right dosage 3) by the right route 4) to the right patient 5) at the right time. (39)

fixation Immobilization of a fractured bone to facilitate healing. (40)

flatus Gas generated in the stomach or intestines. (26)

flexion The act of bending a joint. (23)

flora The normal growth of organisms within the environment of body tissues. (21)

flow sheet A chart or graph used to record specific factual information. (15)

fluid overload A situation in which there is a larger quantity of fluid in the circulatory system than the body can manage. (25)

fluid volume deficit Inadequate fluid in the body. (30)

fluid volume excess Too large a volume of fluid in the body. (30)

fluoroscopy A radiologic diagnostic test using a device that gives serial images of the appearance and function of an organ. (38)

focusing A facilitating response in which the person is helped to concentrate on pertinent factors. (13)

food additive A substance added to food for purposes of either preserving, enhancing food value, or adding cosmetic properties. (25)

force fluids To encourage a person to drink a large amount of fluid. (25)

formal group A group with a planned structure and manner of operating. (14)

formal operational stage Piaget's term for the cognitive stage of the 11-year-old, during which abstract thought is first possible. (17)

formulation of a plan One part of the planning phase of the nursing process during which nursing actions are determined. (11)

free foods Those foods that have a minimal number of calories and therefore can be eaten without limit by those on a weight-reduction diet. Examples are celery, lettuce, and diet carbonated beverages. (25)

frequency The need or desire to void at more frequent intervals than usual. (27)

frigidity Inability of the female to become sexually aroused. (37)

fungus A moldlike low form of plant life that inhibits the subduing of pathogens. (21)

functional health patterns An organizing framework for assessment developed by Marjory Gordon. (9)

functional nursing A system of nursing care delivery in which work assignments are based on tasks to be accomplished, rather than on clients needing care. (1)

functional residual capacity The volume of air that remains in the lungs after a normal expiration. (28)

future orientation A belief that what is to happen is more important than the present or past. (36)

gait The manner in which a person walks. (23)

gastrocolic reflex A reflex urge to empty the rectum caused by the presence of food in the stomach. (26)

gastroenteric reflex Peristalsis of the intestine caused by the ingestion of food. (26)

gastrostomy A surgical opening directly into the stomach through the abdominal wall. A gastrostomy tube is placed into the opening for the purpose of instilling fluid. (25)

gate-control theory Melzack and Wall's theory of how pain impulses are transmitted. (32)

gay Homosexual. (37)

gender An individual's sex, male or female. (37)

gene Part of a chromosome that determines hereditary characteristics. (17)

General Adaptation Syndrome (GAS) Hans Selye's formulation of the common response to all stressors, composed of the alarm reaction, the stage of resistance, and the stage of exhaustion. (6)

general anesthesia Creating a loss of all sensation and perception through action on the central nervous system. (40)

general leads Facilitating responses composed of single words or noncommital sounds. (13)

generativity Erikson's term for the task of the middle years of forming ideas and plans for the next generation. (19)

generativity vs. stagnation stage The seventh of Erikson's stages of psychosocial development seen in the middle adult. (19)

genetic Hereditary. (17)

genetic defect An abnormality caused by defective genes. (17)

geriatrics The specialty in health care dealing with the aged patient. (20)

gerontology A broad field of study of old age. (20)

gestures Movements of the hands and arms that are designed to communicate. (13)

gigantism Excessive physical growth, usually related to hormonal oversecretion. (17)

glaucoma A disease of the eye, frequently afflicting older adults, that is characterized by an increase in intraocular pressure. (20)

global community The peoples of the world considered together. (33)

glucosuria The presence of abnormally high sugar in the urine. (27)

glomerulofiltration The process by which water and waste products are filtered and released by the glomeruli to produce urine. (27)

glycosuria Sugar or glucose in the urine. (27)

goal The purpose or aim; the desired outcome. (8, 11, 14)

goniometer A device for measuring the angle of a joint. (23)

"Good Samaritan" law A statute that provides immunity from claims of malpractice for health care professionals who render care in an emergency situation outside the health care facility. (3)

grief Sometimes used interchangeably with mourning. Feelings of despair that begin when a person perceives a loss. (41)

group Three or more people united for a common purpose. (14)

group process The manner in which a group works together that includes who speaks, to whom they speak, and the way in which they handle their tasks. (14)

growth Enlargement of the human structure, tissues or organs. (17)

guaiac A natural resin used as a reagent to test for blood in specimens.

guilt 1) A feeling of remorse over having done something wrong 2) Erikson's term for the unsuccessful outcome of early childhood in which the child is remorseful for having done something wrong.

gunnysacking Mentally saving grievances against another person and then "dumping" them all at one time, rather than dealing with each individual situation as it arises. (13)

gurgles A bubbling sound of moisture in large airways heard upon auscultation of the lungs. (28)

hair follicle The cavity out of which a hair grows. (22)

halitosis Unpleasant mouth odor. (22)

hallucinations The experiencing of sounds, sights, or smells that do not exist. (31)

healing Restoring to health. (6)

health An optimal state of homeostasis. (7)

health belief model A framework describing three factors that affect the chronically ill person's adherence to the prescribed regimen: how the severity and complications of the illness affect daily living, the person's ability to perform what is required, and the person's perception of the benefits to be derived from the care. (42)

health care team All those individuals of a variety of health occupations who work together to provide care to individuals. (2)

health deviation self-care requisites In Orem's theory, those unique needs created by illness, disability, or health problem. (9)

health maintenance Actions to preserve a state of health. (7)

health maintenance organization (HMO) An organization that provides all health care for a set prepaid fee. (2)

health promotion Efforts directed at improving an individual's state of health. (7)

heat loss Loss of heat from the body by any of four processes: radiation, conduction, convection, or evaporation. (4)

Heimlich maneuver An emergency procedure devised to expel foreign bodies from the air passageways. (28)

helminthic infections Infections caused in a person by the infestation of parasitic worms. (21)

hematocrit A measurement of the percentage of red blood cells in whole blood expressed as a volume per 100 ml. (29)

hematuria Blood in the urine. (27)

hemiplegia Paralysis of one side of the body. (23)

hemodialysis The process of circulating a patient's blood through a kidney machine for the purpose of removing wastes and excess fluid. (27)

hemoglobin The iron-containing, oxygen-carrying component of the blood; measured as the weight of the hemoglobin contained in the red blood cells in 100 ml of blood. (28)

hemoglobin saturation The percentage of oxygen being transported by the hemoglobin molecule. Normal is 90–100%. (28)

hemolytic reaction An adverse reaction to a blood transfusion in which red blood cells are broken down (hemolyzed). (30)

hemorrhagic exudate Fluid containing blood that is secreted into an area of inflammation. (6)

hepatitis An inflammatory condition of the liver. (22)

hernia The protrusion of an organ from its normal position through the wall that contains it. (26)

herpes A group of infections which can affect mucous membrane and nerve tissue in various locations of the body; mouth, skin, and genital organs. (21)

heterosexual Pertaining to sexual preference for members of the opposite sex. (37)

hexachlorophene An odorless white powder used in preparations as a bactericidal agent. (22)

hierarchy of needs Maslow's ascending ranking of needs, in which primary or physiologic needs are at the bottom and secondary or nonphysiologic needs are at the top. (5)

high-level wellness A term used by Dunn to describe a state of optimal balance and energy within an individual. (7)

Hinduism An ancient religion originating in India that teaches that one can become a part of a universal life force through correct actions. (36)

Hispanic Designating several groups of people who speak Spanish or Portuguese. (33)

histamine A protein product, found in all tissues of the body, that plays an active role in the inflammatory process by dilating blood vessels. It also causes constriction of bronchioles and increases secretion of gastric acid. Histamine production is increased when the body comes into contact with products to which it is sensitive. (6)

holistic healing Restoration of total or holistic health. (7)

holistic nursing Nursing that focuses on all body systems and psychosocial aspects of the person. (7)

Holy Communion A sacrament of Christians in which bread and wine (or grape juice) are taken as symbols of Christ's death and resurrection. (36)

homeodynamics Homeostasis. (4)

homeostasis The tendency of all living tissue to restore and maintain itself in a condition of balance or equilibrium. (4)

homosexual Pertaining to sexual preference for members of the same sex; gay. (37)

hopelessness A subjective state in which an individual sees limited or no alternatives or personal choices available and is unable to mobilize energy on own behalf. A NANDA diagnosis. (35)

hospice A philosophy of care and a system of delivery of care for the terminally ill and their families. (2, 41)

host The person in or on whom a pathogen lives. (7)

hostility A feeling of antagonism toward another in which the other is perceived as an opponent. (34)

huff cough A cough accomplished with the glottis open to prevent the buildup of intrathoracic pressure. (28)

human dignity The intrinsic worth that each individual has. (34)

human response patterns In the NANDA taxonomy, the overall framework for organizing nursing diagnoses. (10)

human serum albumin A protein component of blood that increases the colloidal osmotic pressure of the blood. (30)

humidification Increasing the amount of water vapor in the air. (28)

humoral immunity A generalized resistance of the whole body to an infecting agent. (6)

hunger A physical sensation of discomfort in the stomach indicating a need for food. (25)

hydrating solution An intravenous solution that primarily provides water, with dextrose or sodium chloride added for tonicity. (30)

hydrostatic pressure The pressure in the capillary that is created by the pressure in the arteries and tends to force fluid out of the capillary into the interstitial spaces. Also called filtration pressure. (30)

hygiene Those practices that bring about personal cleanliness, comfort, and feelings of well-being. (22)

hypalgesia Decreased perception of pain. (31, 32)

hyperalgesia Increased perception of pain. (31, 32)

hyperalimentation A method of providing complete nutrients via an intravenous line, usually into a subclavian vein; also called *total parenteral nutrition (TPN)*. (25)

hypercalcemia An excessive amount of calcium in the serum, greater than 5.5 mEq/L. (30)

hyperesthesia Increased sensation. (31)

hyperextension The act of straightening a limb to its position of maximal extension. (23)

hyperglycemia High blood sugar, above 120 mg/100 ml. (25)

hyperkalemia An excessive amount of potassium in the blood, greater than 5 mEq/L. (30)

hypernatremia An excessive amount of sodium in the blood, greater than 145 mEq/L. (30)

hyperpnea Very deep and rapid respirations. (28)

hypertension An elevated blood pressure, usually above 160 systolic and/or 100 diastolic. (29)

hypertonic 1) Designating excessive muscle tone. 2) Having an osmolality (number of particles per liter) greater than 300 mOsm/L of blood. (30)

hyperventilation Deep, rapid respiration. (28)

hypesthesia Decreased sensation. (31)

hypnosis A process of inducing a passive state in which the usual objective abilities are decreased and the person is abnormally suggestible. (32)

hypnotic Drug used to induce sleep. (24)

hypocalcemia A deficit in calcium in the blood, less than 4.5 mEq/L. (30)

hypoglycemia Low blood sugar. (38)

hypokalemia A deficit of potassium in the blood, less than 3.5 mEq/L. (30)

hyponatremia A deficit of sodium in the blood, less than 136 mEq/L. (30)

hypostatic pneumonia Pneumonia due to lack of movement. (28)

hypotensive Having a lower than normal blood pressure—in the adult, a systolic below 100. (29)

hypothermia A condition in which body temperature is lower than that necessary for body processes to function adequately. (40)

hypotonic 1) Designating lessened muscle tone. 2) Having an osmolality (number of particles per liter) less than 300 mOsm/L of blood. (30)

hypoventilation Shallow respirations. (28)

hypoxemia Low blood oxygen level, usually a PaO_2 of less than 55 mm Hg. (28)

hypoxia An oxygen deficiency of body tissues. (28)

hysterectomy The surgical removal of the uterus. (37)

iatrogenic Injury or illness caused by some aspect of health care. (21)

id As defined by Freud, the more primitive self. (17)

identification The adoption of attitudes and behaviors of an admired or cared-for person. (34)

identity Erikson's phrase for the adolescent's task of becoming independent as a person and beginning to set goals. (18)

identity vs. role confusion stage The fifth of Erikson's stages of psychosocial development seen in the adolescent. (18)

ileostomy A surgically created opening of the ileum onto the abdominal wall. (26)

illicit drugs Drugs which are possessed unlawfully. (39)

illusion The misinterpretation of real sights, sounds, or smells. (31)

imagery A healing technique that consists of helping people to visualize the inner working of their bodies in relationship to their illness and the treatment regimen. (7)

immobility Inability to move. (23)

immune response The reaction of the body to substances identified as foreign. (6)

immune system A group of tissues that react to pathogens and defend the body. (6)

immunity A condition of heightened responsiveness to an antigen, enabling the body to destroy the antigen and not contract the disease. *Active* immunity is produced by previous contact with the antigen in which the body develops the ability to produce an antibody against the antigen. *Passive* immunity is conferred temporarily by providing the body with an antibody produced elsewhere. (6)

immunoglobulins Antibodies. (6)

immunopathy A condition in which the immune system attacks the body's own cells, generating an autoimmune disease. (7)

immunosuppression Suppression of the body's natural immune system by drugs or other agents. (7)

impaction Lodging of compressed material in a confined space—for example, of hardened feces in the bowel. (26)

impaired adjustment The state in which the individual is unable to modify his/her life style/behavior in a manner consistent with a change in health status. A NANDA diagnosis. (34)

implementation The third step in the nursing process—carrying out the nursing plan through nursing intervention. (8, 11)

impotence The inability of the male to produce or maintain a penile erection. (37)

incident report A written record of the objective circumstances of untoward happening in a health care facility. (3) (15)

incipient pressure ulcer An area where pressure has interfered with the blood supply and cell damage has begun, but an open sore is not present. (22)

incontinence Involuntary urination or defecation. (26)

independence The ability to function alone without relying on anyone else. (18)

independent Competent and capable of managing one's own life. (18)

independent functioning Taking actions based on personal decision-making. (2)

independent role A function or position in which one acts based on one's own decision making. (1)

indirect contact The transmission of pathogens from one area to another by means of an object. (21)

industry Erikson's term for the task of middle childhood in which the child increases physical activity, develops competitiveness, and deals with authority. (18)

industry vs. inferiority stage The third of Erikson's stages of psychosocial development seen in the school age child. (18)

infectious agent A pathogen or a disease-causing microorganism. (21)

inferiority Erikson's term for the unsuccessful outcome of middle childhood in which the child feels inadequate. (18)

inflammation Localized heat, redness, swelling, and pain as a result of irritation, injury, or infection. (21)

influence Power to sway or affect another. (14)

informal group A group without a planned structure and manner of operating. (14)

informed consent A decision to accept treatment based on knowledge of both the potential benefits and the potential risks of the proposed treatment. (3)

infradian rhythms Body processes that occur on a regular monthly cycle. (24)

inhibitory ejaculation The inability to ejaculate semen or delay in the ejaculation of semen. (37)

initial plan The first comprehensive plan for medical care made by the physician. (15)

initiation stage The first stage in the life of a group during which the group members begin to establish a relationship. (14)

initiative Erikson's term for the task of early childhood of engaging in assertive interaction with family and peers. (18)

initiative vs. guilt stage The third of Erikson's stages of psychosocial development seen in the preschool child. (18)

inoculate To introduce agents into the body in order to bring about an active immunity. (6)

input Anything put into a system or expended in its operation. (2)

in-service education Classes and courses offered by an employer or taken by a person working in the field. (2)

insomnia The inability to sleep. (24)

inspiration The taking in of air. (28)

inspiratory capacity The maximum volume of air that can be inspired after a maximal expiration. (28)

inspiratory reserve The volume of air that can be inspired with maximal effort after a normal inspiration. (28)

instinctual theory of sleep The theory that sleep is an instinct of all persons. (24)

institutionalized racism Perpetuation of racism within institutions through various practices, including discriminatory employment policies. (33)

instrumental role The collection of behaviors that serve to assist in the accomplishment of tasks. (13)

integrative therapy Therapy in which feelings of loss are expressed and integrated through drawing, poetry, music, and the arts. (41)

integrity Erikson's term for the goal of the later years of developing a feeling of being complete and in contact with others in the environment. (19)

integrity vs. despair stage The eighth of Erikson's stages of psychosocial development seen in the older adult. (19)

interaction The total process of communication between two individuals. (13)

interdependence mode In Roy's assessment system, the responses of those in the individual's support system. (9)

interdependent functioning Taking actions based on joint decisions arrived at through consulting with others. (2)

interdisciplinary team 1) A group of health care workers representing different occupations who work together to provide comprehensive care. 2) In the hospice approach, a team of professional care providers who work together to meet the needs of dying persons. (41)

interferon A group of small proteins produced by the body that are released by cells invaded by a virus and other agents, causing noninvaded cells to form a protein to protect against invasion. (21)

intermittent fever A fever in which the temperature rises each day but sometime during each twenty-four-hour period returns to normal. (4)

intermittent positive pressure breathing (IPPB) A treatment performed intermittently by a machine delivering air or oxygen under pressure to cause maximum inflation of the lungs. (28)

internal girdle Those muscles of the abdomen, back, and hips that provide support to the abdominal contents and the pelvis. (23)

internal influences on learning Those factors within the individual that affect ability to learn. (16)

internal respiration Exchange of gases at the cellular level. (28)

interpersonal factors Those factors affecting the individual that originate in relationships between the individual and others. (34)

interpreting A blocking response in which meaning is ascribed to behavior. (13)

intershift report A verbal report given by a nurse finishing a shift to nursing staff beginning a shift of all significant information regarding patients. (15)

interstitial fluid The body fluid found in the spaces between the cells. (30)

intervention An action that is capable of altering an outcome. (7)

interviewing A sequenced question-and-answer process. (9, 13)

intimacy Erikson's term for the young adult's goal of establishing a close emotional relationship with another. (19)

intimacy vs. isolation stage The sixth of Erikson's stages of psychosocial development seen the young adult. (19)

intracellular fluid All the body fluid found inside the cells of the body. (30)

intraoperative The time period during which a surgical procedure is being done. (40)

intraventricular analgesia The administration of narcotics directly into the ventricles of the brain for purposes of pain relief. (32)

introductory phase The period during which a relationship is established. (13)

intromission Insertion. (37)

invasive A term used to describe any procedure in which a needle, catheter, or instrument enters the body. (38)

inversion The act of turning a limb in an inward direction. (23)

ion An electrically charged particle. (30)

ischemia Lack of blood supply to the tissue. (32)

Islam A religion based on the teachings of Mohammed, who lived in 600 AD in the Middle East. (36)

isolation 1)Erikson's term for the unsuccessful outcome of young adulthood in which the young adult feels separated or set apart from others. 2) A procedure for establishing physical barriers to the spread of microorganisms. (19) (21)

isometric exercises Exercises in which muscles are contracted tightly and held contracted without movement of body parts. (23)

isotonic Having the same osmolality as another fluid; a fluid (such as normal saline) having the same osmolality as blood, 300 mOsm/L. (30)

isotonic exercises Any exercises in which movement takes place. (23)

jaundice A yellowish tinge to the skin and other tissues caused by the deposit of bile salts. (22)

jejunostomy A surgical opening directly into the jejunum from the skin surface on the abdomen. (25)

Judaism The religion of the Jews, based on the Torah and the Talmud. (36)

keratin The hard protein substance that makes up the cells of the nails and the shafts of the hair. (22)

ketogenic diet A diet with a high percentage of calories in fats and proteins that produces a mild ketoacidosis. (25)

kinesis Movement. (4) (23)

kinesthetic feedback The perception of extent and direction of movement and of the position of body parts. (35)

kinetic Pertaining to movement. (23)
knowing In the NANDA taxonomy, a human response pattern of meaning associated with information. (10)
knowledge deficit A nursing diagnosis that refers to a condition in which an individual lacks knowledge or skill that is needed. (16)
Korotkoff sound The characteristic sound, heard on auscultation of the artery, produced by the blood as it forces its way into the artery during systole after the artery has been occluded. It is used to measure blood pressure. (29)
kosher food Food prepared and served in accord with Jewish dietary laws. (25)
Kussmaul's respirations Deep and rapid respirations that cause a "blowing" sound. (28)
kyphosis An abnormal convexity in the curvature of the thoracic spine, often seen in the elderly. (19)

labile Unstable with the tendency to change. (29)
lactase An enzyme found in the kidney, liver, and gastric mucosa that allows the digestion of lactose, a common component in milk products. (25)
lactovegetarian See vegetarian. (25)
ladder concept A general philosophy of providing accessibility from one level of education to another without loss of credit or repetition. (1)
laissez-faire A form of group rule in which there is no designated leader and no formal process for decision-making. (14)
laity The members of a religious group who are not designated as clergy. (36)
laparotomy A surgical procedure in which the abdomen is opened. (40)
laser A device that produces light of specific frequencies focused into very narrow bands that may be used for dissecting tissue in surgery. (40)
lassitude A feeling of lethargy or exhaustion. (24)
latency period Freud's psychosexual stage of the 6- to 11-year-old, when sensual needs are satisfied without overt identification with the parent of the opposite sex. (18)
learning A change in behavior not due to growth or fatigue. (16)
learning need A need for a change in behavior. (16)
learning style The manner of presentation in which an individual most effectively learns. (16)
leave-taking The process of terminating an interpersonal relationship. (13)
legitimizing Establishing an illness or disability as real and acceptable to others. (42)
leisure ethic A belief that the most valuable activities are those that one chooses for pleasure or enrichment. (36)
lesbian A homosexual woman. (37)
lethargy Sleepiness or somnolence. (31)
level of awareness The degree to which a person is responsive to environmental stimuli. (31)
liability insurance Insurance designed to pay legal costs for defense against a suit and damages awarded. (3)
libel Any written, printed, or pictorial statement that damages a person by exposing him or her to ridicule. (3)
libido Sexual desire. (37)
licensed practical nurse (LPN) An individual with a legal credential attesting to a minimum level of competence and permitting the practice of practical nursing for pay. (1)
licensure The acquisition of a license, or legal credential. (1) (3)
licensure by endorsement The acquisition of a license in an additional state after licensure by examination in the initial state. (1) (3)
licensure law The law that specifies the requirements for obtaining, renewing, and removing a professional license. (1) (3)
life change units A measure, developed by Holmes and Rahe, of the relative amount of stress created by any particular change that may occur in a person's life. (6)
life continuum The life span. (17)
life review A process of grieving for the patient and family in which one reflects about the past and reviews family events. (41)
lifestyle The values one holds and the manner in which one's life is conducted. (36)
Local Adaptation Syndrome (LAS) Body responses to localized threats that establish the conditions to restore homeostasis. (6)
local anesthesia Creating a loss of all sensation and perception in a limited area of the body through action on local sensory nerves. (40)
long-term care (LTC) Health care for a condition that requires treatment of a less extensive nature for a prolonged period of time. (2, 20)
long-term care facilities Health care facilities designed to care for individuals for periods of weeks, months, or years. These include rehabilitation centers, nursing homes, assisted living facilities, and congregate care centers. (20)
love-and-belonging needs In Maslow's hierarchy, the needs just above safety needs. (5)
lumen The inner open space of a needle, tube, or vessel. (29)

maceration The softening of tissue caused by prolonged contact with moisture. (22)
macronutrient A food substance needed in large quantities. (25)
macrophage system A group of cells that move throughout the body to engulf and destroy invading microorganisms. (6)
magnetic resonance imaging (MRI) A noninvasive procedure using a powerful magnetic field and radiofrequency pulses to produce images of body tissue on films. (38)
mal de ojo The affliction of the "evil eye," viewed as a cause of illness among some Hispanic people. (33)
malaise A vague feeling of weakness or discomfort. (23)
malingering A conscious exaggeration of symptoms to gain rewards. (7)
malnutrition A state in which the body is poorly nourished because of a general dietary lack of many nutrients or a specific lack of one essential nutrient. (25)
malpractice Failure to act as a reasonably prudent professional person would act in a similar situation. (3)
mandatory continuing education Continuing education that is a prerequisite for relicensure. (3)
mandatory licensure A requirement that a legal credential be obtained to practice an occupation. (1)
markers Substances that can be detected in blood or body

fluid that indicate the presence of abnormal cell growth or disease. (38)

mastectomy Removal of a breast. (35)

masturbation Self-stimulation for the purpose of eliciting sexual pleasure. (37)

maturation The changes in an individual which include changes in growth and development. (17)

maturational crisis A developmental crisis. (34)

means of transmission The route or vehicle by which pathogens move from one person to another. (21)

mediator A chemical that causes certain body processes to take place. (6)

Medicaid A federal and state government system for financing care for individuals meeting financial or disability requirements. (2)

medical diagnosis A statement of a disease state or pathology that is identified and treated by a physician. (10)

medical ethics The area of ethics that relates to health care. (3)

medical experimentation The administration of drugs or performance of treatments or procedures to test knowledge of their validity. (3)

medical healing Bringing about the cessation of symptoms without surgical intervention. (7)

medical plan of care The physician's plan for treating the disease process and its symptoms. (11)

medically indigent Designates an individual without resources to pay for health care. (2)

Medicare A federal government system for financing health care primarily for those 65 or older. (2) (20)

meditation A technique for shutting out stimuli and producing the relaxation response by sitting quietly and focusing the mind on a neutral topic. (6)

membranous exudate A secretion onto an area of inflammation that forms a thin, pliable layer on the tissue. (6)

menopause The cessation of menstruation and the end of reproduction in the woman. The term is sometimes used broadly to indicate lessening of reproductive ability in both men and women. (19)

menses Menstruation. (18)

mental health A situation in which the individual possesses the cognitive and emotional patterns necessary for feelings of well-being and effective functioning in a particular culture. (34)

mental illness A situation in which the individual does not possess the cognitive and emotional patterns necessary for effective functioning and feels distress. (34)

mentation Thinking or cognition. (31)

message That which is communicated. (13)

metabolic acidosis A state in which the blood pH is greater than 7.45 because of a bicarbonate deficit. (30)

metabolic alkalosis A state in which the blood pH is less than 7.35 because of a bicarbonate excess. (30)

metabolic water Water produced by the body in the process of metabolism. (25, 30)

micronutrient A food substance needed in minute quantities. (25)

microorganisms Extremely small animals and plants. (21)

micturition Urination or voiding. (27)

migrants Those individuals who periodically move from one place to another to find work, primarily farm workers. (33)

milliequivalent (mEq) A measure of combining power or electrical charges of a given substance. (30)

milliosmole (mOsm) A measure of osmolality (number of particles) in a solution. (30)

mineral An inorganic compound used by the body in building tissue. (25)

minimum daily requirements (MDR) The lowest amount of a nutrient needed for the body to maintain appropriate functioning. (25)

minority A group smaller than the main group within a society. (33)

mistrust Erikson's term for the unsuccessful outcome of infant development in which the infant fears others or the environment. (18)

modes of adaptation According to the Roy Adaptation Theory, these are areas in which the individual adapts. They include physiologic mode, self concept mode, role function mode, and interdependence mode. (9)

modified Brompton's mixture See Bromptom's mixture. (32)

monoamine oxidase (MAO) inhibitors A class of drugs used primarily for depression (39)

moral development The development of the conscience, which determines principles of right and wrong. (17)

morbidity An illness or the rate of incidence of an illness. (7)

mourning The normal psychological process that follows a loss and accompanies feelings of grief. (41)

Moro reflex An infant's normal response to a loud noise, in which the body jerks and the arms abduct; also called the startle reflex. (18)

motivation An internal drive or desire. (16)

motor aphasia The inability to form words due to lack of innervation of the muscles of speech. (31)

motor impulses Messages conveyed to the brain regarding movement. (23)

mottled Descriptive of irregular, discolored blotches on the skin. (22)

mouth-to-mouth resuscitation Providing respiration to the nonbreathing individual by blowing into the mouth to inflate the lungs and allowing the natural recoil of the chest to empty them; rescue breathing. (29)

moving In the NANDA taxonomy, a human response pattern of activity. (10)

moxibustion The burning of substances for the purpose of enhancing healing. (33)

mucous membrane The tissue that secretes mucus and lines the cavities of the body that open to the outside. (22)

mucus The viscous suspension of mucin, water, cells, and inorganic salts that is secreted as a protective lubricant coating by glands in the mucous membranes. (22)

muscle tone The degree of basic contraction of the muscles that serves to make them prepared for action. (23)

Muslim A person of the Islamic faith. (36)

mutation A change in the genetic material, such as the chromosomes or genes. (7)

myotonia A state of contraction of a muscle group. (23)

NANDA (North American Nursing Diagnosis Association) An organization of nurses that studies and approves nursing diagnosis statements for clinical trial, research, and communication. (8)

narcolepsy A non–life-threatening sleep disorder in which the person may fall asleep for many very short periods throughout each day. (24)

narrative charting A style of patient record keeping in which the nurse records information in a storylike form on the nurses' notes. (15)

nasogastric tube feeding A nutritious formula instilled through a tube that passes from the nose through the esophagus to the stomach. (25)

native American American-born Indians or Eskimos.

natural death acts Statutes passed by a number of states to allow a person to legally determine the extent of use of extraordinary measures to prolong life. (41)

natural immunity Resistance to a specific microorganism acquired through infection with that microorganism. (6)

nausea A subjective feeling of discomfort in the stomach and throat that indicates a potential for vomiting. (25)

nebulization The producing of a fine spray of moisture in the air. (28)

necrosis Breakdown or death of tissue. (6)

need That which is necessary or required for optimal functioning. (5)

need for full functioning As defined by Carl Rogers, the basic need of human beings to realize their full potential. (5)

need to know/understand In Maslow's hierarchy, a higher level need to gain knowledge. (5)

negative feedback A process whereby a rising level of a substance or increased rate of a process signals the system producing the substance or controlling the process to shut off. (6)

negligence The failure to act as a reasonably prudent person would act in a similar situation, resulting in harm to another. (3)

negotiation stage The second state in the life of a group during which members develop a pattern for relating and decision-making. (14)

neonate Newborn infant, usually applied for the first month of life. (18)

neuro signs A brief assessment of neurologic status, usually including pulse, respiration, blood pressure, level of awareness, pupillary response, and muscle strength. (31)

neuroendocrine system The complex interactions of the nervous system and the endocrine system. (6)

neurogenic bladder Partial paralysis of the bladder musculature because of a spinal cord injury that prevents complete emptying. (27)

neurogenic pain Pain originating from stimulation or irritation of a nerve. (32)

neurohormonal theory of sleep A theory attributing sleep to the increased presence of the neurohormonal substance serotonin. (24)

nociceptor A nerve receptor that responds to painful stimuli. (32)

nocturia Urination during the nighttime hours. (27)

noncompliance Failure to adhere to therapeutic recommendations. NANDA diagnosis: A person's informed decision not to adhere to a therapeutic recommendation. (34)

nondirective comments Facilitating responses that open the conversation but do not direct its flow. (13)

noninvasive A procedure that does not involve a needle, catheter, or instrument entering the body. (38)

nontraditional healing Approaches to supporting the body's ability to heal that are outside of the official health care system. The use of a variety of healing methods including those that may be considered without a scientific base. (7)

nonverbal communication Relating to communication through body signs and facial expressions. (13)

normal flora Beneficial microorganisms that inhibit the growth of pathogens within a certain area of the body. (21)

normal saline A solution of sodium chloride with the same osmolality or tonicity as body fluid, usually given as 0.9 percent. (30)

normalizing A response to chronic illness in which the person tries to create the impression of being a completely normal person without disability. (42)

norms the standards for behavior within a group. (14)

nosocomial infections Designating hospital-acquired infections. (21)

novice A person new to an activity or endeavor. (8)

NPO "non per ora" or nothing by mouth. (39)

Nurse Practice Act The statutory law that defines nursing and specifies the requirements for obtaining, renewing, and revoking a license to practice nursing. (3)

nurse anesthetist An advanced practice registered nurse who administers anesthetic agents and provides related care. (40)

nurse practitioner A registered nurse with special education who provides primary health care. (1, 2)

nursing actions Those activities carried out by the nurse to prevent or alleviate problems, including interviews, observations, and interventions. (11)

nursing care plan A written, detailed approach to providing nursing care in which problems are identified, desired outcomes or goals are set, and nursing actions are specified. (8)

nursing diagnosis A statement of a patient problem that the nurse, by virtue of education and experience, is able to identify and treat. It includes the etiology when known. (8, 10)

nursing history A structured interview designed to establish a data base for nursing care. (9)

nursing home A facility designed to provide long term comprehensive care for individuals who are dependent or need skilled care. (20)

nursing interventions Those activities carried out by the nurse in an attempt to prevent or alleviate a problem. (8)

nursing observations Those activities carried out by the nurse to gather objective data. (8)

nursing orders Directions for nursing care for a specific patient written by a nurse. (2, 11)

nursing process A problem-solving approach to planning care that includes the four steps of assessment, planning, implementation, and evaluation. (8)

nutrition All of the processes involved in taking in and using food, including ingestion, digestion, absorption, and metabolism. (25)

obesity Excessive body weight, usually considered to be 15%

to 20% over average weight for sex, age, height, and bone structure. (25)

objective A specific desired outcome. It is often used interchangeably with *goal;* however, the term *goal* is sometimes used to indicate a broader, less specific outcome. (11, 16)

objective data Information based on observable phenomena. (9)

observation The act of systematically noting phenomena. (9)

occult blood Hidden blood, such as blood in the stool. (26, 27, 38)

oedipal conflict Freud's psychosexual stage of the 4- to 5-year-old, when the parent of the opposite sex is the object of sensual satisfaction. (18)

oliguria Scanty formation of urine by the kidneys. (27)

open system A system in which input comes from a variety of sources and output may occur in different ways. (2)

operation stage The third stage in the life of a group during which work is accomplished. (14)

operative period The time during which surgery is performed. (40)

opisthotonos position An abnormal backward, flexed, bridgelike configuration of the body which may accompany decerebration. (31)

opposing responses Setting oneself up in a conflicting position with another. (13)

oral irrigator A device using a high-pressure stream of water, commonly used to clean the teeth. (22)

oral stage A psychosexual stage of development described by Freud during which the infant's mouth is the center of gratification. (18)

orchidectomy Removal of the testicle in the male. (37)

orders Directions for care. (11)

orgasm Sexual climax. (37)

orientation stage The first stage in the life of a group during which members establish themselves as a group. (14)

orthopnea Difficulty in breathing that is relieved by sitting up or standing. (28)

orthopneic position An upright sitting or standing position used to relieve difficulty in breathing. (28)

orthostatic (postural) hypotension A drop in blood pressure caused by a change in position. (23)

osmolality A measure of the number of particles per liter of solvent. (25, 30)

osmolarity A measure of the number of particles per kilogram of a solvent. The term is often used interchangeably with osmolality but is exactly the same only when the solvent is pure water at 3.8°C. (30)

osmosis The diffusion of water across a semipermeable membrane from an area where there are relatively fewer particles to one where there are relatively more particles. (30)

osteoarthritis Degeneration and pain of the joints often associated with aging. (20)

osteoporosis A metabolic failure to replace bone tissue. It causes bones to become thin, porous, and easily fractured. (20)

otitis media Inflammation or infection of the middle ear; frequently occurs in children. (31)

outcome criteria Specific standards by which to evaluate results of nursing care. (11)

output 1) Anything that results from the operation of a system. 2) The fluid excreted by the body—urine, perspiration, vomitus, and so on. (27)

outreach A system whereby care is provided outside of the institutional setting. (2)

ovolactovegetarian See vegetarian. (25)

oxygenation Treating, combining, or infusing with oxygen. (28)

pacing The rate of speaking and pauses in an interaction. (13)

packed red blood cells Components of blood that remain after the majority of the plasma is removed from the whole blood. (30)

pain cocktail An oral liquid medication containing a pain medication and other agents helpful to the patient, such as a tranquilizer or antiemetic. (32)

pain interpretation Comparing the sensation of pain to other experiences and identifying type and severity. (32)

pain perception Recognition by the brain that the stimulus is pain. (32)

pain reaction The response of the individual to pain. (32)

pain receptor The nerve ending that receives the pain stimulus. (32)

pain response The physiologic changes, behaviors, and feelings that occur in the person as a result of pain perception. (32)

pain threshold The amount of painful stimulation needed for pain to be perceived. (32)

palliative For purposes of comfort. (32)

pallor A lack of the red color tones normally given to the skin by oxygen-rich blood. (28)

palsy Paralysis. (23)

panic A state of overwhelming anxiety in which the individual is unable to function. (34)

paradoxic sleep Another name for REM sleep, based on the contradiction between the relaxation of the muscles and the extreme activity of the brain. (24)

paralysis Loss or impairment of the ability to move or have sensation in a body part as a result of injury to or disease of its nerve supply. (23)

paralytic ileus An abnormal loss of bowel motility. (26)

paraorgasm The experiencing of orgasmic equivalents in body areas other than the genitalia. (37)

paraplegia Paralysis of the lower portion of the body. (23)

parasitic worms Long, soft-bodied invertebrates that survive only by feeding off a host. (21)

parasympathetic nervous system The division of the autonomic nervous system that decreases stimulation of smooth muscle and glands. (4)

parenteral nutrition Essential nutrients administered intravenously. (25)

paresis Muscular weakness due to partial interruption of stimuli to that muscle or a group of muscles. (23)

paresthesia A distortion of sensation such as itching, tingling, crawling, or prickling. (31)

passive exercise Any type of exercise in which another person provides the energy and moves the individual. (23)

passive immunity Resistance to a specific microorganism acquired from the administration of antibodies. (6)

paternalism The practice of governing or treating people in a fatherly fashion. (3)

pathogens Disease-producing microorganisms. (7, 21)

patient autonomy The right of the patient to make decisions and determine treatment. (3)

patient care coordinator An individual whose job is to plan for nursing care for those being discharged from an acute care facility. (15)

patient-controlled analgesia (PCA) A method of administering intravenous narcotics through a programmed pump that allows the patient to determine when a dose is needed. (32)

patient outcome Specific results from the patient's care. (11)

patients' rights Those powers or privileges to which the health care consumer has an established moral claim. (3, 11)

peer review organization (PRO) An organization designated by Medicare to evaluate the appropriateness and effectiveness of medical care. (12)

peer A person having equal status or belonging to the same group such as a friend or classmate. (18, 41)

perceiving In the NANDA taxonomy, a human response pattern of reception of information. (10)

perception Becoming aware of the message communicated in an interaction. (13, 31)

perceptual feedback Information about the self gained through touch. (31, 35)

perioperative period The entire period surrounding a surgical procedure including the preoperative, intraoperative, and postoperative phases. (40)

peripheral arterial insufficiency A condition in which circulation to the extremities is inadequate. (29)

peripheral nervous system (PNS) The division of the nervous system that includes all structures and nerves other than the brain and spinal cord. (31)

peripheral venous insufficiency A condition in which return circulation from the extremities is inadequate. (29)

peristalsis Wavelike muscular contractions that propel contained matter along the alimentary canal. (26)

peritoneal dialysis Removal of waste products from the body by the instillation and removal of a dialyzing solution into the peritoneal cavity. (27)

permissive licensure A legal credential that may be obtained to attest to competence but that is not required for practice. (1)

personal identity The consciousness of one's self as a distinct and unique person. (35)

pH A measure of the acidity or alkalinity of a solution, in a range of 1 to 14—7.0 is neutral, numbers below that are acidic, and numbers above that are alkaline. (30)

phallic stage Freud's psychosexual stage of the 3- to 4-year-old, when the genital region provides greatest sensual satisfaction. (18)

phantom pain Pain perceived in a body part that is no longer present, such as an amputated leg. (32)

pharmacotherapeutics The use of drugs to treat disease and/or improve an individual's health. (39)

phlebitis An inflammation of a vein. (29)

phobia An irrational fear. (34)

physical dependence A state in which the body has physiologically adapted to a chemical substance and requires its presence in order to maintain function. (32)

physical needs The external factors necessary for an individual or group to function, including space, light, comfortable temperature, and seating. (5, 14)

physician's assistant An individual who works with a physician performing routine parts of the physician's role such as caring for patients with common illnesses and injuries. (2)

physiologic homeostasis A state of balance or equilibrium within all the physiologic processes of respiration, circulation, and metabolism. (4)

physiologic mode In Roy's assessment system, nine areas of physiologic functioning. (9)

physiologic needs Maslow's lower level needs that are essential to life. (5)

physiologic status The status of the body with regard to the meeting of physiologic needs. (16)

pitting edema An excess of fluid in the interstitial spaces such that pressure from a finger on the surface displaces fluid, creating a depression that refills slowly. (30)

pituitary theory of sleep A theory that the pituitary, a small gland at the base of the brain, is a sleep regulator. (24)

placebo An inert substance given in place of an active agent to which the body reacts as if it were the active agent. (32, 39)

placebo effect A positive response to a substance or treatment that is caused by trust and an attitude of expectation rather than a reaction to the substance or treatment itself. (32, 39)

placental barrier The normal barrier, formed by the semipermeable membrane of the placenta, that selectively admits or inhibits the passage of substances into the fetal circulation. (17)

planning The second stage in the nursing process, which includes setting goals or objectives and establishing a detailed scheme for nursing actions. (8)

plateau 1) A stable state or leveling. 2) The second stage of the sexual response as described by Masters and Johnson in which further vasocongestion of the pelvis and genital area occurs. (18)

pleural rub A chest sound of rubbing or grating as the pleurae rub together. (28)

podiatrist Specialist in the care of the feet. (22)

point of maximal impulse The place on the chest where the heartbeat is most clearly palpated and auscultated, usually the midclavicular line at the fifth intercostal space. (29)

polyuria Increased formation of urine by the kidneys. (27)

portal of entry The portal or opening by which a pathogen enters a susceptible host. (21)

portal of exit The place where a pathogen leaves a reservoir or susceptible host. (21)

positron emission tomography (PET) A computer-based imaging procedure that uses inhaled or injected radioactive material to produce an image of an organ's functional processes. Blood flow and metabolism can both be identified. (38)

postanesthesia recovery room (PARR) An area of the health care facility that provides specialized care for the person in the immediate postoperative period until the patient has recovered from the anesthesia. (40)

postconventional level Kohlberg's level of moral development in which moral decision making is based on issues rather than family, friends, or social authority. (19)

postoperative period The time after a surgery is performed until recovery is complete. (40)

postural blood pressures Blood pressure measured consecutively in the lying, sitting, and standing positions. (29)

postural drainage A procedure for the purpose of draining secretions from the lungs by placing the person in a variety of positions. Percussion or tapping may also be done. (28)

postural (orthostatic) hypotension Low blood pressure that occurs when one changes from a lying to an upright position; orthostatic hypotension. (23, 29)

posture The position of body parts in relationship to one another. (23)

power The ability to exercise control, for example, within a group. (14)

practice Carrying out an activity in order to learn to do it more accurately, effectively, or efficiently. (16)

precaution Step taken to protect. (21)

preconventional level Kohlberg's level of moral development in which moral decision-making is based on consequences to self, often of a physical nature. (17)

preformed water Water found in food substances. (25)

prejudice Adverse judgments or opinions without knowledge or facts; bias. (33)

premature ejaculation Ejaculation of semen by the male generally within 30 to 60 seconds after intromission. (37)

prenatal Before birth. (18)

preoperational stage Piaget's cognitive stage of the 2- to 7-year-old, which incorporates the increasing mastery of symbols and language. (17)

preoperative period The time after a surgery is planned until it occurs. (40)

presbyopia Difficulty accommodating the eyes to near objects. (19)

prescription A written instruction by a physician, most commonly referring to a medication. (11, 39)

present orientation A belief that the current time is more important than either past or future. (36)

pressure ulcer An open sore or lesion of superficial tissue caused by pressure. (22)

preventive health care Intervention that prevents either injury or illness.(7)

primary care The initial source of health care through which a person may obtain entry into other facets of the health care system. It includes health examinations, treatment of illness, and referral when necessary. (2)

primary group The intimate personal group of which one is a part, usually the family unit. (14)

primary nurse The nurse who assumes overall responsibility for a patient. (1)

primary nursing See primary nurse. (1)

primary prevention Actions taken to prevent illness from occurring. (16)

primary role A role that one possesses without choice, such as woman or man, or person of a specific age. (34)

principle A basic rule concerning the functioning of a natural phenomenon that indicates cause and effect. (11)

priority That which takes precedence by virtue of importance or urgency. (11)

probing A blocking response in which one asks detailed personal questions not pertinent to current care needs. (13)

problem A difficulty that arises when a need is not met. (5)

problem list The combined index and table of contents for the problem-oriented record that identifies all notes and problems and when they were resolved. (15)

problem-oriented record (POR) A patient's chart organized around the problems that are present. (15)

problem-solving approach An organized, thoughtful method of seeking a solution to a difficulty, usually outlined in steps. (8)

process The way a group works to meet its goal, including who speaks, the type of contribution of each person, and the feelings expressed; the "how" of group life. (14)

process criteria Specific standards by which to evaluate the methods used in nursing care. (15)

proctoscopy The direct visualization of the rectum and distal portion of the colon using a specialized endoscope. (26)

productivity The quality of being useful through producing something. (14)

professional role A function or position in which one's actions are based on the requirements of the occupation. (1)

progress notes An ongoing record of what is happening to the patient in relationship to the problems presented. (15)

progressive relaxation A technique for achieving the relaxation response in which parts of the body are relaxed in a gradual manner until the whole body is relaxed. (6)

projectile vomiting The forceful expulsion of stomach contents to a distance from the person. (25)

projection Placing one's own feelings, ideas, or attributes onto another. (34)

prophylactic Preventive. (21)

proprioception The ability to identify the location of one's body parts. (23)

proprioceptor Sensory nerve that responds to position of body parts. (23)

prospective reimbursement A system of payment for health care in which the payment is made in advance of the services rendered. (2)

protein A complex compound composed of carbon, hydrogen, oxygen, and nitrogen that is essential for building body tissue and can be broken down to provide energy. (25)

protein reserve The body's stores of amino acids and proteins that can be used for healing and tissue repair. (25)

proteinuria The abnormal presence of protein in the urine; albuminuria. (27)

Protestantism The branch of Christianity that arose during the Reformation in reaction to what were seen as abuses in the Roman Catholic Church. (36)

protocol A set of directions for nursing actions to accomplish a specific task. (11)

pseudoprofessional comments A blocking response involving inappropriate attempts to use psychological terms or methods in an interaction. (13)

psychological equilibrium A state of emotional and mental balance; homeostasis. (4)
psychologic homeostasis A state of balance within the psychologic processes of the person that creates mental well-being and is reflected in being able to maintain equilibrium in the face of stressors. See psychologic equilibrium. (4)
psychological needs Those internal factors that must be provided for a group to function. (5)
psychomotor learning A type of learning related to acquiring technical skills. (16)
psychosexual Designating the psychological aspect of sexuality. (17)
psychosocial needs Those needs that are emotional or that involve others. (5)
psychosocial tasks Havighurst' theory that designated tasks have to be learned at each stage of the life in order to satisfactorily progress. (17)
psychosurgery Surgery performed to change a person's thinking or behavior. (34)
psychotherapy Treatment of psychological disorders. (34)
puberty Freud's psychosexual stage of the 11- to 14-year-old, when there is integration of sensual tendencies from previous stages. (18)
pulmonary edema An excess of fluid in the interstitial spaces of the lungs. (30)
pulmonary embolism An object that moves through the veins to lodge in the lungs. (28)
pulse The pressure wave produced in the artery by the force of the heart's contraction. (29)
pulse deficit The difference in rate between apical and radial pulses. It represents the number of weak, ineffective heartbeats per minute. (29)
pulse pressure The difference between systolic and diastolic blood pressure. It represents the pressure produced by each heartbeat. (29)
pulse rate The number of pulse waves per minute. (29)
pulse rhythm The pattern of the pulse beats, whether regular or irregular. (29)
pulse strength The power felt in each pulse beat. (29)
purulent Containing or secreting pus. (6, 21)
purulent drainage See purulent exudate.
purulent exudate A secretion, produced by inflammation, that contains pus. (6)
pyrexia Fever. (21)
pyuria Pus in the urine. (27)

quad cough A cough that is enhanced by pressure to the abdomen and against the diaphragm to augment the effectiveness of the cough in those with weakened or absent neuromuscular control. (28)
quadriplegia Paralysis of all four extremities. (23)
quality assurance Programs for evaluating health care and its delivery. (2, 12, 39)
quality management Mechanisms used to monitor function and ensure positive outcomes in an organization. (12)
quality of life The extent to which life provides those attributes that are valued by the individual. (42)
quiet room A place in a hospital where individuals may go when a private, quiet atmosphere is desired. (36)

rabbi The clergy or teacher in the Jewish faith. (36)
radiating pain Pain that spreads from its point of origin to other areas. (32)
radiopaque substance A compound that blocks x-rays and therefore creates an image on radiologic exposure; also called contrast material. Used to make soft tissue visible on x-ray. (38)
radiation Heat loss to another object without contact. (4)
râles A bubbling chest sound as air moves through moisture or secretions in the lungs. (28)
range-of-motion exercises (ROM) Exercises in which joints are moved through the full range or extent to which they can be moved. (23)
rapid eye movement sleep (REM) An essential stage in the sleep cycle involving high cortical activity and characterized by the rapid horizontal movement of both eyes, profound muscular relaxation, and vivid dreaming. (24)
rationale Those definitions, facts, and principles that form the fundamental reasons for nursing action. (11)
rationalization Identification of intellectual reasons for behavior and feelings; also called *intellectualization*. (34)
reaction formation Adopting of ideas and beliefs that are the opposite of those held by an individual or group that one dislikes or wishes to be independent of. (34)
reader The individual in the Christian Science Church who provides advice and teaching. (36)
readiness to learn The stage brought about by the combined effect of internal influences on learning. (16)
reasonably prudent nurse A nurse who behaves in accordance with what can be established as the standard for nursing practice in the local community. (3)
receiver The person trying to understand the message in an interaction. (13)
reciprocity A procedure by which a state will grant a license without examination to a person who is licensed in another state. (3)
recoil The ability of the lung to spring back during expiration. (28)
Recommended Dietary Allowances (RDA) The amounts of foods needed to provide an adequately nutritious diet for activity, growth, and repair in most people as determined by the Food and Nutrition Board of the National Research Council. There are different recommendations for each age group and for pregnant and lactating women. (25)
referral form A form used to provide information to another care provider who is being asked to assume responsibility for some portion of the patient's care. (15)
referred pain Pain perceived as originating in a place other than where the stimuli occurred. (32)
reflecting A facilitating response in which a person's statement is simply repeated as a question. (13)
refractory stage According to Masters and Johnson, a stage of sexual response after orgasm during which subsequent performance by the male is not possible. (37)
regional anesthesia Creating a loss of all sensation and perception in a region of the body through action on regional sensory nerves. (40)
regeneration Healing in which the original type of tissue is restored in structure and function. (6)
registered nurse (RN) An individual who has met the edu-

cational and testing requirements for licensure to practice registered nursing as defined in the Nurse Practice Act. (1)

regression Acting in a manner characteristic of a younger age. (7, 34)

rehabilitation The process of restoring an individual to maximum independence and well-being through education and therapy. (2, 7, 42)

reinforcement A reward given to a learner for making the desired responses. (16)

rejecting A blocking response in which a person is unwilling to hear feelings or concerns. (13)

relating In the NANDA taxonomy, a human response pattern of establishing bonds. (10)

relaxation response A state characterized by decreases in sympathetic nervous system activity, muscle tone, blood pressure, pulse rate, respirations, and pupillary constriction. (6)

religious medals Small amulets with religious symbols on the surface. (36)

REM rebound A term used for unusually long periods of REM sleep that occur after the discontinuation of many of the hypnotics. (24)

remedios Traditional folk medicine in the Hispanic culture. (33)

REM sleep See rapid eye movement sleep. (24)

remiss To improve or cease causing symptoms. (7, 42)

remission The phase of a chronic illness in which there are minimal or no symptoms. (42)

remittent fever A fever that rises and falls within a constantly elevated range. (21)

renal calculi Mineral salts that have precipitated out of the urine within the urinary tract, also called renal stones. (27)

renal failure Total absence of the formation of urine by the kidneys. (27)

renal suppression A state in which the kidneys are unable to adequately filter the blood and produce urine. (27)

replacement Filling or finding a substitute for a loss. (41)

replacement solution An intravenous solution containing electrolytes in the same proportion as a body fluid (such as gastric fluid) being secreted in excessive amounts. (30)

report A verbal or written summary of pertinent information regarding the patient, such as that given by one shift to another. (15)

repression Unconsciously putting unpleasant or stressful thoughts completely out of awareness. (34)

reservoir A place where pathogens, under certain conditions, grow and multiply. (21)

resident A person who lives and is cared for in a long-term care facility. (20)

residual volume The amount of air left in the lungs after a maximal expiration. (28)

resignation Passive submission to a situation. (41)

resistance The second stage of Selye's General Adaptation Syndrome during which the body mobilizes its resources and resists the threat. (6)

resistive exercise Movement performed against a resistance such as a weight. (23)

resolution Taking action to accommodate to a loss.(41)

resource A person, organization, or place that can provide needed assistance. (15)

respiratory acidosis A condition characterized by hypoventilation and decreased levels of carbonic acid in the blood, resulting in a blood pH of less than 7.35. (28, 30)

respiratory alkalosis A condition characterized by hyperventilation and increased levels of carbonic acid in the blood, resulting in a blood pH or greater than 7.45. (28, 30)

respite care Care given to a dependent individual to provide temporary relief for the usual caregiver. (41, 42)

restating A facilitating response in which a receiver rephrases the statement of the sender. (13)

restitution Making life changes or responses to the recognition that a death has occurred. (34, 41)

retention The holding of urine within the bladder due to inability to void. (27)

reticuloendothelial system The network of tissues and cells throughout the body that are able to phagocytize particles. (6)

retirement residences Apartments within the community designed for the elderly and which provide limited services. (20)

retraction An abnormal pulling in of soft tissue of the chest on inspiration, commonly seen in the supraclavicular, intercostal, and substernal areas. (28)

retrospective reimbursement A system of payment for health care services in which the payment is made for the exact services that have been given after services are rendered. (2)

retrospective review An evaluation process that takes place after the patient's discharge, usually done by examining records. (8)

reversibility A property of cognitive development described by Piaget in which a child has the ability to perceive an image in a previously presented form; for example, the child recognizes as torn paper as one previously intact. (18)

reviewing A facilitating response in which the interaction is reviewed. (13)

rhonchi Bubbling or wheezing chest sounds indicative of moisture in larger airways. (28)

rigid endoscope A specialized endoscope that cannot be bent, usually made of metal. (38)

risk state for a medical problem A situation in which a person has a high probability of developing a specific problem that will require intervention by a physician. (10)

role The behaviors that characterize a function or position. (34)

role ambiguity A type of role strain in which there are unclear expectations about appropriate role behavior. (34)

role conflict A type of role strain in which the various roles a person must perform require conflicting or incompatible behaviors. (34)

role confusion Erikson's term for the unsuccessful outcome of adolescence in which the adolescent is unable to identify self in relation to others. (18)

role function mode In Roy's assessment system, the ability of the person to function within the primary, secondary, and tertiary roles he or she occupies. (9)

role performance The ability to carry out those behaviors appropriate to any particular role one has in life. (35)

role strain A situation in which a person experiences problems in carrying out any role in life. (34, 41)

Roman Catholicism A branch of Christianity with a central organization based on the leadership of the Pope in Rome. (36)

rotation A circular movement around a fixed axis. (23)

sacraments In the Christian church, any of several religious rituals or rites instituted by Jesus. (36)

safety needs In Maslow's hierarchy, needs related to protecting the self, which constitute the level just above basic or physiologic needs. (5)

sandwich generation Those middle-aged people who are care providers for two generations, their children and their aging parents. (19)

sanguineous exudate A secretion, produced by inflammation, that contains blood. (6)

satiety A feeling of having eaten a sufficient amount of food. (25)

scientific process A method for the acquisition of knowledge that includes: identification of the problem, data collection, formulation of the hypothesis, selection of a method for testing the hypothesis, testing the hypothesis, interpreting the results, and evaluating the hypothesis. (8)

scope of practice The breadth of opportunity to function within a specific occupational field. (1)

scripture A body of religious writings—for Christians, the Bible; for Muslims, the Koran; etc. (36)

scrub nurse The nurse who has performed a surgical scrub, donned sterile garments, and works within the operative field assisting the surgeon. (40)

sebaceous glands Small ducted glands located in the skin and hair follicles that secrete sebum (body oil). (19)

second intention healing Healing of a wound in which granulation tissue fills in the area between non-approximated wound edges. (6)

secondary groups Any group other than the primary group. (14)

secondary health care Care to which the individual has been referred by a primary care individual or agency. (2)

secondary prevention Actions taken to detect disease in its early stages so that it is curable. (16)

secondary role A role that is ascribed to the individual by society but which may be altered by the individual such as wife, friend, member of a religious body. (34)

seeking clarification A facilitating response in which one asks the sender to further explain the message. (13)

self-actualization The fifth level in Maslow's hierarchy of needs, described as "being true to oneself." (5, 34)

self-care Independently participating in activities which promote one's own physiological or psychological well-being. (23)

self-care deficits Those areas in which the person is not able to meet own needs. (10)

self care requisites According to the Orem Self-Care Theory these are the basic requirements (needs) of the individual. They include those that are universal to all people (universal self-care requisites), those that are specific to developmental level (developmental self-care requisites), and, those that are specific to the individual's health problem (health deviation self-care requisites). (9)

self-concept The total view an individual has of the self. (34, 35)

self-concept mode In Roy's assessment system, the person's view of both the physical and personal self. (9)

self-esteem The setting of positive values on the self. (34, 35)

self-help A technique for alleviating or overcoming physical or emotional problems through self-awareness. It is often combined with group dynamics. (34)

self-hypnosis A process of inducing in oneself a passive state in which the usual objective abilities are decreased and one is abnormally suggestible. (6)

self-understanding The ability to recognize the factors in one's own life that cause feelings and behavior. (34)

semen The transport fluid for the sperm. (37)

semicoma A condition in which a person shows some spontaneous movement but is difficult to arouse. (31)

semiformal group A group that has some planned aspects of structure or manner of operating, but other aspects that are not planned. (14)

semipermeable membrane A membrane with openings large enough to permit some particles to pass but too small for the passage of large particles. (30)

sender The person in an interaction who is giving the message. (13)

senile Referring to old age or the process of aging. (20)

sensation A perception created through the sensory organs. Often used to refer to the sensation of touch when examining an extremity for neurovascular function. (31)

sensorimotor stage Piaget's stage of cognitive development in which a child learns the properties of things in the environment, primarily through using the senses. (17)

sensory aphasia Difficulty with speech due to the inability to receive and understand what others are saying. (31)

sensory deprivation A lower level of sensory input than the individual needs for optimal functioning. (31)

sensory input All the messages and impressions that are transmitted to the brain by any of the five senses. (31)

sensory level The optimal level of sensory input to which the individual can respond appropriately. (31)

sensory overload The presence of more sensory stimuli during a given period than can be tolerated. (19, 31)

sensory receptors Nerve cells in the skin and mucous membrane that send messages of sensation to the brain. (31)

sensuality Pleasure perceived through the senses. It may or may not be sexual. (37)

sequence The order in which information is taught. The following sequences facilitate learning: known to unknown, normal to abnormal, simple to complex, and wellness to illness. (16)

seropositive Having a positive reaction to a test of serum for some specific entity. Commonly used to refer to persons who have developed antibodies to the HIV virus. (37)

serous exudate A secretion, produced by inflammation, that contains clear serum. (6)

serum hepatitis An inflammatory viral disease of the liver that is transmitted through blood products, injections, and contact with body secretions such as saliva and semen; hepatitis B. (30)

shaman A healing priest of the native American culture. (33)

shared housing Members of the more independent older

population sharing private housing in order to decrease expenses and share household tasks. (20)

sheltered care A living environment providing supportive service for those not able to live independently but allowing maximum independence. (2)

shock A disturbance of homeostasis caused by a sudden, unexpected emotional threat. (34)

siblings Children of the same parents; brothers and sisters. (17)

side effect an effect of a drug or treatment other than that which is the principal reason for its use. (39)

sigmoidoscopy Direct visualization of the sigmoid portion of the colon using an endoscope.(26)

sighing Deep breaths with long exhalation. (28)

sign An objective bodily manifestation that indicates the presence of a health problem. (9)

signing A system of communication for the deaf in which the position of the hands is used to convey words or phrases. (31)

singultus Hiccoughs. (28, 40)

situational crisis A period in which the coping behaviors that were effective in the past are not adequate to resolve the problems created by current life events. (34)

skilled nursing facility (SNF) A long-term care setting with sufficient licensed personnel (LPNs and RNs) to provide skilled care, the kind that demands knowledge and training and is not merely custodial. (20)

slander The utterance of defamatory statements injurious to the reputation or well-being of a person. (3)

sleep apnea Cessation of breathing during sleep, usually caused by obstruction of the respiratory passages. (24)

sleep cycle A sequence of five stages during sleep. (24)

sleep deprivation A smaller amount of sleep over a period of time than a particular individual needs. (24)

sleep stage A stage of the sleep cycle with unique characteristics and a distinct electroencephalographic pattern. (24)

sliding scale A prescription for a variable drug dosage to be administered based on specific criteria. Example: A sliding scale for insulin is used to vary dosage based on specific blood glucose levels. (39)

smegma A thick, whitish substance composed of epithelial cells and mucus that is found around external genitalia. (22)

SOAP The form in which progress notes are written for the problem-oriented medical record; S = subjective information; O = objective information; A = assessment or analysis of data; P = plan for care. (15)

social role A position in which one's actions are based on one's personal relationships with others. (1)

socialization A process of learning appropriate role behaviors through informal contacts in daily living. (34)

socializing Conversation that focuses on nonpersonal social topics. (1)

somnambulism Sleepwalking. (24)

somnolence Lethargy or sleepiness. (24)

sordes Accumulation of dried secretions and bacteria in the mouth caused by not eating, mouth breathing, and inadequate oral hygiene. (22)

special senses Hearing, vision, taste, smell, and touch. (31)

specific gravity The density of a solution. (27)

sphincter A circular muscle that controls an internal or external orifice. (26, 27)

spinal anesthesia A process for producing the absence of pain in the lower trunk and legs by injecting an agent into the lower spinal canal. (40)

spores Dormant bacteria with thick, resistant walls. (21)

sputum Expectorated matter that contains secretions from the lower respiratory tract. (28)

stance Posture in the standing position. (23)

standing orders A physician's order that is ongoing and usually applies to a group of patients with similar medical problems. (39)

starvation Total intake of calories and other nutrients inadequate to maintain life. (25)

State Board of Nursing The official body appointed by state governments to oversee and administer the Nurse Practice Act. (1, 3)

station See stance. (23)

statutory laws Those laws enacted by a legislative body. (3)

steatorrhea A condition characterized by stools containing large amounts of fat. (26)

stereotyped comments Common social phrases that tend to block communication. (13)

stereotyping Presuming a form or pattern often attributed to a group and applying it to an individual or to all members of the group. (33)

sterile technique A technique designed to make areas or objects free of all pathogens and to minimize pathogens on people. (21)

stimuli Agents that can evoke a response in the person. *External* stimuli originate outside the body; *internal* stimuli originate within the individual. (35)

stimulus control therapy (SCT) A therapy used in treatment of insomnia in which the bedroom is reinstated for only sleep behavior so that the environment acts as a sleep stimulus. (24)

stoicism A response to pain or other stressors in which behavior that would demonstrate the distress is suppressed. (32)

stoma A surgically created opening onto the body surface of any organ, for example, a colostomy, in which the colon is opened onto the abdomen. (26)

stool Feces. (26)

stress A generalized body response to a threat. (6)

stressor Any agent or stimulus that poses a real or perceived threat to the person. (4, 6, 7)

stretch reflex An involuntary reflex that causes the bladder to contract and the internal sphincter to relax, thus releasing urine. (27)

stridor A "crowing" sound due to constriction in the larynx. (28)

structure The pattern of organization of a group. (14)

structured interview A question-and-answer interaction in which the questions are preplanned. (9)

stupor A condition in which a person may be drowsy and fall asleep in the middle of a conversation. (31)

subjective data Information elicited from a patient/client through an interview. (9)

subjective symptom An indication of illness that is perceived and reported by the individual experiencing it. (9)

sublimation Unconsciously redirecting energy from one goal or endeavor toward another. (34)
submission Putting the views and opinions of another before one's own. (13)
subpoena A summons by the court for a witness to appear to offer testimony. (3)
substitution A consciously planned redirection of energy from a blocked goal to another goal. (34)
sudden infant death syndrome (SIDS) A fatal syndrome afflicting very young children, associated with some type of sleep pathology; also known as *crib death*. (24)
sulfonamides A group of synthetic drugs with a similar chemical structure (benzene rings) that have an antibacterial effect. (39)
superego According to Freud, the expressive self that controls behavior; the conscience. (17)
superficial pain Pain located in surface tissues of the body. (32)
supination The act of turning or placing the hand and forearm so that the palm is upward. (23)
support system Those persons or groups who offer emotional and physical assistance to an individual. (6)
suppository A solid medication that is designed to melt in a body cavity other than the mouth. (26, 39)
suppressants Cough medications that eliminate cough by suppressing the cough center in the medulla. (28)
suppression 1) Withdrawn from conscious thought. 2) Urinary suppression: Total absence of formation of urine by the kidneys; anuria. (27, 34)
suppuration The formation of pus. (21)
surgicenter An ambulatory care facility providing surgery as its primary service. (40)
surrogate mother A woman who becomes pregnant through artificial insemination with the specific intent of providing the infant for adoption by the biologic father and his wife. (3)
susceptible hosts Persons who are less able than most to defend against pathogens and thus will become ill on contact with pathogens. (21)
symbolic language Drawings used to express thoughts and feelings. (41)
symmetrical Balanced or even. (9, 23)
sympathetic nervous system The division of the autonomic nervous system that increases stimulation of smooth muscle and gland. (4)
sympathy Feelings of sorrow or concern for another person. (13)
symptom *See* subjective symptom. (9)
synthesis Combining information from more than one source to develop a broader perception and understanding. (16)
system A group of interrelated, interreacting, or interdependent elements forming a collective entity. (2)
systolic Pertaining to the period of time when the heart muscle is contracting the propelling blood through the arteries. (29)

tachycardia An abnormally rapid heartbeat, usually defined as over 100 beats/min in the adult. (29)
tachypnea Very rapid respirations. (28)
tactile Pertaining to the sense of touch. (31)
tactile input Input received through the sensory neurons of the skin; touch. (31)
Taoism One of the religions of China, based on the teachings of Lao-tse, a philosopher of the sixth century BC. (36)
taxonomy An organizing framework or pattern. (10)
teaching–learning process All of the actions of the teacher and the learner. (16)
team conference A meeting of a health care team (either nursing or multidisciplinary) in which patient care problems are discussed, goals set, and plans for action established. (15)
team nursing A way of organizing the nursing staff around teams composed of persons with different levels of education and ability. The team leader organizes the work of the entire team, and the team members provide the care that requires their ability. (1)
teleologic approach An ethical approach in which consequences of an act are considered the most important factor. (3)
terminal pain pain caused by an illness that is expected to end in death. (32, 41)
termination phase The ending period of an interaction. (13)
termination stage The final stage in the life of a group during which the group is ended. (14)
territoriality The need of an individual or a group to have emotional "space" to be comfortable. (33)
tertiary prevention Actions taken to prevent complications of an existing illness. (7)
tertiary role A role that is freely chosen and can be transient such as an occupation, a member of a jury, or a student. (34)
testosterone A male sex hormone produced in the testicles which controls secondary sex characteristics. (37)
theory A group of concepts, their definitions, and statements regarding the relationships between those concepts, identified for some purpose. (1)
therapeutic environment A setting that provides support and an atmosphere conducive to meeting an individual's needs. (35)
therapeutic interaction An interpersonal conversation in which the professional focuses on assisting the patient/client in coping with problems. (13)
therapeutic touch A process of using focused, intentional touch to enhance well-being and healing. (13)
third-party payer A group or organization that does not receive or provide health care but contracts to pay costs. Insurance companies, Medicaid, and the armed services (CHAMPUS) are examples of third-party payers. (2)
thoracotomy A surgical procedure that involves opening the chest (thorax). (40)
thrombus A blood clot. (29)
tidal volume The amount of air that can be exchanged with a single breath. (28)
time sequence The order in which events occur. (8)
tolerance A situation in which an increased dosage of a drug is necessary to achieve the same effect. (32)
tonic stage The stage of a seizure that involves stiffening of the body and clenching of the jaws. (31)

tonicity The state of a solution measured in regard to the number of particles in solution. (30)
torsion Twisting. (23)
tort A violation of civil law resulting in harm to another individual. (3)
total parenteral nutrition (TPN) Providing all essential nutrients via an intravenous line; also called *hyperalimentation.* (25)
total patient care A method of organizing nursing care whereby one individual handles all care for a single patient. (1)
total lung capacity The maximum volume of air that the lungs are able to hold. (28)
toxic Poisonous. (21)
toxoid A toxin that has been attenuated but maintains its ability to stimulate the production of antibodies. (21)
trace elements Minerals needed as micronutrients. (25)
tracheostomy A surgically devised opening into the trachea from the surface of the neck. (28)
trajectory One's perception of the course or path of an illness. (41)
transcultural nursing A nursing specialty focused on the adaptation of nursing to multicultural needs. (33)
transcutaneous electrical nerve stimulator (TENS or TNS) A battery-powered electrical device with electrodes placed on the skin that produces an electrical stimulation that can interfere with transmission of pain impulses. (32)
trauma Injury. (7)
tremor Involuntary shaking of a part, extremity, or head. (23)
trigger words Words or phrases that have particular meanings to certain cultural or ethnic groups that arouse feelings of distress and anger. (33)
trocar A large-bore needle, often with an inner stylet; used for aspiration or biopsy. (38)
trust Erikson's term for the infant's goal of developing reliance and a feeling of being safe with others. (13, 18)
trust vs. mistrust stage The first of Erikson's stages of psychosocial development seen in the infant. (18)
truth telling The bioethical issue of what rights a person has to be given medical knowledge related to treatment, condition, and prognosis. (3)
tube feeding Nutrients in a liquid form administered through a tube directly into the gastrointestinal system. (25)
turgor The degree of resiliency of the skin caused by the pressures of interstitial and intracellular fluid. (22)

UA Urinalysis. (38)
ultradian Body rhythms that occur in cycles of less than 24 hours. (24)
unconscious mind According to Freud, that part of one's emotional life that is not apparent to the person. (17)
unhealthy health Tillich's description of multidimensional health in which one can maintain overall health even when one system is unhealthy. (7)
uricosurics A classification of drugs that block reabsorption of uric acid crystals and increase urinary secretion. (27)
urinary diversion A surgically created change in the anatomy of the urinary system resulting in the urine flowing to a pseudobladder or to a stoma on the abdomen. (27)
urinary suppression The absence of urine caused by the inability of the kidneys to function. (27)
universal blood and body fluid precautions A frequently used type of protection against infectious diseases which are transmitted by blood and body fluid. Consists of the wearing of protective garb when there is the possibility of exposure to fluids when caring for any patient. (21)
universal self-care requisites In Orem's theory, those needs that are common to all people regardless of age or state of health. (9)
unstructured interview A question-and-answer interaction in which the questions arise from the response and are not specifically planned. (9)
urgency The inability to postpone urination. (27)
urimeter An instrument used for determining the specific gravity of urine. (27)
urinalysis The chemical analysis of urine, which commonly checks for color, clarity, pH, specific gravity, and the presence of glucose, RBCs, casts, and WBCs. (38)
urination The act of excreting urine. (27)
utilitarianism A belief that ethical behavior is that behavior which results in the greatest good for the most people. (3)
utilization review A mechanism for evaluating whether health care was of the right type, in the right setting, and of appropriate length for the needs of the individual patient. (15)
uvulopalatophrayngoplasty (UPPP) A surgical procedure for adult sleep apnea in which the soft palate is restructured to prevent respiratory obstruction during sleep. (24)

vaccine Attenuated or dead microorganisms, administered to produce an active immunity to a disease. (21)
vaginismus Pain caused by severe spasm of the vaginal orifice, usually with attempted intercourse. (37)
validation Checking with the sender to verify that your understanding of the message is correct. (13)
Valsalva maneuver Using expiration with force against a closed glottis, such as bearing down to defecate; often accompanied by grunting. (26)
values Principles or standards of life that are highly prized. (36)
valuing In the NANDA toxonomy, a human response pattern of assigning relative worth. (10)
vascular theory of sleep The theory attributing sleep to a periodic drop in blood pressure. (24)
vasoconstriction The narrowing of the lumen of the arteries by contraction of the muscles in the artery wall. (29)
vasodilatation The widening of the lumen of the arteries by relaxation of the muscles in the artery wall. (29)
vectors Insects or animals that can carry disease. (21)
vegetarian Pertaining to a diet containing only plant products. A *lacto vegetarian* diet also includes milk and milk products; an *ovo lacto vegetarian* diet also includes eggs, milk, and milk products. (25)
verbal Pertaining to the words exchanged in an interaction. (13)
verbal feedback 1) Explanations from another individual rel-

ative to a problem or process. 2) Descriptions of the body and its function from another person. (35)

violence Physical actions that have the potential for causing injury to another person. (34)

virulence The potency or ability of a pathogen to cause disease. (21)

virus A single-celled microorganism, the smallest of all pathogens. (21)

visceral (internal) pain Pain originating deep within body tissue. (32)

visual feedback 1) Visible results of a process. 2) Visual identification of body parts and their structure to clarify body image. (31, 35)

visual input Images received through the eyes; sight. (31)

vital capacity The largest possible amount of air that can be exchanged by the lungs. (28)

vitamins Organic compounds that are essential to metabolic processes. (25)

vocabulary level The level of difficulty of the words and terms used and/or understood. (16)

voice quality Loudness or softness of speaking. (13)

voice tone The quality of the speaking voice that conveys feeling. (13)

voiding Emptying urine from the bladder through the urethra; urinating; micturating. (27)

voluntary association An organization established to support a specific goal, for example, the American Heart Association. (15)

vomiting The ejection of stomach contents through the mouth. (25)

walking rounds Conferences held by the health care team at the bedsides of one client after another on a unit. (15)

wheezing A whistling sound heard upon auscultation of the lungs and indicating constriction of airways. (28)

work ethic A belief that work has intrinsic value and that the value of the person is related to the work the individual does. (36)

working phase The time during an interaction in which goals are accomplished. (13)

working stage The stage in the life of a group during which decisions are made and tasks accomplished; the middle stage of a three-stage process that encompasses negotiation and operation. (14)

worried well Those people who are overly fearful of becoming ill, primarily because of media emphasis on the prevalence of health problems. (7)

yang The male, active, dominant cosmic element in Chinese dual philosophy. Foods designated "hot" in terms of healing properties (not temperature) are classified as yang by some Asians. (33)

yeast A type of fungi. Pathogenic types may cause infections of moist, warm areas such as the mouth, moist skin folds, and the vagina. (21)

yin The female, passive cosmic element in Chinese dual philosophy. Foods designated "cold" in terms of healing properties (not temperature) are classified as yin by some Asians. (33)

Photo Credits

Fig. 19-3: © Marcia Keegan/Peter Arnold, Inc., New York, NY
Fig. 21-6: © Alex Webb/Magnum Photos, New York, NY
Fig. 33-2: Indian Health Service, USPHS, DHHS
Fig. 6-4, 7-8, 17-3, 21-5 Chapter 4 opener: Bob Kramer, South Boston, MA
Fig. 5-2, 5-3, 17-1, 17-4, 18-3, 20-4, 27-4: Larry Pezzato, Magnolia, NJ

Photo Reasearchers, Inc. (New York, NY):
Fig. 20-3: Stephanie Dinkins/Photo Researchers, Inc.
Fig. 41-2: Ray Ellis/Photo Researchers, Inc.
Fig. 16-2: Russ Kinne/Danbury Hospital/Photo Researchers, Inc.
Fig. 20-6: Russ Kinne/Photo Researchers, Inc.
Fig. 6-6: Susan Oristaglio/Photo Researchers, Inc.
Fig. 31-7: Lily Solmssen/Photo Researchers, Inc.

Fig. 42-3: Ann Chwatsky/Phototake (New York, NY):
Fig. 7-5, 14-3, 14-4, 23-2, 26-6, 29-6, 33-5: H. Armstrong Roberts, Inc., Phila, PA
Fig. 10-1, 16-5, 18-4, 18-5, 20-2, 22-9, 24-7, 26-4, 31-9, 33-3: Kathy Sloane, Oakland, CA

Stock, Boston (Boston, MA):
Fig. 18-6: Anestis Diakopoulos/Stock, Boston
Fig. 41-9: Gabor Demjen/Stock, Boston
Fig. 20-1: Ellis, Herwig/Stock, Boston
Fig. 13-2: Hazel Hankin/Stock, Boston
Fig. 25-3, 28-4: Jean-Claude Lejeune/Stock, Boston
Fig. 41-5: Ann Kaufman Moon/Stock, Boston
Fig. 41-1: Frank Siteman/Stock, Boston
Fig. 41-8: Carol Wolinsky/Stock, Boston

The Picture Cube, Inc. (Boston, MA):
Fig 3-2: © Read D. Brugger/The Picture Cube
Fig. 19-1: © Alice Grossman/The Picture Cube
Fig. 29-2: © Carolyn Hine/The Picture Cube
Fig. 36-2: © Emilio Mercado/The Picture Cube
Fig. 23-1: © David S. Strickler/The Picture Cube
Fig. 17-2: © Steve Takatsuno/The Picture Cube
Fig. 1-5: © Richard Wood/The Picture Cube
Fig. 42-2: Courtesy of the Nursing Department, Thomason Hospital, El Paso, Texas

Fig. 36-3: Wide World Photos, Inc., New York, NY

Appendices

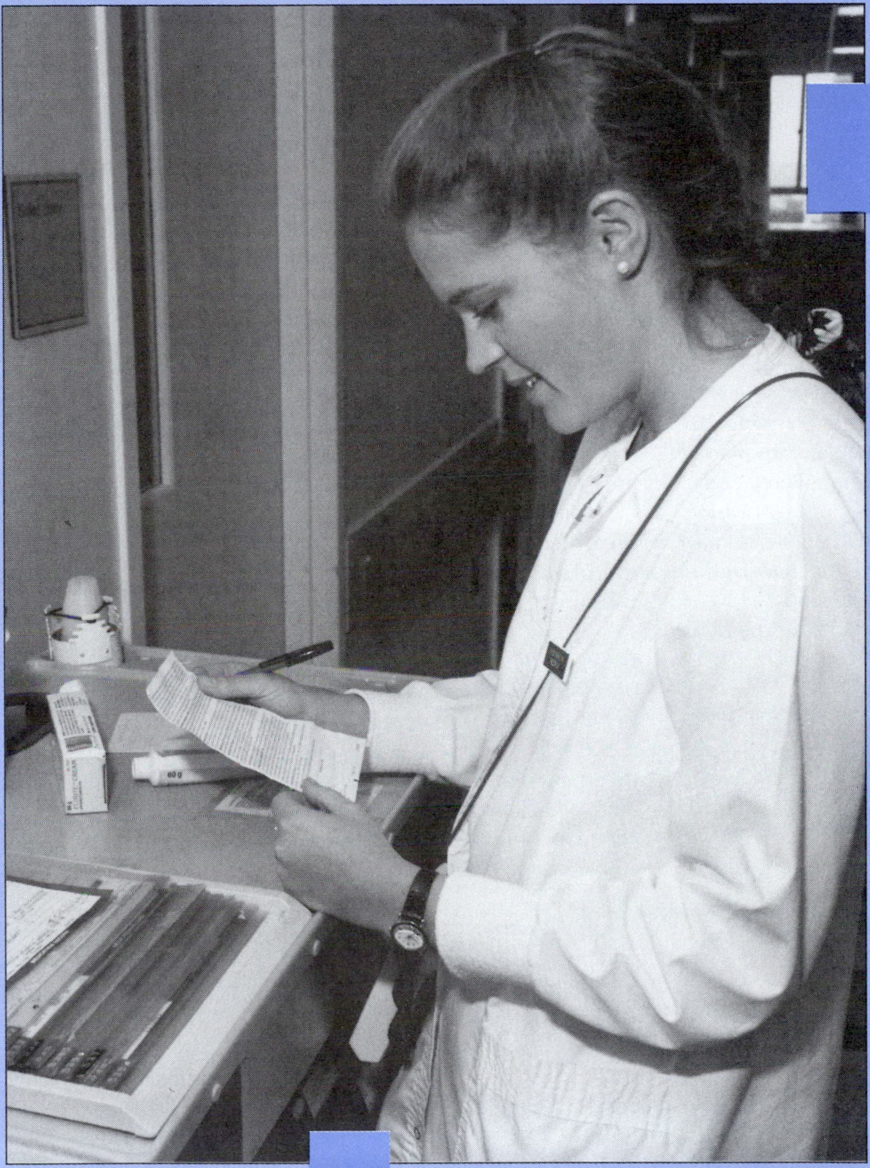

A Definitions of NANDA-approved Diagnoses

B Common Abbreviations

C Abbreviations of Medical Conditions

D Combining Forms

E Voluntary Associations

F Level I Screen from the Nutrition Screening Initiative

Appendix A

Definitions of NANDA-approved Nursing Diagnoses

The North American Nursing Diagnosis Association (NANDA) taxonomy approved in 1992 is found in Chapter 10. A quick reference alphabetized list is found on the inside of the front cover. Here the nursing diagnoses are alphabetized based on the major topical term in the diagnosis. The descriptive terms—altered, decreased, disturbed, dysfunctional, and so forth—and other modifiers are placed after the major topical term. All definitions come from the work of NANDA. When an example of the nursing diagnosis as used in care planning can be found in the text, a reference to that particular care plan is provided. *High Risk* nursing diagnoses are not covered separately unless the high risk problem is the only one appearing in the taxonomy. NANDA has indicated that *high-risk* may be an appropriate modifying phrase in any nursing diagnosis. The numbered position in the taxonomy and the year when the diagnosis was approved are included after the definition.

Activity Intolerance—A state in which an individual has insufficient physiologic or psychological energy to endure or complete required or desired daily activities. (6.1.1.2; High risk state 6.1.1.3, 1982) Examples Chapters 19 and 23.

Adjustment, Impaired—The state in which the individual is unable to modify his/her lifestyle/behavior in a manner consistent with a change in health status. (5.1.1.1.1, 1986) Example Chapter 34.

Airway Clearance, Ineffective—A state in which an individual is unable to clear secretions or obstructions from the respiratory tract to maintain airway patency. (1.5.1.2, 1980) Example Chapter 27.

Anxiety—A vague uneasy feeling whose source is often nonspecific or unknown to the individual. (9.3.1, 1973, revised 1982) Example Chapter 33.

Aspiration, High Risk for—The state in which an individual is at risk for entry of gastrointestinal secretions, oropharyngeal secretions, or solids or fluids into tracheobronchial passages. (1.6.1.4, 1988)

Body Image Disturbance—Disruption in the way one perceives one's body image. (7.1.1, 1973) Example Chapter 35.

Body Temperature, High Risk for Altered—The state in which the individual is at risk for failure to maintain body temperature within normal range. (1.2.2.1, 1986)

Bowel Incontinence—A state in which an individual experiences a change in normal bowel habits characterized by involuntary passage of stool. (1.3.1.3, 1975)

Breast-feeding, Ineffective—The state in which a mother, infant, or child experiences dissatisfaction or difficulty with the breast-feeding process. (6.5.1.2, 1988)

Breast-feeding, Effective—The state in which a mother–infant dyad/family exhibits adequate proficiency and satisfaction with breast-feeding process. (6.5.1.3, 1990)

Breast-feeding, Interrupted—A break in the continuity of the breast-feeding process as a result of inability or inadvisability to put baby to breast for feeding. (6.5.1.2.1, 1992)

Breathing Pattern, Ineffective—A state in which an individual's inhalation and/or exhalation pattern does not enable adequate pulmonary inflation or emptying. (1.5.1.3, 1980) Example Chapter 28.

Cardiac Output, Decreased—A state in which the blood pumped by an individual's heart is sufficiently reduced that it is inadequate to meet the needs of the body's tissues. (1.4.2.1, 1975) Example Chapter 28.

Caregiver Role Strain—A caregiver's felt difficulty in performing the family caregiver role. (3.2.2.1; High risk state 3.2.2.2, 1992)

Constipation—A state in which an individual experiences a change in normal bowel habits characterized by a decrease in frequency and/or passage of hard dry stools. (1.3.1.1, 1975) Example Chapter 26.

Constipation, Colonic—The state in which an individual's pattern of elimination is characterized by hard, dry stool which results from a delay in passage of food residue. (1.3.1.1.2, 1988)

Constipation, Perceived—The state in which an individual makes a self-diagnosis of constipation and ensures a daily bowel movement through abuse of laxatives, enemas, and suppositories. (1.3.1.1.1, 1988)

Coping, Defensive—The state in which an individual repeatedly projects falsely positive self-evaluation based on a self-protective pattern which defends against underlying perceived threats to positive self regard. (5.1.1.1.2, 1988)

Coping, Ineffective Family: Compromised—A usually supportive primary person (family member of close friend) is providing insufficient, ineffective, or compromised support, comfort, assistance, or encouragement which may be needed by the client to manage or master adaptive tasks related to his or her health challenge. (5.1.2.1.2, 1980)

Coping, Ineffective Family: Disabling—Behavior of significant person (family member or other primary person) that disables his or her own capacities and the client's capacities to effectively address tasks essential to either person's adaptation to the health challenge. (5.1.2.1.1, 1980)

Coping, Ineffective Individual—Impairment of adaptive behaviors and problem-solving abilities of a person in meeting life's demands and roles (5.1.1.1, 1978) Examples Chapters 19 and 34.

Coping, Family: Potential for Growth—Effective managing of adaptive tasks by family member involved with the client's health challenge, who now is exhibiting desire and readiness for enhanced health and growth in regard to self and in relation to the client. (5.1.2.2, 1980)

Decisional Conflict (specify)—The state of uncertainty about course of action to be taken when choice among competing actions involves risk, loss, or challenge to personal life values. (5.3.1.1., 1988)

Denial, Ineffective—The state of a conscious or unconscious attempt to disavow the knowledge or meaning of an event to reduce anxiety/fear to the detriment of health. (5.1.1.1.3, 1988)

Diarrhea—A state in which an individual experiences a change in normal bowel habits characterized by the frequent passage of loose, fluid, unformed stools. (1.3.1.2, 1975) Example Chapter 26.

Disuse Syndrome, High Risk for—A state in which an individual is at risk for deterioration of body systems as the result of prescribed or unavoidable musculoskeletal inactivity. (1.6.1.5, 1988)

Diversional Activity Deficit—The state in which an individual experiences a decreased stimulation from or interest or engagement in recreational or leisure activities. (6.3.1.1, 1980)

Dysreflexia—The state in which an individual with a spinal cord injury at T7 or above experiences a life-threatening uninhibited sympathetic response of the nervous system to a noxious stimulus. (1.2.3.1, 1988)

Family Processes, Altered—The state in which a family that normally functions effectively experiences a dysfunction. (3.2.2, 1982)

Fatigue—An overwhelming sustained sense of exhaustion and decreased capacity for physical and mental work. (6.1.1.2.1, 1988)

Fear—Feeling of dread related to an identifiable source which the person validates. (9.3.2, 1980)

Fluid Volume Deficit—The state in which an individual experiences vascular, cellular, or intracellular dehydration. (1.4.1.2.2.1; High risk state 1.4.1.2.2.2., 1978) Example Chapter 30.

Fluid Volume Excess—The state in which an individual experiences increased fluid retention and edema. (1.4.1.2.1, 1982) Example Chapter 30.

Gas Exchange, Impaired—The state in which the individual experiences a decreased passage of oxygen and/or carbon dioxide between the alveoli of the lungs and the vascular system (1.5.1.1, 1980) Example Chapter 28.

Grieving, Anticipatory—Potential loss of significant object; expression of distress at potential loss; denial of potential loss; guilt; anger; sorrow; choked feelings; changes in eating habits; alterations in sleep patterns; alterations in activity level; altered libido; altered communication patterns. (9.2.1.2, 1980)

Grieving, Dysfunctional—Verbal expressions of distress at loss; denial of loss; expression of guilt; expression of unresolved issues; anger; sadness; crying; difficulty in expressing loss; alterations in: eating habits, sleep patterns, dream patterns, activity level, libido; idealization of lost object; reliving of past experiences; interference with life functioning; developmental regression; labile affect; alterations in concentration and/or pursuits of tasks. (9.2.1.1, 1980) Example Chapter 41.

Growth and Development, Altered—The state in which an individual demonstrates deviations in norms from his/her age group. (6.6, 1986)

Health Maintenance, Altered—Inability to identify, manage, and/or seek out help to maintain health. (6.4.2, 1982)

Health-Seeking Behaviors (specify)—A state in which an individual in stable health is actively seeking ways to alter personal health habits, and/or the environment to move toward a higher level of health. (5.4, 1988)

Home Maintenance Management, Impaired—Inability to independently maintain a safe growth-promoting immediate environment. (6.4.1.1, 1980)

Hopelessness—A subjective state in which an individual sees limited or no alternatives or personal choices available and is unable to mobilize energy on own behalf. (7.3.1, 1986)

Hyperthermia—A state in which an individual's body temperature is elevated above his/her normal range. (1.2.2.3, 1986)

Hypothermia—The state in which an individual's body temperature is reduced below normal range. (1.2.2.2, 1986, revised 1988)

Infant Feeding Pattern, Ineffective—A state in which an infant demonstrates an impaired ability to suck or coordinate the suck swallow response. (6.5.1.4, 1992)

Infection, High risk for—The state at which an individual is at increased risk for being invaded by pathogenic organisms. (1.2.1.1, 1986) Example Chapter 20.

Injury, High Risk for—A state in which the individual is at risk of injury as a result of environmental conditions interacting with the individual's adaptive and defensive resources. (1.6.1, 1978) Examples Chapters 20, 31, and 38.

Knowledge Deficit (specify)—Verbalization of the problem; inaccurate follow-through of instruction; inaccurate performance of test; inappropriate or exaggerated behaviors, *e.g.*, hysterical, hostile, agitated, apathetic. (8.1.1, 1980) Examples Chapters 15 and 39.

Management of Therapeutic Regimen (Individuals), Ineffective—A pattern of regulating and integrating into daily living a program for treatment of illness and the sequelae of illness that is unsatisfactory for meeting specific health goals. (5.2.1, 1992)

Noncompliance (specify)—A person's informed decision not to adhere to a therapeutic recommendation. (5.2.1.1, 1973) Example Chapter 42.

Nutrition: Less Than Body Requirements, Altered—The state in which an individual experiences an intake of nutrients insufficient to meet metabolic needs. (1.1.2.2, 1975) Chapter 25.

Nutrition: More Than Body Requirements, Altered—The state in which an individual is experiencing an intake of nutrients which exceeds metabolic needs. (1.1.2.1, 1975) Example Chapter 25.

Oral Mucous Membranes, Altered—The state in which an individual experiences disruption in the tissue layers of the oral cavity. (1.6.2.1.1, 1982)

Pain—A state in which an individual experiences and reports the presence of severe discomfort or an uncomfortable sensation. (9.1.1, 1978) Example Chapter 31.

Pain, Chronic—A state in which the individual experiences pain that continues for more than 6 months in duration. (9.1.1.1, 1986) Example Chapter 31.

Parental Role Conflict—The state in which a parent experiences role confusion and conflict in response to crisis. (3.2.3.1, 1988)

Parenting, Altered—The state in which a nurturing figure(s) experiences an inability to create an environment which promotes the optimum growth and development of another human being. (3.2.1.1.1; High risk state 3.2.1.1.2, 1978)

Peripheral Neurovascular Dysfunction, High Risk for—A state in which an individual is at risk of experiencing a disruption in circulation, sensation, or motion of an extremity. (6.1.1.1.1, 1992)

Personal Identity Disturbance—Inability to distinguish between self and nonself. (7.1.3, 1978)

Physical Mobility, Impaired—A state in which the individual experiences a limitation of ability for independent physical movement. (6.1.1.1, 1973) (Suggested functional level classification: 0 = Completely independent; 1 = Requires use of equipment or device; 2 = Requires help from another person, for assistance, supervision, or teaching; 3 = Requires help from another person and equipment or device; 4 = Dependent, does not participate in activity. Adapted from E. Jones. *Patient Classification for Long-Term Care: Users' Manual.* HEW, Publication No. HRA-74–3107, November 1974.)

Poisoning, High Risk for—Accentuated risk of accidental exposure to or ingestion of drugs or dangerous products in doses sufficient to cause poisoning. (1.6.1.2, 1980)

Post-Trauma Response—The state of an individual experiencing a sustained painful response to an overwhelming traumatic event(s). (9.2.3, 1986)

Powerlessness—Perception that one's own action will not significantly affect an outcome; a perceived lack of control over a current situation or immediate happening. (7.3.2, 1982)

Protection, Altered—The state in which an individual experiences a decrease in the ability to guard the self from internal or external threats such as illness or injury. (1.6.2, 1990)

Rape Trauma Syndrome—Forced, violent sexual penetration against the victim's will and consent. The trauma syndrome that develops from this attack or attempted attack includes an acute phase of disorganization of the victim's lifestyle and a long-term process of reorganization of lifestyle. (9.2.3.1, 1980)

Rape Trauma Syndrome: Compound reaction—Force, violent sexual penetration against the victim's will and consent. The trauma syndrome that develops from this attack or attempted attack includes an acute phase of disorganization of the victim's lifestyle and a long-term process of reorganization of lifestyle. (9.2.3.1.1, 1980)

Rape Trauma Syndrome: Silent reaction—Forced, violent sexual penetration against the victim's will and consent. The trauma syndrome that develops from this attack or attempted attack includes an acute phase of disorganization of the victim's lifestyle and a long-term process of reorganization of lifestyle. (9.2.3.1.2, 1980)

Relocation Stress Syndrome—Physiological and/or psychosocial disturbances as a result of transfer from one environment to another. (6.7, 1992)

Role Performance, Altered—Disruption in the way one perceives one's role performance. (3.2.1, 1978)

Self-care Deficit

Bathing/Hygiene—A state in which the individual experiences an impaired ability to perform or complete bathing/hygiene activities for oneself. (6.5.2, 1980) Example Chapter 22.

Feeding—A state in which the individual experiences an impaired ability to perform or complete feeding activities for oneself. (6.5.1, 1980) Example Chapter 24.

Dressing/Grooming—A state in which the individual experiences an impaired ability to perform or complete dressing and grooming activities for oneself. (6.5.3, 1980)

Toileting—A state in which the individual experiences an impaired ability to perform or complete toileting activities for oneself. (6.5.4, 1980)

Self-esteem, Chronic Low—Long-standing negative self evaluation/feelings about self or self-capabilities. (7.1.2.1, 1988)

Self-esteem, Situational Low—Negative self-evaluation/feelings about self which develop in response to a loss or change in an individual who previously had a positive self-evaluation. (7.1.2.2, 1988) Example Chapter 35.

Self-esteem Disturbance—Negative self-evaluation/feelings about self or self-capabilities, which may be directly or indirectly expressed. (7.1.2, 1978, Revised 1988)

Self-mutilation, High Risk for—A state in which an individual is at high risk to perform an act on the self to injure, not kill, which produces tissue damage and tension relief. (9.2.2.1, 1992)

Sensory/Perceptual Alterations (specify) (visual, auditory, kinesthetic, gustatory, tactile, olfactory)—A state in which an individual experiences a change in the amount or patterning of oncoming stimuli accompanied by a diminished, exaggerated, distorted, or impaired response to such stimuli. (7.2, 1978)

Sexual Dysfunction—The state in which an individual experiences a change in sexual function that is viewed as unsatisfying, unrewarding, inadequate. (3.2.1.2.1, 1980) Example Chapter 37.

Sexuality Patterns, Altered—The state in which an individual expresses concern regarding his/her sexuality. (3.3, 1986)

Skin Integrity, Impaired—A state in which the individual's skin is adversely altered. (1.6.2.1.2.1; High risk state 1.6.1.2.1.2.2, 1975) Example Chapter 22.

Sleep Pattern Disturbance—Disruption of sleep time causes discomfort or interferes with desired lifestyle. (6.2.1, 1980) Example Chapter 24.

Social Interaction, Impaired—The state in which an individual participates in an insufficient or excessive quantity or ineffective quality of social exchange. (3.1.1, 1986) Examples Chapters 23 and 33.

Social Isolation—Aloneness experienced by the individual and perceived as imposed by others and as a negative or threatened state. (3.1.2, 1982) Example Chapter 41.

Spiritual Distress—(Distress of the human spirit) Disruption in the life principle which pervades a person's entire being and which integrates and transcends one's biologic and psychosocial nature. (4.1.1, 1978) Example Chapter 36.

Suffocation, High Risk for—Accentuated risk of accidental suffocation (inadequate air available for inhalation). (1.6.1.1, 1980).

Swallowing, Impaired—The state in which an individual has decreased ability to voluntarily pass fluids and/or solids from the mouth to the stomach. (6.5.1.1, 1986)

Thermoregulation, Ineffective—The state in which the individual's temperature fluctuates between hypothermia and hyperthermia. (1.2.2.4, 1986)

Thought Processes, Altered—A state in which an individual experiences a disruption in cognitive operations and activities. (8.3, 1973) Example Chapter 20.

Tissue Integrity, Impaired—A state in which an individual experiences damage to mucous membrane, corneal, integumentary, or subcutaneous tissue. (1.6.2.1, 1986)

Tissue Perfusion, Altered (specify type) (renal, cerebral, cardiopulmonary, gastrointestinal, peripheral)—The state in which an individual experiences a decrease in nutrition and oxygenation at the cellular level due to a deficit in capillary blood supply. (1.4.1.1, 1980) Example Chapter 29.

Trauma, High Risk for—Accentuated risk of accidental tissue injury, *e.g.*, wound, burn, fracture. (1.6.1.3, 1980)

Unilateral Neglect—A state in which an individual is perceptually unaware of and inattentive to one side of the body. (7.2.1.1, 1986)

Urinary Elimination, Altered—The state in which the individual experiences a disturbance in urine elimination. (1.3.2, 1973)

Urinary Incontinence, Functional—The state in which an individual experiences an involuntary, unpredictable passage of urine. (1.3.2.1.4, 1986) Example Chapter 26.

Urinary Incontinence, Reflex—The state in which an individual experiences an involuntary loss of urine, occurring at somewhat predictable intervals when a specific bladder volume is reached. (1.3.2.1.2, 1986)

Urinary Incontinence, Stress—The state in which an individual experiences a loss of urine of less than 50 ml occurring with increased abdominal pressure. (1.3.2.1.1, 1986)

Urinary Incontinence, Total—The state in which an individual experiences a continuous and unpredictable loss or urine. (1.3.2.1.5, 1986)

Urinary Incontinence, Urge—The state in which an individual experiences involuntary passage of urine occurring soon after a strong sense of urgency to void. (1.3.2.1.3, 1986)

Urinary Retention—The state in which the individual experiences incomplete emptying of the bladder. (1.3.2.2, 1986) Example Chapter 26.

Ventilation, Inability to Sustain Spontaneous—A state in which the response pattern of decreased energy reserves results in an individual's inability to maintain breathing adequate to support life. (1.5.1.3.1, 1992)

Ventilatory Weaning Response, Dysfunctional—A state in which a patient cannot adjust to lowered levels of mechanical ventilator support, which interrupts and prolongs the weaning process. Further characterized as *mild, moderate,* or *severe.* (1.5.1.3.2, 1992)

Verbal Communication, Impaired—The state in which an individual experiences a decreased or absent ability to use or understand language in human interaction. (2.1.1.1, 1973)

Violence, High Risk for: Self-directed or Directed at Others—A state in which an individual experiences behaviors that can be physically harmful either to the self or others. (9.2.2, 1980)

Appendix B
Common Abbreviations

Abbreviation	Latin Meaning	English Meaning
@		at
abd.		abdomen
a.c.	ante cibum	before meals
ADLs		activities of daily living
ab lib.	ad libitum	at will
adm.		admitted
amp.		ampule
amt.		amount
ax.		axillary
b.i.d.	bis in die	twice a day
BM		bowel movement
BP		blood pressure
BRP		bathroom privileges
$\bar{c}$	cum	with
cap.		capsule
c/o		complains of
CSF		cerebral spinal fluid
DAT		diet as tolerated
d.c.		discontinue
Δ (Greek delta)		change
disch.		discharge
DOA		dead on arrival
dsg. or drsg.		dressing
Dx		diagnosis
et	et	and
ext.		extremity
fl.		fluid
Fr.		French
Frax., Fx.		fractional, fracture
gtt.	gutta/guttae	drop/drops
h.	hora	hour
H/P		history and physical
h.s.	hora somni	hour of sleep (bedtime)
ICN		intensive care nursery
ICU		intensive care unit
I&D		incision and drainage
IM		intramuscular
incont.		incontinent
IV		intravenous
KVO		keep vein open (with intravenous infusion)
liq.		liquid
LLQ		left lower quadrant (of abdomen)
LUQ		left upper quadrant (of abdomen)
N/A		not applicable
NPO	non per ora	nothing by mouth
n.r.	non repetatur	not to be repeated

Abbreviation	Latin Meaning	English Meaning
"o"		orally
o.d.	omne die	every day
OD	oculus dexter	right eye
OOB		out of bed
OS	oculus sinister	left eye
OT		occupational therapy
OU	oculi uterque	each eye
p.c.	post cibum	after meals
p.o.	per ora	by mouth
p.r.n. (PRN)	pro re nata	when needed
PT		physical therapy
q.d.	quaque die	each day
q.h.,	quaque hora	every hour,
q2h.,		every 2 hours,
q3h., etc.		every 3 hours, etc.
q.i.d.	quater in die	four times a day
q.o.d.	quaque altera die	every other day
q.s.	quantum sufficit	sufficient quantity
RLQ		right lower quadrant (of abdomen)
R/O		rule out
ROM		range of motion
RUQ		right upper quadrant (of abdomen)
$\bar{s}$	sine	without
SNF		skilled nursing facility
s.o.b.		short of breath
s.o.s.	si opus sit	if necessary
spec.		specimen
SSE		soapsuds enema
stat.	statim	immediately
sub q.		subcutaneous
tab.		tablet
t.i.d.	ter in dies	three times a day
TKO		to keep open (intravenous infusion)
TLC		tender loving care
TPR		temperature, pulse, and respiration
TWE		tap water enema
UA		urine analysis
ung.	unguent	ointment
WC		wheelchair

Appendix C
Abbreviations of Medical Conditions

AIDS	acquired immune deficiency syndrome
AK Amp.	above-knee amputation
ARDS	adult respiratory distress syndrome
ASCVD	arteriosclerotic cardiovascular disease
ASHD	arteriosclerotic heart disease
BE	bacterial endocarditis
BK Amp.	below-knee amputation
BPH	benign prostatic hypertrophy
Ca	cancer (carcinoma)
CF	cystic fibrosis
CHD	coronary heart disease
CHF	congestive heart failurc
COPD	chronic obstructive pulmonary disease
CVA	cerebral vascular accident
D&C	dilation and curettage (of uterus)
DIC	disseminated intravascular coagulation
DTs	delerium tremens
FUO	fever of undetermined origin
GB	gall bladder
GC	gonococcal infection
HCVD	hypertensive cardiovascular disease
IDDM	insulin dependent diabetes mellitus
LTB	laryngotracheobronchitis
MI	myocardial infarction, mitral insufficiency
MODM	maturity onset diabetes mellitus
MRSA	methicillin resistant *Stapholococcus aureus*
MS	multiple sclerosis
PAP	primary atypical pneumonia
PID	pelvic inflammatory disease
PVD	peripheral vascular disease
RDS	respiratory distress syndrome
RF	rheumatic fever
RHD	rheumatic heart disease
RIND	reversible ischemic neurologic deficit
SBE	subacute bacterial endocarditis
SIDS	sudden infant death syndrome
STD	sexually transmitted disease
T&A	tonsillectomy and adenoidectomy
TB or Tbc	tuberculosis
TIA	transient ischemic attacks
TURB	transurethral resection of the bladder
TURP	transurethral resection of the prostate
URI	upper respiratory infection
UTI	urinary tract infection
VD	venereal disease

Appendix D
Combining Forms

The combining form may appear at the beginning of, within, or at the end of a term. By identifying the meaning of each combining form contained in a word, one can often discern the meaning of the word. A dash preceding the form indicates that it is most commonly a suffix (appearing at the end of a term); a dash following the form indicates that it is most commonly a prefix (appearing at the beginning of a term).

Form	Meaning
a-, an	without
ab-	away from
ad-	to, toward
adeno-	gland
-algia	pain
ambi-	on two sides
angio-	vessel
ano-	anus
ante-	before, forward
arterio-	artery
arthro-	joint
bis-	two
broncho-	bronchus
cardi-, cardio-	heart
-cele	hernia, tumor, protrusion
-centesis	puncture
cepha-, cephalo-	head
cerebro-	cerebrum of brain
cervico-	neck
chole-	bile
cholecysto-	gall bladder
chondro-	cartilage
circum-	around
cranio-	head
cysto-	sac, cyst, bladder (most often urinary bladder)
-cyte	cell
derm-	skin
dys-	abnormal, painful
-ectasis	expansion, dilation
-ectomy	excision
-emia	blood
encephalo-	brain
endo-	within, inner layer
entero-	intestines
ex-	out, out of, away from
exo-	outside, outer layer
gastro-	stomach
hem-, hema-, hemo-, hemato-	blood
hemi-	half
hepato-	liver
histo-	tissue
hyper-	excessive
hypo-	low, lesser
hystero-	uterus
-iasis	condition, formation of, presence of
ileo-	ileum (part of small intestine)
ilio-	ilium (part of pelvic bones)
intra-	within
-itis	inflammation of
laparo-	loin, flank, abdomen
laryngo-	larynx
latero-	side
sympho-	lymph
-lysis	dissolution, breaking down
macro-	large
mal-	bad, poor
-malacia	softening
masto-	breast
medio-	middle
-megaly	enlargement
meningo-	meninges
micro-	small, microscopic
mono-	single
myelo-	bone marrow, spinal cord
myo-	muscle
naso-	nose
neo-	new
nephro-	kidney
neuro-	nerve
non-	not
oculo-	eye
odonto-	tooth
-oma	tumor
oophoro-	ovary
ophthalmo-	eye
orchio-, orchido-	testes
oro-	mouth
-orrhaphy	suture/repair of
os-	bone, mouth
-osis	condition, disease, increase

Form	Meaning
osteo-	bone
-ostomy	artificially created opening into an organ
oto-	ear
-otomy	incision into
ovario-	ovary
para-	beside, along with
-pathy	disease
-penia	deficiency, decrease
peri-	around
-pexy	suspension, fixation
pharyngo-	pharynx
phlebo-	vein
-plasty	surgical correction, plastic repair of
-plegia	paralysis
pneumo-	lungs, breath
post-	after
pro-	in front of, before
procto-	rectum
pseudo-	false

Form	Meaning
-ptosis	falling, drooping
pyo-	pus
retro-	behind
rhino-	nose
salpingo-	Fallopian tube
sclero-	hard
-spasm	involuntary contraction
spleno-	spleen
sterno-	sternum
super-, supra-	above, more than
teno-	tendon
thoraco-	thorax, chest
thyro-	thyroid
tracheo-	trachea
trans-	across, throughout
urethro-	urethra
uro-	urine, urinary
utero-	uterus
vaso-	blood vessel
veno-	vein

Appendix E

Voluntary Associations

Aging

Alzheimer's Disease International (ADI)
919 N. Michigan Avenue, No. 1000
Chicago, IL 60611 (312) 335 5777

Provides educational and support systems regarding a variety of disorders for patients, families, and other interested persons. Seeks to destroy the myth that senility is a natural part of aging by stressing that some problems can be treated and by assuring those with irreversible conditions that help is available.

American Association of Retired Persons (AARP)
601 E St. NW
Washington, DC 20049 (202) 434 2277

Large organization devoted to sponsoring broad-based community service programs. Addresses travel, investment, and insurance opportunities and a variety of concerns of those who are retired.

American Society on Aging (ASA)
833 Market St., Suite 512
San Francisco, CA 94103 (415) 882 9210

This organization is composed of health care providers, educators, persons from the business community, students, and elders. Works to enhance the quality of life for older individuals; also offers continuing education programs related to issues surrounding aging.

Gerontological Society of America (GSA)
1275 K St. NW, Suite 350
Washington, DC (202) 842 1275

A group of professionals who promote the scientific study of aging, publish information, and bring together groups interested in older people.

Gray Panthers
1424 16th St. NW, Suite 602
Washington, DC 20036 (202) 387 3111

An organization seeking to combat ageism. Local chapters hold programs, monitor policy toward the aged, and offer a variety of services. A newsletter is available.

National Caucus and Center on Black Aged (NCCBA)
1424 K Street NW, Suite 500
Washington, DC 20005 (202) 637 8400

Focuses primarily on housing, employment opportunities, and social issues of the black elderly. Promotes legislation addressing concerns of this group.

Alcohol and Drug Abuse

Alcoholics Anonymous World Service (AA)
475 Riverside Drive
New York, NY 10163 (212) 686 1100

Large organization devoted to helping persons toward abstinence from alcohol. Local self-help groups operate on a "buddy system," with associated problems for spouses and children of alcoholics. Issues numerous publications.

Narcotics Anonymous (NA)
PO Box 9999
Van Nuys, CA 91409 (818) 780 3951

Local groups, patterned after those of AA (see above), provides self-help and group support to become drug free as well as support for family and friends.

National Council on Alcoholism and Drug Dependence (NCAAD)
12 W. 21st St.
New York, NY 10010 (212) 206 6720

Acts as an advisory council on improved drug therapy for the government, the scientific community, and the public. Conducts monitoring for the FDA. Holds conferences for the public.

Birth Defects

March of Dimes Birth Defect Foundation (MDBDF)
1275 Mamaroneck Ave.
White Plains, NY 10605 (914) 428 7100

Seeks to prevent birth defects through supporting research. Offers public and professional health education and community action programs to improve maternal and neonatal health.

United Cerebral Palsy Associations (UCPA)
7 Penn Plaza Suite 804
New York, NY 10001 (212) 268 6655

National organization with regional and local affiliates. Promotes various programs for those disabled from cerebral palsy and their families. Issues several publications.

Death and Dying

Compassionate Friends Inc.
PO Box 3696
Oak Brook, IL 60522–3696 (708) 990 0010

A support group of parents for parents who have experienced the death of a child. Local chapters offer self-help through groups as well as individual help. Publishes newsletter.

Candlelighters Childhood Cancer Foundation (CCCF)
1312 18th St. NW, No. 200
Washington, DC 20036 (202) 659 5136

Composed of parents who have lost a child through cancer. Provides emotional support through groups. Assists in providing equipment and devices needed during illness. Conducts parent group meetings, bereavement services.

National Sudden Infant Death Syndrome Alliance (NSIDSA)
10500 Little Patuxent Pkwy., No. 240
Columbia, MD 21044 (410) 964 8000

Local groups assist bereaved parents through self-help groups and counseling. Offers a public education program. A variety of articles and publications are available.

National Hospice Organization (NHO)
1901 N. Moore St., Suite 901
Arlington, VA 22209 (703) 243 5900

Promotes principles of hospice care for the terminally ill for the public and its member organizations. Acts as a liaison and clearing house for information. Develops educational projects for professionals and the public and monitors legislation.

Health Maintenance

American Health Foundation (AHF)
320 E. 43rd St.
New York, NY (212) 953 1900

Devoted to promoting preventive medicine. Conducts research disseminates information. Emphasizes nutrition and nontraditional health care. Newsletter.

Center for Attitudinal Healing
49 Main Street
Tiburon, CA 94920 (415) 435 5022

Established to supplement traditional health care by providing programs for adults and children with life-threatening illnesses. The center defines healing as inner peace.

Center for Well-Being of Health Professionals (CWBHP)
21 W. Colony Place, Suite 150
Durham, NC 27707 (919) 489 9167

A group of professionals who promote the physical and mental well-being of health care workers through preventive education designed to increase awareness of stresses and of ways to improve and maintain functional integrity.

National Migrant Resource Program (NMRP)
2512 S, IH-35, Suite 220
Austin, TX 78704 (512) 447 0770

Seeks to promote quality primary health care to migrant families in the United States. Maintains a system of networking so that migrant persons can find and have medical records transferred. Coordinates staff for migrant health areas.

National Minority Health Association (NMHA)
PO Box 11876
Harrisburg, PA 17108 (717) 234 3254

Focuses on the health needs of minorities. Involved in research and better training of health care practitioners. Provides information to professional organizations and pharmaceutical and insurance companies.

National Women's Health Network (NWHN)
1325 G St. NW
Washington, DC 20005 (202) 347 1140

Composed of professionals and laypersons interested in women's health. Monitors federal health policies as they affect women. Presents public programs.

Recovery
802 N. Dearborn St.
Chicago, IL 60610 (312) 337 5661

In an approach based on a self-help model, local groups of formerly mentally ill persons meet weekly to prevent relapses. Prints bimonthly publication.

Injury and Perceptual Impairment

American Council of the Blind (ACB)
1155 15th St. NW, Suite 720
Washington, DC 20005 (202) 467 5081

Large professional and lay membership. Provides multiple services such as information on vision research, libraries, insurance, and employment opportunities.

Deafpride
1350 Potomac Ave. SE
Washington, DC 20003 (202) 675 6700

Brings together the hearing impaired and hearing persons to provide opportunities for the development of full potential. Protects the human rights of the hearing impaired.

National Association of the Deaf (NAD)
814 Thayer Ave.
Silver Spring, MD 20910 (301) 587 1788

Services deaf adults and children. Provides educational films. Maintains legal services for the hearing impaired and encourages eliminating communication barriers for the hearing impaired.

National Spinal Cord Injury Association (NSCIA)
600 W. Cummings Park, Suite 2000
Woburn, MA 01801 (617) 935 2722

Informs and educates professionals and the public about the spinal cord-injured person. Establishes treatment centers and encourages individuals to meet their personal goals. Issues several publications.

Professional Organizations

American Holistic Nurses Association (AHNA)
4101 Lake Boone Trail, Suite 201
Raleigh, NC 27609 (919) 787 5181

Membership consists of registered and practical nurses as well as student nurses. With an emphasis on holistic nursing, the organization examines new directions in health care delivery. Maintains a library and awards scholarships.

American Nurses Association (ANA)
2420 Pershing Rd.
Kansas City, MO 64108 (816) 474 5720

Professional organization of professional nurses. State and local groups. Sponsors education, political action, recognition, and standards of practice.

American Public Health Association (APHA)
1015 15th St. NW
Washington, DC 20005 (202) 789 5600

Large professional organization that promotes broad programs in personal and environmental health. Works to establish standard practices in controlling communicable disease as well as to improve community sanitation. Offers numerous publications.

National League for Nursing (NLN)
350 Hudson St.
New York, NY 10014 (212) 989 9393

Composed of leaders in nursing, other health care professionals, and individuals interested in solving problems in health care. Looks at nursing needs and ways to improve nursing preparation and delivery of services. Is responsible for testing new graduates and accrediting new programs in nursing.

National Student Nurses Association (NSNA)
555 W. 57th St., No. 1325
New York, NY 10019 (212) 581 2211

Encourages programs for nursing students in state-approved schools. Sponsors recruitment and civic and community programs on nursing. Has regional groups; offers several publications.

National Center for the Advancement of Blacks in the Health Professions (NCABHP)
PO Box 21121
Detroit, MI 48221 (313) 345 4480

Disseminates information regarding positions in health care. Demonstrates recruitment projects and provides information for networking various organizations. Conducts skills workshops. Computer service to link applicants to centers of higher education.

Specific Disorders

American Cancer Society (ACS)
1599 Clifton Rd. NE
Atlanta, GA 30329 (404) 320 3333

Supports education and research in the prevention, diagnosis and treatment of cancer. Provides special services to cancer patients and their families. Wide variety of publications available.

International Association of Laryngectomies
A program of the American Cancer Society to assist persons who have had a laryngectomy. Offers classes in speech alteration, self-help groups, psychological support to patients and families.

Reach to Recovery
A program of the American Cancer Society to help women who have had mastectomies. Volunteers are former patients.

American Diabetic Association (ADA)
PO Box 25757, 1660 Duke St.
Alexandria, VA 22314 (703) 549 1500

Composed of professionals and laypersons for the education and free exchange of information about diabetes. Holds, classes and self-help groups. Numerous publications.

American Heart Association (AHA)
7320 Greenville Ave,
Dallas, TX 75231 (214) 373 6300

Broad based organization supported by contributions. Research on prevention, diagnosis, and treatment of heart disease and stroke. A variety of publications are available.

American Pain Society (APS)
5700 Old Orchard Road, 1st Fl.
Skokie, IL 60077–1024 (708) 966 5595

Regional groups. Conducts research and public education regarding acute and chronic pain. Also offers individual counseling and family support.

American Parkinson Disease Association (APDA)
60 Bay St., Suite 401
Staten Island, NY 10301 (718) 981 8001

Provides information and counseling services to those who have Parkinson's disease and their families. Encourages research and publishes numerous pamphlets and brochures.

Amyotrophic Lateral Sclerosis Association (ALSA)
21021 Ventura Blvd., Suite 321
Woodland Hills, CA 91364 (818) 340 7500

Solicits funds for research and provides patient–family counseling program. Promotes education. Publishes newsletter and handbook.

Anorexia and Related Eating Disorders (ANRED)
PO Box 5102
Eugene, OR 97405 (503) 344 1144

Offers classes and information for people with anorexia or bulimia. Holds workshops and other educational sessions for community groups. Acts as a resource center, produces articles and papers.

Autism Society of America (ASA)
8601 Georgia Ave., Suite 503
Silver Spring, MD 20910 (301) 565 0433

Professional and lay membership. Seeks to promote better understanding of the problems of autistic children and adults. Serves as a centralized source of information on autism.

Cystic Fibrosis Foundation (CFF)
6931 Arlington Road, No. 200
Bethesda, MD 20814 (301) 951 4422

Local groups. Supports research, public education, and care centers to provide services to patients and their families. Sponsors legislation. Publishes newsletter.

Epilepsy Foundation of America (EFA)
4351 Garden City Drive
Landover, MD 20785 (301) 459 3700

Local groups. Promotes education and research into the causes and treatment of epilepsy. Encourages employment and social opportunities for those who are afflicted with a seizure disorder. A variety of publications are available.

Muscular Dystrophy Association (MDA)
3561 E. Sunrise Dr.
Tucson, AZ 85718 (602) 529 2000

Local groups. Fosters research and sponsors conferences. Provides patient and family counseling. Offers publications.

National Association for Sickle Cell Disease (NASCD)
3345 Wilshire Blvd., Suite 1106
Los Angeles, CA 90010–1880 (213) 736 5455

A group of professionals and lay persons who work to promote information and research into sickle cell disease. Holds seminars and publishes a newsletter.

National Hypertension Association (NHA)
324 E. 30th St.
New York, NY 10016 (212) 889 3557

Dedicated to the prevention and effective treatment of hypertension. Sponsors seminars and gives information on effects of cholesterol. Public school program.

National Kidney Foundation
30 E. 33rd St., Suite 1100
New York, NY 10016 (212) 889 2210

National and local groups. Conducts service and educational activities. Active in facilitating a kidney organ donor program. Prints several publications.

National Multiple Sclerosis Society
733 3rd Ave
New York, NY 10017 (212) 986 3240

Local chapters. Supports research and offers educational programs and counseling to patients and families. Provides publishing and other programs for education through the media.

National Psoriasis Foundation (NPF)
6443 SW Beaverton Hwy., Suite 210
Portland, OR 97221 (503) 297 1545

Offers support to persons with psoriasis, their families and friends. Participates in research at various universities. Provides literature to schools and libraries. Pamphlets and brochures are available.

Scoliosis Association (SA)
PO Box 51353
Raleigh, NC 27609–1353 (919) 846 2639

Sponsors spinal screening programs, films, seminars, and other educational activities. Publishes newsletters and articles.

United Ostomy Association (UOA)
36 Executive Park, Suite 120
Irvine, CA 92714 (714) 660 8624

Local groups. Serves persons who have lost part of the bowel and have diversional appliances. Provides mutual aid and support groups and educational programs. Works to end job discrimination.

Rehabilitation

National Rehabilitation Association (NRA)
633 S. Washington St.
Alexandria, VA 22314 (703) 836 0850

Composed of health care professionals and other persons who are interested in the rehabilitation of the physically and mentally disabled. Publishes a newsletter and a journal.

Sexual Identity

National Lesbian and Gay Health Foundation (NLGHF)
PO Box 65472
Washington DC 20035 (202) 797 3578

Gay and nongay persons, interested in better accessibility of health care for the gay community. Promotes research regarding health issues for gay persons. Maintains a speaker's bureau.

National Gay and Lesbian Task Force (NGLTF)
1734 14th St. NW
Washington, DC 20009–4309 (202) 332 6483

Local groups. Promotes elimination of discrimination against persons because of sexual preference. Works to ensure fair treatment of gay and lesbian people by the media as well as in employment practices and other areas of society. Monitors legislation concerning gay rights.

Appendix F

Level I Screen from the Nutrition Screening Initiative

Level 1 Screen

Body Weight

Measure height to the nearest inch and weight to the nearest pound. Record the values below and mark them on the Body Mass Index (BMI) scale to the right. Then use a straight edge (ruler) to connect the two points and circle the spot where this straight line crosses the center line (body mass index). Record the number below.

Healthy older adults should have a BMI between 24 and 27.

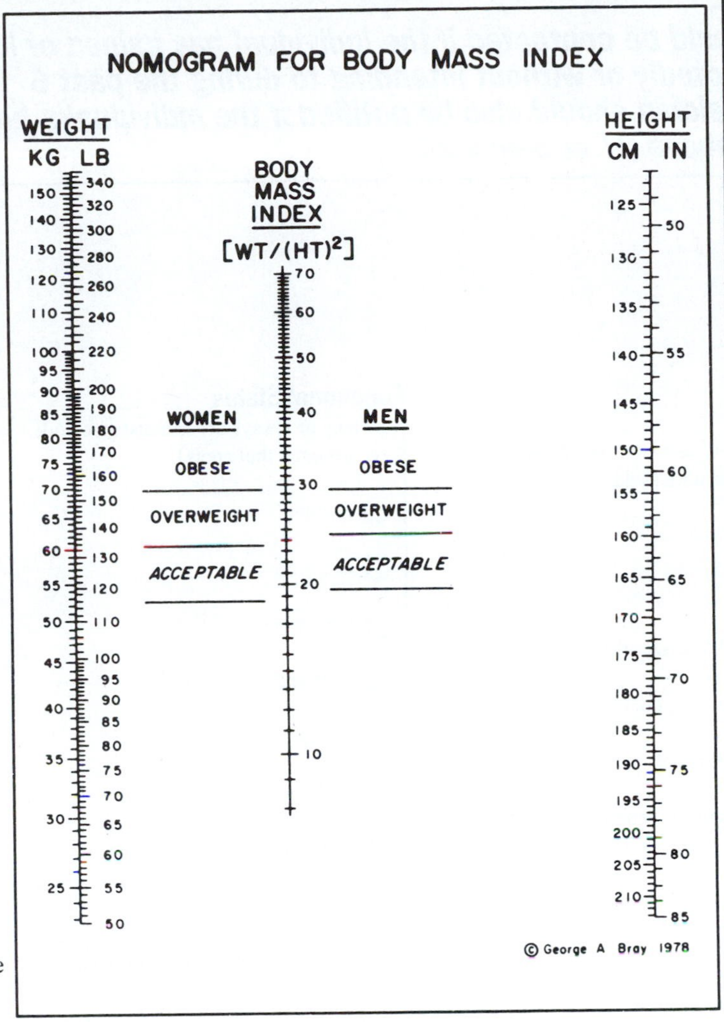

Height (in):_______________

Weight (lbs):_______________

Body Mass Index:_______________

(number from center column)

Check any boxes that are true for the individual:

- ❑ Has lost or gained 10 pounds (or more) in the past 6 months.
- ❑ Body mass index <24
- ❑ Body mass index >27

For the remaining sections, please ask the individual which of the statements (if any) is true for him or her and place a check by each that applies.

Eating Habits

- ❑ Does not have enough food to eat each day
- ❑ Usually eats alone
- ❑ Does not eat anything on one or more days each month
- ❑ Has poor appetite
- ❑ Is on a special diet
- ❑ Eats vegetables two or fewer times daily
- ❑ Eats milk or milk products once or not at all daily
- ❑ Eats fruit or drinks fruit juice once or not at all daily
- ❑ Eats breads, cereals, pasta, rice, or other grains five or fewer times daily
- ❑ Has difficulty chewing or swallowing
- ❑ Has more than one alcoholic drink per day (if woman); more than two drinks per day (if man)
- ❑ Has pain in mouth, teeth, or gums

LEVEL I SCREEN

Name:

Date:

Reprinted with permission by the Nutrition Screening Initiative, a project of the American Academy of Family Physicians, The American Dietetic Association, and the National Council on the Aging, Inc. and funded in part by a grant from Ross Laboratories, a division of Abbott Laboratories.

A physician should be contacted if the individual has gained or lost 10 pounds unexpectedly or without intending to during the past 6 months. A physician should also be notified if the individual's body mass index is above 27 or below 24.

Living Environment

- ❑ Lives on an income of less than $6000 per year (per individual in the household)
- ❑ Lives alone
- ❑ Is housebound
- ❑ Is concerned about home security
- ❑ Lives in a home with inadequate heating or cooling
- ❑ Does not have a stove and/or refrigerator
- ❑ Is unable or prefers not to spend money on food (<$25-30 per person spent on food each week)

Functional Status

Usually or always needs assistance with (check each that apply):

- ❑ Bathing
- ❑ Dressing
- ❑ Grooming
- ❑ Toileting
- ❑ Eating
- ❑ Walking or moving about
- ❑ Traveling (outside the home)
- ❑ Preparing food
- ❑ Shopping for food or other necessities

If you have checked one or more statements on this screen, the individual you have interviewed may be at risk for poor nutritional status. Please refer this individual to the appropriate health care or social service professional in your area. For example, a dietitian should be contacted for problems with selecting, preparing, or eating a healthy diet, or a dentist if the individual experiences pain or difficulty when chewing or swallowing. Those individuals whose income, lifestyle, or functional status may endanger their nutritional and overall health should be referred to available community services: home-delivered meals, congregate meal programs, transportation services, counseling services (alcohol abuse, depression, bereavement, etc.), home health care agencies, day care programs, etc.

Please repeat this screen at least once each year--sooner if the individual has a major change in his or her health, income, immediate family (e.g., spouse dies), or functional status.

These materials developed by the Nutrition Screening Initiative.

Reprinted with permission by the Nutrition Screening Initiative, a project of the American Academy of Family Physicians, The American Dietetic Association, and the National Council on the Aging, Inc. and funded in part by a grant from Ross Laboratories, a division of Abbott Laboratories.

Index

Page numbers in italics *indicate illustrations; those followed by* t *indicate tables; and those followed by* d *indicate display material. Page numbers in* **boldface** *indicate where glossary terms are defined in the text. All* **boldface** *entries are defined in the glossary.*

455 LBIC
7/8/94 Y10-2 17 CLB